Swenson's Pediatric Surgery

Fifth Edition

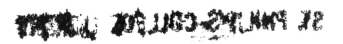

Swenson's Pediatric Surgery

Fifth Edition

Edited by
John G. Raffensperger, MD
Surgeon-in-Chief
The Children's Memorial Hospital
Chicago, Illinois

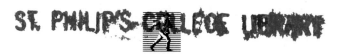

APPLETON & LANGE
Norwalk, Connecticut

Notice: Our knowledge in clinical sciences is constantly changing. As new
information becomes available, changes in treatment and in the use of drugs
become necessary. The author and the publisher of this volume have taken
care to make certain that the doses of drugs and schedules of treatment are
correct and compatible with the standards generally accepted at the time of
publication. The reader is advised to consult carefully the instruction
and information material included in the package insert of each drug or
therapeutic agent before administration. This advice is especially
important when using new or infrequently used drugs.

Copyright © 1990 by Appleton & Lange
A Publishing Division of Prentice Hall
Copyright © 1980 by Appleton-Century-Crofts, New York;
Under the title *Pediatric Surgery* by Orvar Swenson,
Copyright © 1969, 1962, 1958 by Appleton-Century-Crofts, New York

90 91 92 93 94 / 10 9 8 7 6 5 4 3 2 1

Prentice Hall International (UK) Limited, *London*
Prentice Hall of Australia Pty. Limited, *Sydney*
Prentice Hall Canada, Inc., *Toronto*
Prentice Hall Hispanoamericana, S.A., *Mexico*
Prentice Hall of India Private Limited, *New Delhi*
Prentice Hall of Japan, Inc., *Tokyo*
Simon & Schuster Asia Pte. Ltd., *Singapore*
Editora Prentice Hall do Brasil Ltda., *Rio de Janeiro*
Prentice Hall, *Englewood Cliffs, New Jersey*

Library of Congress Cataloging-in-Publication Data
Swenson's pediatric surgery.—5th ed. / edited by John G.
  Raffensperger.
      p.   cm.
  Includes bibliographies and index.
  ISBN 0-8385-8757-7
  1. Children—Surgery.   I. Swenson, Orvar.   II. Raffensperger,
John G., 1928–   III. Title: Pediatric surgery.
  [DNLM: 1. Surgery—in infancy & childhood.   WO 925 S9744]
RD137.S85   1989
617.9'8—dc20
DNLM/DLC
for Library of Congress   89–6762
                                                      CIP

Acquisitions Editor: William R. Schmitt
Production Editor: Elizabeth C. Ryan
Designer: Michael J. Kelly

PRINTED IN THE UNITED STATES OF AMERICA

Contributors

Richard J. Andrassy, MD, FACS, FAAP
A.G. McNeese Professor of Surgery and Pediatrics
Surgeon-in-Chief, University Children's Hospital
Hermann and M.D. Anderson Cancer Hospital

Bruce S. Bauer, MD
Associate Professor of Surgery
Northwestern University Medical School
Chief, Division of Plastic Surgery
Children's Memorial Hospital
Chicago, Illinois

Edward S. Baum, MD
Attending Physician
Division of Hematology and Oncology
Professor of Clinical Pediatrics
Northwestern University School of Medicine
Children's Memorial Hospital
Chicago, Illinois

C. Thomas Black, MD
Assistant Professor of Surgery and Pediatrics
University of Texas Medical School at Houston
Attending Pediatric Surgeon,
University Children's Hospital
Hermann and M.D. Anderson Cancer Center
Houston, Texas

John D. Burrington, MD
Director of Surgical Education
The Children's Hospital of Denver
Professor of Clinical Surgery
University of Colorado
Denver, Colorado

A. Todd Davis, MD
Head, Division of General Academic and Emergency
    Pediatrics
Children's Memorial Hospital
Professor of Pediatrics
Northwestern University Medical School
Chicago, Illinois
Evanston Hospital
Evanston, Illinois

Stephen E. Dolgin, MD
Chief, Pediatric Surgery
Assistant Professor, Surgery and Pediatrics
Mt. Sinai School of Medicine
New York, New York

Mark I. Evans, MD
Director, Division of Reproductive Genetics
Associate Professor, Department of Obstetrics and
    Gynecology
Department of Molecular Biology and Genetics
Hutzel Hospital, Wayne State University
Detroit, Michigan

Neil R. Feins, MD
Director of Pediatric Surgery, Boston City Hospital
Professor of Surgery and Pediatrics, Boston University
    School of Medicine
Surgeon-in-Chief, Franciscan's Children's Hospital
Boston, Massachusetts

Orville C. Green, MD
Chief, Division of Pediatric Endocrinology

Children's Memorial Hospital
Professor of Pediatrics
Northwestern University
Chicago, Illinois

Yoon S. Hahn, MD
Chief of Pediatric Neurosurgery
Children's Memorial Hospital
Professor of Neurosurgery and Pediatric Neurosurgery
Loyola University School of Medicine
Chicago, Illinois

Lauren D. Holinger, MD
Director of Pediatric Otolaringology
Children's Memorial Hospital
Professor of Otolaryngology
Northwestern University Medical School
Chicago, Illinois

Babette Horn, MD
Assistant Professor of Clinical Anesthesia
Northwestern Memorial Hospital
Attending Anesthesiologist
Children's Memorial Hospital
Chicago, Illinois

Farouk S. Idriss, MD
Professor of Surgery,
Northwestern University Medical School
Division Head, Cardiovascular-Thoracic Surgery
Evanston, Illinois

Michel N. Ilbawi, MD
Associate Professor of Surgery
Northwestern University Medical School
Attending Cardiovascular-Thoracic Surgeon
Evanston, Illinois

Juda Z. Jona, MD
Assistant Clinical Professor of General and Cardiothoracic Surgery
Medical College of Wisconsin
Milwaukee, Wisconsin

Frederick M. Karrer, MD
Assistant Professor of Surgery,
Section of Pediatric Surgery and Transplantation
University of Colorado School of Medicine
Denver, Colorado

Bruce H. Kaufman, MD
Assistant Clinical Professor of General and Cardiothoracic Surgery
Medical College of Wisconsin
Milwaukee, Wisconsin

Susan R. Luck, MD
Associate Professor of Clinical Surgery
Northwestern University Medical School
Children's Memorial Hospital
Chicago, Illinois

Donald G. Marshall, MD, FRCS(C), FAAP
Clinical Professor of Pediatric General Surgery
Chief of Pediatric Surgery
St. Joseph's Hospital
Attending Pediatric Surgeon,
Victoria Hospital, Westminster Campus
London, Ontario

David G. McLone, MD, PhD
Division Head, Pediatric Neurosurgery
Children's Memorial Hospital
Professor of Surgery
Northwestern University Medical School
Chicago, Illinois

David P. Meagher, Jr., MD
Associate Clinical Professor of Surgery
University of Colorado Health Sciences Center
Attending Surgeon
The Children's Hospital
Denver, Colorado

Elaine R. Morgan, MD
Associate Professor of Pediatrics
Northwestern University School of Medicine
Attending Pediatric Hematologist and Oncologist
Children's Memorial Hospital
Chicago, Illinois

Henry L. Nadler, MD
President and Chief Executive Officer
Michael Reese Hospital and Medical Center
Professor of Pediatrics
University of Illinois
Chicago, Illinois

Jay M. Pensler, MD
Assistant Professor of Surgery
Northwestern University School of Medicine
Attending Plastic Surgeon,
Children's Memorial Hospital
Chicago, Illinois

William J. Pokorny, MD
Associate Professor of Surgery and Pediatrics
Baylor College of Medicine
Chief of Pediatric Surgery
Ben Taub General Hospital and Jefferson Davis Hospital
Houston, Texas

Randall W. Powell, MD
Head, Division of Pediatric Surgery
University of South Alabama Medical Center
Associate Professor, Departments of Surgery and Pediatrics
University of South Alabama College of Medicine
Mobile, Alabama

John G. Raffensperger, MD
Surgeon-in-Chief
Children's Memorial Hospital
Professor of Pediatric Surgery
Northwestern University Medical School
Chicago, Illinois

Marleta Reynolds, MD
Assistant Professor of Clinical Surgery
Northwestern University School of Medicine
Children's Memorial Hospital
Chicago, Illinois

Richard Ricketts, MD
Chief of Surgery
Egleston Children's Hospital
Associate Professor of Pediatric Surgery
Emory University School of Medicine
Atlanta, Georgia

Alan J. Sacks, MD
Director, Division of Obstetric and Gynecologic Imaging
Assistant Professor, Wayne State University School of Medicine
Detroit, Michigan

Louise Schnaufer, MD
Associate Professor, Pediatric Surgery
University of Pennsylvania School of Medicine
Senior Surgeon, Children's Hospital of Philadelphia
Philadelphia, Pennsylvania

Frank L. Seleny, MD
Chairman, Department of Pediatric Anesthesia
Children's Memorial Hospital
Professor of Clinical Anesthesia
Northwestern University Medical School
Chicago, Illinois

James A. Stockman, III, MD
Professor and Chairman, Department of Pediatrics
Northwestern University School of Medicine
Physician-in-Chief, Children's Memorial Hospital
Chicago, Illinois

Orvar Swenson, MD
Surgeon-in-Chief, Retired
Children's Memorial Hospital
Chicago, Illinois

Jessie L. Ternberg, MD
Attending Surgeon
St. Louis Children's Hospital
Professor of Surgery and Pediatrics
Washington University School of Medicine
St. Louis, Missouri

Gabriel F. Tucker, Jr., MD†
Professor, Department of Otolaryngology, Head and Neck Surgery
Northwestern University School of Medicine
Head, Division of Bronchoesophagology/Otolaryngology, and Department of Communicative Disorders
Children's Memorial Hospital
Chicago, Illinois

Robert J. Winter, MD
Associate Professor of Pediatrics
Northwestern University School of Medicine
Director of Medical Education
Children's Memorial Hospital
Chicago, Illinois

☐ Contents

☐ Introduction

The first edition of Swenson's textbook *Pediatric Surgery* was published 31 years ago in 1958. Although operative techniques have continued to evolve and operations are now being performed that were unheard of at that time, the general principles of care remain the same. The greatest advances have come in the areas of pre- and postoperative care and anesthesia. Our knowledge of the physiologic responses of newborn infants has broadened dramatically. Total intravenous nutrition allows infants with catastrophic gastrointestinal anomalies to survive. The techniques of nutritional support first developed in neonates are now being applied to older children with a variety of diseases which cause malnutrition. Miniturization and refinement of respirators save the lives of countless infants who would have died from respiratory failure. Chemotherapy of childhood tumors was not mentioned in the first edition. Today, drug therapy, more than any other single factor, has radically improved the prognosis of children with malignancies. Descriptions of new diagnostic techniques appear in medical journals every month. Roentgenograms and the recording of innumerable scans and assays can almost become an end in themselves, yet they may allow rapid delineation of many lesions. Pre- and postoperative changes can be followed critically and with ease.

The pediatric surgeon must be more than a skilled and delicate technician. Along with being well versed in the many implications of pediatric disease and the optimum utilization of the appropriate specialists, he must also be sensitive to the psychological and emotional needs of his young patients. With these responsibilities in mind, the editor has emphasized a problem-oriented approach which attempts to reflect the actual presentation of a pediatric patient. Both the pediatric surgeon and the general surgeon will find that this perspective facilitates the recognition and management of the great variety of problems encountered in surgical practice.

Every child born with a surgically correctable anomaly should be able to survive. Life can be prolonged almost indefinitely with total intravenous nutrition and artificial ventilation. This technical ability raises a moral and ethical dilemma because there are infants with incurable defects or chromosomal abnormalities who will remain crippled or retarded regardless of our efforts. The surgeon must look to his own ethical and religious background in order to counsel the parents of such children.

Ideally, all major operations upon high risk infants and children should be performed in a pediatric center. Obviously, this is not always possible. Any surgeon may be called upon to care for a sick child. This book is intended to help every surgeon in the diagnosis and treatment of pediatric surgical disease.

The authors are all active practiconers who treat sick children every day. This book reflects their experience and of course their personal prejudices.

The bibliography is not all inclusive. Articles were selected as references that are current and easily available in most medical libraries. They are to be consulted for further information on a specific topic.

Dr. Orvar Swenson, the first author and editor of this text continues to maintain an active interest in pediatric surgery and continues to follow his old patients. He spends his summers sailing on Penobscot Bay in Maine and winters in Florida, where he has just taken up fishing.

John G. Raffensperger
Chicago, Illinois, 1989

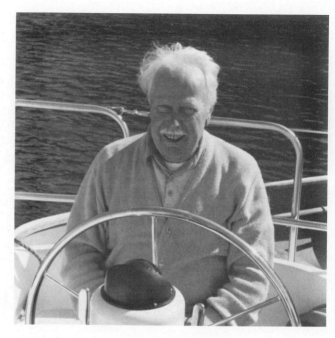

Orvar Swenson, MD

SECTION I

Assessment and General Considerations in the Care of the Pediatric Surgical Patient

The operation is only a brief phase in the continuing care of the pediatric surgical patient. To achieve success, the proper diagnosis must be made and the child must be in the best possible physical and emotional condition before the operation. This requires that we personally obtain a history and perform a physical examination. The time spent with the child will reassure the parents and will aid the surgeon in evaluating the patient as well as the family. In the preoperative evaluation, it is the surgeon's responsibility to find and correct underlying diseases or abnormalities that may complicate the operation. A careful history will eliminate many pitfalls by turning up a potential coagulation disorder, an allergy to drugs, or perhaps a familial history of hyperthermia in reaction to certain anesthetic agents.

With the many techniques available for artificial feeding, any patient can be brought into an optimum nutritional state to ensure sound wound healing and rapid recovery. When there is any question in the surgeon's mind about the diagnosis or the patient's general condition, the surgeon should not hesitate to obtain the help of a consultant. In some patients, such as diabetics, it is extremely helpful to work closely with a medical specialist. However, the surgeon must bear the entire responsibility for the patient's preoperative and the postoperative care.

The operating room is a relatively dangerous place. In this section, we have avoided adding the traditional chapter on anesthesia but have included a discussion on care of the child in the operating room. Here there is a division of responsibility: the anesthesiologist must maintain a steady, safe plane of anesthesia, monitor the

patient, administer transfusions and other fluid therapy, and at the end awaken the patient. Surgeons must be aware of the many hazards facing a pediatric patient, especially a newborn infant, from the time he or she is first brought into the operating room. The surgeon must watch the temperature in the room itself and work with the anesthesiologist and nurses in preventing hypothermia, contamination, and electrical burns. Often the surgeon must provide vascular access to aid the anesthesiologist in monitoring and in administering fluid therapy.

We often overlook our responsibility to rehearse a new or complicated operation with the nursing team; it is our own fault if at a critical time during the procedure a specific suture or instrument is lacking.

Beware of routine postoperative orders! No patient, least of all a baby, is "routine." All drug dosages must be calculated carefully by taking into consideration the infant's weight, age, and metabolic requirements. The hospital pharmacist and reference books must be consulted if there is doubt about the correct dosage of any medication. Similar care is taken with fluid therapy and in determining the need for antibiotics. When the child is settled in the recovery area, we have an obligation to explain our procedure in detail to the child's parents. We must gain the parents' confidence by providing them with accurate information at each phase of their child's care. This is particularly important when dealing with birth defects or tumors when we want long-term follow-up studies to evaluate our work. Several chapters in this section are written by medical specialists because we recognize their expertise in important areas of pediatric surgical care. As surgeons, we must understand the fundamentals of blood coagulation, but when we are faced with unexplained hemorrhage, most of us require assistance from a pediatric hematologist. We must be able to provide specialists with the proper information and have the ability to interpret their findings.

Finally, we have included a chapter on genetics because at some point every parent of a deformed child will ask, "Why did this happen?" We must be prepared to formulate a logical answer and know how and where to find further consultation so that the family can obtain accurate information.

1
History and Physical Examination

Attention to detail in taking the patient's history and in performing a complete pediatric examination is the cornerstone of diagnosis and treatment. Diagnostic errors rarely result from misinterpretation of laboratory results or from not ordering appropriate tests. The responsible surgeon must verify for himself or herself the particulars of the history and physical examination. It is not enough to rely on a medical student's examination or even that of a distinguished referring physician. The child and the surgeon have an opportunity to become acquainted during the initial interview and physical examination; it is a mistake for the surgeon to deny the child this period of accommodation and to proceed brusquely with the examination. Haste may provoke the child into being uncooperative and may make it difficult to perform the examination and evaluate the findings.

Even in emergency situations, there is usually time for introductions and an opportunity to learn something about the child's interests. The history itself should be obtained from both the parents and the child. Frequently, when asked the nature of the child's problem, the mother will state the diagnosis as given to her by another physician. One must not be tempted by this shortcut. She should be asked to explain the problem in her own words, commencing with the first symptom. The written history should begin, "The mother saw an inguinal bulge 2 months ago." The inguinal bulge may or may not be a hernia, but it is important to record the mother's own observations. When the recent history has been completed, the examiner should continue to obtain information about earlier illnesses, operations, responses to anesthetics, bleeding tendencies, allergies, and medications. The examiner should inquire specifically about a family history of tuberculosis, allergies, blood dyscrasias, and congenital anomalies. For younger children, a detailed history of the mother's pregnancy and delivery is also important.

Obviously the complexity of the presenting complaint determines the extent of the history-taking process. Many surgical diseases are straightforward. The surgeon is primarily interested in learning if there are any factors that might influence the choice of anesthetic agents and the decision whether the child should be hospitalized or treated as an outpatient. Chronic problems, such as abdominal pain and constipation, require detailed medical, emotional, and social history. Divorce, the birth of a sibling, or a death in the family may precipitate psychosomatic symptoms that mimic surgical diseases.

The examination of a child is different from that of an adult. Occasionally, during conversation between the parents and the physician, the child will of his own accord approach the physician. This is an indication that the child has confidence in the doctor and may be cooperative. When children have been prepared for the experience by their parents, they are more likely to confront the surgeon without fear. They enjoy being the center of attention. If the examiner keeps this fact in mind, he is likely to have more success with young patients. Children are proud of new articles of clothing and their toys, and they are usually willing to show off these items. When a child seems friendly, the situation can be made more secure by inquiring about brothers, sisters, and pets. Obviously, children of different ages require different handling. Frequently, the entire examination of an infant can be carried out while the mother or nurse holds the baby on her lap. The older child is likely to cooperate without difficulty, but the 2- to 5-year-old child is a rebel. Sometimes it is not possible to complete the examination of a crying and uncooperative child. Rather than forcing the issue or becoming angry, the examiner should calmly tell the parents that it is not possible to perform an adequate examination. Some insight into the child's behavior may be gained by discussion with the parents. Sometimes a child can be brought back for another visit after having been properly prepared. In an acute situation, sedation may be indicated. Even a minimally apprehensive child is difficult to examine. Voluntary wincing may be misinterpreted as abdominal tenderness, and unless the child is completely relaxed, it is possible to overlook an abdominal tumor. On the other hand, a stoic child may lead the examiner to underestimate painful reactions.

Observation of appearance and reactions is very valuable. Does the child move briskly about the room, or does abdominal pain cause him or her to walk stooped over? Is the child pale and puny from a chronic illness, or does he or she look considerably more healthy than expected from the parents' recitation of symptoms? The examiner should watch the child's face and talk during the examination. Is the child normally responsive for his or her age, retarded, or unusually frightened? The child who smiles during abdominal palpation is unlikely to have an acute condition of the abdomen; on the other hand, the stoic who disclaims pain but winces a little may have peritonitis.

Careful handwashing before the examination not only helps prevent the spread of nosocomial infections but also warms the hands for the child's comfort. It does not hurt to warm the stethoscope as well. In older children, one may perform the traditional top-to-bottom examination, but in younger or uncooperative children, one must take the opportunity to examine whatever the child will allow. A bottle or pacifier often will calm an infant so that the examiner can listen to the heart and lungs and palpate the abdomen. However, the examiner should insist that the child be completely undressed. It is amazing how often parents expect the surgeon to examine only the area for which he or she is being consulted. It is impossible to properly examine a child for an inguinal hernia between trousers that have been dropped an inch or two and a shirt pulled up to the umbilicus. Of course, the child should have some covering; infants may be covered with a blanket to prevent a chill, and older children appreciate a sheet or gown.

SKIN

Complete inspection may very well lead to a diagnosis. Superficial hemangiomas may be associated with visceral lesions causing gastrointestinal bleeding. Pigmented spots on the mucous membranes and palms are part of the Peutz-Jeghers syndrome. Café au lait spots are the tipoff to von Reicklinghausen's disease, and observation of Schönlein-Henoch purpura may prevent a needless laparotomy for abdominal pain. Cyanosis and jaundice are easily overlooked in children with pigmented

skin, but observation of the eyes and mucous membranes will reveal these signs. The skin is also an excellent indicator of the state of hydration. Edema, first noted in the eyelids, may be a sign of overhydration. Dehydration is accompanied by loss of tissue turgor and may be demonstrated by pinching a fold of abdominal skin; the fold will remain elevated, only slowly sinking back to a flat surface.

LYMPH NODES

Small, shotty, discrete, nontender lymph nodes up to 3 to 5 mm in diameter in the cervical, axillary, epitrochlear, inguinal, and occipital areas are normal. Until the age of 12 years, normal lymph nodes may range up to 1 cm in diameter. Larger isolated nodes or those that are fixed, indurated, or reddened should cause concern. Skin infections, such as impetigo, frequently explain larger nodes.

HEAD AND NECK

A glance is usually sufficient to determine if the head is of normal size and shape. Alopecia may be caused by hair swallowing, which can result in a trichobezoar. Asymmetry of the head accompanies torticollis. Dermoid cysts, malignant tumors, or metatases from a neuroblastoma often occur as localized scalp lesions. A bulging fontanelle is one of the first clues to increased intracranial pressure. Low-set ears are associated with chromosomal defects. Examination of the auditory canal often must be deferred to last in younger children, and restraint may be necesary. The mother should hold the child's arms over his or her head to keep the hands out of the way and the head immobilized. Tenderness in the external auditory canal may be caused by a furuncle or otitis externa. In the infant, the auditory canal is directed downward, and in order to visualize the eardrum, the auricle must be pulled down, whereas in the older child, it is pulled up and back.

Absence of the iris is seen in some children with Wilms' tumor. An absence of red reflex is seen with retinoblastoma. With a little practice, one can learn to visualize the retina. Abnormal facies can be another indication of chromosomal defects. Down's syndrome is recognized easily on the basis of the epicanthal folds, protruding tongue, and flat occiput.

If possible, the child's mouth should be examined without the use of a tongue blade. No one enjoys being gagged. If the examiner promises not to use the blade, the child will usually say "Ah." One should look for pallor and dryness of the mucous membranes and for

Candida infection. Decayed teeth often are the source of infection that can cause enlarged upper cervical lymph nodes. A painful superficial ulcer surrounded by erythema and edema may be the lesion of herpes simplex, which causes fever, anorexia, and occasionally vomiting in infants. Koplik's spots, the prodromal sign of measles, are bluish white and about the size of a grain of sand. They are scattered about the buccal mucosa at the level of the lower teeth and within the lower lip. It is important to take a careful look at the throat in a child with acute abdominal pain, because tonsillitis and pharyngitis may mimic appendicitis.

Thyroglossal duct sinuses and cysts as well as branchial cleft remnants are usually obvious. Teenage girls frequently have prominent thyroid glands. The thyroid should be carefully palpated for isolated nodules. One should always check for cervical motion in acutely ill children because meningitis can cause fever and abdominal pain. Meningitis can be an unsuspected postoperative complication.

CHEST WALL

The breasts of both boys and girls remain enlarged for a month or two after birth. In girls, normal breast development commences at about 12 years of age, although it is not uncommon to see a bud of breast tissue beneath the areola in younger girls. This must not be biopsied! It is perfectly normal, and removal of this bud of tissue is the equivalent of a mastectomy in older patients. Teenage boys frequently note tender buds of breast tissue as well. They need reassurance that this is normal and will disappear in about 6 months. However, real gynecomastia requires investigation and occasionally removal for cosmetic purposes.

LUNGS

The normal respiratory rate decreases from 40 respirations per minute at birth to 16 or 20 at 6 years of age and 14 to 16 at puberty. Rapid shallow respirations are seen with peritonitis and dehydration, as well as acute pulmonary disease. Slow breathing accompanies increased intracranial pressure. Infants breathe primarily with the diaphragm, and they become distressed when increased intraperitoneal pressure elevates and restricts diaphragmatic movement. One should look specifically for retractions, asymmetry, and paradoxical motion in any child with respiratory distress. The chest x-ray may be more accurate than auscultation and percussion, especially in younger children; however, the stethoscope is immediately available in emergencies. A normal exami-

nation eliminates the need for a routine preoperative chest roentgenogram. Physical findings that suggest mediastinal shift or elevation of the diaphragm, as well as absence of breath sounds or abnormal breath sounds, demand a chest x-ray.

CARDIOVASCULAR SYSTEM

Congenital heart disease is so frequently associated with other birth defects that the surgeon who operates on children must recognize cardiac abnormalities. The heart rate at birth is 140 beats per minute. It decreases to 80 to 140 beats per minute at 1 year of age and 80 to 130 at 2 years, and it reaches 70 to 115 by 3 years. Blood loss, heart failure, dehydration, fever, and anxiety all increase the pulse rate. The normal blood pressure in a newborn infant is approximately 75/40 mm Hg. It gradually increases to 85/60 mm Hg by 4 years and reaches 100/65 mm Hg by 10 years of age. The proper blood pressure cuff should cover one half to two thirds of the upper arm. A larger cuff may give lower readings, and a smaller cuff may give higher readings. The pneumatic cuff and stethoscope are accurate in older children, but in many infants only the systolic pressure can be determined by palpation or auscultation of the brachial or radial artery as the cuff is deflated. The Doppler ultrasound sensor for measuring blood pressure has proved simple and reliable. The examiner must not neglect to palpate the pulses in each extremity. Diminution or absence of the femoral pulses suggests the diagnosis of aortic coarctation. Since current intravascular monitoring techniques may lead to thromboembolism, pulses must be palpated and recorded daily in ill infants. A change in pulse amplitude with respiration, which is more easily detected while deflating a blood pressure cuff, indicates pulsus paradoxicus. This is seen most commonly with cardiac tamponade. Observation and palpation of the veins provide considerable information on the patient's cardiovascular status. Collapsed, or guttered, veins in the feet or hands are diagnostic of hypovolemia, whereas distended neck veins are seen with heart failure or fluid overload.

When the physician takes the time to carefully auscultate the heart in every child, he or she soon learns to recognize deviations from normal. Consultation with a pediatric cardiologist will save the embarrassment of having an elective operation cancelled at the last minute. Repeat examinations are important. During the first weeks of life, a lesion, such as a patent ductus arteriosus or a ventricular septal defect, may not cause a murmur, but as pulmonary vascular resistance falls, a left-to-right shunt will develop, with the appearance of a murmur.

Echocardigraphy is a noninvasive, superbly accurate

technique to diagnose congenital heart disease in doubtful cases.

ABDOMEN

The abdominal wall must be inspected for abnormal venous patterns and umbilical drainage. The abdomen in the older child is slightly scaphoid, and minimal distention or obvious masses can be best appreciated by sighting across the abdomen. However, a scaphoid abdomen in an infant is suggestive of a Bochdalek diaphragmatic hernia with all the intestine in the thoracic cavity. Peristaltic waves from left to right in the upper abdomen suggest a pyloric or high duodenal obstruction. Sometimes a succussion splash can be heard in such a child. Peristaltic waves may also be seen without intestinal obstruction. Palpation of a child's abdomen is an art that requires patience and practice. Sometimes a child can be distracted with a patter of cheerful conversation. Sometimes it may help to tell the child that one can guess what he or she had for lunch by feeling the tummy. Warm hands and gentle examination are essential. The examiner should first palpate well away from any area of suspected pathology to avoid frightening the patient. A light touch with two or three fingers, commencing in the flank and then sweeping over the abdomen, will locate areas of tenderness and enlarged organs. When the child relaxes, one may cautiously palpate more deeply. The spleen and liver edges are found by having the child inhale while the examiner approaches the costal margins from the lower abdomen. Bimanual palpation of each flank is performed to evaluate the kidneys and to search for retroperitoneal tumors. Light percussion is helpful in outlining the liver and spleen and detecting abnormal masses and shifting dullness. Any tenderness detected depends on the examiner's subjective evaluation of the child's reactions. If definite tenderness is found on light palpation, deeper prodding will only cause unnecessary pain. Nothing is to be gained by testing for rebound tenderness because the normal child will wince at the sudden change of pressure. When tenderness is found on light palpation, there is no need to hurt the child further. When it is impossible to distinguish between tenderness and general fussiness in a crying or upset child, it is helpful to use a mild nonnarcotic sedative. If the child awakens from sleep when the examiner touches the sore spot, there can be little doubt about the finding.

Auscultation of the abdomen may be performed before palpation so that the child will become accustomed to a light touch. One should listen to the abdomen in every child to recognize the continuous musical sounds of normal peristalsis. A total absence of intestinal sounds is ominous; this suggests peritonitis or gangrenous bowel.

An early intestinal obstruction results in frequent high-pitched sounds. Later, when the intestine is overdistended and worn out, peristalsis is infrequent, with low-pitched sounds. It is necessary to listen for as long as 5 minutes before deciding whether peristaltic sounds are really absent or merely infrequent.

Abdominal ultrasonography should be used liberally in the evaluation of abdominal problems. This procedure has become almost a routine extension of the physical examination in children with abdominal pain.

INGUINAL AREA

An inguinal hernia is usually obvious. With coughing or crying, a bulge appears just above and lateral to the symphysis pubis. When the sac is completely open, the bulge will extend down into the scrotum. An ovary that prolapses into the inguinal canal is palpable as a small mass that, with manipulation, will pop back into the abdomen. If the hernia is not obvious, the older child can jump up and down or strain. One must always count the testicles; it is embarrassing to miss an undescended testicle, especially when it is intra-abdominal and twisted, simulating appendicitis. Anxiety or application of cold hands can excite a strong cremaster reflex, leading the unwary examiner to misdiagnose cryptorchidism.

SPINE AND EXTREMITIES

It takes only a minute to check for scoliosis and to look for sinus tracts or masses over the lumbosacral spine. In babies, one should flex the hips and feel for the "click" of a dislocated hip. After carefully examining many normal children, one can quickly spot an abnormal finding, even if the exact diagnosis is not immediately apparent.

RECTAL AREA

A properly performed rectal examination will cause no more trauma than a look at the tonsils. The abdominal examination is incomplete unless the pelvic structures and rectum are palpated. A rubber glove and surgical lubricant are required. The child should be lying supine, with hips and knees flexed to facilitate a bimanual examination. The fifth finger is used for infants, but the index finger is satisfactory for older children. The examiner should ask the child to push down as if having a bowel movement; at the same time the examiner is very gently applying pressure to the sphincter. As the sphincter relaxes, the finger is slowly advanced, then rotated 360° to palpate all areas. The examiner should check particularly for sphincter tone, presacral tumors, and fecal impactions, as well as for ovaries in girls. One can also evaluate the inferior extension of a large abdominal mass.

2
Preoperative Evaluation and Preparation

_____ *Susan R. Luck*

In terms of preoperative physical status, the patient may be categorized in one of three ways: the previously healthy child who requires an elective operation; the child who has an acute surgical emergency; or the chronically ill child.

THE WELL CHILD

When a surgically correctable lesion is found during the course of a routine pediatric examination, an operation is merely another event in overall health care. Aside from measures necessary to confirm the diagnosis, the only preoperative studies required are a complete blood count and urinalysis. In non-Caucasian children, a sickle cell test is essential. There is no indication for any other laboratory tests or for a chest roentgenogram. Ideally, the pediatrician or family practitioner should discuss any health problems with the surgeon. Many elective operations are now performed on an outpatient basis, and laboratory tests may be obtained up to a month before the proposed operation. If the child has not had comprehensive care, the preoperative evaluation should include a review of the family situation as well as a review of physical and emotional development. It may be necessary to arrange for further pediatric consultation, immunizations, and counseling to ensure continued health care in the postoperative period.

If outpatient surgery is elected, it must be made clear to the parents that the child cannot have anything to eat or drink on the morning of the operation. It also is wise to tell the parents that the operation will have to be cancelled if symptoms of an upper respiratory infection develop.

THE ACUTELY ILL CHILD

Acute surgical emergencies are some of the most interesting and most difficult problems encountered in pediatric surgery. Trauma, intraabdominal catastrophies, the aspiration or ingestion of foreign objects, and acute infectious conditions fall into this category. Preoperative care for specific diseases is discussed in later chapters. Here we discuss some general principles that are important and that can be applied in many situations.

A clear and open airway with efficient pulmonary exchange is essential. Respiratory insufficiency or airway obstruction can quickly follow obtundation from central nervous system depression or shock. Ventilatory assistance can be instituted with a bag and mask, followed by endotracheal intubation. An emergency tracheotomy is necessary only when facial, laryngeal, or tracheal trauma makes intubation impossible. Pulmonary parenchymal compression by a pneumothorax or by blood, pus, or herniated intestine must be relieved immediately by a thoracostomy drainage or operation.

Rapid vascular collapse can result from hemorrhage or from depletion of body fluids secondary to peritonitis, burns, vomiting, or diarrhea. The signs of shock in a child are more difficult to appreciate than in an adult.[1] Vasoconstriction will maintain the blood pressure until approximately 5 percent of the intravascular volume is lost. Pallor, tachycardia, collapsed veins, and an obtunded sensorium are more important signs of shock than is hypotension. Rapid access to a vein is essential; a cutdown must be performed if percutaneous venipuncture is impossible. Hypovolemia is initially treated with lactated Ringer's solution (20 ml/kg body weight) given as rapidly as possible. Further infusions of crystalloids, colloid, or blood depend on the clinical response and on the type of fluid to be replaced.[2] Volume infusion should be continued until skin color and capillary filling improve. A urinary catheter should be placed in the patient; in the absence of renal failure, urine flow should be at least 1 ml/kg body weight per hour. Rapid bolus administration of measured increments of fluid is preferred to continuous infusion. The effect of each bolus load on volume expansion must be monitored in order to gauge the need for continuing or cutting back fluids.

Initial improvement in vital signs followed by deterioration is clinical evidence of continued occult bleeding or fluid loss. Except in cases of exsanguinating hemorrhage, every effort should be directed toward achieving at least temporary normovolemia by rapid fluid infusion. Children with peritonitis from gangrenous bowel or intestinal perforation may require several hours of resuscitation before they can be anesthetized safely. Anesthetic agents will cause vasodilatation and sudden hypotension in any patient with a contracted blood volume. A central venous line measuring venous pressure is especially helpful in gauging acute fluid shifts. Additional therapy aimed at the correction of acid–base imbalance and electrolyte disturbances must be guided by the status of blood pH, Po_2, Pco_2, and electrolytes. As a general rule, fluid losses owing to burns, peritonitis, and intestinal obstruction should be replaced with lactated Ringer's solution and colloid that approximate the electrolyte concentration of the sequestered fluid. Loss of gastric juice alone requires saline with additional potassium chloride to replace the large amounts of chloride lost with gastric acid.

Temperature control is particularly important. Hypothermia accompanies shock and exposure in small infants and contributes to the development of apnea and acidosis. Fever complicates dehydration and infections. Elevation of body temperature increases caloric expenditure and oxygen use, as well as the amount of drugs necessary for sedation or anesthesia. Hyperthermia during administration of an anesthetic may lead to convulsions. Preoperative measures include rehydration, rectal administration of acetaminophen, and sponging with tepid water. Extreme surface cooling is limited by shivering, which increases heat production and consumption. After the correction of hypovolemia, heavy sedation with narcotics and phenothiazines will reduce shivering if surface cooling is necessary.[3]

THE CHRONICALLY ILL CHILD

Chronic illness can result in emotional depression, malnutrition, chronic hypovolemia, anemia, and growth retardation. Many children in this category have immunologic or coagulation abnormalities as a result of disease or drug therapy. Preoperative transfusions of packed cells or plasma are necessary to restore normal blood volume and to elevate the hemoglobin level to 13 or 14 g/dl. The plasma protein level should be at least 5 g/dl. If the gastrointestinal tract is functioning, judicious tube feedings may be helpful in improving nutrition. In the face of chronic gastrointestinal obstruction, inflammatory disease, or malabsorption, total intravenous nutrition is essential. Every child should be brought into positive nitrogen balance and should demonstrate weight gain before an elective operation. Vitamins, especially ascorbic acid, should be supplied in dosages two to three times the minimum daily requirements. Specific electrolyte and coagulation defects must be corrected before operation. By planning ahead, platelets, fresh frozen plasma, and fresh whole blood can be available on the day of surgery.

SPECIFIC PROBLEMS

Central Nervous System Disease
Children with hydrocephalus who have ventriculoperitoneal or ventriculoarterial shunts often are poorly nourished and are always at risk of developing infection around the shunt tubing. Consequently, cultures should be taken of the skin, throat, and stool to guide preoperative and postoperative antibiotic therapy. Children with meningomyeloceles require repeated corrective operations and are prone to develop urinary tract infections and increasing renal impairment. Renal status is monitored by observing the blood urea nitrogen (BUN) and creatinine levels and the creatinine clearance, as well as urine cultures. Children with convulsive disorders must be continued on parenteral medications after oral intake is stopped. Both phenytoin (Dilantin) and phenobarbital, the most commonly used anticonvulsants, have long half-lives. Effective blood levels will remain for 4 to 5 days. Phenobarbital may be given intramuscularly, but phenytoin is poorly absorbed unless it is given intravenously. In order to prevent cardiac arrhythmias, the calculated dose of phenytoin should be diluted to 100 ml and given over 5 to 10 minutes intravenously while the electrocardiogram is being monitored.

Cardiac Disorders
Children with congenital heart disease, particularly those who have had prosthetic valves or patches, systemic pulmonary shunts, or a prolapsed mitral valve with insufficiency, require antibiotic prophylaxis before many surgical procedures.[4] The standard regimen for children who are to undergo dental work, oral surgery, or upper airway endoscopy requires only penicillin. If the antibiotic can be taken orally, 1 g of penicillin V is given 1 hour before and 500 mg 6 hours after the procedure to children who weigh less than 60 pounds. Older children

are given 2 g before and 1 g after the operation. When the operation prevents the child from taking oral medications, 50,000 units/kg of aqueous penicillin G is given 1 hour before and half the dose is repeated 6 hours after the operation. If the child is allergic to penicillin, either erythromycin or vancomycin is used. High-risk patients, such as those with a prosthetic valve or those undergoing operations on the genitourinary or gastrointestinal tract, are given a combination of 50 mg/kg of ampicillin and 2 mg/kg of gentamicin 1 hour before the operation and again 8 to 12 hours later.

A child with more serious heart disease should be admitted to the hospital several days before the operation for reevaluation by a pediatric cardiologist. The dosage of digitalis may be accurately controlled by determining blood levels and by repeated electrocardiography.[5] Vomiting and poor feeding may be signs of digitalis intoxication, whereas excess perspiration, cool extremities, facial edema, and oliguria are signs of heart failure. The liver size is a good gauge of heart failure in children. Serum electrolytes may be abnormal and may require correction if the patient has been on a salt-restricted diet or has been treated with diuretics.

Pulmonary Disease

Cystic fibrosis of the pancreas and asthma are the most common chronic lung diseases in children, although tuberculosis and fungal infections are still seen. Infants who have recovered from hyaline membrane disease or who have required prolonged ventilation may have bronchopulmonary dysplasia, which increases the risk of atelectasis and carbon dioxide retention. Radiation therapy to the lungs may cause severe pulmonary fibrosis. Simple observation of the child's activities together with a history of his or her exercise tolerance usually will be sufficient to permit estimation of pulmonary reserve. A current chest roentgenogram, sputum cultures, and blood gas determinations will provide more information. A child over 3 years of age can cooperate well enough to permit satisfactory determination of vital capacity and forced expiratory volume.[6] If these studies indicate bronchopulmonary obstruction or reduced function, intensive preoperative care is indicated to reduce secretions and bronchospasm. Children with cystic fibrosis produce copious amounts of tenacious purulent sputum. They are usually malnourished and are poor operative risks. However, much can be done to improve physical status in such patients. Several days of vigorous preoperative therapy consisting of postural drainage, chest percussion, and humidification combined with specific antibiotic therapy will improve lung function. Bronchoscopic aspiration and bronchial lavage also can decrease secretions.[7] Saline lavage can be carried out through an endotracheal tube during general anesthesia for an operative procedure. Atropine thickens tracheobronchial secretion; it

should be given intravenously in small amounts during the induction of anesthesia only if necessary to decrease vagal tone.

Fortunately, children with allergies or asthma often are asymptomatic preoperatively because of environmental control, diet, and drug therapy. All these factors must be considered in planning an elective operation. A time of year must be chosen such that environmental allergens will be minimal. The parents should be allowed to remove objects from the hospital room and substitute pillows or blankets brought from home that may be less allergenic. The administration of xanthine derivatives, sympathomimetic drugs, tranquilizers, and aerosols should be continued at appropriate dosages until the immediate preoperative period. These should then be replaced by similar agents that can be given rectally or parenterally. The anesthesiologist must know precisely what drugs the child has been taking. This is particularly true of corticosteroids. If these agents are being given currently or have been used during the previous 12 months, they must be continued or restarted just before the anesthetic and then tapered during the postoperative period.

Liver Disease

Neonatal hepatitis, biliary atresia, cystic fibrosis, and infectious hepatitis may all result in chronic liver disease. Chemotherapeutic agents and abdominal irradiation also may injure the liver. Any child with a history suggesting liver disease or injury requires baseline liver function and coagulation tests. Edema and ascites should be treated with sodium restriction, diuretics, and salt-poor albumin infusions. If there is no evidence of ammonia intoxication, amino acids can be infused along with carbohydrates and vitamin supplements to ensure an anabolic state. Preoperative administration of vitamin K and fresh frozen plasma and intraoperative infusion of freshly drawn blood will at least partially correct coagulation abnormalities. The anesthesiologist must choose those agents that are least metabolized by the liver. The blood levels of such drugs as nafcillin, erythromycin, chloramphenicol, and acetaminophen, which are partially metabolized and excreted by the liver, must be carefully monitored. With optimum attention to detail, children with severe liver disease will tolerate major operations, such as portosystemic shunts, with minimal difficulty.

Kidney Disease

Calculations of preoperative and postoperative fluid requirements are predicated on normal kidney function. A number of factors may precipitate acute renal failure in a child with borderline renal function: the usual withholding of oral fluids before operation, the tissue breakdown associated with trauma, as well as operative dissection, infections, and blood transfusions. Therefore, it is essential to screen every child who is to have an operation for renal disease. Specific renal function studies must be carried out for any child with a history of abnormal fluid intake and urine output or any child with edema, hypertension, anemia, or unexplained growth failure. An infant with a single umbilical artery, an imperforate anus, or the VATER (vertebral, atresia, trachea, esophagus, rectum) syndrome may have dysplastic or obstructed kidneys. Unfortunately, children with dysplastic kidneys, ureteral reflux with chronic pyelonephritis, and low-grade ureteral obstructions may have severe impairment of renal function with few symptoms.

The urinalysis is the usual screening test. Protein, blood cells, or casts in the urine or inability to produce concentrated urine suggests renal disease. Elevations of BUN and creatinine levels and a decrease in creatinine clearance provide further evidence of renal impairment. Intravenous pyelograms, cystograms, renal radionuclide scans, and ultrasonography furnish information on the anatomy and differential functioning of the kidneys and collecting systems.

A child with abnormal renal function should be admitted to the hospital several days before an elective operation. An accurate record of normal oral intake and urine output, with determination of baseline urine electrolytes, will guide the calculation of preoperative and postoperative fluid therapy. The urine-concentrating mechanisms often are impaired in children with renal dysplasia or obstructive uropathy. Consequently, these children ingest large amounts of fluid and salt to compensate for an obligatory increase in urinary output. These children can become dehydrated very quickly if restricted to nothing by mouth without supplementary intravenous fluids. Serum electrolytes, including calcium, phosphorus, and bicarbonate, should be monitored. If the child is acidotic, sufficient sodium bicarbonate must be given to increase the serum bicarbonate level to 20 to 22 mEq/liter. The extracellular space is equivalent to 0.3 times the body weight in kilograms. The calculated bicarbonate deficit (serum bicarbonate level subtracted from 20 or 22) is multiplied by 0.3 and then by the body weight to find the milliequivalents of bicarbonate required for correction.

Hyperkalemia, hyperphosphatemia, and acidosis are ominous signs of advanced renal failure. In these cases, potassium-containing fluids, such as lactated Ringer's solution, must be withheld. When serum potassium levels rise above 6 or 6.5 mEq/liter, immediate intervention is indicated. Rapid intravenous administration of sodium bicarbonate (up to 2 mEq/kg body weight over a 5- to 10-minute period) will temporarily reduce the serum potassium level. Ten percent glucose (10 to 20 ml/kg), which contains 17 units of regular insulin per 500 ml, also will reduce the serum potassium level. Intravenous calcium gluconate will counter the cardiac toxicity of hyperkalemia, but the electrocardiogram should be monitored while calcium gluconate is being administered. The dose of calcium gluconate may be as much as 0.5 ml of a 10 percent solution/kg of body weight given over a period of 2 to 4 minutes. The measures mentioned drive potassium ions intracellularly, removing them only transiently from the intravascular space. A negative total-body potassium balance must be established either by the use of ion-exchange resins (Kayexalate, 1 g/kg up to every 3 hours, orally or as a retention enema) or by hemodialysis or peritoneal dialysis.[8]

Hemoglobin levels as low as 5 to 6 g/dl occur in uremic children because of bone marrow depression and losses from the gastrointestinal tract. With skilled induction of anesthesia and careful hemostasis, operations may be carried out at these levels. When transfusions are necessary, packed red blood cells are recommended to prevent volume overloading. If there is any possibility of future renal transplantation, pretransplantation blood transfusion may enhance survival of the kidney graft.[9]

Diabetes Mellitus

Juvenile diabetics require close control to prevent wild fluctuations in blood sugar levels during and after operation and the complications of dehydration or ketosis. Management requires cooperation among the pediatrician, the surgeon, and the anesthesiologist.[10]

The child should be admitted to the hospital before an elective procedure. His or her insulin needs and metabolic state must be determined by frequent checks of urine and serum glucose and electrolyte levels. For accurate comparison, the patient should empty the bladder 30 minutes before a meal, and then immediately before eating, another voided specimen should be collected and tested with Clinitest and Acetest tablets. Simultaneous blood glucose levels should be performed to determine the renal threshold for glucosuria. When possible, an operation, such as superficial biopsy or abscess drainage, should be performed under local anesthesia so that the child's normal routine of eating and taking insulin remains undisturbed.

Although some physicians prefer 6-hour management for any child who is to undergo an operation with general anesthesia, many procedures will interfere with no more than one or two meals. More stable management is achieved by giving the child two thirds of the usual dose of immediate-acting insulin before an early morning operation. Intravenous glucose should be provided until the patient can take sufficient carbohydrate-containing liquids in the postoperative period. Frequently, normal food intake can be resumed within 6 hours after the operation, with no additional insulin being required until the next usual dose. For more serious operations, regular insulin should be given on a 6-hour schedule. A controlled diabetic is most likely to become hypoglycemic during general anesthesia, and the aftereffects of hypoglycemia are more dangerous than those of hyperglycemia and must be avoided. From 1 to 2 g of glucose/kg of body weight should be given as a 5 or 10 percent solution to a maximum of 50 or 60 g every 6 hours. Urine and blood glucose levels must be used to determine insulin dosage at each 6-hour interval. An indwelling catheter should not be used routinely because of the danger of infection. The dosage of insulin may be predicted roughly on the basis of the child's preoperative needs.

Vigorous preoperative preparation will be necessary for many diabetic patients with acute surgical emergencies. Sepsis and fever increase insulin requirements. Interference with normal food intake by anorexia or vomiting further increases ketosis and dehydration. Initially, the intravascular volume should be restored with insulin at 20 ml/kg body weight. One half of the insulin dose should be given intravenously and one half subcutaneously. Insulin should never be added to a bottle of intravenous fluid because it adheres to the glass, and an unpredictable amount reaches the patient. Vigorous medical management is essential, but the surgical problem must be corrected as soon as possible in order to restore normal oral intake and treat sepsis.

ANESTHETIC EVALUATION

The pediatric anesthesiologist has an immense responsibility for the child's welfare during an operation. He or she monitors vital signs, maintains an even state of anesthesia, and administers appropriate fluids, blood, and medications. The surgeon can then concentrate on his or her own work without having to worry. In assuming this responsibility, the anesthesiologist must have exact knowledge of the patient's physical and emotional condition and considerable input into the preoperative evaluation and preparation. The anesthesiologist must review the history and physical examination the day before the operation. The surgeon should consult the anesthesia service well in advance of complicated procedures to ensure planning for optimum care. There are several specific areas of concern in preparing for any anesthesia. A history of prior complications in the patient or family may alert the anesthesiologist to an increased risk of bleeding problems or hyperpyrexia or an unusual sensitivity to succinylcholine.[11,12] Postoperative right upper quadrant pain together with jaundice may be a clue to halothane sensitivity.[13] Knowledge of prior drug therapy is particularly important. Specifically, prior chronic use of steroids, reserpine, chlorpromazine, or propranolol may result in intraoperative hypotension.[14-16]

Postintubation laryngotracheal edema can be severe in a child with an upper respiratory tract infection. It may be difficult to determine if a mild clear rhinorrhea

results from crying, from a chronic allergy, or from the prodrome of a respiratory infection. The child and the family are emotionally keyed up, and it is difficult to decide to cancel an operation at the last minute. If the family and the referring physician agree that the child has a mild allergic rhinitis, and if he or she is afebrile, with clear lungs, throat, and ears, it is probably safe to proceed with the planned operation. However, the surgeon should gracefully acquiesce to the anesthesiologist's decision to cancel the proposed operation if there is any sign of an upper respiratory infection.

Vomiting and aspiration are major anesthetic hazards. Every effort should be made to empty the child's stomach before the operation. Irrigation and aspiration through a large-bore oral or nasogastric tube will remove some of the stomach's contents, and these measures are particularly important in any patient with an intestinal obstruction or an ileus. For elective operations scheduled for morning, the usual regimen of nothing by mouth after midnight is satisfactory for children over 3 years of age. Infants and some older children may become irritable, mildly dehydrated, and even febrile if oral fluids are withheld until an afternoon operation. Therefore, it is wise to schedule the youngest children early in the morning. If this is impossible, clear liquids, such as glucose and water, apple juice, or a soft drink, should be allowed up to 4 hours before the operation. Infants under 6 months of age are particularly prone to dehydration. A special effort should be made to awaken them for a 2 AM feeding of clear liquids even if they are to be operated on in the early morning.

PREOPERATIVE MEDICATION

No matter how carefully a child has been prepared for the operation, the final separation from parents, the trip to the operating room, and the strange sights and sounds are frightening. Preoperative sedative drugs are almost universally recommended in order to reduce this fear and anxiety and make the induction of anesthesia easier. Ideally, the drug chosen for this purpose should provide sedation and amnesia without respiratory depression. Obviously the perfect drug has not yet been found, since only about 75 percent of children arrive in the operating room in a relaxed and cooperative state.[17] Narcotics such as meperidine hydrochloride (Demerol) and morphine, antihistamines, barbiturates, and a variety of tranquilizing drugs such as the phenothiazines have potential hazards as well as advantages. Morphine provides tranquility and is a definite advantage in children with cardiac disease. Unfortunately, when morphine is used routinely, there are occasional disastrous errors in dosage. An inexperienced nurse may easily misinterpret 1 mg as 10 mg, particularly if orders are not written clearly. Morphine also appears to cause more nausea and vomiting preoperatively and postoperatively than other agents. Narcotics usually are given subcutaneously 45 minutes to 1 hour before the operation. Since the maximum effect of atropine occurs at the same time as that of the narcotic, both may be given in the same syringe.

Rita et al. compared the effectiveness of morphine and pentazocine as premedication agents in a double-blind study.[18] Sixty percent of the 150 children premedicated with morphine (0.1 mg/kg) were calm while awaiting surgery, and about half became excited during the induction of anesthesia. The results with pentazocine (1.2 mg/kg) were better; 80 percent were calm before and during the induction of anesthesia. There were no significant differences in other parameters, such as pulse, blood pressure, and respirations.

Children are fearful of needles, and they are often more upset than sedated by an injection. Rectal administration of drugs, either by suppository or small enema, is not sufficiently dependable. Root and Loveland have evaluated many oral agents in an attempt to find a substitute for parenteral premedication.[19] They found that 10 mg of Demerol with 0.375 mg of scopolamine hydrobromide/ml in a syrup given orally was as effective as a comparable parenteral dose. Also, they found that 0.2 mg of diazepam and 0.25 mg of scopolamine per pound of body weight provided better hypnosis and amnesia than the same drugs given intramuscularly. At the time of induction, there were no differences in the volumes of gastric juice in the group of children given oral medication and the group given parenteral drugs. Oral medication can be successful only when the surgical schedule will allow 1 to 1.5 hours between drug administration and the operation. Dosage schedules of the various sedative drugs used for premedication are given in Table 2–1. However, these dosage schedules are merely a rough guide; the anesthesiologist must evaluate each patient in order to tailor the drug dosage to fit the patient. An obese or chronically ill child will require less drug on a weight basis than a slender and obviously well patient. On the other hand, a hyperactive and apprehensive youngster will require more sedation.

Anticholinergic agents are given to dry secretions and block vagal activity. Usually, atropine is given subcutaneously or intramuscularly 45 minutes to 1 hour before surgery. However, for outpatient operations many anesthesiologists prefer to give this drug intravenously just after induction of anesthesia. Atropine may cause an alarming, transient red rash, and it is often blamed for an elevated body temperature.

REFERENCES

1. Stiehm EH: Recognition and management of shock in pediatric patients. Curr Probl Pediatr 3:4, 1973
2. Rowe MI, Arango A: The choice of intravenous fluid in shock resuscitation. Pediatr Clin North Am 22:269, 1975
3. Dundee JW, Mesham PR, Scott WEB: Chlorpromazine and the production of hypothermia. Anaesthesia 9:296, 1954
4. Shulman S: Prevention of bacterial endocarditis. Pediatrics 75:603, 1985
5. Krasula RW, Pellegrino PA, Hastreiter AR, Soyka LF: Serum levels of digoxin in infants and children. J Pediatr 81:566, 1972
6. Spector SL, Minden P, Farr RS: Surgery in the allergic child. In Gaus SL (ed): Surgical Pediatrics, New York, Grune & Stratton, 1973, p 313
7. Altman RP, Kulczycki LL, Randolph JG, McClenathan JE: Bronchoscopy and bronchial lavage (BBL) in children with cystic fibrosis. J Pediatr Surg, 8:809, 1973
8. Lewy PR: Renal failure and related disorders in clinical pediatric urology. In Kelalias PP, King LR (eds): Clinical Pediatric Urology, Philadelphia, Saunders, 1976, vol 2, p 769
9. Opelz G, Terasaki PI: Improvement of kidney graft survival with increased numbers of blood transfusions. N Engl J Med 299:799, 1977
10. Traisman HS: The Management of Juvenile Diabetes Mellitus. St. Louis, Mosby, 1971
11. Aldrete JA, Padfield A, Solomon CC, Rulbright MW: Possible predictive tests for malignant hyperthermia during anesthesia. JAMA 215:1465, 1971
12. Lehman A, Liddell J: Human cholinesterase (pseudocholinesterase) genetic variants and their recognition. Br J Anaesth 41:235, 1969
13. Carney FMT, Van Dyke RA: Halothane hepatitis: A critical review. Anesth Analg (Cleve) 51:135, 1972
14. Vandam LD: Effects of prior drug therapy on the course of anaesthesia. In Eckenhoff JE (ed): Science and Practice of Anesthesia. Philadelphia, Lippincott, 1962, p 21
15. Alper MH, Flacke W, Krayer O: Pharmacology of reserpine and its implications for anesthesia. Anesthesiology 24:524, 1963
16. Bourgeois-Gavardin M, Nowill WK, Margolis G, Stephens CR: Chlorpromazine, a laboratory and clinical investigation. Anesthesiology 16:829, 1955
17. Smith RM: Anesthesia for Infants and Children. St Louis, Mosby, 1968
18. Rita L, Seleny FL, Levin RM: A comparison of pentazocine and morphine for pediatric premedication. Anesth Analg (Cleve) 49:377, 1970
19. Root B, Loveland JP: Pediatric premedication with diazepam or hydroxyzine: oral versus intramuscular route. Anesth Analg (Cleve) 52:717, 1973

TABLE 2–1. PREOPERATIVE MEDICATION

Morphine, 0.1 to 0.2 mg/kg

Meperidine, 1.0 to 1.5 mg/kg

Pentobarbital, 2 to 3 mg/kg intramuscularly or orally, 5 mg/kg rectally

Pentazocine, 1 mg/kg

Diazepam, 0.4 mg/kg

Chlorpromazine, 0.5 mg/kg

Atropine, 0.03 mg/kg (maximum 0.6 mg/kg)

3
Emotional Preparation

The craft of surgery involves more than an assembly line of operations accompanied by a ritual of preoperative and postoperative care. Needless emotional trauma can leave a terrified child who will have temper tantrums and will wet the bed long after a successful operation. Distorted fantasies about such simple procedures as the drawing of blood may affect his or her reactions to physicians for years. In fact, Shuster has suggested that the horror story *Dracula* was inspired by the emergence of long-repressed anxiety relating to the author's childhood experience with a surgeon.[1] Concern over the adverse psychologic effects that hospitalization and illness can have on children has been evident in both medical and popular literature for some time.[2-9]

Vernon et al. reported the behavior of 387 children, ages 1 month to 16 years, after hospitalization.[10] General apathy, aggression towards authority, and changes in sleeping and eating habits were noted frequently. Many children temporarily regressed to nail-biting, soiling and incontinence, and the use of pacifiers. Separation anxiety was most marked, as indicated by demands for parental attention and anxiety when left alone. Separation appeared most upsetting to children between the ages of 6 months and 4 years. Interestingly, a small group of children benefited emotionally from hospitalization. For some children who came from emotionally deprived homes, a stay in the hospital was a positive experience.

An extensive study of 1020 English children who were hospitalized during their early years provided strong evidence that even one admission to the hospital of more than a week's duration before 5 years of age was associated with increased risk of behavior disturbance and poor reading ability in adolescence.[11] The factor of early separation had a strong influence, since children admitted to hospitals with a policy of unrestricted visiting were less likely to show adverse emotional changes. There was considerable evidence that children who suffered long-term disturbances were insecure before hospital admission. It was found that the risk of disturbed behavior could be reduced if children who were highly dependent on their mothers and children known to be under increased stress because of a death, divorce, or birth in the family had their elective hospital admissions postponed. Although it was a factor difficult to study, there was evidence that maternal separation was detrimental even to newborns and young infants. Separation of the neonate from the mother may interfere with normal bonding and may result in child–parent disturbances. Young infants have an increased incidence of feeding difficulties and more fretfulness when separated from their mothers. Older children, particularly teenagers, are not so concerned about separation from their families as about physical injury or mutilation. When one considers the well-known anxieties of teenagers concerning facial acne, it is easy to imagine how devastating it must be to undergo an amputation or a genital operation or to be faced with a permanent ileostomy stoma.

Since hospitalization and surgery involve painful and unpleasant experiences, it is not possible to completely avoid emotional trauma. However, one can encourage the child to overcome his or her fears. The approach to each child and to the family must be individualized. In each case, it is essential to be honest with the child, including the child in the discussions about the operation and explaining what will happen. The child's level of comprehension will determine the amount of detail he or she can absorb without increasing fears. Perhaps most important is that the parents understand the procedure so that they can answer their child's questions at home. Timing is important. At the first visit with the surgeon, the parents should be told simply and factually about the disease process, the operation, and the details of the hospitalization procedure. It is helpful to include in this explanation a drawing of the anatomy and the proposed operation. Knowing how much information to present is difficult. Their confidence must be won without inflicting additional worry into an already tense situation. Discussion of long-term results and potential complications must not be omitted. The child should be present during the initial discussion and consultation with the surgeon so that he or she may have an opportunity to ask questions. The family must be encouraged to be perfectly honest. Older children may need several days or even weeks to discuss a forthcoming operation with their families. Children less than 3 years of age may become more anxious if told too soon; they may be better prepared if they are told the day or evening before their hospitalization.

The preexisting attitudes of the parents toward doctors and surgery have a potent influence on the behavior of the child. If the surgeon senses unusual anxiety or hostility, he or she should make every effort to draw out the family's feelings. The problem may be as simple as reassuring them that open-drop ether with its nauseous sequelae is no longer employed in pediatric anesthesia. Frequently, the parents' sense of inadequacy and fear prevents them from being truthful. The child must not be misled but should be told truthfully that he or she is going to the hospital and that some pain will be involved. The child must not be led to feel that any part of the experience is a punishment. An unprepared child will feel that parents and doctor have lied when attacked by strangers with syringes and needles. It is no wonder that some patients create havoc on the ward, refuse to eat, and cry uncontrollably during the induction of anesthesia. It should be emphasized repeatedly that the surgeon's ability to communicate with the parents is most important in helping them to develop a healthy attitude toward their child's treatment. They can then better help their child accept the operation and all that goes with it. Parents best remember information that is accompanied by a drawing and written instructions.[12] They become confused and upset if not given definitive answers to their questions.

A single overall explanation may not be sufficient to relieve stress at certain critical points in the hospital experience. Specific preparation of the young child may be helpful before each of the following events: admission to the hospital, venipuncture, injections, the withholding of food and drink, transport to the operating room, induction of anesthesia, and the immediate postoperative recovery period.[13] Motion pictures and booklets designed to explain various procedures to the child are helpful.[14] Although it is not necessary to tour the operating room with the child before the operation, it is better for the child to know what to expect than to fantasize. Some children really think that all their blood will be removed during venipuncture. A specially trained nurse or other psychologically oriented individual can relieve anxiety

by a simple explanation just before the procedure. The child may be less upset if allowed to handle a syringe and give a doll an injection. This type of play therapy also may be carried on with puppets before elective operations to give children an opportunity to become familiar with the operating room equipment and the caps and masks worn by surgeons and nurses. However, there comes a time when explanations and games fail. At that point, it is necessary to firmly but gently impose restraint on the child, preferably by the mother, and get on with the venipuncture or induction of anesthesia.

The development of an overall program to reduce psychologic trauma to children in hospitals is a group responsibility. The admission of the child must be handled in a warm and friendly manner by an individual who is gentle and patient. The child's introduction to his or her room should be made by a nurse who is willing to help the child and the family become accustomed to the hospital. Playrooms, bright colors, and toys and articles brought from the child's home are also helpful.[15] Physicians must be discreet in their discussions during rounds in front of patients. Children, as well as their parents, are anxious for every scrap of information, and they are likely to misinterpret clinical discussions that are unrelated to their case.

The shortest hospitalization is the best. Many operations are performed on an outpatient basis so that the child is separated from the family only while in the operating room. As much preoperative workup as possible should be done on an outpatient basis. The previously held attitude that children were better off in wards with minimal interference from their parents is definitely wrong.[15–17] It is better for the parents to spend as much time as possible with their child, and it is also helpful for them to be with their child during times of particular stress, such as during painful procedures. One mother put it very simply: "When he wakes up at night crying, I am right there to love him back to sleep."

The following statement was written by a 9-year-old boy who had undergone radical excision of his bladder and rectum for a sarcoma a few years earlier, with apparent cure.

> Feelings about my surgeries might be helpful to other children. When I found out I had to go to the hospital, I had many worries. One of the worries was were the doctors nice. Another one was how much would it hurt. I also worried about having a nose tube because it felt strange when they took it out. I worried about the doctor making a mistake. It helped to bring my favorite stuffed toy to the operating room at the time of the first surgery. I thought that the lights were drills. I don't remember any pain after surgery. I liked it best when a nurse I knew came with me.
>
> But I wished my mother could come with me down the surgery hall and be with me.

REFERENCES

1. Shuster S: Dracula and surgically induced trauma in children. Br J Med Psychol 46:259, 1973

2. Davenport HT, Werry JS: The effects of general anesthesia surgery and hospitalization upon the behavior of children. Am J Orthopsychol 40:806, 1970

3. Belmont HS: Hospitalization and its effects upon the total child. Clin Pediatr 9:472, 1970

4. Fagin CM: The case for rooming in when young children are hospitalized. Nurs Sci 2:324, 1964

5. Jessner L, Blom GE, Fogel SW: Emotional implications of tonsilectomy and adenoidectomy on children. In Eissler RS, et al (eds): The Psychoanalytic Study of the Child. New York, International Universities Press, 1952, pp 126–169

6. Prugh DG, Staub E, Sands HH, Kirshbaum RM, Lenihan E: A study of the emotional reactions of children and families to hospitalization and illness. Am J Orthopsychol 23:70, 1953

7. Schaffer HR, Callender WW: Psychologic effects of hospitalization in infancy. Pediatrics 24:528, 1959

8. Stott DH: Infantile illness and subsequent mental and emotional development. J Genet Psychol 94:233, 1956

9. Vernon DTA, Foley JM, Sipowics RR, Schulman JL: The Psychologic Responses of Children to Hospitalization and Illness: A Review of the Literature. Springfield, Ill, Thomas, 1965

10. Vernon D, Schulman J, Foley J: Changes in children's behavior after hospitalization. Some dimensions of response and their correlates. Am J Dis Child 111:581, 1965

11. Douglas JWB: Early hospital admissions and later disturbances of behavior and learning. Dev Med Child Neurol 17:456, 1975

12. Kupst MJ, Dresser, BS, Schulman JL, Paul MH: Improving physician–parent communication. Clin Pediatr 15:27, 1976

13. Visitaniner MA, Wolfer JA: Psychological preparation for surgical pediatric patients: The effect on children's and parents' stress responses and adjustment. Pediatrics 56:187, 1975

14. Vernon DT, Bailey WC: The use of motion pictures in the psychological preparation of children for induction of anesthesia. Anesthesiology 40:68, 1974

15. Lindquist I: Play as therapy. Paediatrician 3:295, 1974

16. Cremancini R, Bonistalli E: Hospitalized children and parental relationships. Minerva Pediatr 25:904, 1973

17. Bivalec LM, Berdman J: Care by parent, a new trend. Nurs Clin North Am 11:109, 1976

4
Care of the Child in the Operating Room

Frank L. Seleny
Susan R. Luck

Each member of the operating team must be alert to potential complications and injuries that can befall pediatric patients. Prolonged and intricate procedures are now possible only because of the high level of sophistication in anesthetic administration, cardiovascular monitoring, fluid and blood replacement, and temperature control. However, technologic advances will never obviate the many possibilities for human error and machine malfunction.

When the child arrives in the operating room suite, he or she is checked for identity and diagnosis. Complete laboratory evaluation and availability of blood are confirmed. The surgeon should review the planned procedure with the operating team to ensure that all necessary instruments and sutures are available. The anesthesiologist will have checked the armamentarium of masks, airways, endotracheal tubes, and laryngoscopes as well as the anesthetic machine and all necessary medications. Noise will arouse even a well-sedated child; consequently, the room must be kept very quiet during induction. The patient should be brought into the operating room only when everything is ready. Infants and small children may be carried; older children may arrive on a cart. The surgeon or assistant, the circulating nurse, and the anesthetist should help make the child comfortable and answer his or her questions. One person must be with the child at every moment to prevent a fall from the operating table. In spite of excellent preoperative preparation, many children will be fearful and apprehensive. The presence of a familiar toy or blanket often is reassuring. Demonstration of pieces of equipment may distract the patient's attention.

INDUCTION OF ANESTHESIA

A skilled pediatric anesthesiologist can allay last-minute apprehension by talking to the child and by gently stroking the child's face. This seems to have an almost hypnotic effect.[1] During this time, the precordial stethoscope, blood pressure cuff, electrocardiogram leads, and pulse oximeter electrode are attached. The child is given a choice of induction by mask or by intravenous injection. If the mask is chosen, the child is told to "blow up the balloon." Otherwise, a 25-gauge needle is inserted into a vein, and thiopental sodium is administered. The technique of induction, the anesthetic agent, and the choice of endotracheal intubation are the anesthesiologist's responsibilities. However, the surgeon must stay with the child to restrain him or her if necessary and to observe the pulse and electrocardiogram while the anesthesiologist is busy securing and maintaining an airway. The anesthesiologist must keep an eye on the pulse oximeter to ensure that the child's O_2 saturation stays between 99 and 100 percent.

Some children are totally unmanageable, resisting all reasonable efforts to obtain their cooperation. They are obviously frightened and disturbed. If this problem is anticipated, midazolam, 0.8 mg/kg, may be given intramuscularly 10 minutes before the patient is brought to the operating room. Schulman et al. found that the mother's presence during induction of anesthesia helped relieve the child's anxiety.[2] However, even with the mother present, the most important factor in a smooth induction appeared to be the anesthesiologist's ability to establish rapport with the child.

The greatest threat to life during induction of anesthesia is failure to establish an airway. Cooperation between the surgeon and anesthesiologist is vital. The surgeon may be required to inject drugs to help break a laryngospasm and must be ready to perform a tracheotomy if there are anatomic problems. It may be impossible to intubate, even with the help of fiberoptic scope, or to maintain a safe oral airway in children with the Pierre Robin syndrome or those with tumors in the mouth or neck. Ventilation by face mask frequently results in visible distention of the stomach. The routine passage of a gastric tube after induction of anesthesia will help prevent postoperative vomiting and aspiration.

CARDIOVASCULAR MONITORING

By means of frequent observation and evaluation of the patient's vital signs, changes in cardiovascular and respiratory homeostasis can be detected and corrected before serious complications arise. Temperature, pulse, blood pressure, electrocardiogram, O_2 saturation routinely, and, when indicated, end-expiratory CO_2 are monitored and recorded. Anesthetic and surgical mishaps may occur at any time. Hypoxia is most likely to occur during induction of anesthesia and intubation, regardless of the type of operation.

Heart tones and breath sounds can be continuously ausculated by a precordial stethoscope attached to a monaural earpiece. When the operative field encroaches on a precordial stethoscope, an esophageal instrument may be substituted after the child is asleep. A battery-powered radiofrequency telemetry instrument can record the electrocardiogram, a digital reading of the pulse rate, and an audible and visible signal with each heartbeat. The electrodes are attached to the shoulders or legs and may be left in place during transfer to the recovery ward. The great advantage of radiotelemetry is the complete isolation of the patient from the hospital power supply, and thus there is less likelihood of electrical injury.[3] No wires connect the patient to the electrical recorder, and this eliminates the possibility of a low-resistance ground with the potential for exit of electrical current and subsequent patient burn. Eliminating these tethering wires also allows greater flexibility in equipment and patient positioning.

Even in newborn infants, blood pressure can be accurately determined with a stethoscope and a pressure cuff that covers two thirds of the upper arm. During complicated operations in which considerable blood loss is anticipated or in which deliberate hypotensive techniques are to be used, a continuous and more precise technique is desirable. Direct arterial cannulation not only provides continuous recording of the blood pressure but also allows rapid sampling for intraoperative determination of blood gas levels and pH. The Doppler ultrasound flowmeter applied over the brachial or radial artery beneath a blood pressure cuff has proved as reliable as direct arterial measurements.[4-6] The Doppler flowmeter also is helpful in detecting air emboli and may be useful in localizing catheter tips in large vessels.[7]

An indwelling urinary catheter connected to a graduated chamber is invaluable in prolonged operations or in any acute situation in which fluid balance and renal function are unstable. The hourly urine output is an excellent gauge of intravascular volume and effective cardiac output. A urinary flow of 0.5 to 1 ml/kg/hour is adequate.

The central venous pressure reflects the filling pressure in the right heart and the capability of the right ventricle to handle the volume of venous return. The right and left atrial pressures and implied ventricular outputs may be approximately equal in children with normal hearts. Cardiac failure or pulmonary disease will change this relationship. Left ventricular output then must be followed by measurement of the left atrial end diastolic pressure. In such patients a flow-directed pulmonary artery catheter (Swan-Ganz) may be indicated to permit accurate adjustment of fluid infusion and pharmacologic support.[8] In older children both central venous pressure catheters and Swan-Ganz catheters can be placed through an upper extremity or the neck. Placement and maintenance of lines are difficult in infants. Veins may be sacrificed that later will be needed for fluid therapy or hyperalimentation.[9]

Regardless of the degree of monitoring, direct physician observation is essential. The surgeon must be constantly alert to any alteration in the clinical picture at all times during the operation. Airway obstruction, hypoxia, and arrhythmias can occur quickly and unexpectedly, especially during induction, intubation, and extubation. The color of the nailbeds or of the blood provides a far more rapid index of oxygenation than a blood gas determination. Any sudden change calls for immediate assessment of the airway, body temperature, and anesthetic agents, as well as factors in the operative field, such as vena cava compression, pneumothorax, and visceral traction.

MONITORING AND CONTROLLING TEMPERATURE

The body temperature of a child is far more labile than that of an adult, and it should be continuously monitored during any operation. The rectum or esophagus is the most common and most convenient site for a monitor probe. The thermistor probe is a heat-sensitive resistor made from compressed metal oxide powders fused into a terminal bead. When used in the rectum, the tip of the probe is covered with a disposable plastic sheath and inserted no more than 3 cm. Flattened metallic probes also may be taped to the skin or held in place with a plastic foam pad. Thermometers powered by battery or by the hospital power source may be used to display the temperatuue on a meter dial or as a digital readout. Many reliable instruments are available. All are sensitive to trauma and should be calibrated frequently against a standard mercury thermometer. In the last few years, the thermistor probe has been incorporated in the esophageal stethoscope, and they became very accurate. They are very useful in rectal or perirectal surgical procedures.

By use of a reliable and continuous monitor, body temperature must be maintained at a normal steady state. Body heat is lost through evaporation, radiation, conduction, and convection.[10] All these factors, but especially radiation and conduction, affect an infant in a cold operating room. The infant's subcutaneous tissues are thin, and anesthesia abolishes muscular activity and causes vasodilation, both of which contribute to heat loss.[11] The proportionately larger surface area in relation to body weight accelerates heat loss in infants and small children. Premature infants have 10 times the surface area per unit weight as adults. Birth defects, such as omphalocele, gastroschisis, and meningocele, further increase the proportion of body surface area. An abdominal or thoracic operation exposes large serous surfaces to the lower humidity and temperature of the environment. The awakened, exposed, full-term newborn responds to a cold environment first by increased muscular activity, which may increase his oxygen consumption by 64 percent.[12] At the same time, norepinephrine excretion is increased. This increased catecholamine excretion decreases the infant's tolerance to further stress imposed by an operaton or sepsis. Hypoglycemia, poor tissue perfusion, and metabolic acidosis all contribute to and are aggravated by hypothermia. The hypothermic infant metabolizes drugs and anesthetic agents more slowly than normal, and this results in slow emergence from anesthesia and the possibility of delayed respiratory depression.[13]

The temperature of the operating room and the area immediately around the operating table must be warmed to the same temperature as the infant. Even a normal recorded temperature is insufficient evidence that the infant's body heat is not being dissipated, since core temperature falls only when stress is so intense as to overwhelm normal physiologic mechanisms. Hey and Katz have determined the range of temperature adequate to provide thermal neutrality for infants weighing 1 to 4 kg and lying naked in a draft-free environment; the temperature decreases with the increasing weight and age.[14]

The infant should be brought to the operating room in a warmed incubator. The extremities should be wrapped in a clear plastic film, and the infant should not be moved to the operating table until the air conditioning is turned off and the operating room temperature is at least 29 to 30C. A thermostatically controlled warming and cooling blanket is standard equipment for every pediatric patient. Some servocontrolled units are regulated through the thermistor probe by the child's temperature. Poorly perfused tissue, such as the skin of the feet, may be burned even by moderate temperature of the heating mattress. Several thicknesses of sheeting should separate the infant from the heating pad. Supportive rolls or a towel should be placed underneath the heating pad, and the electrocautery plate should be as small as possible so as not to unduly insulate the infant from the heating mattress. Intravenous fluids should be passed through a warmer before they enter the vein, especially if the surgery is prolonged. Many other systems for warming infants in the operating room have been described.[15-17] The choice of method is not too important; what is important is persistence in maintaining a normal temperature with whatever method is used.

The body temperature may drop 2 to 3C during induction of anesthesia, insertion of the intravenous lines, and skin preparation. Supplemental heat from an infrared lamp can help keep the child warm before the drapes are placed. The open infrared-heated infant bed can be used as an operating table. There is no place for prolonged skin preparation with small infants, and volatile antiseptics are to be avoided. The sterile drapes should be applied immediately after rapid skin preparation with a warmed solution. An adherent plastic sheet will protect the child's body from soaking with irrigation fluid and help hold the heat from the warm mattress. At this point, if the infant is normothermic, the lamps can be turned off. They contribute to dehydration of exposed tissues, and there is experimental evidence of increased intestinal adhesions after exposure to infrared heat.[18] Minimal exposure of intestines and other organs to the atmosphere is good surgical technique, and it also helps reduce heat loss. An additional measure to prevent hypothermia is to warm blood and intravenous and irrigating fluids to body temperature.

An increase in tissue oxygen requirement occurs with elevated body temperatures. A febrile child should be treated with rectal acetaminophen, intravenous fluids, tepid sponging, and even external cooling before induction of anesthesia. Some children, particularly those with peritonitis, can be cooled more rapidly in the operating room under general anesthesia. Body temperature will drop on exposure to a cool, air-conditioned room. An additional cooling mattress, covered with a blanket, may be placed over the lower extremities, or ice bags covered with towels may be applied to the axillae and groin. Cooling can be continued during the operation by pleural or peritoneal irrigation.

MALIGNANT HYPERTHERMIA

Malignant hyperthermia is a rare complication of general anesthesia that is seen in susceptible patients. It is characterized by an acutre hypercatabolic state of the muscles. Tachycardia, tachypnea, rapidly rising end expiratory CO_2 tension, rising cardiac output, ventricular arrhythmias, bigemini, and ventricular tachycardia are the most common symptoms. Rigidity is not always present and can be gradual. Fever is usually a late reaction, and it is caused by biochemical breakdown of the muscles.[19] Death or major neurologic and renal complications will ensue if fever is not promptly recognized and treated.[20]

The pathophysiology involved in malignant hyperthermia has been intensively investigated.[21,22] The precipitating agents [various inhalation anesthetics and depolarizing muscle relaxants (succinylcholine)] trigger an accumulation of calcium within the myoplasm. The excess calcium is channeled from the sarcoplasmic reticulum because of a primary defect in the cell membrane or the mitochondia. An increase in cellular catabolism results, with breakdown of glycogen, release of lactate and carbon dioxide, and increased hydrolysis of adenosine triphosphate (ATP). With further membrane instability, intracellular potassium, magnesium, and myoglobin are released. The patient who is not paralyzed responds to the resulting acidosis and hypercarbia with tachypnea. Cyanosis and darkening of blood in the operative field appear after increased extraction of oxygen in the peripheral tissue. Hyperkalemia and acidosis lead to frequent arrhythmias. Myoglobin discolors the urine and precipitates within the tubules. Other clinical signs may include muscle rigidity, skin mottling, and high fever.

The unexpected or sudden appearance of any of these signs demands evaluation. Arterial blood gases and electrolytes will document the metabolic changes. The anesthetic should be terminated at once, and the operation must be completed rapidly or abandoned. Every operating room should be prepared to deal effectively with this emergency.[23,24] Vigorous therapy must be instituted, first by removing any triggering agent; ideally, the entire anesthetic machine should be replaced. Patients must be hyperventilated 3 to 5 times normal values to remove excess CO_2 produced in the muscles[19] with 100 percent oxygen and $NaHCO_3$ to combat acidosis and hyperkalemia. The drug of choice for immediate correction is dantrolene, 1 to 10 mg/kg intravenously given at a rate of 1 mg/kg/minute, which can be repeated after 15 minutes if necessary. The body must be cooled by packing it in ice or by ice saline lavage of body cavities or stomach or bladder. Cardiopulmonary bypass with heat exchange may be feasible in some instances, but it should not be necessary in most children.[24] Diuretics should be administered. Fluid infu-sion and alkalinization will expedite myoglobin excretion and thus prevent acute renal failure. A Foley catheter should be inserted to monitor urine color, pH, and volume. Hypoglycemia must be prevented by infusing hypertonic glucose.

Procainamide will correct arrhythmias and increase calcium transfer from the myoplasm into the sarcoplasmic reticulum. The dose must not exceed 1/mg/kg because the myocardium is already compromised. Measurement of serum K every 15 minutes is imperative, first to detect an increase then a fall of serum K. The former should be treated with regular insulin in 50 percent glucose, the latter with large and prolonged doses of intravenous potassium.

Preoperatively, the diagnosis of malignant hyperthermia must be suspected in any patient with a myopathy, unexplained fever, a history cf muscle cramps or weakness, or a suggestive family history. The maximum incidence occurs between the ages of 3 and 30. The disease is more common in males than in females among teenagers. A specific phenotype has been described in children: A male of short stature with cryptorchidism, pectus carinatum, and spinal deformities.[25] An autosomal dominant mode of inheritance has been described, but most reported cases are not familial. The diagnosis can be confirmed only by in vitro demonstration of muscle contracture potentiation by caffeine, which is further potentiated by halothane. Many, but not all, of these patients will have elevated serum levels of creatine phosphokinase (CPK). The results of electromyography and histopathology of muscle tissue are nonspecific.

ELECTRICAL HAZARDS IN THE OPERATING ROOM

Skin burns, cardiac arrest, and explosions are some of the tragedies that can result from faulty or improperly handled electrical equipment. The electrosurgical unit consists of a spark-gap radiofrequency generator that produces localized tissue coagulation and hemostasis by means of heat at the cautery tip. The vacuum-tube oscillator produces an undamped single-frequency current that rapidly produces a cut by means of dissolution of tissue.[26] A ground plate completes the circuit between the patient and the unit, dissipating the electrical energy concentrated at the operative site. If the plate does not make adequate contact, or if there are alternate pathways for the current through electrocardiogram leads or through contact with any grounded metal, a severe full-thickness burn can result. Rigid ground plates are not recommended; they may touch only a small portion of the child's body, and they may cause pressure sores if placed beneath bony prominences. A flexible disposable plate or conductive surface surrounded by adhesive foam is easy to mold around the buttocks or thigh. The ground plate should not be applied to the back of the chest or the arms. Ventricular fibrillation may occur if the current passes through the heart.[27] Two insulated ground wires connect the plate to the electrosurgical unit; electrocardiogram leads, temperature probes, catheters, and intravenous lines must be kept well away from the ground plate and wires so as not to become alternate pathways for the current and cause skin burns.[28] Skin preparation solution, irrigating fluid, and blood should not be allowed to accumulate under the child because the moisture may create an electrical contact between the child's body and the operating table. The surgeon should begin the operation using the minimum satisfactory current output, which is gradually increased to an optimum level. When the electrosurgical unit does not coagulate well, it is dangerous to increase the current to more than 30 or 35 μA. Its malfunctioning may be caused by a short in the system, and the connections must be rechecked before the unit is used again. Component failure has resulted in ventricular fibrillation with current as low as 20 μA.[29]

Electrical safety depends on factors that are beyond the control of the surgeon. Strict electrical codes and laws should require manufacturers to submit their equipment to approved testing organizations.[30] Frequent maintenance inspections are necessary to detect potential malfunctions. Duncalf and Parker reviewed a 6-month experience with 66 electrical operating room instruments.[31] A specially trained electronics technician routinely tested each instrument every week, and 34 defects that had not been suspected by the surgical or nursing staff were found and repaired.

SKIN PREPARATION AND DRAPING

Applying an antiseptic solution to the skin and draping the area of the operative site with sterile linen have the historic function of excluding skin bacteria from the operative wound. Each surgeon develops routines for these procedures, but some thought must be given to their side effects and hazards. Soaking the skin with soap and water or applying volatile solutions, such as alcohol, that rapidly evaporate contributes to body heat loss. Water or antiseptic solutions can run down under the patient, increasing the electrical hazard. An alcoholic solution that remains on the skin may become ignited by electrocautery. Many systems of skin preparation provide adequate protection against skin bacteria. Povidone (polyvinylpyrrolidone) combines with iodine to form an organic water-soluble preparation that is effective against bacteria, fungi, viruses, and spores. This preparation has been used safely on the skin of patients with known

sensitivity to iodine and has been used in open body cavities and wounds with minimal ill effect.[32,33] When it was applied as a wet soak to patients with 30 percent body burns, there was a 20 percent rise in protein-bound iodine, which returned to normal within 4 to 6 days after discontinuation of the dressings.[34] For these reasons, povidone-iodine is used widely in pediatric surgery. In our experience, there has been no increase in the incidence of wound infection when only a 10 percent preparation solution has been applied to the skin. This technique eliminates the soap-and-water scrub, and consequently the solution must be vigorously applied with gauze sponges held by a ring forceps. Simply painting the skin is insufficient to achieve mechanical as well as chemical cleansing. Towels should be applied about the area to catch the excess solution and prevent soaking of the underlying sheet.

Plastic adhesive drapes serve several functions: they effectively prevent the spread of bacteria from the skin to the wound, they hold the sterile linen in place, and they protect the skin surface from cold wet towels.[35] French et al. studied bacterial contamination of wounds during total hip replacements that were performed in a laminar-flow operating room.[36] The only source of wound contamination was the patient's own skin. A 60 percent incidence of deep wound contamination occurred with the use of cloth drapes, but only 6 percent of wounds became contaminated when the plastic adhesive drape was added.

Operations on the rectum frequently require both an abdominal approach and a perineal approach. Each area should be draped separately, and different sets of instruments should be used to prevent cross-contamination from the perineum to the abdomen. Disposable paper gowns and surgical drapes are impervious to water and bacteria, but they may shed cellulose lint into the wound and cause a distinctive foreign-body reaction. Therefore they should not be used.[37]

PEDIATRIC SURGICAL INSTRUMENTS

The special child-size operating table designed by Swenson is narrow so that the surgeon and his assistant may stand close to the patient. This table will accommodate children up to 14 years of age, but it is particularly suited to operations on small infants. The underlying receptacle for an x-ray plate and attachments for stirrups increase its versatility. Suitable instruments are necessary for any operation, but instruments of the correct size are essential in pediatric surgery. Skin hooks and small shallow retractors are helpful in carrying out herniorrhaphies and other superficial operations, but various small retractors, including "baby" Deaver retractors and miniature Finochietto retractors, are necesary to expose deeper organs in the abdominal and thoracic cavities. Fine-tipped hemostats that crush a minimum of tissue are superior to the standard-size Kelly forceps. Long hemostats with delicate tips are helpful in clamping vessels in deep cavities. Light delicate needle holders that will hold securely but will not bend or abrade small needles are required for fine anastomoses. Metzenbaum scissors with fine curved points are useful for most dissections, but tenotomy scissors with slender tips are best for delicate work in small infants. Potts-Smith scissors with delicate pointed blades are excellent for sharp dissection in deep cavities.

A fiberoptic headlight provides extraordinarily bright illumination in deep, inaccessible cavities. When the surgeon anticipates the need for such lighting, the head attachment can be fitted and the light beam focused before he scrubs. Magnification can be of considerable value in performing cutdowns in small premature infants and in accurate suturing of vascular and intestinal anastomoses. One should select a magnifying loupe that fits and practice with it until one becomes familiar with the limited depth of field.

A reliable bipolar nerve and muscle stimulator can help identify nerves in the head and neck and can facilitate accurate location of the external rectal sphincter in a child with an imperforate anus.

The choice of suture material is more likely to be based on the surgeon's training, experience, and prejudice than on the biologic interaction between the suture material and the host's tissues. There is no single perfect suture material; the best suture for a specific purpose in each case must be selected. The time required for tissue healing varies among species and among different organs in the same species. Biochemical and histologic studies have suggested that wound healing is accelerated in younger patients.[38] In general, there is a lag phase in healing during the first 5 days, when tensile strength depends entirely on the sutures. Fibroplasia lasts up to 14 days, and the wound slowly matures, gaining strength for several months. Poor nutrition, steroid therapy, cancer chemotherapy, and contamination or infection retard normal healing. Animal experiments designed to detect the influence of the suture material itself on wound healing have yielded conflicting results. Catgut produces milder inflammatory reactions in dogs and lasts longer in the tissues than in either rats or rabbits.[39] Van Winkle et al. found no mechanical, biochemical, or histologic differences in skin wounds sutured with polypropylene silk, Merselene, chromic catgut, plain catgut, and polyglactin up to 28 days after operation.[40] At 70 days, wounds sutured with nonabsorbable sutures demonstrated a higher rate of infection and were weaker than those closed with absorbable sutures. In these studies, the suture material had no effect on collagen synthesis. Most investigations have indicated that during the

first 7 days after implantation, all suture materials produce an intense inflammatory reaction. Thereafter, the reaction to monofilament suture is minimal, and the reaction to absorbable suture continues until the material has disappeared.

Absorbable sutures have their greatest value in contaminated wounds; silk, cotton, and the multistrand polyesters form draining sinus tracts that cannot heal until the suture is extruded. These draining sinus tracts are most annoying in children, because the removal of a deep suture is a painful process that occasionally requires a general anesthetic. Unfortunately, catgut has several disadvantages. The prolonged tissue reaction to catgut may be a factor in the development of intestinal adhesions, and the rate of dissolution of catgut is unpredictable. In clinical studies, Haxton et al. determined that 6 percent of 0 chromic catgut sutures in fascia gave way on the second postoperative day. Thirty-five percent of the sutures broke by the fifth day. This study and others have indicated that catgut may not be safe for closure of abdominal fascia. Catgut dissolves even more rapidly in mucosa. This fact is of considerable clinical importance, since we have observed chromic catgut to disappear 3 days after repair of an imperforate anus, with separation of the suture line. However, catgut is preferred in urinary tract work because nonabsorbable sutures rapidly form a nidus for stone formation.[42]

Synthetic absorbable sutures made of polyglycolic acid have been studied in animals and in controlled clinical trials.[43,44] There are conflicting data on the tissue reaction to polyglycolic acid sutures in comparison with catgut and on the tensile strength of this suture. Varma et al. found no statistical difference in tissue reactions to silk, Merselene, catgut, and polyglycolic acid.[45,46] In one report, the incidence of dehiscence and infection was the same as in abdominal wounds closed with nonabsorbable suture.[47] The major difference was the absence of prolonged drainage from sinuses in wounds closed with the synthetic absorbable suture. In our experience, polyglycolic acid sutures have remained at an anastomosis of rectum to anal skin for several weeks. The skin reaction to subcutaneous sutures is as great as with catgut.

There are three types of nonabsorbable sutures. Silk, cotton, and linen are natural materials composed of multifilament strands. These popular suture materials retain their strength for prolonged periods of time; they are pleasant to handle, and their knots are reliable. The synthetic polyester fibers, such as Dacron or Teflon-coated material, are stronger than silk. The Teflon eventually flakes off, and they become multifilament sutures, with reactions to infection the same as or perhaps worse than that of silk.[48] Any multifilament suture is contraindicated in infected or potentially contaminated wounds. Bacteria remain in the interstices of the suture and in the large knots required for safe tying of the polyesters.

A draining sinus in a wound closed with these sutures will not heal until the suture extrudes spontaneously or is removed. In an adult this complication is a nuisance; in a frightened child it can be traumatic.

Thus, we have continued to search for the perfect suture material for use in pediatrics. Nonabsorbable sutures all have disadvantages; even though steel wire and other monofilaments hold up well in the face of infection, they may leave painful subcutaneous knots in thin patients. Therefore, we have concentrated on the new monofilament absorbable sutures. Polydioxanone is completely absorbed within 180 days by hydrolysis but will maintain satisfactory strength in a wound for up to 6 weeks. It proved to be safe and reliable in a series of abdominal wounds in poor-risk patients.[49] This was our suture of choice for several years, although the material is stiff and difficult to handle because of kinking. Monofilament polyglyconate also maintains its strength in wounds for prolonged periods of time and eventually is completely absorbed. This is now our suture of choice for abdominal and thoracic wound closure, hernia repair, and mucosal anastomosis. We have compared subcuticular monofilament polyglyconate with 5–0 chromic catgut sutures. There appear to be less tissue reaction and induration to the monofilament, with no increase in wound complications. The more prolonged wound support provided by the polyglyconate may result in an improved cosmetic appearance of wounds on the neck and chest. Flat square knots are essential when using any fine material. Monofilament sutures must be tied with supreme care, or they will untie. They hold nicely with a square knot on top of a surgeon's knot or with four square throws.[50]

We still use 5–0 or 6–0 polyester vascular sutures for intestinal and esophageal anastomosis, although there is some evidence that polyglycolic acid absorbable sutures may provide superior results in esophageal anastomosis.[51]

TECHNIQUE

Good pediatric surgical technique requires meticulous application of established surgical principles. The surgeon should plan each step of the operation; he should have alternative plans to deal with unexpected pathology and should be prepared to deal with emergencies.

Concern for the patient's tissue commences with carefully rinsing and wiping all traces of starch from gloves. The cornstarch used to lubricate surgical gloves can cause a granulomatous reaction that is particularly troublesome in the peritoneal cavity.[52–54] When this happens, some patients complain only of a low-grade fever and abdominal pain; others develop adhesive intestinal obstruction. Dixon and Beck reported a fatal case involv-

ing an infant who was operated on twice for an adhesive obstruction.[55] At autopsy, the peritoneal cavity was found to be obliterated by adhesions that contained collections of starch and gauze particles.

The incision must be planned to provide optimum exposure without excessive retraction, which injures tissues and retards healing. Skin incisions placed parallel to Langer's lines have a better cosmetic appearance, with a much lower incidence of keloid formation. Transverse abdominal incisions are also less likely to dehisce than are vertical wounds. Campbell and Swenson reviewed 2692 laparotomies performed over a 10-year period, all closed with an interrupted silk technique.[56] They found that 3.37 percent of vertical midline incisions and 1.46 percent of paramedian incisions eviscerated. Evisceration occurred in only 0.2 percent of transverse incisions, and no eviscerations were seen in muscle-splitting McBurney-type incisions. The single evisceration in a transverse incision occurred in a child whose rectus muscles were disconnected from the pubis. She also had a postoperative intussusception.

The incision line should be marked off either on the patient or in the mind of the surgeon so that it can be opened from one end to the other without having to waste time extending the incision. Assistants should apply pressure and traction along the margins of the incision until the first layer of fascia has been divided. By then, oozing from small vessels will have stopped, and by eversion of the skin, the remaining bleeders may be coagulated. Muscle bundles, such as the rectus, latissimus, and serratus, should be divided with needle-point electrocautery. By alternating between the cutting current and coagulation current, muscles can be divided and vessels coagulated with a minimum of tissue destruction. In older children, the intercostal and inferior epigastric arteries should be clamped and ligated. Almost all other vessels in thoracic and abdominal incisions can be controlled with electrocautery. Larger vessels within the operative field should be ligated with 5–0 or 4–0 silk or polyester. Heavier ligatures are required only for pulmonary or major intestinal vessels. Sharp dissection by spreading scissor points at right angles to vessels in anatomic tissue planes allows identification and coagulation or ligation of vessels before they are divided. This technique is critically important when dissecting arteries near the aorta. When the scissors are opened parallel to these vessels, at right angles to the aorta, there is less likelihood that an artery will be sheared off and cause troublesome hemorrhage.

Sudden hemorrhage is always a possiblity when removing large, well-vascularized tumors or when dissecting near the great vessels. Blind attempts to clamp the bleeding point frequently result in more damage and considerable blood loss. Firm digital pressure will control almost any hemorrhage. Nothing further should be done until the patient's vital signs are stable and a large volume of blood is available for transfusion. The first assistant should provide optimum exposure and lighting and make certain that the suction is functioning. The bleeding point should then be cautiously exposed; if possible, it should be clamped and ligated. Frequently, it is necessary to obtain proximal and distal control or to apply a vascular clamp if there is a tear in the vena cava or aorta. The laceration may then be closed with vascular sutures. No attempt should ever be made to clamp or suture the bleeding point until the exposure, lighting, and equipment are optimal. This may even require the help of an additional surgeon or assistant. The control of hemorrhage from large oozing surfaces is a vexing problem. Electrocautery, suture ligatures, and packing with oxycellulose or Avitene may all be employed. Every surgeon must learn, usually by bitter experience, that the wound must be dry before it is closed or it will be reopened that night.

The 6–0 and 5–0 sutures used for the esophagus, bowel, and vessels require a delicate touch because inept handling of the needle will result in unnecessary damage. Tissue adjacent to an anastomosis should be handled with forceps only if there is no other way to stabilize it against the needle. The surgeon's elbow and upper arm should be held against his or her body. After the needle is passed through the tissue, it must be grasped with a tissue forceps before it turns and is lost. Adoption of the palm grip and opening the needle holder with the thenar eminence instead of the fingers will improve suturing accuracy and reduce fumbling for the needle. At all times during the operation, only the structures that require the surgeon's attention should be exposed. The wound edges, organs, and tissues should be covered with warm moist pads. Dry gauze should never cover the intestine because drying damages the serosa, and bits of lint escape and further contribute to adhesion formation. The least reactive sutures and ligatures should be used in the peritoneal cavity to further reduce adhesion formation.

Before closing the incision, the surgeon and the assistant must carefully inspect the wound for lost sponges or instruments and for bleeding. Tubes and drains must be placed accurately and secured before the wound is closed. Saline irrigation will remove loose particles of fat and blood clot from the wound. There is considerable evidence that irrigation with antibiotics helps prevent wound infection in contaminated wounds. The peritoneum should be everted so that a smooth surface will be presented to the abdominal cavity. When an old incision has been used, it is probably better to close with interrupted figure-eight sutures that take both the peritoneum and fascia. Thoracic incisions and extremity incisions may be closed with continuous polyglyconate monofilament sutures, but in the neck or on the face,

fine interrupted nonabsorbable sutures give the best results. Wherever possible, the child's skin should be closed with subcuticular sutures and sterile adhesive strips. In most instances, the adhesive strips are the only dressing necessary.

REFERENCES

1. Bothe A, Galdston R: The child's loss of consciousness: A psychiatric view of pediatric anesthesiology. Pediatrics 50:252, 1972
2. Schulman JL, Foley JM, Vernon DTA, Allan D: A study of the effect of the mother's presence during anesthesia induction. Pediatrics 39:111, 1967
3. Hickman DM: Telemetry in monitoring practice. Clin Anesth 9:85, 1973
4. Lowry RL, Lighti EL, Eggers GWN Jr: The Doppler: Aid in monitoring blood pressure during anesthesia. Anesth Analg (Cleve) 52:531, 1973
5. Janis KM, Kemmerer WT, Hagood CO: Doppler blood pressure measurement in infants and small children. J Pediatr Surg 6:70, 1971
6. Janis KM, Kemmerer WT, Kirby RR: Intraoperative Doppler blood pressure measurements in infants. Anesthesiology 33:361, 1970
7. Carden E, Doll W: A Doppler flowmeter for detecting air and other emboli, incorporating a simple method of screening against interference. Anesthesiology 33:551, 1970
8. Pace NL: A critique of flow-directed pulmonary arterial catheterization. Anesthesiology 47:455, 1977
9. Talbert JL, Heller JA: Technique of central venous pressure monitoring of infants. Am Surg 32:767, 1966
10. Hey EN: Thermal regulation in the newborn. Br J Hosp Med 8:51, 1972
11. Silverman WA, Sinclair SC, Scopers JW: Regulation of body temperature in pediatric surgery. J Pediatr Surg 1:321, 1966
12. Stern W, Lees MD, Leduc J: Environmental temperature, oxygen consumption and catecholamine excretion in newborn infants. Pediatrics 36:367, 1965
13. Roe CF, Santulli TV, Blair CS: Heat loss in infants during general anesthesia and operations. J Pediatr Surg 1:266, 1966
14. Hey EN, Katz G: The optimum thermal environment for naked babies. Arch Dis Child 45:328, 1970
15. Poulos P, D'Alessandro E, Barbara A, Falla A, Groff DB: Operating room infant warmer: Modification of a commercially available unit. J Pediatr Surg 9:521, 1974
16. Shaw A, Franzel I, Bordiuk J: Prevention of neonatal hypothermia by a fiber optic "hot pipe" system: A new concept. J Pediatr Surg 6:354, 1971
17. Russell HE Jr, Otherson HB Jr, Hargest TS: Thermal regulation of pediatric patients in the operating room by means of a fluidized bed. Ann Surg 38:111, 1972
18. Arima E, Fonkalsrud EW: The relationship of intestinal adhesions to infrared heating lamp exposure. J Pediatr Surg 10:231, 1975

19. Britt BA: Malignant hyperthermia. Can Anaesth Soc J 32:666, 1985
20. Britt BA: Malignant hyperthermia. Mod Med Can 31:511, 1976
21. Britt BA, Kalow W, Gordon A, et al: Malignant hyperthermia: An investigation of five patients. Can Anaesth Soc J 20:431, 1973
22. Britt BA: Malignant hyperthermia: A pharmacogenetic disease of skeletal and cardiac muscle. N Engl J Med 290:1140, 1974
23. Fraser JG, Crumrine RS, Izant RJ: A preplanned treatment for malignant hyperpyrexia. Anesth Analg (Cleve) 55:713, 1976
24. Ryan JF, Donlon JV, Malt RA, et al: Cardiopulmonary bypass in the treatment of malignant hyperthermia. N Engl J Med 290:1121, 1974
25. Kaplan AM, Bergeson PS, Gregg SA, Curless RG: Malignant hyperthermia associated with myopathy and normal muscle enzymes. J Pediatr 91:431, 1977
26. McLean AJ: The Bovie electrosurgical current generator. Arch Surg 18:1863, 1929
27. Mitchell JP, Lumb GN: The principles of surgical diathermy and its limitations. Br J Surg 50:314, 1962
28. Finlay B, Couchie D, Boyer L: Electrosurgical burns resulting from use of miniature ECG electrodes. Anaesthesiology 41:263, 1974
29. Brunner J: Workshop on electrical hazards in hospitals. Anaesthesiology 29:1071, 1968
30. Monks PS: Safe use of electro-medical equipment. Anaesthesia 26:264, 1971
31. Duncalf D, Parker B: A program to prevent defects in electronic equipment in the operating room. Anesth Analg (Cleve) 52:222, 1973
32. Sindelar WF, Mason R: Irrigation of subcutaneous tissue with povidone-iodine solution for prevention of surgical wound infections. Surg Gynecol Obstet 148:277, 1979
33. Faddis D, Daniel D, Boyer J: Tissue toxicity of antiseptic solutions. J Trauma 17:895, 1977
34. Connell JF Jr, Rousselot CM: Povidone-iodine, extensive surgical evaluation of a new antiseptic. Am J Surg 108:849, 1964
35. Maxwell JG, Ford CR, Peterson DE, Richards RC: Abdominal wound infections and plastic drape protectors. Am J Surg 118:844, 1969
36. French ML, Eitzen HE, Ritter M: The plastic surgical adhesive drape: An evaluation of its efficacy as a microbial barrier. Ann Surg 184:46, 1976
37. Tinker MA, Burdman D, Deysine M, Teicher I, Platt N: Granulomatous peritonitis due to cellulose fibers from disposable surgical fabrics: Laboratory investigations and clinical implications. Ann Surg 180:831, 1974
38. Viljanto J, Raekallio J: Wound healing in children as assessed by the cellastic method. J Pediatr Surg 11:43, 1976
39. Van Winkle W Jr, Hastings JC: Considerations in the choice of suture material for various tissues. Surg Gynecol Obstet 135:113, 1972
40. Van Winkle W Jr, Hastings JC, Barker E, Hines D, Nichols W: Effect of suture materials on healing skin wounds. Surg Gynecol Obstet 140:7, 1975
41. Haxton HA, Clegg JF, Lord MG: A comparison of catgut and polyglycolic acid sutures in human abdominal wounds. J Abdom Surg 16:239, 1974
42. Yudofsky SC, Scott FB: Urolithiasis on suture materials: its importance, pathogenesis and prophylaxis: An introduction to the microfilament Teflon suture. J Urol 102:745, 1969
43. Echevarria E, Jimenez J: Evaluation of an absorbable synthetic suture material. Surg Gynecol Obstet 131:1, 1970
44. Allman FL Jr: Polyglycolic acid suture in routine sports injury surgical practice. Surg Gynecol Obstet 131:1, 1970
45. Varma S, Ferguson HL, Breen H, Lumb WV: Comparison of seven suture materials in infected wounds: An experimental study. J Surg Res 17:165, 1974
46. Postlethwaite RW: Further study of polyglycolic acid suture. Am J Surg 127:617, 1974
47. Gallitano AL, Kondi ES: The superiority of polyglycolic acid sutures for closure of abdominal incisions. Surg Gynecol Obstet 137:794, 1973
48. Postlethwaite RW, Willigan DV, Vlin A: Human tissue reactions to sutures. Ann Surg 101:144, 1975
49. Schoetz D, Coller J, Veidenheimer M: Closure of abdominal wounds with polydioxanone: A prospective study. Arch Surg 123:72, 1988
50. Magilligan DJ, De Weese JA: Knot security and synthetic suture materials. Am J Surg 127:355, 1974
51. Spitz L, Kiely E, Brereton R: Esophageal atresia: Five-year experience with 148 cases. Pediatr Surg 22:103, 1987
52. Ignatius JA, Hartmann WH: The glove starch peritonitis syndrome. Ann Surg 175:388, 1972
53. Holmes EG, Eggleston JC: Starch granulomatous peritonitis. Surgery 71:85, 1972
54. Aarons J, Fitzgerald N: The persisting hazards of surgical glove powder. Surg Gynecol Obstet 138:385, 1974
55. Dixon MF, Beck JS: Multiple peritoneal adhesions related to starch and gauze fragments. J Pediatr Surg 9:531, 1974
56. Campbell DP, Swenson O: Wound dehiscence in infants and children. J Pediatr Surg 7:123, 1972

5
Immediate Postoperative Care

Postoperative care commences as soon as the last stitch is tied. The child should be responding and extubated before removal of the monitoring devices. If respirations are inadequate, the child must be observed in the operating room until he or she has improved. It may be preferable to leave the endotracheal tube in place in the recovery area until breathing is satisfactory. If the body temperature has dropped during the procedure, the child may again be exposed to infrared heating lamps when the drapes have been removed. In addition, he or she should be covered with a prewarmed blanket for transport to the recovery room. The patient should be placed on his or her side on the cart or stretcher to lessen the danger of aspiration.

Postoperative orders must be individualized for each child; however, there are some general guidelines. Children who have had operations on the skin, subcutaneous tissues, or extremities or have undergone hernia repair will require only the simplest of care. Respiration and vital signs must be monitored until the patient is fully awake. This recovery time varies with the anesthetic technique, but rarely is it longer than 30 minutes to 1 hour. Intravenous fluids are not required, and clear liquids may be offered by mouth as soon as the effects of the anesthetic have worn off. By the evening, most children who have had operations of this magnitude will be up and about and will be able to take their usual diet. Rarely, a child will have continuing nausea and vomiting. Medications are seldom helpful. Food and fluids should be withheld for 2 hours; then 10 to 15 ml of clear liquids should be offered at half-hour intervals. Solid food should not be started until the next day. Full activity may be allowed by the next day or as soon as incisional pain has subsided.

GASTROINTESTINAL CARE

The recovery of the child after an abdominal operation depends on how much his illness or operation has disturbed the gastrointestinal tract. Procedures, such as elective splenectomy or nephrectomy, may be performed with minimal manipulation of the stomach and intestine; consequently there should be little postoperative intestinal ileus. Children, especially infants, tend to swallow considerable amounts of air while crying, so that even a minimal degree of ileus can result in gastric distention. For this reason, any child who has had a major laparotomy should have a nasogastric tube inserted either before or during anesthesia. We have used a soft plastic size 12 double-lumen Anderson sump tube for the past 18 years, with no complications referable to the tube. It is inserted through the mouth in the newborn infant because the newborn breathes exclusively through the nostrils. Intermittent suction may be applied to the tube, or it may be left on gravity drainage. With either technique, the nurse should inject 5 to 10 ml of air into the tube every 2 hours and aspirate all air and fluid with a syringe. When the gastrointestinal tract has not been disturbed, the tube is often removed the following morning. Otherwise, it is left in place until there is no longer bilious drainage and the abdomen is soft and scaphoid, with normal intestinal sounds. Diminution in gastric drainage and passage of stool or flatus are other welcome signs of returning peristalsis. When there has been peritonitis, major abdominal trauma, or an extensive gastrointestinal tract resection, the ileus will be prolonged. There should be a gradual decrease in tenderness, diminution in abdominal distention, and resumption of peristaltic sounds. After removal of the gastric tube, oral feedings should be withheld until it is clear that the child's intestinal tract will handle its own secretions and swallowed air. Feedings should be resumed gradually with measured amounts of clear fluids. No more than 1 to 2 ounces should be given at first because, if offered unlimited amounts of liquid, some children will again become distended and will vomit. When limited liquid feedings are tolerated without distress, the volume of fluid may be increased until all the patient's maintenance water requirements are satisfied. Then solid food is offered, and the patient is advanced to a diet suitable for age. It is wise to continue intravenous fluids until the gastrointestinal tract will tolerate a full fluid load.

Most children will tolerate oral feedings the day after a thoracic operation. However, even when there has been no manipulation of the vagus nerve or abdominal viscera, acute gastric dilatation is still a postoperative threat. If distention is detected on physical examination or if the gastric air bubble is prominent on the chest x-ray, a nasogastric tube should be inserted. Prolonged bilious drainage from the tube after an intestinal anastomosis suggests obstruction at the anastomotic site. This often results from a mechanical problem such as kinking, but in newborn infants prolonged dysfunction is more often secondary to overdistended intestine proximal to the anastomosis. These patients require meticulous nutritional support, with intravenous alimentation and intravenous replacement of the fluids and electrolytes lost from the gastrointestinal tract. The decision to reoperate on patients with this complication is extremely difficult. Sufficient time should elapse to allow spontaneous resolution of edema about the suture line. If there is continued high gastric output with radiologic evidence of obstruction for an interval of 2 to 3 weeks, reexploration is indicated.

An intestinal obstruction that develops after a period of normal intestinal function is a completely different problem. A small intestinal intussusception is the most common etiology for an early postoperative obstruction. The initial operation may not have been related to the gastrointestinal tract.

Following the usual period of ileus, there will be decreases in intestinal drainage, in the passage of flatus or stool, and in normal peristaltic sounds. The child may tolerate feedings for a day or two, then will become distended and vomit, and roentgenograms will demonstrate dilated loops of small intestine. In contrast with the previously described clinical picture, in which a repeat operation may be delayed, an immediate operation is indicated in these circumstances.

PAIN RELIEF

Medication to relieve pain is as important in children as in adults, but it is amazing how few children complain specifically of pain. They cry and seem unhappy, but they are as disturbed by intravenous lines and catheters as by incisional pain. Pain may affect the recovery of even small infants. We have observed decreases in arterial oxygen saturation and an increase in pulmonary vascular resistance in response to painful stimuli. These responses are abolished by small, frequent doses of narcotics.

Pain relief commences in the operating room, with the liberal use of nerve blocks and local wound infiltration with bupivicaine. The maximum dose is 3 mg/kg, which may be given as a 0.5 or 0.25 percent solution, depending on the size of the child. Small incisions, such as are used for herniorrhaphy, orchiopexy, pyloromyotomy, or splenectomy, may be completely blocked. This provides 6 to 7 hours of pain control; by then the child often can take fluids and oral pain medication. It is more difficult to achieve total pain control by infiltration in larger abdominal incisions, but intercostal nerve blocks are useful in thoracic and some upper abdominal incisions.

When complete pain relief is not possible with local anesthesia, intravenous narcotic analgesia is the next best choice. In the recovery room or intensive care atmosphere, with continuous observation and monitoring, an intravenous infusion of 0.1 mg/kg/hour of morphine provides excellent pain control without respiratory depression. For general use, however, there are too many opportunities for errors in the morphine dosage. A misplaced decimal point can have tragic results. Demerol, at 1 mg/kg, is safe and the dosage is easy to remember. This dose may be given at 4-hour intervals, but pain control is better when half that amount is given intravenously every 2 hours. This concept is supported with experience in the use of patient-controlled analgesic systems. When the child has control of his own pain relief, he or she tends to use less analgesia overall but uses smaller amounts more frequently.[1]

When the child can take oral medications, acetaminophen either alone or in combination with codeine is effective. Pain relief must always be balanced against the danger of respiratory depression, especially after a thoracic or upper abdominal operation that inhibits coughing. Demerol may be diluted to a concentration of 1 mg/ml solution and then given in increments of 0.25 to 0.5 mg/kg until the child is more comfortable. Often, after the pain has been relieved, the child can be encouraged to breathe deeply and cough and then will be able to sleep undisturbed for several hours.

Efficient pain control allows earlier ambulation and quicker recovery in older children. Pain control is no less important in younger patients, who will recover more quickly when they and their parents are more tranquil.

REFERENCE

1. Rodgers B, Webb C, Stergios D, et al: Patient-controlled analgesia in pediatric surgery. J Pediatr Surg 23:259, 1988

6
Postoperative Infections in Surgical Patients

_____ *A. Todd Davis*

Postoperative infections can be categorized broadly as those that remain localized at the site of the operation, those that start at the wound site but disseminate to distant sites, and those that are hospital-acquired (nosocomial infections) without relation to the surgical procedure.

SURGICAL INFECTIONS

Surgical infections usually are divided into the following categories: those occurring in clean, uncontaminated wounds, those following procedures in a clean/contaminated area, and those following operations in an obviously contaminated body site. The acceptable rates of infection and the kinds of bacterial species involved differ in each of these three categories.

Clean surgical cases are those in which the surgeon operates in a sterile body cavity. No inflammation is encountered, and no break in aseptic technique occurs during the procedure. In such cases, postoperative infection rates should be well under 1 percent. When infections do occur, they are likely to be caused by gram-positive cocci, such as *Staphylococcus aureus* and Group A beta-hemolytic streptococci. The occurrence of postoperative infection in a clean case provides convincing evidence that a break in technique occurred during or soon after the surgical procedure. A sudden outbreak of wound infections in several clean cases is ominous, suggesting a common source. Such outbreaks have been traced to operating room personnel who are heavy shedders of *S. aureus* from the anterior nares.[1] Several such outbreaks caused by Group A beta-hemolytic streptococci

have been traced to anorectal carriage of the organism by operating room personnel.[2,3]

Clean/contaminated cases are those in which surgery is performed in areas that are known to have a bacterial population, but where no acute inflammation was noted and no major break in technique occurred. One does not ordinarily expect these procedures to result in infection. However, it is not too surprising when infections do occur, caused by bacteria that normally inhabit or are in close proximity to the site operated on. Anaerobic organisms susceptible to penicillin normally inhabit the oropharynx and nasopharynx. Potential aerobic pathogens sometimes found in the indigenous flora of the upper respiratory tract include *S. aureus*, *Streptococcus pneumoniae*, *Haemophilus influenzae*, and *Streptococcus pyogenes*. Such skin bacteria as *S. aureus* and, at times, *S. pyogenes* can infect lacerations and other superficial wounds. Anaerobes and aerobic gram-negative enteric bacteria are the normal inhabitants of the lower gastrointestinal tract.

Contaminated cases are those in which an operation is performed in the presence of acute inflammation, on a traumatic wound more than 8 hours old, to drain an abscess, or in which a major break occurs in aseptic technique. Postoperative infections are not uncommon in such cases. When an infection does occur, the offending organisms are almost always those that normally inhabit that site. For example, an infection following treatment for a ruptured appendix usually is caused by bacteria normally present in the gut. There are 600 to 700 different species of anaerobic organisms that account for 95 percent of the entire bacterial flora of the colon.[3] Aerobic gram-negative rods, such as *Escherichia coli*,

Klebsiella-Enterobacter, Pseudomonas aeruginosa, and enterococci, comprise the other 5 percent.[4] Abdominal infections in contaminated cases are usually polymicrobic. It is often difficult to determine which bacteria are pathogens and which are innocent bystanders.

The infection rate in neonates requiring an operation is higher than in older children. In Sharma and Sharma's series from India, 13.75 percent of 160 neonates developed infections.[5] The frequency of infection was higher in patients who were considered clean/contaminated or contaminated from the beginning, but the rate was still 5 percent in clean cases. The incidence of infection in neonates from another series was 26.3 percent.[6] This higher rate of infection in newborn infants may be related to the presence of a contaminated umbilicus near the incision as well as to the poor immunity demonstrated by newborn infants. In these series, wound infections also were more common when patients spent a week or more in the hospital before the operation and when operations were on an emergency basis.

PROPHYLACTIC ANTIBIOTICS

Prophylactic antibiotics are inappropriate for those clean cases in which the incidence of infection is low (<1 percent). In excess of 99 percent of patients would be unnecessarily exposed to antibiotics. The use of prophylactic antibiotics might obscure the presence of infections and delay recognition of the cause of a common source outbreak.

The use of prophylactic antibiotics in clean/contaminated cases depends on the surgical lesion and the extent of expected contamination at the time of operation.

The role of prophylactic antibiotics in surgery has been best studied in clean/contaminated abdominal surgery in adults.[7] Experimental and clinical studies suggest that antibiotics must be present in tissue at the time of operation and for a few hours thereafter.[8,9] For example, Galland et al. administered tobramycin and clindamycin before surgery and again 8 hours later to adults undergoing colon surgery.[10] Of the treated patients, 8.1 percent developed wound infections, compared with 42 percent in the control group. Similar results were obtained with gentamicin/clindamycin or gentamicin/metronidazole for 3 to 5 days postoperatively.[11] Therefore, extending the period of antibiotic usage after operation did not further reduce the wound infection rates. Other studies also have implied that continuing administration of prophylactic antibiotics for several days after an operation is unwarranted.[12] Further, this practice may predispose patients to colonization by bacteria that are resistant to multiple antibiotics.[13]

Anaerobic bacteria appear to be the most important pathogens controlled by prophylactic antibiotics in abdominal surgical procedures. Studies have shown that metronidazole (Flagyl) is an effective prophylactic agent.[14] This antibiotic has activity against many anaerobes but virtually no aerobes. However, metronidazole is no more effective than oral erythromycin plus neomycin, or parenterally administered cephalosporins.[15,16]

The role of prophylatic antibiotics in the repair of congenital heart defects and genitourinary tract surgery has not been well studied. Most cardiovascular surgeons use a prophylactic antistaphylococcal agent, although the incidence of postoperative endocarditis seems to be much lower in children following repair of congenital defects than in adults following valve replacement. If prophylaxis is to be undertaken in genitourinary surgery, knowledge of the organism(s) colonizing the patient's genitourinary tract could be helpful in deciding an appropriate antibiotic strategy. However, the value of prophylaxis in genitourinary tract surgery remains unproven.

For surgical procedures of the head and neck, the surgeon must be aware of the penicillin-sensitive anaerobes that inhabit the mouth and pharynx. *S. aureus* can be found in more than 85 percent of the anterior nares of normal children. Other potential pathogens include Group A beta-hemolytic streptococci, which in the fall and winter are found in 15 to 25 percent of children. There have been few controlled studies to assess the efficacy of prophylactic antibodies for head and neck procedures in children. If prophylaxis is undertaken, a semisynthetic penicillin (such as nafcillin, methicillin, or oxacillin) may be most effective insofar as most anaerobes are sensitive to these agents. Penicillin prophylaxis would be theoretically very effective in eradicating Group A streptococci and hindering the development of anaerobic infections. However, in the last decade or so, the majority of community-acquired *S. aureus* strains have been resistant to penicillin.[17]

In contaminated cases, antibiotics are required for therapeutic, not prophylactic, purposes. The choice of antibiotic depends on the expected normal bacterial flora of the body site involved. In contaminated abdominal cases, one can generally anticipate the presence of such anaerobes and gram-negative enteric aerobes as *E. coli, Klebsiella,* and *P. aeruginosa.* A combination of clindamycin, which is effective against *Bacteroides fragilis* and all other anerobes, and an aminoglycoside such as kanamycin or gentamicin is most useful. There are very few species of bacteria that are not susceptible to this antibiotic combination. Among the exceptions are the enterococci, also known as *Streptococcus faecalis* and Group D streptococci. The precise role of enterococci in the pathogenesis of infections after ruptered abdominal viscus is unclear. Clindamycin and gentamicin are almost always effective in such infections, suggesting that the enterococci are innocent bystanders rather than important causative pathogens. If an enterococcal infection is suspected, ampicillin should be added to the regimen.

EVALUATION AND TREATMENT OF POSTOPERATIVE INFECTIONS

The clinical and laboratory investigation of a child suspected of having an infection after surgery is dependent on the child's age and the clinical presentation of the illness. Infants less than 1 month old are much less able to localize infections than are older infants and children.

Neonates

Neonatal infections frequently occur with such nonspecific symptoms as lethargy, irritability, respiratory distress, apnea, jaundice, and convulsions.[18] Any of these symptoms mandates a search for infection, as well as for such metabolic problems as hypoglycemia and hypocalcemia.[19] Appropriate laboratory investigation of a neonatal infection includes cultures of the blood, the urine, the spinal fluid, and the wound.

Administration of antibiotics must often be started immediately after cultures are obtained from neonates (Table 6–1). Broad-spectrum coverage must be obtained rapidly with the antibiotics most appropriate for the suspected pathogen until specific cultures and sensitivity reports are available. Thus all neonates should be treated with an aminoglycoside and ampicillin or a semisynthetic penicillin (the latter should be used if staphylococcal infection is suspected). The choice of gentamicin or amikacin is dependent on the percentage of gram-negative enteric organisms susceptible to gentamicin in a particular hospital, along with the likelihood of a *Pseudomonas* infection. It should be recognized that many *P. aeruginosa* strains are resistant to gentamicin. Amikacin and carbenicillin or ticarcillin or ceftazidime (one of the extended-spectrum cephalosporins) are useful in this situation.[20]

In the past, cephalosporins had little to offer the sick neonate. Many gram-negative enteric organisms were resistant. The cephalosporins rarely crossed the blood–brain barrier in concentrations necessary for efficacy. *P. aeruginosa* strains were rarely susceptible to the first- and second-generation cephalosporins. However, the development of newer cephalosporins, the so-called second- and third-generation agents, have obvi-

TABLE 6–1. ANTIBIOTIC DOSAGES FOR NEONATES

Antibiotic	Route	Daily Dosage and Intervals[a]	
		0–7 Days of Age	*> 7 Days of Age*
Amikacin	IM,IV	15 mg/kg/day div q12h	15.0–22.5 mg/kg/day div q8h
Ampicillin	IM,IV		
Meningitis		100–200 mg/kg/day div q6–8h	200–400 mg/kg/day div q6–8h
Other indications		50–75 mg/kg/day div q8–12h	75–100 mg/kg/day div q6–8h
Ceftazidime	IM,IV	100 mg/kg/day div q8–12h	150 mg/kg/day div q8h
Ceftriaxone	IM,IV	50 mg/kg/day once daily	50–75 mg/kg/day once daily
Meningitis		50–80 mg/kg/day	80–100 mg/kg/day
Cephalothin	IV	40–60 mg/kg/day div q12h	60–80 mg/kg/day div q6–8h
Gentamicin	IM,IV	5 mg/kg/day div q12h	7.5 mg/kg/day div q8h
Kanamycin	IM,IV	15–20 mg/kg/day div q12h	20–30 mg/kg/day div q8h
Methicillin	IM,IV	50–75 mg/kg/day div q8–12h	75–200 mg/kg/day div q6–8h
Nafcillin	IV	50–100 mg/kg/day div q8–12h	100–200 mg/kg/day div q6–8h
Penicillin G	IM,IV		
Meningitis		200,000–300,000 U/kg/day div q6–8h	200,000–400,000 U/kg/day div q6–8h
Other indications		50,000 U/kg/day div q8–12h	75,000–100,000 U/kg/day div q6–8h
Ticarcillin	IM,IV	200–300 mg/kg/day div q8h	200–400 mg/kg/day div q6–8h

[a] The smaller doses and longer intervals are for infants weighing less than 2000 g.
Adapted from Nelson.[21]

ated many of these problems. In general, the spectrum of coverage has broadened with each succeeding generation of drugs, the concentration required for inhibition or killing of gram-negative species has diminished, and some third-generation agents have activity against *P. aeruginosa*. It was hoped initially that the very low mean inhibitory bactericidal concentrations required for many gram-negative organisms would lead to superior therapeutic results, particularly in central nervous system (CNS) infections. This has not proven to be the case.[21]

Thus, a cephalosporin, such as cefotaxime, may be substituted for an aminoglycoside in the initial therapy of suspected sepsis, but results will likely be equivalent to an aminoglycoside plus ampicillin. Moreover, it should be noted that each succeeding generation of cephalosporins tends to have less antistaphylococcal activity than first-generation agents, such as cephalothin.

Older Children

Older children with intact host-defense mechanisms are much less likely to have disseminated infections than are neonates. Therefore, only wound and blood cultures are required in the febrile postoperative child. Other cultures (or cerebrospinal fluid or urine, for example) need be taken only when specific clinical findings or symptoms point to the involvement of the related organs. The decision on the antibiotic should be based on which pathogen(s) is the most likely cause of the infection (Table 6–2).

NOSOCOMIAL INFECTIONS

Nationwide, about 5 percent of all hospitalized patients acquire nosocomial infections. The incidence in pediatric hospitals appears to be approximately the same as in adult hospitals.[22] However, there are unique problems in children's hospitals or wards posed by such diseases as measles, chickenpox, Group A streptococcal pharyngitis, and bacterial or viral diarrheas. Some other nosocomial infections that occur in hospitalized children and adults are pneumonia, urinary tract infections (particularly those associated with indwelling urinary catheters), sepsis caused by contaminated intravenous fluids, and

TABLE 6–2. ANTIBIOTIC DOSAGES FOR CHILDREN MORE THAN 1 MONTH OLD

Generic Name	Route	Total Daily Dose	Dosage Interval
Amoxicillin	PO	40 mg/kg/day	q8h
Ampicillin	IM,IV	100–200 mg/kg/day	q4–q6h
Carbenicillin	IM,IV	400–600 mg/kg/day	q4–q6h
Dicloxacillin	PO	25–50 mg/kg/day	q6h
Penicillin V	PO	20–50 mg/kg/day	q6–q8h
Penicillin G	IV	200,000–400,000 U/kg/day	q4h
Procaine penicillin	IM	25,000–50,000 U/kg/day	q12–q24h
Nafcillin	IV	100–200 mg/kg/day	q4–q6h
Methicillin	IM,IV	100–200 mg/kg/day	q4–6h
Oxacillin	PO	50–100 mg/kg/day	q6h
	IV	100–200 mg/kg/day	q4–q6h
Cephalothin	IM,IV	75–150 mg/kg/day	q4–q6h
Cefazolin	IM,IV	50–100 mg/kg/day	q8h
Cefaclor	PO	40 mg/kg/day	q8h
Ceftazidime	IM,IV	100–150 mg/kg/day	q8h
Meningitis		150 mg/kg/day	
Ceftriaxone	IM,IV	50–100 mg/kg/day	q12–q24h
Meningitis		100 mg/kg/day	q12h
Cefuroxime	IM,IV	100–150 mg/kg/day	q8h
Meningitis		200–250 mg/kg/day	q6h
Clindamycin	PO	15–25 mg/kg/day	q6h
	IM,IV	25–40 mg/kg/day	q6–q8h
Amikacin	IM,IV	15–22.5 mg/kg/day	q8–q12h
Gentamicin	IM,IV	5–7.5 mg/kg/day	q8h
Kanamycin	IM,IV	15–30 mg/kg/day	q8h
Sulfisoxazole	PO	120–150 mg/kg/day	q4–q6h
Trimethoprim-sulfamethoxazole	PO	8–16 mg TMP/40–80 mg SMX/kg/day	q12h
Nitrofurantoin	PO	5–7 mg/kg/day	q6h
Prophylaxis		2–3 mg/kg/day	q12–24h

septic thrombophlebitis from IV catheters left in place too long.

All children admitted to a hospital should be screened carefully for recent exposure to infectious diseases. Despite such precautions, children will frequently develop bacterial diarrhea or one of the childhood exanthems following admission. It is crucial to recognize and isolate such illnesses so as to decrease the chance of spread within the hospital. Susceptible patients exposed to the same disease may be isolated together. Hospital personnel responsible for infection control should be promptly notified about all actual and potential nosocomial infections.

Nosocomially acquired pneumonias are particularly problematic for patients requiring mechanical ventilation who are housed together in intensive care units.[23] Gram-negative enteric bacteria are prominent causes of such infections. The risk of such infection can be minimized by strict attention to aseptic techniques while suctioning the artificial airway, the judicious use of narrow-spectrum antibiotics, and careful attention to handwashing by medical, nursing, and respiratory therapists providing medical care.

Every effort should be made to prevent nosocomial infections associated with IV cannulae and urinary catheters. IV cannulae for the routine administration of fluids and medication should not be left in place for more than 48 hours if they are made of polyvinylchloride or polyethylene.[24] Small Teflon catheters are preferred because of the decreased risk of infection.[25] Teflon catheters should be changed every 72 hours along with the IV fluid delivery set. Clinical circumstances sometimes dictate that IV cannulae need remain in place longer than 3 days. When this is anticipated, the initial insertion should be made with sterile technique, including the use of gown, gloves, and mask. The dressing site should be inspected daily.

Open urinary catheter drainage systems are totally unacceptable. Even with closed systems, as many as half of all patients will develop bladder infections within 8 days.[26] The likelihood of developing a urinary catheter-associated infection can be decreased by scrupulous aseptic precautions when the catheter is placed or manipulated. There have been a number of outbreaks of *Serratia marcescens* urinary tract infections in which personnel manually transferred the organisms from one patient to another.[27]

Contaminated intravenous fluid is an infrequent source of sepsis. An unexpected episode of sepsis in a child, particularly if the offending organism belongs to the *Klebsiella-Enterobacter* group or is an unusual gram-negative species, suggests the diagnosis.[28] The intravenous fluid, bottle, administration set, and cannulae should be immediately replaced and sent to the laboratory for culture. Even though sepsis in many such cases will resolve spontaneously once the contaminated intravenous fluid has been replaced, it is nonetheless advisable to institute antibiotic therapy.

CULTURING TECHNIQUES

Blood Cultures
The skin should be prepared either with an iodophor cleanser or by rubbing the area with 70 percent alcohol for at least 60 seconds. After aseptically drawing the blood, a new needle should be substituted before inoculating the collection tube or bottle. A ratio of 1 ml of blood to 10 to 20 ml of media appears to be optimal. Anaerobes are best recovered from blood cultures when no air is present in the syringe while drawing the blood and when no air has been introduced into the anaerobic blood culture bottle. Blood culture bottles especially designed to remove antibiotics should be used for patients on antimicrobial therapy.

Urine Cultures
Obtaining meaningful urine cultures in infants can be quite difficult. Culture data obtained from bag-collected urine is reliable only if the culture is sterile. A positive bag culture must be confirmed by either a clean-catch specimen or suprapubic aspiration, since bag urine cultures are contaminated so often. Greater than 100,000 colonies/ml in clean-catch voided urine usually indicates infection. Any number of colonies in a suprapubic aspiration culture is meaningful.

In children who are toilet trained, a clean-catch midstream urine specimen obtained after cleansing the external genitalia is the preferred method of urine collection. Catheterization should be used only in special circumstances, with the awareness that about 1 percent of intermittent catheterizations result in a urinary tract infection.

Wound Cultures
A gram stain of wound exudate is essential for the evaluation of a possible wound infection. Careful attention to the collection of specimens for anaerobic cultures of wounds or abscesses is particularly important. Whenever possible, material should be aspirated into a syringe, the needle inserted into a stopper, and the specimen sent to the laboratory. Swab cultures for anaerobes should be made with special collection tubes. Usually a pair of oxygen-free test tubes are provided, one of which contains a swab. After use, the swab should be rapidly inserted into the second oxygen-free test tube and then sent to the laboratory.

ANTIMICROBIAL AGENTS IN PEDIATRIC SURGERY

When properly performed, in vitro antibiotic susceptibility tests can be of great use in choosing an appropriate
antibiotic. As a general principle, a narrow-spectrum
antibiotic should be used to decrease the probability of
superinfection with a resistant bacterium. For example,
when treating a staphylococcal infection, a semisynthetic
penicillin, such as nafcillin, methicillin, or oxacillin, is
preferable to a cephalosporin, which acts not only on
gram-positive cocci but on many gram-negative rods as
well.

Moreover, antibiotics must be used only when indicated in order to prevent the development of resistant
strains in the patient and in the hospital. An outbreak
of a resistant *Klebsiella* infection, including meningitis,
occurred several years ago on a neurosurgical unit. The
organism was eliminated from the unit only when all
antibiotic usage was halted.[29]

ANTIMICROBIAL THERAPY FOR COMMON INFECTIOUS DISEASES OF CHILDREN

Otitis media in children 3 months of age or older is
almost always caused by *S. pneumoniae*, *H. influenzae*,
or *Branhamella catarrhalis*. Unusual isolates include *S.
aureus*, *Staphylococcus epidermidis*, *S. pyogenes*, *Pro-
pionibacterium*, and anaerobes. Amoxicillin at 40 mg/
kg/day given every 8 hours is the most appropriate choice
for initial therapy.[30] In the child allergic to penicillin,
cefaclor (Ceclor), erythromycin ethylsuccinate and sulfisoxazole acetyl (Pediazole), trimethoprim-sulfamethoxazole (Bactrim or Septra) may be used.

The diagnosis of Group A streptococcal pharyngitis
must always be made by a positive throat culture or a
positive rapid test employing an antigen detection
system.[31] Appropriate therapy consists of a 10-day course
of oral penicillin or erythromycin.

The therapy of a urinary tract infection depends
in part on the causative organism and whether the infection appears to involve the kidneys or the lower urinary
tract alone. For mild, uncomplicated urinary tract infections acquired outside the hospital, sulfisoxazole, nitrofu-
rantoin, and amoxicillin are all effective agents. Urinary
tract infections occurring in hospitalized patients present
more difficulties in choosing initial therapy. In contrast
to community-acquired infections, which are almost always caused by *E. coli* susceptible to most antibiotics,
hospital-acquired urinary tract infections are often caused
by other pathogens with varying antibiotic resistance.
If the child is not particularly ill, it is often best to
await culture and sensitivity reports before initiating

therapy; for more seriously ill children, a broad-spectrum
agent, such as gentamicin or amikacin, often is indicated
initially. When susceptibility results are known, a less
expensive, more easily administered, and less toxic antibiotic should be substituted if possible.

REFERENCES

1. Nahmias AJ, Godwin JT, Updyke EL, Hopkins WA: Postsurgical staphylococcic infections: Outbreak traced to an
individual carrying phage strains 80/81 and 80/81/52/52A.
JAMA 174:123, 1960
2. Schaffner W, Lefkowitz LB Jr, Goodman JS, Koenig MG:
Hospital outbreak of infections with Group A streptococci
traced to an asymptomatic anal carrier. N Engl J Med
280:1224, 1969
3. McKee WM, DiCaprio JA, Roberts CE Jr, Sherris JC:
Anal carriage as probable source of streptococcal epidemic.
Lancet 2:1007, 1966
4. Finegold SM, Flora DJ, Attebery HR, Sutter VL: Fecal
bacteriology of colonic polyp patients and control patients.
Cancer Res 35:3407, 1975
5. Sharma L, Sharma P: Postoperative Wound Infection in
a Pediatric Surgical Service. J Pediatr Surg 21:889, 1986
6. Doig C, Wilkinson A: Wound Infection in a Children's
Hospital. Br J Surg 63:647, 1976
7. Kaiser AB: Antimicrobial prophylaxis in surgery. N Engl
J Med 315:1129, 1986
8. Burke JF: The effective period of preventive antibiotic
action in experimental incisions and dermal lesions. Surgery 50:161, 1961
9. Burke JF: Preventive antibiotics in surgery. Postgrad Med
58:65, 1975
10. Galland RB, Saunders JH, Mosley JC, Darrell JH: Prevention of wound infection in abdominal operations by preoperative antibiotics or povidone-iodine: A controlled trial.
Lancet 2:1043, 1977
11. Feathers RS, Sagor GR, Lewis AAM, et al: Prophylactic
systemic antibiotics in colorectal surgery. Lancet 2:4, 1977
12. Stokes EJ, Waterworth PM, Franks V, et al: Short-term
routine antibiotic prophylaxis in surgery. Br J Surg 61:739,
1974
13. Selden R, Lee S, Wang WLL, et al: Nosocomial *Klebsiella*
infections: Intestinal colonization as a reservoir. Ann Intern
Med 74:657, 1971
14. Willis AT, Ferguson IR, Jones PH, et al: Metronidazole
in prevention and treatment of *Bacteroides* infections in
elective colonic surgery. Br Med J 1:607, 1977
15. Clarke JS, Condon RE, Bartlett JG, et al: Preoperative
oral antibiotics reduce septic complications of colon operations: Results of prospective, randomized, double-blind
clinical study. Ann Surg 186:251, 1977
16. Lau WY, Fan ST, Yiu TF, et al: Prophylaxis of postappendi-
cectomy sepsis by metronidazole and cefotaxime: A randomized, prospective and double-blind trial. Br J Surg
70:670, 1983
17. Musher DM, McKenzie SO: Infections due to *Staphylococcus aureus*. Medicine (Baltimore) 56:383, 1977

18. Klein J, Marcy S: Bacterial sepsis and meningitis. In Remington JS, Klein JO (eds): Infectious Diseases of the Fetus and Newborn Infant, 2nd ed. Philadelphia, Saunders, 1983

19. Davis AT: Approach to the febrile pediatric patient. In Youmans G, Patterson P, Sommers H (eds): The Biologic and Clinical Basis of Infectious Disease, 3rd ed. Philadelphia, Saunders, 1985

20. Odio CM, Umana MA, Saenz A, et al: Comparative efficacy of ceftazidime vs. carbenicillin and amikacin for treatment of neonatal septicemia. Pediatr Infect Dis 6:371, 1987

21. Nelson J: 1987–1988 Pocketbook of Pediatric Antimicrobial Therapy, 7th ed. Baltimore, Williams & Wilkins, 1987

22. Gardner P, Carles DG: Infections acquired in a pediatric hospital. J Pediatr 81:1205, 1972

23. Stevens RM, Teres D, Skillman JJ, Feingold DS: Pneumonia in an intensive care unit. Arch Intern Med 134:106, 1974

24. Goldmann DA, Maki DG, Rhame FS, et al: Guidelines for infection control in intravenous therapy. Ann Intern Med 79:848, 1973

25. Maki DG, Ringer M: Evaluation of dressing regimens for prevention of infection with peripheral intravenous catheters: Gauze, a transparent polyurethane dressing, and an iodophor-transparent dressing. JAMA 258:2396, 1987

26. Garibaldi RA, Burke JP, Kickman ML, Smith CB: Factors predisposing to bacteriuria during indwelling urethral catheterization. N Engl J Med 291:215, 1974

27. Maki DG, Hennekens CH, Bennett JV: Prevention of catheter-associated urinary tract infection: an additional measure. JAMA 221:1270, 1972

28. Edwards KE, Allen JR, Miller MJ, et al: *Enterobacter aerogenes* primary bacteremia in pediatric patients. Pediatrics 62:304, 1978

29. Price DJE, Sleigh JD: Control of infection due to *Klebsiella aerogenes* in a neurosurgical unit by withdrawal of all antibiotics. Lancet 2:1213, 1970

30. Paradise JL: Otitis media in infants and children. Pediatrics 65:917, 1980

31. Denny FW: Current problems in managing streptococcal pharyngitis. J Pediatr 111:797, 1987

7
Hematologic Evaluations

James A. Stockman, III

Normal hemoglobin levels vary widely throughout infancy and childhood. The mean hemoglobin level of cord blood is 17.5 g/dl. Approximately 95 percent of all cord hemoglobin values fall between 13.7 and 20.1 g/dl. In the presence of a normal reticulocyte and nucleated red cell count, a value of 13.6 g/dl may be considered the lower limit of normal for a newborn.[1] This initial cord hemoglobin level will decline over the first 4 to 8 weeks of life. The lower limits of normal for a term infant at 8 weeks are approximately 9.8 g/dl. Preterm infants may have values as low as 7 g/dl, depending on the degree of prematurity. After this nadir is reached, the hemoglobin gradually rises again throughout the first year of life[2] (Table 7–1). After the first year of life, the hemoglobin values gradually rise until the onset of puberty, when adult hematologic data are achieved[3] (Fig. 7–1).

It has been generally accepted that a hemoglobin value of 10 g/dl is considered a safe minimum level for anesthesia. Since the lower limit of normal hemoglobin may be less than this figure in very early infancy, it is not clear if an increased anesthestic risk would exist in such infants who fall within the range of normal for age. Certainly, a transfusion may be indicated to raise the oxygen-carrying capacity to higher levels if the type of surgery to be undertaken is major.

The minimum evaluation of anemia in infancy and childhood requires a complete blood count, including all erythrocyte indices, a reticulocyte count, a platelet count, and an examination of the peripheral blood smear. This is done, of course, in conjunction with a complete history and physical examination. Children with microcytic anemias generally have such anemias on the basis of iron deficiency. The same findings may be seen in thalassemia trait disorders, especially if the red cell count is within the normal range. In children, iron deficiency most commonly represents inadequate iron intake rather than blood loss. Such children rarely require transfusion and respond well to correction of diet and iron supplementation. Among older children, however, blood loss on a chronic basis can be a cause of iron deficiency. Such blood loss may result from bleeding into the stool, hemosiderinuria, idiopathic pulmonary hemosiderosis, epistaxis, or occult internal bleeding. Anemias associated with an increased mean corpuscular volume (MCV) are uncommon in children. These may be caused by folic acid deficiency, liver disease, hyperthyroidism, leukemic states, aplastic anemia, and, rarely in children, vitamin B_{12} deficiency. Normal newborns have macrocystosis, and most children with Down's syndrome can be expected to be macrocytic.

The reticulocyte count is important in the evaluation of any child with anemia. An elevation of reticulocyte counts suggests a hemolytic process or recent blood loss. Anemia in the presence of a low reticulocyte count suggests bone marrow failure, especially if the MCV is normal or increased. The anemia of chronic diseases in children generally is normocytic and normochromic.

Correction of anemia before surgery using transfusions can be accomplished by the use of packed red cells in an amount of 10 to 15 ml/kg body weight, administered over 3 to 5 hours. This is best done a day before surgery to allow reestablishment of a normal blood volume after transfusion. With currently available anticoagulants, effective oxygen release properties of stored red blood cells are maintained for approximately 7 days. Following that, erythrocyte 2,3-diphosphoglycerate lev-

TABLE 7–1. NORMAL VALUES OF HEMOGLOBIN (g/dl), HEMATOCRIT (%), ERYTHROCYTE COUNT (10^12/liter), MEAN CORPUSCULAR HEMOGLOBIN (pg), MEAN CORPUSCULAR VOLUME (fl), AND MEAN CORPUSCULAR HEMOGLOBIN CONCENTRATION (g/dl)[a]

n	Age (months)						
	0.5 (n = 232)	1 (n = 240)	2 (n = 241)	4 (n = 52)	6 (n = 52)	9 (n = 56)	12 (n = 56)
Hb (mean ± SE)	16.6 ± 0.11	13.9 ± 0.10	11.2 ± 0.06	12.2 ± 0.14	12.6 ± 0.10	12.7 ± 0.09	12.7 ± 0.09
−2 SD	13.4	10.7	9.4	10.3	11.1	11.4	11.3
Hct (mean ± SE)	53 ± 0.4	44 ± 0.3	35 ± 0.2	38 ± 0.4	36 ± 0.3	36 ± 0.3	37 ± 0.3
−2 SD	41	33	28	32	31	32	33
RBC count (mean ± SE)	4.9 ± 0.03	4.3 ± 0.03	3.7 ± 0.02	4.3 ± 0.06	4.7 ± 0.05	4.7 ± 0.04	4.7 ± 0.04
−2 SD + 2 SD	3.9–5.9	3.3–5.3	3.1–4.3	3.5–5.1	3.9–5.5	4.0–5.3	4.1–5.3
MCH (mean ± SE)	33.6 ± 0.1	32.5 ± 0.1	30.4 ± 0.1	28.6 ± 0.2	26.8 ± 0.2	27.3 ± 0.2	26.8 ± 0.2
−2 SD	30	29	27	25	24	25	24
MCV (mean ± SE)	105.3 ± 0.6	101.3 ± 0.3	94.8 ± 0.3	86.7 ± 0.8	76.3 ± 0.6	77.7 ± 0.5	77.7 ± 0.5
−2 SD	88	91	84	76	68	70	71
MCHC (mean ± SE)	314 ± 1.1	318 ± 1.2	318 ± 1.1	327 ± 2.7	350 ± 1.7	349 ± 1.6	343 ± 1.5
−2 SD	281	281	283	288	327	324	321

[a] These values were obtained from a selected group of 256 healthy term infants followed at the Helsinki University Central Hospital who were receiving continuous iron supplementation and who had normal values for transferrin saturation and serum ferritin. Values at the ages of 0.5, 1, and 2 months were obtained from the entire group. and those at the later ages from the iron-supplemented infant group after exclusion of iron deficiency. (Saarien and Siimes,[2] with permission.)

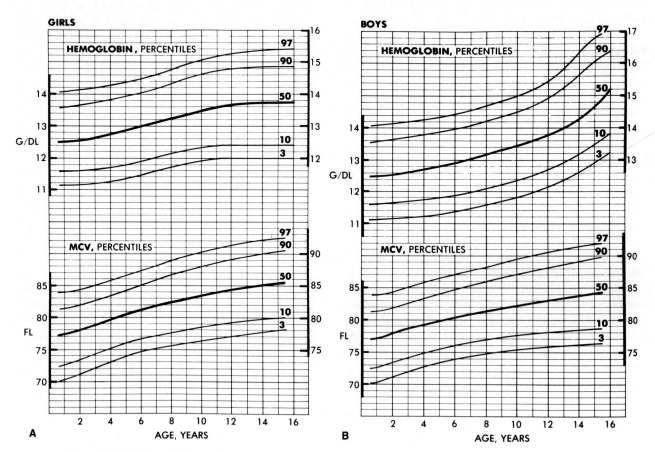

Figure 7–1. A. Hemoglobin and MCV percentile curves for girls. **B.** Hemoglobin and MCV percentile curves for boys. These figures were obtained from populations of nonindigent white children residing in either Northern California or Finland. Hemoglobin values were derived from a total of 9946 children and MCV values from 2314 children. The reference population excluded subjects with laboratory evidence of iron deficiency, thalassemia minor, or hemoglobinopathy. (Dallman and Siimes,[3] with permission.)

els will decline, resulting in an increased oxygen affinity at any given hemoglobin concentration.

SICKLE CELL DISEASE

Children with sickle cell anemia and other sickling hemoglobinopathies may be at risk of serious complications from anesthesia and surgery. In this country, approximately 8 percent of American blacks have sickle cell trait, and slightly under 1 percent will have some form of severe sickle syndrome (SS, SC, S-thalassemia).[4] Children with sickle cell trait are not at an unusual risk from anesthesia unless they experience episodes of severe hypoxia or acidosis.

Among the more common surgical procedures performed in children with sickle cell anemia are splenectomy and cholecystectomy. Splenectomy usually is indicated in a child who has had two or more episodes of sequestration crisis involving the spleen. By age 18 years, as many as 42 percent of patients with sickle cell anemia will develop gallstones.[5] The majority of individuals with sickle cell anemia will ultimately develop cholelithiasis or cholecystitis sometime during their lifetime.

The anesthetic risk to patients with sickle hemoglobinopathies is based on the risk of hypoxia and acidosis during a surgical procedure. Such risk can be reduced by preoperative transfusion programs designed to replace circulating sickle cells with normal hemoglobin cells.[6] Several transfusions beginning some weeks before surgery of 10 ml of packed cells/kg of body weight usually will successfully reduce the sickle hemoglobin concentration below 30 percent. A sickle hemoglobin concentration between 20 and 30 percent appears to be relatively safe for even the most complex of surgical procedures. If necessary, preparation for surgery can be expedited with an exchange transfusion.

It is not clear that all children with serious sickle hemoglobinopathies require such preoperative transfusion preparation. Many centers now will perform minor to moderately complex surgical procedures without attempting to reduce significantly the percentage of sickle hemoglobin. It is advisable, however, to at least raise the hemoglobin concentration of the patient to greater than 10 g/dl.[7] Meticulous attention must be paid during such surgical procedures to maintain adequate oxygenation and to avoid any potential acidosis. Anesthetic complications have been described in patients who have not been prepared preoperatively with transfusion, although these probably are rare if appropriate care and attention are given to providing the anesthesia. Anesthetic complications have been described, including deaths, as a result of surgery on patients with sickle cell trait. This risk is very low, and it is not necessary to preoperatively transfuse such patients. All black pa-

tients, however, should have a screening test for sickle hemoglobin before general anesthesia. Positive tests should be followed by hemoglobin electrophoresis in order to determine the exact nature of the sickle hemoglobinopathy.

BLEEDING PROBLEMS IN THE PEDIATRIC SURGICAL PATIENT

The Normal Hemostatic Process

Normal hemostasis involves a complex mechanism. When vascular endothelium is damaged, platelets aggregate around the site, and thrombin is formed on the surface of the platelets. Ultimately, cross-linked fibrin will cause the platelets to aggregate irreversibly. The generation of thrombin is the final common pathway from the stimulation of aggregation either by the intrinsic coagulation process or the extrinsic pathway.

Activation of the intrinsic coagulation pathway is triggered by the exposure of basement membrane collagen to blood (Fig. 7–2).[8] Factor XII (Hageman factor) will bind to subendothelial structures. This results in activation of factor XII, which then hydrolizes prekallikrein (Fletcher factor) and factor XI, as well as plasminogen, thus activating the kinin-generating, coagulation, and fibrinolytic mechanisms all at one time. Factor XI, once activated, will interact with factor IX (Christmas

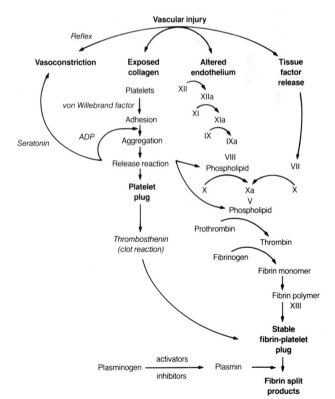

Figure 7–2. Diagrammatic representation of the hemostatic mechanism.

factor), which is converted to a serine protease factor IXa (activated factor IX). The amounts of factor IX present vary widely with age, and factor IX is one of the major liver-dependent factors in the coagulation scheme. When factor IXa is formed, it will convert factor X to factor Xa. The activation of factor X by factor IXa must occur at a rapid rate and be well localized to the site of hemostatic injury. This is accomplished by the action of factor VIII, the antihemophilic factor. Factor VIII circulates within the blood complex found with von Willebrand's factor. Von Willebrand's factor functions by binding to specific platelet receptors and is thought to mediate the adhesion of platelets to subendothelial structures.

Activation of the extrinsic coagulation cascade is initiated by the exposure of blood to tissue factor. This substance is present on the surface of many different cells. Tissue factor is able to form a stable complex with the plasma protein, termed factor VII (also a liver-dependent factor). Activation of factor VII ultimately will result in activation of factor X. It is activated factor X that is the final common product produced by stimulation of both the intrinsic and extrinsic pathways.

The common pathway of clotting is triggered when prothrombin is activated to thrombin. The presence of factor V markedly augments the ability of prothrombin to be converted to thrombin. Thus, it is apparent that many critical events must happen for the final formation of thrombin and its interaction with platelets at the sites of vessel injury. Ultimately, once this interaction has occurred, fibrinogen activation will take place, and a fibrin clot will form.

There are several major inhibitors of the coagulation scheme present in both children and adults. These include the antithrombins, protein S, and protein C. Absence of these may result in a hypercoagulable state. Excessive clot formation also can occur if there is inhibition of the normal fibrinolytic mechanism.

Preoperative Evaluation of the Surgical Patient

The initial evaluation of the surgical patient for potential bleeding disorders includes a history and physical examination. The history to be elicited for bleeding disorders should begin in the neonatal period.[9] Bleeding at the time of circumcision, excessive formation of cephalohematomas, unexplained anemia, and unexplained jaundice are all potential manifestations of bleeding from inherited disorders. Bleeding at the site of separation of the umbilical cord from the skin at several days or a week or more of life is suggestive of an inherited deficiency of factor XIII (fibrin-stabilizing factor).

Some children with inherited coagulation defects and some children with disorders of platelet function will have bleeding at the time of eruption of their deciduous or permanent teeth. It is mandatory to take a careful dental history related to bleeding. Patients with hemophilia often have deep tissue bleeding and joint bleeding. Mucosal bleeding is much more common with von Willebrand's disease.

Patients with coagulation factor abnormalities and those with inherited platelet disturbances may have exacerbation of their bleeding when they ingest medications or other substances that affect platelet function. This is particularly true of aspirin ingestion in patients with von Willebrand's disease.

Most coagulation abnormalities are autosomal recessive. This is not true of classic hemophilia (factor VIII deficiency) or Christmas disease (factor IX deficiency), which are X-linked in inheritance. Von Willebrand's disease may show either a dominant or a recessive pattern. In most instances, the degree of abnormality in a particular family member will be similar in other family members. Approximately 25 to 40 percent of patients with hemophilia may give no positive family history of this disorder.

ROUTINE LABORATORY TESTING OF THE SURGICAL PATIENT

Except for minor surgical procedures, routine preoperative coagulation screening testing is now performed, including platelet count, bleeding time, prothrombin time, and partial thromboplastin time.

Platelet Count

Although the bleeding time becomes abnormal when the platelet count falls to between 50,000 and 100,000 cells/dl, surgical bleeding usually is not significant until the platelet count falls below 50,000 cells/dl. Wherever possible, the platelet count should be artificially raised to greater than 100,000 cells/μl before surgery. At platelet counts between 20,000 and 50,000, surgical bleeding can be expected. Spontaneous bleeding may occur when the platelet count falls below 20,000 cells/dl. If a platelet count cannot be determined before a surgical procedure, a careful examination of the peripheral blood smear should suffice to determine if there are adequate numbers of platelets present.

Bleeding Time

Prolongation of bleeding times can result from intrinsic platelet defects, a decrease in platelet number, vascular abnormalities, or deficiencies in von Willebrand's factor as in von Willebrand's disease. There are a variety of tests currently available to determine bleeding time. Previously, a stab incision in the ear lobe (Duke method) or a similar stab in the forearm (Ivy method) was employed,[10,11] but these have proven relatively difficult to reproduce with a high degree of accuracy. Alternative tests using a template have been devised, which have been simplified further into a test known as the "simplate" test that appears to be quite reproducible.[12,13] The normative values for bleeding time vary somewhat from laboratory to laboratory. With the use of the simplate bleeding time, most hospital laboratories use an upper limit of normal of 8 minutes for the detection of prolonged bleeding times.

Partial Thromboplastin Time

The partial thromboplastin time (PTT) provides the most useful indicator of abnormal coagulation in most instances.[14] Since the PTT reflects activation of the intrinsic pathway and ultimately results in the formation of a fibrin clot, it is theoretically able to detect any of the intrinsic and common pathway factor deficiencies. In practice, however, the PTT may not be sufficiently sensitive to detect mild to moderate deficiencies of prothrombin or fibrinogen. The PTT also may fail to detect mild depressions of the first-stage coagulant factors, which is probably of no clinical significance, since such mild depressions would not be expected to result in surgical bleeding. Because the PTT is unable to detect with a high degree of sensitivity the common pathway factors, a prothrombin time should also be determined.

Prothrombin Time

A prothrombin time should be considered part of the routine screening tests before surgery.[15] In addition to indicating many coagulation deficiencies detected by abnormal PTT, the prothrombin time is considered to be more sensitive than the PTT for deficiencies of prothrombin. It also will detect factor VII deficiency, whereas the PTT will not. It should be noted that neither the prothrombin time nor the PTT is capable of detecting factor XIII deficiency, which is usually screened for with the urea clot solubility test. Also, specific factor assays are available for factor XIII. The prothrombin time is considered the most sensitive test for screening for evidence of liver dysfunction. A combination of both the prothrombin time and the PTT should be considered complementary in preoperative testing.

Thrombin Time

The thrombin time is determined by the addition of thrombin to recalcified plasma. Specifically, the test is intended to detect deficiencies of fibrinogen, and thrombin time basically measures the conversion of fibrinogen to fibrin. Therefore, it will also detect functional abnormalities of fibrinogen (the dysfibrinogenemias) and any inhibitor of the conversion of fibrinogen to fibrin. In many laboratories, the thrombin time is not a routine procedure, since they prefer to measure fibrinogen levels directly.

Other Screening Tests of Hemostasis

There are many other tests that are available for studying coagulation abnormalities, and some of these may even be considered screening tests. However, other than the bleeding time, prothrombin time, and PTT, these tests are not routinely employed. As noted, the thrombin time will detect levels of hypofibrinogenemia and dysfibrinogenemia as well as inhibitors of the conversion of fibrinogen to fibrin, the most common of which are elevated levels of fibrin degradation products in patients who have disseminated intravascular coagulation. Some laboratories routinely screen for factor XIII deficiency in preoperative screening testing, since no commonly employed test, such as the prothrombin time or PTT, will detect factor XIII deficiency. The urea clot solubility test will detect factor XIII deficiency and is very inexpensive; however, factor XIII deficiency is an extremely rare disorder.

Specific Coagulation Factor Assays

Assays are available for all known factor deficiencies. Specific assays are not indicated unless screening tests are abnormal. The only exception to this rule is the PTT, which may not be sufficiently sensitive to detect the very mild depressions of factor deficiency that might be diagnostic of a disorder, such as von Willebrand's disease; e.g., the PTT may be normal when coagulant factor VIII is in the range of 45 percent of normal,[16] which is abnormal but not associated with bleeding tendencies. A level in this range, however, could be consistent with a diagnosis of von Willebrand's disease, and to be completely satisfied that a patient does not have von Willebrand's disease, it would be necessary to add factor assays for procoagulant factor VIII, factor VIII antigen, and von Willebrand's factor. If a PTT is abnormal and the prothrombin time is normal, it may be necessary to quantitate the amounts of factors VIII, IX, XI, and XII. Currently, von Willebrand's disease is the most common disorder producing prolongations of the PTT in otherwise healthy individuals. A deficiency of Hageman factor (factor XII) is the next most common disorder. Patients who have a normal PTT and an abnormal prothrombin time may have an isolated deficiency of factor VII, and specific assays for this would be indicated by the coagulation profile. When both the prothrombin time and PTT are abnormal, assays for factors I, II, V, X, or a combination of these should be considered.

Platelet Function Studies

The single best screening test for platelet functional abnormalities is the bleeding time. Tests of platelet aggregation are certainly excellent studies to detect qualitative platelet dysfunction, but these are reserved for patients who have abnormal bleeding times.[17] Platelet aggregation tests are based on the principle that when a platelet-aggregating agent is added to platelet-rich plasma, the platelets will clump, and the optical density of the plasma will be decreased, allowing for increased light transmission. Several agents are used as aggregating agents in these tests, the most common being the natural physiologic stimulator of platelet aggregation, adenosine diphosphate (ADP).[18] Other aggregating agents include epinephrine, collagen, and thrombin. Patients with von Willebrand's disease may demonstrate platelet aggregation with the antibiotic ristocetin. This form of aggregation testing is included as part of the diagnostic evaluation of von Willebrand's disease. Specific diagnoses may be made depending on the pattern of aggregation abnormality. For example, prolonged bleeding times caused by aspirin ingestion will result in an abnormal aggregation pattern in which a second wave of aggregation produced by low concentratons of ADP is not seen.

MANAGEMENT OF PATIENTS WITH KNOWN BLEEDING DISORDERS

Hemophilia

The term hemophilia is generally reserved for patients with congenital deficiencies of factor VIII (classic hemophilia or hemophilia A), factor IX (hemophilia B or Christmas disease), or factor XI. The first two usually occur in a similar fashion, and both are inherited as X-linked recessive disorders. Factor XI deficiency is usually inherited as an autosomal recessive disorder. With each of these disorders, the bleeding manifestations correlate best with the level of deficiency of the factor. Less than 1 percent activity is associated with severe bleeding, 1 to 5 percent activity is associated with moderate bleeding, and 6 to 25 percent is associated with mild bleeding. Deficiencies of factors may exist between 25 and 50 percent of normal but usually are not associated with clinical bleeding. Patients with mild hemophilia may actually give a negative history of bleeding and are diagnosed only at the time of preoperative surgical testing.

Patients with factor VIII or factor IX deficiency will be detected with prolonged PPT on routine screening. Quantitation of the specific level of factor deficiency is mandatory. These diagnoses can be made at any age, since neither factor VIII nor factor IX crosses the placenta.

Patients with virtually any type of inherited bleeding disorder as a result of factor deficiency can undergo surgical procedures with adequate supervision. Cryoprecipitate became available in the 1960s and is capable of correcting factor VIII-deficient plasma to virtually any level necessary before surgery. Cryoprecipitate may be used as a replacement source of fibrinogen.[19] Soon after the introduction of cryoprecipitate, factor concentrates

became commercially available and generally remain the mainstay of factor replacement for most patients with severe forms of hemophilia.[20] Any patient with factor VIII or factor IX deficiency who is about to undergo surgery must have a preoperative screening test to determine if there is a circulating inhibitor present. Approximately 1 patient in 7 with hemophilia will develop an anticoagulant (or inhibitor) some time during their lifetime. Patients with circulating anticoagulants are poor candidates for surgery and may require special treatments before surgery depending on the level of inhibitor.

In the overall management of patients with hemophilia, careful attention should be paid to what otherwise might seem to be minor points of management. For example, dressing changes, suture removal, intramuscular injections, endoscopy, and other relatively noninvasive procedures may cause significant bleeding. Even simple lumbar puncture should not be performed without prior factor replacement. Venipuncture may be performed as long as it is done carefully. Intramuscular injections may be given if indicated without factor replacement in most instances. Certainly all patients must avoid the ingestion of such agents as aspirin or other compounds that inhibit platelet function.[21]

One unit of factor VIII administered per kilogram of body weight will raise the factor VIII level 2 percent. The same amount of factor IX will increase the plasma level of factor IX 1 percent. For surgical preoperative correction, the patient should have the factor deficiency corrected to 100 percent activity, which should be determined after administration of the factor concentrate by specific assay. Postoperatively, it is ideal to have the patient's level of factor remain at or above 40 to 50 percent. This will require factor VIII-deficient patients to receive factor concentrate every 8 to 12 hours in an amount of 20 to 30 units/kg for the first several days after surgery. This may be administered as a continuous infusion. Usually by the third to fifth postoperative day when the wounds have begun to heal, either the dose of factor VIII is decreased or the interval between infusions is increased. Factor IX has a longer biologic half-life than factor VIII, and factor IX-deficient hemophiliacs usually can be treated with 30 to 50 units/kg of factor IX every 12 hours for the first several days. Following that, 50 units/kg may be given just once a day. The type of replacement management is very much dependent on the nature of the surgical procedure performed. Patients undergoing intracranial surgery will require much closer management of these factor levels than patients undergoing more simple procedures, such as herniorrhaphy. A failure to respond to factor therapy may indicate development of a circulating inhibitor, and assays should be performed immediately.

It is well understood that the use of factor concentrate replacement is associated with complications. Contamination of blood products with the human immunodeficiency virus (HIV) was first noted as early as 1978.[22] Within the last several years, all factor concentrate products have been screened for HIV antibody positivity and also are heat treated. Currently, it is believed that heat treatment of factor concentrates is adequate to prevent transmission of HIV.[23] Heat treatment also may decrease the risk of hepatitis B, but its effect on non-A, non-B hepatitis transmission is not well understood.[24] The risk of contamination by type of product varies. Single donor cryoprecipitate would appear to be the safest product in most instances, although convenience and cost may preclude its use. Factor concentrates are known to alter immune function exclusive of any contamination with HIV. The presumption is that the multiple antigenic exposure by foreign protein will alter T cell function and number. Each single lot of concentrate is produced from as many as 22,000 different donors. In order to obviate this problem, new methods of purifying factor VIII concentrates have been developed using murine monoclonal antibodies and affinity chromotography.[25] This technology produces a relatively pure concentrate of factor VIII, devoid of many of the contaminating foreign proteins. Currently, such preparations are available but are several times more expensive than standard heat-treated concentrates. It is anticipated that recombinant human factor VIII will be available some time in the next several years and will prevent most of the known complications of currently used factor concentrates.

One must take into account the blood type of the patient who is to receive large doses of factor concentrate replacement. Patients with blood types A, B, or AB may receive significant quantities of isohemagglutinins with the concentrate. This can produce a mild hemolytic anemia. Low-titer isohemagglutinin concentrates are available on specific request.

Factor IX concentrates have a tendency to manifest prothrombotic complications. Thrombotic complications have been seen in patients undergoing operations, particularly those with underlying liver disease.[26]

Patients who have factor VIII inhibitors usually can be managed with standard factor concentrate if the amount of inhibitor present in the plasma is of low titer. When the amount of inhibitor present is quite high, activated complexes often are needed. As noted previously, factor IX contains activated amounts of factor materials and may be suitable for administration to patients who have inhibitors against factor VIII in subjects with classic hemophilia. In addition to factor IX concentrates, intentionally activated concentrates, such as Autoplex or FEIBA, are available for such purposes. Porcine factor VIII concentrates also may be used.[27]

OTHER COAGULATION FACTOR DEFICIENCIES

Most of the other coagulation factor deficiencies are inherited in an autosomal recessive manner and thus can affect both males and females. This is true of congenital factor deficiencies of factor II, V, VII, X, and XII as well as fibrinogen deficiencies. Depending on the level of factor deficiency, each of these may result in clinical bleeding, with the exception of factor XII.

For most of these factor deficiencies, replacement with fresh frozen plasma at 10 to 20 ml/kg of body weight may be necessary. Because this may result in large volumes of plasma administered, it may be necessary to consider plasma exchange in patients who must undergo prolonged periods of factor replacement. Fibrinogen deficiency usually can be corrected with the administration of cryoprecipitate. Prothrombin complex concentrate (factor IX concentrate) contains varying levels of factors II, VII, IX, and X and may be useful in the management of selected patients with such deficiencies. Because of the high risk of hepatitis associated with prothrombin complex concentrates, fresh frozen plasma usually is indicated unless correction of the factor deficiency is higher than what can be achieved with fresh frozen plasma. The basic management of these factor deficiencies varies somewhat because of differences in half-life of the transfused material. With factor XIII deficiency (fibrin-stablizing factor), fresh frozen plasma is indicated for surgery. Congenital factor XIII deficiency usually has a classic triad consisting of bleeding at the time the umbilical cord falls off, rebleeding after cessation of initial bleeding, and poor wound healing because of defective clot formation. In this instance, fresh frozen plasma is given in an amount of 5 to 10 ml/kg of body weight.

von Willebrand's Disease

Von Willebrand's disease is not a single diagnostic entity. In most instances, this disorder is inherited as an autosomal disorder, with the most severely affected patients having inherited a genetic abnormality from both parents.[28] In most instances, patients with von Willebrand's disease have a prolonged bleeding time and a prolongation of the PPT, with low procoagulant activity for factor VIII, reduced factor VIII-related antigen, decreased ristocetin-induced platelet aggregation, and diminished levels of factor VIII von Willebrand's antigen.

Wide variability in clinical expression is to be expected. Patients who have severe bleeding histories can be expected to have significant problems in surgery. Management usually includes the infusion of cryoprecipitate, although fresh frozen plasma will suffice if lower levels of factor are needed. Although factor concentrates will raise the factor VIII level, they will not predictably reduce the prolonged bleeding time. Cryoprecipitate may do this, but for a much shorter period of time than the half-life of the factor VIII itself. In most instances, it is not necessary to have full correction of the bleeding time to achieve surgical hemostasis. Since some patients with von Willebrand's disease have induction of endogenous synthesis of factor VIII with the administration of cryoprecipitate, replacement therapy should begin 24 to 48 hours before surgery. This may allow the patient to produce adequate levels of endogenous factor VIII without excessive factor VIII replacement for the surgery itself. The amount of factor VIII necessary in the plasma to achieve hemostasis is the same as for classic hemophilia.

Platelet Disorders

Platelet disorders usually are separated into two categories: thrombocytopenia and thrombocytopathy.

Thrombocytopenias usually are caused by either accelerated destruction of platelets or bone marrow production failure states. Generally, surgery can be adequately performed as long as the platelet count is above 50,000 to 60,000 cells/μl. In those conditions associated with defective platelet production, platelet transfusions usually are adequate for preoperative management. The dosage required is based on the observation that 1 unit of platelets/5 kg of body weight should result in a rise in the platelet count of 50,000 to 100,000 cells/μl. It is necessary to monitor posttransfusion platelet counts closely to maintain the platelet count above 50,000 cells/μl. If adequate platelet counts are not achieved with the standard dose, one must look for acquired platelet antibodies, splenomegaly, and situations, such as fever, that reduce platelet survival. Patients exposed to repetitive administration of foreign platelet antigens usually will develop platelet antibodies within 2 weeks of exposure to multiple units of platelets. In such instances, the use of HLA-matched platelets will result in appropriate responses to platelet concentrate administrations.

Patients with intrinsic platelet functional defects usually can be managed with the administration of platelets. Patients with functional platelet disorders that produce prolonged bleeding times may have life-threatening hemorrhage at the time of surgery. Almost all of these disorders are hereditary. Thrombasthenia probably is the most significant bleeding problem in this group and is inherited as an autosomal recessive disorder.[29] Patients with this entity frequently have spontaneous gum bleeding, purpura, epistaxis, and often gastrointestinal bleeding. The diagnosis of these disorders is made easily by platelet aggregation studies.

DIAGNOSIS AND MANAGEMENT OF THE PATIENT WITH UNEXPECTED BLEEDING

Intraoperative bleeding as a consequence of coagulation factor abnormalities or platelet functional abnormalities is rare if preoperative screening testing is carried out. However, some patients with these disorders will not be detected with preoperative screening, and one must be prepared to manage virtually any potential type of bleeding disorder in the course of a surgical procedure.

Intravascular Coagulation

Disseminated intravascular coagulation (DIC) may follow episodes of hypoxemia, trauma, hypotension, infection, malignancy, burns, intravascular hemolysis, extracorporeal circulation, and a variety of neonatal insults. The end process of the pathophysiologic mechanism resulting in DIC is the formation of a hypercoagulable state and depletion of certain of the coagulation factors and platelets. Among the factors that are consumed easily during the process of clotting are factors II, V, VIII, X, and XIII. In addition, fibrinogen may be diminished to dangerously low levels. The platelet count usually is subnormal, and the diagnosis of DIC almost invariably is associated with the presence of a microangiopathic hemolytic anemia easily detected by a review of the peripheral blood smear. Most patients will have prolongations of the prothrombin time and PTT. The thrombin time will be abnormal because of hypofibrinogenemia and elevated levels of fibrin degradation products.

There is no one treatment of DIC. All studies to date have shown that the best management is treatment of the underlying cause of the disorder. While this is being attempted, replacement therapy with fresh frozen plasma and platelet concentrates may be indicated. Studies have failed to show any demonstrable evidence of efficacy of heparinization. This is not true of the thrombotic thrombocytopenic purpura, in which heparin may be life saving.

Vitamin K Deficiency

Vitamin K, which is a fat-soluble vitamin, is necessary for the activation of the final carboxylation of factors II, VII, IX, and X.[30] It also may be important in a lesser manner for other factors. It is derived both from the diet and from intestinal flora. Deficiency of vitamin K is rare in adequately fed patients. It may occur if an infant is solely breast-fed and has not received vitamin K prophylactically at the time of birth.[31] Indeed, vitamin K deficiency should be suspected as a cause of hemorrhage in any newborn who has not received prophylactic vitamin K at birth. Deficiencies of vitamin K are seen in many of the malabsorption syndromes, particularly cystic fibrosis, and in patients who have hepatobiliary disorders.

Vitamin K deficiency is usually suggested when prolongations of prothrombin time and PTT are seen. Usually, the prothrombin time is disproportionately prolonged with respect to the prolongation of the PTT. A simple assay for prothrombin will usually be indicative of a deficiency state consistent with vitamin K deficiency. If the deficiency is caused by absence of vitamin K, correction is very simple, with the intravenous administration of 1 to 2 mg of vitamin K_1 oxide. The response time is rapid (4 to 6 hours). Patients who have severe liver dysfunction may respond to the administration of vitamin K, but the results are less predictable. Patients with obstructive hepatobiliary disease should be treated on a chronic basis with water-soluble vitamin K preparations. Some patients may require periodic parenteral administration of vitamin K.

Acquired Platelet Abnormalities

Acquired thrombocytopenia most often is a consequence of severe underlying bone marrow dysfunction or a result of a naturally occurring platelet antibody. Either of these two states can result in a severe level of thrombocytopenia, resulting in bleeding at the time of surgery.

The single most important diagnostic test to determine the cause of thrombocytopenia is the bone marrow examination. If a bone marrow shows no evidence of malignancy and megakaryocytes are present in adequate numbers, it is likely that there is peripheral destruction of platelets. This may be consistent with an autoimmune thrombocytopenic state, and platelet transfusions are of little value, since donor platelets will be quickly destroyed. If a patent must undergo a surgical procedure and has active ongoing autoimmune thrombocytopenia, every attempt should be made to raise the platelet count. Although steroids may be effective in elevating the platelet count, the most prompt rise in platelet count will occur after the administration of intravenous gamma globulin.[32] In general, the dose range has varied from 0.5 g/kg daily for 4 days to as much as 1 g/kg daily as a single administration or administered 2 days in a row. The platelet count frequently will begin to rise within a matter of hours after the use of intravenous gamma globulin.

BLOOD COMPONENT THERAPY

In most instances, packed red cells may be used both preoperatively and operatively to correct bleeding. Whole blood may be administered if bleeding is brisk, although it is often preferable to administer packed red blood cells in association with fresh frozen plasma. In situations in which patients must go immediately to surgery and anemia has developed over a long period of time, patients may require partial red cell exchange transfusion if the anemia is not a result of blood loss. It is usually not necessary to use fresh blood (less than 24 hours old). Although fresh blood offers the advantages of higher levels of intracellular 2,3-DPG and better tissue oxygenation, with current storage techniques (CPD-adenine-stored blood), oxygen-carrying characteristics usually are preserved for up to 7 days. When replacement therapy is needed intraoperatively, it is best given in conjunction with fresh frozen plasma, which is a good source of all coagulation factors that may be consumed during surgery or lost through excessive bleeding. As noted, cryoprecipitate may be used under specific indications, such as for factor VIII deficiency, fibrinogen deficiency, and von Willebrand's disease. Other factor concentrates are likewise reserved for specific indications.

Platelet concentrates remain the most effective component therapy for correcting thrombocytopenia, although in the postoperative state, the turnover rate of platelet concentrates is extremely high. Intraoperative thrombocytopenia may result from massive transfusion of blood component therapy that is platelet poor. For this reason, patients who are receiving massive transfusional therapy may be in need of periodic platelet concentrate replacement.

It is recognized that if fresh frozen plasma is not being used as part of replacement therapy for large-volume blood losses, at least 1 unit of fresh frozen plasma should be given for every 5 units of blood that are replaced. This would be expected to maintain a minimum level of 20 percent of all factors.

Current blood banking techniques preoperatively screen donors for a variety of infectious agents, including hepatitis B virus, HIV antibody, and alanine aminotransferase activity (to detect most cases of non-A, non-B hepatitis). In some instances, it is desirable to ascertain that transfused blood is not likely to transmit cytomegalovirus (CMV). Specifically, severely immunocompromised recipients, including those with malignancy, inherited disorders, or underlying immunocompromised states, should be afforded the benefit of CMV-free blood. This may be achieved with the use of frozen or washed red cells, since the virus is contained in leukocytes. In most instances, however, this is most readily accomplished by CMV antibody screening of donor units of blood. CMV contamination of blood component therapy is the single most common cause of the postprefusion syndrome. To date, problems related to Epstein-Barr virus contamination of blood products have not been a major issue.

One should be aware that if blood component therapy is given that contains viable leukocytes, graft-versus-host disease may be a problem if the recipient is severely immunocompromised. This problem may be avoided by the use of irradiated blood products. Some have recommended the use of irradiated blood products for all premature infants, since graft-versus-host disease has been described in patients after intrauterine transfusions and postnatal exchange transfusions.

REFERENCES

1. Oski FA, Naiman JL: Hematologic Problems in the Newborn, 2nd ed., Philadelphia, Saunders, 1972, p 11
2. Saarien UM, Siimes MA: Developmental changes in red blood cell counts and indices of infants after exclusion of iron deficiency by laboratory criteria and continuous iron supplementation. J Pediatr 92:414, 1978
3. Dallman PR, Siimes MA: Percentile curves for hemoglobin and red cell volume in infancy and childhood. J Pediatr 94:28, 1979
4. Wiesenfeld SL: Sickle-cell trait in human biological and cultural evolution. Science 157:1134, 1967
5. Sarnaik S, Slovis TL: Incidence of cholelithiasis in sickle cell anemia using ultrasonic gray-scale technique. J Pediatr 96:1005, 1980
6. Burrington JD, Smith MD: Elective and emergency surgery in children with sickle cell disease. Surg Clin North Am 56:55, 1976
7. Homi J, Reynolds J: General anesthesia in sickle cell disease. Br Med J 1:1599, 1979
8. Nathan D, Oski F: Hematologic Disorders of Infancy and Childhood. Philadelphia, Saunders, 1987, p 1294
9. Ingram GIC: Investigation of a long-standing bleeding tendency. Br Med Bull 33:261, 1977
10. Duke WW: The relation of blood platelets to hemorrhagic disease. JAMA 55:1185, 1910
11. Ivy AC, Shapiro PF: The bleeding tendency in jaundice. Surg Gynecol Obstet 60:71, 1935
12. Harker LA, Slichter SJ: The bleeding time as a screening test for evaluation of platelet function. N Engl J Med 287:155, 1972
13. Abildgaard CF, Simone JV: von Willebrand's disease: A comparative study of diagnostic tests. J Pediatr 73:355, 1968
14. Proctor RR, Rappaport SI: The partial thromboplastin time with kaolin. Am J Clin Pathol 36:212, 1961
15. Kuick AJ: Hemorrhagic Diseases and Thrombosis, 2nd Ed. Philadelphia, Lea & Febiger, 1966
16. Zimmerman TS, Ratnoff OD: The immunologic differentiation of classical hemophilia (factor VIII deficiency) and von Willebrand's disease with observation on combined deficiencies of antihemophilic factor and proaccelerin (factor V) and on an acquired anticoagulant against antihemophiliac factor. J Clin Invest 40:24, 1971
17. Born GVR, Cross MJ: The aggregation of blood platelets. J Physiol (Lond) 168:178, 1963
18. Claesson AG, Malmsten C: On the inter-relationship of prostaglandin endoperoxide G_2 and cyclic nucleotides in platelet function. Eur J Biochem 76:277, 1977
19. Lewis JH, Spero JA: Transfusion support for congenital clotting deficiencies other than hemophilia. Clin Haematol 13:119, 1984
20. Colombo M, Mannucci PM, Carnelli V, et al: Transmission of non-A, non-B hepatitis by heat-treated factor VIII concentrate. Lancet 2:1, 1985
21. Kaneshiro MM, Mielke CH, Kasper CK, et al: Bleeding time after aspirin in disorders of intrinsic clotting. N Engl J Med 281:1039, 1969
22. CDC Update: Acquired immunodeficiency syndrome (AIDS) in persons with hemophilia. MMWR 33:589, 1984
23. Levy JA, Mitra G, Mozen MM: Recovery and inactivation of infectious retroviruses from factor VIII concentrates. Lancet 2:722, 1984
24. Gerety RJ, Eyster ME: Hepatitis among hemophiliacs in non-A, non-B hepatitis. In Gerety RJ (ed): Non-A Non-B Hepatitis, New York, Academic Press, 1981, pp 97–117
25. Levine PH, Brettler DB, Sullivan JL, et al: Heat-treated factor VIII purified by use of affinity chromatography. XI International Congress on Thrombosis and Haemostasis. Satellite symposium. Brussels, Thromb Res (Suppl 7):61, 1987
26. Blatt PM, Lundblad RL, Kingdon HS, et al: Thrombogenic materials in prothrombin complex concentrate. Ann Intern Med 81:766, 1974
27. Gatti L, Mannucci PM: Use of porcine factor VIII in the management of 17 patients with factor VIII antibodies. Thromb Haemost 51:379, 1984
28. Wahlberb TB, Blomback M, Ruggeri ZM: Differences between heterozygous dominant and recessive von Willebrand's disease type I expressed by bleeding symptoms and combinations of factor VIII variables. Thromb Haemost 50:864, 1983
29. Hardisty RM, Dormandy KM, Hutton RA, et al: Thrombasthenia: Studies on three cases. Br J Haematol 10:371, 1964
30. Prydz H: Vitamin K-dependent clotting factors. Semin Thromb Hemost 4:1, 1977
31. Goldman HI, Deposito F: Hypoprothrombinemic bleeding in young infants. Am J Dis Child 111:430, 1966
32. Imbach P, d'Apuzzo V, Hirt A, et al: High-dose intravenous gamma globulin for idiopathic thrombocytopenic purpura in childhood. Lancet 1:1228, 1981

8
Genetics in Surgery and Prenatal Diagnosis

Henry L. Nadler
Alan J. Sacks
Mark I. Evans

The pediatric surgeon commonly is involved in the care of children with congential malformations, as well as in the management of children with chronic diseases who may develop surgical complications. Increasingly, these disorders are being diagnosed prenatally, allowing for very early surgical intervention and, in selected instances, even prenatal surgical attempts at correction.[1] Knowledge of genetic disorders and malformation syndromes commonly associated with surgical problems can be of great benefit in predicting outcome and in planning the most appropriate course of management (both pre- and postnatal) for an individual patient. In addition, familiarity with the principles of human genetics is helpful in counseling the family of a child with a birth defect.

PATTERNS OF INHERITANCE IN HUMANS

Thousands of genes are located on each chromosome. In the case of the autosomes (nonsex chromosomes), each gene is matched by a corresponding gene for the same characteristic on the other chromosome of the pair, and the different gene forms are called alleles. If the genes present at a specific location on a pair of chromosomes are similar, the individual is homozygous. Homozygous individuals can produce only one type of gamete with respect to this gene, whereas heterozygous individuals will produce equal numbers of gametes with each type of gene.

The X chromosome contains a full complement of genes, but no corresponding genes are present on the Y chromosomes. Clearly, some genes are present on the Y, particularly those dealing with the development of male sexual characteristics, but these have no corresponding match on the X chormosomes. In the female, therefore, those genes carried on the X chromosomes are present in pairs, whereas in males they are not.

Almost 4000 disorders in humans have been attributed to a single mutant gene. These are the disorders that follow the classic mendelian patterns of inheritance. In many cases, the specific gene product is unknown or cannot be measured, although pedigree studies clearly indicate a specific inheritance pattern.

AUTOSOMAL DOMINANT INHERITANCE

The term *dominant* implies that only one of the two genes in a pair needs to be abnormal for the individual to be affected with a particular disease. Autosomal dominant disorders are transmitted from generation to generation by affected individuals of both sexes; males and females are equally affected. In any pregnancy, the risk to an affected individual of having an affected child is 1 out of 2. Except in the unusual circumstance in which an autosomal dominant gene exhibits incomplete penetrance, unaffected family members have essentially no risk of passing the disorder on to their offspring.

The manifestations and severity of an autosomal dominant disorder may vary considerably among affected individuals in the same family, which is referred to as *variable expressivity.* Usually, an individual who has the gene for an autosomal dominant disease has that disease, and one who is completely free of the disorder can be assumed not to be a carrier of the gene. One factor that has been related to an increased incidence of autosomal dominant disorders involving new mutations is advanced paternal age.

A child who clearly has an autosomal dominant disorder can be born to two parents who are normal and have no family history of other affected family members. When false paternity is excluded, the disorder can be assumed to reflect the new mutation of a normal gene to the mutant form in one of the germ cells or in the zygote. In some instances, particularly with severe disorders, the majority of cases are fresh mutations. Parents of a child with an autosomal dominant disorder secondary to a new mutation have essentially the same (nearly zero) risk as the general population of having an affected child in a subsequent pregnancy. The affected individual, on the other hand, has a 50 percent risk of passing the mutant gene on to each of his or her offspring.

One note of caution should be entered here. Before any autosomal dominant disorder is assumed to represent a new mutation, the parents, siblings, and occasionally other family members must be carefully examined. It is well known that the manifestations of many autosomal dominant disorders are quite variable and may be so subtle as to be overlooked unless carefully sought.

Examples of autosomal dominant disorders that may come to the attention of the surgeon are detailed in Table 8–1.[2,3]

Ehlers-Danlos Syndrome

One autosomal dominant disorder commonly encountered by the surgeon is the Ehlers-Danlos syndrome, a generalized disorder of connective tissue. Individuals with this disorder typically exhibit hyperextensible skin and joints and may bleed or bruise easily because of lax connective tissue in the vascular walls. They may come to the surgeon with hernias or unexplained gastrointestinal bleeding. Because of the abnormal connective tissue, repair may be difficult, and wound healing may be prolonged.

The Ehlers-Danlos syndrome actually is a constellation of disorders, with well-characterized varieties. Among these are dominant, recessive, and X-linked inheritance patterns. The basic defect is known for some varieties, the most important of which is type IV, the ecchymotic variety, in which there is marked skin fragility and bruising. Death from arterial rupture, aortic dissection, or intestinal perforation is relatively common, particularly in pregnancy. The disorder is associated with a deficiency of type III collagen and has relatively minimal or absent skin hyperextensibility and joint hypermobility as compared to the other types of Ehlers-Danlos syndrome.

Osteogenesis Imperfecta

Osteogenesis imperfecta (OI) can be divided into four types. Type 1, which is most common, is an autosomal dominant inherited disorder of connective tissue with the major feature of bone fractures from very mild traumas. Over the past several years, there has been a huge increase in available information on the molecular basis of OI. The fundamental understanding is that there are defects in the characteristic repeating sequence of collagen on the chains, or the combining of the chains is improper. For reasons that are incompletely understood, as the patients move past puberty, their tendency to sustain fractures is reduced considerably. A characteristic feature of OI includes blue sclera.

Type 2 OI is an autosomal recessive disorder in which multiple fractures and limb deformities are seen in utero, and the disease process usually is lethal. The diagnosis of OI type 2 in the third trimester can be the source of much medical, legal, and ethical debate covering how aggressive to be in delivery. Vaginal delivery may hasten neonatal death but reduce maternal risks and complications. Is it ethically appropriate to do "everything for the baby" if the diagnosis is certain?

Type 3 is the so-called progressive deforming variety and is more severe than type 1 but is compatible with life.

Type 4 is milder and also dominantly inherited. Type 4 individuals may have significant bowing of long bones and growth deficiency in addition to their fractures. Both types 1 and 4 often are accompanied by dentinogenesis imperfecta. All the dominant forms of OI would appear to be a heterogeneous group of mutations in type 1 collagen. The correlation between their biochemistry and the clinical phenotype is not yet completely understood.

Patients with OI often come to the attention of the pediatric surgeon or pediatric orthopedist because of their multiple fractures and bone formation.[4]

Marfan's Syndrome

Marfan's syndrome is an autosomal dominant disorder characterized by a distinct phenotype of a tall, lanky person with reduced upper/lower-body ratio, often with

TABLE 8–1. AUTOSOMAL DOMINANT CONDITIONS OFTEN ENCOUNTERED BY THE PEDIATRIC SURGEON

Marfan's syndrome
Neurofibromatosis
Achondroplasia
Osteogenesis imperfecta
Ehlers-Danlos syndrome

a pectus excavatum, long fingers and toes, a high arched palate, floppy mitral valve, laxity of the ligaments, dislocated lenses, hyperextensible joints, and, most important, a very high frequency of dissecting aortic aneurysms that result from structurally imperfect connective tissue within the aortic trunk (Fig. 8–1). Recent reports have suggested impairment of pyridinium crosslinks between collagen fibrils as perhaps the underlying structural defect in the connective tissue. There are many potential ways in which interference with the crosslinking may occur, but at present there is still no clear understanding of the pathogenesis of the disorder.

It is well appreciated that the degree of aortic dilatation is correlated with the prognosis for risk of dissecting aneurysm. This appears to be particularly so in pregnancy. Patients with significant aortic dilatation entering pregnancy have as much as a 50 percent maternal mortality rate. For patients without evidence of dissecting aneurysm, pregnancy under careful observation can be considered relatively safe.

Neurofibromatosis (von Recklinghausen's Disease)

Neurofibromatosis (NF) is an autosomal dominant disorder occurring in approximately 1 in 3000 patients. Diagnosis is characterized by café au lait spots and freckles in the axilla and multiple neurofibromas on the limbs and trunk. Other features include pseudoarthrosis of the tibia, scoliosis, and neoplasms, including meningiomas, gliomas, pheochromocytomas, and neurofibromas. Approximately 50 percent of all cases are spontaneous mutations. Patients with neurofibromatosis may have compression of the spinal cord from neurofibromas or may need facial reconstruction because of fibromas. Cosmetic surgery often is unrewarding, however, since the fibromas tend to return. Acoustic neuromas can be seen in patients with NF or may appear as a distinct entity.

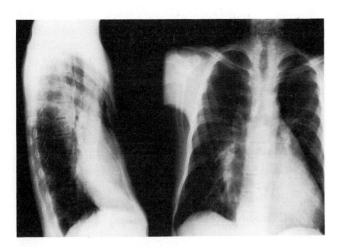

Figure 8–1. Chest roentgenogram of a teenage boy with Marfan's syndrome, showing pectus excavatum.

Because of the high incidence of bilateral tumors, which can result in deafness if untreated, such patients often come to the attention of the pediatric neurosurgeon.

Achondroplasia

Achondroplasia is an autosomal dominant disorder characterized by short stature, large head, prominent forehead, midface hypoplasia, genu varum, trident hands, and lumbar lordosis. Characteristics visible on x-ray include decreasing intrapedicular distance from the thorax to the lumbar spine, rounded iliac crests, a narrow sacrosciatic notch, horizontal acetabular roof, and oval translucency of the proximal femur. Children with achondroplasia require close orthopedic supervision to ensure maximum bone growth and to prevent excessive lordosis. Neurosurgery occasionally is required to prevent compression of the cisterna magna. Because of the potential for compression, there is debate in the obstetric literature about the advisability of delivering known achondroplastic babies by cesarean section to reduce the risk of trauma that occurs during vaginal delivery.

Although the autosomal dominant genetics of achondroplasia are well understood, approximately 80 percent of all cases are new mutations for which there is an association with advanced paternal age.

Achondroplasia must be differentially diagnosed from other similar conditions, such as metatrophic dysplasia, diastrophic dysplasia, and acromesomelic dwarfism, all of which are nonlethal, autosomal recessives, and spondyloepiphyseal dysplasia, hypochondroplasia, and pseudoachondroplasia, which can be either autosomal dominant or recessive.

AUTOSOMAL RECESSIVE INHERITANCE

Autosomal recessive genes are located on the autosomes and exert an effect only if both genes are abnormal. Such disorders occur with equal frequency in males and females and often occur in multiple siblings born to normal parents. The parents, if normal, are by definition carriers of the disorder. Unlike autosomal dominant conditions, which tend to show vertical transmission, autosomal recessive pedigrees are often horizontal, with multiple affected members within the same generation. Other affected family members usually are not found. Two carriers of an autosomal recessive disorder face a risk of 1 in 4 in each pregnancy of having an affected child. Of the normal siblings, 2 in 3 are carriers like the parents, and 1 in 3 is not a carrier (Fig. 8–2). It is important for such parents to recognize that each pregnancy represents a new event and that the outcome is not altered by the outcomes of previous pregnancies.

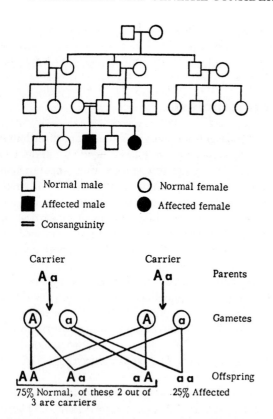

Figure 8–2. Top. Autosomal recessive inheritance. **Bottom.** Off-spring who are both carriers of an autosomal recessive disorder. A, normal genes; a, mutant recessive genes.

Siblings of individuals with an autosomal recessive disorder often request genetic counseling about their risks of having children with the same disorder. Although such individuals have a 2 in 3 chance of being a carrier of the disorder, their risk of having affected children usually is quite low. Essentially, the risk is always less than 1 percent, since it depends on their mating with someone who is also a carrier. The precise risk depends on the frequency of carriers for the disorder in the general population, but even the most common autosomal recessive genes have a carrier frequency of 1 in 20 or less.

Examples of autosomal recessive disorders include cystic fibrosis, sickle cell anemia, beta-thalassemia, and Tay-Sachs disease. It is generally accepted that every individual is the carrier of at least four or five deleterious autosomal recessive genes. Because these genes are individually quite rare, it is unusual for two people carrying the same gene to have children together. The birth of an affected child is usually the first indication to either parent that he or she is a carrier of a specific gene. Under certain circumstances, such as consanguinity, this event is more likely to occur than one would expect. In general, the rarer the condition, the more likely consanguinity will be a factor.

Certain autosomal recessive disorders occur dispro-

portionately within certain racial or ethnic groups. Tay-Sachs disease, for example, occurs most commonly in the Ashkenazi Jewish population, and sickle cell anemia occurs most commonly in the black population. All disorders can occur in any population, but at times the common occurrence in one specific group can increase the index of suspicion for a given disorder. In the United States today, however, there are more non-Jewish than Jewish Tay-Sachs babies because (1) despite the lower frequency, there are multifold more non-Jewish babies, and (2) most Jewish couples are screened.

X-LINKED RECESSIVE INHERITANCE

An X-linked recessive gene is not manifested as long as it is balanced by a normal gene on the other X chromosome. Thus, females who have a mutant gene on one X chromosome and a normal gene on the other are usually but not always completely normal. Males, on the other hand, have no genes on the Y chromosome to match those on the X. Thus, all of the genes on the X chromosome of the male, whether dominant or recessive, are exposed and exert their full effect.

It should be clear that such disorders occur almost exclusively in males and are transmitted through the family by carrier females who themselves are usually normal. A female carrier of such a disorder faces a risk of 1 in 4 in any pregnancy of having an affected child, but this risk is 1 in 2 if the child is a male and essentially 0 if it is a female; 1 out of 2 daughters will be a carrier. This risk figure is not affected by the male unless he happens to be affected by the X-linked recessive disorder in question.

The normal sisters of males with an X-linked recessive disorder generally have a 1 in 2 chance of being a carrier. Their risk of having an affected child in any pregnancy is thus ½ × ¼ = ⅛—or ¼ if the child is a male and essentially 0 if it is a female, although some of the daughters also might be carriers. The only exception to this rule occurs in the family with only one affected male who has developed the disorder as the result of a new mutation. In such an instance, other family members may not be at increased risk of having affected children. One can never automatically assume, however, that an isolated case actually represents a new mutation.

Occasionally an X-linked recessive disorder may be observed in a female. This may occur by one of any number of different mechanisms. A female with Turner's syndrome (45,X), for example, will exhibit all of the traits coded by genes on her one X chromosome in the same way as in the male. Alternatively, if a male with an X-linked recessive disorder mates with a female who is a carrier of the same disorder, they may have a daughter with the recessive gene on both of her X chromosomes.

These are extraordinarily rare events unless the parents are blood relatives.

Examples of X-linked recessive disorders include hemophilia A and B, Duchenne muscular dystrophy, hemolytic anemia related to glucose-6-phosphate dehydrogenase deficiency, and deutan color blindness. Screening methods are now available for the detection of carriers of some of these disorders in families at risk, and prenatal diagnosis is available for many.

X-LINKED DOMINANT INHERITANCE

X-linked dominant genes exert their effects in both males and females, since only a single dose of the mutant gene need be present for the disorder to be manifested. The feature that distinguishes X-linked dominant inheritance from autosomal dominant inheritance is the absence of male-to-male transmission. An affected father obviously cannot pass the gene to his sons, since he gives his sons the Y chromosome instead of the X. An affected female has a risk of 1 in 2 in any pregnancy of having an affected child, and the risk is the same if the child is a male or a female. An affected male, on the other hand, always passes the disorder on to his daughters (since they receive his X chromosome) and never to his sons. As a result, X-linked dominant disorders are twice as common in females as in males.

Examples of X-linked dominant disorders, which are actually quite rare, include familial hypophosphatemic vitamin D-resistant rickets, pseudohypoparathyroidism, ornithine transcarbamylase deficiency (a urea cycle defect), and incontinentia pigmenti. Some of these disorders are much more severe in the male than in the female and may actually be lethal in the male. Males with ornithine transcarbamylase deficiency usually die in the neonatal period, whereas affected females frequently survive. Incontinentia pigmenti is virtually never seen in the male and presumably results in the loss of male fetuses early in gestation.

MULTIFACTORIAL INHERITANCE

There are a number of familial disorders, including some of the most common isolated congenital malformations, that cannot be attributed to the effect of a single mutant gene but to the additive effects of several mutant genes and environmental factors. Such disorders are said to exhibit multifactorial inheritance. Congenital malformations within this group include neural tube defects, cleft lip and palate, clubfoot, congenital hip dislocation, and some types of congenital heart disease.

Several basic principles separate disorders with multifactorial inheritance from single gene defects. First degree relatives of an affected individual, including parents, siblings, and offspring, are all equally likely to be affected. For example, a couple who has had a child with cleft lip and palate face a risk of about 4 percent that the next child also will be affected. Similarly, if one parent has a cleft lip and palate, the risk is about 4 percent that the first child will be affected. Recurrence rates for malformations with multifactorial inheritance tend to cluster in the range of 3 to 7 percent. The risk of recurrence is increased if there are more than one affected family members. Many multifactorial disorders, such as pyloric stenosis, are more common in one sex than in the other, implying that more mutant genes may be required for the malformation to be manifested in the less commonly affected sex. Risk may be affected also by maternal factors. Preliminary data suggest that the recurrence risk of neural tube defects (anencephaly and spina bifida) may be reduced by preconceptual folate administration.[5]

GENETIC DISORDERS MANIFESTED IN CHILDHOOD

Chromosomal Abnormalities

Alterations in the normal number or structure of chromosomes are not rare in the young child. Numerous cytogenetic studies of consecutive newborn infants have documented an incidence of gross chromosomal abnormalities of about 1 in 150 despite the availability of prenatal diagnosis. Even with rapidly increasing use of the prenatal diagnostic techniques of amniocentesis and chorionic villus sampling, most chromosomally abnormal babies are born to low-risk women who were not offered testing.

Most chromosomal epidemiology studies were performed with conventional techniques of cytogenetic analysis. With current, more sophisticated banding techniques, more subtle chromosomal aberrations can be identified. It is possible that the true incidence of significant chromosomal abnormalities may actually be somewhat higher than previously reported.

Karyotypes are ordinarily derived from actively dividing cells during the portion of meiosis referred to as metaphase, when the chromosomes are most dense and line up in the center of the cell in preparation for cell division. The tissues most commonly used for chromosome analysis in children are peripheral lymphocytes and cultivated skin fibroblasts. In prenatal diagnosis, amniotic fluid cells or chorionic villi or fetal blood is used.

The normal number of chromosomes, which in humans is 46, is referred to as the diploid number (Fig. 8–3). The haploid number is 23, the number present in the gametes. The presence of additional complete

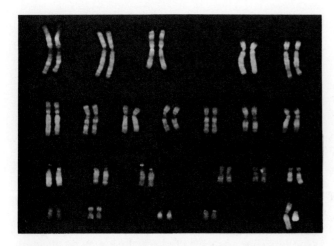

Figure 8–3. Normal male karyotype using quinacrine fluorescent banding.

sets of chromosomes within a cell is referred to as polyploidy, e.g. triploid=69, tetraploid=92. Aneuploidy refers to an abnormality in chromosome number resulting from the presence or absence of a single chromosome or several chromosomes. The most common example of this is trisomy, in which an extra chromosome is added to a given pair, and monosomy, in which only one member of the pair is present. Occasionally, one encounters in a given individual two or more populations of cells, each of which contains a different chromosome complement. This is mosaicism and presumably results from an accident in cell division, or mitosis, occurring in the zygote after fertilization.

The most commonly encountered internal structural abnormality is a translocation in which part or all of a particular chromosome is attached to another chromosome. This is referred to as "balanced" if the appropriate amount of chromosomal material is present and as "rearranged" and "unbalanced" if there is part of a chromosome missing or extra. In reality there is probably no such thing as a completely balanced translocation, since translocations are the result of chromosome breakage followed by recombination. The amount of material lost apparently can be so small as to be insignificant. Breakage of a chromosome with complete loss of the broken segment gives rise to a deletion. A ring chromosome is the result of breakage of both ends of a chromosome with subsequent fusion. More complex structural abnormalities, such as inversions and duplications, also occur but to date have been of limited clinical significance and are beyond the scope of this chapter.

Chromosome analysis clearly is indicated when a specific chromosomal abnormality (such as Down's syndrome) is suspected. It is also indicated in infants with multiple congenital anomalies of unknown etiology and in infants who have neurologic abnormalities in combination with physical anomalies that may be subtle.

AUTOSOMAL ABNORMALITIES

The most common autosomal abnormalities observed in the neonate are trisomies 21, 18, and 13. Patients have been reported who are trisomic for one of the other autosomes, but most other autosomal trisomies are incompatible with fetal survival. In spontaneous abortus tissue, many other aberrations are seen.

Down's Syndrome

Down's syndrome is by far the most common and most widely known abnormality of the autosomes. The clinical syndrome was recognized and well delineated long before its cytogenetic basis could be established. It is now known that the clinical features of this syndrome are related to the presence of an extra dose of chromosome 21 in the cells of the affected individual.

The major features of Down's syndrome are listed in Table 8–2, along with the frequency with which they occur.[2] Most affected individuals are readily recognizable on the basis of the characteristic facial features (Fig. 8–4). Clinical recognition may be somewhat more difficult in the neonatal period, since overall appearance at this age is not always typical. Ultrasonographic findings even in the midtrimester, such as excess nuchal folds, may heighten suspicion and precipitate invasive studies, but the data dealing with true relative risks are controversial.

The most significant problem associated with Down's syndrome is mental retardation, which is invariably present, although some variation in IQ within the retarded range may be observed. The average individual

TABLE 8–2. THE MAJOR CLINICAL FEATURES OF DOWN'S SYNDROME

Feature	Frequency of Occurrence (% of cases)
Mental retardation	100
Hypotonia (neonatal period)	95
Flat facial features	90
Slanted palpebral fissures	80
Flat occiput	78
Short, broad hands with short fingers	70
High arched palate	70
Dysplastic pelvis on x-ray	67
Open mouth with protruding tongue	65
Short fifth middle phalanx	62
Brushfield spots in iris	50
Abnormal ears	50
Clinodactyly	50
Congenital heart disease	40–60
Simian crease	48
Increased space between first and second toes	45
Epicanthal folds	40
Single flexion crease, fifth finger	20
Strabismus	20
Duodenal atresia	8

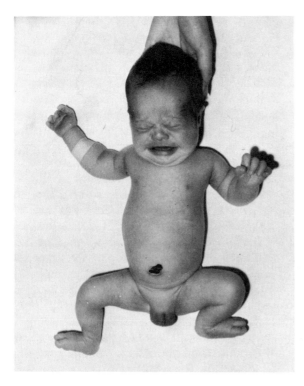

Figure 8–4. An infant with Down's syndrome.

with Down's syndrome ultimately is able to walk, dress himself or herself, say some words, and learn other simple tasks, but the person is never able to become self-sufficient. More severely retarded individuals are not uncommon.

In addition to the characteristic physical features of the disorder, several life-threatening anomalies occur with an increased incidence in Down's syndrome. It has been calculated that 40 to 60 percent of affected individuals have congenital heart disease, the most commonly encountered lesions being endocardial cushion defect and ventricular septal defect. Duodenal atresia and Hirschsprung's disease both occur with increased frequency in the neonate with Down's syndrome, and there appears to be an increased incidence of leukemia of a variety of types in children with Down's syndrome.

In the absence of serious physical anomalies, the life span of the individual with Down's syndrome may be normal or comparable to that of other retarded individuals, many of whom are institutionalized in adulthood if not before. Approximately 25 percent of infants with Down's syndrome do not survive beyond the first year of life, and another 25 percent die by the age of 8 or 10 years. Most of these deaths are related to the complications of congenital heart disease.

As previously mentioned, the underlying defect in Down's syndrome is the presence of an extra dose of chromosome 21. In about 95 percent of patients with

Down's syndrome, chromosome analysis reveals the presence of 47 chromosomes in each cell, the extra one being a number 21 (Fig. 8–5). This finding gives rise to the descriptive term for the disorder, trisomy 21. Trisomic states are thought to result from an accident in meiosis during the formation of the egg or the sperm. When the two members of a chromosome pair fail to segregate appropriately during meiosis, an event referred to as nondisjunction, both may be included in the gamete. When this combines with the normal gamete, a zygote trisomic for that chromosome pair results.

The factors responsible for the occurrence of nondisjunction are not completely understood. It is certainly a common event, as evidenced by the observation of numerical chromosomal abnormalities in spontaneous abortuses and by the relatively high incidence of Down's syndrome and other chromosomal abnormalities in the general population. One factor that has definitely been associated with an increased incidence of chromosomal abnormalities (and thus presumably of nondisjunctional events) is advanced maternal age; this is best illustrated by Down's syndrome.

A second factor that appears to increase the likelihood of a nondisjunctional event in a given individual is its previous occurrence in the same individual. Once a couple has had a child with trisomic Down's syndrome, for example, they are at increased risk in subsequent pregnancies of having another affected child, when compared to couples of comparable age in the general population. The exact risk is dependent on age but is generally 3 to 6 times higher than that of other couples in the same age group. The reasons for this phenomenon are not clear.

Approximately 5 percent of individuals with classic Down's syndrome do not have 47 chromosomes and thus cannot be said to have typical trisomy 21. Although such individuals are found to have 46 chromosomes, they

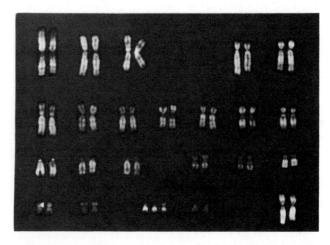

Figure 8–5. Karyotype of Down's syndrome female by quinacrine fluorescent banding (note three copies of chromosome 21).

have the equivalent of 47, with the extra number 21 chromosome being attached to another chromosome. This is the translocation type of Down's syndrome and is clinically indistinguishable from the trisomic type. The only difference between the two is in the packaging of the extra chromosome material. The extra chromosome is most commonly attached to a D group chromosome in a D/G or D/21 translocation. Alternatively, it may be attached to another G group chromosome, either number 21 or number 22.

Although there are no clinical differences between the trisomic and the translocation forms of Down's syndrome, the finding of a translocation has great significance in terms of genetic counseling. When a child is diagnosed to have the translocation form of Down's syndrome, chromosome analyses must be performed on both of the parents. In about one third of the cases, one of the parents will be found to have 45 chromosomes, with a balanced translocation between a number 21 and one of the D or G group chromosomes. The importance of this finding is that it gives the carrier a substantial risk of having additional children with Down's syndrome, since the attached chromosomes cannot segregate normally at meiosis. The theoretical risk to a D/G translocation carrier of having a child with Down's syndrome is 1 in 3 for any pregnancy. In practice, the risk is substantially lower than this and is dependent for some balanced translocations on whether the male or the female is the carrier of the translocation. Female carriers of a D/G translocation have a risk of about 10 to 15 percent in any pregnancy of having a child with Down's syndrome regardless of the age of the translocation carrier, equivalent to the risk of nondisjunctional trisomy 21 for a 47-year-old woman. For male carriers, the risk is about 2 to 3 percent. The reasons for the discrepancy between theoretical and actual risk values are not clear but may include decreased viability of embyros with unbalanced chromosomal complements and decreased fitness of sperm with abnormal complements.

Trisomy 18

Trisomy 18 is the second most common autosomal abnormality, occurring with an incidence of about 1 in 3500 live births. Females are affected three times more commonly than males. This is a disorder that is readily recognizable in the neonatal period on the basis of the multiple malformation pattern observed, which includes, among others, mental retardation, growth retardation, congenital heart disease, abnormal hearing, prominent occiput, high arched palate, micrognathia, rocker-bottom feet, and a single umbilical artery. Recognition at this time is of utmost significance because of the prognostic implications. Fifty percent of affected infants die by 2 months of age, and 90 percent die by 1 year of age. The survivors

are uniformly severely retarded. The physician should, therefore, take these facts into consideration before instituting extraordinary measures for prolongation of life.

The exact cause of death in affected infants often is unknown. Apneic episodes are common in the neonatal period, and poor sucking commonly leads to severe feeding problems. A large number of trisomy 18 fetuses exhibit significant intrauterine growth retardation from early in the third trimester, and a large proportion of trisomy 18 babies are delivered by emergency cesarean section for fetal distress.

Trisomy 13

Trisomy 13 is the third most frequent major autosomal abnormality observed in the neonatal period. It occurs with an incidence of about 1 in 5000 births. As with trisomy 18, this disorder usually is clinically recognizable on the basis of the malformation pattern observed, which includes growth and mental retardation, cryptochordism in males, hypertelorism, abnormal ears, congenital heart disease, and renal and brain anomalies. Again, variability is the rule, and many other abnormalities may be observed.

Anomalies of the midface, eye, and forebrain are characteristic of the trisomy 13 syndrome. The presence of holoprosencephaly, varying from cyclopia or cebocephaly to less severe forms, in combination with extracephalic anomalies should suggest this diagnosis (Fig. 8–6). In other infants, polydactyly and the triad of microphthalmia, cleft lip, and palate should bring the diagnosis to mind.

The prognosis for this disorder is extremely poor; 44 percent of affected infants die within the first month of life, and 80 percent die within the first year. The survivors have severe mental retardation and failure to thrive. Once again, the physician should consider these facts before initiating extraordinary methods of life support in the neonatal period.

Autosomal Deletion Syndromes

A number of clinical syndromes have been associated with a deletion of chromosome material from one of the autosomes. With the current widespread use of banding techniques, there is no doubt that additional deletion syndromes will be described. It is beyond the scope of this chapter to describe in detail the features of the specific syndromes recognized to date. Again, there is great variability in these disorders, and an example is given of one of the more commonly encountered deletion syndromes. Chromosome analysis is indicated in the parents of any child who is found to have a chromosomal deletion or translocation, since the possibility of a familial translocation has great implications for genetic counseling.

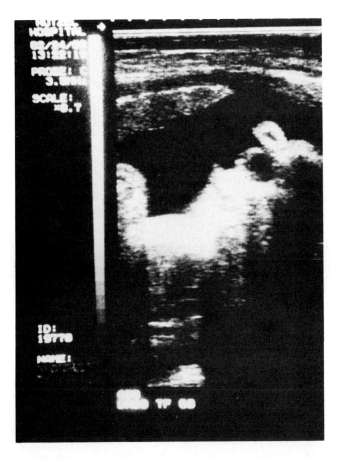

Figure 8–6. Profile of fetal face with holoprosencephaly. Note the proboscis apparently superior to the orbits.

Cri du Chat Syndrome

The cri du chat syndrome is a clinically recognizable disorder associated with a deletion of the short arm of chromosome 5. Affected infants are typically small for gestational age, grow poorly, and have a peculiar catlike cry in infancy. Most are hypotonic and exhibit microcephaly, hypertelorism, epicanthal folds, downslanting palpebral fissures, and simian creases. About 30 percent have congenital heart disease of variable type. A variety of other anomalies occasionally are noted. Although most infants with this disorder survive the neonatal period, the prognosis is for severe mental retardation, with the average IQ in the 20 to 30 range.

The deletion of the short arm of chromosome 5 is a sporadic occurrence in most cases of the cri du chat syndrome. The etiologic factors related to its occurrence are unknown. In 10 to 15 percent of cases, however, a balanced chromosomal translocation is found in one of the parents, with the deleted material from the short arm of chromosome 5 being attached to another chromosome. When this is the case, the recurrence risk for this syndrome is quite high. Such individuals obviously

might have an increased risk of having offspring with other unbalanced chromosomal abnormalities, depending upon the nature of the translocation.

Wolf-Hirschhorn Syndrome

Before chromosome banding was available, the cytogenetic appearance of a short arm B chromosome deletion was seen in a very clinically different combination, characterized by microcephaly, protruding frontal bossing, and profound mental retardation. Subsequent improvement of cytogenetics has revealed this picture with a 4p− rather than the 5p−, as seen in cri du chat.

SEX CHROMOSOME ABNORMALITIES

Abnormalities of the sex chromosomes are relatively common in liveborn infants, occurring in approximately 1 in 400 births. They are twice as common in phenotypic males as in phenotypic females. In general, most children with sex chromosome abnormalities are not recognized as such in the neonatal period. Multiple major anomalies are not the rule in such disorders. The major stigmata of sex chromosomal abnormalities tend to revolve around body habitus, ultimate stature, and sexual development. Mental retardation and other somatic abnormalities are seen with an increased frequency in some of these disorders, but not to the same extent as in the autosomal abnormalities. Abnormalities of this chromosome pair seem, in general, to have less widespread implications than the abnormalities of the autosomes. Both numerical and structural anomalies of the sex chromosomes may be observed.

Turner's Syndrome

Turner's syndrome (45,X) is the only monosomic chromosomal abnormality seen with any frequency in humans. It occurs with an incidence of about 1 in 3000 newborn females and is the most common significant sex chromosomal abnormality in females. The incidence of the 45,X karyotype in the newborn does not reflect the true occurrence of this condition in the zygote, since the vast majority of 45,X fetuses are spontaneously aborted. This observation suggests that the presence of a second sex chromosome (X or Y) may be far more critical in early fetal life than it is in postnatal life.

Because the most obvious stigmata of the disorder—short stature and failure of secondary sexual development—are not apparent until later in life, many infants with Turner's syndrome are not recognized. Occasionally, however, suggestive features may be noted in the neonate, the most common of which is lymphedema of the dorsum of the hands and feet. Any female infant with this finding should be suspected of having this disor-

TABLE 8–3. THE MAJOR CLINICAL FEATURES OF TURNER'S SYNDROME

Feature	Frequency of Occurrence (% of cases)
Short stature	100
Ovarian dysgenesis	95
Congenital lymphedema of the hands and feet	80
Shield chest with widely spaced nipples	80
Low posterior hairline	80
Abnormal ears	80
Cubitus valgus	70
Narrow, hyperconvex nails	70
Renal anomalies, usually minor	60
Perceptive hearing loss	50
Excessive pigmented nevi	50
Webbed neck	50
Short fourth metacarpal or metatarsal	50
Epicanthal folds	40
Congenital heart disease (usually coarctation of aorta)	20
Ptosis	16
Mental retardation	10

der. A rare patient also will exhibit swelling of the nape of the neck. Webbing of the neck or coarctation of the aorta in a female infant may alert the physician to this diagnosis (Table 8–3).

XO/XX, XO/XY, and more complex forms of mosaicism also are seen with a Turner phenotype. In addition, a significant number of patients with the clinical stigmata of Turner's syndrome have been reported who are 46,XX but have a structural abnormality of one of the X chromosomes. Such patients often have a normal percentage of Barr bodies on buccal smear. Any patient suspected of having Turner's syndrome or any other sex chromosmal abnormality should have a complete chromosome analysis.

The 45,X karyotype is thought to result from the loss of a sex chromosome during the early meiotic divisions in the zygote after fertilization. It is presumably not a result of meiotic nondisjunction in either of the parents. Thus, parents of an affected child are not at substantially increased risk in subsequent pregnancies for having children with this or any other chromosomal abnormality.

Klinefelter's Syndrome

Klinefelter's syndrome, or XXY syndrome, affects 1 in 500 newborn males and is thus the single most common sex chromosome abnormality in humans. Similar to the XXX syndrome, it is almost never suspected in the neonatal period, since most affected infants appear grossly normal. The most significant features of the disorder are hypogonadism and infertility. Indeed, this represents the most common single cause of genetic infertility in the adult male. Testes that are significantly smaller than

normal are noted in the neonate. Without hormonal therapy, the penis and testes remain prepubertal, since testosterone production is almost invariably inadequate. Occasionally, an affected individual will exhibit cryptorchidism and hypospadias.

The second major feature of Klinefelter's syndrome is tall stature related to the pubertal hypogonadism, with a low upper/lower body segment ratio. The average IQ is reduced in this disorder, and 15 to 20 percent of patients are mentally retarded. Other features may include radioulnar synostosis and multiple minor anomalies, such as dermatoglyphic abnormalities.

In most cases, the Klinefelter's syndrome presumably is the result of meiotic nondisjunction in one of the parents. A maternal age factor has been demonstrated. As with other nondisjunctional abnormalities, parents of an affected child are at increased risk in subsequent pregnancies. The magnitude of this increased risk is not currently known.

ISOLATED CONGENITAL MALFORMATIONS

It has been estimated that as many as 4 of every 100 newborn infants have at least one congenital malformation. Although minor and insignificant malformations often are included in such estimates, major malformations clearly are not uncommon. Certain basic principles must be kept in mind in evaluating an infant who is found to have a congenital anomaly at birth. The first is that any infant who has had one major malformation or a combination of minor malformations has an increased risk of having other malformations. Thus, once a single anomaly has been identified, others must be carefully sought. Children who have multiple malformations may have a chromosomal abnormality, some of which have been described, or a recognizable malformation complex. In other instances, the etiology has not been established, but the specific recurrence risks have been calculated and the natural history has been documented. In evaluating the infant with multiple malformations, every effort should be made to establish a specific diagnosis. This has obvious significance in terms of predicting the long-term prognosis for the affected infant and for providing precise genetic counseling.

In some instances, the presence of a specific anomaly will prompt a search for specific disorders in which that anomaly is a common component. For example, it has been demonstrated that about 11 percent of infants born with an omphalocele have Beckwith's syndrome. The other common features of this disorder, including large size for gestational age, macroglossia, neonatal hypoglycemia, visceromegaly, and unusual ear creases, occasionally may be overlooked or disregarded if the physician is unfamiliar with the syndrome. The implications of making this diagnosis are obvious. First, affected infants should have their blood sugar carefully monitored. Second, the recurrence risk for Beckwith's syndrome, presumably an autosomal recessive disorder, is 1 in 4, whereas for an isolated omphalocele it is less than 1 percent.

A number of infants born with anencephaly or an encephalocele will have other malformations compatible with the diagnosis of Meckel's syndrome (another autosomal recessive disorder). Other significant abnormalities associated with this disorder include microphthalmia, cleft palate, polydactyly, and polycystic kidneys. Here again, the recurrence risk for this disorder is 1 in 4, as opposed to the recurrence risk of 4 to 5 percent for isolated neural tube defects.

Cleft lip and palate, which occurs with an incidence of 1 or 2 per 1000 live births, is one of the most common congenital malformations in humans. About 10 percent of people with this anomaly have recognizable malformation syndromes, some of which are attributable to a single mutant gene. Genetic counseling obviously will be different in these cases than it will be for isolated cleft lip and palate.

Certain types of congenital malformations, although not part of a specific syndrome, are known to commonly occur together. The association of low-set or abnormally formed ears with renal anomalies is well known, and every infant with this type of finding should have renal studies. An infant with one or more features of the VATER association should be examined carefully for the other anomalies in this group, which include vertebral anomalies, anal atresia, tracheoesophageal fis-

tula, renal anomalies, radial dysplasia, and congenital heart lesions. Such associations, although they are not strictly malformation syndromes, represent the nonrandom association of specific anomalies. Many more such associations could be cited.

In some circumstances, information from the prenatal history may prompt a search for specific types of malformations in the newborn. Chronic alcoholism, for example, has been associated with a high incidence of specific abnormalities in the neonate.[6] These abnormalities may include growth deficiency, short palpebral fissures, and microcephaly. Other teratogenic drugs (such as methotrexate, warfarin, and diphenylhydantoin) and teratogenic viruses (such as rubella) have been identified.

It is a common but incorrect assumption that infants with multiple malformations will also inevitably exhibit mental retardation; this is a concern invariably expressed by the parents of such infants. Indeed, many disorders associated with physical anomalies are associated with mental retardation, and any infant with significant birth defects is at increased risk of also having abnormalities of the central nervous system. This, however, is by no means always the case. Many malformation complexes can be cited that are usually associated with normal intelligence. In such instances, the establishment of a specific diagnosis can be most reassuring to the parents and physician and can guide them toward vigorous rehabilitative efforts for the affected infant.

When a newborn has been carefully examined and a single isolated congenital malformation has been detected, genetic counseling can be provided for that anomaly. The etiology of most of the more common isolated malformations in humans is very poorly understood. Many of these exhibit multifactorial inheritance, as previously described. For these disorders, data and recurrence risks are tabulated from studies of large numbers of families with affected individuals. The recurrence risks for some common congenital malformations are listed in Table 8–4.

It is important, as always, to elicit a careful family history before providing counseling. Multiply affected family members may imply a higher risk of recurrence than in the isolated case. Examination of other family members, especially the parents and siblings, may be indicated. Certain types of isolated congenital heart lesions, for example, occasionally are inherited in a dominant fashion even though the majority of cases show multifactorial inheritance. Affected individuals may be unaware of the presence of a clinically insignificant lesion.

As with other genetic disorders, it is a good general rule in dealing with congenital malformations to collect as much information as possible via all possible routes before providing genetic counseling. Precise and accurate counseling always is based on accurate diagnosis and knowledge of the disorder with which one is dealing.

TABLE 8–4. RECURRENCE RISKS FOR SOME COMMON CONGENITAL MALFORMATIONS[a]

Malformation	Risk for Each Subsequent Child (%)
Cleft lip with or without cleft palate[b]	
One affected child	4
Two affected children	9
One affected parent	4
One affected parent + one affected child	17
Cleft palate only	
One affected child	2
Two affected children	10
One affected parent	6
One affected parent + one affected child	15
Neural tube defects (anencephaly, myelomeningocele, encephalocele)	
One affected child	4–5
Two affected children	12–15
Congenital heart disease	
Ventricular septal defect	5
Atrial septal defect	3
Patent ductus arteriosus	4
Pulmonic stenosis	3
Aortic stenosis	2
Tetralogy of Fallot	3
Transposition of great vessels	2
Coarctation of aorta	2
Clubfoot	3
Congenital hip dislocation	4–5
Pyloric stenosis	
One affected child	3
Mother affected	16
Father affected	5

[a] Data compiled from multiple sources.
[b] All of the risk figures in this category are somewhat increased if the affected individual is female or if the cleft is severe.

PRENATAL DIAGNOSIS

The advent of increasingly sophisticated prenatal diagnostic techniques, including ultrasonography, and techniques for sampling fetal tissues, including amniocentesis, chorionic villus sampling, percutaneous umbilical cord blood sampling, and fetal tissue biopsy either by ultrasound-guided needle procedures or by fetoscopy, have allowed the prenatal diagnosis of hundreds of disorders. Some of these may have a better prognosis when recognized prenatally for both early postnatal correction and, in some limited instances, prenatal correction of anomalies.[1]

Invasive Techniques

Amniocentesis has been the mainstay of prenatal diagnosis for 15 years. In the most experienced hands, the risk of this procedure causing an abortion or any significant fetal damage has been reduced to approximately 1 in 300 to 400. The diagnosis of chromosomal and hundreds of metabolic disorders can be expected with high reliability. The advent of molecular DNA technology that uses the gene itself as opposed to the gene product

as the basis of diagnosis has allowed diagnosis before pathophysiology has occurred for disorders, such as cystic fibrosis, for which the fundamental defect is not understood.

The procedure involves the transabdominal needle aspiration of about 20 ml of amniotic fluid, usually aided by ultrasound guidance. The procedure usually is performed at about 16 to 17 weeks from the first day of the last menstrual period, and chromosome results usually are available in 2 to 3 weeks. Metabolic and molecular diagnosis normally requires another 7 to 10 days.

Chorionic Villus Sampling

One of the principal complaints about prenatal diagnosis has been the late stage of gestation at which diagnoses are available. Two alternatives are now available to move most diagnoses toward the first trimester.

Chorionic villus sampling (CVS) usually is performed between 9 and 12 weeks as a transvaginal–transcervical placental biopsy (Fig. 8–7). In some instances, the procedure is performed transabdominally, similar to an amniocentesis. Even with a slightly higher complication rate (about 0.5 to 1%) as worldwide CVS experi-

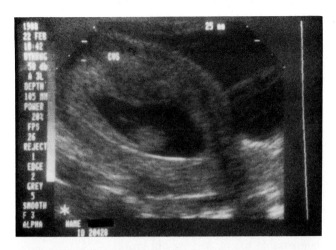

Figure 8–7. Ultrasound scan showing chorionic villus sampling procedure. Catheter is inserted from right to left, and the left tip of the catheter is in the middle of the placenta.

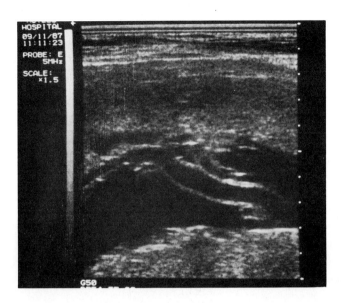

Figure 8–8. Ultrasound scan of umbilical cord coming off anterior placenta. A needle can be passed through the placenta and into the lumen of the umbilical vein to obtain specimens for cytogenic, biochemical, or molecular testing.

ence approaches 50,000 cases, the advantages of first trimester diagnoses are substantial, including earlier diagnoses, shorter wait between procedure and result, parental privacy of results before the pregnancy is visible, and the psychologic advantage of having results before quickening. If there is an abnormality and the couple elects a termination, first trimester methods are safer, quicker, less expensive, and generally less emotionally traumatic than second trimester techniques.

There are further advantages for metabolic and molecular diagnoses, since even the smallest solid tissue villus specimen has multifold more cells than an amniotic fluid specimen. Thus these diagnoses often are possible 7 to 10 days from the time of the procedure.

Early Amniocentesis

An emerging alternative to CVS is late first and early second trimester amniocentesis. With improved laboratory cell culture techniques and with increasingly sophisticated ultrasonography to guide needle entry, early amniocentesis results are encouraging and suggest the procedure as being practical in experienced hands.

Percutaneous Umbilical Cord Sampling

Despite the effectiveness of amniotic fluid and chorionic villus analysis, specific fetal tissues, such as blood or skin, sometimes are needed for diagnosis, and certain therapeutics, such as transfusions, are required (Fig. 8–8). Experience with percutaneous umbilical cord sampling in a few centers has suggested the general risk of fetal injury from 1 to 2 percent, but great advantages of direct access to the fetal circulation. Before recent advances in ultrasonography, direct fetal biopsies were performed in the past decade by fetoscopy, which requires a considerably larger instrument and has relatively poor visualization and a higher complication rate.

Ultrasonography

Perhaps nowhere in medicine has technology evolved at a faster rate than in prenatal ultrasound imagery. Normograms for fetal development are possible at ever decreasing gestational age, as is recognition of anatomic defects. Some authors have suggested ultrasonographic anatomic markers for chromosomal disorders, although there is great controversy surrounding their sensitivity and specificity. A few abnormalities, such as holoprosencephaly and single umbilical artery, clearly are associated with a significant risk of chromosomal and other defects. More subtle findings, such as femur/biparietal diameter (BPD) ratios and excess nuchal folds, are less accepted as being significantly predictive of abnormalities and prompting invasive techniques to assess chromosomal status.

Changes in obstetric management, such as where, when, and how to deliver a baby, can be anticipated by ultrasound diagnosis. Common examples include ventral wall defects, such as gastroschisis and omphaloceles (Fig. 8–9). Experience dictates a better neonatal prognosis when such babies are delivered in tertiary care centers with the pediatric surgery team waiting.

Another area of intense interest is in cardiac anatomy and function. The development of Doppler applications allows concomitant assessment of both anatomy and functions. Some recent examples of neonatal cardiac transplantation have been possible secondary to accurate assessment of pathology prenatally.

It can be anticipated that the physiology of other systems will be delineated in the next few years, giving

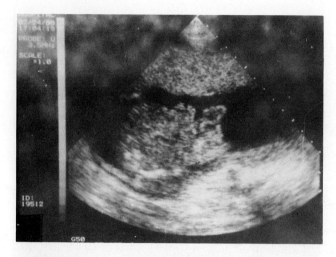

Figure 8–9. A transverse scan through the abdomen of a fetus with gastroschisis, demonstrating fetal intestines free floating in the amniotic fluid.

clues to pathology that will allow both earlier and more precise neonatal medical and surgical interventions.

Alpha-Fetoprotein Screening

Invasive techniques for prenatal diagnosis are the routine methods of diagnosis for patients in high-risk groups. Yet in absolute terms, far more babies are born with congenital abnormalities, such as neural tube defects or chromosomal abnormalities, from low-risk groups than from high-risk groups. Perhaps 97 percent of neural tube defects occur in families with no known history, and only 12 percent of infants with Down's syndrome are born to women over 35.

Alpha-fetoprotein (AFP) is an oncofetal protein produced by the liver. Fetal serum levels rise through the first trimester and then fall toward term. Amniotic fluid levels are markedly elevated in fetuses with anencephaly or open spina bifida; thus amniocentesis to measure amniotic fluid AFP and acetylcholinesterase (ACHE) is offered to all women at high risk.[7]

To detect the majority of defects, amniocentesis would have to be offered to all women, which is impractical. Levels of AFP in maternal serum (MS) have been shown to be an effective screen to delineate low-risk from high-risk patients. Patients with two elevated MSAFP values, optimally drawn at 15 to 17 weeks, can be offered amniocentesis to measure amniotic fluid AFP and ACHE. Whereas ultrasonography can detect many of the neural tube defects, in our experience, ultrasonography alone may miss as much as 25 percent of the anomalies.

There are many determinants to the interpretation and effectiveness of MSAFP screening, such as gestational age, maternal weight, multiple gestations, and diabetes.

In 1984, another use of MSAFP screening was recognized. There is an association between abnormally low MSAFP values and an increased risk of chromosome abnormalities. Maternal age risk counseling has now evolved from a unitary function to essentially the product of the a priori age risk and how low the MSAFP value is. We define a low value as one for which the adjusted risk for the specific pregnancy is at least equal to that of a 35-year-old woman, i.e., 1 in 200. Therefore, the MSAFP lower cutoff varies with maternal age, and a younger woman has to have a lower MSAFP to be low than does an older woman. In our own program, cytogenetic abnormalities have been found at a rate of over 1 percent of specimens obtained for low MSAFP and are comparable to our 35-year-old group.

The offering of MSAFP screening to all women has become standard practice in the United States. It is estimated that 90 percent of neural tube defects and 40 to 50 percent of chromosome abnormalities could be detected if screening and follow-up were universal. The next frontier will be to move screening earlier in gestation than the current 15-week minimum to permit earlier diagnosis of abnormalities.

FETAL THERAPY

At the very least, the prenatal recognition of defects allows for changes in the obstetric management of certain patients, whether it be recognition of a problem that will require postnatal attention, one that may alter obstetric management, or one that presents an option of abortion. Beyond the routine, however, the increasing sophistication of prenatal diagnosis now allows for attempts to correct defects in utero. Although still in its infancy, fetal therapy holds exciting possibilities for expanding neonatal outcomes in specific situations.

Surgical Therapy

Obstructive uropathies form a group of anomalies for which in utero intervention may improve the prognosis significantly. One of the most common etiologies for obstructive uropathies is a posterior urethral valve in males. Such obstruction can lead to a prune-belly syndrome and destruction of the kidneys with a Potter sequence-like presentation. Analysis of the data from the Fetal Surgery Registry of the International Fetal Medicine and Surgery Society reveals that there have now been approximately 100 attempts at in utero correction of obstruction by placement of a double pig-tailed vesicoamniotic shunt (Fig. 8–10).[8] Before any prenatal intervention is attempted, it is critical to rule out concomitant disorders, such as chromosome anomalies, that would alter the desirability of attempting intervention.

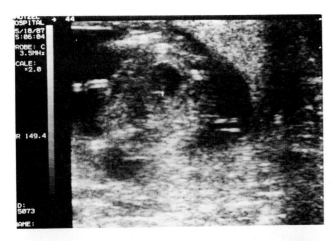

Figure 8–10. Ultrasound scan showing bladder shunt in place. Arrow points to the tip of the catheter in the bladder, and the outside of the catheter can be seen in the amniotic cavity.

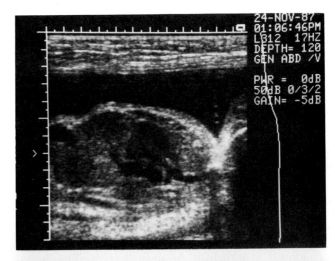

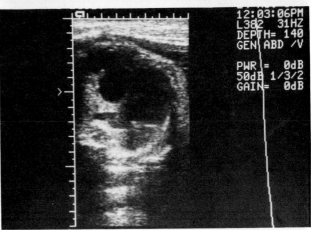

Figure 8–11. Top. Parasagittal view through a fetus with a diaphragmatic hernia demonstrating abdominal contents within the posterior aspect of the thorax. **Bottom.** Transverse view through the fetal thorax demonstrating a large, echolucent structure adjacent to the heart. This is the stomach and duodenum in a fetus with a diaphragmatic hernia.

Obstructive hydrocephalus, ventriculomegaly, and spina bifida are similarly diagnosable by ultrasonography and measurement of amniotic fluid AFP and ACHE. Great enthusiasm surrounded attempts early in the 1980s to reduce obstructive hydrocephalus through the placement of ventricular amniotic shunts. Assessment of the data from the Fetal Surgery Registry, however, has been very disappointing, and there has been a de facto moratorium on the use of these shunts in the past few years. A large proportion of patients had other anomalies in addition to the obstructive hydrocephalus, suggesting the futility of attempts in many of these fetuses. More recent data, however, have shown that, contrary to earlier expectations, the natural history of in utero diagnosed ventriculomegaly was far worse than had been originally believed when compared to neonatally diagnosed ventriculomegaly. Thus, the outcomes in attempts at correction of isolated ventriculomegaly may not have been as dismal as originally thought. Current thinking is that it may be appropriate to renew attempts in a very limited number of centers to test the efficacy of this therapy.

Open fetal surgery has been attempted on a very limited number of cases that required more serious intervention. Most notably, there have been several attempts at in utero correction of diaphragmatic hernias (Fig. 8–11). Work by Harrison et al. has shown that the prognosis for neonatally diagnosed diaphragmatic hernia is extremely poor, and early attempts at in utero repair revealed that a major prognostic factor at the time of surgery was the presence of the liver in the left side of the chest.[8] Repair of a fetus in whom the liver was not in the left side of the chest was technically easy and was considered successful. It can be anticipated that in a very limited number of instances such surgery may be appropriate and beneficial.

Medical Therapies

There is now a large experience with pharmacologic fetal therapy. Several cardiac drugs administered to the mother are known to cross the placenta and can be made to correct fetal arrhythmias. In the evaluation of potential therapeutic candidates, a detailed fetal echocardiogram is essential, since about 14 percent of patients with arrhythmias have underlying cardiac structural anomalies.

Documented prevention of external genital masculinization has been achieved in 21 hydroxylase deficiency congenital adrenal hypoplasias. Maternally administered dexamethasone beginning at 9 weeks crosses the placenta, suppresses the fetal adrenal, and allows proper female development.

Gene Therapy

The near future holds the prospect of the introduction of genetic material to give the fetus or neonate without the capability of making an enzyme the ability to do so. Examples of disorders for which gene therapy would be highly desirable include the hemoglobinopathies and storage disorders, such as Tay-Sachs disease.

SUMMARY

It is clearly unrealistic to expect the surgeon to recognize all of the innumerable genetic disorders and malformation syndromes associated with surgical problems in childhood. It is realistic, however, to expect him or her to view the overall child with an eye for underlying disease or multiple problems and not to focus on a single surgical event. The surgeon should be prepared to join a team of physicians providing diagnosis, management, and counseling for children with multiple malformations and chronic genetic disorders. It is hoped that this chapter will provide a basis for the understanding of the complex problems that may be encountered.

REFERENCES

1. Evans MI, Schulman JD: In Avery GB (ed): Neonatology, Pathophysiology, and Management of the Newborn, 3rd ed. Philadelphia, Lippincott, 1987, pp 130–138.
2. Smith DW: Recognizable Patterns of Human Malformation. Genetic, Embryologic, and Clinical Aspects, 2nd ed. Philadelphia, Saunders, 1982
3. Baraitser M, Winter R: A Colour Atlas of Clinical Genetics. London, Wolf Medical, 1984
4. Wynne-Davies R, Hall CM, Appley AG: Atlas of Skeletal Dysplasias. Edinburgh, Churchill-Livingstone, 1985
5. Smithells, RW: Prevention of neural tube defects by vitamin supplements. In Dobbing J (ed): Prevention of Spina Bifida and Other Neural Tube Defects. London, Academic Press, 1983, p 53
6. Abel E, Sokol RJ: Social and environmental risks in pregnancy: alcohol. In Evans MI, Fletcher JC, Dixler AO, et al. (eds): Fetal Diagnosis and Therapy: Science, Ethics and the Law. Philadelphia, Lippincott, 1989
7. Evans MI, Belsky RL, Grebb A, et al: Maternal serum alpha-fetoprotein screening. Clin Immunoassay 10:210, 1988
8. Adzick N, Harrison M, Glick P, et al: Diaphragmatic hernia in the fetus: Prenatal diagnosis and outcome in 94 cases. J Pediatr Surg 20:357, 1985

SECTION II

Critical Care

Critical care is the latest term used to describe the pre- and postoperative management of very sick or injured patients. In itself, it is not a new specialty but is the close monitoring of sick children and the application of physiologic principles to reverse their pathology and make them well. This phase of care is an extension of the operation or an episode of trauma that is as much the surgeon's responsibility as closing the incision. The various components of critical care originated because of the increasing complexity of surgical operations. Mechanical endotracheal ventilation originally was required for the anesthetic management of the open chest during thoracic surgery. Long-term endotracheal ventilation was then taken up in Scandinavia during the last episode of paralytic poliomyelitis. This technique was then quickly adapted in this country during the late 1950s to the management of the postoperative cardiac surgical patient and for the care of patients with flail chest caused by trauma.

In those days, we knew that a new era was at hand because general surgical residents had to carry screwdrivers and wrenches to keep the old piston respirators going. Continuous electrocardiographic monitors were introduced first into the operating room and then the postoperative recovery room for the observation of cardiac surgery patients. The concept of total intravenous nutrition was introduced by surgeons in the 1950s but was not widely used until reliable central venous lines became available for the newborn infant.

Although the most advanced technology is used to aid in the care of our sickest patients, the most valuable tool in the care of these people is an inquiring, alert mind. Each time we see a very sick patient we should keenly observe for such things as skin color, tissue turgor, and venous collapse or distention. If the patient's foot is pink and warm and one can easily see veins on the dorsum and palpate a dorsalis pedis pulse, we can take these signs as an indication that the person has good peripheral circulation and good cardiopulmonary function. Observation of chest motion and bilateral auscultation of the lungs is as good a way as any to determine the proper placement of endotracheal tubes and to see if the lungs are being ventilated satisfactorily.

Other simple but important observations include the hourly urinary output, frequent body weights, and daily calculation of the caloric, protein, and vitamin intakes. It is too easy to become bogged down in laboratory results and the apparent complexity of such things as ventilatory management and intravenous nutrition. There are specialists and technicians who would like to make us believe that these modes of treatment are extremely complex and should be in their domain. This is simply not so. Continuity of care by the surgeon and the surgeon's team is superior to having the patient managed by multiple specialists.

Continuity of care and the continued and personal interest of the surgeon are particularly important as the child is getting well and plans must be made for his long-term nutritional, physical, and psychologic support. We must always keep in mind that the surgical operation and the immediate postoperative care are simply a point on the road to making the child well again.

9
Vascular Access

_____ *Susan R. Luck*

Children are afraid of needles, and most will squirm when a well-meaning physician attempts to draw blood or start an intravenous infusion. Unfortunately, venipuncture is the procedure most frequently performed on pediatric surgical patients. To decrease trauma to the veins, every effort should be made to sample blood through the same needle that is to be used for fluid therapy. Another plan is to use the antecubital veins for sampling and the veins of the forearm or hand to give fluids. Blood samples may be obtained from an antecubital or scalp vein by the following technique. One assistant restrains the baby while another holds a syringe that is attached to a 21- or 23-gauge scalp vein needle (butterfly) with plastic tubing. The site is prepared with several applications of povidone-iodine solution. Once the skin is penetrated, the assistant applies gentle suction to the syringe; as soon as the vein is entered, blood will flow into the plastic tubing. Almost any movement by the patient will dislodge a needle directly attached to a syringe. The scalp vein needle fixed to flexible tubing usually stays intraluminal. A peripheral artery can be aspirated in a similar fashion.

When other sites for blood sampling cannot be used because of obesity, shock, or other reasons, an experienced physician may use the femoral vein. The child is restrained, with the thighs extended. After palpation of the femoral artery with the middle and index fingers of one hand, a 23-gauge scalp vein needle is inserted through the skin just medial to the index fingertip. The needle is angled in a cephalad direction, with gentle suction on the syringe. There is no chance for the needle to penetrate the hip joint. One insertion usually is sufficient, but if blood is not obtained immediately, the needle is withdrawn all the way to the skin and then redirected.

ROUTINE VASCULAR ACCESS

A plastic cannula can be inserted percutaneously into a peripheral vein of most children while under general anesthesia, before surgery. With practice, a hand or scalp vein of even a newborn can be cannulated with a 20- or 22-gauge size. This single venipuncture, if well-secured, should remain in place for several days, providing venous access for the administration of drugs and for fluid therapy. Teflon and Silastic catheters are well tolerated. Complications, such as phlebitis and local infection, are not significantly related to the duration of cannulation but to the type of fluids and drugs administered. Concentrated glucose solutions, nafcillin, and the aminoglycosides are associated with a higher incidence of phlebitis.[1]

A small nick made at the insertion site with a separate metal needle will eliminate skin traction on the plastic cannula and prevent damage to the soft tip. In awake patients, a skin wheal should be raised with a local anesthetic. The needle and plastic cannula are inserted until blood is aspirated or flashes back, then the cannula alone is advanced into the vein. Further advancement sometimes is facilitated if fluids are running through the cannula. The catheter should be secured to the skin with a sterile clear plastic film, reinforced with tape. The insertion site and the skin over the needle tip can be visualized without changing the dressing. The tissues above the infusion site must be uncovered for constant

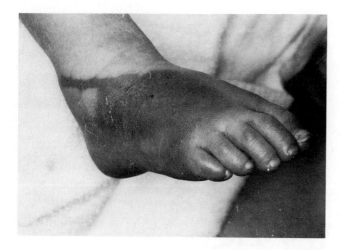

Figure 9–1. Parenteral nutrition fluid infiltrated into a dorsal vein on this infant's foot, and the pump continued to run. Eventually, a skin graft was required to repair the defect.

inspection because pumps that inject fluid at a constant rate may continue the infusion even though the solution is infiltrating tissue outside the vein. Infiltration of intravenous fluids must be treated promptly with injections of hyaluronidase and with warm wet applications to avoid skin sloughing (Fig. 9–1).

Emergency Vascular Access

Skill with percutaneous techniques has reduced the need for peripheral venous cutdowns in children in shock from trauma or dehydration, obese patients, and the occasional child who has run out of veins but urgently requires intravenous therapy. The saphenous vein at the ankle is easily found and cannulated just anterior and superior to the medial malleolus. Although commonly used, especially during an emergency, this venous site does present disadvantages. During an operation, while hidden under the drapes, the tubing connections may separate or the catheter may infiltrate into tissue, without the knowledge of the anesthetist. Furthermore, a lower extremity cutdown is useless for transfusion during an operation for abdominal trauma or for tumor resection. The incidence of septic phlebitis is higher in lower extremity veins. Some patients have been found to have developed varicose veins at long-term follow-up.[2]

The cephalic vein at the wrist, which is prominent medial and dorsal to the radial styloid process, is ideal for an elective venesection (Fig. 9-2). With the forearm in pronation, this vein crosses the center of the snuffbox and pursues a course straight up to the lateral side of the elbow. Light, fine-tipped tissue forceps and sharp iris scissors are indispensable for any cutdown. The sur-

geon should sit during the procedure so that his forearms may rest on the operating table for increased steadiness. The infant's forearm and hand are securely taped to a padded arm board. A sterile field is blocked with towels and clips after the skin has been prepared from the elbow to the fingertips. The vein may be seen or palpated, or its position may be inferred from a confident knowledge of topical anatomy. A short vertical incision made directly over the vein will give far better exposure than a larger transverse incision. Proximal extension will expose additional length if the vein is accidentally transected or injured. The catheter should be attached to a syringe containing sterile injectable saline before opening the vein and must be placed close enough to the sterile field that the operator can pick up the catheter without looking away from the vein once the venotomy is made. The vein always should be cut tangentially. The venotomy can be dilated gently with scissors tips or a plastic catheter introducer. Slow infusion of saline will dilate the vein while the catheter is advanced. When in good position, the catheter can be secured to the vein with absorbable sutures. The incision is approximated with a subcuticular suture and sterile tape strips. A small sterile plastic film secures the catheter and covers the incision.

The child who is in shock from trauma and the infant who has had massive gastrointestinal fluid losses present the most difficult vascular access problems. The peripheral veins are often in such severe spasm that they are difficult or impossible to find and cannulate. Once a catheter is in place, vasospasm and a small cannula diameter restrict the rapid administration of large volumes of fluid. Additional resuscitation efforts, such as endotracheal intubation, limit access to the neck or upper extremities. In these situations, the saphenous vein at the groin should be used. The femoral area is quickly prepared with povidone-iodine, and a transverse incision is made 1 to 2 cm below the inguinal ligament and medial to the femoral triangle. The saphenous vein is found below Scarpa's fascia. Any type of long vascular catheter can be threaded to the right atrium through a venotomy or direct venous puncture. The atrial position bypasses abdominal sites of blood loss and allows for measurement of the central venous pressure if desired.

Fluids for emergency resuscitation can be infused directly into the bone marrow.[3] The medullary cavity is composed of a network of venous sinusoids that drain into the venous system. The most accessible site is the proximal tibia. Up to age 5 or 6 years, the broad and flat portion of the tibia just below and medial to the tibial condyle can be punctured with a short stiff needle. An 18-gauge intravenous needle may be used in infants, but, in older children, a 13- to 16-gauge bone marrow needle is easier to insert. This route should be used until intravenous access is established.

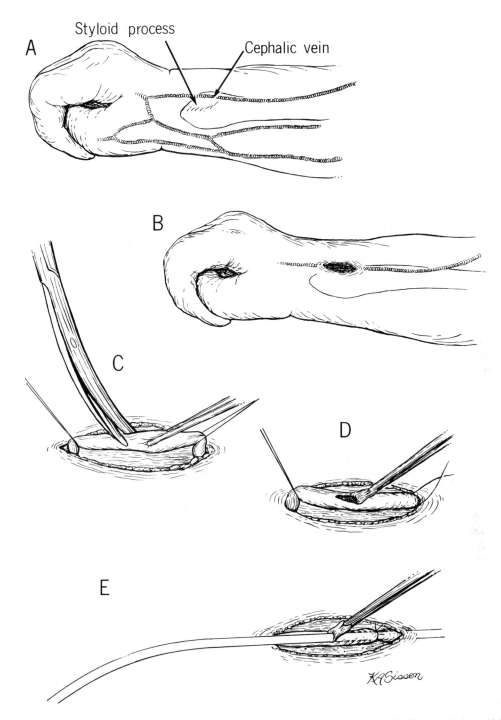

Figure 9–2. A wrist cutdown is preferable to one at the ankle for surgical patients. **A.** The vein is located just dorsal and proximal to the radial styloid. **B.** A vertical incision allows much better exposure of the vein. **C.** The vein is ligated distally and then held up with a proximal ligature while it is opened at an angle to create a flap (**D**). **E.** The cannula may exit from the same wound or may be tunneled away from the incision.

CENTRAL VENOUS CATHETERIZATION

A Silastic catheter with a Teflon felt cuff buried under the skin 1 cm from the exit site is used whenever there is need for long-term vascular access. The most common indication is for parenteral nutrition. Double- and even triple-lumen catheters are used when multiple access ports are required. These multilumen catheters are particularly valuable in children with malignant tumors who require both parenteral nutrition and chemotherapy. Larger double-lumen catheters may be used for hemodialysis in children with renal failure.

Catheters may be passed into the superior vena cava via the basilic, subclavian, and internal and external jugular and facial veins.[4,5] Percutaneous catheterization of the subclavian vein is a popular and relatively uncomplicated procedure in adults. This vein provides rapid access to the superior vena cava for infusion of large volumes of fluids and for measurement of central venous pressure. The potential hazards of hemorrhage, pneumothorax, perforation of the myocardium, and catheter embolism should restrict the use of this technique to situations in which other infusion methods are impractical or impossible. Before attempting subclavian puncture in children, the surgeon should perfect his technique in adults. We prefer to limit the use of subclavian catheters to children weighing at least 5 kg. A general anesthetic with good control of the airway is safer in many cases than heavy sedation and restraint. Complications are minimized by adherence to the following technique. The child is placed in the Trendelenburg position with a folded sheet between the shoulder blades, with the head turned to the opposite side. The neck and chest are carefully prepared and draped. If the child is awake, the skin is infiltrated with lidocaine just beneath the junction of the middle and medial thirds of the clavicle. A variety of introducer and catheter sets is available in various sizes. Single-, double-, and triple-lumen catheters of Silastic or Teflon can be placed by this technique. The needle is inserted, aiming deep into the sternal notch. When blood is withdrawn into the syringe, a guidewire is threaded into the superior vena cava (SVC) or right atrium. After this position is confirmed by radiograph of fluoroscopy, the needle is removed. A plastic dilator and sheath are introduced into the vein over the guidewire. After the wire and dilator are removed, the catheter is advanced through the sheath. The sheath is withdrawn and removed, leaving the catheter in final position. If long-term use is intended, the catheter can be tunneled from a separate incision on the anterior chest before being passed through the sheath. Silastic catheters are less likely to perforate a large vein or the heart than are those of firmer polyethylene or Teflon.

An external jugular venesection is a safe and reliable route to the superior vena cava. This procedure is regarded as a major operation and is performed in the operating room or the intensive care unit with meticulous aseptic technique. Patient movement is not as hazardous as with subclavian puncture. Sedation and local anesthesia can be used in small infants and some older children. The infant is restrained, with arms at the sides, and the head turned to the opposite side (Fig. 9–3). The skin of the anterior chest, neck, and scalp is prepared and draped into a sterile field. The drapes are held away

from the baby's face by a Mayo stand. An assistant continually observes the infant's respirations and can quiet him or her with a pacifier. The skin over the external jugular vein is infiltrated with 0.5 percent lidocaine. The vein is isolated and encircled with a 5-0 ligature. If the vein is carefully mobilized to just behind the clavicle, lateral traction can be applied, thus straightening the angle between the external jugular vein and the subclavian vein. A steel ventricular puncture cannula is used to tunnel beneath the skin down over the chest wall. The Silastic catheter is then inserted through the subcutaneous tunnel and into a tangential incision in the vein. The position in the superior vena cava or right atrium must be verified by a radiograph or fluoroscopy while the baby is still on the operating table. The catheter is secured to the skin at the exit site with nonabsorbable sutures and sterile adhesive tape. Povidone-iodine ointment is applied to the catheter exit site, which is covered with a clear plastic film. The cervical incision is closed with subcuticular sutures and sterile tape strips.

It is often necessary to use the internal jugular vein in tiny premature infants. The skin incision is centered over the lower portion of the sternocleidomastoid muscle, and the clavicular and sternal heads of the muscle are separated to widen the space. The carotid sheath is seen immediately, and the internal jugular vein is isolated and encircled with two ligatures. In older infants, the catheter can be inserted through a small venotomy and secured by a pursestring suture, avoiding vein ligation. The percutaneous insertion of size 2.7 Silastic catheters through a 19-gauge needle has almost elminated the need for cutdowns in many tiny infants. Peripheral scalp or extremity veins can be cannulated, threading the catheters to the right atrium.[6]

Complications

Central venous catheters can be left in place for months or even years without difficulty. Complications are reduced or eliminated by the use of Silastic catheters, careful aseptic technique, fixation with Teflon pledgets, and the use of heparin in all administered fluids. Parents can learn how to care for lines at home. Broken catheters can be repaired and need not be removed. The catheter position should be verified by radiographs from time to time, and if there is catheter obstruction, an echocardiogram may demonstrate an atrial clot. Such clots can be dissolved with urokinase, thus salvaging obstructed catheters. Thrombosis of major veins is now rare, since all fluids are heparinized. This complication still occurs when multiple catheters are inserted through various veins into the superior vena cava or sclerosing medications are infused into subclavian veins.

Sepsis is of particular concern in oncology patients who become neutropenic with long-term chemotherapy.[7,8] When a central catheter is the only sus-

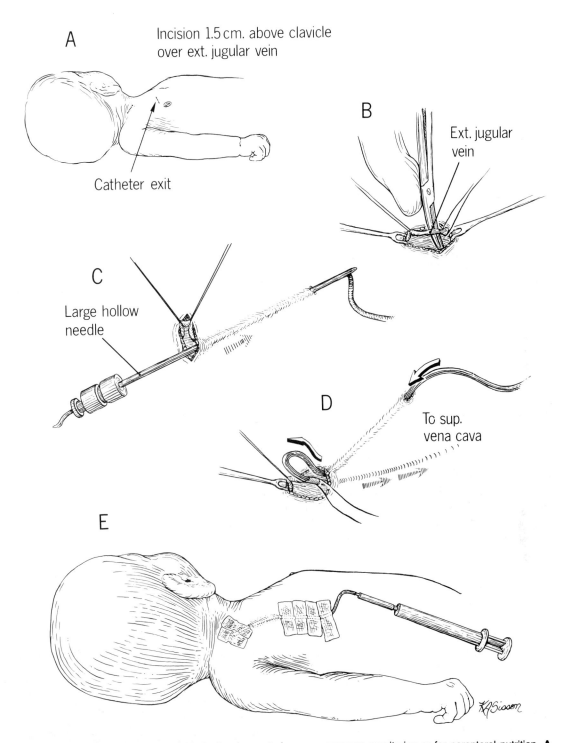

A — Incision 1.5 cm. above clavicle over ext. jugular vein

Catheter exit

B — Ext. jugular vein

C — Large hollow needle

D — To sup. vena cava

E

Figure 9–3. Central venous catheterization for central venous pressure monitoring or for parenteral nutrition. **A.** The infant is positioned with his shoulders elevated and his neck extended. The entire neck, chest, and upper arm are prepared with a soap scrub, alcohol, and povidone-iodine. **B.** The vein is isolated just above the clavicle. **C.** A ventricular needle is an excellent tunneling device. **D.** The tube is first tunneled, then placed in the vein. **E.** The catheter is secured with sutures and multiple Micropore tapes.

pected source of infection, it may be left in place while the patient is treated with specific antibiotics. If blood cultures become negative after 72 hours of therapy, the line may be kept in place while therapy is continued.[9]

UMBILICAL VESSEL CANNULATION

The umbilical cord provides easy access to both the central venous and arterial systems in infants less than 24 hours of age. The usual aseptic skin preparations and sterile field are made, and the cord is transected beneath the tie. The vein is a thin-walled oval structure, and the arteries appear as small dots of blood clot. Visible clot is removed, and then a soft No. 5 French plastic catheter attached to a saline-filled syringe is inserted into the vein. The catheter must traverse the ductus venosus and the left hepatic vein to enter the inferior vena cava. If an obstruction is met, the tip has most likely entered the left or right branch of the portal vein. When blood cannot be aspirated freely, the catheter is removed rather than flushed to avoid pushing a clot into the right heart, liver, or spleen. The catheter tip position in the right atrium must be confirmed by a radiograph. The umbilical vein may be catheterized from inside the peritoneal cavity during an abdominal operation if there is need for rapid transfusion. When the cord is dried, this vein may also be isolated extraperitoneally just below the fascia through a small midline incision above the umbilicus.

The umbilical artery can be catheterized during the first 24 hours of life for monitoring blood gases and arterial pressure and for fluid infusion. This route also may be used for cardiac catheterization or angiography. The complications of umbilical artery catheterization include tissue or organ infarction after thrombosis of the renal, superior mesenteric, gluteal, or hypogastric artery, as well as aortic thrombosis.[10,11] Perforation and hemoperitoneum have been reported.

A No. 3.5 French soft plastic catheter with an end hole and a rounded tip is connected to a saline-filled syringe. The umbilical artery is located in the cord; clot is removed, and the vessel is dilated with forceps or with the tips of iris scissors. During insertion of the catheter, obstruction may be encountered at the level of the abdominal wall near the bladder. Gentle continuous pressure usually will overcome the first resistance, but an injection of 0.5 ml of 1 percent lidocaine may relax vessel spasm at the junction of the umbilical and hypogastric arteries. With aspiration, blood will be obtained just at the hypogastric junction. The tip of the catheter is advanced to above the diaphragm or to a position below the renal arteries. Final position is documented by a radiograph; a location opposite the third lumbar vertebra is ideal. A continuous dilute heparin infusion helps prevent thrombosis. If blood cannot be aspirated, the catheter must be removed rather than flushed. Blanching of the leg or buttock area indicates a peripheral position of the catheter tip and is an indication for immediate removal. Although umbilical catheters have been maintained in place for as long as 3 weeks, they should be removed as soon as possible to prevent sepsis and thrombosis. Filston and Izant have recommended tunneling the umbilical artery to a new site lateral to the umbilicus and away from an abdominal incision.[12]

PERIPHERAL ARTERIAL CANNULATION

Although transcutaneous oxygen monitors accurately reflect arterial Po_2 within established limits, the sampling of arterial blood and continuous blood pressure monitoring are essential in the management of seriously ill children. Percutaneous catheterization of arteries is now almost routine during major operations, particularly during the neonatal period. Unfortunately, arterial puncture in a baby with vasoconstriction and poor peripheral perfusion may trigger thrombosis and gangrene[13] (Fig. 9–4). The radial artery is cannulated, with the wrist held in dorsiflexion. The skin just proximal to the volar wrist crease is penetrated, holding the cannula parallel to the palpated artery to add stability to the system. The cannula should cross 1 cm of soft tissue before the artery is entered. When blood returns in the catheter, the cannula

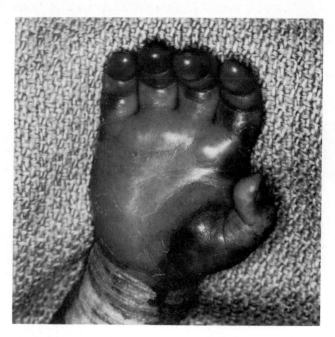

Figure 9–4. Vascular compromise following radial arterial cannulation for monitoring in an infant who was in shock with poor perfusion before the cannulation.

is advanced over the needle, and the needle is withdrawn. The cannula is then held in place with sterile tape strips or with a suture.

A dilute solution of saline containing 100 units of heparin/100 ml is infused slowly into any arterial line. All connections must be made with Luer locks to prevent separation and hemorrhage. A system with three-way stopcocks allows continuous flushing of the catheter, arterial pressure monitoring, and blood sampling.

IMPLANTABLE VENOUS ACCESS DEVICE

Catheters that exit from the skin limit bathing, prevent many normal childhood activities, and are always liable to sepsis. A completely implantable venous infusion device minimizes these problems. A Silastic catheter is connected to a chemically inert reservoir, which is buried subcutaneously. The rubber diaphragm injection port of the reservoir is self-sealing and can be penetrated repeatedly through the skin by a needle without leakage. This system is most suitable for children with malignant tumors who require long-term chemotherapy. Routine intravenous fluids also can be given through the device, and blood may be withdrawn for sampling. In our hands, the implantable device has not been successful in children with coagulation defects, such as hemophilia, because bleeding and hematoma formation occur at the injection site. A careful injection procedure is essential. If the silicone diaphragm is not entered precisely and blood is aspirated before injection, extravasation and serious tissue damage occur about the device. The jugular, cephalic, and proximal saphenous veins are all suitable for insertion.

Technique

General anesthesia is preferred. The entire neck and chest are prepared and draped as for insertion of any central venous line. A transverse incision is made over the chest wall above or below the breast but away from the nipple. A subcutaneous pocket is created above the pectoralis fascia by sharp dissection. Hemostasis must be perfect within this pocket. The external jugular or cephalic vein is isolated through a separate incision. The Silastic catheter is tunnelled from the pocket to the cervical incision. Venotomy and central venous catheterization are performed as previously described. The base of the reservoir is sutured to the pectoral fascia within the pocket, and the incision is closed. The injection site must be well away from the incision. During the procedure, the reservoir is filled with saline to prevent blood from backing up into the catheter. The system is flushed with a heparinized solution at the end of operation. Golladay and Mollitt have described a technique for the percu-

taneous insertion of the catheter into the subclavian vein rather than the external jugular.[14] The exact injection site can be marked by a small skin tattoo. Scrupulous sterile injection technique is required. The needle is inserted straight into the Silastic membrane after careful palpation of the ring. Blood is aspirated, and 5 ml of sterile saline is flushed through the catheter before and after the injection of any medication. If there is resistance to flushing, 2 ml of heparin, 100 units/ml, is injected. Clots may be dissolved with the instillation of 1 ml of urokinase into the catheter, and then the system is again flushed with heparin and saline. A right-angled needle whose hub parallels the skin is easy to stabilize for prolonged fluid administration.

Complications are extrusion of the device through the skin in poorly nourished children, extravasation at the injection site, occlusion of the catheter, and infection of the catheter or the injection site and pocket. Implantation of the device beneath the pectoralis muscle has been attempted, but the injection site is difficult to puncture. In one study of 39 pediatric oncology patients, only five children required removal of the system because of complications.[15]

REFERENCES

1. Nelson D, Garland J: The natural history of Teflon catheter-associated phlebitis in children. Am J Dis Child 141:1090, 1987
2. Schuster SR, Laks H: Varicose veins following ankle cutdowns. J Pediatr Surg 8:245, 1973
3. Spivey W: Intraosseous infusion. J Pediatr 111:639, 1987
4. Pietsch JB, Nagaraj HS, Groff DB: Simplified insertion of central venous catheter in infants. Surg Gynecol Obstet 158:91, 1984
5. Prince SR, Sullivan RL, Hackel A: Percutaneous catheterization of the internal jugular vein in infants and children. Anesthesiology 44:170, 1976
6. Durand M, Ramanathan R, Martinell B, Tolentino M: Prospective evaluation of percutaneous central venous Silastic catheters in newborn infants with birth weights of 510 to 3920 grams. Pediatrics 78:245, 1986
7. Shapiro E, Wald E, Nelson K, et al: Broviac catheter-related bacteremia in oncology patients. Am J Dis Child 136:679, 1982
8. Wang E, Prober C, Ford-Jones I, et al: The management of central intravenous catheter infections. Pediatr Infect Dis 3:110, 1988
9. Olson T, Fischer G, Lupo M, et al: Antimicrobial therapy of broviac catheter infections in pediatric hematology oncology patients. J Pediatr Surg 22:939, 1987
10. Vailas GN, Brouillette RT, Scott JP, et al: Neonatal aortic thrombosis: recent experience. J Pediatr 109:101, 1986
11. O'Neill JA Jr, Neblett WW III, Born ML: Management of major thromboembolic complications of umbilical artery catheters. J Pediatr Surg 16:972, 1981
12. Filston HC, Izant RJ Jr: Translocation of the umbilical

artery to the lower abdomen: An adjunct to the postoperative monitoring of arterial blood gases in major abdominal wall defects. J Pediatr Surg 10:225, 1975

13. Miyaska K, Edmonds JR, Conn AW: Complications of radial artery lines in the pediatric patient. Can Anaesth Soc J 23:9, 1976

14. Golladay E, Mollitt D: Percutaneous placement of a venous access port in a pediatric population. J Pediatr Surg 21:683, 1986

15. Wallace J, Zeltzer P: Benefits, complications and care of implantable infusion devices in 31 children with cancer. J Pediatr Surg 22:833, 1987

10
Fluids and Electrolytes

Accurate fluid, electrolyte, and nutritional therapy is essential in pediatric surgery. By calculating maintenance requirements, estimating preexisting deficits, and measuring ongoing abnormal losses, we can accurately manage fluid and electrolyte problems in patients ranging from the premature infant to the teenager with massive burns. Innumerable formulas and rules have been applied to what appears to be a complex therapeutic problem. Fortunately, most patients have normal kidneys and will tolerate remarkably different forms of therapy. Best results are obtained by beginning with a knowledge of physiologic principles, then applying clinical and laboratory observations in the individual patient.

The volume of total body water and the rate of fluid exchange vary with age (Fig. 10–1). A child's metabolism is altered by the trauma of an operation. Consequently, the methods of managing pediatric medical patients and adult surgical patients are not necessarily applicable in pediatric surgery. The differing approaches to correcting dehydration are good examples: it is not uncommon to correct dehydration in a child with diarrhea over a period of 24 to 48 hours, but the patient with an intussusception or a perforated appendix must have the deficits corrected within a few hours so that he or she may safely undergo anesthesia and operation. Surgical patients frequently have fluid sequestered in injured tissue. These large volumes of plasmalike fluid can be estimated on purely clinical grounds.

The maintenance needs of a patient are that amount of fluid and electrolytes required for insensible losses through respiration and skin evaporation and to maintain a normal urine output. In most patients, the fluid and electrolytes required for normal maintenance are arrived at through simple calculations based on metabolic needs, which in turn are related to body weight or surface area.[1] These maintenance requirements are altered by such factors as fever, tachypnea, environmental temperature and humidity, and the patient's clinical state.

THE FULL-TERM NEONATE

Before birth, the nutritional needs of the fetus are met through the placental circulation. The normal full-term infant has a built-in fluid reserve to tide him or her over the transitional period to full oral feeding of breast milk. The neonate has a total body water content of 75 percent and an extracellular fluid volume that is 35 to 40 percent of body weight (Fig. 10–2). By 1 year of age, the total body water has dropped to 60 percent, and thereafter it decreases only slightly. The extracellular fluid volume falls to 27 percent by 1 year and represents only 20 percent of body weight by adolescence. The intracellular fluid space constitutes 35 to 40 percent of a newborn infant's birth weight, and this increases slightly with age.[2,3] The total blood volume of a newborn infant may be as high as 8.5 percent of body weight. This increased level, as compared with levels seen in older patients, reflects the infant's hematocrit, which may be as high as 60 percent. Immature infants have even higher percentages of total body water and extracellular fluid.[4]

In the neonate, the kidney has a slow diuretic response to a water load and cannot maximally dilute urine until 5 days of age.[5] The maximum urine osmolality is only 600 to 700 mOsm/kg, in comparison with 1200

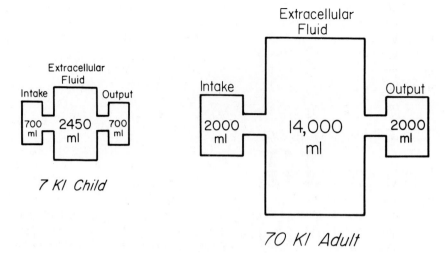

Figure 10–1. A child weighing less than 10 kg requires an intake of 100 ml of water/kg. This high water turnover progressively decreases with increase in age and weight.

mOsm/kg in older patients. The urine volume for normal infants gradually increases from zero to 68 ml on the first day of life to 40 to 302 ml by 7 days.[6] Fasting newborn infants will tolerate a loss of 13 percent of body weight with only minimal elevations of blood urea nitrogen and sodium concentrations when all fluid is withheld for 72 hours. When given 50 ml of water per kilogram per day there is still an 8 percent decrease in body weight.[7] This weight loss is accompanied by a period of negative nitrogen balance. Milk feedings induce positive nitrogen balance and weight gain by the end of the first week. Wilkinson et al. found that when infants were offered unlimited amounts of breast milk during the first few days of life, they still lost weight, had minimal urinary output, and had negative nitrogen balance.[8]

These metabolic studies confirm clinical observations; the normal newborn is inactive, has no appetite, and becomes interested in food only on the third or fourth day. The fluid volume taken by a breast-fed infant slowly increases from the second day of life to approximately 150 ml/kg by the fifth to the seventh days. Feedings of 150 ml of breast milk per kilogram provide 100 to 110 calories/kg.[9] The logical conclusion to be drawn from these data is that the newborn infant has endogenous water to carry him over the first few days of life until his mother has sufficient milk to satisfy his needs. One of the most frequent errors is to administer too much fluid to the newborn during his first 2 or 3 days of life. The small urine volume is normal and is not indicative of dehydration.

Fifty milliliters of maintenance fluid/kg per day is sufficient for the first 2 days, provided there are no abnormal losses. This volume is increased stepwise to 100 ml/kg by the fifth day. Initially, 10 percent glucose is administered because any form of stress can precipitate hypoglycemia.[10] After the second day, glucose is given in 0.2 percent saline with potassium to provide sodium at 2 to 3 mEq/kg/day and potassium at 2 mEq/kg/day. Frequently, supplemental calcium must be added to prevent tetany. Cold, stress, or exposure to heating lamps in an open bed will increase insensible fluid losses, but if the infant is kept in a closed isolette with humidity, fluid requirements will be diminished.

Fluid sequestered in the peritoneal or thoracic cavity at birth, as with urine or meconium peritonitis, has already been replaced by the placental circulation. Losses incurred by postnatal vomiting may be accurately estimated by comparing the infant's birth weight and current weight. After the infant comes under observation, all abnormal gastrointestinal, urine, and serous exudative

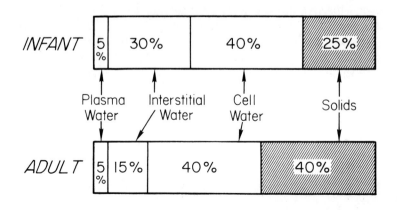

Figure 10–2. Comparison of the fluid spaces in infants and adults. The total body and interstitial water spaces are larger in the small child.

losses are carefully measured and replaced at intervals of 4 to 12 hours, depending on their volumes. While the newborn infant is on conventional short-term fluid therapy, he or she should lose 10 to 15 g/day. An increase in weight over that produced by replacement of preexisting deficits must represent edema fluid.

THE PREMATURE INFANT

Premature infants have a large surface area in relation to body weight, and their insensible water losses are up to four times greater than in full-term babies. Most of this increased water loss is through the thinner stratum corneum in the premature infant, which offers less passive resistance to the diffusion of water from the skin capillaries to the environment.[11] These skin losses are proportional to decreased gestational age and are greatest during the first postnatal day but decrease with increasing age.[12] These losses may reach 129 ml/kg/24 hours during the first postnatal day in an infant with a gestational age of 25 to 27 weeks. These insensible losses are further increased by exposure of the infant to phototherapy and infrared heating lights.[13,14] The high insensible skin losses are decreased by nursing premature infants in a closed incubator with maximum humidity; unfortunately, since most of these babies require intensive care and ventilator therapy, they are kept in open beds with radiant warmers.[15] Infants weighing less than 1500 g should be wrapped in a clear plastic film to decrease evaporative water losses and to prevent surface cooling from convection currents stirred up by air in the nursery. Even though these plastic films reduce evaporative losses, premature infants require larger volumes of maintenance fluid.

During the first day of life, a premature infant who is in a high humidity incubator may require only 50 ml/kg/24 hours of maintenance fluid. This is increased up to 100 to 120 ml on succeeding days. The small infant in a radiant-heated bed who is receiving phototherapy may require as much as 100 ml/kg during the first 24 hours and 150 to 170 ml/kg/24 hours on succeeding days. Volumes over this amount may result in fluid overload, congestive heart failure, and reopening of a closed ductus arteriosus.[16] The sodium requirements in a premature infant are also increased to 5 mEq/kg/day in babies born before 30 weeks gestation.[17]

We commence fluid therapy in premature infants with 10 percent glucose but switch to glucose in 0.2 percent saline, which provides 3.6 mEq of sodium and chloride per 100 ml. This solution usually is adequate for maintenance, but these infants must be closely monitored. They must be assessed several times a day for edema, fontanelle depression, and abdominal distention. The urine output and urine osmolality should be monitored and maintained at 1 to 2 ml/kg/hour and the osmolality between 270 and 290.[18] Body weight is measured at 8 hourly intervals, and fluid volumes are adjusted. Rapid changes in body weight reflect water loss or gain as accurately as any other measurement. The serum sodium will increase with unreplaced evaporative losses; thus, hypernatremia is a good index of dehydration. All body fluids lost through stomas, chest tubes, or gastric tubes are measured and replaced at 4 hourly intervals. It is a good idea to send an aliquot of all lost fluid for electrolyte measurement. During the postoperative period and when there is fluid loss caused by peritonitis, at least some of the replacement fluid should be either fresh frozen plasma or serum albumin in doses of 10 to 20 ml/kg. It is necessary to measure and replace blood lost through sampling every 2 or 3 days. One-half normal saline with an additional 10 to 15 mEq of potassium per liter is used to replace pure gastric losses, whereas lactated Ringer's solution with additional potassium is more suitable for losses secondary to a high small intestinal obstruction.

SHORT-TERM MAINTENANCE THERAPY IN OLDER INFANTS AND CHILDREN

Any child who is not expected to take oral fluids for 24 hours because of an operation or illness should be given parenteral fluids. In addition, fluids are administered during anesthesia to provide a route for emergency medications. When it becomes apparent that a patient's nutritional needs are unlikely to be met by the oral route within 5 to 7 days, routine maintenance fluid therapy should be changed to total intravenous nutritional support. At best, short-term therapy maintains a balance between intake and output of fluids and electrolytes. Calories supplied in 5 or 10 percent glucose provide minimal energy, with some sparing of body protein.

Holliday and Segar developed curves relating body weight to caloric requirements of hospitalized children.[19] By considering their weight groups, this information may be summarized and remembered as follows:

0–10 kg = 100 calories kg
10–20 kg = 1000 calories + 50 calories/kg for each kilogram over 10 kg
20 kg and over = 1500 calories + 20 calories/kg for each kilogram over 20 kg

The following values for electrolytes are suggested for maintenance:

Na: 3 mEq/100 calories
Cl: 2 mEq/100 calories
K: mEq/100 calories

Thus a 15-kg child would require 10 × 100 or 1000 calories for his first 10 kg plus 5 × 50 or 250 calories, for a total of 1250 calories/day. Fever increases caloric requirements by 12 percent for each degree Celsius, and the stress of trauma or an operation with consequent wound healing increases caloric, protein, and vitamin requirements even more.

The metabolic expenditure of 100 calories forms the basis for calculating water requirements. Maintenance fluid provides for insensible water losses—water lost through skin, lungs, and urine. The afebrile child in an environmental temperature of 26.5 to 29.5C loses 30 ml/100 calories through skin evaporation and 15 ml through expired air.[20] Fever or an elevated environmental temperature that induces sweating increases these losses. With starvation, there is still an obligatory renal solute load consisting of electrolytes and the nitrogenous breakdown products of protein metabolism. The calculations for maintenance fluid presuppose normal renal function. The combined osmotic load of these substances is about 12 to 16 mOsm/100 calories. By allowing 55 ml/100 calories for excretion of the expected solute load, urine osmolarity is in the range of 220 to 290 mOsm/liter.

Children with chronic renal disease who are unable to concentrate urine can avoid dehydration only by increasing their intake of free water or by decreasing the solute load by limiting protein intake.[21]

The following is a summary of the components of maintenance water requirements:[22]

> Insensible (skin and lungs): 45 ml/day/100 calories
> Urine: 50–75 ml/day/100 calories
> Sweat: 0–25 ml/day/100 calories
> Stool: 5–10 ml/day/100 calories

The water of oxidation provides approximately another 12 ml of water per kilogram. Consequently, when there are no abnormal losses, 100 ml of water is required for each 100 calories expended. Infants up to 10 kg in body weight require 100 calories and 100 ml of water per kilogram; an additional 50 ml/kg is given for patients weighing between 10 and 15 kg, and an additional 20 ml/kg for patients weighing between 15 and 20 kg. In calculating fluids for older children, it must be remem-

bered that caloric water requirements per kilogram decrease after the first 10 kg of weight. Fever and hyperventilation increase water requirements, but placing a child in high humidity decreases lung and skin losses by approximately 10 percent.

Normal kidneys will handle widely varying concentrations of sodium, chloride, and potassium in the diet. Intravenous solutions, which contain sodium chloride and potassium at 2 to 3 mEq/ml in 5 or 10 percent dextrose, are satisfactory for short-term maintenance therapy in children and most infants (0.2 percent saline in 5 percent dextrose with 20 mEq of potassium chloride added per liter).

Obviously, this short-term therapy cannot provide sufficient calories, fat, and protein for basal requirements. A patient with sufficient stores of fat and muscle can tolerate a short period of negative nitrogen and caloric balance without undue harm.

DEFICIT REPLACEMENT

Intestinal obstruction, peritonitis, diarrhea, burns, hemorrhage, empyema, and crushing injuries of the extremities all cause abnormal losses of intravascular volume, electrolytes, and protein. Iatrogenic derangements of body fluids are induced by surgical trauma, by withdrawal of pleural or ascitic fluid, and by administration of enemas or hyperosmolar contrast material.

The first clinical signs of dehydration are dry oral mucous membranes and skin pallor. Further dehydration results in loss of tissue turgor, a rapid and thready pulse, collapsed veins, and sunken eyes (Fig. 10–3). If the fontanelle is open, it will also be sunken. By comparing current body weight with last known weight, external losses can be closely estimated. The number of times a child has voided or has wet diapers can confirm the clinical impression of fluid deficits. Laboratory evaluation will reveal a rising hematocrit, high urinary specific gravity, and ketonuria. Determinations of serum and urine osmolarity and the blood urea nitrogen are useful in assessing hydration.

The volume and character of gastrointestinal losses may be partly assessed on the basis of the history and

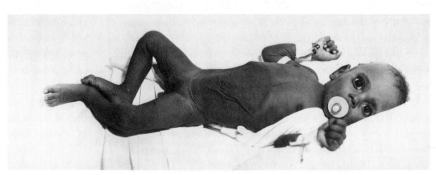

Figure 10–3. Severe dehydration seen in an infant with hypertrophic pyloric stenosis. Poor tissue turgor indicates 10 percent fluid loss.

observations of diarrhea, stool, and vomitus. The electrolyte composition of vomited fluid depends on the level of obstruction. Pure gastric juice, vomited by an infant with hypertrophic pyloric stenosis, contains 120 to 140 mEq of chloride per liter, with 10 to 12 mEq of potassium and 60 to 75 mEq of sodium. On the other hand, bile and pancreatic juice contain 120 to 140 mEq of sodium, up to 100 mEq of chloride, and approximately 10 to 12 mEq of potassium per liter. With distal obstruction, the combined gastric and duodenal losses of sodium exceed the losses of chloride. Diarrhea and ileostomy losses contain approximately 40 mEq each of sodium, potassium, chloride, and bicarbonate per liter.

Fluid sequestration in dilated loops of intestine and in the peritoneal cavity is to be expected when there is abdominal distention with tenderness. Third-space losses obviously occur in burned children and in crush injuries. We have found losses of 3.5 to 4.5 g of protein per 100 ml of peritoneal fluid in children with intestinal obstruction who have been resuscitated solely with lacerated Ringer's solution. At least one third of the fluid used to resuscitate hypovolemic children in these clinical situations should consist of serum albumin or plasma.

With a few exceptions, which will be noted later, the usual child with an acute surgical illness is isotonically dehydrated. Thus, a replacement solution that resembles extracellular fluid is indicated for deficit replacement. Lactated Ringer's solution is ideal for children with peritonitis, intestinal obstruction, trauma, or burns. Mild to moderate dehydration is treated with 15 to 20 ml/kg body weight given as a push during the first 30 minutes of therapy. Further therapy after this initial bolus of fluid may be calculated according to the clinical evaluation.

Filston et al. have described a practical plan for the estimation of third-space losses in the peritoneal cavity.[23] They give an additional one fourth of the child's maintenance volume for each quadrant of the abdomen involved in an inflammatory process. Thus, a 20-kg child who would have a maintenance requirement of 1350 ml/day would be given an additional one fourth of this amount, or approximately 350 ml, if he or she had an early appendicitis localized to the right lower quadrant. The same child with generalized peritonitis that involved the entire cavity would require an additional 1350 ml for replacement. This scheme tends to overestimate fluid requirements in the postoperative period.

Minimal dehydration, detected only by dry mucous membranes, represents 5 percent dehydration and requires 50 ml/kg for replacement. Shock or obvious hypovolemia may require up to 150 ml/kg for total deficit repair. Obviously, fluid therapy of this magnitude must be carefully monitored. Improvements in skin color, pulse volume, and venous filling are clinical indications that the blood volume is returning to normal. A urinary output of 0.5 ml/kg/hour is minimally acceptable, but an output of 2 ml/kg/hour indicates excellent tissue perfusion.

Electrolyte deficiencies ordinarily will be corrected by volume replacement, provided kidney function is normal. However, deficits of sodium or chloride may be corrected according to the following calculation. The sodium required equals the deficits multiplied by the extracellular fluid volume. Thus, in a 6-kg child with a serum sodium concentration of 120 mEq/liter, the calculation is as follows.

$$Na^+ = (138 - 120)(35\% \times 6)$$
$$= 18 \times 2.1$$
$$= 37.8 \text{ mEq}$$

Unless the deficit is quite severe, replacement of sodium and chloride may take place over 24 hours with lactated Ringer's solution or saline with additional sodium bicarbonate. Potassium deficits are most likely to occur when long-standing gastrointestinal losses have not been properly replaced. Serum potassium deficits are rare in acute surgical problems, possibly because catabolism releases considerable intracellular potassium. Any decrease in the serum potassium concentration reflects a major deficit in total body potassium and should be corrected by adding potassium at 40 mEq/liter to the repair solution.

Hypochloremic dehydration with metabolic alkalosis occurs in infants with pyloric stenosis. In this clinical situation, lactated Ringer's solution is contraindicated, since it does not supply an excess of chloride nor sufficient potassium. The proper repair solution is normal saline or 4.5 percent saline with additional potassium chloride at 20 to 40 mEq/liter (Table 10–1).

Fluid losses from low intestinal fistulas or ileostomies can lead to hypertonic dehydration because water losses exceed electrolyte losses. In severe cases, fluid leaves the cells in an attempt to maintain equal osmolarities in the intracellular and extracellular compartments. With the resulting increase in blood viscosity and endothelial cellular damage, intravascular thrombosis may develop, with extremity gangrene and renal infarcts. Treatment consists of rehydration with 4.5 percent saline. Bicarbonate losses may initiate metabolic acidosis, which requires correction with sodium bicarbonate or with lactated Ringer's solution.

TABLE 10–1. REPLACEMENT OF GASTROINTESTINAL LOSSES

Gastric (clear): 4.5% normal saline, 20–40 mEq/liter KCl
Gastric and duodenal (bile-stained, green): lactated Ringer's solution, 20–40 mEq/liter KCl
Ileostomy: lactated Ringer's solution
Diarrhea: 4.5% normal saline, KCl, or lactated Ringer's solution and KCl

INTRAOPERATIVE FLUID MANAGEMENT

Although fluid management during an operation is the responsibility of the anesthesiologist, this phase cannot be separated from pre- and postoperative treatment. During most operations, a normovolemic child requires sufficient fluid to make up for the fact that he or she was given nothing by mouth for several hours and for fluid lost during evaporation from the site of operation. This can be considerable during major abdominal or thoracic operations but, in most cases, is replaced by giving 10 ml/kg/hour of lactated Ringer's solution in 5 percent dextrose in water. In addition, blood loss is estimated by weighing sponges and by measuring the accumulation in suction bottles. The actual blood lost is more because of blood in the operative field and drapes. In general, when the child starts with a normal hemoglobin level, either whole blood or packed red blood cells are transfused when the blood loss equals 10 percent of the blood volume. Fresh frozen plasma or albumin may be given when there is preexisting peritonitis or intestinal obstruction or when there is extensive dissection without blood loss.

In an emergency, such as an operation for trauma or gastrointestinal bleeding, it is necessary to continue the preoperative resuscitation with rapid transfusion during the operation. During any operation on a neonate and during other lengthy operations, our anesthesiologists monitor the urinary output, the serum electrolytes and blood glucose, the hematocrit, and the blood gases. Some neonates, especially premature infants, will become hyperglycemic and will not tolerate intravenous glucose. Unfortunately, fluid loss during long operations is often overestimated, and excessive volumes are given intraoperatively. The surgeon must critically evaluate the amount of fluid given and make allowances for intraoperative fluids when planning postoperative therapy.

Several authors have advocated hemodilution to reduce blood lost during major tumor resections.[24,25] With this method, blood is withdrawn from the patient at the beginning of the operation, and the volume is replaced with three times as much lactated Ringer's solution or hetastarch. This may be combined with mild hypothermia and deliberate hypotension to reduce operative blood loss. The patient's own blood is then retransfused at the end of the operation, and diuretics are given to remove the excess volume of crystalloid. Although this technique can reduce the amount of donor blood transfused, there have been complications because of bowel edema sufficiently severe to interfere with abdominal closure. This technique may be of most use in patients who are Jehovah's Witnesses.

POSTOPERATIVE FLUID MANAGEMENT

With optimum replacement and maintenance therapy before and during operation, the child should enter the postoperative period in fluid and electrolyte balance. He or she then will require only daily maintenance plus replacement of ongoing losses. Immediate postoperative serous or bloody drainage from chest tubes or intraperitoneal drains is measured and replaced with blood or plasma. Dressings may be removed and weighed. Plastic bags fixed to the skin about drainage sites allow for more precise collection and measurement of fluid losses. All gastrointestinal drainage is collected and measured, and an aliquot is sent to the laboratory for electrolyte determination. Usually, there is a mixture of gastric juice and biliary and pancreatic secretions, but the electrolyte concentrations vary tremendously. The measured volumes are replaced at intervals of 4 to 12 hours, depending on the clinical situation. Usually, the nurse measures the gastric drainage and then adds an equal volume of either lactated Ringer's solution or 4.5 percent saline with 15 to 20 mEq of potassium chloride per liter to the intravenous fluids by the piggyback technique.

Satisfactory oral intake usually is established within 3 to 5 days after even the most complex pediatric operation. When a complication, such as continued anastomotic obstruction or leakage, sepsis, untoward ileostomy drainage, or malabsorption, precludes oral alimentation, total parenteral alimentation is indicated.

The following case history provides an example of fluid therapy in a 3-kg infant with duodenal atresia:

A 2-day-old infant was transferred from another hospital because of bilious vomiting that had begun at 12 hours of age. His birth weight was 3400 g. After his stomach was emptied of dark green fluid, his weight was 3000 g. Approximately half of this weight loss could be physiologic; consequently, half his weight loss, or 200 g, must represent fluid lost by vomiting. His mucous membranes were dry, but skin turgor was only minimally decreased. Roentgenograms demonstrated the classic double bubble of duodenal atresia. He was losing all of his gastric and duodenal secretions. A bolus of lactated Ringer's solution (20 ml/kg) was infused over the first hour through a scalp vein. He was given an additional 120 ml over the next 3 hours and was nursed in a warm humidified isolette. His mucous membranes became moist, and he had wet his diapers. Serum electrolyte levels determined after the first 60 ml of fluid replacement were within normal limits. The initial hematocrit was 58 percent.

During the operation, which lasted 2 hours, he was given 60 ml of lactated Ringer's solution (maintenance of 10 ml/kg/hour of anesthesia). His estimated blood loss of 20 ml was replaced with 30 ml of 5 percent albumin. During the next 24 hours, he was given maintenance fluids of 10 percent glucose in 0.2 percent saline with potassium at 20 mEq/liter (providing water at 75 ml/kg/day, sodium at 2.5 mEq/kg/day, and potassium at 1.5 mEq/kg/day). The gastric aspirate was dark green and measured 150 ml for the first 24 hours, with chloride at 110 mEq/liter, sodium at 120 mEq/liter, and potassium at 12 mEq/liter. Replacement of these losses was continued with lactated Ringer's solution with an additional 10 mEq of potassium chloride per liter.

Over the following 3 days, maintenance fluids were increased to 100 ml/kg. Gastric losses were measured and replaced at 8-hour intervals. On the fifth day, the gastric drainage turned a light yellow, resembling a pure gastric juice. Replacement fluid was changed to half-strength saline with addition of potassium chloride at 20 mEq/liter to make up a solution containing sodium at 75 mEq/liter, chloride at 95 mEq/liter, and potassium at 20 mEq/liter.

After an initial weight gain of 150 g, his weight stabilized, then dropped 15 g/day. Tissue turgor remained good, mucous membranes remained moist, and urine output was satisfactory. Serum electrolytes were rechecked and were normal. On the third and fifth postoperative days, 5 percent albumin was infused at 20 ml/kg.

By the sixth day, the gastric drainage was minimal; the tube was removed. Half-strength formula was started. As oral intake increased over the next 4 days, the intravenous fluids were correspondingly decreased, until the ninth postoperative day, when he was on full oral intake.

REFERENCES

1. Oliver WM, Graham BD, Wilson JL: Lack of scientific validity of body surface as basis for parenteral fluid dosage. JAMA 167:1211, 1967
2. Friss HB: Body water compartments in children, changes during growth and related changes in body composition. Pediatrics 28:169, 1961
3. Edelman IS, Leibman J: Anatomy of body water and electrolytes. Am J Med 27:256, 1959
4. Weil WB Jr, Helmrath TA: Chemical composition. In Barnett HL (ed): Pediatrics, 15th ed. New York, Appleton, 1972, p 29
5. McCance RA, Naylor NJB, Widdowson EM: The response of infants to a large dose of water. Arch Dis Child 29:104, 1954
6. Edelman CM, Barnett NL: Role of the kidney in water metabolism in young infants. J Pediatr 56:154, 1960
7. Hansen JD, Smith CA: Effects of withholding fluid in the immediate postnatal period. Pediatrics 12:99, 1953
8. Wilkinson A, Stevens L, Hughes E: Metabolic changes in the newborn. Lancet 1:983, 1962
9. Foman SJ: Infant Nutrition, 4th ed. Philadelphia, Saunders, 1974, p 359
10. Shelley H, Heligan CS: Neonatal hypoglycemia. Br Med Bull 22:34, 1966
11. Doyle L, Sinclair J: Insensible water loss in newborn infants. Clin Perinatol 9:453, 1982
12. Hammarlund K, Sedin G, Stromberg B: Transepidermal water loss in newborn infants. Acta Paediatr Scand 72:721, 1983
13. Baumgart S: Radiant energy and insensible water loss in the premature infant nursed in a radiant warmer. Clin Perinatol 9:483, 1982.
14. Bell EF, Neidrich G, Cashore W, et al: Combined effect of radiant warmer and phototherapy on insensible water loss in low birthweight infants. J Pediatr 94:810, 1979
15. Harpin V, Rutter N: Humidification of incubators. Arch Dis Child 60:219, 1985
16. Bell E, Warburton D, Stonestreet B, et al: Effect of fluid administration on the development of symptomatic patent ductus arteriosus and congestive heart failure in premature infants. N Engl J Med 302:598, 1980
17. Al-Dabhan J, Haycock GB, Chantler C, et al: Sodium homeostasis in term and preterm neonates. Arch Dis Child 58:335, 1983
18. Rowe M, Lloyd D, Lee M: Is the refractometer specific gravity a reliable index for pediatric fluid management? J Pediatr Surg 21:580, 1986
19. Holliday MA, Segar WE: Parenteral fluid therapy. Pediatrics 19:823, 1957
20. Darrow DC: A Guide to Learning Fluid Therapy. Springfield, IL, Thomas, 1964, p 52
21. Siegler EE, Fomon SJ: Fluid intake, renal solute load, and water balance in infancy. J Pediatr 78:561, 1971
22. Winters RW: The Body Fluids in Pediatrics. Boston, Little, Brown, 1973, p 124
23. Filston H, Edwards C, Chatwood W: Estimation of postoperative fluid requirements in infants and children. Ann Surg 196:76, 1982
24. Schaller R, Schaller J, Furman E: The advantages of hemodilution anesthesia for major liver resection in children. J Pediatr Surg 19:705, 1984
25. Adzick N, deLorimer A, Harrison M: Major childhood tumor resection using normovolemic hemodilution anesthesia and hetastarch. J Pediatr Surg 20:372, 1985

11
Nutrition and Metabolism

Susan R. Luck

The technique of parenteral nutrition is one of our most significant medical advances and has saved countless lives. Nutritional depletion was long recognized as fatal to those children and adults who were unable to take oral feeding. The obvious loss of skeletal muscle is paralleled by a decrease in visceral protein mass. The starving patient suffers impairment of vital organ function, immunologic incompetence, and poor wound healing. Plasma, amino acids, ethyl alcohol, and 20 percent dextrose were administered to patients even before 1950 through a plastic catheter inserted into the superior vena cava.[1] However, the techniques of total parenteral nutrition (TPN) did not become popular until Dudrick et al. demonstrated that intravenous amino acids and glucose would support growth and development of infants who were unable to take sufficient oral feedings.[2] Since these early efforts, many publications have attested to the effectiveness of intravenous nutrition in a wide variety of clinical conditions, including inflammatory bowel disease, trauma, cancer, chronic diarrhea, malabsorption, and even anorexia nervosa.

TPN has become a routine clinical tool, but some questions remain for the basic physiologist and for the clinician providing daily patient care, for example (1) the role and required amounts of trace elements, (2) the best regimen of administration of solutions for specific pathologic conditions, and (3) the etiology and prevention of TPN-associated cholestatic jaundice. Babies and older patients with a variety of severe handicaps who require indefinite support raise ethical questions that tax the conscience of the physician, the family, and society at large.

ENERGY REQUIREMENTS

Recommendations for protein and amino acid requirements are subject to the limitations of extrapolation from healthy or starved adult determinations. However, the values listed in Table 11–1 are generally accepted as baseline in the growing but unstressed child.[3–5] Prematurity and the degree of preexisting malnutrition alter basal figures for both calories and protein. The energy needs per unit of body weight of infants and small children are much greater than those of adults. The maintenance of body temperature is more costly in small patients because of the larger surface area/weight ratio. Smaller nutrient stores are available, especially in premature infants. Nutritional needs after trauma are increased, particularly those for protein.[6,7] On the other hand, Witte et al. have shown that some critically ill pediatric patients, sedated and supported with mechanical ventilation, may not have increased caloric needs.[8] Precise measurement of metabolic activity and caloric requirement can be accomplished by indirect calorimetry even in premature infants. The resting energy expenditure can be calculated from the measured oxygen consumption and carbon dioxide production.[9]

NUTRITIONAL ASSESSMENT AND FOLLOW-UP

Assessment of the child's nutritional state before and during TPN allows anticipation of unusual protein requirements and objective interpretation of weight

TABLE 11–1. ESTIMATED DAILY REQUIREMENTS FOR PROTEIN AND CALORIES

	Protein (g/kg/day)		Calories (cal/kg/day)	
	Enteral	*Parenteral*	*Enteral*	*Parenteral*
Premature	4–6	2.5–3.5	150	85–130
Full-term neonate	1.8–2.0	2.5	100–110	Approximately the same
1 year old	1.5	1.5–2.0	80–135	Approximately the same
Adolescent	0.85–1.0	1.0–1.5	50–60	Approximately the same

changes. Height, weight, and head circumference should be plotted on a growth curve and followed at monthly or more frequent intervals. Daily weight changes may reflect only alterations in body water, but weight gain or loss averaged over several days indicates growth trends. Data from normal breast-fed infants indicate that the following are ideal daily growth rates: 10 g/kg from 8 to 28 days of age, 6.5 g/kg at 1 to 2 months, 3.5 g/kg at 3 to 4 months, and 1 g/kg at 1 year of age.[10] Anthropomorphic measurements (triceps skinfold and arm circumference) can predict the amount of subcutaneous fat and muscle mass. Established percentiles correlate with normal heights and weights.[11] The serum albumin should be 3.5 g/dl (2.5 g/dl in an infant). Severe nutritional deficits can cause depression of cell-mediated immunity. The total lymphocyte count should be greater than 1500. Intact immunity is indicated by a normal skin test reaction to any one antigen used to assess delayed cutaneous hypersensitivity (i.e., mumps, *Candida*, or purified protein derivative, PPD). More detailed evaluation includes determination of bone age and bone mineralization, specific levels of vitamins and minerals, and the levels of those visceral proteins with rapid turnover rates (prealbumin and retinol-binding protein).[12,13]

TECHNIQUES OF TOTAL PARENTERAL NUTRITION

TPN requires the infusion of glucose, amino acids, an emulsified fat solution, minerals, vitamins, and trace elements in various combinations and concentrations. The goal of this therapy is to promote the maintenance of body tissue, appropriate growth, and the healing of wounds. The initial weight gain is slower in starved patients as excess body water is lost and replaced with muscle and fat. Metabolic complications are the direct result of the infusion solutions and their rate of administration. Stable patients who are free from other medical complications will tolerate a variety of regimens without difficulty. However, the metabolic consequences of TPN

become critical in those children who are very small or very sick.

Glucose

Nonprotein carbohydrate and fat allow adequate use of amino acids for protein synthesis and prevent undue muscle catabolism and urea production. Glucose is the direct energy source for the central nervous system, erythrocytes, retina, renal medulla, and intestinal mucosa. Anhydrous glucose contains 3.4 calories/g and is metabolized at the rate of 0.4 to 1.5 g/kg/h.[14] Glucose is the major osmolar component of TPN solution.[15] The caloric content and osmolarity of various concentrations are shown in Table 11–2. Any solution with a glucose concentration greater than 5 percent is hypertonic. With constant infusion of 20 percent glucose, as much as 27 g/kg/day will be well tolerated in full-term neonates without the addition of insulin.[16] Sanderson and Deitel found initial rises in both blood glucose and serum insulin levels. Within 6 hours after beginning steady infusion, serum insulin levels were 4 to 6 times basal levels.[17] Insulin responses to glucose are impaired in premature infants.[18] Some small stressed infants are unable to tolerate more than a 12.5 to 15 percent glucose concentration, especially in the immediate postoperative period. In these infants, TPN should be started with the infusion of a 10 percent glucose solution, followed by 2.5 percent daily increments to allow equilibrium with insulin and metabolic requirements. Intraventricular hemorrhage

TABLE 11–2. CALORIC AND OSMOLAR CONTENT OF ANHYDROUS GLUCOSE SOLUTIONS

Glucose Concentration (%)	Glucose		
	g/ml	*cal/ml*	*mOsm/L*
5	0.05	0.17	253
10	0.1	0.34	505
20	0.2	0.68	1010
30	0.3	1.02	1515

can develop in hyperglycemic neonates and premature infants.[19]

The major complication of glucose infusion is hyperosmolar diuresis, which can progress to coma. When the renal tubular threshold for glucose (approximately 180 mEq/L) is exceeded, glucose appears in the filtrate and acts as an osmotic diuretic. The renal threshold for glucose is lower in neonates who may have glycosuria with normal serum glucose levels.[20] Following trauma, insulin levels are disproportionately low in relation to plasma glucose levels.[21] The same is probably true in those patients with sepsis. Some urine sugar spillage is safe, but prolonged or severe glycosuria may herald the development of hyperosmolar diuresis. The concentration of glucose or the rate of infusion must be reduced. The currently infusing solution need not be discarded. The rate is decreased, and a supplementary solution of 5 percent glucose with maintenance electrolytes is infused concomitantly to provide fluid volume. Glucose tolerance must be assessed several times each day when TPN is initiated and in small babies and critically ill patients. Serum screening methods using Dextrostix (Ames Division, Miles Laboratories, Inc., Elkhart, Ind.) or Chemstrip by (Bio-Dynamics, Indianapolis, Ind.) supplement specific chemical determinations. The presence of glycosuria is monitored with Chemstrip.

Protein

Proteins are polymers of amino acids linked by aminocarboxyl peptide bonds.[22] The stereoisomer form of 20 amino acids is found in most proteins (glycine is the only stereosymmetrical amino acid). Essential amino acids, those whose carbon skeleton cannot be synthesized in adequate amounts by the living organism, vary between neonates and older humans. Histidine, cystine, and tyrosine are essential in young infants. Taurine probably also is essential for these babies. In aqueous solution, amino acids can act as a weak acid or base depending on the numbers of carboxyl (acidic) or amino (basic) groups available for ionization. Amino groups bind with positively charged cations (i.e., sodium, calcium), and carboxyl groups bind with negatively charged anions (chloride, hydrochloride, phosphate, acetate, and lactate). Metabolism of those amino acids with an excess of carboxylic groups releases an excess of anions that demand protons [H$^+$] for stabilization, resulting in acidosis. The opposite occurs during metabolism of the anionic amino acids.

During TPN, all essential amino acids must be provided; 125 to 150 nonprotein calories (carbohydrate or fat) per gram of nitrogen are required to prevent metabolism of the amino acids for energy, sparing them for protein synthesis.[23] Commercially available standard crystalline L-amino acid products contain variable proportions of 15 amino acids.[24] The total amino acid content varies from 3.5 to 10 percent. The crystalline amino acid profile, total amino acid content, and solution osmolality vary among commercially available products (Table 11–3). A 3.5 percent solution is slightly hypertonic (300 to 500 mOsm/L), and more concentrated solutions should be administered into a central vein.

All metabolic complications will be magnified if more amino acids are administered than the patient requires. The crystalline amino acid solutions introduced in the early 1970s contained amino acids precipitated solely as chloride or hydrochloride salts. Metabolism liberated hydrochloric acid, and patients developed hyperchloremic metabolic acidosis.[16] The substitution of acetate-precipitated amino acids or the addition of sodium and potassium acetate or lactate can prevent this acidosis. On the other hand, the administration of a chloride-wasting diuretic to a patient receiving a low chloride solution can precipitate metabolic alkalosis.

Glycine and serine are ammoniogenic amino acids. Also, hyperammonemia may be related to arginine deficiency, which decreases the efficiency of the urea cycle and the conversion of ammonia to urea. Excess ammonium ions bind to protons in the kidney, increasing acid excretion, leading to alkalosis. Additional arginine is now added to commercial solutions. Whenever the amino acid solution is changed, altering the amino acid profile, the overall TPN formulation and concomitant medications must be reevaluated. Specific amino acid products have been developed for some patients with complicated conditions.

Neonates and Premature Infants

Although human breast milk contains only 0.8 to 0.9 g/100 ml of true protein, 45 percent of this high-quality protein is essential amino acids.[25] The plasma amino acid profile seen after a breast feeding is assumed to be one that best promotes protein synthesis and growth in infants. Neonates maintained on standard adult formulations develop deficiencies of cysteine, taurine, and tyrosine and elevations of methionine, phenylalanine, and glycine.[26] The serum profile of breast-fed babies can be duplicated by the use of specifically formulated pediatric preparations.[27] When compared with a standard formula (FreAmine III), TrophAmine has promoted better weight gain and nitrogen balance in neonates and good weight gain with lower than the usually recommended amounts of protein and calories.[28]

Renal and Hepatic Failure

Solutions that contain only the essential amino acids can be combined with 70 percent glucose to give essential protein and adequate calories with minimal fluid to patients in renal failure. However, deficiencies of nonessential amino acids can develop with prolonged therapy.[29] Standard preparations can be used in patients who are

TABLE 11–3. REPRESENTATIVE AMINO ACID COMMERCIAL PRODUCTS (VALUES CALCULATED *DRUG INFORMATION*, AMERICAN HOSPITAL FORMULARY SERVICE[22])

Amino Acid	Characterization	Aminosyn 10% (Abbott)	TrophAmine 6% (Kendall McGaw)	FreAmine HBC 6.9% (Kendall McGaw)
Essential		1000 mOsm/L	525 mOsm/L	620 mOsm/L
Isoleucine	BCAA	7.2%	+	↑
Leucine	BCAA	9.5	↑	↑ ↑
Lysine	Cationic	7.2	+	+
Methionine		4.0	+	+
Phenylalanine		4.4	+	+
Threonine		5.2	+	↓
Tryptophan		1.6	+	+
Valine	BCAA	8.1	+	↑
Essential in infants				
Cystine	Anionic	−	Minute amount	Minute amount
Tyrosine		0.4	↑	−
Histadine	Cationic	3.0	+	+
Taurine		−	+	−
Nonessential				
Alanine		12.9	↓ ↓	↓ ↓
Arginine	Cationic	9.9	↑	+
Proline		8.7	↓	+
Serine	Ammoniogenic	4.2	+	+
Glycine	Ammoniogenic	12.9	↓ ↓	↓ ↓
Glutamic acid	Anionic	−	+	−
Aspartic acid	Anionic	−	+	−

BCAA, branched-chain amino acid.
+, amino acid present in solution; −, amino acid absent.
↑ or ↓, percentage of amino acid increased or decreased by 2–5%, as compared to Aminosyn.
↑ ↑ or ↓ ↓, percentage of amino acid increased or decreased 5% or more, as compared to Aminosyn.

on dialysis. Protein losses are increased by dialysis, and increased amounts must be provided in these patients.

The serum amino acid pattern of patients with cirrhosis and acute liver failure is characterized by low levels of the branched-chain amino acids (BCAA), leucine, isoleucine, and valine.[30] A similar amino acid pattern is seen in patients with severe sepsis. Increased catabolism of these amino acids in skeletal muscle to provide energy may explain these deficiencies. The infusion of solutions with increased amounts of the BCAA can improve or reverse hepatic encephalopathy and improve survival of patients with hepatic failure. The amino acid profile can be normalized in these patients and in those with severe sepsis. Improved survival has been shown in septic patients by some authors.[31]

Lipids

Half of the caloric requirement in milk-fed infants is derived from fat. Linoleic acid, linolenic acid, and arachidonic acid are essential fatty acids for normal growth in all humans. Deficiencies in the essential fatty acids cause poor wound healing, thrombocytopenia, increased susceptibility to bacterial infection, and scaly dermatitis. These deficiencies formerly became clinically evident in infants given fat-free TPN for longer than 3 months. Premature infants have limited fat stores and may de-

velop biochemical evidence of essential fatty acid deficiency in a few days.[32] The requirements for essential fatty acids can be provided by intravenous fat emulsions, in the amount of 0.5 to 1 g/kg/day.[4] Fat emulsions can deliver a high concentration of calories in a smaller volume than glucose solutions and are well tolerated when given by peripheral vein.[33] The use of fat emulsions is particularly advantageous in the very sick hypermetabolic patient or premature infant, neither of whom can tolerate high glucose loads. Neonates are able to use intravenous fat as a source of energy on their first day of life.[34] However, small-for-gestational-age infants may have a limited ability to use fat,[35] and sepsis may decrease fat tolerance in the neonate.[36]

Intralipid (Kabibitrum, Alameda, CA) provides 1.1 calories/ml, has an osmolarity of 280 μOsm/liter, and contains 54 percent linoleic, 26 percent oleic, 9 percent palmitic, and 8 percent linolenic acid. Intralipid is cleared from the bloodstream by lipoprotein lipase activity, similar to the activity of natural chylomicrons. The normal newborn metabolizes intravenous fat to triglycerides, which are hydrolyzed in turn to glycerol and free fatty acids. When Intralipid is infused into full-term neonates over a 4-hour period, the concentrations of serum triglycerides and free fatty acids rapidly rise. Infants with a gestational age of less than 33 weeks clear lipids more slowly. Fat emulsions should be started at a dose of 0.5 g/kg/day in premature infants and 1 g/kg/day in term babies. If the serum triglyceride levels remain within normal limits (less than 150 to 200 mg/dl) and if there are no signs of hypersensitivity, such as an allergic skin rash or fever, the dose is increased by 0.25 g/kg/day to a maximum of 3 g/kg/day in prematures and 4 g/kg/day in full-term and older infants.

The administration of fat emulsions to jaundiced infants is controversial because fatty acids and bilirubin compete to bind with albumin. The displacement of bilirubin by fatty acids may contribute to the development of kernicterus. It may be reasonable to use fat as a source of up to only 4 percent of caloric intake in a jaundiced baby. Fat droplets have been found within the pulmonary capillaries of animals who had received a large bolus of a fat emulsion.[37] Similar findings have been noted at autopsy in low birth weight infants who died after prolonged intravenous lipid therapy.[38] There is no evidence, however, that these fat deposits interfere with gas exchange. Therefore, intravenous fat is administered to infants with decreased pulmonary function at our hospital.

Minerals

Normal serum levels of sodium, chloride, and potassium are maintained easily in the stable patient who is well nourished at the onset of TPN. Difficulties arise when there are large and upredictable gastrointestinal tract losses. When possible, these lost fluids are collected, measured, and analyzed for their electrolyte content, then replaced through a separate intravenous line or piggybacked into the TPN solution. In a patient with prolonged and predictable losses from a gastric tube, for example, additional sodium, potassium, and chloride can be added to the TPN fluid. The potassium requirement during TPN may be higher than that recommended in routine intravenous feeding because of the increased cellular uptake of glucose and protein.

The bones and teeth contain 99 percent of the bodily stores of calcium at birth. Consequently, the serum calcium level not only fails to reflect total body calcium but may even be maintained at the expense of bone calcium. The normal oral intake of calcium is approximately 1 g/day, of which only 15 to 20 percent is retained.[39] The usual daily requirements are, therefore, met by the gastrointestinal absorption of 15 mEq/day. Rickets (the inadequate mineralization of bones) has been recognized in premature infants who have been breast or formula fed but is particularly common in low birth weight babies who have been maintained on TPN with a low calcium intake. It is difficult or impossible to supply enough calcium with TPN to maintain normal bone mineralization because calcium and phosphorous precipitate in the solution as their concentrations are increased.

TABLE 11–4. AMOUNTS OF TRACE ELEMENTS ADMINISTERED IN TPN SOLUTIONS, CHILDREN'S MEMORIAL HOSPITAL

Element	Patient Weight		
	<3 kg	3–50 kg (μg/kg per day)	> 50 kg (mg/L administered)
Zinc	300	100	5
Copper	20	0.01[a]	1
Manganese	5	2.5	0.5
Chromium	0.75	0.1	0.01

[a] An additional 100 μg are added to each 1000 ml of TPN solution

Calcium salts given through peripheral veins cause severe tissue necrosis if the solution infiltrates. Every effort should be made to give the maximum amount possible of calcium; as much as 20 mEq/L of fluid can stay in solution.

Zinc is a crucial component of several essential enzyme systems and is necessary to cellular function and division and to cell membrane stability. Wound healing is retarded in zinc deficiency, since zinc is an obligatory participant in collagen synthesis. The risk of zinc deficiency is increased in low birth weight infants, whose stores of zinc are low at birth and who are additionally endangered by excessive intestinal fluid losses. These babies require up to 300 μg/kg/24 hours (10 times the adult requirement) to prevent zinc deficiency.[40] Copper also is an essential trace element. Deficiencies are found only after the prolonged use of parenteral nutrition because the initial stores of copper in the liver are sufficient for several months.[41] Chromium and manganese are added routinely to the TPN solution (Table 11–4).

Administration

The TPN and fat solutions are infused by constant flow pumps. The two solutions are infused simultaneously, the fat emulsion entering the TPN solution near the infusion site but distal to a check valve that prevents backflow into the main line. Ideally, replacement fluids, blood products, and other medications are administered through a separate intravenous line to prevent contamination. However, this method becomes difficult, if not inhumane, in those patients with fragile and small veins. At our hospital, medications and blood products are given through the TPN catheter after flushing the TPN/fat emulsion through the tubing with saline. Replacement solutions, such as Ringer's lactate, can be infused simultaneously with the TPN.

TPN can be administered through peripheral veins when the concentration of glucose is lowered to 10 percent. Caloric requirements are met by increasing the volume of the solution to 150 ml/kg/day or more and by adding Intralipid. Some infants are unable to tolerate more than 100 ml of fluid per kg per day, and peripheral sites become difficult to maintain. Despite these complications, weight gain can be promoted with peripheral TPN. This route can be used in patients who require short-term TPN or nutritional supplement to enteral feedings and in those who require removal of a central venous catheter during episodes of sepsis.

Once the patient can tolerate full amounts of glucose and fat, the daily TPN solution can be ordered by determining (1) the number of grams of protein/kg/day required by the patient's age, estimating additional needs, (2) the grams of fat desired (up to 3 g/kg/per day), and (3) the concentration of glucose in the remaining tolerated volume of fluid that will provide the estimated caloric requirement. Electrolytes, vitamins, and heparin are added in varying amounts according to the child's age and clinical condition. Calcium and phosphorus are added in those amounts that will remain in solution. Measurement of electrolytes, urea, glucose, calcium, phosphorus, and serum osmolarity may be necessary on even a daily basis during the initiation of TPN, after any change in formulation, and whenever the clinical condition of the patient is unstable. These studies can be obtained much less frequently in a stable patient. Trace elements, liver function studies, and the serum albumin are followed at intervals in those children who require long-term TPN.

COMPLICATIONS OF TPN

The venous thrombosis and sepsis associated with TPN are complications of vascular access (Chapter 9). Cholestatic jaundice is now recognized as the most serious complication of TPN. Liver disease was observed very soon after the introduction of TPN[42–45] and is more common in premature infants who require major intestinal resections and are unable to tolerate any oral nutrition. The serum alkaline phosphatase and bilirubin gradually rise in these infants but will return to normal levels when oral feedings are given. Microscopic examination of liver biopsies from these patients have shown early cholestasis, with only minimal hepatocellular damage.[46] Cholestasis was observed in fasted neonates even before the use of parenteral nutrition.[47,48] When severe intestinal dysfunction precludes enteral feeding and prolonged parenteral nutrition is necessary, cholestasis progresses to liver fibrosis, cirrhosis, and finally liver failure. We have observed inflammatory cell infiltrates in liver biopsies obtained from children as long as 6 years after the cessation of TPN. One of our patients, whose birth weight was 1000 g, required TPN for 395 days. He developed a hepatocellular carcinoma in his cirrhotic liver at 26 months of age.[49]

No definite cause and effect relationship has been found between any specific component of the parenteral nutrition solutions and liver disease. Amino acids have come under the most suspicion.[50,51] Taurine, choline, or carnitine deficiencies in premature infants also have been implicated. Taurine conjugates bile salts and stimulates bile salt secretion, but when taurine intake is low, more bile salts are conjugated into glycine.[52] In animals, the administration of taurine prevents cholestasis.[53] Hughes et al. carried out serial enzyme studies and percutaneous liver biopsies in seven premature infants born at 27 to 33 weeks gestation to follow the course of TPN cholestasis.[54] Jaundice became clinically apparent within 22 to 57 days. In one infant who died, the common bile duct was obstructed by plugs of dark green biliary sludge. In this study, cholestasis was seen without extensive hepatocyte damage. The electron microscopic features were nonspecific and resembled those documented in association with any form of cholestasis. These authors concluded that TPN cholestasis is multifactorial in etiology but that the absence of gastrointestinal hormone stimulation of bile flow played a major role in pathogenesis.

Further evidence for the importance of enteral feedings came from the work of Balistreri et al.[55] These authors have observed a physiologic delay in establishing the enterohepatic circulation in animals. There is also a normal phase of physiologic cholestasis, particularly in the premature human infant. This phase can be continued and accentuated by a variety of insults, such as hypoxia, sepsis, bowel disease, and TPN. A lack of intraluminal nutrients will blunt the release of gastrointestinal hormones, the normal stimulants to bile flow. The fetal and neonatal enterohepatic circulation is functionally incompetent. Bile salts are passively, rather than actively, reabsorbed from a jejunal site with the result that there is an excess loss of bile acids in the feces. Circulating bile acids remain elevated in normal infants during the first 6 to 8 months of life. Physiologic cholestasis thus seems to be a normal phase that may persist when normal enteral feeding must be withheld. Ultrasonographic examination of the gallbladder and bile ducts in fasted patients often demonstrates bile sludge after several days of fasting. The delayed development of gallstones in children who have received TPN is further evidence for this diminution of bile flow.

When oral feedings cannot be given because of continued gut dysfunction, cycling of TPN may simulate the circadian rhythmicity of the gut hormones.[56,57] The relative hypoglycemia that develops during a short cessation of TPN infusion may increase the secretion of glucagon, which acts as a choluretic. We begin cycling when TPN is first initiated. Even premature babies are able to tolerate 45 to 60 minutes without glucose before the serum glucose drops to 40 mg/dl. The cycle time without caloric infusion gradually is increased. Infants several months of age can tolerate 6 to 8 hours off calorie solutions, and older children can tolerate 10 to 12 hours. When the cycle times must be short, the TPN can be discontinued several times each day. During the cycle, all calories are discontinued, including fat and any glucose in replacement or medication diluent solutions. The catheter can be capped with a heparin lock or infused with Ringer's lactate or 0.5 normal saline. Blood contains approximately 3 percent glucose and cannot be substituted as a cycle fluid. After the cycle is increased to 3 hours or longer, the infusion rate of the glucose-containing TPN is reduced by one half for 30 minutes before and immediately after the cycle period. We have not observed a single case of prolonged or serious cholestasis in a surgical patient since this policy of cycling was instituted at our hospital in 1983.

ENTERAL NUTRITION

Whenever possible, the gastrointestinal tract should be used for caloric intake by oral feedings or by feeding through a nasogastric tube, gastrostomy, or jejunostomy tube. Standard infant formulas are designed to meet the nutritional needs of infants up to 1 year of age and provide a caloric intake that is 50 percent fat and 10 to 12 percent protein, approximating the composition of human milk.[58] The usual concentration of infant formulas provides 20 calories per ounce (0.67 calorie/ml). More concentrated solutions, 24 calories/oz (0.81 calorie/ml), can be given without an undue increase in the renal solute load to the child with normal renal function and fluid tolerance. The full-strength enteral formulas designed for adults usually provide 30 calories/oz. Additional vitamins and minerals may be needed for children who receive these formulas. Chemically defined formulas are available that are readily absorbed by infants with damaged or short guts. An example of such a formula is Pregestimil (Meade Johnson & Co., Evansville, Ind.), which contains casein hydrolysate with added cystine, tyrosine, and tryptophan. Forty percent of the fat in Pregestimil is from medium-chain triglycerides. Special formulations that contain increased BCAA or essential L-amino acids can be used for patients with compromise of renal or hepatic function.[59]

The colloid oncotic pressure of plasma, dependent on serum proteins, especially albumin, attracts interstitial water across the capillary membrane into the intravascular space. The decreased oncotic pressure of the hypoalbuminemic patient leads to peripheral and visceral edema and gut dysfunction. Andrassy has shown a statistically significant improvement in gastrointestinal feeding tolerance in young children whose serum albumin levels are kept within the normal range by periodic albumin replacement.[60] Albumin deficits can be calculated by the following formula[61]:

$$3.5 - \text{patient serum albumin in g/dl} \times \text{patient's weight (kg)} \times 3$$

Both malnutrition and a lack of enteral feeding are thought to contribute to the translocation of bacteria across the gut, with an increased incidence of sepsis and endotoxemia. Children will tolerate very early postoperative feedings with enteral formulas, and these may replace or supplement parenteral nutrition.[62]

METABOLIC RESPONSE TO STRESS

A review of the hormonal controls and the intermediary metabolism of unstressed starvation is important to the appreciation of the body's response to limited trauma and to major trauma or sepsis.[63] The early implementation of TPN was predicated on the principles of starvation, recognizing increased energy needs for growth and healing of traumatized tissue. The metabolism of humans is adapted to maintain glucose homeostasis despite cycles of feeding and fasting and varying levels of activity. Normal serum glucose levels are maintained by insulin and glucagon, which have opposing effects on the liver, muscle, and adipose tissue.[64] Insulin is the hormone of energy storage and protein conservation. Ingested food that is not immediately used for energy production and protein synthesis can be converted to carbohydrate (glycogen) and stored in the liver and muscles or be converted to fat. Insulin promotes hepatic glucose uptake, synthesis of glycogen and fat, glucose and amino acid entry into muscle, and the synthesis of new protein. Glucagon, the hormone of energy release or catabolism, is responsible for increased glucose production from glycogen and the breakdown of amino acids and triglycerides for energy production.

When the serum glucose level falls, glycogen in the liver is metabolized rapidly and released as glucose. However, the limited hepatic stores are depleted within hours. Muscle glycogen is metabolized slowly and with less efficient production of energy. Glucagon now stimulates gluconeogenesis within the liver. Amino acids released from protein breakdown are used first; then glycerol from fat. Protein exists within the body only as essential cellular or structural components, and any protein loss is detrimental. Therefore, long-term survival during starvation depends on the body's adaptation to glucose production from fat and on the ability of the brain to use ketone bodies for energy (Fig. 11–1).

Injury and sepsis initiate neural and hormonal stimuli that promote glucose release and protein catabolism.[31,65] ACTH, glucocorticoids, and epinephrine are released in addition to glucagon. These hormones remain abnormally elevated as long as the stress continues. The result is a persistent release of amino acids from muscle and lipolysis. Insulin production is sup-

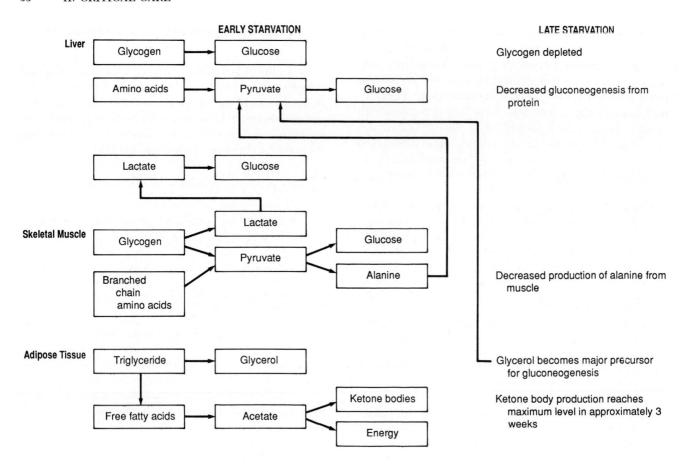

Figure 11–1. Metabolism in unstressed starvation.

pressed even when serum glucose levels are high. The adaptive mechanisms outlined in Figure 11–1 are blocked by this hormonal response. The hypermetabolic demands of a stressed patient are met by the catabolism of BCAA within the muscle, released as alanine and glutamine, for gluconeogenesis.[66] This autocatabolism can persist even when exogenous glucose and fat are provided.

Major trauma, sepsis, and multiple organ failure go hand in hand with malnutrition in the critically ill patient. The complications of increased catabolism can be blunted and sometimes reversed with specific nutritional support in addition to appropriate surgical therapy. Exogenous BCAA have been shown to serve as an energy substrate for skeletal muscle. The absolute amounts of protein provided in the TPN solution should be increased. Reduction of the calorie/nitrogen ratio will decrease hyperglycemia and further energy expenditure. The stress response to an operation or to trauma is directly related to the severity of injury. An operation, such as an inguinal herniorraphy, that is followed by normal activity and normal food intake results in minimal surgical stress and no change in hormonal metabolism.

It has been difficult to translate the results of studies in stressed adults to neonates and young children. The young infant has limited stores of fat and muscle and must divert energy to growth and organ maturation. Thus, it is particularly disadvantageous for the neonate to experience prolonged catabolism. Anand et al. developed a scoring system to evaluate the immediate responses of the neonate to surgery.[67,68] This score is based on the duration of the operation, the amount of blood lost, and the degree of visceral handling. A score of 0 to 5 represents a minimal operation, such as a herniorrhaphy or a pyloromyotomy. An intestinal resection or repair of a malrotation would be moderate stress, with a score of 6 to 10. More severe stress would be rated at 11 to 20. Blood glucose concentration increased significantly and remained elevated for 12 hours postoperatively in all patients. There also were increases in lactate, pyruvate, ketones, and catecholamines in all patients. An increase in insulin levels was not found until 12 hours after surgery. Neonates given pentothal had a greater hyperglycemic response than those given halothane, and those with the most stressful operations had the most significant responses. This severe hyperglycemic response is probably the result of epinephrine release without an inhibition of corresponding increase in serum insulin response. Hyperglycemia during operation increases serum osmolality, which can cause a confusing urinary diuresis and may lead to cerebral hemorrhage.[69] The serum glucose should be monitored during prolonged operations on the neonate and in the immediate postoperative period. If there is hyperglycemia, glucose-free solutions are given.

REFERENCES

1. Dennis C, Grosz CR: A quarter century of intracaval feeding. Surg Gynecol Obstet 135:883, 1972
2. Dudrick SJ, Wilmore DW, Vars HM, Rhoads JE: Long-term total parenteral nutrition with growth, development, and positive nitrogen balance. Surgery 64:134, 1968
3. Committee on Dietary Allowances, Food and Nutrition Board: Recommended Dietary Allowances, 9th ed. Washington, DC, National Academy of Sciences, 1980
4. Committee on Nutrition, American Academy of Pediatrics: Commentary on parenteral nutrition. Pediatrics 71:547, 1983
5. Zlotkin SH, Stallings VA, Penchary PB: Total parenteral nutrition in children. Pediatr Clin North Am 32:381, 1985
6. Phillips R, Ott L, Young B, et al: Nutrition support and measured energy expenditure of the child and adolescent with head injury. J Neurosurg 67:846, 1987
7. Winthrop AL, Wesson DE, Pencharz PB, et al: Injury severity, whole body protein turnover, and energy expenditure in pediatric trauma. J Pediatr Surg 22:534, 1987
8. Witte MKM, Lough M, Reed MD: Energy expenditure in critically ill infants and children (Abstr). Pediatr Res 23:237A, 1988
9. Dechert R, Wesley J, Schafer L, et al: Comparison of oxygen consumption, carbon dioxide production, and resting energy expenditure in premature and full-term infants. J Pediatr Surg 20:792, 1985
10. Foman SJ, Ziegler EE, Filer LJ Jr, et al: Growth and serum chemical values of normal breast-fed infants. Acta Paediatr Scand (suppl) 273:1, 1978
11. Walker WA, Hendricks KM: Nutritional assessment. In Manual of Pediatric Nutrition. Philadelphia, Saunders, 1985
12. Helms RA, Miller JL, Burckart GL, et al: Clinical outcome as assessed by anthropomorphic parameters, albumin and cellular immune function in high-risk infants receiving total parenteral nutrition. J Pediatr Surg 18:564, 1983
13. Helms RH, Dickerson RN, Ebbert ML, et al: Retinol-binding protein and prealbumin: useful measures of protein repletion in critically ill, malnourished infants. J Pediatr Gastroenterol Nutr 5:586, 1986
14. Geyer RP: Parenteral nutrition. Physiol Rev 40:150, 1960
15. Amercian Society of Hospital Pharmacists, Inc: Drug Information, Bethesda, MD, American Hospital Formulary Service, 1988, p 1427
16. Heird WC, Winters RW: Total parenteral nutrition: the state of the art. J Pediatr 86:2, 1975
17. Sanderson I, Deitel M: Insulin response in patients receiving concentrated infusions of glucose and casein hydroly-

sate for complete parenteral nutrition. Ann Surg 179:387, 1974
18. Grasso S, Messina A, Saporito N, Reitano G: Serum insulin response to glucose and amino acids in the premature infant. Lancet 2:755, 1968
19. Thomas DB: Hyperosmolality and intraventricular hemorrhage in premature babies. Acta Paediatr Scand 65:429, 1976
20. Cowett RM, Oh W, Pollak A, et al: Glucose disposal of low birth weight infants: steady state hyperglycemia produced by constant intravenous glucose infusion. Pediatrics 63:389, 1979
21. Meguid MM, Ann F, and Soeldner JS: Temporal characteristics of insulin:glucose ratio after varying degrees of stress and trauma in man. J Surg Res 25:389, 1978
22. Valgeirsdottir K, Munro HN: Protein and amino acid metabolism. In Fischer JE (ed): Surgical Nutrition. Boston, Little, Brown, 1983, p 129
23. Moore FD: Metabolic Care of the Surgical Patient. Philadelphia, Saunders, 1959, pp 460–461
24. American Society of Hospital Pharmacists, Inc.: Drug Information. Bethesda, MD, American Hospital Formulary Service, 1988, p 1421
25. Gaull GE, Young VR: Proteins. In Pediatric Nutrition Handbook. Evanston IL, Committee on Nutrition, American Academy of Pediatrics. 1979, p 2
26. Das JB, Filler RM: Amino acid utilization during total parenteral nutrition in the surgical neonate. J Pediatr Surg 8:193, 1973
27. Heird WC, Dell RB, Helms RA, et al: Evaluation of an amino acid mixture designed to maintain normal plasma amino acid patterns in infants and children receiving parenteral nutrition. Pediatrics 80:401, 1987
28. Helms RA, Johnson MR, Christensen ML, et al: Altered caloric and protein requirement in neonates receiving a pediatric amino acid formulation (Abstr). Pediatr Res 21:429, 1987
29. Motil KJ, Harmon WE, Grupe WE: Complications of essential amino acid hyperalimentation in children with acute renal failure. JPEN 4:32, 1980
30. Nachbauer CA, Fischer JE: Nutritional support in hepatic failure. In Fischer JE (ed): Surgical Nutrition. Boston, Little, Brown, 1983, p 551
31. Cerra FB: Hypermetabolism, organ failure, and metabolic support. Surgery 101:1, 1987
32. Friedman Z, Danon A, Stahlman M, et al: Rapid onset of essential fatty acid deficiency in the newborn. Pediatrics 58:640, 1976
33. Phelps S, Cochran E, Kemper C: Peripheral venous line infiltration in infants receiving 100 percent dextrose, 10 percent dextrose/amino acids, 10 percent dextrose/amino acids/fat emulsion (Abstr). Pediatr Res 21:67A, 1987
34. Andrew F, Chon G, Schiff D: Lipid metabolism in the neonate. J Pediatr 88:273, 1976
35. Pereira C, Fox W, Stomley C, et al: Decreased oxygenation and hyperlipemia during intravenous fat infusions in premature infants. Pediatrics 66:26, 1980
36. Park W, Peust H, Brosicke H, et al: Impaired fat utilization in parenterally fed low-birthweight infants suffering from sepsis. JPEN 10:627, 1986

37. Greene H: Effects of intralipid on the lungs. In Winters R, Hasselmeyer R (eds): Intravenous Nutrition in the High Risk Infant. New York, Wiley, 1975, p 370

38. Friedman Z, Marks K, Maisels J, et al: Effects of parenteral fat emulsion on the pulmonary and reticuloendothelial systems in the newborn infant. Pediatrics 61:694, 1978

39. Committee on Nutrition, American Academy of Pediatrics: Calcium requirements in infancy and childhood. Pediatrics 62:826, 1978

40. Suita S, Ikeda K, Hayashida K, et al: Zinc and copper requirements during parenteral nutrition in the newborn. J Pediatr Surg 19:126, 1984

41. Henkin R, Schulman G: Changes in total non-diffusible and diffusible plasma zinc and copper during infancy. J Pediatr 82:831, 1973

42. Peden VH, Witzleben CL, Skelton MA: Total parenteral nutrition. J Pediatr 78:180, 1971

43. Touloukian RJ, Dowing SE: Cholestatis associated with long-term parenteral hyperalimentation. Arch Surg 106:58, 1973

44. Touloukian RJ, Seashore JH: Hepatic secretory obstruction with total parenteral nutrition in the infant. J Pediatr Surg 10:353, 1975

45. Rodgers BM, Hollenbeck JI, Donnelly WH, et al: Intrahepatic cholestasis with parenteral alimentation. Am J Surg 131:149, 1976

46. Bernstein J, Chang CH, Brough AJ, et al: Conjugated hyperbilirubinemia in infancy associated with parenteral alimentation. J Pediatr 90:361, 1977

47. Rager R, Finegold MJ: Cholestasis in immature newborn infants: is parenteral alimentation responsible? J Pediatr 86:264, 1975

48. Nakai H, Landing BH: Factors in the genesis of bile stasis in infancy. Pediatrics 27:300, 1961

49. Vileisis RA, Sorensen K, Gonzalez-Crussi F, Hunt CE: Liver malignancy after parenteral nutrition. J Pediatr 100:88, 1982

50. Black D, Suttle E, Whitington P, et al: The effect of short-term total parenteral nutrition on hepatic function in the human neonate: A prospective randomized study demonstrating alteration of hepatic canalicular function. J Pediatr 99:445, 1981

51. Vileisis RA, Inwood RJ, Hunt CE: Prospective controlled study of parenteral nutrition associated cholestatic jaundice and effect of protein intake. J Pediatr 96:893, 1980

52. Jarvenpao A, Rassin O, Kuitunen P, et al: Feeding the low birthweight infant: diet influences bile and metabolism. Pediatrics 72:677, 1983

53. Dorril N, Yausef M, Tuchweber B, et al: Taurine prevents cholestasis induced by lithocholic acid sulfate in guinea pigs. Am J Clin Nutr 37:221, 1983

54. Hughes CA, Talbot IC, Ducker DA, et al: Total parenteral nutrition in infancy: effect on the liver and suggested pathogenesis. Gut 24:241, 1983

55. Balistreri WF, Heubi JE, Suchy FJ: Immaturity of the enterohepatic circulation in early life: factors predisposing to "physiologic" maldigestion and cholestasis. J Pediatr Gastroenterol Nutr 2:346, 1983

56. Maini B, Blackburn GL, Bistraian BR, et al: Cyclic hyperalimentation: An optimal technique for preservation of visceral protein. J Surg Res 20:515, 1976

57. Jacopy-Lanza S, Sitren HS, Stevenson NR, et al: Changes in circadian rhythmicity of liver and serum parameters in rats fed a total parenteral nutrition solution by continuous and discontinuous intravenous or intragastric infusion. JPEN 4:496, 1982

58. Academy of Pediatrics, Committee on Nutrition: Commentary on breastfeeding and infant formulas, including proposed standards for formulas. Pediatrics 57:278, 1975

59. Moore MC, Greene HL: Tube feeding of infants and children. Pediatr Clin North Am 32:401, 1985

60. Ford EG, Jennings LM, Andrassy RJ: Serum albumin (oncotic pressure) correlates with enteral feeding tolerance in the pediatric surgical patient. J Pediatr Surg 22:597, 1987

61. Hardin TC, Page CP: Rapid replacement and maintenance of serum albumin in patients receiving total parenteral nutrition. Surg Gynecol Obstet 163:359, 1986

62. Andrassy RJ, Dubois T, Page CP, et al: Early postoperative nutritional enhancement utilizing enteral branched-chain amino acids by way of a needle catheter jejunostomy. Am J Surg 150:730, 1985

63. Orten JM, Neuhaus OW: Human Biochemistry. St. Louis, Mosby, 1982, p 663

64. Levenson SM, Seifter E: Starvation: Metabolic and physiologic responses. In Fischer JE (ed): Surgical Nutrition. Boston, Little, Brown, 1983, p 423

65. Hasselgren P, Pederson P, Sax H, et al: Current concepts of protein turnover and amino acid transport in liver and skeletal muscle during sepsis. Arch Surg 123:992, 1988

66. Finley R, Inculet R, Pace R: Major operative trauma increases peripheral amino acid release during the steady-state infusion of total parenteral nutrition in men. Surgery 99:491, 1986

67. Anand K, Brown M, Cavson N: Can the human neonate mount an endocrine and metabolic response to surgery. J Pediatr Surg 20:41, 1985

68. Anand K, Aynsley-Green A: Measuring the severity of surgical stress in newborn infants. J Pediatr Surg 23:297, 1988

69. Finberg L: Dangers to infants caused by changes in osmolar concentrations. Pediatrics 40:1031, 1961

12
Respiratory Support

Babette Horne
Marleta Reynolds

Airway obstruction, hypoventilation, atelectasis, aspiration, and pneumonia are potential threats to any sick infant or child. The factors responsible for one complication frequently lead to another, since irritation and drying of the airways result in thickened secretions that are not cleared because the cough reflex is depressed by pain or medications. Most respiratory complications can be prevented by good nursing care combined with simple adjuncts, such as humidity and chest physiotherapy. In the immediate postoperative period, the child should be positioned on his or her side to prevent soft tissue obstruction of the pharynx by the relaxed tongue. Bedridden infants and children should be turned from side to side at frequent intervals. The common practice of restraining a patient flat on the back invites atelectasis and aspiration pneumonia. Small infants should be stimulated to cry, and older children should be encouraged to breathe deeply and cough to mobilize secretions and improve ventilation. A painful abdomen or chest can be splinted by hands or pillows. A good cough is encouraged after four or five deep breaths. Considerable urging with an occasional bribe usually will produce an effective cough. Nasopharyngeal suctioning will stimulate a cough in reluctant children, although nasotracheal suctioning may be necessary. Early ambulation stimulates deeper breathing in children who are old enough to walk.

HUMIDIFICATION AND MIST THERAPY

The mucous membranes of the nasopharynx warm and humidify inspired air before it reaches the larynx and trachea. This process is facilitated by a large mucosal surface area as well as turbulence of the airstream as it passes over the turbinates.[1] Breathing unhumidifed gases or bypassing the nasopharynx with an endotracheal tube or tracheostomy dries and thickens secretions, interferes with ciliary function, and damages respiratory epithelium. In experimental animals, inhalation of dry gas for only 30 minutes damages the ciliated epithelium and increases the desquamation of cells into the lumen.[2,3] Humidification thins secretions and serves as a lubricant to protect the tracheal mucous membranes from the constant motion of endotracheal and tracheotomy tubes.

Humidity is water vapor, or water in the gaseous state. Absolute humidity is the maximum amount of water possible in the gaseous state at a given temperature. If gas is delivered at 100 percent absolute humidity at body temperature (37C), the gas contains 44 mg of water per liter of gas. If this gas is allowed to cool to room temperature, it will contain only 18 mg of water at 100 percent absolute humidity. If this gas then returns to the body where it is warmed to 37C, it will have only 50 percent relative humidity. Thus, to provide better humidity to the airway, the humidifier and its delivery circuits should be heated so that the gas arrives at the airway with the maximum amount of water.

Mist therapy involves the nebulization of water whereby droplets rather than gaseous water are supplied to the airway. These larger particles do not pass the nasopharynx. However, the ultrasonic nebulizer produces smaller, uniform droplets from 1 to 3 μ in diameter that are more effective in thinning secretions in the lower trachea and bronchi.[4]

Humidity or mist therapy may be delivered via tent, head hood, or face mask or through mechanical ventilation systems with either room air or an increased concentration of oxygen. Humidification is most helpful in those children who have difficulty mobilizing secretions after an operation and is most useful when combined with cough stimulation or respiratory physical therapy.

Complications of Mist Therapy

A mist-filled tent hampers nursing observation and care, and the isolation may frighten an already ill child. Stagnant water encourages the growth of bacteria. Meticulous sterilization and frequent changing of equipment are necessary to prevent the transmission of infections. Ultrasonic nebulization increases airway resistance in patients with obstructive airway disease.[5] Some children develop bronchospasm, with wheezing and squeaky breath sounds during mist therapy. This problem disappears when the mist is discontinued or the concentration of water is reduced.

The most serious complication of ultrasonic mist therapy is overhydration from water absorption through the respiratory tract. Small infants with an endotracheal tube are most susceptible to this problem. This is doubly important because both postoperative respiratory failure and the process of mechanical ventilation increase the tendency for the lung to retain water, which in turn worsens the respiratory failure. Fluid restriction and diuretic therapy may be indicated. Simple humidification is less risky, since supersaturated solutions are not used.

OXYGEN THERAPY

Hypoxia is a broad term indicating that the demand for oxygen is less than the available supply at the cellular level. The signs of hypoxia are cyanosis, restlessness, tachypnea, diaphoresis, and tachycardia. In infants, lethargy also is a sign of hypoxia.

Room air contains 21 percent oxygen. At a barometric pressure of 760 torr, this percentage represents a partial pressure of 159 torr of oxygen in the inspired air. However, dilution with water vapor and carbon dioxide reduces the Po_2 in the alveoli to about 100 torr. There is a small tension differential between alveolar gas and arterial blood, resulting in a normal arterial Po_2 of about 90 torr (96 percent saturated).

The most common immediate postoperative respiratory complication is hypoxemia secondary to hypoventilation caused by depression of the respiratory center by residual anesthetic agents or muscle relaxants. Increasing the oxygen content in the inspired air through a mask or head hood will improve mild hypoxemia. Oxygen supplementation is required until the child awakens and is able to breathe deeply. Careful observation is essential

during this time because hypoventilation will not respond to oxygen therapy but requires mechanical ventilation. For long-term therapy in infants, oxygen may be supplied through a tent or head hood. A nasal catheter is almost never used in a small child. The most effective way to deliver a consistent concentration of oxygen to a spontaneously breathing infant is through a plastic head hood. Nursing care is easily continued with the baby in an open, heated bed or in an isolette. A head hood can be set up with a heated humidifier so the air–oxygen mixture is delivered warm and fully saturated with water at body temperature. A flow rate of 12 L/min is required for small head hoods and 15 L/min for larger ones. The concentration of oxygen can be accurately controlled from 21 percent to 100 percent by changing the oxygen/air ratio. Orders for oxygen therapy must include the concentration desired expressed as a fraction of inspired gas (F_iO_2). The delivered oxygen concentration is then monitored continuously. However, the only accurate guide to the oxygenation of the patient's blood is measurement of the arterial or capillary blood gases. During recovery, the F_iO_2 is reduced in increments of 5 to 10 percent until room air is tolerated.

Oxygen Toxicity

Although its therapeutic benefits are undisputed, oxygen exposure is not innocuous. The lungs and the retina are two target organs that appear unusually susceptible to oxygen toxicity.

Retrolental fibroplasia (RLF) was first reported in newborns in the early 1950s and appeared to be associated with oxygen administration. The incidence of RLF is highest in infants born prematurely, hence the more descriptive term retinopathy of prematurity (ROP). The immature retina responds to hyperoxia with vasoconstriction and subsequent capillary necrosis. When normoxia resumes, marked endothelial proliferation arises from residual vascular complexes adjacent to closed capillaries. This exudative reaction leads to retinal hemorrhage, detachment, scar formation (cicatrix), and blindness. Maturity of the nasal retina is achieved by 8 months' gestation, but temporal retinal maturity is incomplete until 46 weeks postconceptual age. The more premature the infant, the more immature the retina and the greater the chance of developing ROP when exposed to oxygen.

Oxygen is not the sole culprit in ROP. Retinopathy has been reported in babies who never received supplemental oxygen, in infants with cyanotic heart disease, and in term infants. Infants exposed to oxygen-enriched environments for many days have survived without ROP, whereas retinopathy has developed in others after only a brief period of hyperoxia. That the severity of ROP has no clear-cut relationship to duration of oxygen exposure or to Pao_2 levels signifies that this is a multifactorial disease.

After reviewing several multicenter reviews of ROP, Lucey and Dangman concluded that the disorder manifests in one of two forms, hyperoxic and nonhyperoxic RLF. Other contributing factors include hypocarbia, exchange transfusion, apnea, sepsis, and vitamin E deficiency.[6] The American Academy of Pediatrics recommends that F_iO_2 levels be maintained as low as possible to ensure that the infant's preductal PaO_2 is 50 to 90 mm Hg.[7] The ability to monitor oxygenation status continuously using transcutaneous electrodes or pulse oximetry has not resulted in fewer cases of ROP.[8]

The lungs also are affected by oxygen therapy. Early damage to type I pneumocytes from oxygen therapy results in pulmonary edema. This is followed by cellular proliferation of type II (surfactant-producing) pneumocytes and capillary endothelial cells. This healing process may result in fibrosis caused by proliferation of fibroblasts and production of collagen. A scarred, low volume, fibrotic lung results.

To avoid pulmonary toxicity Deneke and Fanburg have made the following recommendations based on animal and human experiments.[9]

1. One hundred percent oxygen, when administered for periods of 24 hours or less, is probably harmless.
2. Forty percent oxygen can be used for long periods of time without apparent danger.
3. If oxygen concentration greater than 40 percent must be used to prevent hypoxia, the lowest concentration possible should be used for the shortest period of time.

Bronchopulmonary dysplasia (BPD) is a chronic lung disease that occurs in premature infants who have had hyaline membrane disease.[10] The radiographic, clinical, and functional criteria include:

1. Assisted ventilation during the first week of life
2. Signs of respiratory distress (tachypnea, rales, retractions) persisting for longer than 28 days
3. Oxygen dependence for longer than 28 days
4. Areas of radiolucency persisting on chest roentgenograms (Fig. 12–1).

Oxygen therapy, positive pressure ventilation, and a prolonged course of hyaline membrane disease contribute to the development of BPD.[11] Clinical trials of vitamin E and superoxide dismutase therapy to prevent BPD have been disappointing.[12–14]

Oxygen is a valuable therapeutic agent that must be used with great caution. The postoperative newborn who requires oxygen therapy may have a right radial arterial line for blood gas monitoring. An umbilical artery line samples postductal blood, which may have deceptively low PaO_2 levels. Capillary blood gas samples accurately reflect arterial values in the range of 50 to 70

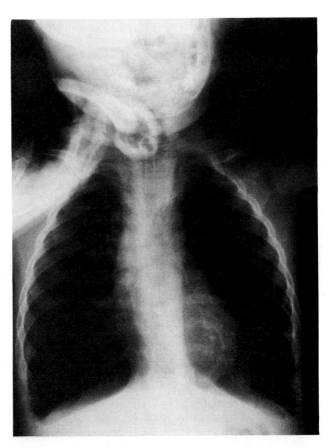

Figure 12–1. Bronchopulmonary dysplasia. There is air trapping and fine hilar infiltrated.

mm Hg provided the infant's peripheral perfusion is good. Capillary samples underestimate arterial PO_2s as the PaO_2 rises and are a poor indicator of hyperoxia. Transcutaneous PO_2 electrodes and pulse oximeters are useful noninvasive monitors of oxygenation. Transcutaneous monitors underestimate PaO_2 values in infants with BPD.[15]

ASSISTED VENTILATION

Mechanical support of ventilation is indicated when other measures fail to maintain adequate arterial blood gases (PaO_2, $PaCO_2$). Apnea obviously is an urgent indication for artificial ventilation. Cyanosis in the absence of an intracardiac right-to-left shunt when a patient is breathing 40 percent oxygen is a clinical sign of respiratory insufficiency. Children with central nervous system injury may require respiratory support because of shallow respirations or periodic apnea. A common postoperative problem is encountered with the infant who is just barely able to maintain normal blood gases and pH by working to breathe with maximum use of his or her accessory muscles. Such an infant may have cardiac or pulmonary disease, but just as frequently the clinical setting involves abdominal distention with restricted diaphragmatic movement. The infant breathes 60 to 80 times a minute with grunting respirations, and the skin is pale or dusky. The breath sounds are diminished or absent over the lower lung fields. In spite of increased atmospheric oxygen and the correction of metabolic acidosis, these infants become exhausted with progressive respiratory failure. Every effort should be made to identify the cause of hypoventilation and to institute assisted ventilation before cardiorespiratory arrest.

Although clinical observations are important, repeated measurements of the arterial or capillary blood gases are essential to determine which patients require mechanical support. The generally accepted guidelines on indications for respiratory assistance in infants and children with respiratory distress syndrome are those suggested by Seleny and by Downes and Raphaely.[16,17] Carbon dioxide elimination is impaired when large areas of pulmonary tissue are diseased or unused (deadspace ventilation). Therefore, a rising Pa_{CO_2} is even more ominous as a sign of severe alveolar hypoventilation. If the Pa_{CO_2} reaches 60 torr and is rising at the rate of 10 torr/hour, respiratory assistance is indicated. Another indication is the infant's inability to maintain an arterial oxygen tension of 50 to 70 torr while breathing 100 percent oxygen. If the Pa_{CO_2} is not rising rapidly and if the arterial pH can be kept above 7.20 with intravenous bicarbonate, ventilation may not be required. The required dose of bicarbonate in milliequivalents is calculated by the following formula.

$$\text{Required mEq NaHCO}_3 = 0.3 \times \text{weight in kg} \times \text{base deficit}$$

Half the calculated dose is given at the rate of 1 mEq/minute diluted by one half, with the remainder allowed to drip in over 1 hour.

Assisted Ventilation with Bag and Mask

Assisted ventilation with a mask and bag is a simple rapid technique that can be used in an emergency for an apneic patient. Hand ventilation is also used before suctioning and again at intervals to support children with borderline respiratory failure. Hand-operated bag ventilators are adaptable to endotracheal and tracheostomy tubes. Ventilation in this manner should precede and follow tracheal suctioning; it is used to "sigh" patients on respirators and will hyperinflate atelectatic segments. The self-inflatable bags, such as the Ambu or Hope units, are most useful in an emergency and during transport, since they do not require a source of compressed air or oxygen. Anesthesia or Rusch bags are more effective and versatile in the intensive care setting (Fig. 12–2). The Rusch bag has the safety features of being nonrebreathing and pressure-relieving. The bags are inflated by the entry of oxygen or compressed air, which can be mixed to provide from 21 to 100 percent oxygen. The mask must fit snugly over the patient's nose and mouth without causing injury to the eyes. One hand elevates the chin and holds the mask in place while the other squeezes the bag with sufficient pressure to visibly expand the thoracic cage. An assistant auscultates the lungs to guage the effectiveness of ventilation.

ENDOTRACHEAL INTUBATION

In many surgical patients, an endotracheal tube is necessary, not only for ventilation but also for optimum tracheal toilet. A full range of pediatric-size endotracheal tubes and laryngoscope blades should be available. Table 12–1 lists the proper sizes of tubes and blades for children of various weights. In general, a newborn infant will take a 3-mm tube, a 5-year-old child a 5-mm tube, and a teenager a 7-mm tube. The tube must be small enough

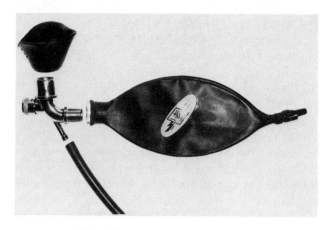
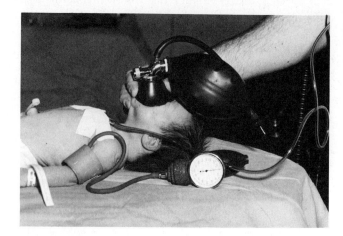

Figure 12–2. Left. The Rusch bag, which can be used for ventilation. **Right.** The mask fits tightly over the baby's face while the chin is elevated.

TABLE 12–1. LARYNGOSCOPE BLADES AND TUBE SIZES RECOMMENDED ACCORDING TO A CHILD'S WEIGHT

Weight of Child (lb)	Weight of Child (kg)	Size of Tube—Internal Diameter (mm)	Laryngoscope Size	Connector Size (mm)	Length of Tube (cm)
5	2	2.5–3		3	10–11
5–10	2.5–5	3.0–3.5		3–4	11–12
10–20	4.5–9.0	3.5	Premature Infant	4	14
20–30	9.0–13.6	5.0		4–4.5–5	15
30–40	13.6–18.1	5.5		4.5–5	17
40–50	18.1–22.6	6.5		5.5–6	19
50–60	22.6–27.2	7.0		5.5–6	20
60–70	27.2–31.7	7.5	Child	6–6.5	20
70–80	31.7–36.2	8.0		6.5–7	22
80–90	36.2–40.8	8.5		7–7.5	22
90–100	40.8–45.3	9.0		7.5–8	22

to allow an air leak between the tube and larynx. A cuffed tube is used in patients 8 years and older.

The technique of endotracheal intubation can be learned only by considerable practice, first at autopsy to learn the anatomy and then under supervision of an anesthesiologist in the operating room. Only the most experienced person available should attempt intubation outside the operating room because fumbling attempts are dangerous to the life of the patient and can needlessly traumatize the larynx and trachea. Figure 12–3 illustrates the proper position for intubation. The head is slightly elevated but not hyperextended. The laryngoscope blade is inserted slightly to the right of the midline, displacing the tongue to the left. No attempt is made to lift the tongue, and if it slips out of control, the blade is withdrawn and another attempt is made. The blade is then advanced, exposing the oropharynx, the hypopharynx,

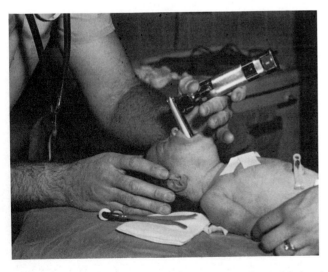

Figure 12–3. During laryngoscopy, the head is elevated but not hyperextended. The blade is inserted, displacing the tongue to the left.

and the epiglottis. If the blade is advanced too rapidly, the esophagus is entered, and all landmarks are lost. The epiglottis of an infant is short, folded on itself (omega-shaped), and easily traumatized. In younger children, the epiglottis is picked up, exposing the vocal cords directly. In older children, the laryngoscope is inserted into the vallecula. The tongue and jaw are then elevated. This maneuver lifts the epiglottis and exposes the larynx. A tube of appropriate size is then inserted to approximately 2 cm below the level of the vocal cords. The tube is connected, and the infant is ventilated with a bag and 100 percent oxygen. Chest movement should be symmetrical, and breath sounds should be present bilaterally, especially at the apices.

Attempts to intubate should not take longer than 30 seconds. Except in emergency situations, the electrocardiogram should be monitored during the procedure, and an assistant should continually palpate the pulse and observe the patient for cyanosis. When the tube is properly positioned, it is marked at the level of the upper lip and held in place while an assistant liberally applies tincture of benzoin to the face and secures the tube with strips of waterproof adhesive tape that extend from ear to ear. The tube position is then checked with an x-ray; ideally it should be midway between the carina and the clavicle.

Any patient with an endotracheal tube in place requires intensive nursing care and close medical observation. A team of respiratory therapists is invaluable in providing chest physiotherapy and performing blood gas analyses. The inspired gases should be warmed and humidified to provide 35 to 44 ml of water vapor per liter of gas flow—80 to 100 percent of the relative humidity in the trachea. Frequent suctioning is vital in keeping small tubes patent and in clearing dependent secretions. This important procedure requires more than one person to ensure sterility and to avoid hypoxia. Secretions can be loosened before suctioning by instilling 0.5 normal saline into the tube. The infant is disconnected from the ventilator and hyperventilated with 100 percent oxygen with a hand bag unless the infant is still at risk for retrolental fibroplasia, in which case he or she is given an increase of only 10 percent more oxygen than he or she was getting from the ventilator. A sterile catheter that fits comfortably through the endotracheal tube is handled with a sterile gloved hand and advanced without force. Suction is applied as the tube is rapidly withdrawn to minimize hypoxia. The entire procedure must take no longer than 5 to 10 seconds. After ventilation by hand for 1 or 2 minutes, the infant is suctioned with the head turned in the opposite direction so that the catheter will pass down the other mainstem bronchus. If bradycardia develops at any time, the procedure is stopped, and the patient is ventilated with 100 percent oxygen. Anderson and Chandra warned of the danger of perforating lung tissue with a suction catheter, and in autopsy studies they determined the distances that a catheter may be passed before hitting the walls of the lower and middle lobe bronchi (Table 12–2).[18]

There is considerable controversy about how long an endotracheal tube may be left in place without causing permanent tracheal damage and scarring. Fisk and Baker found mucosal ulceration in the trachea and bronchi in babies dying after only 1 week of intubation.[19] Squamous metaplasia has been found in the tracheas of infants dying 7 to 108 days after intubation. Arytenoid and posterior commissure ulcerations and cartilage erosion may cause long-term hoarseness as well as airway obstruction.[20] The most unfortunate complication of endotracheal intubation is subglottic stenosis, which is not apparent until the endotracheal tube is removed and the baby develops airway obstruction. A tracheostomy or anterior cricoid split may then be necessary.[21] Milder degrees of tracheal stenosis may become evident only with an intercurrent respiratory infection. The incidence of subglottic stenosis

TABLE 12–3. GUIDELINE FOR RACEMIC EPINEPHRINE

Weight (kg)	R.E. 2.25% cc (0.05 ml/kg)	Normal Saline cc Diluent	Total cc	Dose (μg/kg/min)
5	0.25	2.75	3.00	112.0
10	0.50	2.50	3.00	112.5
15	0.75	2.25	3.00	112.4
20	1.00	2.00	3.00	112.5
25	1.25	1.75	3.00	112.2
30	1.50	1.50	3.00	112.5

has been reduced markedly, and the duration of safe intubation has been increased in our own intensive care units by the use of nonirritating Silastic tubes that fit loosely enough to allow an air leak. The continued presence of the air leak is confirmed several times a day.

Every aspect of endotracheal tube care is important in preventing subglottic stenosis. The tube must be inserted atraumatically, fixed to prevent motion against the glottis, and removed as soon as possible. In small infants, endotracheal tubes can be left in place for several months with minimal difficulty.

Postextubation subglottic edema may occur immediately after an operation, as well as after a patient has been intubated for many months. The patient is hoarse and may have a croupy cough and stridor. These symptoms usually abate with mist therapy alone. However, at the onset of symptoms, it is wise to give intravenous dexamethasone at 1 to 2 mg/kg even though there is little proof of the efficacy of this drug. The administration of nebulized racemic epinephrine will further relieve the child's edema and airway obstruction (Table 12–3).[22] Although the drug can be administered with intermittent positive pressure breathing (IPPB), there is greater patient acceptance when the drug is nebulized for the child to breath.[23]

Established endotracheal tube injuries may be treated by the removal of granulation tissue via a bronchoscope and the direct injection of triamcinolone into the area of injury. Systemic steroids are administered, and a smaller endotracheal tube is placed. It is then important to sedate the child and to immobilize the head and neck with sandbags. Otherson successfully used this technique to avoid tracheotomy in 15 children with acute endotracheal tube injuries.[24]

CONTINUOUS POSITIVE AIRWAY PRESSURE

Distressed infants grunt or finish their expiration against a closed glottis, which increases airway pressure and raises the arterial oxygen tension in a spontaneously breathing baby. Maintaining positive end expiratory pressure opens collapsed alveoli and improves the distri-

TABLE 12–2. MAXIMUM CATHETER MEASUREMENTS FOR ENDOTRACHEAL SUCTION MEASURED FROM THE GINGIVAL MARGIN*

Patient Weight (gm)	Catheter Length (cm)
<500	7.0
600–1000	8.0
1100–1500	9.0
1600–2000	10.0
2100–2500	11.0
2600–3000	12.0
3100–3500	13.0
3600–4000	14.0

* Measure catheter along appropriate line for weight. Add the length of the E-T tube which is sticking out of mouth. This is the maximum safe distance for insertion of a suction catheter through an E-T tube.

bution of gases within the lungs. Insertion of an endotracheal tube makes this auto-continuous positive airway pressure (CPAP) maneuver impossible.

In the CPAP system developed by Gregory et al., a suitable flow of warmed, humidified gas is brought to a T adapter attached to an endotracheal tube.[25] The opposite side of the T is connected by way of a large-bore tube to a 500 ml reservoir bag. A screw clamp on the tail of the bag regulates the system's pressure, which is recorded in centimeters of water on a pressure gauge. The rebreathing of expired gas is prevented by a high flow through the system (not more than 5 L/min). When originally described, the system included an underwater pop-off to prevent pressure from rising beyond 30 cm of water. Currently, a valve on the tail of the bag can be set accurately to limit the pressure (Fig. 12–4). At the beginning of therapy, the pressure is set at 6 cm of water. If this fails to improve the Pa_{O_2}, the pressure is progressively increased up to 15 cm of water until an optimum end-expiratory pressure is reached that is deemed most beneficial to the patient.[26,27]

When the arterial oxygenation improves, the inhaled oxygen concentration is reduced, and the pressure is diminished gradually in 1 cm increments until the infant is weaned from support.

The CPAP system is of most value to patients who are breathing spontaneously and in patients in whom hypoxia owes primarily to decreased functional residual capacity of the lungs. This simple system should be the first form of respiratory care; if it fails, mechanical ventilation is indicated. CPAP has been used successfully for postoperative support in children under 3 years of age who have undergone open heart surgery. In this group of patients, the work of breathing was reduced, atelectasis was prevented, and excellent oxygenation was

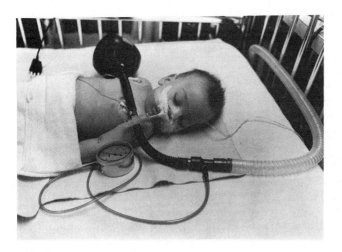

Figure 12–4. A simple apparatus to provide continuous positive airway pressure with a bag, oxygen source, pressure monitor, and tube.

maintained.[28,29] Haller et al. further used CPAP as an alternative to mechanical ventilation in neonates with thoracic and abdominal surgical emergencies.[30] In experimental animals subjected to increased intraabdominal pressure, CPAP reduced cardiac output; there was, however, still an improvement in blood gases.[31] Adverse effects of positive end-expiratory pressure (PEEP) therapy include barotrauma, decreased cardiac output, and decreased urine output.

MECHANICAL VENTILATION

Mechanical ventilation is necessary when the patient is unable to perform the work of breathing alone, with resultant hypercarbia, hypoxemia, and acidosis. Because of the enormous size variation in pediatric patients, as well as the wide range of cardiorespiratory problems encountered in pediatric intensive care, there is no single ideal ventilator. The following factors must be evaluated when considering a particular ventilator for use in a pediatric intensive care setting:

1. Is the machine pressure preset or volume preset?
2. Are there alarms that indicate both loss of volume and loss of pressure?
3. For what size range of patient can the ventilator be used effectively?
4. Can PEEP be given?
5. Is there an intermittent mandatory ventilation (IMV) mode?
6. Can the inspired gases be humidified?
7. Is there an oxygen analyzer?

Most ventilators can be classified as either volume or pressure preset. Examples of the former are the Siemens-Elema Servo 900, Bear, Bennett MA-1, Engstrom, and Emerson models. These machines deliver a preset tidal volume regardless of the pressure. The peak inspiratory pressure (PIP), therefore, becomes a useful tool to monitor changes in lung mechanics. Increases in PIP are caused by either a decrease in pulmonary parenchymal compliance or an increase in airway resistance (kinked endotracheal tube, secretions, pneumothorax). Decreases in PIP are seen when the patient's condition improves or if a leak develops either around the endotracheal tube or within the ventilator system. Volume preset machines are useful for the majority of patients beyond the neonatal period. The air leak often found around the endotracheal tubes of newborns makes the delivery of an accurate preset tidal volume difficult.

Pressure preset ventilators (Bird, Bourns BP-200, Sechrist, Healthdyne) deliver breaths to a predetermined positive pressure. Mechanical characteristics of the patient's respiratory system (airway resistance and lung compliance) determine the volume of each breath. These machines can be used to deliver rapid rates over a wider range of I:E (inspiratory/expiratory) ratios. They are, therefore, useful in the management of newborn infants with hyaline membrane disease. However, the rapid changes in pulmonary compliance that occur in hyaline membrane disease may result in the delivery of inconsistent tidal volumes from pressure preset machines, leading to hypo- or hyperventilation.

To initiate mechanical ventilation using a volume preset machine, it is necessary to select a respiratory rate and tidal volume. The appropriate rate usually depends on the patient's age.

Age	Rate (Breaths/Minute)
Newborn	30–35
1 Year	25–30
2 Years	20–25
5 Years	15–20
10 Years	12–15
15 Years	10–12

A tidal volume of 10 ml/kg is commonly used. The internal compression volume of the circuit, including hoses, humidifier, and water trap, must be taken into consideration when setting the tidal volume.

Once the patient is connected to the ventilator system, it is imperative to auscultate both lungs, visually inspect chest excursion and patient appearance, and check PIP. Of course, the final verification of the adequacy of ventilation lies in the analysis of arterial blood gas tensions.

With pressure preset machines, one choses a respiratory rate and a pressure maximum (P_{max}), the airway pressure at which inspiration is terminated. Healthy newborns can be ventilated adequately with a P_{max} of 20 cm H_2O and a rate of 25 breaths/minute. The presence of underlying pulmonary pathology makes individual titration of rate and P_{max} necessary, with frequent blood gas sampling to ensure adequacy of ventilation.

Morray has presented some general guidelines to assess readiness for weaning from mechanical ventilation (Table 12–4).[32] Most volume preset ventilators have an IMV circuit incorporated into them. This provides a continuous flow of fresh gas, enabling the patient to breathe around the ventilator-supplied breaths. The IMV

TABLE 12–4. SUGGESTED GUIDELINES FOR INITIATION OF WEANING FROM MECHANICAL VENTILATION

Positive nitrogen balance
Metabolic stability
Cardiovascular stability
Maximum inspiratory force > 20 cm H_2O
Vital capacity > 10–15 ml/kg
Acceptable Po_2 with $F_iO_2 \leq 0.5$ and PEEP < 8–10 cm H_2O
Absence of muscle relaxants or high-dose sedatives or relaxants

breaths are gradually withdrawn as the patient takes more spontaneous breaths. Synchronized IMV (SIMV) circuits allow better coordination of machine-delivered breaths with the patient's spontaneous breaths. Ultimately, the patient takes over the full work of breathing and is then given CPAP therapy for a period of time before extubation.

Monitoring of the patient receiving mechanical ventilation includes frequent chest auscultation, mucous membrane inspection, and arterial blood gas analysis. The need for frequent arterial blood gas analysis has diminished somewhat with the development of pulse oximetry[33] and transcutaneous oxygen monitoring.[34] These techniques provide a continuous real-time display of either arterial hemoglobin oxygen saturation or skin oxygen tension. Agreement with arterial Sao_2 or Pao_2 is fairly good in most instances.

Ventilator support of infants and children should not be undertaken unless the physicians and nurses are completely familiar with the equipment. Ideally, a respiratory therapy service takes responsibility for setting up, maintaining, and sterilizing all equipment. The physician's responsibilities include writing orders for oxygen concentration, humidity or mist therapy, respiratory rate, tidal volume, and pressure limits.

RESPIRATORY FAILURE

Respiratory failure in children can be the result of direct or secondary injury to the lungs. When the injury results in increased permeability of the alveolar–capillary membrane and pulmonary edema, it is referred to as adult respiratory distress syndrome (ARDS). Although originally described in adults, ARDS can occur in children as young as 2 weeks of age. Mortality rates for ARDS reach 59 percent.[35]

After an acute pulmonary injury, a period of apparent stability ensues and lasts 6 to 48 hours. The child may be tachypneic, and the chest roentgenogram may show a fine reticular infiltrate. As acute respiratory failure develops, the child becomes hypoxemic and refractory to oxygen therapy. Diffuse infiltrates develop on chest roentgenograms, and there is a decrease in the pulmonary compliance. Increased pulmonary vascular resistance with intrapulmonary shunting is in a large part responsible for the persistent hypoxemia.

Any child with impending respiratory failure must be transferred to the intensive care unit for monitoring and ventilator support. Arterial catheters for monitoring blood pressure, pulse, and arterial blood gas tensions should be used in conjunction with pulse oximetry or transcutaneous oxygen and carbon dioxide monitoring. In an older child, a Swan-Ganz catheter may be useful in measuring cardiac output and systemic and pulmonary vascular resistance.

PEEP is the mainstay of therapy for ARDS. The PEEP is increased to a level that maximizes the benefits by improving tissue oxygen delivery with the lowest F_iO_2. Intravascular volume expansion and positive inotropic drugs may be needed to offset the effects of high levels of PEEP on cardiac output. Clinical trials of high-frequency jet ventilation have not shown consistent benefit in ARDs.[36] Extracorporeal membrane oxygenation may offer some improvement in outcome for the children who do not respond to conventional methods.

Extracorporeal Membrane Oxygenation

Extracorporeal membrane oxygenation (ECMO) is being used with increasing frequency to support infants and children with reversible respiratory and cardiac failure. ECMO is prolonged extracorporeal cardiopulmonary bypass using a membrane oxygenator. The initial clinical trials of ECMO in the early 1970s were unsuccessful, but in 1975, Bartlett reported the first successful use of ECMO in a neonate.[37] Since that time, the technique, equipment, and use of ECMO have been refined and expanded. A number of centers have successfully used ECMO to treat infants and children with respiratory failure or cardiac failure following open heart surgery.

Patient selection criteria for neonatal ECMO vary from institution to institution. All are based on a predicted 90 percent mortality. Krummel et al. use an alveolar-arterial oxygen gradient ($AaDo_2$) of >620 for 12 hours.[38] Hirschl and Bartlett use the oxygenation index [$OI = (MAP \times F_iO_2 \times 100)/Pao_2$] of greater than 40 to predict mortality.[39] Contraindications to the use of ECMO include weight less than 2.0 kg, age more than 7 days, gestational age less than 35 weeks, renal failure, intraventricular hemorrhage, or major associated anomalies. The majority of neonates treated with ECMO have respiratory failure secondary to meconium aspiration. Other diagnoses for which ECMO is used include persistent fetal circulation or persistent pulmonary hypertension of the newborn, congenital diaphragmatic hernia, pneumonia, sepsis, and respiratory distress syndrome. Babies with congenital diaphragmatic hernia represent a special group of patients. Some centers select only those babies who they believe to have adequate pulmonary parenchyma (based on a $Po_2 > 100$ at any time or the presence of a honeymoon period postoperatively) as ECMO candidates. Others accept all babies with congenital diaphragmatic hernia as candidates for ECMO.

Success with neonatal ECMO has rekindled interest in the use of ECMO for cardiorespiratory failure in older children and adults. Some centers currently are using ECMO to support children after cardiac surgery.[40] Reversible pulmonary conditions, such as aspiration pneumonia, viral and bacterial pneumonia, and ARDS have been treated with ECMO. An 80 to 100 percent predicted mortality ($AaDo_2$ greater than 610, shunt greater than 30 percent, or Pao_2 less than 60 on F_iO_2 of 100 percent) is used as the selection criterion. The efficacy of ECMO in this group of patients is not yet determined.

ECMO can be accomplished with two methods, venoarterial (VA) or venovenous (VV). VV bypass does not provide cardiac support and is, therefore, not used as frequently as VA bypass in neonates. The development of an adequate single-lumen catheter may increase the use of VV bypass. VA bypass is instituted using cannulas placed into the right atrium through the right internal jugular vein and the aortic arch through the right common carotid artery. A standard roller pump is used at most centers, although a few are using centrifugal pumps. A membrane oxygenator with a separate heat exchanger usually is used. Systemic heparinization is maintained and monitored with the activated clotting time (ACT) averaging 220. Pre-ECMO head ultrasonograms and echocardiograms are obtained on each ECMO candidate to rule out preexisting lesions. Head ultrasonograms are repeated daily and when clinically indicated. While on ECMO, the lungs are allowed to rest and are ventilated with low airway pressures (20 to 25 cm of H_2O), an F_iO_2 of 30 percent, and a rate of 10. Recent studies by Keszler et al. indicate that higher levels of PEEP reduce the time on ECMO and encourage lung recovery.[41] Chest physiotherapy and suctioning are continued as indicated. The chest roentgenogram usually shows complete opacification shortly after beginning bypass. After several days of ECMO, the lungs will appear clear on the chest roentgenogram as the compliance improves. The usual ECMO run lasts 3 to 6 days.

Problems that develop on ECMO are related to technical failures and patient-related complications. Bleeding is the most common complication, and the need for systemic heparinization makes this complication difficult to avoid and treat. In the recent report from the ECMO Registry, intracranial hemorrhage occurred in 197 of 1492 patients. To prevent extension of the hemorrhage, the patient must be weaned from bypass. Forty-nine percent of babies weaned from bypass because of intracranial hemorrhage ultimately survived. Bleeding from other sites occurs in 16 percent of patients. Lowering the ACT levels to 200 and increasing the platelet count to greater than 100,000 may help control some bleeding. Other major complications include renal failure, seizures, sepsis, and hypertension. Technical problems can occur at any time. Failure of the membrane, pump, and heat exchanger and tubing rupture are not uncommon and, unless identified promptly, may lead to death.

The ECMO Registry has compiled data on 1492 patients supported with ECMO from 1973 to 1988.[42] Table 12–5 lists the diagnoses and associated outcomes

TABLE 12–5. NEONATAL ECMO REGISTRY

	Number	% Survival
Meconium aspiration	611	90.8
Respiratory distress syndrome	206	77.2
Congenital diaphragmatic hernia	221	64.7
Persistent fetal circulation	234	84.6
Sepsis	138	74.6
Cardiac conditions	17	52.9

Bartlett[42]

TABLE 12–6. NEONATAL ECMO REGISTRY: MAJOR COMPLICATIONS

	Number	% Survival
Intracranial hemorrhage	197	48.7
Gastrointestinal hemorrhage	64	62.5
Surgical site hemorrhage	169	69.2
Seizures	250	63.6
Creatinine > 3	22	54.5
Positive cultures	80	75
Hypertension	156	80.1

Bartlett[42]

for these children. Some of major patient complications are listed in Table 12–6. A heparin-bonded system and other advances in equipment and techniques should improve survival by decreasing the complication rate.

REFERENCES

1. Walker JEC, Wells RE: Heat and water exchange in the respiratory tract. Am J Med 30:261, 1961
2. Marfatia S, Donahoe PK, Hendren A: Effect of dry and humidified gases on the respiratory epithelium in rabbits. J Pediatr Surg 10:583, 1975
3. Chalon J, Loew D, Malebranche J: Effects of dry anesthetic gases on tracheobronchial ciliated epithelium. Anesthesiology 37:338, 1972
4. Avery ME, Galina M, Nachman R: Mist therapy. Pediatrics 39:160, 1969
5. Cheney FW, Butler J: The effects of ultrasonically produced aerosols on airway resistance in man. Anesthesia 29:1099, 1968
6. Lucey JF, Dangman B: A reexamination of the role of oxygen in retrolental fibroplasia. Pediatrics 73:82, 1984
7. Guidelines for Perinatal Care. Elk Grove Village, Ill., The American Academy of Pediatrics and The American College of Obstetricians and Gynecologists, 1983, pp 212–216
8. Yu UYH, Hookham DM, Nave JRM: Retrolental fibroplasia: Controlled study of 4 years' experience in a neonatal intensive care unit. Arch Dis Child 57:247, 1982
9. Deneke SM, Fanburg BL: Oxygen toxicity of the lung: an update. Br J Anaesth 54:737, 1982
10. Northway WH, Rosan RC, Porter DY: Pulmonary disease following respiratory therapy of hyaline membrane disease. N Engl J Med 276:357, 1967
11. Philip AG: Oxygen plus pressure plus time: The etiology of bronchopulmonary dysplasia. Pediatrics 55:44, 1975
12. Saldanha RL, Cepeda E, Poland RL: The effect of vitamin E prophylaxis on the incidences and severity of bronchopulmonary dysplasia. J Pediatr 101:89, 1982
13. Ehrenkranz RA, Ablow RC, Warshaw JB: Prevention of bronchopulmonary dysplasia with vitamin E administration during the acute stages of respiratory distress syndrome. J Pediatr 95:873, 1979
14. Rosenfield W, Evans H, Concepcion L, et al. Prevention of bronchopulmonary dysplasia by administration of superoxide dismutase in preterm infants with respiratory distress syndrome. J Pediatr 105:781, 1984
15. Rome ES, Stork EK, Waldemar AC, Martin RJ: Limitations of transcutaneous Po_2 and Pco_2 monitoring in infants with bronchopulmonary dysplasia. Pediatrics 74:217, 1984
16. Seleny FL: Respiratory failure, part II: The child. Curr Probl Anesth Crit Care Med 1:24, 1978
17. Downes JJ, Raphaely RC: Pediatric intensive care. Anesthesiology 43:238, 1975
18. Anderson KD, Chandra R: Pneumothorax secondary to perforation of sequential bronchi by suction catheters. J Pediatr Surg 11:687, 1976
19. Fisk GC, Baker W: Mucosal changes in the trachea and main bronchi of newborn infants after naso-tracheal intubation. Anaesth Intensive Care 3:209, 1975
20. Hengerer AS, Strome M, Jeffe BF: Injuries to the neonatal larynx from long-term endotracheal tube intubation and suggested tube modification for prevention. Ann Otol Rhinol Laryngol 84:764, 1975
21. Johnson DC, Jones R: Surgical aspects of airway management in infancy and childhood. Surg Clin North Am 56:263, 1976
22. Jordan WJ, Graves GL, Elwyn PA: New therapy for postintubation laryngeal edema and tracheitis in children. JAMA 212:585, 1970
23. Taussig LM, Castro O, Beaudry PH, et al: Treatment of laryngotracheobronchitis (croup). Use of intermittent positive-pressure breathing and racemic epinephrine. Am J Dis Child 129:790, 1975
24. Otherson HB: Intubation injuries of the trachea in children. Ann Surg 189:601, 1979
25. Gregory AG, Phibbe RH, Kitterman JA, et al: Treatment of the idiopathic respiratory distress syndrome with continuous positive airway pressure. N Engl J Med 284:1333, 1971
26. Berman L, Fox WW, Downes JJ: Optimal levels of CPAP for tracheal extubation of newborns. J Pediatr 89:109, 1976
27. Suter PM, Fairley HB, Isenberg MD: Optimum end-expiratory airway pressure in patients with acute pulmonary failure. N Engl J Med 292:284, 1975
28. Crew AD, Varkonyi PI, Gardner LG, et al: Continuous positive airway pressure breathing in the postoperative management of the cardiac infant. Thorax 29:437, 1974
29. Stewart S, Edmunds LH, Kirklin JW, et al: Spontaneous breathing with continuous positive airway pressure (CPAP) after open intracardiac operations in infants. J Thorac Cardiovasc Surg 65:37, 1973
30. Haller JAS, White JJ, Moynihan PC, Galvis AG: Use of continuous positive airway pressure breathing in the im-

proved management of neonatal emergencies. J Pediatr Surg 8:669, 1973

31. Buyukpanukcu N, Hicsonmez A: The effect of CPAP upon pulmonary reserve and cardiac output under increased abdominal pressure. J Pediatr Surg 12:49, 1977

32. Morray JP (ed): Pediatric Intensive Care. Norwalk, CT, Appleton & Lange, 1987, p 130

33. Barker SJ, Tremper KK: Pulse oximetry: applications and limitations. Anesthesiol Clin 25:155, 1987

34. Cassady G: Transcutaneous monitoring in the newborn infant. J Pediatr 103:837, 1983

35. Royall JA, Levin DL: Adult respiratory distress syndrome in pediatric patients. I. Clinical aspects, pathophysiology, pathology, and mechanisms of lung injury. J Pediatr 112:169, 1988

36. Royall JA, Levin DL: Adult respiratory distress syndrome in pediatric patients. II. Management. J Pediatr 112:335, 1988

37. Bartlett RH: Extracorporeal membrane oxygenation (ECMO) cardiopulmonary support in infancy. Trans ASAIO 22:80, 1976

38. Krummel TM, Greenfield LJ, Kirkpatrick BV, et al: Clinical use of an extracorporeal membrane oxygenation in neonatal pulmonary failure. J Pediatr Surg 17:525, 1982

39. Hirschl RB, Bartlett RH: Extracorporeal membrane oxygenation (ECMO) support in cardiorespiratory failure. Adv Surg 21:189, 1987

40. Kanter KR, Pennington DG, Weber TR: Extracorporeal membrane oxygenation for postoperative cardiac support in children. J Thorac Cardiovasc Surg 93:27, 1987

41. Keszler M, SivaSubramanian KN, Smith YA, et al: Pulmonary management during extracorporeal membrane oxygenation. Proceedings of the Fourth Annual CHNMC ECMO Symposium, February 1988, Snowmass, Colorado. Washington D.C., National Children's Medical Center

42. Bartlett RH: Personal Communication. Neonatal ECMO Registry. Ann Arbor, MI, 1988

13
Shock

_____ *Michel N. Ilbawi*

The word shock previously was applied loosely to describe a variety of life-threatening situations in which the patient manifested pallor, weakness, apathy, and poor circulation. Information gained from recent major wars and from extensive laboratory investigations helped in defining shock as a specific syndrome that can result from several etiologies but has a common and unique pathophysiology.

DEFINITION

Shock is defined as a decline in vital organ function caused by inadequate tissue oxygen delivery and metabolic exchange at the capillary level. It is a condition in which circulation fails to meet the nutritional needs of the cell and to remove metabolic wastes, resulting in an imbalance between metabolic demands and blood flow. Consequently, there are alterations in cellular function and structure and eventually cell death. Although diminished tissue perfusion in shock is preceded often by systemic hypotension, the two are not synonymous, and not all patients with low blood pressure are in shock. The hypotensive state may not last long enough for a significant diminution in tissue flow to occur, or compensatory increases in cardiac output or peripheral vascular resistance may maintain metabolic integrity. Conversely, patients in shock may not be hypotensive. Severe peripheral vasoconstriction might maintain normal systolic blood pressure at the expense of significant decrease in peripheral tissue perfusion.[1]

CLASSIFICATION

In spite of a pathophysiologic pattern common to all types of shock, this syndrome may be divided into four broad categories based on the underlying causes.

I. Hypovolemic shock (Table 13–1). The cause of inadequate systemic perfusion is related to loss of effective intravascular volume.
II. Cardiogenic shock (Table 13–2). The primary underlying cause of circulatory collapse is cardiac pump failure.
III. Septic shock. The etiology of the disturbance in circulation is related to release of endotoxins or exotoxins, with secondary changes in intermediary metabolism.
IV. Vasogenic shock (Table 13–3). The changes in circulation are brought about by specific disorders that result in decreased peripheral vascular resistance.

Although this classification is helpful in identifying the underlying causes of shock and, therefore, is essential for directing the initial treatment, it is important to emphasize that shock is caused basically either by a decrease in effective blood volume (as in types I and IV), by myocardial failure (as in type II), or by a combination of the two (as in type III). Moreover, although the etiologies vary, these different types of shock blend into one another and progress along a common pathophysiologic pathway, which, if untreated, would eventually lead to cell death.

TABLE 13–1. HYPOVOLEMIC SHOCK IN CHILDREN

A. Whole blood loss
   1. External or internal hemorrhage
B. Plasma Loss
   1. Burns
   2. Inflammation/sepsis
   3. Nephrotic syndrome
   4. Intestinal obstruction
   5. Hypoproteinemia
C. Fluid and electrolyte loss
   1. Vomiting and diarrhea
   2. Excessive sweating
   3. Pathologic renal loss
D. Endocrine causes
   1. Adrenal insufficiency
   2. Diabetes insipidus
   3. Diabetes mellitus
E. Relative losses
   1. Vasodilatation
      a. Medications, e.g., morphine
      b. Sepsis
      c. Neurogenic

TABLE 13–2. CARDIOGENIC SHOCK IN CHILDREN

A. Primary myocardial failure
   1. Idiopathic myopathies
   2. Infectious myopathies
   3. Ischemic disease
      a. Anomalous coronary arteries
      b. Kawasaki disease
   4. Obstructive or insufficiency lesions
   5. Postoperative factors
   6. Trauma
B. Arrhythmias
C. Mechanical
   1. Cardiac tamponade (fluid or air)
   2. Venae cavae obstruction
   3. Tension pneumothorax
   4. Pneumomediastinum

TABLE 13–3. VASOGENIC SHOCK IN CHILDREN

A. Spinal cord injuries
B. Anaphylactic shock
C. Neurogenic reflexes
D. Anesthetic agents

PATHOPHYSIOLOGY

Pathophysiologic Changes Common to All Types of Shock

All types of shock result in a failure of the circulation to deliver a sufficient amount of oxygen and other nutrients to satisfy the requirements of the tissues. As a consequence, shock alters cellular metabolism and energy production, which in turn leads to changes in cell function and structure. Eventually, if the shock state is not treated, the cell dies and releases proteolytic enzymes and other toxic products that further destroy the neighboring viable cells, resulting in irreversible vasodilatation, excessive permeability of the cell membrane and vascular bed, and eventual organ death.

Because of the progressive nature of these pathophysiologic events, they can be divided into two phases.

Compensated Shock. At this stage of shock, the integrity of vital organs is maintained by the different compensatory mechanisms of the body that aim at redistributing blood flow preferentially to these organs (Fig. 13–1). Among the most important of these mechanisms is catecholamine release caused by adrenergic discharge. This maintains cardiac output by increasing myocardial contractility through increasing shortening of muscle fibers and shifting the Starling curve to the left and by increasing heart rate. It also displaces the blood back to circulation by constricting the capacitant veins and venules and protects vital structures by selective systemic arteriolar vasoconstriction. Hyperventilation is another mechanism for improving cardiac output during shock. It results from direct neurogenic regulation and from progressive acidemia caused by poor peripheral perfusion. It increases the negative intrathoracic pressure and, as a consequence, displaces blood into the heart and lungs.

Other hormonal changes that accompany shock also help in sustaining vital circulation. Renal vasoconstriction from catecholamines decreases perfusion to the kidneys and leads to release of renin, activation of angiotensin mechanism, and secretion of aldosterone. This, in turn, results in retention of sodium and water and maintains blood pressure. Hypovolemia decreases the stretch on atrial wall baroreceptors and induces the release of vasopressin once 10 percent or more of blood volume is lost. Adrenal release of corticosteroids protects the integrity of the cell membrane and promotes metabolic changes necessary for organ viability. In addition, the decrease in cardiac output and the severe arteriolar vasoconstriction in shock state cause hypoperfusion of the capillary bed and lower intravascular hydrostatic pressure. This, in combination with hyperosmolality from hyperglycemia and hemoconcentration, helps to shift the fluids back into the vascular compartment from the insterstitial space.

Decompensated Shock. If the stimulus for shock persists and no attempt at controlling it is made, the shock syndrome progresses to an uncompensated state. At this stage, perfusion to vital organs is compromised. The precapillary arteriolar sphincter relaxes from excessive metabolic acidosis. Postcapillary venular constric-

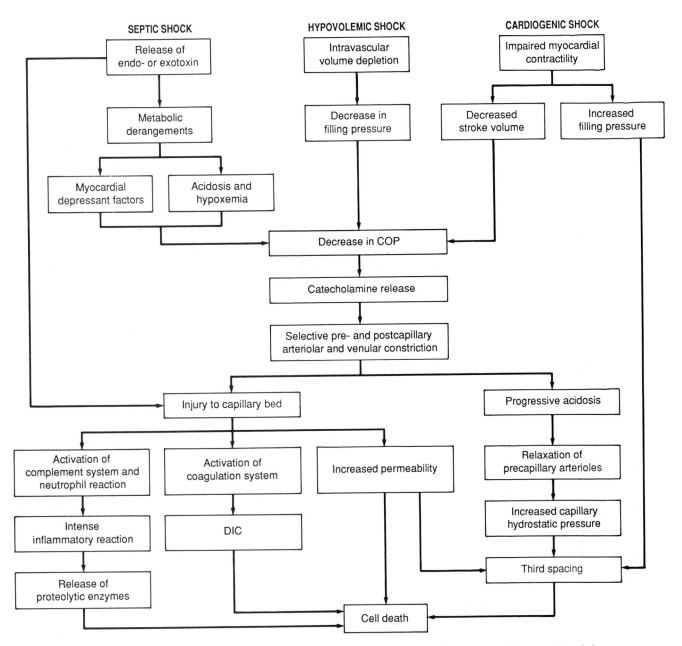

Figure 13–1. Pathophysiology of shock (COP, cardiac output; DIC, disseminated intravascular coagulopathy).

tion, however, continues. Consequently, capillary hydrostatic pressure increases, leading to loss of fluids into the interstitial space across the already injured capillary membrane.[2] Resting cell membrane potentials decrease because of lack of adenosine triphosphate (ATP) production, and sodium and fluids move into the cell, causing further cell dysfunction and fluid depletion of the intravascular space. Damaged cells release their toxic contents, including myocardial depressant substances, which exaggerate the shock state by causing myocardial dysfunction. Ischemic or toxic injury to endothelium leads to activation of clotting mechanism and disseminated

intravascular coagulopathy (DIC), which usually indicates an irreversible terminal stage.

Specific Pathophysiology and Clinical Picture of Different Types of Shock

Hypovolemic Shock. The most common type of shock encountered by surgeons, hypovolemic shock, is caused by loss of blood or any other body fluids in quantities sufficient to reduce venous return to the heart and, therefore, decrease cardiac output. The loss of fluid may be apparent, as in external bleeding or gastrointestinal hemorrhage, or may be less appreciated, as in evaporation from skin after burns, profuse sweating, or infiltration into the traumatized muscle. Peritonitis, pancreatitis, or intestinal obstruction may result in severe loss of protein-rich fluids into the retroperitoneal space or intestine, resulting in severe hemoconcentration with a fall in intravascular volume. Disease of the endocrine glands, such as uncontrolled diabetes mellitus (water and salt loss), diabetes insipidus (free water loss), or adrenal insufficiency (salt loss), can cause varying degrees of hypovolemic shock.

In mild hypovolemia (loss of 10 percent or less of blood volume), the clinical signs are related primarily to adrenergic constriction of cutaneous blood vessels. Skin is pale, extremities are cool with damp sweat, and the superficial veins are collapsed. Adequate compensatory mechanisms usually maintain cardiac output, and the urine output, blood pressure, and sensorum are not grossly affected.

In moderate hypovolemia (10 to 20 percent), there is a definite decrease in cardiac output and blood pressure despite generalized vasoconstriction and increased levels of renin–angiotensin and antidiuretic hormones. Dysfunction of the kidneys becomes apparent, and urine output decreases. Tachycardia and hyperventilation are obvious, and the patient is diaphoretic, apprehensive, and restless.

In severe hypovolemia (loss of more than 20 percent), the pulse becomes thready and weak. The blood pressure is low, and urine output stops. The child becomes agitated, restless, or obtunded.

Cardiogenic Shock. Cardiogenic shock is the state in which an abnormality of cardiac function is responsible for failure of the cardiovascular system to meet the metabolic needs of the body. The common denominator is depressed cardiac output as a result of decreased myocardial contractility, mechanical factors affecting heart performance, or arrhythmias. A frequent cause of cardiogenic shock in children is impaired performance after intracardiac surgery and is associated with significant mortality and morbidity in the early postoperative period. Other causes of cardiac decompensation in pediatric patients are dysrhythmias, drug intoxication, hypoxic or ischemic episode, acidemia, hypothermia, hypoglycemia, and primary or secondary myopathies. Extrinsic inflow or outflow obstruction, such as tension pneumothorax, pneumopericardium, pneumomediastinum, and pericardial tamponade, can lead to profound cardiac dysfunction.[3] Intrinsic congenital obstructive or insufficiency lesions, such as severe aortic stenosis or congenital mitral insufficiency, might lead to myocardial fibrosis and decompensation if timely treatment is not instituted.

As in other types of shock, the low output of the failing heart initiates the previously mentioned compensatory responses. These responses, however, have more deleterious effects in patients with cardiogenic rather than other forms of shock. The increase in pulmonary and systemic vascular resistance they produce leads to a significant rise in ventricular work and oxygen consumption of an already compromised myocardium, depresses further the cardiac function, and accelerates tissue injury. The severe peripheral vasoconstriction also results in metabolic acidosis, which exaggerates myocardial failure. Compensatory mechanisms also exaggerate sodium and water retention, which increases the preload (ventricular filling) and causes cardiac distention and impairment of subendocardial perfusion.

Because of this self-perpetuating cycle, compensated phases of cardiogenic shock rarely are observed, and frequently only one cardiorespiratory pattern, in varying degrees of severity, is seen.[4] The patients have poor peripheral perfusion, with pallor or cold sweat. They are apprehensive or agitated, with low blood pressure and urine output, tachycardia, and tachypnea. Cardiac output is decreased, but the venous pressure or pulmonary wedge pressures are high. Systemic and pulmonary vascular resistance is elevated.

Septic Shock. Septic shock is frequent and is associated with high mortality in children.[5] It is caused by microorganisms or their products in the blood. In the majority of cases, it is caused by gram-negative bacilli. Occasionally, however, gram-positive bacterial, rickettsial, fungal, or viral infections can lead to sepsis. In 10 to 20 percent of patients, no site or etiology for infection is firmly established.

The precise mechanism(s) causing circulatory collapse in septic shock is not well delineated. It is primarily related to endotoxin release (a lipopolysaccharide with a molecular weight of 10^6) and its effect on different organs.[6,7] Among these effects is derangement of intermediary metabolism, with inability to use existing metabolic substrates effectively and resultant energy failure.[8,9] Another effect is increased arteriovenous shunting, impaired oxyhemoglobin dissociation, and direct depression of cellular respiration at the mitochondrial level.[10] These events cause a decrease in oxygen consumption and result in anaerobic glycolysis with lactate production and metabolic acidosis, which is a hallmark of impending sepsis.[11] A third effect of endotoxins, mediated by the Hageman factor, is the production of secondary metabolites from activated protein cascade systems. These include complement, coagulation, and bradykinin systems.[12–14] Complement activation results in the generation of anaphylotoxins and intense inflammatory reaction. Initiation of coagulation and fibrinolysis cascades leads to DIC, with resultant consumption of clotting factors and tissue ischemia. Formation of bradykinins exaggerates the inflammatory process and causes vasodilatation. A fourth effect of endotoxins, which is also a hallmark of septic shock, is endotoxin-incited hormonal and cellular insults to the vascular endothelium.[15] This results in a diffuse capillary permeability as manifested by total body vascular leak. The transcapillary escape rate of albumin may rise by more than 300 percent and can result in significant intravascular volume depletion.[16]

Thus, the various initial manifestations of gram-negative or gram-positive sepsis do not relate to a perfusion defect but rather to metabolic and toxic derangement.[17] However, the shock state that appears subsequently is caused by intravascular volume depletion, peripheral vasodilatation, and myocardial depression, all of which are secondary to the endotoxemia. The differences in presentation of gram-positive shock from that of gram-negative shock are minor and reflect only different hemodynamic and clinical manifestations of the same pathophysiology.

The clinical picture that characterizes septic shock in humans varies considerably but, in general, has two phases. The earlier hyperdynamic phase, or warm shock, is characterized by irritability, confusion, feeding difficulties, warm and dry extremities, oliguria, hyperventilation, hypoxemia, respiratory alkalosis, metabolic acidosis, hypothermia, or fever.[17,18] The cardiac output is increased, systemic vascular resistance is low because of peripheral vasodilatation and arteriovenous shunting, and there is venous pooling in the peripheral and splanchnic circulation. Despite the increase in cardiac output, tissue injury continues secondary to impaired cellular metabolism. Increased capillary permeability leads to intravascular volume depletion and progressive elevation in systemic vascular resistance. This, in addition to myocardial ischemia from impaired metabolism, sets the stage for the second phase of septic shock, the hypodynamic phase, or cold shock. The latter is characterized by cold extremities, poor peripheral perfusion, poor pulses, diminished urine output, hypotension, and narrow pulse pressure. Cardiac output is decreased, and systemic and pulmonary vascular resistance is elevated. Progressive respiratory failure with depressed neural function appears, and this cycle of poor tissue perfusion, decreased oxygen use, and myocardial dysfunction leads to progressive acidosis, multiple organ failure, and eventual death. Variables that determine at which phase septic shock becomes obvious include the duration of sepsis (warm shock occurs only in the very early phase of endotoxemia), the status of intravascular volume at the onset of sepsis (hypovolemic patients are likely to manifest the second phase directly), and the type of causative organism (the first phase is more likely to appear with gram-negative rather than gram-positive organisms).

Vasogenic Shock. Vasogenic shock is brought about by specific disorders in systemic vascular resistance. There is a decrease in arteriolar resistance (tone) and pooling of the blood in the periphery, especially the systemic venules and small veins. Right ventricular filling pressure decreases, and as a result the stroke volume and systemic cardiac output drop. Spinal cord injuries cause a decrease in vascular tone secondary to loss of sympathetic control. Neurogenic reflexes precipitated by acute pain produce profound peripheral pooling of blood. Several medications, including vasodilators, dilate systemic and pulmonary vascular beds. Anaphylactic shock, a hypersensitivity reaction to certain medications or compounds to which the patient has been sensitized, is one form of vasogenic shock caused by a sudden release of potent chemical mediators and vasodilators. These include histamine, leukotreins, kallikreins, and serotonin.[19] The resultant peripheral pooling, increased vascular permeability, bronchial constriction, and negative inotropic action lead to profound cardiopulmonary decompensation. Autonomic dysfunctional states, such as Shy-Drager syndrome, constitute a special form of vasogenic shock. Characteristically, most of the patients with vasogenic shock remain warm and vasodilated, at least in the initial phases.

Effect of Shock on Other Organs

Shock, regardless of etiology, is a multiorgan disease. Prolonged, profound, or poorly treated shock may result in transient or permanent damage to any organ. The organ injury tends to be progressive and interrelative, such that worsening function of one organ affects multiple systems.[1] It is these complications that may eventually be the cause of death in patients with shock.

Myocardium. Untreated shock, regardless of etiology, will cause reduced cardiac function because of the poor tolerance of the heart to diminished perfusion and ischemia. This is because autoregulatory mechanisms for coronary blood flow are lost when mean arterial pressure drops below 50 to 60 torr, at which point coronary flow becomes solely dependent on arterial pressure.[20] Significant and sustained drop in coronary perfusion leads to severe cardiac derangement and depletion of glycogen stores. The glycolytic state shifts the myocardium from lactate use to lactate production. Moreover, a variety of substances released from damaged tissue during shock and labeled as myocardial depressant factors (MDF) have been identified as causing a significant reduction in myocardial contractility.[21] In addition, intracellular acidosis and increased afterload from peripheral vasoconstriction can result in, or exaggerate, pump failure.

Lungs. The pathophysiology of respiratory distress syndrome, seem frequently after shock, starts with ischemic injury or endotoxin insult to the endothelium of pulmonary capillaries. Subsequent complement activation and leukocytes and platelet aggregation lead to intravascular coagulopathy and intense inflammatory reaction, with release of neutrophil by-products of phagocytosis, release of proteolytic enzymes, and destruction of collagen and fibronectin.[22] Humoral mediators, such as bradykinins, kallikreins, leukotreins, and tissue thromboplastin, exaggerate vascular permeability. Increased capillary leak causes alveolar atelectasis and interstitial pulmonary edema, with consequent decrease in lung compliance and signifiant arteriovenous shunting. Hormonal factors, such as prostaglandins and thromboxane, may contribute to cell damage. Qualitative and quantitative injury to pulmonary surfactant further impairs the function of gas exchange units. High concentrations of inspired oxygen and barotrauma from mechanical ventilation exaggerate the parenchymal destruction.[23] Increased lung water, hypoxemia, and acidosis result in pulmonary vasoconstriction and increased pulmonary vascular resistance.

Clinically, respiratory distress syndrome follows a period of apparent stability of the cardiovascular system. It is characterized by progressive hypoxemia, tachypnea, and increased respiratory effort over and above that secondary to lactic acidemia.[24] Later, diffuse respiratory rales and rapidly progressive signs of interstitial and intraalveolar infiltrates appear. The correct diagnosis of permeability pulmonary edema is made by measuring a low or normal left atrial or pulmonary wedge pressure in combination with a high protein content of the edema fluid.[25] These findings establish that the edema is pulmonary, not cardiac, in origin. Evaluation reveals a progressive decrease in pulmonary compliance, increased respiratory dead space, and increased pulmonary arteriovenous shunting, as evidenced by a progressive rise in airway pressure and a fall in arterial Po_2.

Kidneys. Ischemic injury is the cause of renal manifestations seen in shock, namely, oliguria and subsequent renal failure. In general, the more pronounced and long-lasting the hypotension associated with shock, the more likely that ischemic renal injury will occur. Structural factors implicated in the pathogenesis of renal failure seen experimentally include leakage of filtrate through damaged tubular endothelium, tubular obstruction with debris and casts, and tubular necrosis.[26] Despite reversal of the shock state, significant renal failure might persist for several days or weeks afterward. Ultimate recovery of renal function, however, is the usual outcome if early hemodynamic stability is achieved.

Nervous System. The decrease in cerebral perfusion pressure from hypotension and acidemia-induced hypocarbia results in progressive decrease in cerebral blood flow and subsequent cerebral hypoxia. This leads to confusion, restlessness, decreased responses, and if

untreated, cerebrovascular accident and permanent brain damage. In infants and small children, intracranial bleeding may occur because of shock-induced DIC.

Gastrointestinal Tract. Severe vasoconstriction from shock decreases perfusion and leads to injury to the intestinal mucosa, which is extremely sensitive to ischemic insult. Initially, ileus occurs, followed by distention and, later, sequestration of large amounts of fluids intramurally.[27] Ischemic injury to gastrointestinal mucosa also allows absorption of bacterial toxins and may lead to sloughing, bleeding, or perforation. Oxygen-free radicals liberated after reversal of ischemia may cause further damage to the intestinal mucosa. Hypoxia and hypotension impair the function of the reticuloendothelial tissue in the liver, predisposing the patient to the risk of infection.[28]

MANAGEMENT OF PATIENTS WITH SHOCK

Once the diagnosis of shock is made, monitoring and therapy must be designed to stabilize and support all involved organs. When a patient has shock, the surgeon may not be able to determine the etiology initially. Even without that knowledge, progress in treatment along certain guidelines should be instituted without delay. Investigations into the etiology should proceed simultaneously with treatment.

Assessment of Patient with Shock

The best initial method of evaluating patients in shock is careful examination. The moisture of mucous membranes and skin turgor reflect the degree of dehydration. The central pulses permit an estimate of arterial pressure, stroke volume, heart rate, and rhythm. The peripheral pulses and skin temperature allow an assessment of cardiac output and vasoconstriction. Discrepancy between the rectal and toe temperatures indicates severe vasoconstriction and heralds the onset of significant decrease in cardiac output. The degree of distention of neck veins reflects the right ventricular filling pressure.

Establishing Secure Intravenous Access

Securing a good intravenous catheter is the most essential step in the early management of pediatric patients in shock. Such access, however, could be difficult in the small pediatric patient, especially a child with severe vasoconstriction. Aggressive use of more central veins, such as the femoral or jugular veins, could be lifesaving.

Assessment of Adequacy of Ventilation

Patients in shock may have inadequate respiratory effort and significant arteriovenous shunting, resulting in hypoxemia and hypercarbia. Supplementary oxygen with or without mechanical ventilation should be provided when needed.

Hemodynamic Monitoring

Adequate monitoring generates information that serves the following purposes: (1) it defines the exact cardiorespiratory status and thus helps in diagnosis and treatment, (2) it permits continuous assessment of vital organs, (3) it evaluates response to therapy, and (4) it helps in early detection of complications. *All* patients in shock should have continuous electrocardiographic display, heart rate monitor, skin or core temperature recording, and intraarterial systemic blood pressure and pulse wave displays. The sphygmomanometer is not helpful in monitoring patients in shock,[29] since it tends to underestimate the blood pressure in the severely vasoconstricted child. Doppler assessment of pulses may allow more accurate measurement of systolic blood pressure. The information obtained from arterial pressure tracings is helpful not only in determining blood pressure but also in assessing grossly the changes in cardiac output (reflected by the area under the pressure curve) and the systemic vascular resistance (reflected by diastolic and mean pressures). The intraarterial catheter also provides quick access to blood sampling.

Central venous pressure should be measured using a long catheter placed into the superior or inferior vena cava. It provides information on the status of intravascular volume in patients without known cardiac or pulmonary disease. However, it often does not reflect the left ventricular function reliably. In patients with left ventricular failure, for example, central venous pressure might be normal in spite of an elevated left ventricular filling pressure. Conversely, the central venous pressure might be extremely high in obstructive airway disease (e.g., asthma), pulmonary vascular disease (primary or secondary pulmonary hypertension), or right ventricular dysfunction despite a normal or even low left atrial pressure.

The use of a balloon-tipped Swan-Ganz catheter in selected pediatric patients can give information essential for diagnosis of hemodynamic derangement in shock. It provides assessment of pulmonary artery wedge pressure, which is usually equal to left ventricular filling pressure except in mitral valve disease or pulmonary hypertension. It also facilitates measurement of cardiac output, oxygen saturation in mixed venous blood, and pulmonary and systemic vascular resistance.[1,30] It is even more helpful in guiding treatment and evaluating the response to different therapeutic interventions.

A Foley catheter to measure urine output accurately should be a part of monitoring patients with shock. Changes in cardiac output are accompanied by changes in urine output.

Two-dimensional echocardiographic and Doppler studies in patients with circulatory collapse can evaluate noninvasively myocardial contractility, ventricular filling pressure, aortic blood flow velocity (reflects changes in systemic cardiac output), and the presence of mechanical problems (such as tamponade).[31]

Serial blood gas determinations can reveal the presence of progressive metabolic or respiratory acidosis and assess the adequacy of ventilation. Lactate levels have been found to be helpful in following a patient in shock and in determining the ultimate prognosis.[32,33]

THERAPEUTIC APPROACH TO SHOCK

The aim of treatment in shock is to improve oxygen and nutrient delivery to the cells. This is accomplished by optimizing blood oxygen content, preload (or myocardial end-diastolic fiber length, determined by the filling volume as related to systemic or pulmonary venous return and estimated by measuring the right and left atrial pressure), myocardial contractility, and afterload (ventricular wall tension during systole, dictated by systemic and pulmonary vascular resistance). From the therapeutic point of view, the etiology of shock can be divided into three major categories: (1) decreased effective intravascular volume, (2) pump failure, and (3) a combination of both (Fig. 13–2).

Decrease in Effective Intravascular Volume

Decrease in effective intravascular volume could be caused by hemorrhagic shock, by increased permeability of septic shock, or by peripheral pooling of septic or vasomotor shock. In these patients, the filling pressures (right and left atrial pressures) are low, the heart size is normal, pulmonary vascularity is decreased on chest x-ray, and the liver is not enlarged. Resuscitation of this category of patients should be aimed primarily at reexpanding the blood and plasma volumes and rehydrating the interstitial space and the cellular compartment.

Intravascular volume is best normalized by administration of whole blood. The red blood cells in blood help in the much needed oxygen delivery to the tissues. Plasma proteins in the transfused blood help to increase the oncotic pressure and thus minimize extravasation of fluids and third-spacing. Hematocrits of 35 to 40 percent are most desirable; higher values increase blood viscosity and impair microcirculation. Blood substitutes, when blood is not available or the hematocrit is inadequate, include crystalloid (saline or lactated Ringer's solution) or colloid (albumin, plasma, hetastarch, or dextran) solutions. Selection among these alternatives can be guided by answering the following questions: What type of fluid has been lost and what is its composition? What are the specific underlying pathophysiologic problems

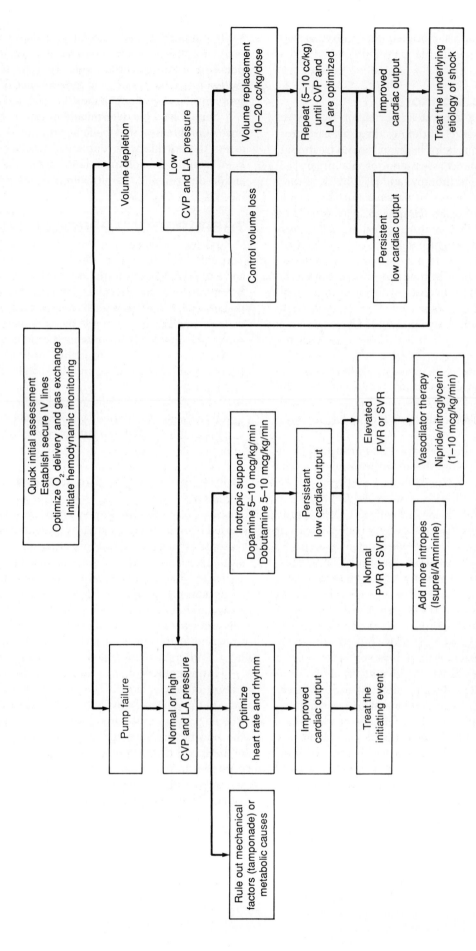

Figure 13-2. Approach to the child in shock (CVP, central venous pressure; LA, left atrial; PVR, pulmonary vascular resistance; SVR, systemic vascular resistance).

of the patient? What are the advantages and disadvantages of the different resuscitation fluids?

The crystalloid solutions in common use are normal saline and Ringer's lactate solution. These fluids remain in the intravascular space only temporarily before passing into the interstitium. As little as 20 percent of the administered fluid remains intravascularly after 4 hours, and thus up to two to five times the amount of volume actually lost has to be given for replacement.[34] Moreover, these fluids, normally restricted to extracellular space, enter the cell during shock because of failure of the cell membrane pump and cause intracellular swelling. Use of lactated solutions in patients with impaired liver function may increase blood lactate and lead to acid-base imbalance. Recently, hypertonic saline solution (sodium concentration in excess of 180 mEq/L) has been used in shock resuscitation. It increases serum osmolality and induces movement of intracellular water into the extracellular space.[35] Its use in pediatric patients has not been established yet, although it is being evaluated in the resuscitation of severely burned children.[4,35]

Available colloid solutions include albumin (5 percent and 25 percent in normal saline), dextran (40 and 70 in normal saline or 5 percent dextrose solution), and hydroxyethyl starch (6 percent solution in normal saline). They contain large molecules that do not pass through the capillary membrane under usual circumstances. As a result, they increase colloid oncotic pressure and achieve and sustain the desired filling pressure quickly and more efficiently. However, numerous studies have demonstrated that these large molecules do leak out of the circulation and exaggerate interstitial edema when the capillary membrane is damaged in the later stages of shock.[36] In addition, they may not correct all of the functional extracellular fluid deficit and may increase the incidence of renal failure and respiratory distress syndrome.[37] Moreover, some of these solutions have complications of their own. Albumin is expensive. Plasma carries the risk of hepatitis and other blood-transmitted diseases. Dextran can cause coagulopathy by decreasing platelet function, nephropathy, or anaphylaxis. Hetastarch, an amylopectin in which hydroxyethyl groups are substituted, seems to be the best plasma expander. It is inexpensive and safe. However, clinical experience with Hetastarch in children is still inconclusive.[38]

Although several studies have demonstrated successful resuscitation using either crystalloid or colloid solutions, the choice of the ideal fluid for volume replacement remains unsettled and is best judged by evaluating the type of fluid lost.[20,39,40] In patients with uncomplicated hypovolemia, a balanced crystalloid solution, in addition to red cells if needed, provides the best volume expansion. The use of colloids is reserved for cases where intravascular volume cannot be maintained with the use of crystalloids alone.

The amount of fluids necessary to restore effective circulating blood volume depends on the preceding deficit and rate of ongoing loss. It is usually more than the estimated loss because of the expanded capacity of the vascular space and dysfunction of cellular membranes.[41] Enough fluid must be given to achieve adequate intravascular volume and to ensure that one determinant of cardiac performance, namely, the filling pressure, has been optimally maximized. In cases of hypovolemia uncomplicated by myocardial dysfunction, fluid resuscitation should be initiated at 10 to 20 ml/kg of fluids per dose and repeated until the patient's blood pressure and heart rate are stabilized, the urine output is adequate (0.5 to 1.0 ml/kg/hour), or the central venous pressure is about 10 to 12 torr and the left atrial pressure (pulmonary artery wedge pressure) is 12 to 14 torr. Lack of significant improvement after what seems to be adequate volume replacement may indicate the presence of associated cardiac failure, and the focus of therapy should shift to pharmacologic manipulation of myocardial contractility.

Pump Failure

The other main cause of shock is pump failure or myocardial failure with inability of the heart to deliver adequate cardiac output in spite of what seems to be optimal preload or filling pressure. This could result from primary myocardial disease, such as in myopathies, congenital heart disease, and coronary artery disease, or be secondary to myocardial depressant factors frequently released in septic or other types of shock.[21] Occasionally, mechanical factors or arrhythmias can decrease cardiac output. The goals of therapy in pump failure are to optimize heart rate, achieve appropriate preload (filling pressure), improve myocardial contractility, and optimize the afterload (systemic vascular resistance).

Administration of antiarrhythmic medications or the use of cardiac pacing or chronotropic drugs restores the normal cardiac rhythm and eliminates brady- or tachyarrhythmias. Achieving adequate filling pressure is accomplished by fluid replacement and is assessed by measurement of right and left atrial pressures. Because of the many factors that affect the absolute measurements of central venous pressure and pulmonary artery wedge pressure, the best use of these values is in evaluating the changes they undergo with fluid challenge. Slow increases in atrial pressures with fluid replacement signal that the optimal filling pressure has not been reached and there is a place for administration of more fluids. On the other hand, rapid increases in these measurements with small fluid challenges indicate limitations in cardiac compliance and signal optimal filling pressure.[42]

Persistence of low cardiac output in spite of adequate preload implies myocardial dysfunction and the necessity for use of inotropic agents to augment myocardial contractility. Among the inotropic agents used for the treatment of myocardial failure and decreased contractility in children is isoproterenol (Isuprel), which is a beta-$_1$- and beta-$_2$-agonist. It increases myocardial fiber shortening and wall tension (inotropic action). It also increases heart rate (chronotropic action) and reduces peripheral vascular resistance by dilating primarily skeletal muscle arterioles.[43] This dual action, namely, improvement in contractility and reduction in afterload, makes isoproterenol an ideal inotrope. However, the marked increase in myocardial oxygen consumption and the decrease in ventricular filling time (from tachycardia) it produces limit its widespread use.[6,44] Dobutamine hydrochloride (Dobutrex) is another agent, which, at doses of 1 to 10 μg/kg/minute, increases myocardial contractility, thus increasing cardiac output and decreasing ventricular filling pressure. It also decreases peripheral and pulmonary vascular resistance with little change in arterial pressure, heart rate, and renal or hepatic blood flow.[44,45] Higher doses of dobutamine (12 to 20 μg/kg/minute) produce a biphasic vasoconstriction–vasodilatation response and may impair renal blood flow.

Dopamine hydrochloride, a third inotropic agent, is among the most commonly used. In small doses (1 to 5 μg/kg/minute), it increases renal, mesenteric, cerebral and coronary blood flow, a distinct advantage in patients with shock. At slightly higher doses (5 to 10 μg/kg/minute), it increases cardiac contractility through beta-$_1$-adrenergic stimulation but without affecting heart rate. At still higher doses (10 to 15 μg/kg/minute), it increases peripheral vasoconstriction by stimulating the alpha-adrenergic receptors and thus might be harmful to patients in shock who are already maximally vasoconstricted. Amrinone lactate (Inocor), a recently introduced inotrope, is a bipyridine derivative with strong positive inotropic effects. Unlike other inotropes, it does not exert its action through beta-$_1$ receptors but rather through inhibition of phosphodiasterase enzyme, with subsequent accumulation of cAMP and potentiation of calcium delivery to the contractile elements of the myocardium. Its main advantages include its potent concomitant peripheral and pulmonry vasodilatation as well as lack of increase in myocardial oxygen consumption.

Digitalis glycosides, used frequently in the past to augment myocardial contractility in the failing heart, tend to be ineffective in the management of acute cardiac dysfunction. Because of the availability of more specific inotropic agents, digitalis is rarely used in acute shock. A less commonly used but very important inotrope is epinephrine hydrochloride. It has potent alpha- and beta-receptors action and, therefore, increases both stroke volume and peripheral and pulmonary vascular resistance, as well as myocardial oxygen consumption. For this reason, epinephrine has been largely supplanted by new agents that are more selective. Its current use in shock is limited mainly to anaphylactic shock, where it decreases bronchospasm and counteracts the pooling of blood in the periphery.[46]

The choice of the appropriate inotrope for patients with cardiogenic failure depends on the individual clinical situation. There is no usual drug or dose in shock; therapy should be continually tailored to the patient's response (Table 13–4). In general, the combination of dopamine in doses of 5 to 10 μg/kg/minute and dobutamine in doses of 5 to 10 μg/kg/minute provides a very effective initial therapy and produces a greater increase in cardiac output and arterial pressure than could be produced by either agent alone. The combination improves myocardial contractility and results in pulmonary, peripheral, and renal vasodilatation with minimal, if any, peripheral vasoconstriction.[47] Persistence of myocardial failure in spite of maximal therapy with dopamine and dobutamine signals significant cardiac decompensation. The addition of isoproterenol if the patient is not severely tachycardic, or preferably amrinone, would further improve myocardial function and decrease the afterload of an already compromised heart.

Special clinical situations may dictate the choice of inotrope. In patients with low cardiac output from severe pulmonary hypertension, such as in newborns with diaphragmatic hernia, avoidance of dopamine in high doses (more than 5 μg/kg/minute) is advisable, since this inotrope could exaggerate the existing pulmonary arteriolar vasoconstriction. Dobutamine, with or without isoproterenol, and amrinone are better choices. In contrast, shock states with marked peripheral vasodilatation (septic or anaphylactic shock) may benefit from the alpha-receptor stimulation and the splanchnic and renal vasodilatation produced by moderate doses of dopamine.[48] On the other hand, in children with significant peripheral vasoconstriction and elevated systemic vascular resistance, dobutamine, amrinone, and isoproterenol are preferable, since they combine the inotropic action with the much-needed peripheral vasodilatation.[49] Isoproterenol usually is contraindicated in cardiogenic shock caused by inadequate coronary blood flow, such as in children with anomalous coronary arteries, because of the significant increase in oxygen consumption it produces.

Persistence of the shock state in spite of adequate filling pressure (preload) and maximal inotropic support may be because of elevated systemic or pulmonary vascular resistance (afterload). Since the dysfunctional ventricle has a decreased ability to increase its contractility against elevated resistance produced by the compensatory mechanisms of shock, reducing the afterload becomes critically important, and vasodilator therapy is

TABLE 13–4. COMMONLY USED INOTROPES

Drug	Mechanism	Usual Dose	Comment
Isoproterenol	Beta agonist	0.05–0.5 µg/kg/min	Inotropic and chronotropic action; peripheral vasodilator; causes arrhythmias and increases myocardial O_2 consumption
Dobutamine	Beta agonist	1–10 µg/kg/min	Inotropic with minimal chronotropic effect (B_1); mild B_2 activity (peripheral vasodilatation); minimal vasoconstriction of pulmonary vascular bed
Dopamine	Alpha and beta agonist Dopaminergic	1–12 µg/kg/min	Small doses—renal vasodilatation; moderate doses—primarily B_1 and B_2 stimulator; can cause pulmonary hypertension
Amrinone	Phosphodiasterase inhibitor	5–15 µg/kg/min	Potent inotrope; no increase in myocardial O_2 consumption; concomitant vasodilatation
Epinephrine	Alpha and beta agonist	0.05–1.0 µg/kg/min	Strong inotropic and chronotropic action; peripheral vasoconstriction; counteracts peripheral pooling of vasogenic shock; increases myocardial O_2 consumption

indicated.[50] Under these circumstances, systemic and pulmonary arteriolar relaxation induced by vasodilators results in an increase in ejection fraction, an increase in stroke volume, and a decrease in systolic ventricular volume and allows the heart to pump more efficiently. Venous relaxation from vasodilators, on the other hand, reduces ventricular filling pressure, decreases myocardial distention, improves coronary perfusion during diastole, and decreases myocardial oxygen consumption.[4] In general, the anticipated improvement in cardiac output often offsets the hypotension that might be associated with vasodilators, and as a result, peripheral, cerebral, and coronary perfusion is maintained. Occasionally, however, excessive hypotension from venous pooling or excessive arteriolar relaxation might result from the use

of dilators and could be readily reversed with administration of fluids.

The mechanism and the site of action vary considerably among the available vasodilators (Table 13–5). Selection of the proper dilator for a particular patient depends on whether persistence of low cardiac output is caused by elevation of pulmonary or systemic vascular resistance or both. Among the most commonly used vasodilators is sodium nitroprusside. It has a short duration of activity that allows titration of the appropriate dose.[51] In doses of 1 to 10 µg/kg/minute, it causes equal dilatation of the systemic and pulmonary arterioles and leads to progressive decrease in arterial impedance. It also causes dilatation of capacitant vessels and therefore a decrease in ventricular filling pressure. However, sodium nitro-

TABLE 13–5. COMMONLY USED VASODILATORS

Drug	Mechanism	Usual Dose	Comment
Sodium nitroprusside	Smooth muscle relaxant	0.5–8.0 µg/kg/min	Balanced arterial and venous dilator; may cause ventilation/perfusion mismatch; toxic, especially in infants; can cause platelet dysfunction
Nitroglycerin	Smooth muscle relaxant	1–10 µg/kg/min	Primarily venodilator and pulmonary vasodilator in small doses (1–3 µg/kg/min); balanced arterial and pulmonary vasodilatation 3–10 µg/kg/min; tachyphylaxis after prolonged use; adsorbs to polyvinylchloride tubing
Amrinone	Smooth muscle relaxant	5–15 µg/kg/min	Balanced pulmonary and arterial vasodilatation; direct inotropic effect; can cause liver toxicity and thrombocytopenia
Hydralazine	Smooth muscle relaxant	0.1–0.5 µg/kg every 3–6 hr	Pure systemic and pulmonary arterial dilator; not for continuous IV use
Priscoline	Histamine release; alpha antagonist	1 mg/kg/dose 1–2 mg/kg/hr	Preferential pulmonary vasodilator; can cause hyperacidity; decreases renal blood flow

prusside can be toxic, especially in infants and small children, and could result in cyanide poisoning and platelet dysfunction. Another frequently used dilator is nitroglycerin, which has action similar to nitroprusside but with less side effects.[52] In small doses (1 to 5 μg/kg/minute), it causes more pulmonary than systemic vasodilatation and, therefore, is very helpful in patients with pulmonary hypertension.[53] At higher doses (5 to 10 μg/kg/minute), however, it provides equal afterload reduction in both systemic and pulmonary vascular beds. It has the distinct advantage of selective coronary vasodilatation and augmentation of effective coronary blood flow. A third vasodilator, amrinone, is becoming more popular. Its effectiveness in pediatric patients with pulmonary hypertension and its concomitant inotropic action make its use very attractive in certain shock states in children. Tolazoline (Priscoline) is a potent pulmonary vasodilator, which exerts its action through histamine release. It can cause gastric acid hypersecretion and may lead to gastrointestinal bleeding or perforation. It offers no advantage over nitroprusside or nitroglycerin. Alpha-adrenergic antagonists, such as phentolamine and phenoxybenzanine, have been used occasionally to counteract the severe vasoconstriction from excessive sympathetic responses seen in shock.[54] Their use, however, has not proved to be effective or more useful than other commonly available dilators.

Cardiac tamponade caused by high intrapericardial pressure from accumulation of air or fluid in the pericardial sac is a special form of pump failure. Its definitive treatment is prompt drainage. However, temporary emergency treatment may include administration of fluids and catecholamine support.[55]

Occasionally, the underlying etiology of the shock state may be due to a combination of pump failure and a decrease in effective blood volume. This condition is most commonly seen in septic shock and in some cases of cardiogenic shock. The therapeutic approach to patients with this combination consists of fluid replacement and treatment of myocardial dysfunction as outlined previously.

Other Therapeutic Interventions

Alpha-adrenergic Agonists. These medications (such as norepinephrine) increase arteriolar resistance and do not necessarily improve tissue perfusion. Their use at the present time is limited to situations where adrenergic tone of the peripheral vascular bed is markedly decreased, as in vasomotor shock. Under these circumstances, administration of alpha-agonists increases the perfusion pressure and improves circulation to vital organs.

Antibiotics. After obtaining appropriate cultures, empiric broad-spectrum bactericidal parenteral antibiotics should be started immediately to enhance survival. They are indicated primarily in patients with septic shock and should be begun using maximum dosages as dictated by the patient's renal and hepatic function. The choice of antimicrobial agent is determined by the spectrum of organisms likely to cause sepsis in the patient's age group. An aminoglycoside with a cephalosporin or penicillinase-resistant penicillin is sufficient in most pediatric surgical patients. The development of new antibiotics recently, such as beta-lactam compounds, with their wide range of antibacterial activity has added to the unsolved controversy of whether the concomitant use of several potent broad-spectrum medications with synergistic action is indicated in patients with gram-negative sepsis.[56] This combination therapy is indicated at present for patients with sepsis secondary to *Pseudomonas aeruginosa* but is not uniformly accepted for other forms of sepsis. The use of clindomycin (Cleocin), metroidazole (Flagyl), or imipenem-cilastatin (Primaxin) for treatment of anaerobic bacteria should be considered in certain gastrointestinal or abdominal infections even though such organisms have not been cultured. Intravenous antifungal treatment might be needed in immunosuppressed patients after organ transplantation because of their susceptibility to *Candida* infections.

Sodium Bicarbonate. Metabolic acidosis is common in shock because of inadequate tissue perfusion. Adverse effects of acidosis include impaired ventilatory response, depressed myocardial function, dysrhythmias, and altered response of autonomic receptors to drugs. Correction is indicated when the pH is less than 7.25. Sodium bicarbonate is given at 1 to 2 mEq/kg and repeated to achieve a pH of more than 7.25. Rapid administration of bicarbonate should be avoided, since it causes a sudden shift in brain and myocardial pH, impairs oxygen delivery to the tissues, and predisposes to intraventricular bleeding in newborns.

Corticosteroids. The use of steroids in shock remains controversial. Evidence supporting their beneficial action is experimental and based on administration of large doses before the onset of shock. Under these circumstances, these drugs stabilize lysosomal and cell membranes, inhibit complement-induced granulocyte aggregation, improve myocardial performance, modulate the release of endogenous opiates, and promote a rightward shift in the oxyhemoglobin dissociation curve.[57] The use of steroids in human subjects, however, has yielded contradictory results and is considered by some as harmful. High doses of corticosteroids (dexamethasone 3 mg/kg or methyl prednisolone 30 mg/kg intravenously) may be justifiable only if given early in the course of septic shock. They are not of proven benefit in other types of shock.

Calcium. Marked decrease in ionizable calcium occurs frequently with any acute hemodynamic deterioration regardless of etiology. The exact underlying cause is unknown but could be related to hypoxic insult to the parathyroid gland. Persistent hypocalcemia can cause significant myocardial dysfunction, acidosis, temperature instability, and motor nerve excitability.[58] Treatment is indicated when the serum ionized calcium level falls below 2.4 mg percent. The dose is 10 to 20 mg/kg given slowly and repeated every 3 hours until the calcium level is within the normal range.

Naloxone. Naloxone hydrochloride, an opiate antagonist, has been used in treating shock.[59] It is thought to counteract the hypotensive and bradycardic effects of endorphins (endogenous opiates) released from the anterior pituitary gland in response to the stress of shock or endotoxemia.[59,60] Although it is only mildly pressor in normal humans, naloxone in intravenous boluses of 0.1 to 10 mg/kg followed by an infusion of 1 to 2 mg/kg/minute will sometimes block and reverse hypotension in shock caused by endotoxins, hypovolemia, or spinal cord injury in experimental animals. Naloxone administration, however, remains experimental, since it has not been shown to improve human survival in shock.

Glucagon. An inotropic agent that stimulates adenylcyclase and increases myocardial levels of cyclic adenosine monophosphate (cAMP), glucagon's ultimate role in shock has not been fully established.

Mechanical Support of Circulation. Intraaortic balloon counterpulsation has been used successfully in the management of cardiogenic shock.[1] It reduces left ventricular afterload (aortic impedance) and end-diastolic volume during systole by creating negative pressure in the descending aorta. It also increases coronary and cerebral perfusion by diverting blood flow primarily to these organs during diastole. As a result, there is improvement in myocardial pump performance and more time for recovery of the cardiac muscle. Blood flow to peripheral tissues increases as cardiac function improves, and the shock state may be stabilized rapidly with this therapeutic modality. Prolonged extracorporeal circulation (EC), which diverts most of the venous return away from the heart, and ventricular assist devices (VAD), which support one or both ventricles with a pneumatic pump, have been used in cases of biventricular failure and in septic shock. The delayed application of these mechanical devices until other measures have failed lim-

its their beneficial effects, since many organs already have been damaged irreversibly. With improvement in the safety and efficacy of these devices, earlier institution of mechanical support of circulation is likely to improve the outcome of patients with shock.

Investigational Therapies

Extensive experimental work has been focused on interventions to counteract the metabolic derangements seen primarily in septic shock. These include administration of endotoxin antiserum, anti-C5 antibody, arachidonic acid inhibitors, fibronectin, and toxic oxygen scavengers. The results of these investigations are still inconclusive.

REFERENCES

1. Billhardt RA, Rosenbush SW: Cardiogenic and hypovolemic shock. Med Clin North Am 70:853, 1986
2. Zeifach BW, Bronek A: The interplay of central and peripheral factors in irreversible hemorrhagic shock. Prog Cardiovasc Dis 18:147, 1975
3. Lappas DB, Powell WMJ, Daggett WM: Cardiac dysfunction in the perioperative period. Pathophysiology, diagnosis, and treatment. Anesthesiology 47:117, 1977
4. Perkins DM, Levin DL: Shock in the pediatric patient (Part I). J Pediatr 101:163, 1982
5. Ayres SM: SCCM's New Horizons Conference on sepsis and septic shock. Crit Care Med 13:864, 1985
6. Zimmerman JJ, Dietrich KA: Current perspectives on septic shock. Pediatr Clin North Am 34:131, 1987
7. Rietschel ET, Zahringer U, Wollenweber HW, et al: Bacterial endotoxins: Chemical structure and biological activity. Am J Emerg Med 2:60, 1985
8. Siegel JH: Cardiorespiratory manifestations of metabolic failure in sepsis and the multiple organ failure syndrome. Surg Clin North Am 63:379, 1983
9. Pollack MM, Fields AI, Ruttiman UE: Sequential cardiopulmonary variables of infants and children in septic shock. Crit Care Med 12:554, 1984
10. Houtchens BA, Westenskow DR: Oxygen consumption in septic shock. Circ Shock 13:361, 1984
11. Pollack MM, Fields AI, Ruttiman UE: Distributions of cardiopulmonary variables in pediatric survivors and nonsurvivors of septic shock. Crit Care Med 13:454, 1985
12. Demling RH, Wong C, Fox R, et al: Relationship of increased lung serotonin levels to endotoxin-induced pulmonary hypertension in sheep. Am Rev Respir Dis 132:1257, 1985
13. Leon C, Rodrigo MJ, Tomasa A, et al: Complement activation in septic shock due to gram-negative and gram-positive bacteria. Crit Care Med 10:308, 1982
14. Rees M, Brown JC, Payne JG, et al: Plasma beta-endorphin immunoreactivity in dogs during anesthesia, surgery, *Eschericia coli* sepsis and naloxone therapy. Surgery 93:386, 1983

15. Heflin AC, Brigham KL: Prevention by granulocyte depletion of increased vascular permeability of sheep lung following endotoxemia. J Clin Invest 68:1253, 1981

16. Fleck A, Hawker, F, Wallace PI, et al: Increased vascular permeability: A major cause of hypoalbuminemia in disease and injury. Lancet 1:781, 1985

17. Mizock B: Septic shock, a metabolic perspective. Arch Intern Med 144:579, 1984

18. Karakusis PH: Considerations in the therapy of septic shock. Med Clin North Am 70:933, 1986

19. Kapin M, Ferguson JL: Hemodynamic and regional circulatory alterations in dog during anaphylactic challenge. Am J Physiol 249:H430, 1985

20. Mosher P, Ross J Jr, McFate PA, et al: Control of coronary blood flow by an autoregulatory mechanism. Circ Res 14:250, 1964

21. Lefer AM: Properties of cardioinhibitory factors produced in shock. Fed Proc 37:2734, 1978

22. Zimmerman JJ, Shelhamer JH, Parrillo JE: Quantitative analysis of polymorphonuclear leukocyte superoxide anion generation in critically ill children. Crit Care Med 13:143, 1985

23. Rinaldo JE, Rogers RM: Adult respiratory distress syndrome: Changing concepts of lung injury and repair. N Engl J Med 306:900, 1982

24. Balk R, Bone RC: The adult respiratory distress syndrome. Med Clin North Am 67:685, 1983

25. Calliford AT, Thomas S, Spencer FC: Fulminating noncardiogenic pulmonary edema. A new recognized hazard during cardiac operations. J Thorac Cardiovasc Surg 80:868, 1980

26. Levinsky NG: Pathophysiology of acute renal failure. N Engl J Med 296:1453, 1977

27. Sobel BE: Cardiac and non-cardiac forms of acute circulatory failure (shock). In Braunwald E (ed): Heart Disease: A Textbook of Cardiovascular Medicine. Philadelphia, Saunders, 1984, pp 578–604

28. MacLean LD: Shock: A century of progress. Ann Surg 201:407, 1985

29. Houston MC, Thompson WL, Robertson D: Shock: Diagnosis and management. Arch Intern Med 144:1433, 1984

30. Goldenheim PD, Kazemi H: Cardiopulmonary monitoring of critically ill patients. N Engl J Med 311:717, 776, 1984

31. Walther FJ, Siassi B, Ramadan NA, Wu PY-K: Cardiac output in newborn infants with transient myocardial dysfunction. J Pediatr 107:781, 1985

32. Broder G, Weil MH: Excess lactate: An index of reversibility of shock in human patients. Science 143:1457, 1964

33. Cowan BN, Burns HJG, Boyle P, Ledingham IMcA: The relative prognostic value of lactate and haemodynamic measurements in early shock. Anaesthesia 39:750, 1984

34. Rackow EC, Falk JL, Fein A, et al: Fluid resuscitation in circulatory shock: A comparison of the cardiorespiratory effects of albumin, hetastarch, and saline solutions in patients with hypovolemic and septic shock. Crit Care Med 11:839, 1983

35. Caldwell FT, Browser FB: Critical evaluation of hypertonic and hypotonic solutions to resuscitate severely burned children. Ann Surg 189:546, 1979

36. Shoemaker WC, Schluchter C, Hopkins JA, et al: Comparison of the relative effectiveness of colloids and crystalloids in emergency resuscitation. Am J Surg 142:73, 1981

37. Bennett WM: Management of acute renal failure in sepsis—clinical considerations. Circ Shock 11:261, 1983

38. Hauser CJ, Shoemaker WC: Volume therapy treatment of hypovolemia. Hosp Phys 16:38, 1980

39. Virgilio RW, Smith DE, Zarins CK, et al: Crystalloid vs. colloid resuscitation: Is one better? Surgery 85:129, 1979

40. Puri VK, Howard M, Paidipaty BB, et al: Resuscitation in hypovolemia and shock: A prospective study of hydroxyethyl starch and albumin. Crit Care Med 11:518, 1983

41. Lucas CE: Resuscitation of the injured patient: The three phases of treatment. Surg Clin North Am 57:3, 1977

42. Weil MH, Henning RJ: New concepts in the diagnosis and fluid treatment of circulatory shock. Anesth Analg 58:124, 1979

43. Kardos GG: Isoproterenol in the treatment of shock due to bacteremia with gram-negative pathogens. N Engl J Med 274:868, 1966

44. Makabali C, Weil MH, Henning RJ: Dobutamine and other sympathomimetic drugs for the treatment of low cardiac output failure. Semin Anesth 1:63, 1982

45. Van Trigt P, Spray TL, Pasque MK, et al: The comparative effects of dopamine and dobutamine on ventricular mechanics after coronary artery bypass grafting: a pressure-dimension analysis. Circulation 70 (suppl I):I112, 1984

46. Perkins R, Anas N: Mechanisms and management of anaphylactic shock not responding to traditional therapy. Ann Allergy 54:202, 1985

47. Richard C, Ricone JL, Rimailho A, et al: Combined hemodynamic effects of dopamine and dobutamine in cardiogenic shock. Circulation 67:620, 1983

48. De La Cal MA, Miravelles E, Pascual T, et al: Dose-related hemodynamic and renal effects of dopamine in septic shock. Crit Care Med 12:22, 1984

49. Jardin F, Sportiche M, Bazin M, et al: Dobutamine: A hemodynamic evaluation in human septic shock. Crit Care Med 9:329, 1981

50. Cohn JN: Physiologic basis of vasodilator therapy for heart failure. Am J Med 71:135, 1981

51. Shine KI, Kuhn M, Young LS, et al: Aspects of the management of shock. Ann Intern Med 93:723, 1980

52. Pomer S, Sarai K, Krause E, Satter P: Hemodynamic equivalence of automated nitroglycerin and nitroprusside infusions combined with dobutamine for augmentation of cardiac output in patients following aorta coronary bypass operation. Int J Clin Pharm Ther Toxicol 22:602, 1984

53. Ilbawi MN, Idriss FS, DeLeon SY, et al: Hemodynamic effects of intravenous nitroglycerin in pediatric patients after heart surgery. Circulation 72 (suppl II):II101, 1985

54. Lillehei RC, Dietzman RH, Motsay GJ, et al: The pharmacologic approach to the treatment of shock. Geriatrics 27:73, 81, 1972

55. Martins JB, Manuel WJ, Marcus ML, et al: Comparative effects of catecholamines in cardiac tamponade: experimental and clinical studies. Am J Cardiol 46:59, 1980

56. Young LS: Combination or single drug therapy for gram negative sepsis. In Remington JS, Swartz MN (eds): Current Clinical Topics in Infectious Diseases. New York, McGraw-Hill, 1982, pp 177–205

57. Melby JC: Systemic corticosteroid therapy: Pharmacology and endocrinologic considerations. Ann Intern Med 81: 505, 1974

58. Perkin RM, Levin DL: Common fluid and electrolyte problems in the pediatric intensive care unit. Pediatr Clin North Am 27:567, 1980

59. Bernton EW: Naloxone and TRH in the treatment of shock and trauma: what future roles? Ann Emerg Med 14:729, 1985

60. Holaday JW, D'Amato RJ, Ruvio BA, et al: Adrenalectomy blocks pressor responses to naloxone in endotoxic shock: Evidence for sympathomedullary involvement. Circ Shock 11:201, 1983

SECTION III

Common Pediatric Surgical Problems

This section includes discussions of the pediatric surgical lesions confronted most often in the surgeon's day-to-day practice. For the most part, these lesions are easily diagnosed by inspection and palpation. Few require any special laboratory tests to confirm the diagnosis. Where it is important, we have included the pathophysiology and embryology as well as simple aids to the diagnosis and the when, why, and how of surgical correction of these lesions. The more common surgical lesions often incite the most controversy over management. For better or worse, the authors have outlined their own techniques, but we readily recognize that other surgeons have equal success with other approaches to the same problems.

Although most of the conditions described in this section are common and relatively simple to treat, there are some dangerous pitfalls. What appears to be a simple inguinal hernia may turn out to be a complicated sliding hernia or a sign of an intersex anomaly. Other lesions described here are often better left alone; hemangiomas in infancy, umbilical hernias, and perhaps long foreskins don't always require an operation. We must be as confident of our judgment when we advise against as when we recommend an operation. With these particular lesions we must take sufficient time to educate the family

so that they don't simply go on to find a more willing surgeon. This is the answer to surgeons who say, "If I don't operate, someone else will."

Sometimes we are uncertain about the correct course of action. With few exceptions, the diseases discussed in this section are elective conditions. If we are uncertain whether a child has a hernia, or doubt the need to biopsy a subcutaneous lump, we feel we should be honest and explain the problem to the family. Parents seem to appreciate being told, "I would like to think this over; come back and see me next week."

From the technical standpoint, one must master the operations for inguinal hernia, excision of neck cysts, and pyloric stenosis so that they can be executed flawlessly. This requires a considerable expenditure of time working with an experienced surgeon in the operating room. First, one must completely understand the anatomy; this can be learned partly from textbooks. Skill in handling tissues and instruments comes only after long practice. Because of their frequency, the common pediatric lesions mentioned here offer the surgeon the opportunity to perfect his ability to dissect delicate tissue, to accurately place sutures, and to tie reliable knots.

14
Inguinal Hernia

Inguinal herniorrhaphy is the most commonly performed pediatric surgical operation. Though it may appear to be simple, in a small infant it is technically demanding and can be difficult even for an experienced surgeon. It is a procedure that must not be taken lightly because an anesthetic or surgical mishap can occur during any operation. A herniorrhaphy may very well be the child's first encounter with a serious medical problem. This experience will color his or her attitude toward doctors and hospitals for the rest of his or her life. Consequently, it behooves us not only to provide expert surgical care but also to make the entire experience as pleasant for the child as possible.

The true incidence of inguinal hernia varies from the estimated 1 percent found in the general pediatric population of England to a startling 30 percent in premature infants with a birth weight of less than 1000 g.[1,2] Inguinal hernias in children are almost invariably indirect and, at least in older children, are more prevalent in boys. There is an increased incidence of congenital hernias in twins and in children with other birth defects.[3] There is a high familial incidence, which seems to indicate an inherited defect.[4] Fifty to 60 percent of inguinal hernias occur on the right side, 30 percent are on the left, and 10 to 20 percent are bilateral.

Fluid in the peritoneal cavity, because of either a ventriculoperitoneal shunt or ambulatory peritoneal dialysis predisposes to inguinal hernias.[5,6] Tauk and Hatch have recommended the injection of contrast material into the peritoneal cavity at the time of catheter insertion in order to identify patients with a processus vaginalis who would develop a hernia. If found, the processus could be ligated at the same time as catheter insertion.

EMBRYOLOGY

In the fifth or sixth week of gestation, the gonads make their appearance on the ventromedial surface of the urogenital ridge, which bulges into the coelom as a slender structure extending caudad from the diaphragm. The trunk of the embryo rapidly elongates, resulting in an apparent shift or descent of the gonads, which at about 10 weeks become situated close to the groin and at 3 months are located near the internal inguinal ring. This process is termed the "internal phase" of the gonadal descent. At about the third month of intrauterine life, the vaginal process appears as a protrusion of the peritoneum into the ventral abdominal wall. In the male, the lower pole of the testes lies near this peritoneal protrusion at the level of the internal ring. The sac evaginates through the ring, and the testes begin their phase of external descent, following the path of the gubernaculum. Between the seventh and ninth months, the testes reach the scrotum, pushing the vaginal sac ahead of them and protruding into its cavity. The vaginal sac normally loses its communication with the peritoneal cavity shortly before or at the time of birth, as the processus vaginalis between the level of the internal ring and the upper level of the scrotum becomes a fibrous cord attached distally to the vaginal sac, which envelops anteriorly the epididymis and the testes. The partial or complete failure of obliteration of this canal predisposes to the formation of indirect inguinal hernias or hydrocele in infancy and childhood. This also accounts for the classification of these hernias and hydroceles as congenital lesions, even though they are not clinically present at birth. The processus vaginalis may fail to close completely, resulting in scrotal hernia, or it may be obliterated at various levels between the abdominal cavity and the vaginal sac in the scrotum, giving rise to indirect inguinal hernias of different sizes. When the opening into the processus vaginalis is too small to admit contents of the abdominal cavity, peritoneal fluid passes through it to give rise to congenital hydroceles. The process of irregular obliteration of the processus vaginalis produces a variety of combinations of hydroceles of the tunica vaginalis, or hydroceles of the cord with and without hernias.[7]

The stimuli to the process of normal descent of the testicle and the causes of failure of the testicle to reach the scrotum or of erring in its location are not well understood. Both mechanical and hormonal factors probably are involved. The role played by the gubernaculum in the external descent of the testis is controversial. It is not clear if the gubernaculum pulls the testis into the scrotum or just prepares the way for its descent. Arey contends that the gubernaculum does not pull the testicle; rather, it prepares the way by providing space for the testicle.[8] Around the seventh month, the gubernaculum ceases to grow and shortens to about half its length; it converts into soft mucoid tissue and becomes as broad as the testes and epididymis. This process may produce dilation of the inguinal canal, preparing the path for the external migration of the testicle. After birth the gubernaculum atrophies.

In the female, the descent of the gonads is similar to that in the male except that the external phase of descent does not exist. This is probably because the uterus is interposed between the ovarian ligament and the round ligament, which appears by the third month as a continuous cord of dense mesenchyme extending from the region of the uterus to the labia majora. A peritoneal pocket—the diverticulum of Nuck, which is related to the round ligament—corresponds to the vaginal process in the male and predisposes to the formation of inguinal hernias in the female.

ANATOMY

The basic anatomy of the inguinal canal is the same in children as in adults.[9, 10] However, it is shorter in relation to body size in infants and children than in adults. The internal ring, which is the inlet to the canal, is located in the transversalis fascia. The external ring is subcutaneous and is formed by a gap in the external oblique aponeurosis adjacent to the pubic spine, through which emerge the spermatic cord structures in the male and the round ligament in the female. The internal ring is superior and lateral to the external ring, providing a protective mechanism so that when there is an increase in the intraabdominal pressure, the posterior wall of the canal is forced against the anterior wall, thus obliterating the

space. The lowermost fibers of the internal oblique and some of the fibers of the transversus muscle arch over the internal ring to form the roof of the canal. The inferior margin of the internal oblique contributes fibers that descend along the cord to form the cremaster muscle. The cord structures rest in a deep gutter on the floor of the canal, which is formed by fibers from the inguinal ligament, the lacunar ligament, and the transversalis fascia, which gives fibers intimately investing the cord structures in a layer called the internal spermatic fascia. In descending through the external ring, the testicle acquires another coat—the external spermatic fascia—from the aponeurosis of the external oblique muscle. In this manner, the testicle and the portion of the spermatic cord outside the inguinal canal acquire their third covering.

The spermatic cord is made up of the vas or ductus deferens, which is a distinct whitish structure lying posteriorly, and the surrounding pampiniform plexus of veins. It is readily identified as a firm structure by rolling the cord between the thumb and index finger. The artery to the vas is a branch of the superior vesicle artery and is applied closely to it, whereas the pampiniform plexus ascends from the scrotum to the abdominal inguinal ring, where it forms the spermatic veins. The internal spermatic artery, a branch of the abdominal aorta, descends anteriorly to the cord in the midst of the pampiniform plexus, and the external spermatic artery is derived from the inferior epigastric and is distributed to the elements of the spermatic sheath. The lymphatics ascend from the testicle to the lumbar and aortic glands at the renal level. The process vaginalis, or ligament, extends from the inguinal ring superiorly, medially, and anteriorly to the cord structures and to the uppermost portion of the tunica vaginalis. The cord in the male and the round ligament in the female curve lateral and anterior to the inferior epigastric vessels.

The inguinal canal in the female is narrow and contains the round ligament and peritoneal process that, if patent, forms the canal of Nuck.

With the exception of children with an extrophy of the bladder or those with a connective tissue disease, few children have any fascial defect or a direct hernia.[11] The only defect is a hernia sac, a patent processus vaginalis that has at some time contained or does contain viscera. With this definition, we can sort out those children who go through life with an asymptomatic processus vaginalis. The processus vaginalis is patent in approximately 60 percent of infants during the first year of life. By 2 years of age, 40 percent of the defects will be open; an appreciable number of asymptomatic adult males show a patent process at autopsy.[12]

By definition, then, a patent process is a potential defect that must not be confused with a clinically evident hernia.

DIAGNOSIS

Most inguinal hernias are found either by the parents or during a well-baby or preschool examination. There usually is a history of a lump appearing intermittently in the groin or scrotum. Hernias are usually asymptomatic. An occasional infant will be fussy and irritable, particularly if the hernia is large and contains loops of intestine. Older children may complain of groin or inguinal pain during exercise. This pain is either vague and chronic or sharp and fleeting; in any case it is difficult to ascribe these symptoms to a hernia. If no hernia is found on careful clinical examination, these children should be reassured and encouraged to continue their activities. This is difficult if another physician has suggested that the symptoms may be caused by a hernia and has advised discontinuing gym at school. The first sign of an inguinal hernia may be an intestinal obstruction secondary to incarceration.

The examination of a child with a possible hernia commences by having the child completely undress, despite the fact that many parents expect us to make a diagnosis between the shirt and the underwear!

With the child supine, first observe for inguinal asymmetry or an obvious mass (Fig. 14–1). An exaggerated cremasteric reflex will produce an inguinal lump that appears at intervals and is often mistaken for a hernia. Consequently, one must be certain that both testicles are descended at the time the inguinal mass appears. Often the mass observed by the mother or by another physician has disappeared by the time the child is brought

in for examination. The diagnosis may be difficult in a chubby infant with an abundance of suprapubic fat. In this situation, one examines the inguinal area for thickening of the cord structures. This is performed by placing the index finger over the cord at the pubic space and moving it from side to side (Fig. 14–2). When the walls of the sac rub against each other, there is a sensation similar to rubbing two layers of silk together. Thickening of the cord structures by a hernia sac is easier to evaluate and is more reliable. Palpation is difficult in fat or ticklish children, but time and patience bring their reward. After this examination, older children are asked to stand and jump up and down. Infants are held upright by their mothers. Crying will increase intraabdominal pressure and should make a hernia more obvious. Often, there is only a sensation of crepitus over the hernia sac. If a bulge in the inguinal area appears during the examination, there is no doubt about the diagnosis. The same maneuvers are then carried out to detect a possible hernia on the opposite side. A hydrocele is differentiated from a hernia by one's ability to palpate above the mass and not feel continuity between the scrotal hydrocele and the inguinal canal. Inguinal lymph nodes are lateral to the canal but can be mistaken for a hernia—especially in a girl, since a lymph node's size and consistency are similar to those of an ovary in the inguinal canal. A hydrocele of the cord may appear to be an incarcerated hernia, but it is neither tender nor moveable. Sometimes, however, an operation is the only way to distinguish a hydrocele from a hernia. Transillumination is of no value because gas in the bowel transilluminates a hernia as

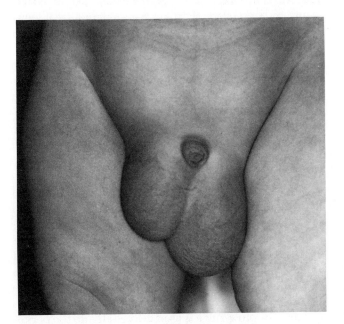 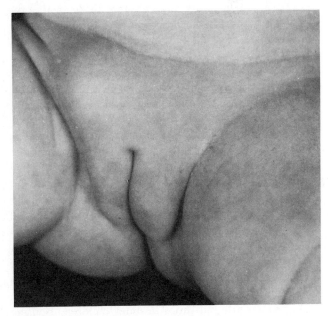

Figure 14–1. Left. Right groin swelling due to a hernia; in addition, the left scrotum is swollen with a hydrocele. **Right.** The right groin bulge is an ovary in a hernia sac.

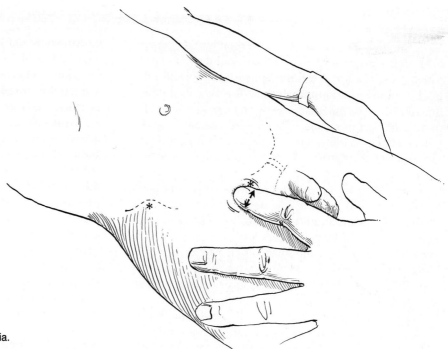

Figure 14–2. Examination for inguinal hernia.

well as a fluid-filled hydrocele. A plain film of the abdomen demonstrating gas in the hernia sac will make the diagnosis (Fig. 14–3).

A diagnosis of a hernia can only be made when a definite bulge or lump is found on physical examination. A slender child with a history of an inguinal mass and palpable thickening of the cord or a "silk sign" is also likely to have a hernia. Palpation of the cord is most unreliable in an infant who has considerable subcutaneous pubic fat. Bronsther et al. reviewed 1000 of their own cases and reviewed the literature to determine the accuracy of physical diagnosis and the incidence of bilateral hernias. In practice, they experienced an accuracy rate of 93.3 percent in detecting a contralateral hernia; in other series the diagnostic accuracy was as low as 46.9 percent.[13] When there is doubt about the diagnosis, it is our policy to advise the family that their child may have a hernia, but that there is no definite indication for an operation. They are warned to observe for an inguinal mass and to return for a repeat examination. This policy has proven satisfactory, since a hernia that is not detectable on careful physical examination is unlikely to incarcerate. Physical examination does have limitations, particularly in attempting to determine if the contralateral side should be operated on. Some surgeons have advocated routine bilateral repairs, particularly in children under 1 year of age. A small patent processus vaginalis will be found in as many as 60 to 70 percent of patients under 2 years of age. The incidence is higher in girls but drops in older children. Routine bilateral repair subjects the child to a longer anesthetic

and increases the risk of damage to the vas deferens and to the testicular vessels. When there is no definite hernia, there is a tendency to undertake a more extensive dissection in order to avoid overlooking a hernia sac. It is our practice to perform a bilateral exploration in girls under 1 year of age and in boys if there is any suggestion of a contralateral thickened cord or a "silk sign." A final examination is carried out when the child is under anesthesia, in addition to the preoperative examination. With this system, approximately half of our patients undergo bilateral exploration. A hernia sac is found in 90 percent of these patients. Very few have returned with an unsuspected contralateral hernia.

Several authors have recommended a herniogram when there is doubt about the diagnosis, or, more importantly, to find out if there is a contralateral hernia.[14–17] A herniogram is contraindicated if there is a ventriculoperitoneal shunt, a history of hypersensitivity to iodine compounds, or a bleeding disorder. The test is performed by injecting dilute Hypaque-M or Renograffin-60 into the peritoneal cavity with a syringe and a 20-gauge needle. There is one case report in which an intramural hematoma of the bowel complicated a herniogram, and in another there was an intestinal perforation with infection and slough of the adbominal wall.[18, 19] Herniograms are never performed in our hospital, and now, most surgeons have abandoned this procedure. The presence of a contralateral hernia can be determined by the injection of air through the open sac.[20] A catheter with an attached asepto syringe is used to force air into the peritoneal cavity. If air can then be palpated in the opposite

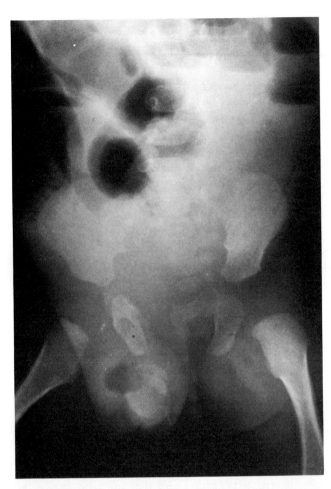

Figure 14–3. There is air in the hernia sac diagnostic of an incarcerated hernia. This will aid in the differential diagnosis of an intestinal obstruction if there is a small hernia and will help differentiate a hernia from a hydrocele.

groin, there is a hernia. Dr. Richard Goldstein has performed this procedure in our hospital in over 5000 cases. Thus far only 24 patients have returned with a contralateral hernia.

TREATMENT

Routine inguinal hernia repairs are performed on an outpatient basis. The physical examination, complete blood count, and urinalysis are performed within a month of the expected date of the operation. Children with other diseases are admitted to the hospital for evaluation at least 1 day before the operation. Premature infants who required ventilator support or any baby with a history of apneic episodes must be admitted to the hospital for careful monitoring. Anesthesia may predispose to more apneic episodes.[21] We prefer local anesthesia with 0.5 percent lidocaine for small premature infants, particularly if the hemoglobin is under 10 g.

Technique

Pediatric surgeons almost always agree on three aspects of inguinal hernia repair: (1) a transverse skin crease incision, (2) high ligation of the hernia sac, and (3) closure of the skin with subcuticular sutures. There are many variations in the actual performance of the operation, but these three points contain the essential elements. The transverse skin incision is placed in an inguinal skin fold midway between the internal and external rings (Fig. 14–4A). The external ring is identified by rolling the thickened cord structures under the index finger. The point at which they can no longer be palpated in the canal marks their disappearance under the external oblique aponeurosis. The skin incision is made with the skin on tension. It need be only 2 or 3 cm long in an infant of average size. The scalpel is carried through the dermis at an exact right angle to the skin. The surgeon and an assistant hold the subcutaneous fat up on outward tension with tissue forceps (Fig. 14–4B). The fat is then spread with scissors at a right angle to the skin. This prevents damage to the one or two vessels that regularly cross the incision. These vessels are ligated or electrocoagulated. The scissors are again spread, retracting the fat to expose the scarpas fascia (Fig. 14–4C). This layer is dense, especially in the infant, and may be mistaken for the external oblique. The scarpas fascia is elevated with tissue forceps and divided. There is another layer of fat beneath the scarpas fascia that must be opened until the loose areolar tissue overlying the external oblique is encountered. When the incision has been placed properly over the external ring, elevation of the lower edge of the incision, with retraction toward the scrotum, will allow exposure of the external ring by separating the scissors blades within the layer of loose areolar tissue. Both sides of the ring must be clearly exposed and definitely identified. Actually, the external ring is not really a ring at all because the fibers of the external oblique continue on as the external spermatic fascia. The tips of the scissors or a curved hemostat are inserted into the external ring to elevate the external oblique for a short incision without injury to the ilioinguinal nerve (Fig. 14–4D, E). An alternate technique is to open the external oblique aponeurosis proximal to the ring. In a small infant, the inguinal canal is so short that a proper high ligation can be performed without opening the external ring, as long as sufficient traction is applied to the sac. Then there is no concern about closing the ring too tightly at the end of the operation. The fibers of the cremaster muscle are drawn into the wound with a tissue forceps, then grasped with a mosquito hemostat that is passed to an assistant. The surgeon then holds up the cremaster opposite his assistant's hemostat and applies counteraction. The cremaster fibers are separated with scissors for 1 to 2 cm to expose the internal spermatic fascia (Fig. 14–4F). The internal spermatic fascia is the final layer that binds the vas deferens and the testicular vessels to the sac (Fig. 14–4G). It is carefully tented up and opened to allow separation of the vessels and vas from the sac. These structures are lateral and posterior to the sac and may be held with a moist sponge while they are being dissected free of the hernia sac. The vas must never be held with an instrument because even pressure with a blunt tissue forceps causes long-term damage to the vas.[22] The vas deferens and testicular vessels are clearly identified both visually and by palpation and are separated from the sac for 1 or 2 cm. The sac is circumscribed at one point (Fig. 14–4H). Great care must be taken to avoid dissecting distally toward the testicle or proximally toward the internal ring until the sac has been completely circumscribed and divided. Sometimes it is necessary to open the sac in order to gain orientation so that one does not inadvertently dissect either proximally or distally until the sac has been completely circumscribed at one point. When the sac is very friable, fibers of the internal spermatic fascia are left attached, and only the vas deferens and the vessels are dissected away. The surgeon applies downward and outward traction on these structures while an assistant holds up the sac (Fig. 14–4I). The separation may be accomplished either by alternately spreading and cutting tissue under direct vision with scissors or by using the tip of a moist sponge held with a tissue forceps to perform a blunt dissection. As soon as a portion of the sac has been separated from the vas deferens and vessels, it should be twisted. This allows one to apply greater trac-

tion and thereby achieve a higher ligation than would otherwise be possible. Properitoneal fat or the thicker fibers of the transversalis fascia mark the neck of the sac. If there is undue thickening or prominent fat at the medial edge, one must make absolutely certain that the urinary bladder is not forming the medial wall of the sac as a sliding hernia. The sac is first closed with a transfixing synthetic absorbable suture and then tied with a second ligature. The cut end of the sac should retract well up under the internal ring (Fig. 14–4J, K). No attempt is made to excise the distal sac, but every small capillary must be either ligated or coagulated to prevent a postoperative scrotal hematoma. One suture is used to approximate the edges of the cremaster. The external oblique aponeurosis is then sutured, making certain that the testicle is in the scrotum. No attempt is made to tighten the external ring (Fig. 14–4L). If anything, it is left slightly loose so that postoperative edema will not compress the testicular vessels. The scarpas fascia is closed with two or three sutures and the skin is approximated with an absorbable running suture and sterile adhesive strips (Fig. 14–4M).

The incision and approach to the hernia sac are the same in girls as in boys. Immediately after identifying and opening the external ring, the entire sac is circumscribed and brought up into the wound. There is often a sizable vessel continuing down into the canal of Nuck which must be ligated or coagulated. In addition, there is often a plexus of small vessels that branch from the inferior epigastric artery and that must be coagulated during dissection of the sac. In approximately 20 percent

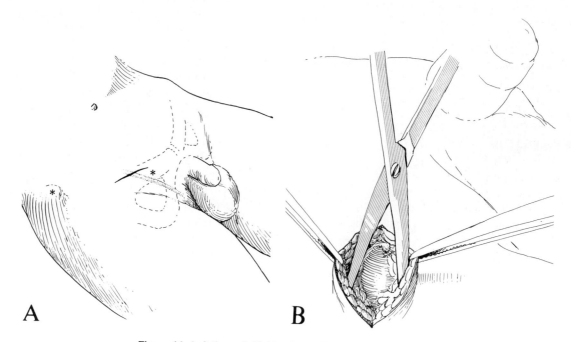

Figure 14–4. A through M. Hernia repair. See text for discussion.

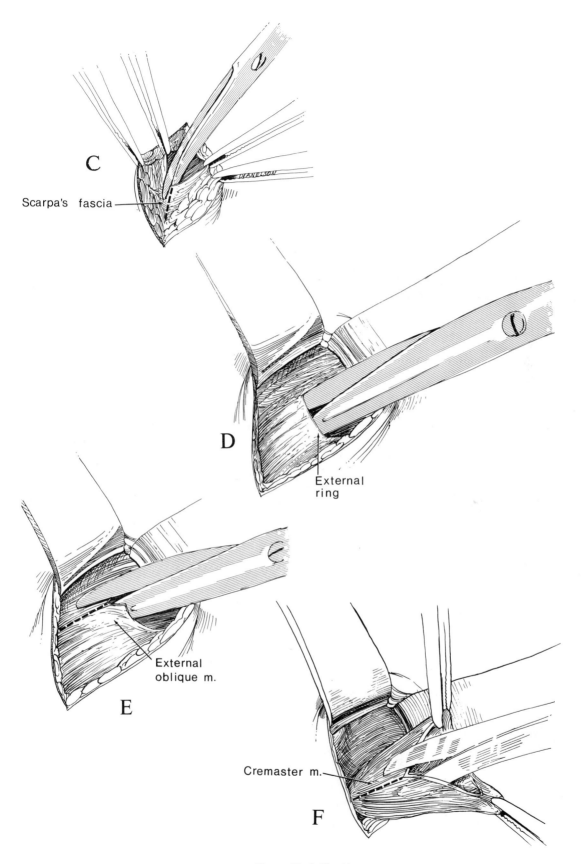

C

Scarpa's fascia

D

External ring

E

External oblique m.

F

Cremaster m.

Figure 14–4. (Cont.)

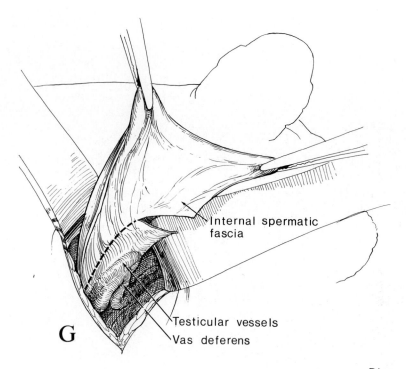

Internal spermatic
fascia

Testicular vessels
Vas deferens

G

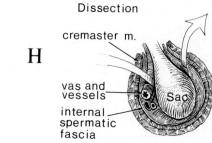

Dissection

cremaster m.

H

vas and
vessels
internal
spermatic
fascia

Sac

Hernia sac

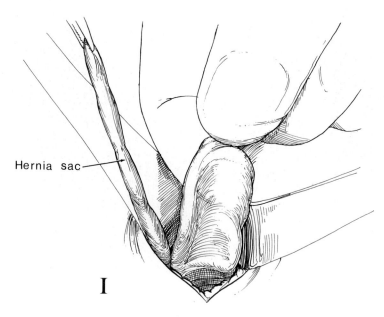

I

Figure 14–4. (Cont.)

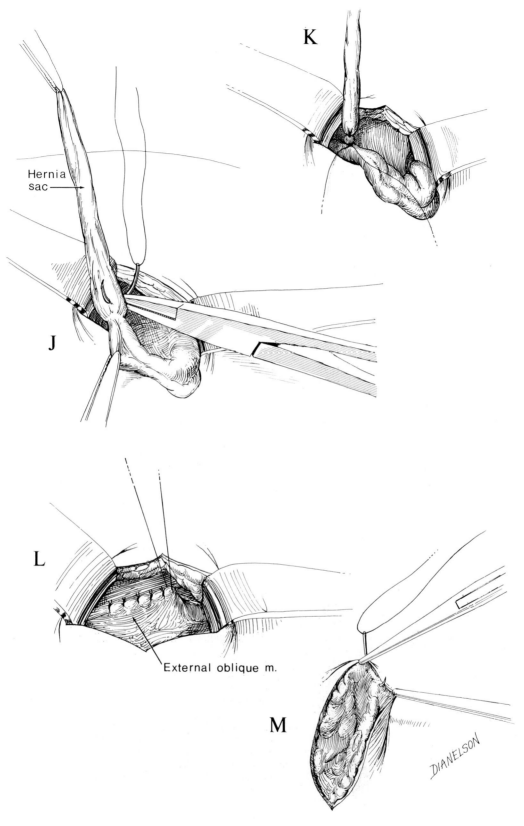

Figure 14–4. (Cont.)

130

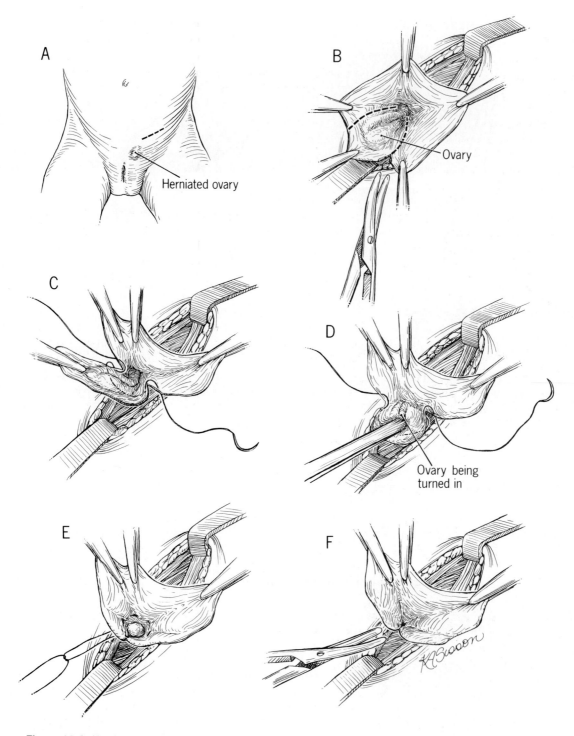

Figure 14–5. Hernia repair in a girl with a sliding ovary. **A.** The ovary is palpable as a lima bean-sized, firm, movable lump in the groin. **B.** The sac is isolated and dissected free from surrounding tissues, then opened. The dotted line marks the incisions that will be made to form a pedicle for the ovary. **C.** A suture is placed at the base of the pedicle, which will close the medial portion of the defect by folding the pedicle back on itself. This prevents injury to the ovarian vessels and the fallopian tube. **D.** The pedicle with the ovary is pushed into the abdominal cavity. **E.** The original suture is passed through the remainder of the sac. **F.** The suture is tied and the excess sac is removed.

of females, the ovary and fallopian tube are attached to the wall of the sac. This is the most common form of sliding hernia encountered in the pediatric age group. No attempt should be made to dissect the ovary and tube away from the wall of the sac because this may injure the blood supply. The ovary may be either inverted into the abdomen with a series of pursestring sutures or dropped into the abdomen with a flap of peritoneum made from the wall of the hernia sac. This technique is performed by holding the ovary and sac up on tension.[23] Incisions parallel to the ovary and tube are made down into the internal ring. With this flap and the sac still held up with hemostats, a suture is placed at the base of the flap, which is then inverted into the abdominal cavity. The suture is tied and then used to suture ligate the remaining sac. (Fig. 14–5).

INCARCERATED HERNIA

The small bowel, cecum, ovary and fallopian tube, or appendix may be caught inside the hernia sac. Initially there is a painful mass in the groin. As symptoms progress, there is an increase in local swelling and tenderness, along with abdominal distention, vomiting, and eventually a fully developed intestinal obstruction. If left untreated, the bowel or other entrapped organs lose their venous return and become gangrenous. In some infants, one encounters signs of an intestinal obstruction, but only very careful palpation will reveal a small knuckle of bowel caught in the hernia sac. Strangulation may occur within as short a time as 6 hours after the onset of symptoms.

Treatment

Any child with an incarcerated hernia is quickly admitted to the hospital. If there is vomiting or abdominal distention, the child is given intravenous fluids and a nasogastric tube is passed. Most hernias can be reduced easily after the child has been sedated with 2 mg/kg of Demerol. In addition, the patient is placed in a deep Trendelenburg position, and ice bags are applied to the scrotum. It is usually necessary to tie the patient's feet to the end of the bed in order to maintain the proper position. Spontaneous reduction usually takes place within an hour. Gentle manipulation may be required, consisting of upward pressure on the scrotum with counterpressure above the internal ring, but an incarcerated hernia must never be reduced forcibly. If reduction has not occurred within an hour or so, an operation is needed. A slightly larger incision than usual is necessary. The hernia sac should be isolated distal to the external ring. The sac is then opened and the bowel inspected. If it is viable, the external ring is widely opened, and the internal ring is dilated with a curved clamp. It is then possible

to replace the bowel back into the abdomen and continue with the hernia repair. Intestine that is obviously gangrenous may be resected through the same incision. The testicle often is swollen and engorged. If the hernia has been incarcerated for some time, there is a 12 to 15 percent incidence of testicular atrophy.[24, 25]

UNUSUAL ASPECTS OF INGUINAL HERNIA

Testicular Feminizing Syndrome

An inguinal hernia with a prolapsed ovary may be the first sign of the testicular feminizing syndrome, especially if the hernia is bilateral and the labia appear larger than normal (Fig. 14–6).[26–28] Afflicted patients have a small, short vagina and though appearing to be feminine have a 46, XY karyotype. This is a familial disorder.[29] As a general rule, any gonad below the inguinal ligament should be considered a testicle until proven otherwise.[30] A buccal smear should be performed for Barr bodies in any child with bilateral hernias with a prolapsing ovary on either side. If the buccal smear is negative for Barr bodies, further workup is indicated, and the gonad is biopsied at the time of hernia repair. If a definitive diagnosis is made, the gonads are excised at the time of herniorrhaphy rather than being moved back into the abdomen. If at operation, an "ovary" is found that is unattached to a fallopian tube, it should be biopsied.

Sliding Hernias

The bladder or an ovary may form the medial wall of the hernia sac, where it is easily injured (Fig. 14–7). The bladder usually can be tucked back with a pursestring suture, but if there is any suspicion that it has been injured, a Foley catheter is placed in the bladder, and a dilute solution of methylene blue is injected. If there is a bladder defect, it is sutured, and the catheter is left in place. The appendix and mesoappendix may be present on the lateral wall of a right-sided hernia, or the appendix may merely appear in the sac. In either case, an appendectomy is indicated. With careful technique, the mesoappendix is ligated, and the appendiceal stump is ligated, coagulated, and inverted. We have seen no complications with this procedure, and Rose and Santulli have reported on 16 patients in whom an appendectomy was performed with no infection in the hernia wound.[31] Other viscera, such as the cecum or sigmoid, are replaced into the abdomen on a pedicle of the sac, as described for a sliding ovarian hernia.

The Absent Vas Deferens

An absent or atrophic vas deferens may be the first clue that the child has either cystic fibrosis of the pancreas

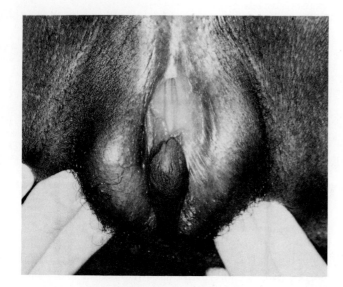
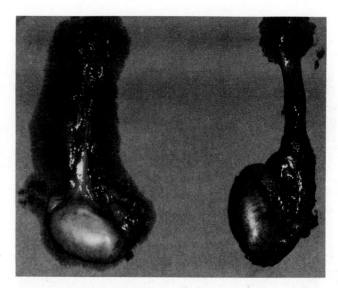

Figure 14–6. Testicular feminizing syndrome. **Left.** External genitalia of a 15-year-old girl with a slightly enlarged clitoris and gonads in each labial fold. **Right.** The resected gonads, which resemble testicles.

or agenesis of one of his kidneys.[32–34] Men with cystic fibrosis have long been known to be sterile. It is thought that the vas is atrophic secondary to viscid secretions or to paralysis of ciliary action during intrauterine life.

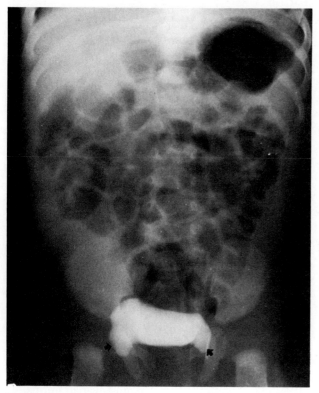

Figure 14–7. Bilateral "bladder ears." It is important to inspect the medial side of the hernia sac for thickening or excess fat, which could represent a sliding bladder hernia. The cystogram demonstrates protrusion of the bladder into bilateral hernia sacs.

Direct Hernia

Some surgeons have described a second or "pantaloon" type of hernia, which involves a second peritoneal sac adjacent to the indirect sac but beneath the inferior epigastic vessels. If such a hernia exists, it should be cured by vigorous traction on the indirect sac, which draws up adjacent peritoneum. Children with extrophy of the bladder have a definite defect in the transversalis fascia and do indeed seem to have a direct hernia, or at least a weak floor (Fig. 14–8). In addition to a high ligation of the sac, the transversalis fascia is sutured to close the defect. Patients with the Ehlers-Danlos syndrome have very fragile tissues and a high rate of recurrent hernia. For this reason, we have repaired the posterior wall of the canal by suturing the transversalis fascia to Pouparts ligament with sutures buttressed with small Teflon felt pledgets. Thus far we have had no recurrences with this technique. Coran and Eraklis observed a 56 percent recurrence rate in children with the Hunter-Hurler syndrome when only a sac ligation was performed, but there were no recurrences when a Bassini or Halsted repair was carried out.[35]

POSTOPERATIVE CARE

Most children who have undergone an uncomplicated hernia repair are up and playing the same day as their operation and are back to full activities within a few days. We have restricted the athletic activities of older boys until complete healing of the skin has occurred.

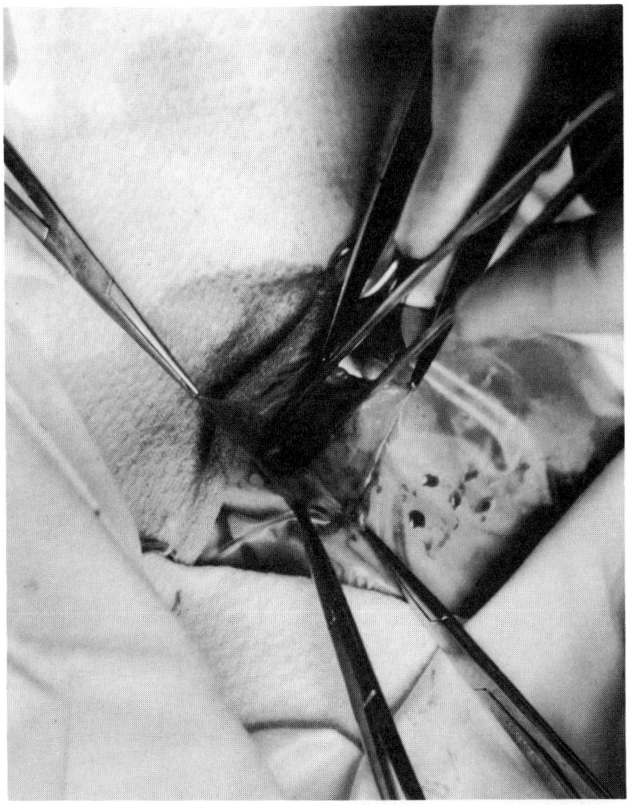

Figure 14–8. The tissue forceps are within the huge internal ring of a child who had an inguinal hernia and an extrophy of the bladder. Some form of posterior wall repair is indicated when the ring is this large.

Complications

The most common immediate complication has been scrotal edema and swelling following incarceration. A hematoma will develop after the repair of a large hernia unless scrupulous care is taken to control every capillary on the cut edge of the distal sac. The incidence of wound infection in our hospital is less than 1 in 1000 cases. All infections have responded to opening of the skin incision, warm compresses, and antibiotic therapy. In several cases, there was extrusion of silk sutures during the ensuing months. This is an annoying complication that requires another anesthetic to remove the offending stitch. For this reason, we now use absorbable synthetic sutures for hernia repair.

A recurrent hernia in a child is the result of either a technical error or a connective tissue defect. Mestel and Turner found that 6 of 7 recurrences occurred within a year of the initial operation.[36] The usual error is a failure to ligate the sac highly enough. We also have observed silk sutures on the lateral wall of a large sac, indicating that the previous surgeon was completely lost.

REFERENCES

1. Knox G: The incidence of inguinal hernia in Newcastle children. Arch Dis Child 34:482, 1959
2. Harper RC, Garcia A, Sia C: Inguinal hernia: A common problem of premature infants weighing 1000 grams or less at birth. Pediatrics 56:112, 1975
3. Bakmin H: Inguinal hernia in twins. J Pediatr Surg 6:165, 1971
4. Weiner BR: Congenital inheritance of inguinal hernia. J Hered 40:219, 1949
5. Tauk ES, Hatch DA: Hernias complicating chronic ambulatory peritoneal dialysis in children. J Pediatr Surg 21:41, 1986
6. Inguinal hernias after ventriculoperitoneal shunt procedures in pediatric patients. Surg Gynecol Obstet 159:570, 1984
7. Burton CC: The embryologic development and descent of the testis in relation to congenital hernia. Surg Gynecol Obstet 107:294, 1958
8. Arey LD: Developmental Anatomy, 7th ed. Philadelphia, Saunders, 1965
9. Ayson BJ, McVay CB: Surgical Anatomy. Philadelphia, Saunders, 1971, vol 1
10. Madden JL, Hakim S, Agorogiannis AD: The anatomy and repair of inguinal hernias. Surg Clin North Am 51:1269, 1971
11. McEntyre RL, Raffensperger JG: Surgical Complications of Ehlers-Danlos syndrome in children. J Pediatr Surg 12: 1977
12. Rowe MI, Copelson LW, Clatworthy HW: The patent processus vaginalis and the inguinal hernia. J Pediatr Surg 4:102, 1969
13. Bronsther B, Abrams M, Elboim C: Inguinal hernia in children: A study of 1,000 cases and a review of the literature. J Am Med Women's Assoc 22:522, 1972
14. Jewett TC, Kuhn JP, Allen JE: Herniography in children. J Pediatr Surg 11:451, 1976
15. Gutman FM, Bertrand R, Ducharne JC: Herniography and the pediatric contralateral inguinal hernia. Surg Gynecol Obstet 135:351, 1972
16. White JJ, Haller JA, Dorst JP: Congenital inguinal hernia and inguinal herniography. Surg Clin North Am 50:823, 1978
17. White JJ: Herniography: A perspective. Surgery 83:363, 1978
18. Butsch J, Kuhn J: Intramural hematoma of the small bowel: A possible lethal complication of herniography. Surgery 83:121, 1978
19. Ducharme J, Guttman F, Polijak: Hematoma of bowel and cellulitus of the abdominal wall complicating herniography. J Pediatr Surg 15:3, 1980
20. Powell R: Intra-operative diagnostic pneumoperitoneum in pediatric patients with unilateral inguinal hernia: The Goldstein test. J Pediatr Surg 20:418, 1985
21. Liu L, Cote C, Goudsouzian N, et al: Life-threatening apnea in infants recovering from anesthesia. Anaesthesiology 58:506, 1983

22. Janik J, Shandling B: The vulnerability of the vas deferens II: The case against routine bilateral inguinal exploration. J Pediatr Surg 17:585, 1982
23. Potts W: The Surgeon and the Child. Philadelphia, Saunders, 1957, p 227
24. Sloman JG: Testicular infarction in infancy, in association with irreducible inguinal hernia. Med J Aust 45:242, 1958
25. Wiklander O: Incarcerated inguinal hernia in childhood. Acta Chir Scand 101:303, 1951
26. Jacobs PA, Baike AG, Court Brown WM: Chromosomal sex in the syndrome of testicular feminization. Lancet 2:591, 1959
27. French FS, Beggeto TB, Van Wyk J, et al: Testicular feminization: Clinical morphological and biochemical studies. J Clin Endocrinol 25:661, 1965
28. Nielsen DF, Bulows S: The incidence of hermaphroditism in girls with inguinal hernia. Surg Gynecol Obstet 172:875, 1976
29. O'Connell MJ, Ramsey HE, Whong-Deng J, et al: Testicular feminizing syndrome in three siblings: emphasis on gonadal dysplasia. Am J Med Sci 265:653, 1975
30. Case records. N Engl J Med 296:439, 1977
31. Rose E, Santulli T: Sliding appendiceal inguinal hernia. Surg Gynecol Obstet 146:627, 1978
32. Gracey M, Campbell P, Noblett H: Atretic vas deferens in cystic fibrosis. N Engl J Med 280:276, 1969
33. Holsclan DS, Perlmutter AD, Jockin H, et al: Genital abnormalities in male patients with cystic fibrosis. J Urol 106:568, 1971
34. Lukash F, Zwiren GT, Andrew HG: Significance of absent vas deferens at hernia repair in infants and children. J Pediatr Surg 10:765, 1975
35. Coran AC, Eraklis AJ: Inguinal hernia in the Hunter-Hurler syndrome. Surgery 61:302, 1967
36. Mestel AL, Turner HA: Recurrent inguinal hernia in infants and children. Int Surg 45:575, 1966

15
Femoral Hernia

Donald G. Marshall

In 1965, Fosberg and Mahin could find records of only 50 children who had had femoral hernias.[1] In my own practice over the past 20 years, I have operated on 12 children with typical femoral hernias. In addition, there was 1 patient with a prevascular femoral hernia and an ectopic testicle. This experience suggests that femoral hernias generally are misdiagnosed and are not as rare in children as is commonly thought.

ANATOMY

Although there is no known congenital sac in the femoral hernia, there is usually a distinct peritoneal sac that passes into the upper thigh beneath the inguinal ligament. Rather than a sac, there may be only a large amount of properitoneal fat in the femoral canal.[2]

The femoral ring is bounded anteriorly by the inguinal ligament, posteriorly by the pectineus fascia and muscle, and laterally by the femoral vein. The medial wall is composed of the fused transversalis fascia and the transversus abdominus aponeurosis as they reflect from the inguinal ligament and insert upon the ileopectineal (Cooper's) ligament. More medial is the sharp edge of the lacunar, or Gimbernat's, ligament. The femoral ring enlarges medially until it is halted by this rigid lacunar ligament. Occasionally, an abnormal obturator artery will be seen to pass around the medial side of the neck of the hernia.

DIAGNOSIS

Our patients have ranged in age from 16 months to 10 years, with 4 years being the average age. There was an equal incidence according to sex. Ten of the 12 hernias were on the right side. One of our patients had bilateral hernias. There is a visible bulge below and lateral to the usual site for an indirect hernia. Thus the pubic spine is above and medial to the visible and palpable swelling.

On palpation, the mass is soft and nontender. Other authors have reported a past history of inguinal hernia repairs.[3–6] None of the patients in our series had a previous inguinal hernia, and all of our patients except the first were given correct preoperative diagnoses. In the misdiagnosed child, the omentum had come through the femoral canal and then turned superiorly to lie at the external ring in the superficial pouch. The preoperative diagnosis was an incarcerated ovary. Only one other of our patients had an incarcerated omentum. The differential diagnosis of a swelling in this area includes consideration of lymph nodes, an abscess, and a saphenous varix. Only a femoral hernia, however, will occur as a soft, nontender swelling. The one saphenous varix we observed showed a bluish discoloration of the overlying skin.

TREATMENT

The treatment is surgical. All are explored through the classic transverse crease incision down to the external oblique. The skin flap is then raised, and the femoral canal is visualized. The sac is identified and freed carefully to avoid venous bleeding. The spermatic cord is now raised, or the round ligament is removed, checking for an indirect sac. The transversalis fascia is opened, leaving an adequate 1 cm flap inferiorly. A fine suture is placed on the cut edges of this layer for later identifica-

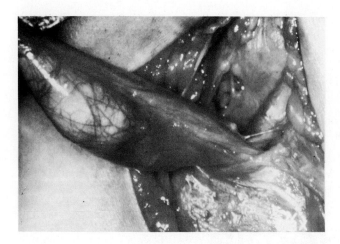

Figure 15–1. Prevascular femoral hernia. This demonstrates the ectopic testicle with the hernia sac emerging from beneath the inguinal ligament in front of the femoral vessels.

tion. Dissection is now carried through the extraperitoneal fat to identify the femoral ring with its sac, which is gently pulled up through the femoral ring. If it is an incarcerated hernia, the sac is first opened above the ring and then below to aid in reducing its contents. The hernial sac is then transfixed and removed. In one patient, there was an abnormal obturator artery around the neck of the sac.

Attention is now given to removing fat from the femoral ring and its clear identification. Although removal of the sac may be adequate for cure, we have in all cases done some sort of repair, most often aimed at trying to reduce the size of the femoral ring. This has been done by using two interrupted sutures of nonabsorbable material between the inguinal ligament in front and Cooper's ligament behind, usually catching the free edge of the transversalis fascia previously marked.

A more formal McVay repair may be performed. Here the transversus muscle and transveralis fascia are sutured to Cooper's ligament, but we tend to catch the free anterior edge of the femoral ring as well. No constant attempt is made to tent the medial edge of the femoral vein with the repair, but the ring always is significantly narrowed.

The lower edge of the transversalis fascia is next approximated to itself superiorly with fine interrupted

sutures. The spermatic cord is replaced in its bed, and the external oblique is closed. One pursestring suture is used to obliterate the dead space in the fat occupied by the femoral sac. The skin wound is then closed with a fine continuous subcuticular suture.

A prevascular femoral hernia occurs when the sac lies in front of rather than medial to the femoral vessels.[7] We encountered a previously unreported variant of a prevascular femoral hernia, in which the sac contained an ectopic testicle (Fig. 15–1). The sac with the testicle was beneath the inguinal ligament but in front of the vessels. This hernia was approached through a standard crease incision. The sac with the testicle was dissected free of the femoral vessels below the inguinal ligament, after which the external oblique fascia and transversalis fascia were opened above the inguinal ligament in order to dissect the sac up to its neck for suture ligation. The spermatic vessels were dissected retroperitoneally until there was sufficient length for the ectopic testis to lie in the scrotum.

RESULTS

There were no immediate postoperative complications in our patients. All patients have been followed up from 4 months to 20 years, and none has had a recurrence.

REFERENCES

1. Fosberg RG, Mahin HP: Femoral hernia in children. Am J Surg 109:470, 1965
2. Cherry JK: Femoral hernia in children. Am J Surg 196:99, 1963
3. Immordino PA: Femoral hernia in infancy and childhood. J Pediatr Surg 7:40, 1972
4. Burke J: Femoral hernia in childhood. Ann Surg 166:287, 1966
5. Fonkalsud EW, deLorimier AA, Clatworthy HH: Femoral and direct inguinal hernias in infants and children. JAMA 192:597, 1965
6. Schulze S, Schmidt PF: Femoral hernia in children. Z Kinderchir 40:287, 1985
7. Marshall DG, Jellie H: Prevascular femoral hernia with ectopic testis in an infant. J Pediatr Surg 16:519, 1981

16
Hydrocele and Varicocele

HYDROCELE

Incomplete proximal obliteration of the processus vaginalis allows entry of peritoneal fluid into the distal sac. This results in a congenital hydrocele, which is usually in the scrotum, enveloping the testicle, but may be anywhere along the course of the spermatic cord. We have observed one large hydrocele around an undescended testicle that appeared as a left lower quadrant abdominal mass (Fig. 16–1). Recurrence after aspiration or simple scrotal excision provides evidence for a connection between the peritoneal cavity and the hydrocele sac. This communication is always present but may be only microscopic.[1] The usual infantile hydrocele appears shortly after birth in the form of soft, fluid-filled sacs about the testicle. These usually disappear spontaneously within the child's first year. They require no treatment unless there is a clinically obvious hernia above the hydrocele. When the distal sac is obliterated but the midportion remains open, the hydrocele involves the spermatic cord above the testicle, which appears as a firm, movable lump several centimeters in diameter. There are several anatomic variations of hydroceles, particularly when there is an associated hernia. The hydrocele may appear to extend up alongside the hernia sac, or there may be several loculi of fluid resembling a chain of lakes along the course of the processus vaginalis.

Diagnosis
A hydrocele may vary in size; as the child is up and about during the day, fluid seeps from the peritoneal cavity into the hydrocele (Fig. 16–2). The hydrocele then becomes tense and larger, but by the next morning, it will have decreased in size. Hydroceles often enlarge or appear during an upper respiratory infection or a bout of the flu. This probably represents generalized serositis. A hydrocele will never disappear completely, however. On physical examination, it is possible to palpate the spermatic cord above the mass of a hydrocele, whereas a hernia will be in continuity with the abdominal cavity. It may be very difficult, however, to palpate above a hydrocele of the cord. In a small child, it is possible to palpate the area of the internal rings through the rectum. If bowel is felt entering the ring, one can make a diagnosis of an incarcerated hernia. One can easily prove a small communication with the peritoneal cavity if gentle squeezing will reduce the size of the hydrocele. Transillumination is mainly of value in ruling out a tumor of the testicle because both a hernia and a hydrocele will transmit light.

Treatment
No treatment is indicated for a hydrocele during the first year of life unless there is a clinically evident hernia. A hydrocele that persists or develops after the first year requires an operation. This operation is exactly the same as that described for an inguinal hernia. Even if no hernia is found, the vas deferens and testicular vessels must be followed up the internal ring, where the proximal portion of the processus vaginalis is identified. Even if there is only a small strand, it must be suture ligated and divided, or the hydrocele will recur. When the processus vaginalis or hernia sac has been ligated and divided, the hydrocele is brought into the incision, either by traction on the distal sac or by manipulation through the scrotum. The cremaster and internal spermatic fibers are dissected off the hydrocele several centimeters away from the cord structures. The sac is then opened and drained. There is no need to excise the sac; in fact, after ligation of the processus vaginalis, aspiration of the sac should be sufficient. An extensive dissection of a hydrocele invites damage to the vas or epididymis

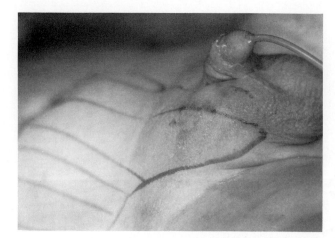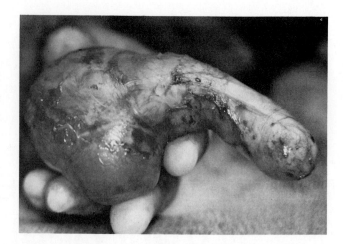

Figure 16–1. An abdominoinguinal hydrocele. **Left.** The mass outlined on the abdominal wall, demonstrating an extension into the inguinal canal. **Right.** The specimen, illustrating the portion of the hydrocele that extended into the canal.

and considerable bleeding from the edge of the sac. A large tense hydrocele that extends up into the inguinal canal will overlie the proximal hernia or processus. The testicular vessels are attenuated and may be difficult to recognize. In addition, if the hydrocele sac is opened, the operative field is obscured with fluid, and often blood, that oozes from the edge of the sac. For this reason, it is helpful to aspirate the hydrocele with a fine needle

through the scrotum just before making the inguinal incision. This simple procedure will return the anatomy to a more normal state so that the surgeon can identify the hernia sac with greater facility.

The postoperative management of a hydrocele is the same as was described for a hernia.

VARICOCELE

A varicocele is a collection of varicose veins in the scrotum, almost always on the left side. This is because of the long route taken by the left vein from the scrotum, up the retroperitoneal space to the renal vein. The varicosities may be caused by either an obstruction in the spermatic or renal veins or an absence of valves in the spermatic vein. In one series of boys studied with venography, 38 were found to have a partial obstruction of the renal vein. This resulted either from compression of the vein between the superior mesenteric artery and the aorta or from a retroaortic course of the vein. Twenty-six of the thirty-eight patients with partial obstruction demonstrated by venography also had elevated left renal vein pressure.[1] The impaired venous drainage increases intrascrotal temperature and causes progressive histologic damage to the testicle.[2,3] In adults, this testicular damage is associated with impaired sperm production and infertility.[4–6] This infertility can be reversed in adults by varicocele ligation and perhaps prevented by treatment during adolescence.[7,8] An early onset of a varicocele may be associated with more severe testicular damage; Kass and Belman documented loss of testicular volume in 20 boys aged 11 to 19.[9] They followed this same group of boys an average of 3.3 years after varicocele ligation and found an average testicular volume increase of 50 to 104 percent.

Figure 16–2. A typical scrotal hydrocele. There is no groin swelling, and palpation reveals a soft cystic mass with transillumination.

Diagnosis

Varicoceles rarely cause pain. Older boys may complain of a dragging or heavy sensation, or they may notice that the testicle on the side of the varicocele is smaller than its mate. The diagnosis may be made by observing the enlarged scrotum, which hangs lower than normal when the boy stands. In the upright position, palpation of the scrotum is like feeling a "bag of worms." The mass of veins disappears when the boy lies down. If the varicosities do not disappear, obstruction of the vein by a tumor is more likely. One should also suspect a tumor or situs inversus if the varicocele appears on the right. Each testicle should be measured, and the relative size of the left to the right testicle should be estimated and recorded. Finally, carefully palpate the flank because on more than one occasion, the varicocele is the first symptom of a renal tumor. Varicoceles are roughly classified into three stages; the first is one that is barely palpable and the testicle is of normal size. Stage two, or moderate-sized, varicoceles are palpable but not particularly noticeable, although the testicle may be smaller than normal. Stage three varicoceles are those that are obvious on inspection.

Treatment

Recent studies of testicular size and histology have changed the approach to these lesions. Formerly, they were merely observed and perhaps were operated on if adult infertility became a problem. It now appears that stage two and three varicoceles should be treated, particularly if there is demonstrable testicular atrophy.

In some centers, varicoceles are being treated with retrograde embolization through the renal vein. However, ligation of the spermatic vein is effective and can be carried out with minimal morbidity on an outpatient basis. The usual approach has been through a standard transverse hernia incision. The cremaster fibers are opened, and the veins of the pampiniform plexus are ligated at the level of the internal ring. This is a messy operation because one must separate and ligate a number of thin-walled dilated veins. A neater approach is through a higher, muscle-splitting incision, which approaches the spermatic vessels in the retroperitoneal space above the inguinal rings. The veins are separated from the artery and ligated, and a segment is excised. The boy should wear a scrotal support until all pain and edema have disappeared. An occasional recurrence seems to be unavoidable, although intraoperative distal venography may identify large collateral veins that also may require ligation.

REFERENCES

1. McKay DG, Fowler R, Barnett JS: The pathogenesis and treatment of hydroceles in infancy and childhood. In Stephens FD (ed): Congenital Malformations of the Rectum, Anus, and Genitourinary Tracts. Edinburgh, London, Churchill-Livingstone, 1963, p 295
2. Gorenstein A, Katz S, Schiller M: Varicocele in children: To treat or not to treat. Venographic and manometric studies. Pediatr Surg 21:12, 1046, 1986
3. Hienz HA, Voggenthale J, Weissbach L: Histological findings in testes with varicocele during childhood and their therapeutic consequences. Eur J Pediatr 133:139, 1980
4. Kass E, Chondra S, Belman G: Testicular history in the adolescent with a varicocele. Pediatrics 79:6:996, 1987
5. Lyon RP, Marshall S, Scott MP: Varicocele in childhood and adolescence: Implication in adult infertility? Urology 19:641, 1982
6. Tuloch WS: Varicocele in subfertility: Results of treatment. Brit Med J 2:356, 1955
7. Howards SS: Varicocele. Fertil Steril 41:356, 1984
8. Steeno O, Knops J, DeClerk L: Prevention of fertility disorders by detection and treatment of varicocele at school and college age. Andrologia 8:47, 1976
9. Kass E, Belman B: Reversal of testicular growth failure by varicocele ligation. J Urol 137:475, 1987

17
Torsion of the Testicle

Torsion of the testicle must be the first consideration in a child with acute scrotal pain. Any delay in the diagnosis increases the risk of infarction and gangrene. The normal testicle is stabilized by an attachment of the epididymis to the posterior lateral wall of the processus vaginalis. When this attachment is incomplete, the testicle is suspended within the processus vaginalis by its blood supply and the vas deferens (Fig. 17–1). This bell clapper type of attachment results in a hypermobile testicle that twists easily. This twisting initially causes venous obstruction and consequent congestion and edema. The inelastic tunic of the testicle increases the pressure on the testicular cells and rapidly compromises arterial flow. Infarction may occur within 4 hours, but viable Leydig cells have been observed in the testicle after a 360° torsion for 30 hours.[1] The Leydig cells are more resistant to ischemia than the seminiferous tubules.[2] An intravaginal torsion of one testicle means that there is another bell clapper type of testicle in the opposite scrotum that also is prone to twist.

Torsion of the testicle at the level of the external ring is better termed "torsion of the spermatic cord." This occurs most commonly in infants or children with hypermobile or undescended testes. The cremaster muscle produces a rotational effect on the cord structures as well as an upward pull during contraction.

DIAGNOSIS

Intravaginal torsion is most common in prepubertal boys, whose rapid testicular growth increases the disparity in size between the testicle and the supporting mesentery. Classically, there is a sudden onset of scrotal pain, which is referred to the lower abdomen, back, and thigh. There may be a history of similar mild episodes in the past, and the onset of pain may even be gradual if the torsion develops slowly, with incomplete venous obstruction. Most boys will be in exquisite pain and will seek medical attention soon after the onset. The symptoms in a newborn or small infant are not so striking. The baby is fussy and in pain, but the diagnosis is not made until the mother or physician notices scrotal swelling. An intrauterine or neonatal torsion may not be noticed until an atrophic testicle is found at the end of a fibrous vas deferens during exploration for an undescended testicle. On examination, the scrotum is red or has a bluish cast and is swollen and exquisitely tender. A twisted testicle is drawn up higher than its mate, in contrast to an inflamed organ, which hangs lower. This will produce a dimple near the bottom of the scrotum. Gentle elevation sometimes relieves the pain of epididymitis, but this has no effect on the pain of testicular torsion. Torsion of a testicle in the inguinal canal produces induration, pain, and tenderness above the scrotum, which easily can be mistaken for an incarcerated hernia.

A twisted intraabdominal testicle simulates appendicitis; the tipoff is the empty scrotum. The differential diagnosis of acute scrotal pain includes acute epididymitis and orchitis. Epididymitis is more likely to be associated with systemic fever and pyuria. Mumps orchitis rarely if ever occurs before puberty and appears within 3 days to a week after the onset of parotid swelling. Torsion of the testicular appendages simulates a testicular torsion. Moharib and Krahn found that 25 of 56 children with acute scrotal pain had a torsion of the testicle or its appendages, whereas Kaplan and King found that 90 percent of children with acute scrotal swellings at the Children's Memorial Hospital had a torsion.[3,4] These studies indicate that torsion of the testis or its appendages is the most common cause of scrotal pain, particularly in prepubertal boys. When there is no doubt about the clinical diagnosis, an operation is indicated as soon as possible. When the symptoms are more suggestive of

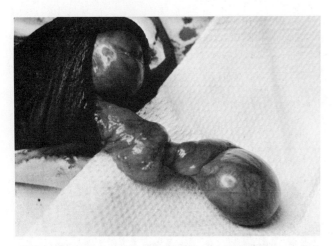

Figure 17–1. Intravaginal torsion of the testicle in a 13-year-old boy. The testicle was suspended within the tunica vaginalis by its blood supply and the vas.

an inflammatory process or are atypical for a torsion, the diagnosis can be made with the Doppler ultrasonic stethoscope, which demonstrates reduced blood flow over the involved testicle.[5,6] Epididymitis should increase the blood flow. Unfortunately, there have been false negative results with the Doppler study in children who have had proven torsion.[7] It is possible that in these cases the inflammatory response to the torsion produced an increased blood flow in the scrotum. Scanning with radioactive technetium-99m has proved to be a reliable diagnostic technique in young adults and teenage boys. When positive, the technetium scan reveals a cold spot

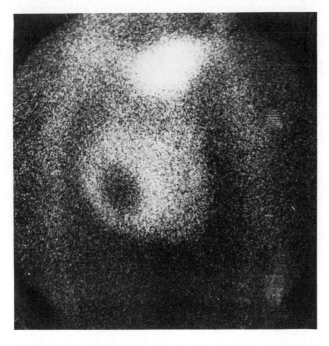

Figure 17–2. Torsion of the right testicle, which produces a cold spot in the scrotum.

or empty space where the testicle should be in the scrotum (Fig. 17–2). Although Riley et al. found this test to be 94 percent accurate, they also found that the test was not reliable in children under 11 years of age whose testicles were small.[8] Hahn et al. also questioned its accuracy in small children.[9] However, in pediatric centers, more refined rectolinear scanning techniques have allowed the diagnosis to be made with greater accuracy.[10] Regardless of the results of either a Doppler examination or a scan, the child should be operated on if there is any doubt about the diagnosis; otherwise in the presence of torsion the testicle will surely die.[11] If there is a reasonable suspicion of torsion by clinical examination, a nuclear scan or Doppler examination should be obtained only if these studies are immediately available.

TREATMENT

The pain in torsion of the testicle may be so great that intravenous morphine is required for relief. An attempt to derotate the testicle may be made in the emergency room while the operating room is being prepared. Betts et al. were able to derotate 8 of 11 cases of torsion in the emergency room. In each of these 8 patients the testicle was rotated toward the thigh on the side of the torsion (clockwise on the left, counterclockwise on the right). In this series, the initial diagnosis as well as successful derotation were determined by Doppler examination.[12]

A scrotal incision is satisfactory for derotation of an intravaginal torsion. A transverse incision is made through the skin, dartos fascia, and tunica vaginalis to expose the testicle. The testicle is then withdrawn from the incision and untwisted. The tunica albuginea is incised to decompress the edematous organ. A row of catgut sutures is then placed through the tunica and the processus vaginalis to stabilize the testicle. The opposite scrotum is opened also, and several sutures are used to fix the other testicle so as to prevent a counterlateral torsion. Ice bags may be used to reduce postoperative pain and to decrease metabolism and oxygen use for several days. Although some authors recommend an ochiectomy if the testicle is obviously gangrenous, it seems logical to leave the testicle in place regardless of appearance. The worst complication of leaving the testicle would be an abscess. Hopefully, some Leydig cells will remain even if there is testicular atrophy. A torsion of the spermatic cord or one involving an undescended testicle is operated on through a transverse hernia type of groin incision. Bartsch et al. determined the late results in 42 patients who had been operated on for testicle torsion in childhood. There were minimal changes in testicular histology when detorsion was carried out within 4 hours. After 8 hours, there was progressive deterioration in testicular

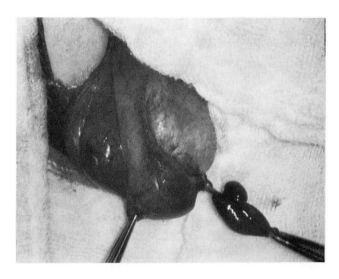

Figure 17–3. Torsion of the appendix testis, which has produced gangrene.

size, semen quality, and histology.[13] This study again emphasizes the urgency of early diagnosis and treatment.

TORSION OF THE TESTICULAR APPENDAGES

There are four testicular appendages: the appendix testis, the appendix epididymis, the vas abernans of Haller, and the paradidymis.[14] The appendix testis is involved in about 90 percent of children with torsion of the appendages (Fig. 17–3). The peak incidence of torsion of the appendix testis occurs between the ages of 10 and 13 years.[15] There is often a history of vigorous play or athletic activity just before the onset of scrotal pain. The pain is not so severe as a torsion of the testicle, but it may not be possible to distinguish between the two unless one can palpate a pea-size tender mass on the testicle. Transillumination may demonstrate a small dark mass. Treatment consists of a scrotal incision with excision of the appendage.

If an operation is performed for a suspected torsion of the testicle and an orchitis is found, the tunica albugi-nea should still be opened to release pressure on the testicle. This is indicated because there is an appreciable incidence of testicular atrophy following mumps orchitis.

REFERENCES

1. Atallah MW, Mazzarino AF, Horton RF: Testicular scan, diagnosis and follow-up for torsion of the testis. J Urol 118:120, 1977
2. Moyad R, Barnett RB, Lapides J, Taub M: Therapy for questionably infarcted testis. Invest Urol 12:387, 1975
3. Moharib NH, Krahn HP: Acute scrotum in children with emphasis on torsion of the spermatic cord. J Urol 104:601, 1970
4. Kaplan CW, King LR: Acute scrotal swelling in children. J Urol 104:219, 1970
5. Levy BJ: The diagnosis of torsion of the testicle using the Doppler ultrasonic stethoscope. J Urol 113:63, 1974
6. Pederson JF, Holm HH, Hald T: Torsion of the testis diagnosed by ultrasound. J Urol 113:66, 1975
7. Nasrallah PF, Manzone D, King LR: Falsely negative Doppler examinations in testicular torsion. J Urol 118:194, 1977
8. Riley TW, Mosborgh PC, Coles JL, et al: Use of radioiso-tope scan in evaluation of intrascrotal lesions. J Urol 116:422, 1976
9. Hahn LC, Nadel NS, Gitter MH, Vernon AR: Testicular scanning of a new modality for the preoperative diagnosis of testicular torsion. J Urol 113:60, 1975
10. Hitch DC, Gilday DL, Shoulding B, Savage JP: A new approach to the diagnosis of testicular torsion. J Pediatr Surg 2:537, 1976
11. Williamson R: Death in the scrotum: Testicular torsion. N Engl J Med 206:338, 1977
12. Betts J, Norris M, Crowie W, Duckett J: Testicular detor-sion using Doppler ultrasound monitoring. J Pediatr Surg 18:607, 1983
13. Bartsch G, Frank S, Marberger A: Testicular torsion: Late results with special regard to fertility and endocrine func-tion. J Urol 124:375, 1980
14. Rolnick D, Kawahove S, Szanto P: Anatomical incidence of testicular appendages. J Urol 100:755, 1968
15. Skoglund RW, McRoberts JW, Rogde H: Torsion of testicu-lar appendages: Presentation of 43 new cases and a collec-tive review. J Urol 104:598, 1970

18
Undescended Testicle

When a boy is found to have an empty scrotum, his father has nagging doubts about his son's future masculinity, the physician is concerned about cancer, and most importantly, the boy is embarrassed and is worried about teasing by his schoolmates. In treatment of a boy with an improperly descended testicle, one must take into account these emotional problems as well as the anatomic factors.

There are unresolved controversies concerning the indications for and the timing of an operation for an undescended testicle. In addition, there are a variety of operative techniques designed to place the testicle in the scrotum. Some of these controversies are resolved by the proper definition of terms. An "undescended testicle" may be located anywhere in the retroperitoneum between the kidney and the scrotum. Most often, the testicle is palpable within the inguinal canal. An "ectopic testicle" is one that has descended beyond the external ring but lies outside the scrotum. It may have passed posteriorly in the buttock area, to the femoral canal, or anywhere in the perineum, including the base of the penis (Fig. 18–1). A retractile, or yo-yo, testicle is not truly undescended but is pulled up into the inguinal canal by a hyperactive cremasteric reflex. When careful palpation fails to reveal a testicle in the inguinal canal or perineum, it is possible that the testicle is congenitally absent or has undergone atrophy as a result of previous torsion. Usually, it is within the peritoneal cavity, adjacent to the internal ring.

INCIDENCE

This problem afflicts 21 percent of premature infants. In full-term newborns, the incidence is 2.7 percent, and at 1 year of age, approximately 1 percent of children have undescended testicles.[1-3] Thus, the testicle almost always spontaneously descends during the first year of life. Whether it continues to descend is open to debate. Some testicles may reach the scrotum during puberty, but the incidences of true maldescent found in 1-year-olds and in young adults is similar. The difference in incidence among various series of patients represents a failure to make a distinction between a retractile testicle and a true maldescent. Careful studies performed by skilled individuals indicate that it is rare for a real undescended testicle to reach the scrotum after the first year of life.[4,5] Undescent of the testicle is more common on the right side, and approximately 10 to 15 percent of children with undescended testicles have bilateral involvement.[6]

PATHOLOGY

The etiology and pathology of true maldescent of the testis are interrelated. There is evidence that testicular descent is under endocrine control. Premature testicular descent may be induced in the rat by injections of gonadotropin, and in mice cryptorchidism may be produced by blocking the production of androgen in the fetus by estrogen administration.[7,8] Atrophy of the Leydig cells in human cryptorchid testes, which is similar to that seen in mice treated with estrogen, has been observed with the electron microscope.[9] If this correlation is correct, androgen produced by the normal Leydig cells may be responsible for normal descent of the testis in humans. In boys with cryptorchidism, there is a deficit in the physiologic early postnatal surge of pituitary luteinizing hormone and testosterone, with reduced responsiveness to the luteinizing hormone-releasing hormone (LHRH), which originates from the hypothalamus. Thus, a partial or transient luteinizing hormone deficiency could be a factor in some cases of cryptorchidism.[10] It

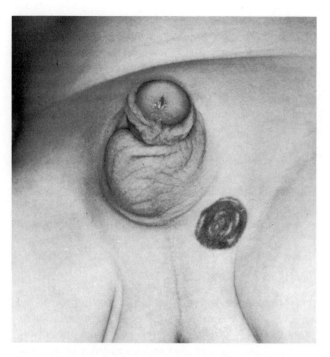

Figure 18–1. An ectopic testicle lateral to and beneath the scrotum.

is not difficult to postulate an endocrine deficiency for bilateral (but not for unilateral) undescended testicles. The unilateral undescended testicle is smaller than its counterpart and has a higher chance of having structural abnormalities. Dickinson found failure of union between the vas deferens and the epididymis or atresia of either the vas or the mesonephric system in three children at the time of orchiopexy.[11] Marshall and Shermeta also observed structural abnormalities in undescended testes that would contribute to infertility regardless of when the testicle was operated on.[12]

The most likely cause of unilateral cryptorchidism is either a defect in the testicle itself, which makes it unable to respond to endocrine stimulation, or a mechanical block to its descent.[13,14] Histologic studies of the undescended testicle have revealed no visible damage to the germinative epithelium during the first 2 years of life.[15] During the third year, there is a drop in the spermatogonia content in the undescended testicle, whereas in a normal testicle, there is an increase in both spermatogonia and tubule diameter, which continues to about 15 years of age. In 14 percent of the cases studied, the undescended testicle demonstrated no spermatogonia. The study also demonstrated a 52.7 percent incidence of decreased spermatogonia in the opposite, normally descended testicle that did not improve with age. This supports the experimental findings in dogs that demonstrate that the cryptorchid testicle damages its normal mate. When the high testicle is brought back down into the scrotum, the lesions in both are reversed.[16] Electron microscopic studies of the undescended testicle

have confirmed the finding of degeneration of the germinal epithelium commencing with the second year of life. However, there are structural changes in the Leydig cells as early as the first year.[17] These may be related to abdominal temperature, which is 1.5 to 2.0F higher than that of the scrotum. The increased incidence of malignant degeneration in the undescended testicle may be another reflection of the fact that the undescended testicle is abnormal from the very beginning.

Practically every cryptorchid testicle is associated with a patent processus vaginalis, and some patients also have a clinical hernia. Defects of the abdominal wall, including omphalocele and gastroschisis, and especially the prune-belly syndrome, frequently are associated with an intra-abdominal testicle. The Noonan, Prader-Willi, Lowess, and Klinefelter's syndromes are all associated with a high incidence of undescended testicles.[18–21] When bilateral cryptorchidism is associated with hypospadias, buccal smears and chromosomal studies are indicated to rule out intersexual disorders.

FUNCTION

Testicular function can be evaluated through endocrine studies, by sperm production, and by the proved fertility rate in married patients who have been treated for an undescended testicle. There are conflicting results among the various studies, but Atkinson found that 76 percent of men treated for unilateral and 44 percent of those treated for bilateral undescent of the testicle had fathered a child.[22] Atkinson also found that 90 percent of men who had been treated for a unilateral undescended testicle had normal plasma androgen levels. However, abnormal gonadotropin levels were found in 15 of 40 men studied.[23] Others have found a significantly higher level of oligospermia in men previously treated for unilateral cryptorchidism.[24,25] Another recent study demonstrated a mean sperm density of only 37 percent in men who had undergone an orchiopexy between 4 and 12 years of age.[26] In addition, these men had a mean follicle-stimulating hormone (FSH) response to synthetic gonadotropin-releasing hormone of more than twice the response of normal men. These same men, however, had normal serum testosterone levels.

DIAGNOSIS

The diagnosis of an undescended testicle commences with the observation that one or both testicles are absent from the scrotum. It is important if the parents can remember or if a physician's record can document the presence of a testicle in the scrotum at the time of birth. If it later disappears, it may be an ascending testicle, which is merely retractile. On the other hand, if there is a history of pain and swelling, the baby may have had a torsion, and the testicle is now atrophic. When the testicle has never been down, the hemiscrotum is small and smooth.

The examination must be unhurried and gentle and accompanied by a patter of conversation with the boy to help him relax. With the child supine, the inguinal canal is examined, commencing at the level of the internal ring. A mobile testicle is difficult to palpate and may pop back and forth out of the abdomen. If a testicle is felt in the canal, attempts should be made with one hand to move it down to the scrotum. If it can be made to reach the upper scrotum, it is grasped with the other hand and demonstrated to the parents. Any testicle that can be manipulated into the scrotum 4 cm or more below the symphsyis pubis is likely to be retractile and does not require an operation. Another test for retractile testicles consists of having the boy sit up, with his hips and knees flexed, grasping his lower legs with his arms. In this position the retractile testicle will enter the scrotum; it may then be held there while the boy slowly extends his legs.[27] Further palpation is performed over the femoral canal and the perineum to find an ectopic testicle. Occasionally, one may palpate a nubbin of tissue in the scrotum that feels like an atrophic testicle; this often turns out to be the gubernaculum, while the testicle is actually at a higher level.

After the child is examined in a supine position, he is asked to stand, or, if the patient is a baby, his mother holds him erect. The internal ring is again palpated while the child coughs and strains. This maneuver frequently causes an intraabdominal testicle to pop out of the internal ring, allowing palpation for a fleeting moment. When the testicle is palpated in the inguinal canal but cannot be brought down into the scrotum, one can make a definitive diagnosis of an undescended testicle.

Preoperative localization of an impalpable testicle is hardly necessary in the usual case. One may argue that surgical exploration is necessary to definitely determine the presence of a testicle regardless of what studies may show, if for no other reason than to insert a Silastic prosthesis. However, if there has been a previous incomplete exploration or if the child has ambiguous genitalia, it may be well to locate or at least to prove the presence of the testicle. Herniography and selective angiography have been recommended in the past. However, these potentially dangerous, invasive tests have been superceded by ultrasonography and computed tomography (CT).[28,29] Either of these techniques in skilled hands can detect masses as small as 1 cm. Their greatest usefulness may be in older patients to detect intra-abdominal testicular tumors. Laparoscopy immediately preceding the surgical exploration can precisely locate intraabdomi-nal testes and, thus, be a valuable guide in the choice of incision. Laparoscopy also is useful in identifying undifferentiated gonads and müllerian duct remnants.[30]

When neither testicle is palpable, it is helpful to determine if there is functioning testicular tissue before exploration. This is accomplished via a human chorionic gonadotropin (HCG)-stimulation test.[31,32] The serum testosterone level is determined before and after the administration of HCG in the amount of 2000 units/day for 4 days. If there are responsive gonads, the plasma testosterone will increase dramatically after stimulation. One may then undertake an extensive retroperitoneal exploration with opening of the peritoneal cavity in an attempt to find the testicles.

TREATMENT

More than 50 years ago, Engle demonstrated increased testicular size and descent in monkeys treated with a hormonal extract.[33] Since then, many investigators have claimed success in achieving testicular descent with injections of HCG. Others have sometimes bitterly objected to these claims on the basis that success with hormonal therapy occurred only in children with retractile testes that would have descended without treatment. An excellent, recently reported clinical trial was conducted in France in which retractile testes were eliminated by careful repeated clinical examination before treatment.[34] There were 109 boys with unilateral and 44 with bilateral maldescended testes. All were age 6 months to 5 years. They were given three injections of HCG weekly for 3 weeks. Each dose ranged from 500 to 1500 units, with the average dose being 2100 IU/m^2 of body surface area. The testicle descended into the scrotum in 12.4 percent. There was some improvement in another 15.6 percent, but in 72 percent, there was no change in the position of the testicle. The best results were when the testicle was originally located in the canal. Only 4 percent of abdominal testes descended. This careful study demonstrated the very limited usefulness of HCG treatment in younger boys.

LHRH may be given intranasally as well as by injection. In two carefully controlled studies of boys with true maldescent, there was no difference between treatment with LHRH and placebos.[35,36] These investigators could find no evidence for a hormonal deficiency in boys with cryptorchidism and considered LHRH treatment useless for impalpable testes. Hormonal evaluation also was of no value in determining in advance which child might respond to treatment. The futility of hormonal therapy was indicated in yet another investigation that compared intranasal gonadotropin-releasing hormone with parenteral HCG.[37] The patients in this study were from 1 to 5 years of age. Descent occurred in 19 percent of patients treated with gonadotropin-releasing hormone, and in 6 percent of those treated with HCG. Testosterone levels increased significantly in both groups. The same authors treated five boys with retractile testes and obtained complete descent in all.

There appear to be two benefits to hormonal therapy in boys with maldescent of the testes. If one cannot determine on physical examination if a testicle is merely retractile or a low but true undescended testicle, a short trial of HCG will cause a retractile testicle to descend. The child with bilateral impalpable testes also presents a special problem. The stimulation test will determine if there are testicles present, and also, preoperative hormonal therapy increases the testicular size and blood supply, to improve the results of surgery.

The results from hormonal therapy in true maldescent are so inconsistent that every effort should be made to position the testicle in the scrotum by operation. The usual reasons given are that an operation will improve fertility and prevent torsion. Also, a developing tumor can be found more easily in the scrotum than in the abdomen. The most important reasons, however, are psychologic. Boys become aware of their bodies at an early age and suffer anxiety over any real or imagined differences between their own genitals and the norm. Furthermore, if schoolmates become aware that one boy is "different," he is mercilessly teased. These same issues influence the timing of an operation. Based on the microscopic studies previously mentioned, one would assume that the child with a definite undescended testicle should be operated on before he is 2 years old. Although the evidence seems to show that age makes little difference in eventual testicular function, Kiesewetter et al.'s serial biopsies indicated improvement of the microscopic architecture of the testicle after an orchiopexy.[38] This finding, along with consideration of the psychologic impact of an undescended testicle and a genital operation, tend to make one think that it is best to perform the operation before 3 years of age.[39] Bilateral undescended testicles, especially if they are just at the internal ring or within the abdomen, should be brought down as soon as possible, certainly by the age of 2 years. In addition, if there is a clinically evident hernia, the operation should be performed at any age.

Operation

The objective of any operation for the cure of cryptorchidism is to position the testicle within the scrotum without tension. This must be accomplished without injury to the blood supply or to the vas deferens. The operative technique varies with the location of the testicle. An inguinal incision is perfectly satisfactory when the testicle is in an ectopic location or when it is easily palpable near the external ring. One that is higher may still be reached through an extended inguinal approach, but either a preperitoneal or a transabdominal operation is preferable in this situation.

Inguinal Orchiopexy

The entire lower abdomen, scrotum, perineum, and upper thighs are carefully prepared and draped to provide scrotal access (Fig. 18–2 A through M). In the usual case, a transverse incision is made in the highest inguinal crease, which may be angled upward toward the anterior superior spine of the ischium. Great care is taken as the incision is made through Scarpa's fascia, since an occasional vas deferens will have prolapsed through the external ring. The external oblique aponeurosis is opened to a point above the internal ring. The testicle usually is found at this time. Loose areolar tissue about the testicle and the cremaster muscle are stripped away until the gubernaculum is isolated, clamped, and divided just distal to the testicle. One hemostat is left attached to the gubernaculum to apply traction on the testicle and spermatic cord. At this point, a finger is gently inserted into the scrotum to gradually make a tunnel. This process is repeated several times during the operation, taking care not to vigorously stretch the scrotum all at once. A forceful thrust will result in postoperative ecchymoses and scrotal swelling. Next, with the testicle held up by an assistant, the cremaster fibers are stripped away, the vas deferens and testicular vessels are then clearly identified, and the overlying internal spermatic fascia is opened. At this point, the vas and vessels may appear to be inside the hernia sac. They can be prominently displayed with traction on the sac. This should allow separation of the vas and vessels so the hernia sac can be divided between clamps. Then, with traction applied upward and laterally on the testicle and medially on the proximal sac, the vas and vessels are dissected up to the peritoneum and just into the retroperitoneal space. The sac is then suture ligated; it should continue to be held with a clamp, since traction on the stump of the sac opens the gateway to the retroperitoneum. The sac and fibers of the internal spermatic fascia are then dissected off the vas and vessels distally to the testicle. The testicle may be left in a pocket of processus vaginalis, but considerable length can be obtained by completely removing all of the sac and the enveloping fascia. At this stage in the operation, the vas and vessels have been freed from all tissue up to and just within the internal ring. This is all that is required in the patient with an ectopic testis or a testis tethered to a short hernia sac.

Greater length can be obtained by further dissection, freeing the vas down to the seminal vesicle and the vessels from the retroperitoneum to their origin. These structures cannot be lengthened, but their course can be straightened. It may be necessary to extend the original skin incision up to the anterior superior spine.

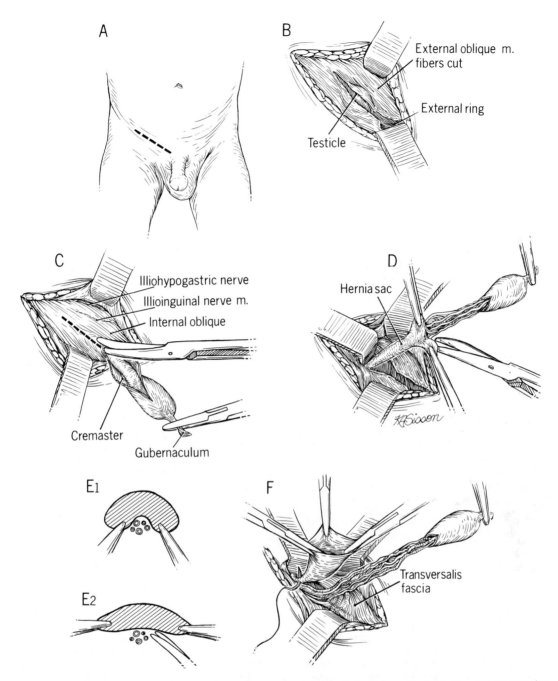

Figure 18–2. Inguinal orchiopexy. **A.** A skin crease incision is made that can be extended to the anterior-superior spine of the ileum if necessary for additional exposure. **B.** The testicle often is just beneath the external oblique fascia and must be protected from damage during the incision. **C.** As the testicle is mobilized, the gubernaculum is divided and grasped with a hemostat for traction. The internal ring may be enlarged at this time for improved exposure of the vessels and the hernia sac. **D.** The hernia sac is found and dissected free from the vas and the vessels. **E.** Occasionally, the vas and vessels appear to be within the hernia sac. This can be confusing and difficult, but if the sac is held on traction between two hemostats or forceps, the vessels and sac will appear to be on the surface of the sac, simplifying their dissection. **F.** The isolated sac is suture ligated. (Continued)

150

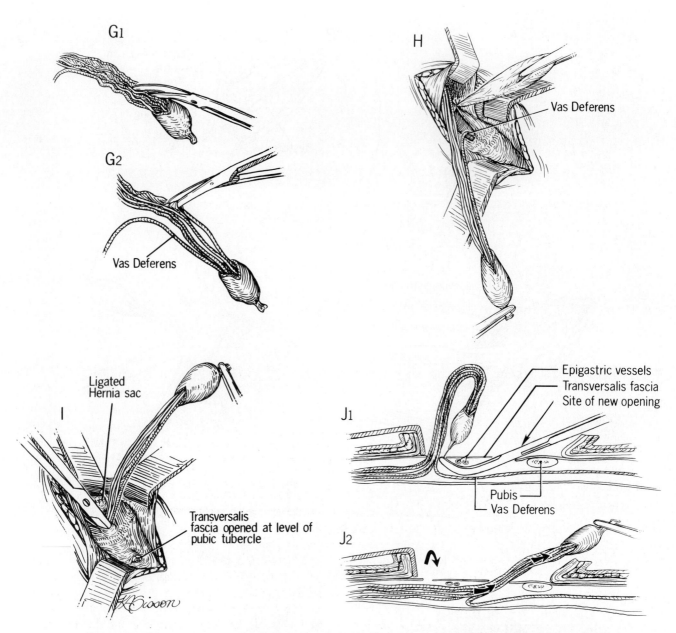

Fig. 18–2. (Cont.) G. At this point, considerable length may be obtained distal to the internal ring by dividing bands of fascia that tether the fold of the vessels together. This must be done with the greatest of care to avoid injury to the vessels. **H.** Further length is obtained by extending the dissection into the retroperitoneum. The hernia sac is held upward and medially with considerable tension. A retractor that elevates the internal oblique muscle opens the gateway to the retroperitoneum, allowing easy dissection and separation of the testicular vessels from the peritoneum and surrounding tissues. This step must be performed with the aid of a good light and with long instruments under direct vision. **I.** The vas and vessels have now been mobilized completely. Still further length is obtained by straightening out the bend around the transversalis fascia and the inferior epigastric vessels. This may be done by dividing the fascia and vessels, but it is much simpler to tunnel into the fatty tissue beneath the fascia and vessels with a curved hemostat down to the pubic tubercle. **J.** This step is demonstrated in cross section—the testicle is brought through the tunnel with an attached suture.

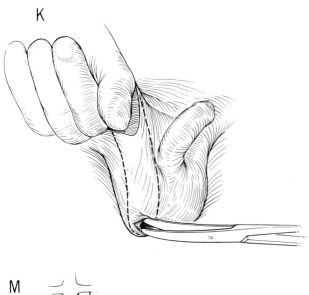

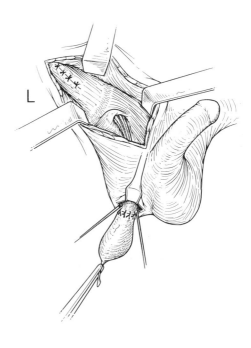

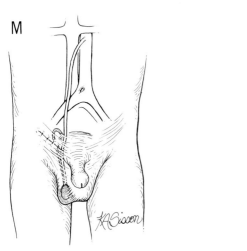

Fig. 18-2 (Cont.) K. The finger is placed into the scrotum and a skin incision is made down to the dartos fascia. The skin is generously undermined to make a pocket between the dartos and the skin. **L.** The testicle is brought through the dartos and placed in the subcutaneous pocket. Three or four sutures are placed through the dartos into the tunica albuginea of the testicle. **M.** The final result; the testicular vessels pursue a straightened course to the testicle, which is secured in its subcutaneous pocket.

In such a case, both the external and internal obliques are opened for 3 to 4 cm. With this accomplished, traction on the end of the hernia sac and blunt dissection with a finger or gauze dissector will allow entry into the loose areolar tissues behind the peritoneum. Curved retractors are then inserted into the incision to allow dissection of the testicular vessels away from the peritoneum. This is accomplished with the aid of a good light, traction on the testicle, and careful separation of the tissues with a long, curved scissors. Small strands of fibrous tissue that fan out from the vessels are divided until they have been freed as high up as possible. With further upward traction, the vas deferens is then traced down to the seminal vesicle. At this point, it becomes evident that attempts to place the testicle in the scrotum result in angulation of the vas and vessels around the edge of the transversalis fascia and the inferior epigastric vessels. Most surgeons divide these structures, but it is simpler and just as effective to tunnel into the loose fatty tissue beneath the transversalis fascia to a point adjacent to the pubic tubercle. This tunnel is opened with a curved forceps, and an incision is made in the fascia adjacent to the tubercle, which allows the testicle to be pulled through beneath the transversalis fascia to exit through a new abdominal ring adjacent to the pubic tubercle. The vessels pursue nearly a straight line from their origin to the testicle. The old internal ring and the transversalis fascia are carefully closed.

There are many techniques for securing the testicle in the scrotum. Formerly, rubberband traction to the inner side of the thigh was popular. I have tried a dental roll, which is sutured outside the scrotal skin and to the testicle. Either of these procedures restricts the boy's postoperative activities and are no more effective than placing the testicle in a subcutaneous position outside the dartos fascia.[40] This is carried out by inserting one's finger into the scrotum. A 1-cm incision is made, only skin deep over the finger. Then, with the finger still in place beneath the dartos, a subcutaneous pouch is created by opening and closing scissors blades beneath the skin. A small incision is then made through the dartos down to the gloved finger. The edges of the dartos are grasped with small hemostats; then another clamp is inserted through the scrotal incision and passed up into the wound to grasp the lower pole of the testicle, which is then drawn down through the dartos incision and placed in the subcutaneous pouch after two or three sutures are inserted between the dartos and the upper pole of the testicle.

The scrotal skin is closed with two or three catgut sutures. Then, after careful hemostasis, the layers of the wound are closed with absorbable, polyglucanate sutures. This operation is carried out on an outpatient basis, and the boys' only restrictions are those self-imposed by pain.

THE HIGH TESTICLE

The impalpable testicle, or one that lies just at the internal ring, presents special problems. One must resist the temptation to skeletonize the vessels or to place the testicle in the scrotum with its blood supply under tension. Testicular atrophy is sure to follow. Previously, I advocated a two-stage procedure, in which the testicle is mobilized as far down in the canal as possible, then brought to the scrotum at a second operation a year later. I now prefer the technique of high vessel division advocated by Stephens and Fowler.[41] These authors demonstrated the vascular anatomy of the undescended testis, which consists of anastomoses between the artery of the vas and the spermatic artery. The testis also receives collateral branches from the scrotal arteries through the gubernaculum. Further evidence for the safety of testicular vessel ligation is the absence of testicular atrophy after ligation of the gonadal vessels during removal of Wilms' tumors. In pigs, division of the testicular vessels does not impair growth, size, or development of spermatogenic epithelium. Further clinical evidence of adequate blood flow to the testicle after this operation has been found on radionuclide studies showing normal circulation to the testicle.

Procedure

Either the standard groin or a preperitoneal incision is used. When the testis is identified, high in the canal or within the abdomen, the hernia sac is found, separated from the vas and vessels, then ligated. The normal point of divergence of the vas and vessels is just superior to the internal inguinal ring. No dissection between the vas or vessels should be carried out distal to this point. The gubernaculum is left intact, but the cremasteric fibers and the internal spermatic fascia must be opened and separated from the testicle and the hernia sac. The testicular vessels are mobilized for several centimeters above the point of divergence from the vas. At that point, they are temporarily occluded with a small, non-crushing vascular clamp. If the color of the testis remains normal and if there is bleeding from a small incision in the tunica albuginea, the vessels may be ligated and

divided. Since the vas is considerably longer than the vessels, the testicle will now easily reach the scrotum, when it can be fixed in a dartos pouch.

Follow-up of our own cases indicates that the testicle remains normal to palpation up to 5 years after operation. In Fowler and Stephens' original article, good results were obtained in 8 of 12 patients.[41] Three of the four failures had atrophic testes at the time of operation. Clatworthy et al. also reported good results with this procedure.[42]

An alternative to ligation of the vessels is microvascular anastomosis between the testicular artery and vein and the inferior epigastric vessels.[43] However, there has been one reported case in which a microvascular anastomosis was performed on one side and ligation on the other. Nine months later, both testes were normal in size.[44]

BILATERAL UNDESCENDED TESTICLES

A transabdominal operation allows the most complete exploration for bilateral nondescent; this operation has its greatest value in children with the prune-belly syndrome.[45] Excellent exposure also may be obtained with a preperitoneal approach, without the hazards of opening the peritoneum. Boley and Kleinhars have recommended the Cheatle-Henry approach to the high testicle and in any situation in which one wishes to explore both sides at once.[46] We prefer the original midline extraperitoneal approach first described by Henry to a transverse incision through the rectus sheath.[47]

For this procedure, the boy is positioned on the operating table with his knees flexed over pillows; the entire abdomen, scrotum, and thighs are prepared and draped. If the bladder is palpable, it is emptied with a catheter. The operation described by Henry uses a midline skin incision, but since this yields a poor cosmetic result, a transverse smile incision is centered halfway between the pubis and the umbilicus and extended toward each iliac crest. The skin and subcutaneous flaps are created by sliding the blades of scissors into the loose areolar tissue that overlies the fascia. By opening the scissors at a right angle to the skin and fascia, small vessels can be easily identified and coagulated. Elevation of two flaps of skin exposes the linea alba from the pubis to the umbilicus. At this point the skin also is dissected up and laterally, first toward the lateral edge of the pubic tubercle and then on into the scrotum. Thus, one starts to open the upper scrotum early in the operation, which facilitates the creation of a new internal and external ring adjacent to the pubis. The midline of the linea alba is sometimes difficult to identify, and often one rectus sheath or the other is opened. This can be avoided by commencing at the upper end of the incision where the recti diverge around the umbilicus; at this point, the fascia is incised down to the peritoneum and thence inferiorly to the pubis. Considerable muscle relaxation is essential for elevation of the fascia and the muscular layers of the abdominal wall, while with finger or gauze dissection the peritoneum is separated from the underlying rectus sheath until the internal ring, inferior epigastric vessels, and the entire back wall of the inguinal canal are exposed.

It is easy to become confused early in the operation because one is not accustomed to seeing the inguinal canal from the inside. The key landmarks are the inferior epigastric vessels and the hernia sac, which extends into the internal ring immediately above and adjacent to the inferior epigastric vessels. Blunt dissection with a bit of gauze held in a forceps will expose the superior, lateral, and inferior portions of the hernia sac. At this point, one must trace the vas to find the testicle. If the testicle is just within the inguinal canal, it is withdrawn into the operative field with traction and dissection about the hernia sac until the entire sac, with the testicle, is brought into the wound. Great care must be taken not to injure the inferior epigastric vessels. If they are in the way, they may be ligated and divided to allow free access to the internal ring. The testicle and sac are then held on traction by a suture through the gubernaculum. The vas and vessels may then be separated from the neck of the sac, which is ligated flush with the peritoneum. After this step, one has complete freedom to strip the testicular vessels away from the peritoneum to their origin, and the vas may be freed to the seminal vesicles. Exposure is obtained by elevating the abdominal wall away from the peritoneum with Deaver retractors. When this has been accomplished, a point just lateral to the pubic tubercle is identified by palpating the abdominal wall with one finger within the pelvis and another beneath the skin. A new ring is then made at that point to enable the testicle and vas to exit from the abdomen into the scrotum. The old internal ring may be completely closed with sutures. At the end of the operation, the vas and vessels pursue a perfectly straight course from their origins to the scrotum. When one side has been completed, the gracious surgeon will relinquish the scissors and forceps and will demonstrate proper retraction technique so that his assistant can have the pleasure of operating on the contralateral side. When both testicles are residing safely and without tension in the scrotum, the midline fascial incision is carefully closed with a figure-eight suture, and the skin is approximated with subcuticular sutures and sterile tapes.

When one finds a vas deferens that ends in a small nubbin of scar tissue, one can be certain that the testicle is absent. Most likely there had been an intrauterine torsion. When no testicle is found after diligent exploration, one has the option of placing a Silastic prosthesis in the scrotum. This is not logical in a child under 5 years of age, when most orchiopexies take place. I prefer to wait until the boy is 9 or 10; then one can insert a prosthesis of an appropriate size for a teenage boy. The prosthesis has a small tab at one pole for suturing to the dartos fascia. After stretching the scrotum, it is inverted into the wound, so that the tab may be sutured deep in the pocket. The entrance to the scrotum must then be closed above the prosthesis to ensure that it stays in place.

RESULTS

Long-term follow-up is necessary to evaluate results in terms of fertility in individual patients. Most studies are flawed because of difficulties in locating patients for evaluation. In one study of fertility, data could be obtained on only 231 of 800 children operated on between 1936 and 1968.[48] In this group, 80 percent of patients with unilateral and 36 percent of those with bilateral cryptorchidism were fertile. Thus, from this study, one can predict normal fertility in children with a unilateral undescended testicle. The age of the child at operation made no difference to ultimate fertility.

Chilvers et al. reviewed 27 articles in a literature review to study adult fertility in terms of sperm density after treatment for undescended testes.[49] They found a 15 percent rate of azospermia and a 30 percent rate of oligospermia (less than 20×10^6/ml) in men operated on for unilateral cryptorchidism. There was no difference between hormonal and surgical treatment and no difference in the age at operation, at least in the range of 4 to 14 years. In this study, it did appear that treatment of bilateral cryptorchidism could produce fertility. In this same study, there were no data to suggest that orchiopexy reduced the ultimate incidence of cancer of the testicle. Thus, boys who have been treated for undescended testicles must be followed throughout their lives for the development of tumors.

REFERENCES

1. Scorer CG: The descent of the testis. Arch Dis Child 39:605, 1964
2. Biogviovanni AM: Diagnosis and treatment: The undescended testicle. Pediatrics 36:781, 1965
3. Spence HM, Culp OS, Glen JF: Panel discussion: Anomalies of external genitalia in infancy and childhood. J Urol 93:1, 1965
4. Pinch L, Aceto T Jr, Mayer-Bahlburg HFL: Cryptorchidism: A pediatric review. Urol Clin North Am 1:573, 1974
5. Scorer CG, Farrington GH: Congenital Deformities of the Testis and Epididymis. London, Butterworths, 1971
6. Gross RE, Jewitt TC Jr: Surgical experiences from 1222 operations for undescended testis. JAMA 160:634, 1956

7. Rejfer J, Walsh PC: Hormonal regulation of testicular descent. Presented at the Annual Meeting of the American Urological Association, Chicago, April 26, 1977

8. Jean C: Croissence et structure des testicules cryptorchides chez les souris nees de meres treitees a l'oestradive pendent la gestation. Ann Endocrinol (Paris) 34:667, 1973

9. Hadziselimovic F, Herzug B: The meaning of the Leydig cell in relation to the etiology of cryptorchidism: An experimental electron-microscopic study. J Pediatr Surg 11:1, 1976

10. Gendrel D, Roger M, Job J: Plasma gonadotropins and testosterone values in infants with cryptorchidism. J Pediatr 97:217, 1980

11. Dickinson TJ: Structural abnormalities in the undescended testis. J Pediatr Surg 8:523, 1973

12. Marshall F, Shermeta D: Epididymal abnormalities associated with undescended testis. J Urol 121:341, 1979

13. Sohvol AR: Testicular dysgenesis as an etiological factor in cryptorchidism. J Urol 72:693, 1954

14. Backhouse KM: The gubernaculum testis: Testicular descent and maldescent. Ann R Coll Surg Engl 35:15, 1964

15. Mengel W, Hienz HA, Sippe WG, Hecker WC: Studies on cryptorchidism: A comparison of histological findings in the germinal epithelium before and after the second year of life. J Pediatr Surg 9:445, 1974

16. Shiran M, Matsushika S, Kagajima H, et al: Histological changes of the scrotal testis in unilateral cryptorchidism. Tohoku J Exp Med 90:363, 1968

17. Hadziselimovic F, Herzug B, Segauchi H: Surgical correction of cryptorchidism at two years: Electron microscopic and morphometric investigation. J Pediatr Surg 10:19, 1975

18. Redman JF: Noonan's syndrome and cryptorchidism. J Urol 109:909, 1973

19. Laurance BM: Hypotonia, mental retardation, obesity and cryptorchidism associated with dwarfism and diabetes in children. Arch Dis Child 42:126, 1967

20. Rudolph AM (ed): Pediatrics, 16th ed. New York, Appleton-Century-Crofts, 1977, p 1305

21. Harris JS, Heller RH: The detection of Klinefelter's syndrome at birth. Clin Pediatr 13:581, 1974

22. Atkinson PM: A follow-up study of surgically treated cryptorchid patients. J Pediatr Surg 10:115, 1975

23. Atkinson PM, Epstein MT, Rippen AE: Plasma gonadotropin and androgens in surgically treated cryptorchid patients. J Pediatr Surg 10:27, 1975

24. Hanson TS: Fertility in operatively treated and untreated cryptorchidism. Proc R Soc Med 42:645, 1949

25. Scot LS: Fertility in cryptorchidism. Proc R Soc Med 55:1047, 1962

26. Lipshultz LJ, Caminos-Torres R, Greenspan C, Synder P: Testicular function after orchiopexy for unilaterally undescended testis. N Engl J Med 295:15, 1976

27. Van Essen W: Undescended testicle. Postgrad Med J 42:270, 1966

28. Madrazo BL, Klugo R, Parks J: Ultrasonographic demonstration of undescended testes. Radiology 133:181, 1979

29. Lee J, Glazer H: Computed tomography in localization of the nonpalpable testis. Urol Clin North Am 9:397, 1982

30. Scott, J: Laparoscopy as an aid in the diagnosis and management of the impalpable testis. J Pediatr Surg 17:14, 1983

31. Grant DB, Laurence BM, Athorden SM: HG stimulation test in children with abnormal sexual development. Arch Dis Child 51:596, 1976

32. Lee PA, Hoffman WH, White JJ: Serum gonadotrophin in cryptorchidism: An indicator of functional testes. Am J Dis Child 127:530, 1974

33. Engle ET: Experimentally induced descent of the testis in the macaque monkey by hormones from the anterior pituitary and pregnancy urine. Endocrinology 16:513, 1932

34. Garagorri J, Job J, Canlorbe P, Chaussain JL: Results of early treatment of cryptorchidism with human chorionic gonadotropin. J Pediatr 101:923, 1982

35. Karpe B, Eneroth P, Ritzen E: LHRH treatment in unilateral cryptorchidism: Effect on testicular descent and hormonal response. J Pediatr 103:892, 1983

36. DeMuinck Keizer-Schrama S, Hazebroek S, Drop F, et al. Hormonal therapy of cryptorchidism. A randomized double-blind study comparing human chorionic gonadotropin and gonadotropin-releasing hormone. Lancet 1:876, 1986

37. Rajfer J, Handelsman D, Swerloff R, et al. Hormonal therapy of cryptorchidism. N Engl J Med 314:466, 1986

38. Kiesewetter WB, Shull WR, Farrington GH: Histologic changes in the testis following anatomically successful orchiopexy. J Pediatr Surg 4:59, 1969

39. Lattimer JK, Smith AM, Dargherty IJ, Beck L: The optimum time to operate for cryptorchidism. Pediatrics 53:96, 1974

40. Penn WJ: The maintenance of maldescended testicles within the scrotum using a dartos pouch. Br J Surg 59:175, 1972

41. Fowler R, Stephens FD: The role of testicular vascular anatomy in the salvage of high undescended testis. In Stephens FD (ed): Congenital Malformations of the Rectum, Anus and Genito-urinary Tracts. London, Edinburgh, Churchill-Livingston, 1963, p 306

42. Clatworthy H, Hollabaugh S, Grosfeld J: The "long loop vas" orchiopexy for the high undescended testis. Am J Surg 38:69, 1972

43. Silber S: Microsurgery for the undescended testicle. Urol Clin North Am 9:429, 1982

44. Hamidinia A, Nold S, Amankwah K: Localization and treatment of nonpalpable testes. Surg Gynecol Obstet 159:439, 1984

45. Flinn RA, King LR: Experiences with the midline transabdominal approach in orchiopexy. Surg Gynecol Obstet 133:215, 1971

46. Boley SJ, Kleinhars S: A place for the Cheatle-Henry approach in pediatric surgery? J Pediatr Surg 1:394, 1966

47. Henry AK: Extensive Exposure. Baltimore, Williams & Wilkins, 1957, p 160

48. Gilhooly P, Meyers F, Lattimer J: Fertility prospects for children with cryptorchidism. Am J Dis Child 138:940, 1984

49. Chilvers C, Dudley N, Gough M, et al: Undescended testis: The effect of treatment on subsequent risk of subfertility and malignancy. J Pediatr Surg 21:691, 1986

19
Circumcision

The most ancient and prevalent operation performed on males recently has become hotly controversial. It has been condemned as the "rape of the phallus" and denigrated as a mere ritual.[1,2] The only long-term medical advantages of routine circumcision are possible reductions in the incidence of penile and cervical cancer among adults.[3,4] Even this relationship is questionable because personal hygiene appears to have more influence on the eventual development of these malignancies than does circumcision.[5,6]

The normal foreskin is adherent to the glans at birth and is not fully retractable in 90 percent of males by 3 years of age. During the first year or so of life, the foreskin protects the glans from being irritated by a wet diaper. Further, an intact foreskin may enhance sensitivity of the glans in later life. The arguments for and against circumcision are rarely considered when a male is circumcised at birth; the parents usually expect circumcision as part of routine newborn care. This is unfortunate, but it is unlikely that the practice will change until the physicians responsible for newborn care discuss the pros and cons of circumcision with the family. Any form of hypospadius is a contraindication to circumcision. Complications following neonatal circumcision include hemorrhage, infection, septicemia, retention of plastic bells, and necrosis of the distal penis.[7-13]

When a child has not been circumcised at birth, the foreskin should be left alone! Some mothers are instructed (usually by a nurse) to retract the foreskin for cleaning. This practice may lead to incomplete return of the foreskin to its normal location and paraphimosis. The foreskin then becomes edematous and requires manual reduction. This can be accomplished by sedating the child and relieving pain with a ring of 0.5 percent lidocaine injected into the skin of the penile shaft proximal to the paraphimosis. An injection of hyaluronidase will help disperse edema. With the pain relieved, it is possible to squeeze out the edema and reduce the foreskin to its proper location. With this technique, it is never necessary to perform a dorsal slit.

We do not advise circumcision for an older child unless there is a definite medical indication, such as a zipper injury, a tight preputial opening that hinders urination, or an episode of paraphimosis. Most families are surprised and often grateful when told that circumcision is not necessary for their son. If the family persists in desiring the operation, they are further warned of potential anesthetic hazards as well as postoperative bleeding and infection. Even with this approach, many parents persist in their desire to have their boy circumcised. Their reasons are usually social. They want their child to look like his father, siblings, and friends. Others desire the operation for religious reasons.[14]

When the operation seems desirable, we use the following technique. The genital area is carefully prepared with povidone-iodine; the foreskin is retracted and cleaned before draping the area. The foreskin is clamped dorsally with a hemostat that extends to within 0.5 cm of the coronal sulcus. Another clamp is applied ventrally, which extends to the frenulum. These clamps are then removed, and with scissors the clamped tissue is cut so that the foreskin now consists of two flaps of skin. These are removed with the scissors, leaving 0.5 cm of skin at the coronal sulcus, taking care to leave the frenulum completely intact. Each bleeding vessel is then clamped and ligated with fine catgut. This must be done with great care because the scissors will temporarily occlude small vessels, which commence to bleed after the child has left the hospital. The electrocoagulation unit must never be used! There is one report in which the distal penis sloughed after a mishap with an electrosurgical unit.[15] After satisfactory hemostasis, the skin edges are approximated with fine catgut or polyglycolic acid sutures. The incision is wrapped with a bit of petrolatum gauze.

Postoperatively, the parents are advised to cover the glans with a bit of petrolatum and avoid using diapers for several days. Postoperative hematuria is diagnostic for a meatal ulcer. This is treated with an antibiotic ointment and spreading of the meatus to prevent a stricture.

REFERENCES

1. Morgan WKC: Rape of the phallus. JAMA 194:309, 1965
2. Bolande RP: Ritualistic surgery: Circumcision and tonsillectomy. N Engl J Med 280:591, 1969
3. Leiter E, Lefkovits AM: Circumcision and penile carcinoma. NY State J Med 75:9, 1975
4. Dagher R, Selzer ML, Lapides J: Carcinoma of the penis and the anticircumcision crusade. J Urol 110:79, 1973
5. Reddy CRRM, Raghavaiah NV, Mouli KC: Prevalence of carcinoma of the penis with special reference to India. Int Surg 60(9):474, 1975
6. Aitken-Swan J, Baird D: Circumcision and cancer of the cervix. Br J Cancer 19(2):10, 1965
7. Kirkpatrick BD, Eitzman DV: Neonatal septicemia after circumcision. Clin Pediatr 13:767, 1974
8. Johnsonbaugh RE, Meyer BP, Catalano JD: Complication of a circumcision performed with a plastic bell clamp. Am J Dis Child 118:781, 1969
9. Rubenstein MM, Bason WM: Complication of a circumcision done with a plastic bell clamp. Am J Dis Child 116:381, 1968
10. Jonas G: Retention of a plastibell circumcision ring: Report of a case. Obstet Gynecol 23:835, 1964
11. Malo T, Bonforte RJ: Hazards of plastic bell circumcisions. Obstet Gynecol 33:869, 1969
12. Peitzsch TT: Fifty consecutive cases of circumcision with the "plastibell" circumcision device. Med J Aust 1:1380, 1971
13. Trier WC, Drach GW: Concealed penis: Another complication of circumcision. Am J Dis Child 125:276, 1973
14. Brown M, Brown C: Circumcision decision: Prominence of social concerns. Pediatrics 80:215, 1987
15. Pearlman CK: Reconstruction following iatrogenic burn of the penis. J Pediatr Surg 11:121, 1976

20
Hemangiomas and Vascular Malformations

Vascular malformations are among the most common lesions observed in the pediatric age group. Most are lumped together under the term "hemangioma" and are found most often on the skin, although they can occur in any organ.

The pathogenesis and natural history of hemangiomas and arteriovenous fistulae are poorly understood but are perhaps comparable to the developing blood supply of an embryonic limb bud.[1,2] Instead of the usual orderly development of arteries, veins, and capillaries, the arteriovenous fistulae (which are normally seen during the early stages of limb development) persist. Thus, a typical capillary angioma represents a localized arteriovenous fistula, whereas a more extensive lesion involves larger vessels and an entire organ or extremity. Although the underlying pathogenesis may be similar, it is useful to classify the various malformations in order to predict which of them will spontaneously involute and to determine at an early stage those lesions that will require active treatment.

Mulliken et al., in a series of important publications, have presented their clinical, microscopic, and research studies of hemangiomas and vascular malformations.[3–6] Hemangiomas in their studies were classified as lesions that grow rapidly during the first months of life, then involute. During the growth phase, there is increased endothelial cell activity, demonstrable by hyperplasia, and the incorporation of [³H]-thymidine into the cells. There is also an increase in the numbers of mast cells during the early growth period. With involution, there is fibrosis and fat deposition with an absence of [³H]-thymidine-labeled endothelial cells. Vascular malformations, on the other hand, are lesions that do not regress, are not hypercellular, but are lined by flat, mature endothelium. The malformations were not proliferative on the basis of an absence of [³H]-thymidine activity. Mulliken has now followed 375 vascular lesions from 1967 to 1981 and was able to classify 96 percent as being either hemangiomas or malformations. This may be a simplified classification, but it allows the clinician to recognize lesions that will in all probability regress and those that will not.

HEMANGIOMA

The typical hemangioma is a strawberry-colored, elevated, irregular lesion that appears during the first few weeks of life (Fig. 20–1). Such lesions may vary in size from small and scarcely noticeable, red, elevated marks to huge grotesque tumors that obscure the facial features. On physical examination, the typical superficial hemangioma is compressible but slowly refills with blood. Most are elevated above the skin surface; a few will be partly covered with normal skin. It is difficult to differentiate between a so-called capillary hemangioma and a cavernous hemangioma. Microscopically, there are numerous dilated vascular spaces within the dermis and subcutaneous tissues in each. A hemangioma often will not appear until the child is several weeks old; then a small red spot grows rapidly for several months, after which its growth plateaus and keeps pace with the rest of the body. The usual superficial hemangioma will begin to involute by 2 or 3 years of age and will disappear by 5 or 6 years of age, leaving only a patch of pale, flaccid skin. The initial rapid neonatal growth possibly results from canalization of adjacent capillaries and systemic vessels, with proliferation of embryonal angioblasts. Regression appears to be caused by progressive thrombosis and sclerosis of vessels, eventually leading to infarction. This course of involution will take place in approximately 85 percent of the common elevated skin hemangiomas.[7,8] The ultimate cosmetic result is superior, and there are fewer complications when the lesion is allowed to pursue

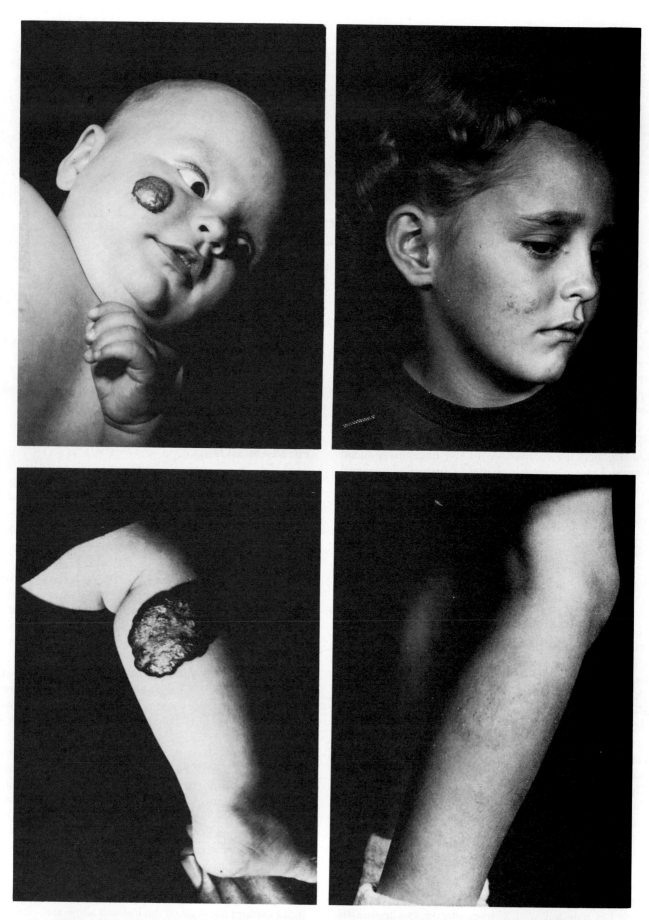

Figure 20–1. Typical capillary hemangiomas. **Upper left.** Hemangioma of the face at 4 months of age. **Upper right.** The same lesion when the girl is 7 years old. There has been almost complete involution. **Lower left.** A hemangioma on the leg of a 5-month-old child. **Lower right.** By 6 years of age, the residual lesion is barely noticeable.

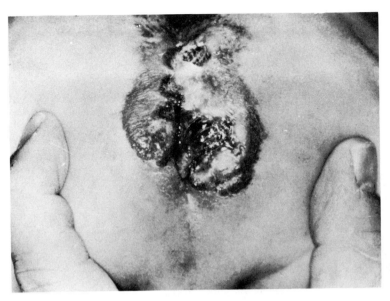 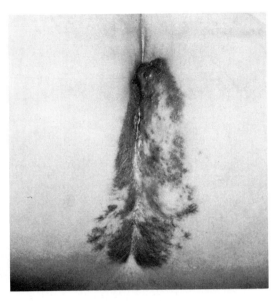

Figure 20–2. Perianal hemangioma with ulceration, bleeding, and infection. **Left.** Before colostomy. **Right.** Two months after colostomy, there has been healing and even some involution.

its normal course than when any form of treatment is undertaken, including surgical excision. There is no need for the injection of sclerosing agents or radiation therapy. The most important treatment consists of reassuring the family that the lesion either will completely disappear or will become smaller in time. It is helpful to demonstrate serial photographs of similar children to doubting parents.

There are some complications that require active treatment. The most common of these is superficial ulceration with a local infection or bleeding. Treatment consists of the application of a topical antibiotic ointment and protection with a dressing. When a small ulcerating lesion bleeds freely, we tend to advise surgical excision unless the hemangioma is in an area where a surgical scar would be cosmetically unacceptable. Small ulcerating lesions on the perineum are particularly difficult to treat conservatively; consequently, they are usually excised. A large perianal hemangioma that ulcerates and bleeds may require a diverting colostomy to allow healing and spontaneous resolution (Fig. 20–2). In other situations, an excellent cosmetic result can be obtained by excision of the lesion (Fig. 20–3). Hemangiomas of the eyelid or medial canthus that interfere with sight in one eye may cause amblyopia, strabismus, or blindness.[9]

This is an indication for the injection of corticosteroids directly into the lesion.[10] The procedure must be performed under general anesthesia, and both dexamethasone and triamcinolone are injected in order to obtain both an immediate and a long-term effect. Steroids also may be given systemically to enhance the injection therapy. Regression of the hemangioma may occur within days. To be most successful, intralesional therapy should be given early during the growth phase. Both intrale-

sional and systemic steroid therapy are indicated in any rapidly growing lesion, which by virtue of its location may interfere with sight, obstruct the airway, or cause problems with any vital function. Steroids also are used with visceral lesions that cause cardiac failure. The response to steroids is unpredictable, but approximately 30 percent of infants treated before 10 months of age for cavernous or mixed hemangiomas will improve. An additional 40 percent may experience equivocal benefit.[11] Edgerton has had wide experience with hemangiomas and has reported a 90 percent dramatic response of capillary cavernous hemangiomas with short course, high-dosage prednisolone therapy; he administered 2 to 4 mg/day. Ulcerations commence to heal within 2 weeks, and if therapy is continued, the lesion shrinks within 30 to 90 days.[12]

Occasionally, hemangiomas will trap platelets and cause a consumption coagulapathy. This syndrome was first recognized by Kasabach and Merritt in 1940.[13] Other investigators subsequently have observed other abnormalities associated with the disseminated intravascular coagulation syndrome.[14–22] The sequestration of platelets in the hemangioma has been confirmed by demonstrating an increased uptake of chromium-51-tagged platelets within the hemangioma.[23,24] Although the exact trigger mechanism that sets off the platelet trapping within the hemangioma is unknown, two thirds of the reported cases have occurred during the first 3 months of life, during the phase of active growth of the lesion. Only 12 percent of the cases were reported as occurring after 1 year of age.[25]

The first sign of hemorrhage usually is a rapid increase in swelling of the hemangioma itself. The overlying skin becomes tense and shining, and there are surround-

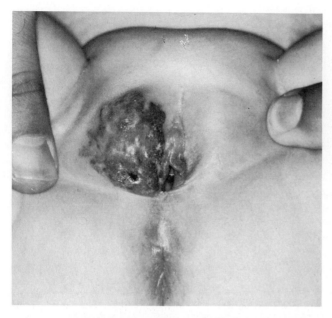
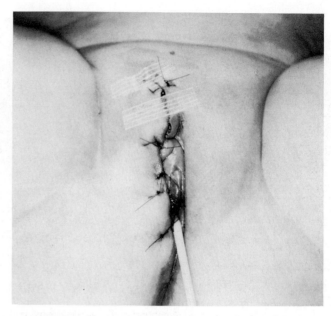

Figure 20–3. Hemangioma of the labia that continually became infected and ulcerated. **Left.** Preoperative appearance after intensive topical therapy. **Right.** Immediate postoperative appearance.

ing areas of ecchymosis and petechiae. Alternatively, bleeding may occur during attempts to remove the lesion or may occur in distant sites. The mortality rate from hemorrhage is approximately 30 percent in such cases.[26] The most important laboratory finding is a decrease in the platelet count. In addition, there is a diffuse intravascular coagulation with decrease in the plasma fibrinogen, increased fibrinolytic activity, prolongation of the bleeding time, and alterations in factors V and VIII and in the prothrombin and thrombin times. Initial treatment consists of heparin, aspirin, fresh blood, platelet transfusions, dipyridamole, and steroids.[27–29] Once the child has become stabilized, surgical excision of the hemangioma results in a prompt return of the platelets and other coagulation factors to normal.[30,31] Whenever possible, this is the treatment of choice. If surgical excision does not appear feasible, long-term treatment with prednisone or a combination of prednisone, heparin, and radiation has been successful.[32,33] Pressure with an elastic bandage also has been helpful, not only in reducing the size of a hemangioma of the extremity but also in increasing the platelet count.[34,35]

In selected, large hemangiomas, arteriography followed by embolization of feeder vessels has reduced the size of the lesions, with improvement in the coagulopathy. One can see just how desperate the Kasabach-Merritt syndrome is by reviewing the multitude of suggested treatments.[36]

There are a number of syndromes involving various combinations of cutaneous and visceral hemangiomas.[37] These include benign neonatal hemangiomatosis, in which there are multiple skin lesions without visceral

involvement. These usually follow a benign uncomplicated course of growth and regression. Disseminated neonatal hemangiomatosis describes infants with multiple skin lesions and involvement of other organ systems, such as the liver, spleen, mouth, and genitourinary tract.[38] Liver involvement is particularly serious, since these babies may be in congestive heart failure or have respiratory distress because of the huge size of the liver (see Chapter 42).

Figure 20–4 illustrates a 16-year-old boy with multiple hemangiomas of the skin, mouth, and gastrointestinal tract. He was anemic and chronically malnourished, and his height and weight were below the 3rd percentile for a 12-year-old boy. The skin lesions were dark blue and easily compressible. He represents an example of the blue rubber bleb nevus syndrome. We removed multiple hemangiomas from his gastrointestinal tract, mouth, and skin. Microscopically, they were cavernous hemangiomas.

There are other rare syndromes, but as a general rule, the associated visceral lesions are most important, although not obvious. For this reason, infants with multiple or unusual skin lesions should first have a complete careful examination looking for an enlarged liver or spleen, or eye problems, a blood count, and stool analysis for blood. CT imaging of the brain and central nervous system is indicated in infants with unusual facial lesions, as is imaging of the spinal cord and kidneys when there are hemangiomas near the rectum or genitalia.

There are some lesions that in the past have been termed "hemangiomas" but do not fit into Mulliken's classification. These are beneath the skin, the vessels

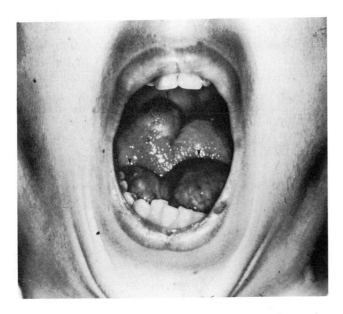

Figure 20–4. This 16-year-old boy had deep cavernous hemangiomas of his gastrointestinal tract, skin, and urinary bladder. These hemangiomas in his mouth interfered with dentition and eating. He developed an exacerbation of platelet trapping with each excision.

are larger, and there is no tendency to spontaneous regression. On physical examination, these deep lesions are firm and barely compressible; they often feel like a bag of worms. The overlying skin usually has a bluish cast, with enlarged skin vessels in the area. Even though deep hemangiomas do not ordinarily undergo spontaneous regression, they should be observed during the first year or 2 of life, especially if they involve the face, parotid gland, or facial nerve (Fig. 20–5). When these lesions persist, whether called cavernous hemangiomas or vascular malformations, they should be excised.

Treatment

A tourniquet may be applied to minimize blood loss in an extremity lesion. However, with care, bleeding during excision of a deep hemangioma can be kept to a minimum. The skin incision may be made directly over the mass, or if there is a residual capillary hemangioma centered over the deeper lesion, an elliptical incision may be made. Most bleeding is from dermal vessels and capillaries encountered in the skin incision. These are controlled with the needle-tipped electrocautery and pressure. The skin is held with hooks away from the mass of blood vessels that make up the tumor. The subcutaneous tissue is separated by spreading the scissor blades at a right

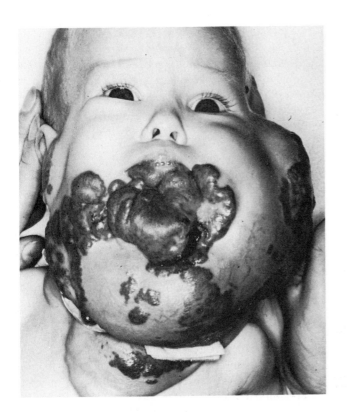

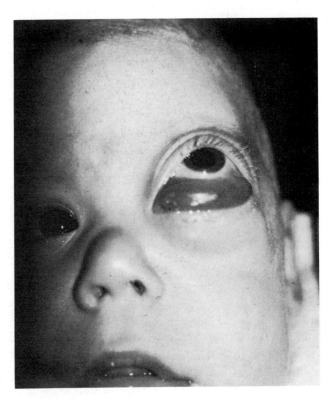

Figure 20–5. Left. There is no satisfactory treatment for an extensive facial hemangioma. A tracheotomy and gastrotomy are necessary, and in a case like this, steroid therapy should be attempted. **Right.** A retroorbital hemangioma causing proptosis. Steroid therapy also is indicated in this situation, where excision would be hazardous.

angle to the mass or parallel to the feeding vessels. Any strand of tissue that fails to separate is either coagulated or clamped and ligated. In this fashion, the tumor is separated from the subcutaneous tissues. In almost every case, there are only one or two larger feeding vessels that must be ligated. The separation from the underlying fascia is usually simple and bloodless. When there is a racemose group of enlarged veins, it is often possible to individually dissect and ligate the larger tortuous channels. Large, persistent buccal hemangiomas have been excised with minimal blood loss by using a carbon dioxide laser beam.[39] Other large facial vascular malformations have been excised with the patient in a state of total circulatory arrest and hypothermia.[40]

THE PORT WINE STAIN

There are many varieties of small flat vascular lesions that have been called "nevus flammeous," "salmon patch," or "intradermal angioma." These must be differentiated from the less common but far more serious port wine stains. They are malformations of the dermal capillaries, and they are permanent and do not involute but grow with the child.

Facial port wine stains are deep red or purple, flat malformations that may cover the cheek or half of the child's face. They may be associated with glaucoma and orbital hemangiomas.[41,42] The Sturge-Weber syndrome consists of a facial port wine stain with a leptomeningeal angioma.[43] These children often are mentally retarded and have seizures. A CT scan is indicated to determine the extent of central nervous system involvement. There is no satisfactory treatment for these lesions. Surgical excision with skin grafting may, in very skilled hands, give satisfactory results. The argon laser produced hypertrophic scarring when used in young children but has been more successful in older patients.[44,45] Cosmetics to cover the lesion may match the child's skin color and may be useful to tide the patient over until he or she is old enough for either laser treatment or surgical excision.

There is a variety of vascular anomalies of the extremities associated with port wine staining. The Klippel-Trenaunay-Weber syndrome describes a variety of these lesions that are associated with venous varicosities, usually on the lateral side of the leg, and limb hypertrophy. The purple discoloration follows dermatomes and may extend onto the buttock, abdomen, chest, and genitalia. The hypertrophy and swelling of the extremity resemble lymphedema. These children may get along for a number of years with little disability except for the necessity of wearing a larger shoe on the affected side. As they grow older, the size and weight of the leg cause difficulties

in sports, and there may be recurrent bouts of painful thrombophlebitis. Varicosities may extend to the bladder, rectum, or colon to cause hematuria and rectal bleeding.[46,47] Resection of the colon or kidney has been necessary.[48]

Venography has demonstrated malformation of the deep venous system, including aplasia, with collaterals to the internal iliac or even the axillary vein.[49] Servelle has studied 78 patients with the Klippel-Trenaunay syndrome and has pointed out the necessity for studying the deep venous system before surgical treatment.[50] He was able to relieve compression on the popliteal or femoral vein in some patients. The varicose veins in this condition provide collateral circulation around the obstructed deep veins. If, however, the deep circulation is intact, resection of the varicose veins on the lateral side of the leg and foot may improve the child's condition.[51] There are large perforating veins, which are ligated at the deep fascia level. The saphenous veins should be left alone.

All children with this syndrome require long-term supportive treatment with elastic stockings, the pneumatic boot, and bedrest with hot packs and antibiotics when they have episodes of thrombophlebitis. In many cases, this is the only necessary or desirable treatment.

ARTERIOVENOUS FISTULA

Congenital communications between arteries and veins proximal to the normal capillary bed may occur anywhere in the body. In children, these lesions are most common in the extremities and in the central nervous system, where they cause intracranial hemorrhage.

Pathophysiology

Studies of amputated limbs have demonstrated that a single fistula is rare. In most cases, there are multiple shunts, some of which are latent and open only after the major fistula has been ligated.[52] Injection studies and arteriography demonstrate a profusion of small, tortuous vessels. During infancy, there may be one or two large fistulae leading into a hemangioma that are large enough to cause heart failure.[53,54] Usually, however, the smaller anastomoses remain closed except in response to growth, activity, or ligation of the main fistula. The shunt may be regarded as a parasitic circuit that deprives the distal extremity of its blood supply. Thus, we have the paradox of an apparently increased flow of blood to an extremity coexisting with possible cutaneous necrosis and ischemic pain. The shunt causes an increased cardiac output, increased blood volume, and, eventually, left heart failure.[55]

Symptoms

Except for heart failure in the neonatal period, there are few early symptoms. There are often associated port wine stains or superficial hemangiomas over the affected leg, which become noticeable during the first few months of life. Later, there is an obvious growth discrepancy because the increased blood flow accelerates growth in the bones and soft tissues. Both the length and girth of the extremity are increased. As the child grows older, there are visible tortuous veins on the surface, which may rupture with severe hemorrhage. In our experience, pain has become a problem only after surgical ligation of the major fistulae, which results in peripheral ischemia. Children with large lesions also seem to experience growth retardation, perhaps because of their borderline or overt cardiac failure. Children with fistulae about the head and neck may complain of a persistent tinnitus or buzzing in the ears. Physical examination will demonstrate the obvious hypertrophy of the extremity with superficial vascular channels. The extremity must be measured in order to accurately record progress. Palpation reveals increased warmth and a palpable bruit. This may be confirmed with auscultation.

The effect of the fistula on the heart can be dramatically demonstrated by eliciting the Nicoladini-Branham sign.[56,57] This is performed by counting the pulse rate and then applying firm pressure to the fistula. A positive sign is a significant slowing of the pulse rate. Further studies include a chest roentgenogram and an electrocardiogram, as well as special x-rays of the extremity to measure leg length. Angiography provides exact information concerning the origin of feeding vessels and the extent of the lesion. This study is necessary before surgical therapy and can be combined with embolization of the lesion.

Treatment

Localized lesions may be excised and cured. We have had most success with excision of small lesions, especially those of the head, neck, and trunk (Fig. 20–6). The feeding artery is first isolated and taped. The remaining vessels, which are thin-walled and tortuous, are dissected away from surrounding tissues, making sure that all feeding vessels are found, divided, and ligated. There is no completely satisfactory treatment for arteriovenous fistulae of the extremities. The goals of therapy should be limb salvage, the prevention or treatment of hemorrhage, prevention of excessive growth, and, if possible, cosmetic improvement. No single form of therapy will achieve all of these goals.

Initial treatment consists of compression with an elastic bandage and a tailor-made elastic stocking. Unfortunately, few children will wear the stockings, they wear out quickly, and, despite the greatest of care, they are

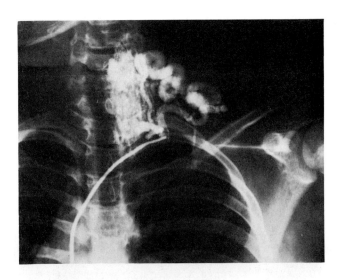

Figure 20–6. Congenital arteriovenous fistula arising from the subclavian artery. This was a localized lesion over the scapula, which was completely excised.

always a bit too tight or too loose. Repeated follow-up visits and continuous supervision are essential for proper fit and patient compliance. The pain of superficial skin and nerve ischemia may be increased by pressure dressings. Proximal ligation of feeding vessels has been attempted for many years.[58,59] The results have been disappointing because after these feeding vessels have been ligated, new collaterals open.[60] Only 4 of 80 patients treated at the Mayo Clinic over a 10-year-period were considered cured after multiple ligations.[61] On the other hand, persistent search for and ligation of recurrent fistulae will prevent hemorrhage and may eventually control the lesion so that the limb may be salvaged.[62] We observed one patient in whom control of rapidly increasing leg length was attained with proximal ligation. However, after the third attempt to ligate all feeding vessels to the femoral artery, the patient experienced peripheral ischemia and severe neuritic pain (Fig. 20–7).

Embolization has proven relatively successful in the management of central nervous and systemic arteriovenous malformations.[62–66] The lesion must first be localized by careful angiography, after which the catheter is advanced into the lesion. Gelfoam, autogenous muscle, and silicone beads have all been used to occlude the multiple vessels within the lesion. The results of embolization thus far appear to be superior to those obtained with multiple ligation. Consequently, this should be the first choice of therapy. With proper planning, the first embolization should take place during the initial angiographic study. Unfortunately, embolization cannot be carried out after the proximal main feeding vessels have been ligated. Thus, embolization should and must precede attempts at surgical control.

164

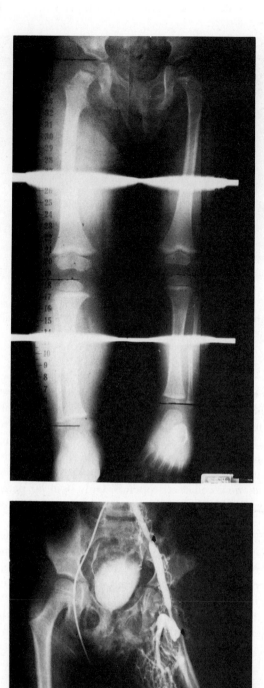

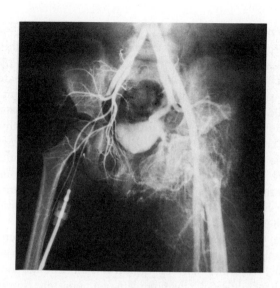

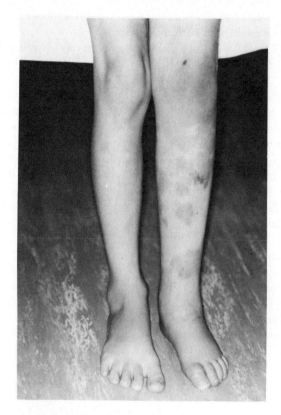

Figure 20–7. An extensive arteriovenous fistula of the leg. **Top left.** Leg length discrepancy at 1 year of age. **Top right.** Arteriogram showing a huge iliac and femoral artery with multiple small vessels in the proximal thigh. **Bottom left.** The first procedure was a banding of the femoral artery. This was followed by ligation of the iliac and finally by femoral artery ligation. Extensive collaterals developed after each of these operations. **Bottom right.** Status of the leg after these multiple procedures. It is still larger than normal, and the superficial port wine stains are visible. The rate of growth has been slowed, however.

REFERENCES

1. Woodard A: The development of the principal arterial system in the forelimb of the pig. Contrib Embryol Carnegie Inst 14:139, 1922
2. Malan E: Vascular Malformations (Angiodysplasias). Milan, Carlo Erba Foundation, 1974
3. Mulliken J, Glowacki J: Hemangiomas and vascular malformations in infants and children: A classification based on endothelial characteristics. Plast Reconstr Surg 69:412, 1982
4. Mulliken J, Zetter B, Folkman J: In vitro characteristics of endothelium from hemangiomas and vascular malformations. Surgery 92:348, 1982
5. Finn M, Glowacki J, Mulliken J: Congenital vascular lesions: Clinical application of a new classification. J Pediatr Surg 18:894, 1983
6. Glowacki J, Mulliken J: Mast cells in hemangiomas and vascular malformations. Pediatrics 70:48, 1982
7. Simpson J: Natural history of cavernous hemangiomata. Lancet 2:1057, 1959
8. Wallerstein R: Spontaneous involution of giant hemangioma. Am J Dis Child 102:233, 1961
9. Haik B, Jakobiec F, Ellsworth R: Capillary hemangiomas of the lids and orbit: An analysis of the clinical features and therapeutic results in 101 cases. Ophthalmology 86:760, 1979
10. Nelson L, Melick J, Harley R: Intralesional corticosteroid injections for infantile hemangiomas of the eyelid. Pediatrics 74:241, 1984
11. Bartosheky L, Bull M, Feingold M: Corticosteroid treatment of cutaneous hemangiomas: How effective? Clin Pediatr 17:625, 1978
12. Edgerton M: The treatment of hemangiomas, with special reference to the role of steroid therapy. Ann Surg 183:517, 1976
13. Kasabach H, Merritt K: Capillary hemangioma with extensive purpura: Report of a case. Am J Dis Child 59:1063, 1940
14. Bachmann F, Vietti T, Kulapongo P: Consumption coagulopathy: Sequential syndrome studies in a patient with Kasabach-Merritt syndrome (Abstr). Blood 28:1016, 1966
15. Beller F, Ruhrmann G: Zur Pathogenes des Kasabach-Merritt Syndroms. Klin Wochenschr 37:1078, 1959
16. Blix S, Aas K: Giant hemangioma, thrombocytopenia, fibrinopenia and fibrinolytic activity. Acta Med Scand 169:63, 1961
17. Inceman S, Tangun Y: Chronic defibrination syndrome due to a giant hemangioma associated with microangiopathic hemolytic anemia. Am J Med 46:997, 1969
18. Lelong J, Alabille D, Habib E, et al: L'hemangioma geant du nourrisson avec thrombopeni. Arch Fr Pediatr 21:769, 1964
19. Saputo V, Vitarelli L, Carrini R: Emangioma con trombocitopenia e ipofibrinogenemia in un neonato. Minerva Pediatr 21:307, 1969
20. Stuber H: Das Syndrom hamangiom, Thrombopenische purpura und Anamie in Sauglingsalter. Helv Paediatr Acta 11:194, 1956
21. Thatcher L, Clatanoff D, Stiehm E: Splenic hemangioma with thrombocytopenia and afibrinogenemia. J Pediatr 93:345, 1968
22. Wacksman S, Flessa H, Glueck H, et al: Coagulation defects and giant cavernous hemangioma. Am J Dis Child 111:71, 1966
23. Brizel H, Raccuqlia G: Giant hemangioma with thrombocytopenia: Radioisotopic demonstration of platelet sequestration. Blood 26:751, 1955
24. Kontras S, Green O, King L, Duran R: Giant hemangioma with thrombocytopenia. Case report with survival and sequestration studies of platelets labeled with chromium 51. Am J Dis Child 105:188, 1963
25. Martins A: Hemangioma and thrombocytopenia. J Pediatr Surg 5:641, 1970
26. Long P, Dubin H: Hemangioma-thrombocytopenia syndrome. A disseminated intravascular coagulation. Arch Dermatol 111:105, 1975
27. Hagerman L, Czapeke E, Donnellon W, Schwartz A: Giant hemangioma with consumption coagulopathy. J Pediatr 87:166, 1975
28. Jona J, Kwaan H, Bjelan M, Raffensperger J: Disseminated intravascular coagulation after excision of a giant hemangioma. Am J Surg 127:588, 1974
29. Koerper M, Addiego J, deLorimer A, et al: Use of aspirin and dipyridamole in children with platelet trapping syndromes. J Pediatr 102:311, 1983
30. Hill G, Longino L: Giant hemangioma with thrombocytopenia. Surg Gynecol Obstet 114:304, 1962
31. Shim W: Hemangioma of infancy complicated by thrombocytopenia. Am J Surg 116:896, 1968
32. Evans J, Betchelor A, Start G, Ultlay L: Hemangioma with coagulopathy sustained response to prednisone. Arch Dis Child 50:809, 1975
33. Carnelli V, Velliui F, Ferrari M, et al: Giant hemangioma with consumption coagulopathy: Sustained response to heparin and radiotherapy. J Pediatr 91:504, 1977
34. Moore A: Pressure in the treatment of giant hemangioma with purpura: Case report and observations. Plast Reconstr Surg 34:606, 1964
35. Miller S, Smith R, Shochart S: Compression treatment of hemangiomas. Plast Reconstr Surg 58:573, 1976
36. Larsen E, Zinkham W, Eggleston J, Zitelli B: Kasabach-Merritt syndrome: Therapeutic considerations. Pediatrics 79:971, 1987
37. Esterly N: Cutaneous hemangiomas, vascular stains and associated syndromes. Curr Prob Pediatr 17:1, 1987
38. Goldberg N, Hebert A, Esterly N: Sacral hemangiomas and multiple congenital anomalies. Arch Dermatol 122:684, 1986
39. Shafir R, Stutzki S, Bornstein L: Excision of buccal hemangioma by carbon dioxide laser beam. Oral Surg 44:347, 1977
40. Mulliken J, Murray J, Castoneda A, Kohon L: Management of vascular malformation of the face using total circulatory arrest. Surg Gynecol Obstet 146:168, 1968
41. Stevenson R, Morin J: Ocular findings in nevus flammeus. Can J Ophthalmol 10:136, 1975
42. Hofeldt A, Zaret C, Jakobiec F: Orbito facial angiomatosis. Arch Ophthalmol 97:944, 1979

43. Alexander G: Sturge-Weber syndrome. In Vinken P, Bruyn G (eds): Handbook of Clinical Neurology. Amsterdam, North Holland, 1972:223–240

44. Yanan A, Fukuda O, Soyano S: Argon laser therapy of port wine stains: Effects and limitations. Plast Reconstr Surg 75:520, 1985

45. Noe J, Barsky S, Geer D: Port wine stains and the response to argon laser therapy: Successful treatment and the predictive role of color, age and biopsy. Plast Reconstr Surg 65:130, 1980

46. Ghahremani G, Kangarloo H, Volberg F, Meyers M: Diffuse cavernous hemangioma of the colon in the Klippel-Trenaunay syndrome. Radiology 118:673, 1976

47. Servelle M, Bastin R, Laggue A, et al: Hematuria and rectal bleeding in the child with Klippel and Trenaunay syndrome. Ann Surg 183:418, 1976

48. Telander R, Kaufman B, Gloviczki P, et al: Prognosis and management of lesions of the trunk in children with Klippel-Trenaunay syndrome. J Pediatr Surg 19:417, 1984

49. Gorenstein A, Shifrin E, Gordon R, et al: Congenital aplasia of the deep veins of the lower extremities in children: The role of ascending functional phlebography. Surgery 99:414, 1986

50. Servelle M: Klippel and Trenaunay's syndrome. Ann Surg 201:365, 1985

51. Lofgren E, Lofgren K: Surgical treatment of cavernous hemangioma. Surgery 97:474, 1985

52. Lawton R, Tidrick R, Brintell E: A clinicopathological study of multiple congenital arteriovenous fistulae of the lower extremity. Angiology 8:161, 1957

53. Ancalmo N, Ochsner J, King T: Congenital arteriovenous fistula of the internal thoracic artery and chest wall. J Pediatr Surg 1:271, 1976

54. Price A, Coran A, Mattern A, Cochran R: Hemangioendothelioma of the pelvis. A cause for cardiac failure in the newborn. N Engl J Med 286:647, 1972

55. Holmon E: Arteriovenous Aneurysm: Abnormal Communications Between the Arterial and Venous Circulations. New York, Macmillan, 1937

56. Branham H: Aneurysma varix of the femoral artery and vein following a gunshot wound. Int Surg 3:250, 1890

57. Nicoladini C: Phlebartericetasie der Reuhten oberen Extremitat. Arch Clin Chir 18:252, 1875

58. Halsted W: Congenital arteriovenous and lymphaticovenous fistulae. Trans Am Surg Assoc 37:262, 1919

59. Holmon E: The physiology of arteriovenous fistula. Am J Surg 89:1101, 1955

60. Szilaqyi D, Elliott J, De Russo F, et al: Peripheral congenital arteriovenous fistulae. Surgery 57:61, 1965

61. Gones M, Becnatz P: Arteriovenous fistula: A review and ten year experience at the Mayo Clinic. Mayo Clin Proc 4:81, 1970

62. Wooley M, Stanley P, Wesley J: Peripherally located congenital arteriovenous fistulae in infancy and childhood. J Pediatr Surg 12:165, 1977

63. Lvessenhop A, Kachmann R, Sherlin W: Clinical evaluation of artificial embolization in the management of large cerebral arteriovenous malformations. J Neurosurg 23:400, 1965

64. Djindjian R, Cophignon J, Theron J: Embolization by superselective arteriography from the femoral route in neuroradiology. Review of 60 cases. Neuroradiology 6:20, 1973

65. Stanley R, Cubillo E: Nonsurgical treatment of arteriovenous malformations of the trunk and limb by transcatheter arterial embolization. Radiology 115:609, 1975

66. Olcott C, Newton T, Stoney R, Ehrenfield W: Intraarterial embolization in the management of arteriovenous malformations. Surgery 79:3, 1976

21
Cystic Hygroma, Lymphangioma, and Lymphedema

Neil R. Feins
John G. Raffensperger

Congenital obstruction of the lymphatic vessels produces defects that vary from the common cystic hygroma to extensive lymphangiomatosis and lymphedema. Although these two lesions are widely different in their clinical presentation, the embryologic basis for their development and pathology is similar.[1,2] Early embryologic studies demonstrated five points of origin for the lymphatic system: the paired sacs in the neck, in conjunction with the jugular vein; a single sac at the root of the mesentery; and paired sacs situated in relation to the sciatic veins.[3,4] The entire system of lymph vessels buds off from these anlagen. Sequestration or obstruction of lymph vessels leads to the various clinical entities, depending on anatomic location. Thus, obstruction of the mesenteric or omental lymphatics causes large intraperitoneal cysts, whereas sequestration or budding of lymph vessels in the neck or other subcutaneous areas results in a typical cystic hygroma. There are a few examples of extensive lymphangiomatosis involving the extremities, bones, and pleural cavities.

CYSTIC HYGROMA

Cystic hygromas are thin-walled cysts lined with flat endothelium and filled with yellowish fluid. One often finds multiple communicating cysts. The cyst wall is exceedingly thin; often it is no more than one or two cells thick. At the periphery of the primary cyst, there invariably are tiny daughter cysts, which infiltrate into muscle and around nerves and vessels (Fig. 21–1). It often seems that the mass has the consistency of water-filled soap bubbles and that there is no end to the infiltration of normal tissue. In spite of the extensive invasion of tissue planes, these are benign lesions. Some cystic hygromas appear to contain hemangiomatous tissue, and on pathologic examination, one often finds fat, strands of muscle, and small lymph nodes. About 75 percent of cystic hygromas are in the neck, 20 percent are in the axilla, and 5 percent are on the trunk or extremity. They may also occur at such unusual sites as the larynx, mouth, tongue, or retroperitoneal areas.[5] Some 50 to 60 percent of cystic hygromas are present at birth, and practically all of them are apparent by two years of age. This is further evidence of congenital origin.

Diagnosis

A cystic hygroma of the neck is soft, watery and easily transilluminated; there is no other lesion that is quite so characteristic. A newborn infant may have massive bilateral swelling of the neck, with involvement of the tongue and larynx, causing an airway obstruction (Fig. 21–2). One must never blame airway obstruction on a cystic hygroma on the outside of the neck, since endoscopy invariably will demonstrate lesions inside the larynx or pharynx. The tongue may be so large that the child cannot close his or her mouth. Later, pressure on the peridontal tissue will result in loss of teeth and overgrowth of the mandible. The tongues in these children not only are large but also covered with infection-prone vesicles 1 to 2 mm in diameter (Fig. 21–3). Cystic hygromas in the axilla and supraclavicular spaces also are characteristically soft and watery. A cystic hygroma on the trunk or extremity may be mistaken for a lipoma, particu-

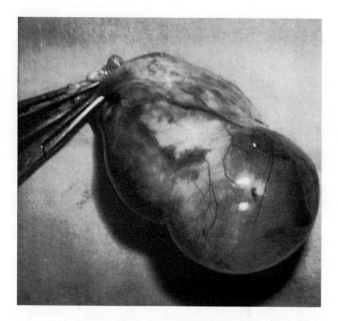
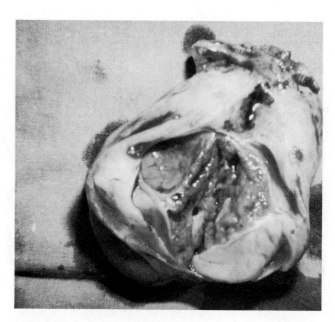

Figure 21–1. A typical cystic hygroma removed from the neck. **Left.** The unopened specimen, which is smooth and translucent. **Right.** The specimen is here shown to be multilocular with many interconnecting cysts.

larly in an older child, but fatty tumors are exceedingly rare in childhood, whereas cystic hygromas are relatively common (Fig. 21–4). A cystic hygroma may be confused with a deep hemangioma, but the hemangioma is firmer, imparting the sensation of a bag of worms, and usually will have a bluish cast and an increased surface vascularity. In the series of 124 cystic hygromas reported by Ninh and Ninh, 16 percent became infected and 12.6 percent showed evidence of hemorrhage.[6] Two hygromas in this series appeared to undergo partial spontaneous regression, whereas in two other patients, new tumors appeared in different locations. In our own experience, a spontaneous regression occurred in a supraclavicular mass after excision of an axillary hygroma. Infection in a cystic hygroma involving the head and neck can be extremely serious. The mass rapidly enlarges, and there is surrounding cellulitis, pain, and tenderness that respond slowly to antibiotic therapy. There is always the possibility that enlargement due to infection

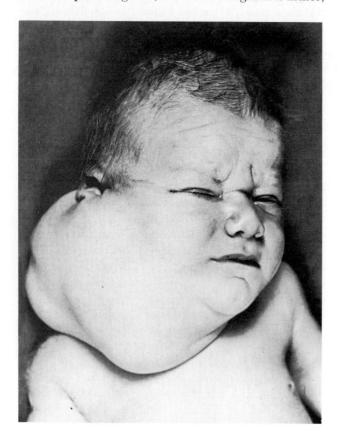

Figure 21–2. Huge cystic hygroma in a newborn infant involving the face, neck, and sublingual areas.

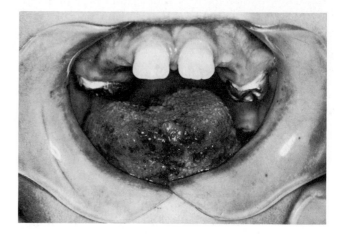

Figure 21–3. Cystic hygroma of the tongue with multiple weeping vesicles, which are prone to frequent infections. The enlarged tongue has pushed the teeth outward and forward.

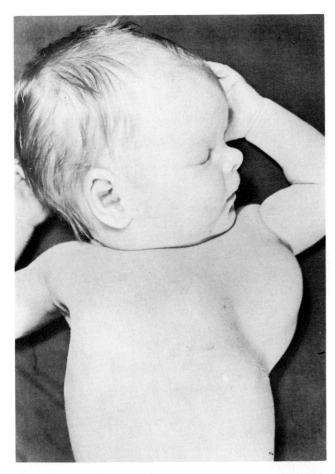
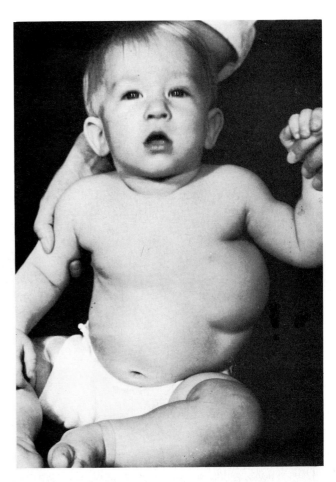

Figure 21–4. **Left.** A cystic hygroma of the axilla. **Right.** Extensive cystic hygroma of the trunk, extending from the dermis down to the fascia and intertwining about the pectoral muscles. When a cystic hygroma occurs in this area in a girl, great care must be taken not to injure the breast bud.

could compromise the airway. Infection leaves fibrosis in the adjacent tissue and destroys the usual planes of dissection through the loose areolar tissue that surrounds most of the hygroma. Any previous infection seriously hampers surgical excision. Sudden hemorrhage into a cystic hygroma produces a tense, painful, hard, and immovable mass. We have seen two of these, and in both cases our preoperative diagnosis was malignant muscle tumor. One child had been examined several months earlier, at which time he had only a vague suggestion of a mass over his shoulder—not even serious enough to recommend excision.

Treatment

A cystic hygroma should be surgically excised when the diagnosis is made, even in the neonatal period. This advice would be modified for a lesion overlying the facial nerve, in which case the risk of facial paralysis outweighs the danger of infection or other complications. If possible, surgery should be delayed for 6 months or a year until the child and the nerve have had an opportunity to grow. When the operation is done, a simple transverse

incision in a normal skin crease is made over the most prominent portion of the tumor. If the mass is on the face or neck, the angle of the mouth and eye must be visible at all times during the operation, so that stimulation of the facial nerve will cause an observable muscle contraction. The skin over the tumor is extremely thin, so the incision must be made gently and with care. Otherwise the main cyst will be entered and drained before the operation gets underway. A solution to this problem is to commence the incision remote from the most prominent portion of the tumor and then, when one is through the skin and subcutaneous tissue, elevate the skin away from the cyst by spreading thin-bladed scissors beneath the skin. When the skin is separated from the cyst, the incision is continued. Hooks are used to elevate the skin flaps to permit sharp dissection over the surface of the hygroma. The cyst itself is never held with the forceps but rather with a moist gauze sponge. Every precaution must be taken to avoid opening the cyst because, if the fluid escapes, one has a difficult time finding the remaining thin endothelial wall.

When the tumor overlies the facial nerve, it is wise

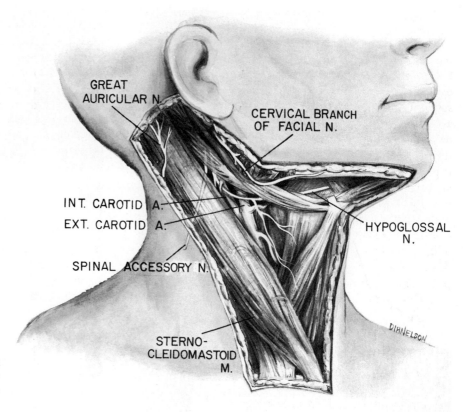

Figure 21–5. Anatomic drawing of the neck demonstrating the nerves commonly encountered in the removal of a cystic hygroma.

to proceed directly to identification of the main trunk. If this is not possible, the mandibular branch is identified and dissected proximally until the main trunk is found. Both the surgeon and his assistant must wear magnifying loops to identify the nerve and its branches. The nerve stimulator must be applied to each strand of tissue. If there is no muscular stimulation, the tissue may be divided. Once the nerve trunks are identified, they can be dissected from the mass and preserved. It is wise to leave small bits of opened cysts attached to nerves and other vital structures rather than risk injury to the facial nerve. The hypoglossal nerve and branches of the brachial plexus also may be involved in a large hygroma. All of these structures must be identified and avoided because this is a benign tumor and recurrences are rare when the main cystic mass is excised (Fig. 21–5). When it has been necessary to leave tissue adjacent to the carotid sheath or major nerve trunks, it is helpful to open any remaining cysts and swab their interior with a dilute solution of iodine. After a minute or so, the iodine is irrigated with normal saline. This technique has successfully eliminated recurrences in cases where it was necessary to leave tissue intertwined about the facial nerve. When dealing with tumors in the neonate, a staged excision often is necessary. First, tissue is removed from one side of the neck, and then a tracheotomy is performed. Attempts are made to remove the remaining tumor 10 days to 2 weeks later. These are terrible,

extensive lesions that almost defy surgical removal. One's goal should be to establish an airway and make it possible for the baby to eat. Barrand and Freeman operated on 9 infants with massive infiltrating cystic hygromas of the neck; 5 experienced respiratory distress in the new-

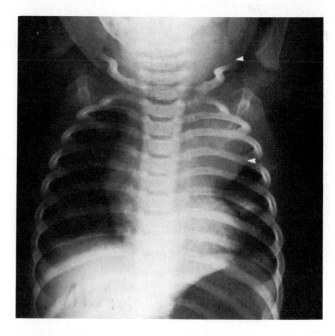

Figure 21–6. This cystic hygroma, involving the left neck and chest, was removed through a cervical and left thoracic incision.

born period, and 4 eventually died of respiratory obstruction.[7]

Meticulous hemostasis may be obtained with the bipolar electrocoagulation unit, but even so there will be an extensive lymph exudate from the wound. Any excess skin should be excised before it is closed with subcuticular sutures. Postoperative fluid collections are avoided by leaving drains in place for a minimum of 5 or 6 days and the application of a bulky compression dressing. A cervical or supraclavicular cystic hygroma may descend into the neck posterior to the subclavian and innominate veins or along the esophagus anterior to the vertebral column or into the anterior mediastinum with the thymus (Fig. 21–6).[8,9] Episodes of infection or hemorrhage into a mediastinal cystic hygroma may follow a simple upper respiratory infection and cause death by airway obstruction.[10] Chylothorax is another potential complication of a mediastinal hygroma.

The surgical approach to a cervicomediastinal hy-groma is dictated by the extent and location of the cervical component as well as by the location of the intrathoracic extension. Computed tomography of the neck and chest accurately localizes these lesions (Fig. 21–7). If possible, the two lesions should be removed at one operation. Mills and Grosfeld have recommended a one-stage removal by extending the transverse cervical incision downward to split the sternum.[11] In their hands, this technique allowed the removal of extensive hygromas from around the trachea and esophagus as well as from the anterior mediastinum. Occasionally, a supraclavicular hygroma may be traced down into the thorax and removed without the necessity of opening the chest. The removal of a mediastinal hygroma interrupts normal lymphatic pathways and invites a postoperative chylothorax. It is essential to ligate every possible lymph channel, give the child a nonfat diet for several days after the operation, and leave the chest tube in place until there is minimal drainage. Lymphangiomas involving the skin

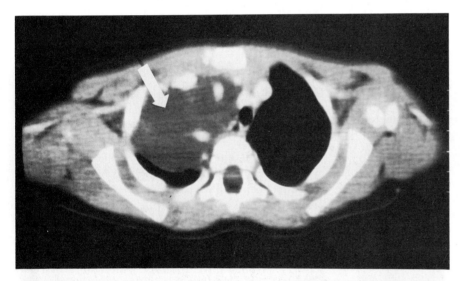

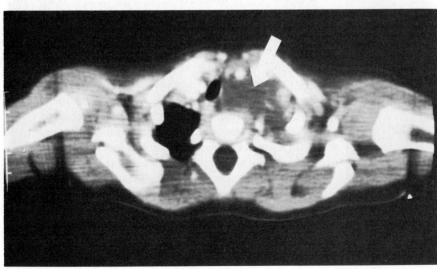

Figure 21–7. CT scan of a cervicomediastinal hygroma. **Top.** Mediastinal component demonstrating tracheal deviation. **Bottom.** The cervical component, extended above the clavicle, was not palpated nor seen on x-ray.

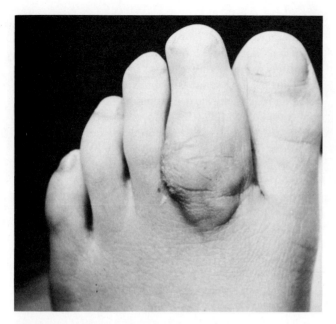

Figure 21–8. A dermal lymphangioma of the toe, with weeping and verrucose changes in the skin.

of the extremities or trunk may be small, simple hygromas situated beneath the skin. In older children, these are thought to be lipomas. The skin overlying a lymphangioma may be covered with fluid-filled vesicles and may initially be thought to be a dermatologic problem.[12] The superficial vesicles may cover several square centimeters of skin. These weep lymphatic fluid, become infected, and occasionally experience hemorrhage. Later, the surrounding skin becomes verrucose in appearance (Fig. 21–8). Beneath the skin there are lymphatic spaces in the subcutaneous tissues. Edwards et al. have demonstrated with lymphangiography that the involved lymphatics in these skin lesions fail to communicate with

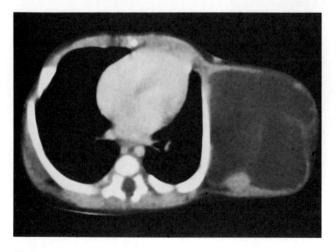

Figure 21–9. CT scan demonstrating chest wall compression by a chest wall hygroma. There is no intrathoracic extension, since these lesions extend into the chest only along vascular planes.

the normal lymphatic channels of the extremity.[13] For this reason, they recommended a wide excision encompassing all of the abnormal tissue. Often, after the excision of a subcutaneous lymphangioma, vesicles will appear on the skin near the incision. Occasionally, these may disappear after coagulation with a needle-tipped electrocautery.

We have observed four newborn infants with huge lymphangiomas involving the chest wall and axilla. In two, the lesion extended down the arm to the wrist, and in one there was a contralateral cervicomediastinal hygroma. Although none extended into the thoracic cavity, the chest wall was compressed, apparently by intrauterine pressure (Fig. 21–9). We attempted reconstruction of the ribcage in one of these children at 3 years of age, without success. She has progressive scoliosis and requires a tracheotomy with ventilator support. Postoperative lymphedema of the arm resulted in further disability of this child as well as in two of the others. These extensive lesions require excision, but their sequelae have defied satisfactory treatment. The parents must be warned about the possibility of significant postoperative complications.

OMENTAL AND MESENTERIC CYSTS

Cysts involving the omentum or mesentery are usually multilocular and filled with a clear serous fluid. They too result from lymphatic obstruction. Chylous cysts are found in the base of the mesentery and are filled with a milky fluid. In our experience, a mesenteric or omental cyst may be huge, with few symptoms other than vague abdominal pain. All we have observed were first considered to be ascites. A good rule to follow is that if a child has no liver, kidney, or heart disease and apparent ascites, he or she probably really has an omented cyst (Fig. 21–10). Of course, a girl could have a huge, thinwalled ovarian cyst. Occasionally, a mesenteric cyst may undergo torsion.[14] We have seen hemorrhage into a mesenteric cyst following a blow to the abdomen. Another of our patients who had an extensive multilocular cyst that involved the mesentery of his sigmoid colon experienced protracted diarrhea with a protein-losing enteropathy (Fig. 21–11). He did not appear to have a generalized intestinal lymphangiomatosis, and his health was improved by resection of the cyst with the adjacent colon.

The most characteristic physical finding in a child with a mesenteric cyst is a protuberant nontender abdomen that is dull to percussion. A cyst may be differentiated from ascites by the facts that the flanks do not bulge when the child is recumbent and that a cyst will seem to follow as the child moves. Plain roentgenograms of the abdomen show the intestinal gas pattern to be pushed forward when there is a mesenteric cyst and backward when the cyst is in the greater omentum.

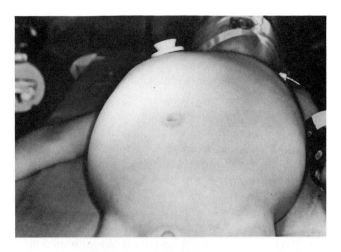
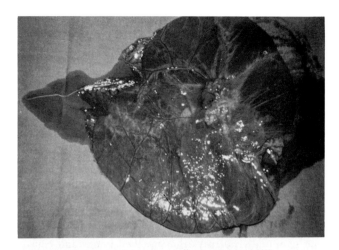

Figure 21–10. Left. This child was thought to have ascites because of his fluid-filled abdomen with bulging flanks. **Right.** The soft, fluid-filled omental cyst. A child who appears to have ascites but has no disease of the heart, kidney, or liver really has an omental cyst.

Ultrasonography is successful in differentiating a cyst from ascites and will also locate the cyst.

Treatment

An omental cyst is removed easily by clamping and dividing the proximal omental tissue—if necessary, flush with

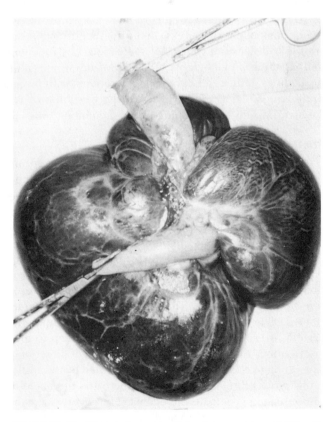

Figure 21–11. Mesenteric cyst involving the mesentery and the sigmoid colon. This patient had a protein-losing enteropathy, possibly caused by the weeping of chyle through the bowel mucosa.

the transverse colon. Cysts that involve the mesentery may be difficult to remove because the blood supply of the bowel must be preserved. However, after the peritoneum is opened, there usually is a plane of loose areolar tissue that lends itself well to easy blunt dissection. It is practically never necessary to resect the bowel.

INTESTINAL LYMPHANGIECTASIA

Obstruction of the lymphatics within the lamina propria, submucosa, or serosa and mesentery of the bowel produces dilated intestinal lymphatics. In such a case, the bowel wall is thickened and edematous, and there is often thickening of the villi. A positive family history of lymphedema often is found, and about a third of children with this disease also have peripheral edema. It would appear that intestinal lymphangiectasis is another expression of congenital lymphatic obstruction, which is determined by an autosomal dominant gene.[15]

The symptoms consist of recalcitrant diarrhea, malnutrition, growth retardation, anemia, and severe hypoproteinemia. The protein loss may result in gross anasarca. The correct diagnosis in 11 of Vardy et al.'s patients was made by peroral duodenal biopsy.[15] Roentgen findings are nonspecific; there is thickening of the jejunal folds, some speculation of the mucosa, and dilatation of loops of small bowel. Lymphocytopenia is an important sign of chyle loss, and some patients show spontaneous chylous ascites or chylothorax as further evidence of their lymphatic block. Treatment consists of a high-protein, fat-free diet with added MCT oil. It may be helpful to start treatment with total intravenous alimentation to more rapidly improve the child's nutritional status. When there is a localized collection of lymphatic cysts in the mesentery, resection may be curative.

When all else fails, the insertion of a high-flow Storz-Denver peritonevenous shunt that drains the peritoneal cavity into the superior vena cava via the saphenous vein may be of benefit. Unfortunately, obstruction of the shunt and clogging of the valves by viscous material are common complications.[16,17]

GENERALIZED LYMPHANGOMATOSIS

This lymphatic abnormality may involve all organs, including the bones, subcutaneous tissues, retroperitoneum, and the thorax.[18–20] This is a generalized disorder of the lymph vessels, with widespread cyst formation that eventually destroys the involved bones and causes peripheral lymphadema and recurrent bouts of chylous ascites and chylothorax. One finds osteolytic bony lesions and, via radioactive scans, filling defects in the liver and spleen. Splenic involvement may lead to a consumption coagulopathy.[21] There is no cure in such cases. Chylous peritonitis can be controlled with a high-protein, low-fat diet, and we have successfully eliminated chylothorax with pleural stripping. Unfortunately, the bone disease and peripheral edema are at this time impossible to treat.

LYMPHEDEMA

Lymphedema is swelling caused by an abnormal collection of lymph in the interstitial tissues resulting from anomalies, functional overload, or both. There are two types: primary or idiopathic and secondary or acquired. Primary lymphedema is classified according to the age of onset; congenital lymphedema is present at birth, carries the poorest prognosis, and is present in 11 percent of cases. Lymphedema praecox, the most common type, is usually discovered during the teens or 20s, often concurrently with a growth spurt. Perhaps growth increases hydrostatic pressure, and the abnormal lymphatics are overwhelmed. The edema may occur after trauma or an infection and, in females, with the onset of menarche. Only 15 percent of patients develop lymphedema after 35 years of age; then it is termed lymphedema tarda. In this age group, it must be differentiated from edema, resulting from other disease or mechanical obstruction.[22,23]

Infants with congenital lymphedema often have a family history. In 1982, Milroy described hereditary edema in 22 patients, 21 of whom had edema at birth.[24] His study included six generations of a family of 97 members. The disease is transmitted as a sex-linked dominant pattern, which fits the concept of the disease as an inborn lymphatic error.[25,26]

Secondary lymphedema is rare in children and most commonly is caused by radical cancer surgery or radiation. Other causes include tumor, inflammation, filariasis, toxins, trauma, and phlebitis. Allen, who classified lymphedema into the primary and secondary types, believed that congenitally underdeveloped lymphatics explained primary lymphedema.[27] Kinmonth confirmed this theory with lymphangiography in over 100 patients. Taylor and Gough modified the classification by adding the term "aplasia" if no formed subcutaneous trunks were found.[28,29] Eighty-seven percent of patients have hypoplastic or smaller and fewer lymphatic vessels. Even when there is unilateral edema, the asymptomatic leg on lymphangiography will have decreased and abnormal lymph vessels.

Varicose, large, tortuous lymphatics with incompetent or absent valves are termed "megalymphatics" and are classified as being hyperplastic. The edema appears to be caused by stagnation and backflow, is more likely to be unilateral and is seen more commonly in males. Chylous reflux, or eruption of intestinal chyle into the limb, is sometimes seen in these patients.[30,31]

In secondary lymphedema, there is proximal acquired obstruction, with secondary dilatation of the vessels. Lymphangiography may demonstrate a backflow of contrast medium into the dermal plexus. Lymphangiography also is the best way to determine if an unaffected limb will develop edema. If there are abnormal lymphatics, there may be future swelling. Follow-up lymphangiograms demonstrate a decrease in the number of channels, probably because of continued stagnation, obstruction, and infection. Phelbograpy rarely shows any venous abnormalities, although I have had four patients with moderate lymphedema and varicosities who were improved by high ligation and stripping of the saphenous vein.

Pathophysiology

Valveless lymphatics of the superficial system appear to drain into a valved subdermal system.[32] Beneath this subdermal system are the subcutaneous lymphatic channels. The deep, muscular system is separated from the subcutaneous lymphatics by the deep fascia, but there are connections at the popliteal and inguinal lymph nodes. These connections may explain the abrupt ending of lymphedema at the knee or groin. In all cases, the fluid is in the subcutaneous tissue, and the muscles are free from lymphedema. This is the key factor in operations designed to deliver lymph to the deep competent system. Muscle action and a valved system deep to the fascia move the lymph fluid in a cephalad direction. The problem of lymphedema is compounded by the accumulation of protein-rich fluid that increases the oncotic pressure, to perpetuate the edema. Moreover, the skin elastic fibers become chronically stretched, and the skin can no longer confine minimal edema without external support.

Clinical Findings

Children usually complain of swelling of one ankle or extremity. There may be a history of recent infection, trauma, insect bite, onset of menses, or a growth spurt. The painless, pitting edema also may involve the genitalia, hand, arm, face, or breast. There is no venous engorgement. Associated findings of yellow nails, a double row of eyelashes, or associated hemangiomas or lymphangiomas may be seen in 10 to 15 percent of patients.[33–35] There is no pain. The differentiation of venous and lymphatic edema is illustrated in Table 21–1. Twenty percent of patients will have severe attacks of cellulitis and lymphangitis in the affected limb. Late changes include dry scaling, stretched skin, firm fibrotic changes, and a warty growth termed "lymphostatic verrucosis." There are rarely ulcerations, such as are seen with arterial or venous disease. Five of my patients had an associated angioma that caused an overgrowth of the extremity. Two required an epiphysiodesis to arrest the overgrowth.

The differential diagnosis of lymphedema includes hemihypertrophy and a condition termed "lipedema," or the "painful fat" syndrome.[36] Four of my patients had this condition. There was symmetrical swelling and aching in both legs, with no evidence of vascular disease. Direct pressure on the swollen tissues produced pain but no pitting, and the feet were not involved. The definitive diagnosis depends on the detection of atypical lipids in the plasma and lipedematous tissue.[37] Surgery had nothing to offer these patients. The clinical diagnosis of lymphedema usually is sufficient. Initially, I performed a variety of invasive tests that only supported the clinical impression. Infection, poor healing, and lymphoria may follow lymphangiography, causing considerable morbidity and delay in treatment. Invasive studies are no longer performed.

I have now treated over 300 patients. All had primary lymphedema except one child whose disease followed a radical groin operation and radiation. The sex ratio is 5 females:3 males.

TABLE 21–1. DIFFERENTIATION OF VENOUS AND LYMPHATIC EDEMA

Variable	Venous	Lymphatic
History	Previous or present phlebitis	None
Examination	Soft, later firm; decreases with overnight elevation	Firmer, does not decrease with elevation
Accompanying	Varicosities, pigmentation, ulcer common	Late skin signs change; ulcer uncommon
Phlebography results	Positive	Negative
Lymphangiography results	Negative	Positive

Treatment

As soon as the diagnosis is made, even at birth, the family must be given a full explanation of the chronicity of the disease, together with the fact that there is no specific curative treatment. Initially, continuous compression is applied to the involved extremity 24 hours a day with an elastic bandage. When the child is 6 months old, he is fitted with a tailor-made stocking. The stocking must apply even pressure, commencing at the foot. Small children rapidly grow out of the stocking. Consequently, new ones must be made at frequent intervals. In most cases, compression therapy, careful attention to skin cleanliness, and topical antibiotic treatment for any skin irritations will prevent the recurrent lymphangitis and cellulitis that plague these patients.

One hundred fifty infants, children, and young adults have now undergone surgery for lymphedema. The indications for surgery include an extremity that is too heavy and cumbersome for daily activities, such as the ability to wear normal clothing and shoes. Another is recurrent episodes of crippling cellulitis and lymphangitis. Resection is not indicated, particulary in young females, for cosmetic improvement. The scarring and contour rarely satisfy these patients. All patients with lymphedema require support hose for life whether or not they undergo surgery. Full activity is encouraged, but they must be taught careful hygienic care of their feet to avoid infections. At any sign of infection, the child is placed on bedrest and intravenous penicillin because the organism is assumed to be a streptococcus even when blood cultures are negative. If there is a history of penicillin allergy, erythromycin is the next drug of choice. Recurrent episodes of infection respond well to excisional surgery. One patient who required bedrest and antibiotics for 10 days each month has not had an attack of cellulitis or lymphangitis since his operation 11 years ago.

In the past, many unsatisfactory operations have been described for the relief of lymphedema. Excision of the skin and subcutaneous tissues was recommended as early as 1911.[38] A year later, Kondoleon excised the deep fascia to allow the superficial lymphatics to drain into the deep vessels.[39] Sistrunk modified this operation by excising extensive amounts of tissue.[40] Seventy-five percent of his patients were improved.

Total excision of the skin and subcutaneous tissues with coverage of the muscle with split-thickness skin grafts was reported in the treatment of tropical elephantiasis, but the grafts were susceptible to breakdown and chronic infection, and the configuration of the leg was bizarre. Homans was the first to excise the subcutaneous tissue and deep fascia and achieve coverage with thin full-thickness skin flaps.[41] Homans reported eight patients with satisfactory results and firmly established this technique. Fonkalsrud advocated staged subcutaneous

176

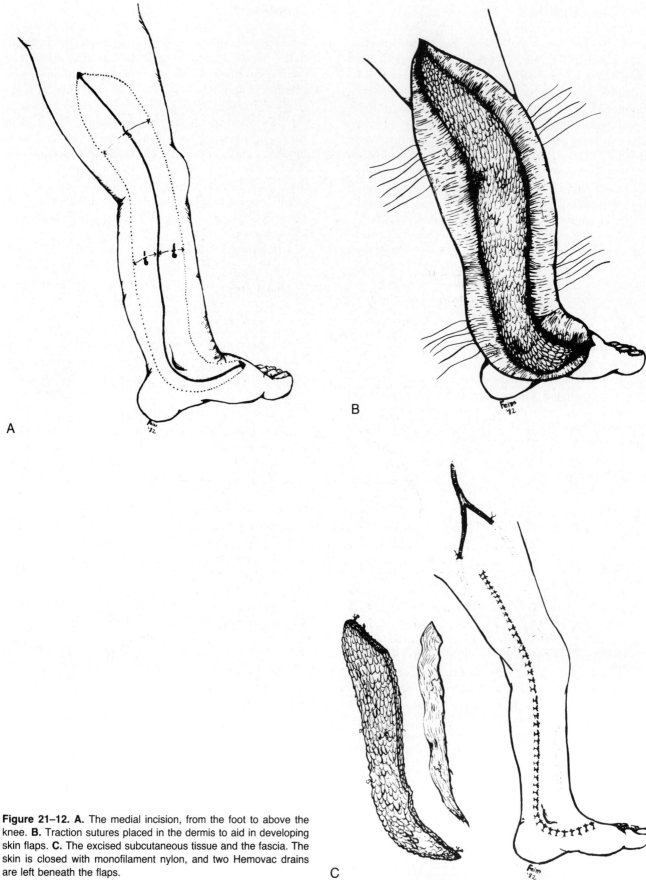

A

B

C

Figure 21–12. A. The medial incision, from the foot to above the knee. **B.** Traction sutures placed in the dermis to aid in developing skin flaps. **C.** The excised subcutaneous tissue and the fascia. The skin is closed with monofilament nylon, and two Hemovac drains are left beneath the flaps.

lymphangiectomy in infants and children and in a follow-up report confirmed the initial good results.[42,43] Others have reported excellent results in managing lymphedema in adults with staged subcutaneous excision. With radioiodinated human serum albumin injections, lymph is 80 percent cleared in 24 hours by a year after surgery.[44]

Surgical Procedure

After evaluation of the available operations, we adopted a modification of the Homans procedure, a staged subcutaneous excision of the lymphedematous tissue.[45,46] The patient is placed on bedrest for 3 to 14 days before surgery. The extremity is painted with povidone-iodine ointment every 8 hours and wrapped with Kerlix. A Jobst air splint is applied and inflated to 30 mm Hg pressure. The pressure is released every 4 hours or as necessary. A plastic cup, stuffed with cotton and placed over the toes, prevents painful squeezing of the foot. This regimen may be instituted at home before admission to the hospital. It results in rapid shrinking of the extremity by mobilization of edematous fluid. One patient lost 54 pounds of lymphedematous fluid with this preoperative treatment. If the edema in the leg involves the foot and continues above the knee, the incision is begun on the medial aspect of the foot, continues behind the malleolus, and goes up the medial aspect of the calf, above the knee, and up the thigh (Fig. 21–12A). If the edema stops at the knee, the incision is gently curved and ends at the medial aspect of the popliteal fossa. Subcuticular silk sutures placed along the entire incision are used for traction during development of the skin flaps (Fig. 21–12B). By holding small groups of traction sutures over the surgeon's index finger, trauma to the skin is avoided, and a thin flap may be developed without buttonholing the skin.

A pneumatic tourniquet and liberal use of electrocoagulation have reduced blood loss and obviated the need for transfusion. The skin flaps are develped one sixth of the circumference of the leg both medially and laterally. These are full-thickness flaps but made as thin as possible. The total size of the two skin flaps must be no more than one third of the leg's circumference to decrease the risk of necrosis. A plane is developed beneath the subcutaneous tissue with a Kelly clamp, then most of the excision is done with blunt finger dissection. The greater saphenous venous system is invariably interrupted, thus an adequate deep venous system must be present. The fascial aponeurosis is removed from the muscles with the coagulation current of the electrocautery. The abrupt edges of the subcutaneous tissue may be tapered, but shoulders at the edge of the dissection mold symmetrically in the postoperative period. After release of the pneumatic cuff, meticulous hemostasis is obtained. One large broviac drain with extra holes is placed beneath each flap and brought out through separate stab wounds in the thigh (Fig. 21–12C). It is only necessary to trim skin edges that appear cyanotic.

The skin is closed with multiple interrupted 4.0 nylon monofilament sutures. The suture line is then covered with povidone-iodine ointment and fluff gauze, the leg is wrapped with Kerlix and the air splint is replaced. The splint is inflated to 30 mm Hg pressure. The Hemovac drains are placed to wall suction for 24 hours and then to regular suction. The patient is kept at complete bedrest, with elevation of the extremity. The air splint is released every 4 hours; every 8 hours, the suture line is redressed and repainted with povidone-iodine ointment. The combination of pressure and suction drains prevents collection of fluid under the flaps and enhances the attachment of flaps to the underlying muscle. Seven days after surgery the drains are removed, and the patient is measured for an elastic stocking with 50 mm Hg pressure. Penicillin, started preoperatively, is discontinued at this time. Tight elastic bandages are applied, and nonweightbearing crutch ambulation is begun. Weightbearing is allowed after 3 weeks, when the custom-made stocking is available. The sutures must be left in for longer than usual because healing is slow. Every other suture is removed at 2 weeks, and the rest are removed as late as 4 weeks. If there is bilateral disease, the second leg may be operated on about 10 days after the first when, after the prolonged bedrest, it is soft, pliable, and ideally prepared for surgery.

Improvement may continue for as long as a year after the first operation. For that reason, if a second stage is indicated, it is delayed until after a year. The second procedure is performed on the lateral side of the leg using the same technique. The fascia near the head of the fibula is left undisturbed, since the peroneal nerve is deep to the fascia and will not be injured. Initially, I attempted to spare the sural nerve, but sacrifice of this nerve causes no long-term sequela.

After operation all patients must wear support hose indefinitely, and many patients continue to use the Jobst air splint at night to control residual edema and to improve the contour of the leg.

Genital Involvement

In females, resection of involved labia is successful. Several techniques described for lymphedema of the male genitalia have proven unsatisfactory. Therefore, the following safe, uncomplicated operation was developed.[47]

The boy is placed on bedrest for 3 days, the genitalia are covered with a thin layer of povidone-iodine ointment, and penicillin is begun before surgery. If shaving of the genitalia is required, this is done in the operating room. A Foley catheter is placed in the urethra and sutured to the glans. A transverse incision is made in the scrotum beneath the base of the penis (Fig. 21–13A). The testes and cord structures are identified and

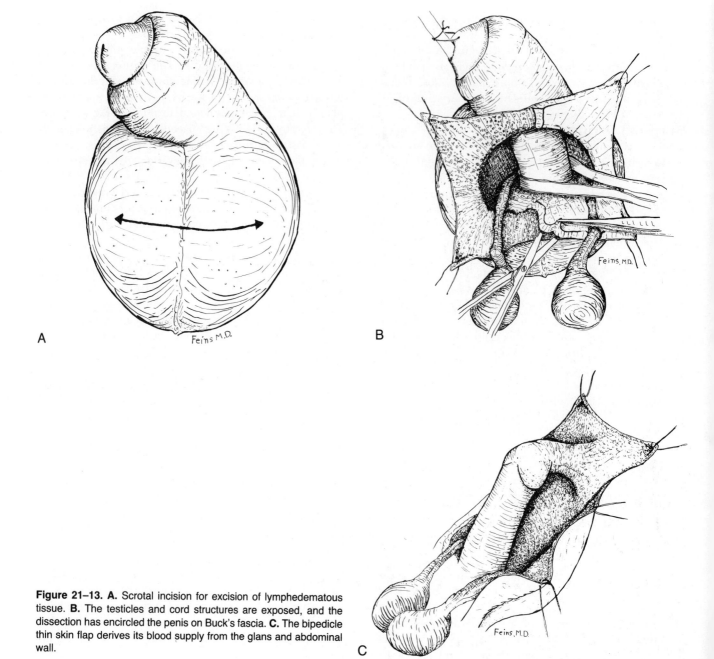

Figure 21–13. A. Scrotal incision for excision of lymphedematous tissue. **B.** The testicles and cord structures are exposed, and the dissection has encircled the penis on Buck's fascia. **C.** The bipedicle thin skin flap derives its blood supply from the glans and abdominal wall.

kept out of harm's way. Next, skin flaps of scrotum are developed and constructed as thin as possible. By grasping the scrotal skin between the thumb and index finger and rolling the skin over the lateral portion of the index finger, the exact depth of the dissection is localized. The subcutaneous tissues of the scrotum are now radically removed. As the base of the penis comes into view, the dissection is begun on Bucks fascia on the ventral side of the penis. It is continued laterally and dorsally around the penis until it is encircled. The base of the penis is now surrounded by a penrose drain to gently invert the penis into the wound (Fig. 21–13B). The dis-

section is continued up to the coronal sulcus of the glans. At this point, the thin skin flap of penile skin receives its blood supply from the corpora, glans, and abdominal wall (Fig. 21–13C). After meticulous hemostasis, two Hemovac drains are placed in the scrotum, with the tip of one along the shaft of the penis. These are brought out a stab wound lateral to the base of the penis. The scrotal skin is closed with interrupted chromic sutures, and the scrotum is supported with a suspensory bridge. The incision is covered with povidone-iodine ointment, and the penis is wrapped with two layers of a transparent, moisture-permeable dressing. The dressing and the Fo-

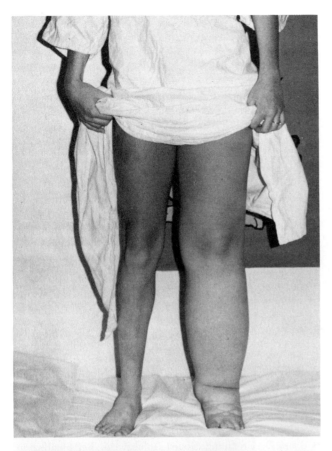

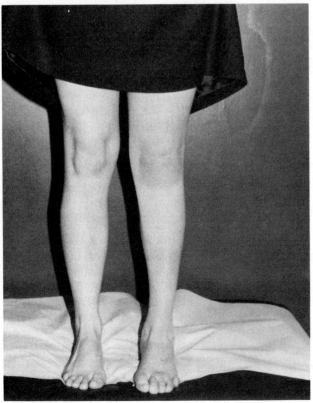

Figure 21–14. Girl with unilateral lymphedema. **Top.** Before surgery. **Bottom.** Postoperative result.

ley catheter are left in place for 1 week. All patients are encouraged to wear an athletic supporter, and a narrow elastic bandage wrapped around the penis helps prevent recurrent edema.

Results

Two patients developed seromas beneath their leg flaps. One was in a patient whose leg was too large to fit in an air splint, and an elastic bandage did not provide evenly distributed compression. The other patient produced such a huge volume of lymph that a larger Hemovac drain was placed. There were no flap sloughs, but two patients had wound separations after early suture removal. One healed spontaneously, but the other had bouts of lymphangitis requiring secondary closure of the granulating wound. Four patients developed keloid scars that were revised, and steroid injections were used in five others who developed keloids.

One half of my patients have required a second procedure to achieve optimum reduction in limb size, and one third of the total need 3-stage operations. Thus far, 20 percent of the 150 patients have require only one excision. Long-term follow-up care is essential with these patients. All require custom-made support hose to apply 50 mmHg pressure. Home use of the air splint with frequent elevation of the limb enhances edema control.

Meticulous skin care is essential, and any minor injury must be treated vigorously to prevent infection. These patients have no limitations on their activities, and 90 percent are pleased with the results of surgery (Fig. 21–14A & B). Most wear normal shoes and clothing. The decrease in attacks of cellulitis and lymphangitis has been most striking.

Overall, the results of the operation and treatment plan have been excellent. The operation itself is tedious, fatiguing, and anatomically unexciting, and the follow-up care requires patience. According to Boston folklore, when John Homans performed surgery for lymphedema, boredom would stimulate him to hum passages from Gilbert and Sullivan operas.

REFERENCES

1. Bill AH Jr, Sumner DS: A unified concept of lymphangioma and cystic hygroma. Surg Gynecol Obstet 120:79, 1965
2. Fonkalsrud EW: Surgical management of congenital malformations of the lymphatic system. Am J Surg 128:152, 1974
3. Rubin FR: The lymphatic system in human embryos, with a consideration of the morphology of the system as a whole. Am J Anat 9:43, 1909
4. McClure CF, Silvester CF: Comparative study of the lymphatico-venous communication in adult mammals. Anat Rec 3:534, 1909

5. Singh S, Babo ML, Pathek LC: Cystic hygroma in children: report of 32 cases including lesions at rare sites. Surgery 69:941, 1971

6. Ninh TN, Ninh TA: Cystic hygroma: A report of 126 cases. J Pediatr Surg 9:191, 1974

7. Barrand KG, Freeman NV: Massive infiltrating cystic hygromas of the neck in infancy. Arch Dis Child 48:523, 1973

8. Camishion RC, Templeton JV: Cervico mediastinal cystic hygroma. Pediatrics 29:831, 1962

9. Feutz ER, Yune HY, Mendelbaum I, Brasher RE: Intrathoracic cystic hygroma: A report of three cases. Radiology 108:61, 1973

10. Nanson EM: Lymphangioma (cystic hygroma) of the mediastinum. J Cardiovasc Surg (Torino) 9:447, 1968

11. Mills NL, Grusfeld JL: One-stage operation for cervico mediastinal cystic hygroma in infancy. J Thorac Cardiovasc Surg 65:608, 1973

12. Easterly NB, Soloman LM: Neonatal dermatology, III: Pigmentary lesions and hemangiomas. J Pediatr 81:1003, 1972

13. Edwards JM, Pearly RD, Kinmouth JB: Lymphangiography and surgery in lymphangioma of the skin. Br J Surg 59:36, 1972

14. Walker AR, Putnam TC: Omental, mesenteric and retroperitoneal cysts: A clinical study of 33 new cases. Ann Surg 178:13, 1973

15. Vardy PH, Lebenthal E, Shwachman H: Intestinal lymphangiectasis: A reappraisal. Pediatrics 55:842, 1975

16. Chang J, Newkirk J, Carlton G, et al: Generalized lymphangiomatosis with chylous ascites treatment by peritoneovenous shunting. J Pediatr Surg 15:748, 1980

17. Guttman F, Montupet P, Bloss R: Re-experience with peritoneovenous shunting for congenital chylous ascites in infants and children. J Pediatr Surg 17:368, 1982

18. Calabrese PR, Frank HD, Taubin HL: Lymphangiomyomatosis with chylous ascites: Treatment with dietary fat restriction and medium chain triglycerides. Cancer 40:895, 1977

19. Murphishi G, Arciuve EL, Krause JR: Generalized lymphangioma in infancy with chylothorax. Pediatrics 46:566, 1970

20. Goldstein MR, Benchimol A, Cornell W, Long D: Chylopericordium with multiple lymphangiomas of bone. N Engl J Med 280:1034

21. Dietz WH, Stuart MJ: Splenic consumptive coaguloapthy in a patient with disseminated lymphangiomatosis. J Pediatr 90:421, 1977

22. Allen EV, Barker NW, Hines EA: Peripheral Vascular Disease, 3rd ed. Philadelphia, Saunders, 1962

23. Kinmonth JB, Taylor GW, Tracy GD, Marsh JD: Primary lymphoedema. Br J Surg 45:1, 1957

24. Milroy WF: An undescribed variety of hereditary oedema. NY State J Med 56:505, 1892

25. Ersek RA, Danese CA, Howard JM: Hereditary congenital lymphedema (Milroy's disease). Surgery 60:1098, 1966

26. Milroy WF: Chronic hereditary edema: Milroy's disease. JAMA 91:1172, 1928

27. Allen EV: Lymphedema of the extremities: Classification, eltiology and differential diagnoses. A study of 300 cases. Arch Intern Med 54:606, 1934

28. Gough MH: Primary lymphoedema: Clinical and lymphangiographic studies. Br J Surg 53:917, 1966

29. Taylor GW: Lymphography in diseases of the lymphatic vessels of the limbs. Minerva Chir 16:704, 1961

30. Kinmonth JB, Taylor GW, Jantet GH: Chylous complications of primary lymphoedema. J Cardiovasc Surg (Torino) 5:327, 1964

31. Kinmonth JB, Taylor GW: Chylous reflex. Br Med J 1:529, 1964

32. Crockett DJ: Lymphatic anatomy and lymphoedema. Br J Plast Surg 18:12, 1965

33. Falls HF, Kertesz ED: A new syndrome combining pterygium colli with developmental anomalies of the eyelids and lymphatics of the lower extremities. Trans Am Ophthalmol Soc 62:248, 1964

34. Robinow M, Johnson GF, Verhagen AD: Distichiasislymphedema: A hereditary syndrome of multiple congenital defects. Am J Dis Child 119:343, 1970

35. Nakielna EM, Wilson J, Ballon HS: Yellow nail syndrome: report of three cases. Can Med Assoc J 115:46, 1976

36. Allen EV, Hines EA Jr: Vascular clinics: lipedema of the legs. A syndrome characterized by fat legs and orthostatic edema. Proc Staff Meet Mayo Clin 15:184, 1940

37. Stallworth JM, Hennigar GR, Jonsson HT Jr, Rodriguez D: The chronically swollen painful extremity: A detailed study for possible etiological factors. JAMA 228:1656, 1974

38. Lanz O: Eroffnung Neuer Abfuhrwege Bei Stauung in Bauch und unteren Extermitaten. Zentralbl Chir 38:153, 1911

39. Kondoleon E: Die operative Behandlung der elephantiastischen Oedema. Zentralbl Chir 39:1022, 1912

40. Sistrunk WE: Conribution to plastic surgery: Certain modifications of the Kondoleon operation for elephantiasis. Ann Surg 85:185, 1927

41. Homans J: The treatment of elephantiasis of the legs: Preliminary report, N Engl J Med 215:1099, 1936

42. Fonkalsrud EW: Congenital lymphedema of the extremities in infants and children. J Pediatr Surg 4:231, 1969

43. Fonkalsrud EW, Coulson WF: Management of congenital lymphedema in infants and children. Ann Surg 177:280, 1973

44. Miller TA, Harper J, Longmire WP Jr: The management of lymphedema by staged subcutaneous excision. Surg Gynecol Obstet 136:586, 1973

45. Feins NR, Rubin R, Crais T, O'Connor JF: Surgical management of thirty-nine children with lymphedema. J Pediatr Surg 12:471, 1977

46. Feins NR, Rubin R, Crais T, O'Connor JF: Treatment of lymphedema in children. In Brooks BE (ed): Controversies in Pediatric Surgery. Austin, University of Texas Press, 1984, pp 186–203

47. Feins NR: A new surgical technique for lymphedema of the penis and scrotum. J Pediatr Surg 15:787, 1980

22
Congenital Cysts and Sinuses of the Neck

Congenital remnants of the ventral portion of the embryonic pharynx and its lateral derivatives, the branchial clefts, are a fascinating group of anomalies that must be considered in the diagnosis of neck masses and cervical infections. The primitive branchial apparatus is of phylogenetic interest to comparative anatomists because, in fish, the branchial clefts, with their corresponding pouches, form the gill slits. Thus, one might say that a persistent branchial sinus tract from the pharynx to the skin is indeed an example of "ontogeny recapitulating phylogeny."

The most common defects arise either from anomalous descent of the thyroid from the floor of the pharynx or from the first and second branchial clefts. There are, however, rare case reports of cysts arising in a persistent ultimobranchial gland, a cervical thymus, or a branchial remnant.[1-3] The diagnosis of these unusual cysts may be made by their location and microscopic appearance.

THYROGLOSSAL CYST AND SINUS

The thyroid anlage develops from an epithelial thickening on the floor of the primitive pharynx between the first and second pharyngeal grooves. The thickening becomes an evagination, which initially lies in contact with the aortic sac of the developing heart.[4] Elongation of the embryo separates the thyroid from its point of origin, which is marked by the foramen cecum at the base of the tongue. During its descent, it passes through or immediately adjacent to the hyoid bone. Normally, the entire thryoglossal duct degenerates during the fifth week of embryonic life, except for a solid cord of tissue that is continuous with the apex of the pyramidal lobe of the thyroid.[5] Persistence of all or portions of the duct results in a cyst or a sinus tract that extends from the midline of the neck to the foramen cecum (Fig. 22–1).

Pathology

Most commonly, a thyroglossal duct cyst is a rounded, firm mass at or just below the hyoid bone. It may be slightly off the midline, but never so far laterally that it would be confused with a branchial cleft cyst. A cyst may also be located at the base of the tongue, where it causes respiratory distress during the newborn period. These cysts are lined by statified squamous, columnar, or transitional epithelium. Figure 22–2 demonstrates multiple arborizing tracts, typical of these lesions. Twenty-four of 45 specimens studied by Soucy and Penning showed multiple tracts, all of which were either anterior to or engulfed in the hyoid bone.[6] The most common complication is infection, which results in an abscess with pain, redness, and fluctuation. After a bout of infection, the epithelium may be destroyed, and there is an increase in the dense fibrous connective tissue surrounding the sac. Malignant degeneration in a thyroglossal duct cyst has been reported in over 100 patients.[7]

Diagnosis

Unless the lesion becomes infected, most thyroglossal duct cysts are asymptomatic firm lumps in the midline of the neck (Fig. 22–3). In our experience, it is unusual for the mass to appear before 1 year of age, although most are observed by the age of 5 years. The cyst is nontender, firm, and under pressure because of its retained secretions, and it moves up and down with swallowing. It is not possible on physical examination to differentiate a thyroglossal duct cyst from a midline ectopic thyroid unless one can definitely palpate thyroid tissue in its normal location. As a rule, if the lesion is a midline ectopic thyroid gland, this will be the child's only thyroid tissue. Removal would leave the child permanently dependent on thyroid medication. For this reason, some authors have recommended a thyroid scan for every child with a possible thyroglossal duct cyst.[8]

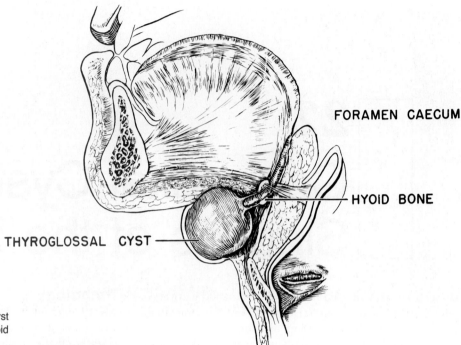

Figure 22–1. A typical thyroglossal duct cyst with a sinus tract extending through the hyoid bone to the foramen cecum.

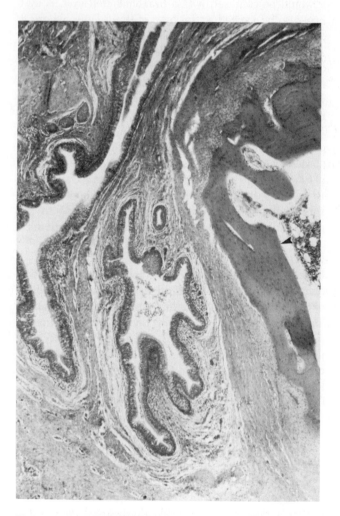

Figure 22–2. A sinus tract lined by columnar epithelium adjacent to the hyoid bone (indicated by arrow).

The midline ectopic thyroid is, however, extremely rare, and one would have to perform a large number of radioactive scans to obtain one positive result. Any surgeon aware of this condition will aspirate or biopsy any midline structure before its removal. The differential diagnosis includes an epidermoid cyst, which is immediately below and attached to the dermis, and a lymph node in the submandibular space. Nodes are movable and often will disappear under observation.

Treatment

An infected cyst must be treated with antibiotics and warm compresses with either aspiration of the pus or incision and drainage. No attempt should be made to surgically excise a previously infected cyst until the inflammatory reaction has subsided.

Operation. The patient is given a general endotracheal anesthetic and positioned so that the chest is elevated and the neck is hyperextended. A transverse incision 3 to 4 cm in length is made over the mass. If there is a fistula to the skin, an elliptical incision is made around the opening. The subcutaneous tissues and the platysma are opened and reflected to expose the sternohyoid muscles beneath the mass. These are opened, and the midline of the neck is examined down to the isthmus of the thyroid. It is possible for a sinus tract to extend inferiorly as well as to the foramen cecum. The dissection on the cyst wall is commenced laterally and inferiorly. Again, one must be cautious at this point to make a positive diagnosis of a cyst. If there is any doubt that the lesion could be thyroid, it must be biop-

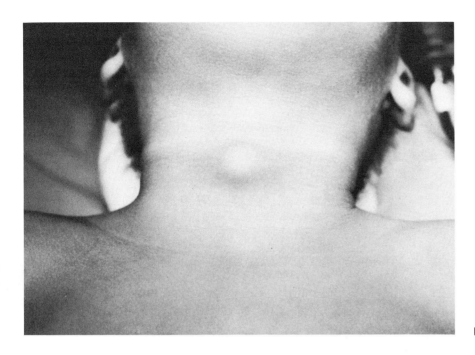

Figure 22–3. Typical thyroglossal duct cyst.

sied. The operative field must be kept free of blood by controlling each vessel with the needlepoint electrocautery. The cautery is also used to separate the sternohyoid muscle from a segment of the hyoid bone on either side of the cyst. When the bone can be elevated from below, scissors are inserted beneath it and spread, at which time the superior portion of the hyoid bone is separated from the geniohyoid muscle. When the bone has been cleared of its muscular attachments, a central portion, 1 cm wide, is removed with the attached cyst (Fig. 22–4). In general, no attempt is made to follow a tiny sinus tract; rather, a generous wedge of tissue is removed from the midline that will encompass any epithelial-lined structure. After removal of the hyoid bone, the dissection must continue up toward the base of the tongue. The exposure is improved if the surgeon himself can reach one hand over the anesthesia screen, insert a finger into the child's mouth, and press forward on the foramen cecum. An assistant can elevate the cyst with the attached hyoid bone, while the surgeon can dissect right to his or her finger within the mouth. A suture ligature is passed through the sinus tract flush with the mucosa of the tongue. The hyoid bone is then reapproximated by suturing together the infrahyoid muscles. It is helpful to leave a small drain in the wound for at least 24 hours.

There is at least a 5 percent recurrence rate, even when the central portion of the hyoid bone is removed.[9] Recurrences may result from multiple branching sinus tracts or even from the presence of more than one cyst. Personally, as I have developed more experience with this seemingly innocuous lesion, I now warn every family of the possibility of recurrence and at operation remove a generous core of tissue. Reoperation is carried out in

identical fashion; more hyoid bone is removed and a large core of tissue is taken from the pyramidal lobe of the thyroid to the base of the tongue.

ECTOPIC THYROID

When a midline ectopic thyroid is found, it is biopsied, hemisected, and placed in the lateral portion of the neck. This is difficult because the mass of tissue is adherent to the hyoid bone, and its blood supply comes through multiple small vessels rather then from a mobile pedicle. This operation should be followed carefully with studies of thyroid function, since as many as 15 percent of patients will be hypothyroid even if there has been no surgical injury to the gland. If the mass is still prominent and presents a cosmetic deformity, it will regress with thyroid extract therapy. Alternatively, the thyroid tissue could be excised, sliced into thin segments, and implanted in muscle. Danis has successfully carried out this procedure in a 6-year-old boy with a large lingual thyroid.[10] Normal thyroid function was maintained after implantation of the gland into muscles of his anterior thigh.

BRANCHIAL CYSTS AND SINUSES

In the 2.5 mm embryo, on the pharyngeal wall, there are paired endodermal pouches that evaginate laterally. Externally, the branchial apparatus is marked by ectodermal clefts. Between each pair of clefts and arches, there is a layer of mesoderm that contains skeletal tissue, nerves, and arches that connect the dorsal and ventral aorta. By the fifth week, four branchial clefts are visible

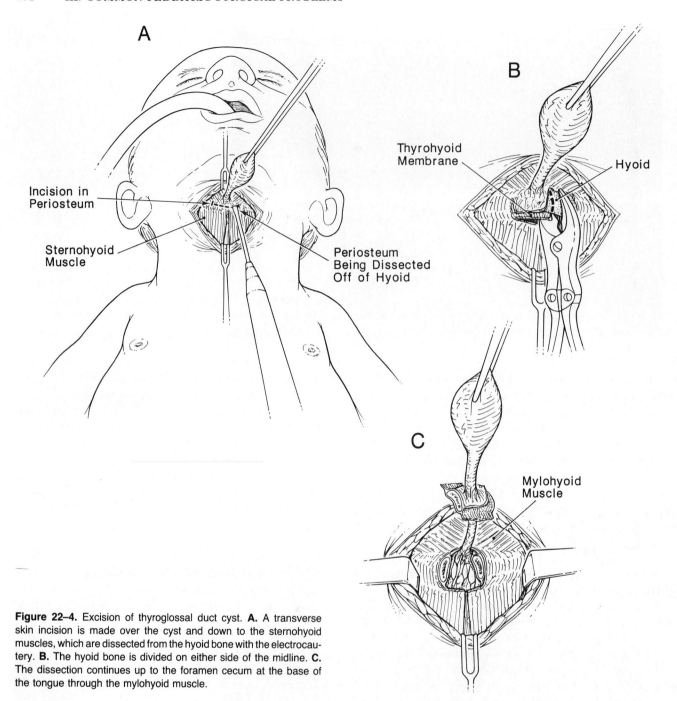

Figure 22–4. Excision of thyroglossal duct cyst. **A.** A transverse skin incision is made over the cyst and down to the sternohyoid muscles, which are dissected from the hyoid bone with the electrocautery. **B.** The hyoid bone is divided on either side of the midline. **C.** The dissection continues up to the foramen cecum at the base of the tongue through the mylohyoid muscle.

from outside the embryo. The dorsal portion of the first cleft remains as the external auditory canal. The other external clefts are obliterated. However, the first, third, and fourth pharyngeal pouches persist as adult organs. The first pouch becomes the eustachian tube, the middle ear cavity, and the mastoid air cells. All that remains of the second pouch is the palatine tonsil and the supratonsillar fossa. The third pouch forms the superior parathyroid, whereas the fourth pouch forms the inferior parathyroid and the thymus.[11] Most branchial fistulae and cysts arise from the second cleft or pharyngeal pouch, which would normally disappear. When complete, a fistula of the second pouch opens in the lower third of the neck at the anterior border of the sternocleidomastoid muscle as a minute skin dimple. The fistula ascends from this opening through the subcutaneous tissue beneath the platysma muscle. Just above the level of the hyoid bone, it turns medially and passes beneath the stylohyoid and digastric muscles, over the hypoglossal and glossopharyngeal nerves, and between the bifurca-

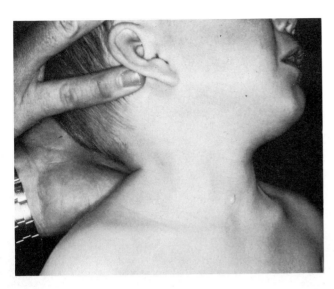

Figure 22–5. A drop of fluid is exuding from a second branchial sinus tract just anterior to the sternocleidomastoid muscle.

tion of the carotid artery. It then enters the lateral wall of the pharynx.[12,13] These lesions are lined by stratified squamous, columnar, or ciliated epithelium and are surrounded by a fairly thick muscular wall. Relatively few children have a complete sinus tract. In 87 patients treated at the Toronto General Hospital, there were only 5 complete sinus tracts, along with 5 incomplete sinuses and 77 cysts.[14]

Diagnosis

A branchial cyst is a painless swelling at the anterior border of the sternocleidomastoid muscle. It is firm and movable and appears to be immediately under the skin. There frequently is a small dimple that occasionally drains a droplet of yellow material (Figure 22–5). The differential diagnosis consists of lymphadenopathy, a mass in the sternocleidomastoid muscle, and a metastatic carcinoma from the thyroid. Lymph node pathology usually is eliminated on the basis of the child's history and a negative response to the usual skin tests. A mass in the sternocleidomastoid muscle often is preceded by a breech delivery. The mass is clearly within the muscle, and the infant has torticollis (Fig. 22–6). If there is any doubt, a period of observation with massage to the mass and exercises to correct the torticollis will make the diagnosis. A complete sinus tract frequently will drain a drop or two of yellowish liquid at intervals, and there is often a crust over the opening. Incomplete sinus tracts are mere dimples in the skin, which are sometimes associated with a bit of ectopic cartilage (Fig. 22–7). Approximately 10 percent are bilateral, and one frequently observes similar lesions in siblings. One child may have a preauricular sinus tract whereas another has the typical cervical lesion. Although some authors have recommended aspiration of the cyst to search for cholesterol crystals or injection of the sinus tract with contrast mate-

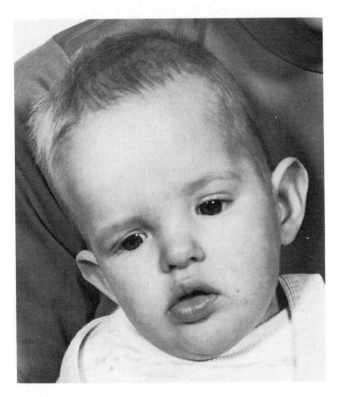

Figure 22–6. A mass in the sternocleidomastoid muscle, which has produced torticollis with asymmetry of the face and head. The head is turned away from the affected muscle.

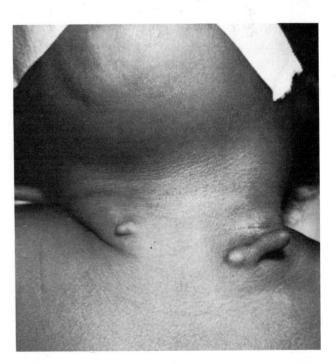

Figure 22–7. Branchial remnants, consisting of skin tags containing a cartilage.

rial, neither of these procedures is desirable or even helpful. Many patients remain asymptomatic for years. The most common complication aside from the cosmetic appearance is infection.

Treatment

All of these lesions should be resected early in life, preferably whenever the diagnosis is made, because surgical excision becomes extremely difficult after there has been a bout of infection.

Operation for a Branchogenic Sinus. The child is positioned on the operating table with the shoulder elevated and head turned away from the side that is to be operated on. The neck is hyperextended. A probe is inserted into the skin opening and up through the tract. A 2-cm transverse incision is made over the probe, through the platysma muscle until the tract is isolated (Fig. 22–8). The tract is dissected distally, and the sinus opening with a tiny ellipse of skin is removed. Traction is then applied to the sinus tract, and it is dissected in an avascular plane between the bifurcation of the carotid artery and its junction with the lateral pharyngeal wall (Fig. 22–9). This final dissection is facilitated by placing a finger in the pharynx with downward and outward pressure.[15,16] Occasionally, the sinus is a short bulbous tract just beneath the skin. A probe can be passed for only a few millimeters. In this case, commence with a small elliptical incision around the sinus opening and follow the probe to the termination of the tract.

Operation for a Branchogenic Cyst. The child is positioned on the operating table in a fashion identical to that for excision of a sinus tract. The incision is placed in the natural skin crease closest to the mass. The dissection is carried down anterior to the sternocleidomastoid muscle and over the carotid sheath. By retracting the muscle laterally, one usually gains sufficient expo-

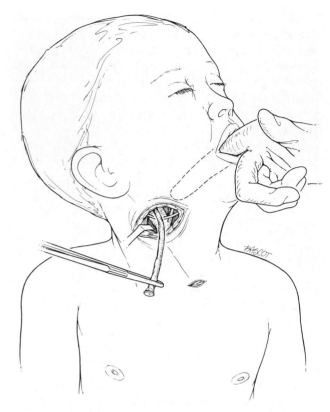

Figure 22–9. Excision of a branchial cleft sinus through one incision, which exposes the sinus tract as it dips deep between the bifurcation of the common carotid artery. The skin opening is excised with a tiny bit of surrounding skin.

sure to keep the dissection in the avascular plane adjacent to the lesion. One must be careful to find an associated sinus tract that communicates with the pharynx. A previous infection that required drainage can make these operations tedious and difficult, with risk of injury to the hypoglossal nerve. Meticulous hemostasis and frequent pauses to identify anatomic structures are advisable.

The First Branchial Cleft. Anomalies of the first branchial cleft are extremely rare and for that reason may be overlooked in spite of classic and predictable signs and symptoms. The first branchial arch gives rise to the upper and lower jaw, the cheek, and the mandibular branch of the trigeminal nerve—the facial nerve, the stapedius, the stylohyoid, and the posterior belly of the digastric muscle are formed from the second arch. Thus any anomalies of the first branchial cleft should arise near the external auditory canal, just below the ear or behind the angle of the mandible, and extend to below the mandible, passing very close to the facial nerve. The important point is that one may expect the tract to pass deep to the nerve, which may be distorted by infection.[17] Dougall described two type of anomalies: one is a cyst lying close to the parotid gland, which usually does not cause symptoms until adulthood; the other is a draining sinus, which is most commonly found

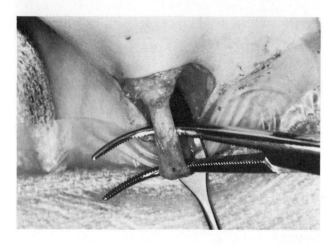

Figure 22–8. The sinus tract is isolated above the skin opening.

in infancy and childhood.[18] Microscopically, the sinus tract is lined with stratified squamous epithelium that may contain skin appendages and strands of muscle. Repeated bouts of infection may destroy portions of the epithelial lining, leaving only granulation tissue. In children, the usual history is one of repeated infections posterior to the ear or near the angle of the jaw. The initial diagnosis may have been lymphadenitis with an abscess or an infected sebaceous cyst. Unfortunately, the infections recur until the proper diagnosis is made. There may be chronic drainage into the external auditory canal, or there may be an area of chronic induration, redness, and crusting over a lesion behind the ear that has failed to heal. The differential diagnosis must include tuberculosis and such chronic infections as actinomycosis. Skin tests and wound cultures should rule out unusual chronic infections. It may be possible to make a correct diagnosis by probing the tract or by the injection of Lipiodol through a fine catheter.

Treatment

Acute infections are controlled with incision and drainage, antibiotics, and warm compresses. However, these measures are of limited help in treating a wound that is chronically indurated and edematous. The entire upper neck, ear, and face must be prepared and draped. An incision is made that removes an ellipse of skin about the fistula; this is extended behind and below the angle of the mandible.[19] Bleeding may be controlled by the prior injection of a solution of epinephrine diluted to 1:100,000. The dissection should stay close to the fistula, but every effort must be made to identify the main trunk and the mandibular branch of the facial nerve; a nerve stimulator will be helpful. The tract may dilate into a cystic cavity behind the angle of the mandible and in the submandibular soft tissues.

PREAURICULAR SINUSES

Small pits anterior to the tragus of the ear probably are not related to a branchial cleft but represent aberrant development of the auditory tubercles. These pits are lined with squamous epithelium and may contain hair and other skin appendages.[20] They extend from the skin surface down through the subcutaneous tissue in close proximity to the superficial temporal artery. The tract is deep and tortuous, reaching the cartilage of the external auditory canal. These lesions are familial and frequently bilateral. They are asymptomatic and have only minor cosmetic importance. Unfortunately, they are prone to develop serious infections, which often point a centimeter or 2 anterior to the skin pit on the face (Fig. 22–10). Incisions and drainage or an inadequate excision leads to a chronic low grade infection that requires wide excision.

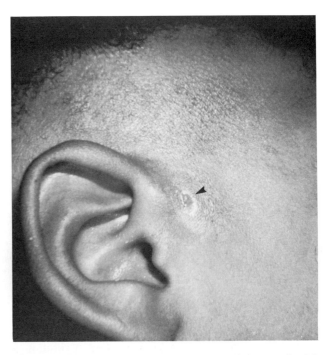

Figure 22–10. An infected preauricular sinus; there is a small patch of chronic granulation tissue at the external orifice.

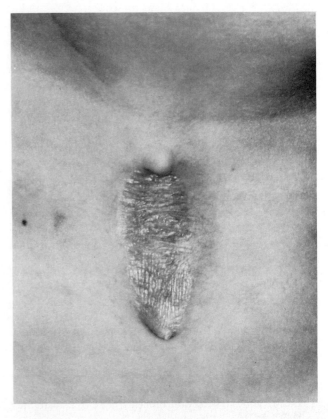

Figure 22–11. A midline cervical fusion defect. The skin over the defect is atrophic, and a sinus tract extends inferiorly.

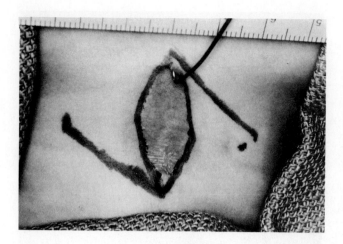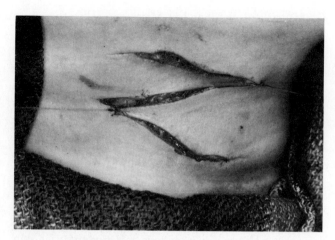

Figure 22–12. Z-plasty to close defect left by excision of midline defect.

Treatment

An uninfected sinus is excised electively whenever the diagnosis is made. It is helpful to inject a solution of epinephrine into the skin around the lesion to obtain a perfectly bloodless operative field. An elliptical incision is made and extended up and down for about 1 cm immediately in front of the ear. The tract is found easily and is traced down to the cartilage. It is often so adherent to the cartilage that one must remove a small portion in order to effect a cure.

MIDLINE SKIN FUSION DEFECT

These are peculiar, midline-depressed scars. They are present in the newborn period and have the appearance of skin that failed to meet in the midline. These lesions are several centimeters long, with a heaped up mound of skin superiorly and a sinus tract that continues beneath the normal skin down to the sternal notch (Fig. 22–11). Pathologically, the dermal layer of the skin is missing. There is only a thin layer of epithelium directly on the platysma muscle. These are unsightly but cause no complications. They are easily removed, but they must be closed with a careful Z-plasty type of repair, or the resultant scar will have a worse appearance than the original lesion. (Fig. 22–12).

REFERENCES

1. Roediger WE, Kalk F, Spitz L, Schmaman A: Congenital thyroid cyst of ultimobranchial gland origin. J Pediatr Surg 12:575, 1977
2. Hanid TK, Johnson AC, Kay L: Cervical thymic cyst. J Pediatr Surg 10:141, 1975
3. Gessendorfer H: Cervical bronchial cyst. J Pediatr Surg 8:435, 1973
4. Arey LB: Developmental Anatomy, 7th ed. Philadelphia, Saunders, 1965, p 215
5. Sqalitzer KE: Contribution to the study of the morphogenesis of the thyroid gland. J Anat 75:389, 1941
6. Soucy P, Penning J: The clinical relevance of certain observations on the histology of the thyroglossal tract. J Pediatr Surg 19:506, 1984
7. Orr R, Kappel D, McConnell D: Carcinoma arising within thyroglossal duct remnants: Case report and review of the literature. Contemp Surg 31:99, 1987
8. Pulito AR, Shaw A: Median ectopic thyroid gland. J Pediatr Surg 8:73, 1973
9. Solomon J, Rangecroft L: Thyroglossal duct lesions in children. J Pediatr Surg 19:555, 1984
10. Danis R: An alternative in management of lingual thyroid: Excision with implantation. J Pediatr Surg 8:869, 1973
11. Gray SW, Skandalakis JE: Embryology for Surgeons: The Embryological Basis for the Treatment of Congenital Defects. Phildadelphia, Saunders, 1972, p 24
12. Lyall D, Stahl WM: Lateral cervical cysts, sinuses, and fistulas of congenital origin. Int Abstr Surg 102:417, 1956
13. Wilson CP: Lateral cysts and fistulas of the neck of developmental origin. Ann R Coll Surg Engl 17:1, 1955
14. McPhail N, Mustard R: Branchial cleft anomalies: A review of 87 cases treated at the Toronto General Hospital. Can Med Assoc J 94:174, 1966
15. Gahr JA, Wesley JR, Woolley MM: Single incision technique for excision of branchiogenic cyst and sinus. Surg Gynecol Obstet 143:805, 1976
16. Buckingham JM, Lynn HB: Branchial cleft csyts and sinuses in children. Mayo Clin Proc 49:172, 1974
17. Gore D, Masson A: Anomalies of the first branchial cleft. Ann Surg 150:309, 1959
18. Dougall AJ: Anomalies of the first branchial cleft. J Pediatr Surg 9:203, 1974
19. Randall P, Royster H: First branchial cleft anomalies: A not-so-rare and a potentially dangerous condition. Plast Reconstr Surg 31:497, 1963
20. Minkowitz S, Minkowitz F: Congenital aural sinuses. Surg Gynecol Obstet 118:801, 1964

23
Umbilical Anomalies

____ *Juda Z. Jona*

The umbilicus to most children is an interesting dimple that assumes near-mystical properties when they learn that it connected them to their mothers before they were born. The umbilicus assumes an even greater importance with a certain type of entertainer.

Anomalies of the umbilicus arise from failure of closure of the fascial ring or from persistence of fetal structures, the omphalomesenteric duct, or the urachus (Fig. 23–1). During fetal life, the umbilicus is the pathway of nutrition from the mother to the fetus. In order to understand its development, as well as to understand the occasional persistence of the omphalomesenteric duct or urachus, it is necessary to review early embryology. The fascinating details of embryonic development are beautifully illustrated in T. S. Cullen's textbook, *The Umbilicus and Its Diseases.*[1]

The developing embryo initially is nourished by a yolk sac, which develops as a posterior projection of the body stalk; this is identifiable in the 0.7 mm embryo. The earliest structure to emerge from the yolk sac is the allantois (Fig. 23–2). The free end of the allantois merges blindly into the umbilical stalk adjacent to the vessels. The other end grows caudally and eventually is incorporated into the hindgut and developing cloaca (Fig. 23–3). With further differentiation of the cloaca, the proximal allantois becomes the urinary bladder, and the remaining portion becomes the urachus. By the 15th week of gestation, the urachus obliterates, leaving a fibrous stalk, the median umbilical ligament. The yolk sac is narrowed as the coelom invaginates at the embryo's crainal and caudal ends. As the coelom continues to grow toward the embryo's midsection, it envelops the developing omphalomesenteric duct, which connects the yolk sac with the gut. As this broad connection is narrowed, the primitive gut is divided into a foregut, a midgut, and a hindgut. By the 3rd fetal week, the omphalomesenteric duct is a slender tube that bridges the gap between the midgut and the shrinking yolk sac (Fig. 23–4). During the same period there is rapid intestinal growth, which during the 6th week results in herniation of the bowel into the umbilical cord. This herniated gut returns to the abdomen with rotation and fixation by the 10th week. By the 16th week of fetal life, the omphalomesenteric duct becomes completely atrophied. There is no trace of this structure in the normal newborn infant. Persistence of portions of the omphalomesenteric duct results in either a Meckel's diverticulum, a complete intestinal fistula, a cyst at the umbilicus, or a fibrous cord that connects the ileum with the umbilicus (Fig. 23–5).

The omphalomesenteric arteries arise as multiple branches of the primitive dorsal aorta and course alongside the omphalomesenteric duct toward the yolk sac. The vessels then become paired, and with resolution of the duct, most of the arteries also disappear. The proximal part of the right artery remains as the superior mesenteric artery, and a small remnant of the omphalomesenteric artery frequently is seen alongside a Meckel's diverticulum (Fig. 23–6). The paired omphalomesenteric veins arise from the yolk sac and course toward the developing liver. The right vein undergoes early atrophy, whereas the left persists and develops into the portal vein.

The actual formation of the umbilical cord as the nutrient channel leading from the chorion is completed with the development of the umbilical vessels as the yolk sac commences to disappear. The two umbilical arteries arise from the primitive dorsal aorta on either

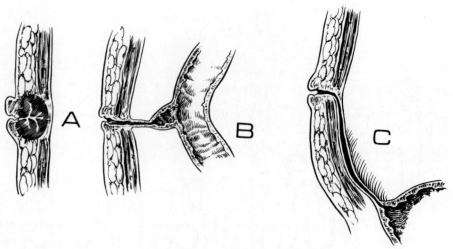

Figure 23–1. A. An umbilical cyst that may contain uroileal or gastric epithelium. **B.** A patent omphalomesenteric duct. **C.** A patent urachus.

side of the hindgut and accompany the allantois to insert into the chorion. Soon after birth, their lumen obliterates; their fibrous remnants become the lateral umbilical ligaments. The umbilical veins are paired in early development and run from the chorion to the liver. By the 6th week, the right vein obliterates, and the left becomes the main venous channel, joining the left portal vein to drain into the sinus venosus. After birth, this vein persists as the ligamentum teres of the falciform ligament.

DEFECTS OF THE OMPHALOMESENTERIC DUCT

Of cases involving vitelline duct remnants, 82 percent show Meckel's diverticulae, 10 percent show a solid cord between the ileum and the abdominal wall, and 6 percent show a patent duct between the ileum and the umbilicus. The remaining 2 percent of cases involve cysts or sinus tracts at the umbilicus (Fig. 23–7).[2]

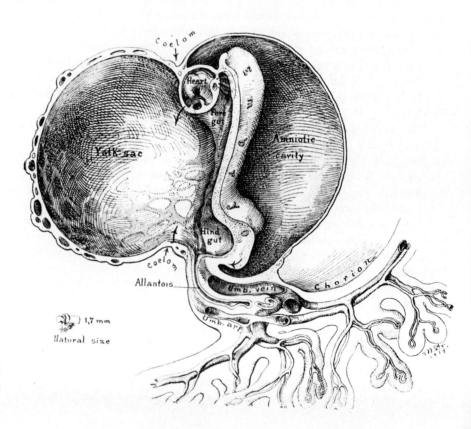

Figure 23–2. The embryo is still an open disc at the 1.7 mm stage; the allantois is visible as a narrow outpouch from the yolk sac. (*Cullen.*[1])

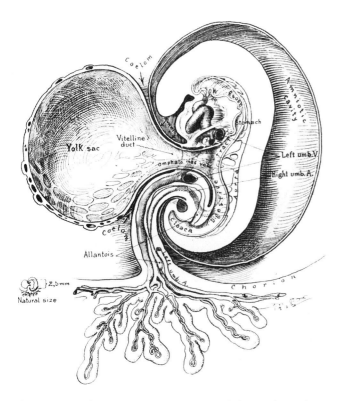

Figure 23–3. The yolk sac is smaller in relation to the embryo, and the allantois has become incorporated into the cloaca. The vitelline duct is seen connecting the midgut with the yolk sac. (*Cullen.*[1])

Persistence of a patent duct may be detected at birth by the presence of a small omphalocele that contains a bit of pouting intestinal mucosa on its surface. After resection of the omphalocele sac, the patent duct is seen to connect with the ileum (Fig. 23–8). If there is no obvious omphalocele, the persistent duct may be ligated with the cord. In such a case it will not become evident until mucus or stool comes through the umbilicus.[3,4] Of the cases reviewed by Kittle et al., 20 percent showed prolapse of the ileum from the umbilical fistula.[5] The diagnosis of a patent omphalomesenteric duct is made by the injection of contrast material that demonstrates communication to the small intestine. Treatment consists of a transverse incision just below the umbilicus into the peritoneal cavity. The duct is dissected free from the abdominal wall and clamped at its junction with the ileum. It is then amputated and the bowel is closed transversely. The distal portion of the duct may persist as a polypoid lesion at the umbilicus (Fig. 23–9). This is found in neonates after the cord has fallen off and is a raised, moist, red lesion consisting of bowel mucosa. There is often a mucous discharge and blood staining of the surrounding skin. The lesion is identical in appearance to the common umbilical granuloma. For this reason, we treat any lesion of this type with several applications of silver nitrate on an outpatient basis before recommending excision.

An umbilical polyp can be removed via a small inci-

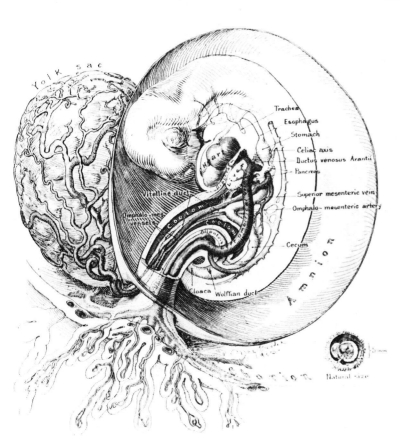

Figure 23–4. A 5-mm embryo. The body stalk has narrowed, but the yolk sac is still present. The vitelline duct is a slender connection between the midgut that is commencing to herniate into the coelom. (*Cullen.*[1])

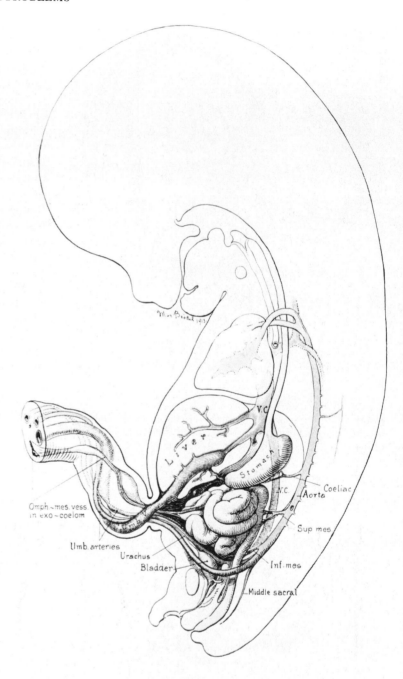

Figure 23–5. The umbilical vein has developed into a large structure that connects through the ductus venosus with the inferior vena cava. The omphalomesenteric duct has disappeared, but remnants of the omphalomesenteric vessels are still visible.

sion through the umbilicus. It is necessary to open the peritoneal cavity to exclude the remnant of the duct that connects with the ileum. The polyp usually consists of ileal mucosa, although gastric or pancreatic tissue also may be found.[6] This is explained by the totipotential differentiation of the primitive omphalomesenteric duct.

When the distal portion of the omphalomesenteric duct perists, one finds an umbilical sinus, which drains mucous and may become infected. A simple test for distinguishing a small draining urachus from an omphalomesenteric sinus is to determine whether the drainage is sticky—intestinal mucus is tenacious, not watery. In-

jection of the sinus tract with contrast material, together with a lateral roentgenogram of the abdomen, will determine the extent of this lesion. Simple excision is all that is required for cure.

Partial persistence of the midportion of the omphalomesenteric duct system may result in an obliterated fibrous band, which may be the fulcrum for a midgut volvulus, or herniation of a loop of intestine between the band and the abdominal wall. In either case, the presenting problem is an intestinal obstruction, with no specific umbilical findings. If there is a lumen with endothelium in the abdominal portion of the duct, one

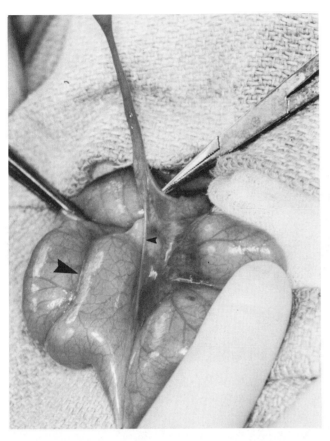

Figure 23–6. The persistent omphalomesenteric artery is marked with a small arrow. It lies alongside a Meckel's diverticulum and is connected to the umbilicus.

will find a vitelline duct cyst. The first symptom is either a mass beneath the umbilicus or an anterior abdominal wall abscess. Lateral roentgenograms will demonstrate loops of intestine that have been separated from the abdominal wall by the cyst. An infection is treated with antibiotics and drainage, after which the cyst can be excised. An infected cyst may appear clinically as an atypical appendicitis.

Hernia of the umbilical cord with persisting omphalomesenteric duct is a rare condition that poses certain obstetric hazards. In this unique situation, a very short omphalomesenteric duct often will fix the involved loop of ileum within the hernia. The gross appearance of the umbilicus may show only minor thickening. The opening of the omphalomesenteric duct is minute in size and is difficult to detect. An unaware obstetrician may clamp the cord through the loop of the bowel and will find to his dismay double stoma above the clamp. When irregular-appearing umbilicus is encountered, it is advised to leave a length of umbilicus intact below the clamp. We have encountered three such anomalies, two with clamped and transected ileum.

THE URACHUS

Failure of obliteration of all of the allantois between the umbilicus and the dome of the bladder results in a completely patent urachus, a sinus tract at the umbilicus, or a urachal cyst.[7]

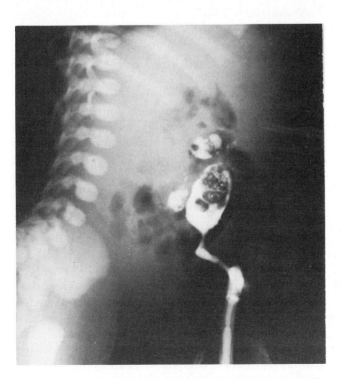

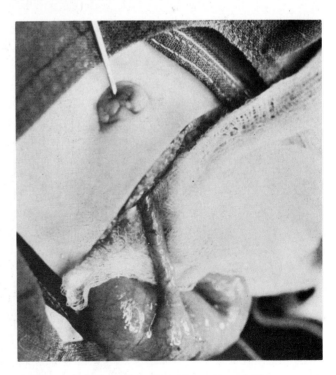

Figure 23–7. A patent omphalomesenteric duct. There is persistent mucuous drainage from the umbilicus, with an occasional bit of stool. **Left.** A roentgenogram. The bowel is demonstrated through injection of the sinus. **Right.** The sinus tract at operation.

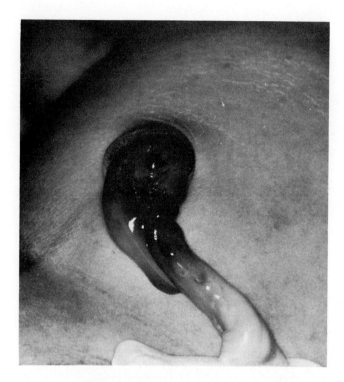

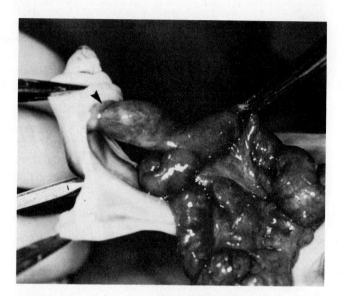

Figure 23–8. Persistent omphalomesenteric duct with omphalocele. **Left.** A small omphalocele, which appears to contain one loop of bowel. **Right.** A widely patent duct, connecting the ileum with the omphalocele sac.

A patent urachus may be obvious at birth because urine will drain onto the abdominal wall. We have observed three children with the prune-belly syndrome whose urine selectively drained from the urachus rather

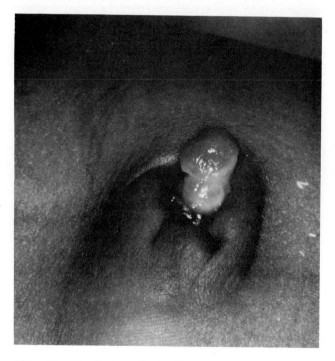

Figure 23–9. A red, elevated polypoid lesion at the umbilicus, consisting of ileal mucosa.

than the urethra. Each had additional urethral anomalies. Therefore, when a patent urachus is found, a voiding cystourethrogram and an intravenous pyelogram must be performed to find other urinary tract anomalies. The connection of the duct with the dome of the bladder can be demonstrated by either injection of the urachus itself or a cystogram with lateral roentgeograms (Fig. 23–10). The urachus must be left open when there is any distal obstruction or vesicoureteral reflux, since free drainage of the urine through the umbilicus prevents further damage to the upper tracts. In the neonatal period, however, continuous urine drainage may result in omphalitis with sepsis. For this reason, the umbilical arteries and veins should be ligated well away from the open urachus, and the area should be kept covered with povidone-iodine dressings until the umbilicus has healed. If there are no other urinary anomalies, the urachus is excised through a subumbilical transverse incision. After separation from the rectus fascia, the urachus is dissected away from the peritoneum to the dome of the bladder, which is closed in two layers with absorbable sutures. The bladder is drained with a catheter for several days.

A urachal sinus occurs when the umbilical portion of the urachus remains patent with no connection to the bladder. The umbilicus remains moist, and there may appear to be a granuloma that resists treatment with silver nitrate. It is rarely possible to probe the small sinus tract or to inject it with contrast material while the infant is awake. A cystogram is indicated to that it is directed toward the bladder. It is then excised through an extraperitoneal infraumbilical incision.

The urachal cyst represents failure of obliteration of the midsection of the urachus. There is no communication with the bladder or umbilicus.[8] Figure 23–11 illustrates a prominent subumbilical mass in a 3-year-old. The first sign of a cyst usually is an infection. Classically, there is a tender lower midline mass with overlying erythema of the skin. Unfortunately, a pyourachus is a serious problem in infants. Only 1 of the 5 cases reviewed by MacMillan et al. had this classic presentation.[9] Of their other patients, 2 had an unexplained peritonitis and 1 had ascites. The cyst may spontaneously drain into the umbilicus, thus masquerading as an omphalitis, or it may cause and perpetuate a chronic urinary tract infection. A cystogram will demonstrate an indentation on the dome of the bladder and perhaps a small connecting sinus tract. An infected urachal cyst must be opened and widely drained, and the accompanying sepsis must be treated with antibiotics. Later, when the inflammatory process has subsided, the cyst is removed through a subumbilical extraperitoneal dissection. This is apt to be a difficult procedure because there will be loops of intestine adherent to the friable peritoneum.

UMBILICAL HERNIA

An umbilical hernia represents a failure of closure of the fascial ring. However, since the peritoneum and skin are intact, this is the mildest anterior wall defect. The diagnosis is obvious; each time the infant cries or strains, the hernia bulges forth with loops of intestine. The mass usually droops inferiorly, although some smaller hernias bulge outward, much like a cauliflower. The fascial size varies from the width of a fingertip to several centimeters in diameter. The defect should be examined while the child is recumbent and again when he or she is standing. In this way, one can determine if the fascial defect is transverse or vertical. The incidence of umbilical hernia is higher in premature infants and is present in 41.6 percent of black children versus 4.1 percent of Caucasians.[10,11] Physicians from Africa have stated that almost every child has an umbilical hernia at birth, which disappears by the teen years. The natural history of an umbilical hernia is, therefore, one of a gradual reduction in the size of the defect, with closure. Some 85 percent close by 6 years of age.[12]

An umbilical hernia frequently is associated with disorders of mucopolysaccharide metabolism, especially Hurler's syndrome (gargoylism). These hernias tend to be huge and are aggravated by the increased intraabdominal pressure of the enlarging liver and spleen. Repair is difficult because of poor tissues and the increased abdominal pressure. An umbilical hernia also may be-

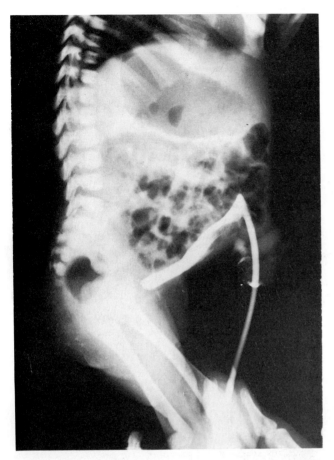

Figure 23–10. Demonstration of a patent urachus and bladder through injection of an umbilical sinus.

rule out a small communication with the blader or other abnormalities. The indication for an operation is the presence of persistent unexplained drainage or a bout of infection. When the infant is asleep at operation, it often is possible to probe the sinus tract and demonstrate

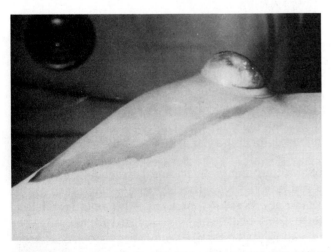

Figure 23–11. A subumbilical mass in a 3-year-old child with a urachal cyst.

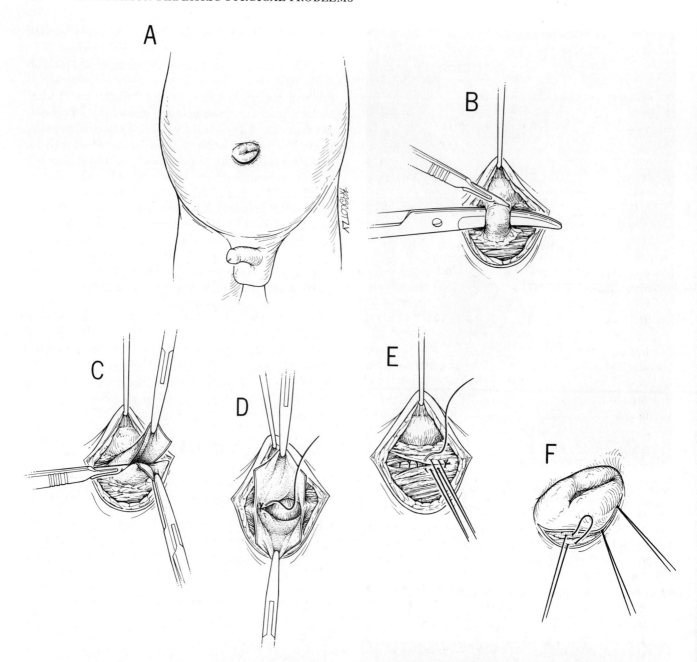

Figure 23–12. Technique for repair of an umbilical hernia. **A.** An incision is made within a skin crease and deepened down to the fascia, which surrounds the hernia sac. **B.** The sac is isolated by dissecting around it with scissors. **C.** The sac is then transected, leaving the distal end attached to skin. The sac is incised down to fascia to make an upper and lower leaf. **D.** Full-thickness mattress sutures are placed, pulled up, and then tied after all have been placed. **E.** A second layer of sutures is placed through all the fascial edges, and one or two are passed through the dermis to invert the skin. **F.** Subcuticular closure.

come a major problem in children with ascites secondary to liver disease. Any umbilical defect should be closed from within the abdomen during an operation for biliary atresia to prevent future problems. There is some controversy over the proper time and the indications for closure of an asymptomatic umbilical hernia. Parents of children with the problem frequently request the operation and

often claim that their chidren have abdominal pain as a result of the hernias. This pain usually is vague and almost always totally unrelated to the umbilical defect. Such pain should not be considered an indication for operation. Haller et al. recommended that a fascial defect of 1.5 cm or more be repaired in girls over 2 years of age and that any hernia that persists after 4 years of age should be repaired to prevent incarceration during adult life.[13] A retrospective review of 590 children with umbilical hernias by Lassaletta et al. revealed a surprisingly high incidence (5.1 percent) of incarceration, strangulation, or evisceration.[14] In this series, hernias with a fascial defect of less than 1.5 cm became incarcerated more frequently than did larger hernias.

In our opinion, there is little indication for an umbilical hernia repair in a child under 2 years of age, regardless of the size of the defect, except when there is a bona fide episode of incarceration. We discourage umbilical hernia repairs before the child is 4 or 5 years of age, but we try to remain reasonably flexible. If the hernia is 1.5 cm or greater in diameter and the mother insists, we will go ahead with a repair. On the other hand, most mothers are willing to wait for spontaneous closure. There is no doubt that an umbilical hernia is a cosmetic defect, particularly since so many sports activities are carried out in rather skimpy attire. It is for this reason rather than any potential problem with incarceration during adult life that we recommend umbilical hernia repair before the child's attendance at school. If the child with an umbilical hernia is to be operated on for an inguinal hernia, we repair both lesions under the same anesthetic.

Treatment

There is no indication for adhesive strapping or any other form of nonoperative therapy.

The operation is performed on an outpatient basis, although slightly more relaxation and deeper anesthesia are required than is needed for an inguinal herniorrhaphy. The technique for umbilical repair is illustrated in Figure 23–12. The curved incision is placed within the umbilical depression, so that the scar will be invisible. The surgeon grasps the apex of the hernia sac with one hand, placing it on a stretch so that the incision is made on tense rather than loose skin. The sac is continually held elevated while an assistant retracts the skin edges with a small sharp rake retractor. Scissors dissection continues until the sac has been completely freed from surrounding tissues. The sac is never dissected free from the skin; a bit of hernia is always left attached to the skin. When the scissors have completely circumscribed the sac, they are left in place (Fig. 23–12B). The sac is then divided over the scissors with a scalpel. The edges of the sac are grasped with hemostats and elevated (Fig. 23–12C). It will be noted that the sac consists of both peritoneum and a thin layer of fascia, which represents the midline fusion of the rectus sheath. The fascia is never separated from the peritoneum but rather is used for a one-layer closure. If the fascial defect is vertical, it is closed with interrupted 3–0 or 2–0 sutures. (Fig. 23–12D, E). If the defect is transverse rather than vertical, we prefer to close the defect with horizontal mattress

sutures, taking bites through the adjacent fascia and peritoneum while the hernia sac is elevated with hemostats. When these are tied down, the defect is approximated transversely. The umbilicus is recreated by inserting sutures through the sac left attached to the skin. One is inserted precisely at the center and sutured to the abdominal fascia below the defect so that when it is tied down, the umbilicus is inverted. The skin is then closed with interrupted subcuticular catgut sutures (Fig. 23–12F). A firm pressure dressing with elastic tape is then applied to prevent an accumulation of blood or serum beneath the skin flap.

RECONSTRUCTION OF A LOST UMBILICUS

Children who have had an omphalocele or gastroschisis repair, or whose umbilicus was for some reason excised, generally feel bereft. They are subject to ridicule by their friends, and their parents are upset. If for any reason further surgery is required, such as the repair of a ventral hernia, a new umbilicus can be created. In older children, the operation can be performed easily under local anesthesia. The exact midline of the abdomen is determined by drawing a line from the xiphoid to the center of the pubis. A skin flap based on healthy skin is then outlined with ink. The flap should be approximately 2.5 cm long and equally wide at its distal end. The base should be about 1 cm wider to ensure good blood supply. The flap is elevated exactly in the midline, based either superiorly or inferiorly. The flap is carefully sutured into a tube with the skin on the *inside*. Interrupted 4–0 chromic catgut sutures mounted on a cutting needle are ideal because the sutures should be placed through the dermis to ensure accurate epidermal approximation. The completed tube, which is closed at its tip, is then sutured down to the fascia in the midline. This results in a skin-lined pit that approximates the size and depth of a real umbilicus. It will now collect lint, sand, and dirt and should be able to hold a 5 karat jewel.

REFERENCES

1. Cullen TS: The Umbilicus and Its Diseases. Philadelphia, Saunders, 1916, pp 1–33
2. Moses WR: Meckel's diverticulum: A report of two unusual cases. N Engl J Med 237:118, 1947
3. Brown KL, Glover DM: Persistent omphalomesenteric duct. Am J Surg 83:680, 1952
4. Moore TC: Omphalomesenteric duct anomalies. Surg Gynecol Obstet 103:569, 1956

5. Kittle CF, Jenkins HP, Dragstedt LR: Patent omphalomesenteric duct and its relation to the diverticulum of Meckel. Arch Surg 54:10, 1947

6. Caberwal D, Kogan SJ, Levitt SB: Ectopic pancreas presenting as an umbilical mass. J Pediatr Surg 12:593, 1977

7. Nix JT, Menville JG, Albert M, Wendt DL: Congenital patent urachus. J Urol 79:264, 1958

8. Constantian HM, Amaral EL: Urachal cyst: Case report. J Urol 106:429, 1971

9. MacMillan RW, Schullinger JN, Santulli TV: Pyourachus: An unusual surgical problem. J Pediatr Surg 8:387, 1973

10. Crump EP: Umbilical hernia: Occurrence of the infantile type in Negro infants and children. J Pediatr 40:214, 1952

11. Evans AG: The comparative incidence of umbilical hernias in colored and white infants. J Natl Med Assoc 33:158, 1941

12. Heifetz CJ, Bilsel ZT, Gaus WW: Observations on the disappearance of umbilical hernias in infancy and childhood. Surg Gynecol Obstet 116:469, 1963

13. Haller JA Jr, Morgan WW Jr, Stumbargh S, White JJ: Repair of umbilical hernias in childhood to prevent adult incarceration. Am Surg 37:245, 1971

14. Lassaletta L, Fonkalsrud EW, Tovard JA, et al: The management of umbilical hernias in infancy and childhood. J Pediatr Surg 10:405, 1975

24

Foreign Bodies in the Gastrointestinal Tract

Toddlers often evaluate their surroundings by tasting and then swallowing new and unusual objects. The variety of ingested materials is limited only by what the child can find in his environment. Most small solid objects, such as buttons, coins, marbles, and pins, are swallowed and excreted without difficulty. When the mother or a sibling sees the child place an object in his mouth or when parents miss some small item that was in the child's vicinity, the diagnosis can be made by the history. Mentally retarded or emotionally disturbed children can ingest an amazing variety of objects. It is not unusual to see 10 or 15 nails, tacks, or coins on x-ray of these children. Fortunately, many ingested foreign bodies are radiopaque, which allows one to diagnose their nature and location. The initial radiologic examination should include the neck, chest, and abdomen. Objects may stop in the esophagus at the level of the cricoid, the aortic arch, or at the esophagogastric junction. They also may lodge at sites of congenital narrowing or at a previous esophageal anastomosis. The combination of poor peristalsis with an inelastic anastomosis for an esophageal atresia will result in food material (such as a bolus of meat) becoming lodged in the esophagus. Initial symptoms of coughing, gagging, excessive salivation, and the inability to swallow food suggest the presence of an esophageal foreign body. These symptoms may disappear if the object does not actually obstruct the lumen, as with a pin or coin. Careful contrast x-rays are indicated if there is any suspicion of a foreign body in the esophagus. General endotracheal anesthesia and esophagoscopy are required for their removal. We have observed three chronic perforations of the esophagus caused by foreign bodies during the past 14 years. In two cases, a coin was visible on x-rays (Fig. 24–1) and covered with mucosa; the coins were removed with an open operation. The third was a nonopaque foreign body that had eroded through the esophagus and trachea

to form a traumatic fistula. Endoscopic removal and tube feedings led to healing of the fistula.

Pop tops from soft drink cans are particularly hazardous because they are almost invisible on roentgenograms. Burrington reported two perforations and one death from an esophageal aorta fistula from these objects.[1] Open safety pins or straight pins may perforate the esophagus to cause a chronic empyema or even a purulent pericarditis.[2] Once a foreign body has entered the stomach, its passage through the rest of the gastrointestinal tract is practically assured. Smooth objects, such as coins, can be safely left in the stomach almost indefinitely without harm to the child. The prolonged gastric retention of a small foreign body may be due to a gastric outlet obstruction; an upper gastrointestinal examination is indicated after 1 month.[3] Attempts should be made to remove the object with the flexible fiberendoscope.[4]

Long, pointed objects have the most difficulty negotiating the sharp duodenal angulations. In our experience, a hat pin once perforated the duodenum just beyond the pylorus, and in another case a hat pin required removal from the duodenojejunal junction. Perforations are exceedingly rare, however. Henderson and Gaston reported only 9 incidences in 800 cases of foreign body ingestion at the Boston City Hospital.[5] Foreign body perforations occur without signs of peritonitis. We observed two asymptomatic patients with straight pins lodged in their spleens, and Abel et al. reported on an 11-month-old infant with a pin in the left lobe of his liver.[6] These pins evidently had perforated the stomach or duodenum and entered the respective organs. In another case, perforation of the stomach by a hairpin led to a left empyema and a pneumothorax, and in yet another patient a whiskbroom bristle penetrated through the duodenum and into the iliac artery, causing a massive gastrointestinal hemorrhage.[7,8] If a pin stays in one place on an abdominal roentgenogram for 5 days or more, it

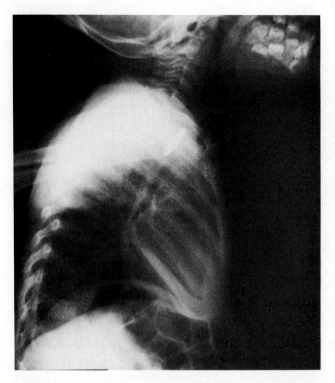

Figure 24–1. Coin lodged in the esophagus for an indeterminate length of time. This coin had slowly perforated the mucosa and come to rest in the esophageal wall.

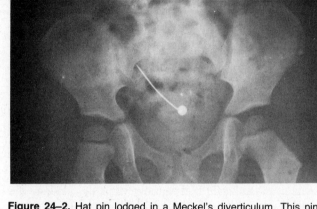

Figure 24–2. Hat pin lodged in a Meckel's diverticulum. This pin remained in one place for 10 days.

has most likely penetrated the wall or is lodged in the appendix or a Meckel's diverticulum (Fig. 24–2).[9] We believe that such objects should be surgically removed even if there are no symptoms. It is wise to take another x-ray just before the proposed operation, so that one is not embarrassed by finding that the object had passed on into the toilet!

Small, easily swallowed disc batteries used to power toys, calculators, and hearing aids are hazardous when ingested. These batteries may contain various toxic chemicals, including potassium hydroxide, or heavy metals, such as mercury or cadmium. Acid gastric secretions corrode and dissolve the casings of these batteries to release their contents. They have eroded through the esophagus to cause death by perforation of the aorta or trachea.[10–12] There is a report of a mercury hearing aid battery that lodged in a Meckel's diverticulum, causing necrosis and peritonitis.[13] Dissolution of fully charged mercuric oxide hearing aid batteries occurs after 24 hours exposure to 0.1 N hydrochloric acid.[14] In this study, discharged cells demonstrated lesser degrees of damage. The addition of standard aluminum- or magnesium-containing antacids protects against dissolution of the casing.

The Long Island Regional Poison Control Center reviewed the problem of battery ingestion and made the following reasonable recommendations.[15] A battery lodged in the esophagus should be removed by endos-

copy as soon as possible. A battery in the stomach may be removed by flexible endoscopy or observed with serial roentgenograms. If the battery rapidly moves down the gastrointestinal tract, observation is continued. During the period of observation a similar battery may be tested for leakage in acid at a ph of 1.4. If the battery remains in the stomach for 24 hours or if there is evidence of gastric irritation, it should be removed by flexible endoscopy if the proper grasping forceps are available or with a magnet attached to a catheter.[16] If the battery continues to move, it is followed with serial roentgenograms. If it stops or if there are either symptoms or radiologic evidence of dissolution of the battery, it should be removed immediately. In one of our children, endoscopic removal from the stomach failed. At operation, the battery was found to be embedded in a shallow ulcer. Based on in vitro evidence, antacids should be given if a course of observation is pursued.

BEZOARS

Children who pluck and eat their own hair must have strange emotional aberrations. Many will deny the habit, but there is no other way to account for children with bald spots on their heads and balls of hair in their stomachs. These children may be perfectly well, although

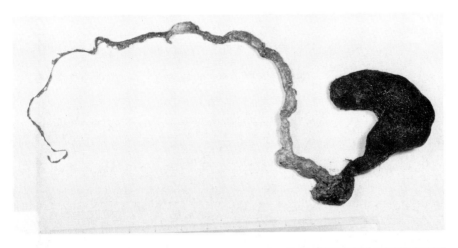

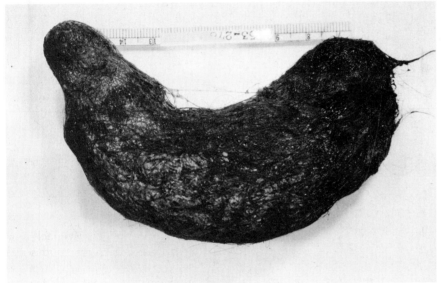

Figure 24–3. Trichobezoar. **Top.** Bezoar obstructing the ileum. **Bottom.** A typical gastric bezoar that conforms to the outline of the stomach.

some have poor appetites and have lost weight. Hair balls and other bezoars rarely if ever obstruct the stomach, although they may completely fill the lumen. We have seen a bezoar impacted into and obstructing the terminal ileum (Fig. 24–3). In such cases, an oblong mass conforming to the stomach outline is almost always palpable in the epigastrium. The diagnosis is confirmed by x-rays of the stomach. Bezoars are easily removed through a gastrotomy incision. The duodenum and small intestine must be carefully palpated for hair balls that may have broken off from the main mass. Although recurrence is rare, children with this problem should undergo psychiatric evaluation and consequent therapy.

REFERENCES

1. Burrington JD: Aluminum pop-tops: A hazard to child health. JAMA 235:2614, 1976
2. Bozer AV, Saylam A, Ersoy V: Purulent pericarditis due to perforation of esophagus with foreign body. J Thorac Cardiovasc Surg 67:590, 1974
3. Mandell GA, Rosenberg HK, Schnaufer L: Prolonged retention of foreign bodies in the stomach. Pediatrics 60:460, 1977
4. Christie DL, Ament ME: Removal of foreign bodies from esophagus and stomach with flexible fiberoptic panendoscopes. Pediatrics 57:931, 1976
5. Henderson FF, Gaston EA: Ingested foreign body in the gastrointestinal tract. Arch Surg 36:66, 1938
6. Abel RM, Fischer JE, Henderson HH: Penetration of the alimentary tract by a foreign body with migration to the liver. Arch Surg 102:227, 1971
7. Esposito G: Left empyema and pneumothorax after perforation of the stomach, diaphragm, and pleura by an intragastric foreign body. Ann Chir Infant 14:413, 20, 1973
8. Grosfield JL, Eng K: Right iliac artery–duodenal fistula in infancy due to a "whisk-broom" bristle perforation. Ann Surg 176:761, 1972
9. Kassner EG, Mutchler RW, Klotz DH, Rose J: Uncomplicated foreign bodies of the appendix in children: Radiologic observations. J Pediatr Surg 9:207, 1974

10. Votteler T, Nash JC, Rutledge J: The hazard of ingested alkaline disc batteries in children. JAMA 249:2504, 1983

11. Blatnick D, Toohil D, Lehman R: Fatal complication from an alkaline battery foreign body in the esophagus. Ann Otol 86:611, 1977

12. Shabino C, Feinberg A: Esophageal perforation secondary to alkaline battery ingestion. J Am Coll Emerg Physicians 8:360, 1979

13. Willis G, Ho W: Perforation of a Meckel's diverticulum by an alkaline hearing aid battery. Can Med Assoc J 126:497, 1982

14. Litovitz T, Butterfield A, Holloway R, Marion L: Button battery ingestion: Assessment of therapeutic modalities and battery discharge state. J Pediatr 105:868, 1984

15. Mofenson H, Greensher J, Caraccia T, Danoff R: Ingestion of small flat disc batteries. Ann Emerg Med 12:88, 1983

16. Ito Y, Ihara N, Sohma S: Magnetic removal of alkaline batteries from the stomach. J Pediatr Surg 20:250, 1985

25
Lesions of the Skin

Bruce S. Bauer
───── *Jay M. Pensler*

The correct diagnosis of most cutaneous and subcutaneous lesions in children can be made by simple physical examination and an understanding of their embryologic origin and histologic characteristics. For any given location, the most common lesion in a child differs from that seen in an adult.

DERMOID CYSTS

Dermoid cysts are the most common cystic lesions in infants and young children. They are predominantly on the face and scalp. It is best to separate them into two groups, those along the craniofacial midline and those occurring laterally. This distinction is most important because of the different embryologic origin of the cysts in these two locations.[1,2] Dermoid cysts are slow-growing congenital hamartomas that occur along embryonic fault lines where developing ectodermal tissue is sequestered. Histologically, they are true cysts with well-defined epidermoid structures, including sebaceous, eccrine, and apocrine glandular elements and rudimentary hair follicles.

Midline Scalp Dermoids
Dermoid cysts overlying the area of the anterior or posterior fontanelle or lambdoid sutures may extend intracranially, but the pattern of extensions varies in each.[3] The anterior fontanelle dermoid cyst may lie directly over a bony defect and attach loosely to the dura directly over the sagittal sinus. These cysts may be filled with clear sweat rather than the typical "cheesy" keratinaceous

material. Deeper extension has not been demonstrated.

The posterior fontanelle dermoid cysts tend to be more firm in consistency and may even be located short distances off the midline. These lesions may extend intracranially through a patent fontanelle to the level of the roof of the third ventricle. Neural elements may be noted in the cyst wall.

A computed tomography (CT) scan is essential to evaluate midline dermoid cysts before surgical extirpation because they may require a craniotomy.

Midline Frontonasal Dermoids
Dermoids of the frontonasal area arise after incomplete obliteration of a tract from the foramen cecum to the nasal tip or the foramen cecum through the frontonasal suture. The dermoid cyst and sinus, glioma, and encephaloceles represent a continuum of lesions of like origin in this region because this tract, or prenasal space, contains a dural projection before closure to the foramen cecum.[1] Any failure of normal obliteration may leave both ectodermal and glial tissue in its path. Fourth-generation CT scans with views in the axial, coronal, and sagittal planes clearly demonstrate the extent of the tract, facilitating identification of those cases that require a combined intra- and extracranial approach for complete excision.[4]

A frontonasal dermoid may be seen at birth or in early infancy as a midline pore, possibly with a protruding hair and with associated widening of the nasal dorsum (Fig. 25–1). Some are first noted at the time of infection within a cyst anywhere from the glabella to the nasal

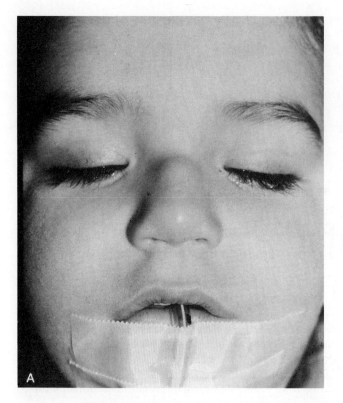 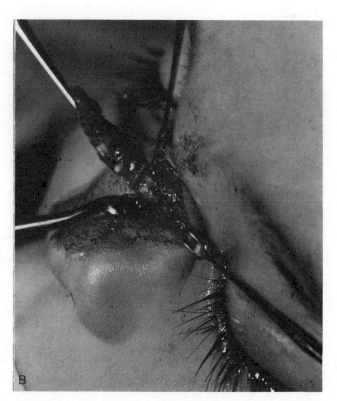

Figure 25–1. **Left.** A frontonasal dermoid cyst, appearing as a punctate opening in the midline of the nose. **Right.** The cyst at operation, demonstrating the sinus tract.

tip. On rare occasions, a brain abscess may be the first indication of a sinus in this area. Those lesions with intracranial extension will course beneath the nasal bones through a widened nasal septum, then through the foramen cecum, or through a widened frontonasal suture to the foramen cecum. In both cases, a bifid crista galli usually is seen on CT scan, and the intracranial portion of the dermoid lies extradurally between the leaves of the falx. Excision of these lesions requires a craniofacial approach by a plastic surgeon and neurosurgeon.

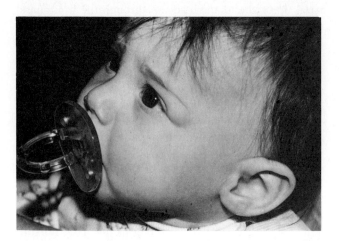

Figure 25–2. This is one of the most common locations for a dermoid cyst. It is a round lesion in the lateral eyelid.

Lateral Frontoorbital Dermoids

Although dermoid cysts occasionally are noted in the frontotemporal region overlying the coronal suture, the most common location is in the lateral brow. These external angular dermoids generally are noted either at birth or within the first 6 months and may increase in size to 2 to 3 cm. Although these cysts may be mobile and extend down onto the upper lid, in almost all cases they are firmly fixed to the periosteum of the orbital rim near the frontozygomatic suture (Fig. 25–2).

Large cysts may lie in a bony depression, split the lateral orbit wall, or extend back toward the temporal fossa. They do not extend intracranially, and a CT scan is unnecessary. Treatment consists of simple careful surgical excision of the entire cyst.[3,5] The incision can vary from just above the lateral eyebrow to just below or even down onto the upper lid, keeping in mind that exposure to the orbital margin is needed in most cases.

CALCIFYING EPITHELIOMA OF MALHERBE (PILOMATRIXOMA)

These common cystic lesions of hair matrix origin occur predominantly on the face or neck but also may arise on the upper extremities. Although they typically occur in early childhood, they may not arise until the early

20s.[6] They may be single or multiple and usually appear as 1 to 2-cm, calcified, deep-seated nodules with a stony-hard lobular consistency and yellowish coloration. However, they may also occur with a history of recurrent inflammation and infection. The overlying skin may be slightly discolored with a reddish blue tint.

Excision should include a portion of the overlying skin when there has been recurrent inflammation or skin surface changes in order to ensure removal of the entire cyst wall.

Histologically, there are sheets of epithelial cells with basophilic shadow cells arranged in irregular bands. Masses of keratin are found interspersed between the cells, with calcification. The latter finding is a late manifestation of cell degeneration.

CONGENITAL NEVOCELLULAR NEVI

Congenital nevocellular nevi (CNCN) are collections of nevus cells in pigmented lesions of the skin that appear in approximately 1 percent of newborn infants. Congenital nevi, 10 cm or more in diameter, are found in 1 of every 20,000 newborns.[7] The management of CNCN is extremely controversial because of the lack of valid data regarding the incidence of malignant change.

Treatment
The primary considerations in treatment are lesion size, location, histology, and patient age. To discuss the surgical approach, we separate them by size.

Small Congenital Nevocellular Nevi.
The incidence of malignant change of 1 to 2.5 cm CNCN is difficult to determine, and there is no convincing evidence that completely quantifies the risk. The work of Rhodes and Melski evaluated patients with melanoma for prior history of a congenital lesion at the site of malignant change and for histologic features of a congenital lesion within the specimen.[8] Based on this work, the cumulative risk of melanoma is 5 percent by the first criterion and 0.8 to 2.6 percent by the latter. Work by Illig et al. demonstrated a risk of malignancy in CNCN of less than 10 cm. The recommendation to excise smaller CNCN is generally made based on these two studies. Since excision removes the risk of malignancy, surgery often is a prudent step when the family has had multiple conflicting and confusing opinions.

Since the risk of malignant change in lesions of this size is extremely low during the first decade, the smaller, less complicated excisions may be delayed until the child is old enough that surgery can be performed under local anesthesia. Intermediate-size lesions and those requiring more complex reconstruction may best be excised in early childhood, since they require general anesthesia

and early excision is well tolerated. Additional benefits include better postoperative scars and complete excision of prominent lesions before an age when peer ridicule related to the lesion becomes a concern.

Large and Giant Nevocellular Nevi.
The association between large and giant CNCN and malignant melanoma has been well established. The magnitude of the risk of malignant transformation is still controver-

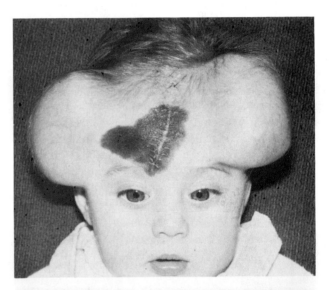

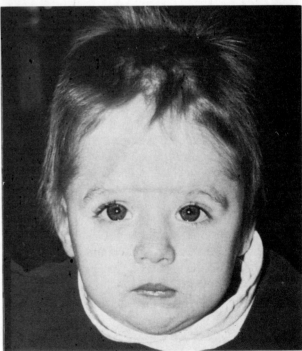

Figure 25–3. A large pigmented nevus of the forehead treated with tissue expansion and excision. **Top.** The tissue expanders are in place and fully expanded. A portion of the nevus was removed at the first stage, with insertion of the two tissue expanders. **Bottom.** Complete excision of the nevus.

sial. Quaba and Wallace, in a review of the subject, placed the widely divergent risk figures (of 1.8 percent up to 42 percent) in perspective.[10] They summarized the prior reviews, discussed the possible reasons for the wide variation in findings, and then calculated an 8.5 percent risk of melanoma developing within nevi larger than 2 percent of the total body surface during the first 15 years of life.

The opinion that complete prophylactic excision of all large and giant CNCN should be accomplished in infancy and early childhood is supported in the literature by evidence that 60 percent of the malignancies developing in giant nevi occur during childhood, and up to 50 percent of melanomas arising in giant nevi were diagnosed in the first 3 years of life. Early recognition of malignant degeneration is difficult, and malignancy in these lesions appears to be uniformly fatal.[10,11] Although complete early prophylactic excision of giant lesions often seems like an insurmountable task, the advent of tissue expansion and early large segment excision and grafting has demonstrated that it is not only possible but has significant benefits.[12]

Complete excision in infancy and early childhood

is best accomplished by recognizing the techniques that are most effective in each body location.[12] These may best be summarized as follows.

Giant Nevi of Head and Neck

1. Tissue expansion is the primary treatment modality for excision and reconstruction of giant nevi of the scalp. Expansion can begin as early as 3 months of age.
2. Tissue expansion of the forehead, neck, and cheek are effective in excision and reconstruction of the face (Fig. 25–3). Full-thickness grafts may be needed in the periorbital region.
3. Combined treatment of scalp and facial nevi may reduce the time required for excision and improve the final result.

Giant Nevi of Trunk

1. Tissue expansion in combination with abdominoplasty and grafting is most effective on the anterior trunk.
2. Giant nevi of the greater part of the back and

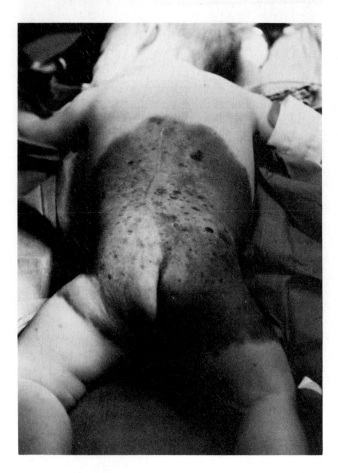 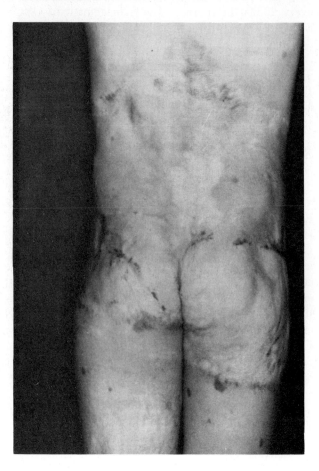

Figure 25–4. Left. A giant nevus of the back and buttocks. A partial midline excision is seen. This lesion was excised and grafted at 4 years of age. **Right.** Postoperative healing of skin grafts. It was necessary to further excise the small lesions at a later date.

buttocks are best treated by early large segment excision and split-thickness skin grafting (Fig. 25–4).

Giant Nevi of Extremities

1. Since most of the giant nevi of the extremity are circumferential, they are best treated by excision and skin grafting (Fig. 25–5).
2. Use of tissue expanders to expand donor sites and harvest large expanded full-thickness skin grafts may provide better coverage and appearance.

By starting surgery in the first 3 to 6 months of life, giant nevi can be excised within the first 2 to 4 years. In addition to the obvious benefit of reducing the risk of malignancy, early excision has significant benefits in terms of the ultimate cosmetic appearance of the affected child.

Older techniques have involved excision of lesions of the back, buttocks, and posterior scalp, since nearly 80 percent of the malignancies that have been reported have occurred in these high-risk areas.[13] Excision in these areas should be carried out to the underlying fascia, since the nevus cells in CNCN often penetrate into the subcutaneous fat and, at times, to the level of the deep fascia.[11,14]

Dermabrasion of giant nevi in infancy, although advocated as a means of decreasing the pigmentation and improving the appearance, may lighten the pigment yet leave nevus cells in all areas. The effect of this procedure on reduction of malignant risk is undetermined.

SEBACEOUS NEVI

The sebaceous nevus of Jadassohn is a congenital hamartoma of sebaceous glands found most commonly on the scalp and face. It appears as a yellowish, waxy, slightly raised plaque without hair. Lesions tend to thicken and become more verrucous with advancing age and characteristically itch and discharge at puberty.[13] These lesions exhibit a 15 to 20 percent malignant potential by the third or fourth decade of life. Ninety-nine percent of the malignancies are basal cell carcinomas.

Excision of the lesions in infancy and early childhood removes the risk of later malignant change and avoids

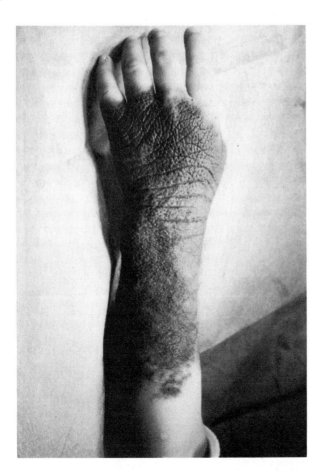
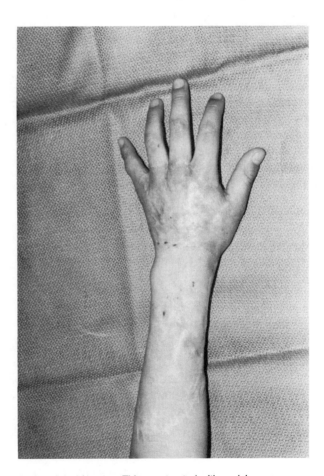

Figure 25–5. Left. Large circumferential pigmented nevus of the hand and forearm. This was treated with excision and coverage with a split-thickness skin graft. **Right.** Two years after excision and grafting.

the problems that occur with increased sebaceous activity in later childhood and adolescence. There appears to be some increased risk of postoperative infection in the scalp when excision is delayed into the period of greater sebaceous activity.

SPITZ NEVUS

The Spitz nevus is a distinct histologic and clinical entity originally misnamed "juvenile melanoma" because of the often bizarre histologic appearance resembling true melanoma.[13] The lesion typically appears in childhood as a firm, raised lesion that at times is mistaken for a hemangioma. This nevus is most easily differentiated by an onset well beyond infancy. At times, the lesion may mimic a raised, pigmented, nonhairbearing compound nevus and demonstrate some variegation of pigment. Most of the lesions are 1 cm or smaller in size, but they may rarely be 10 cm. These are not true melanomas despite the often wild appearance on histologic examination. The predominant appearance is one of epithelioid and spindle cells, often demonstrating heavy pigmentation and frequent mitotic figues. Failure to gain an adequate margin at the time of excision results in recurrence of the lesion with often a more atypical histologic picture. Recurrence is minimized by correct early diagnosis and careful attention to ensure adequate margins during surgical excision.

KELOIDS

Keloids may result from any skin injury, particularly in pigmented children. One of the most common sites for a keloid is the ear lobe after the ears have been pierced to hold earrings. An early keloid may, as with a burn, surgical, or acne scar, be treated with injections of triamcinolone. A 26-gauge needle with a tuberculin syringe is used to inject 0.5 to 1 ml of the solution. The injection is initially painful and difficult, but the scar commences to soften after one or two injections. Fully developed keloids (as in the earlobe) are excised with meticulous gentle technique, and the V-shaped defect is closed with subcuticular sutures. Triamcinolone solution (0.5 ml) is injected into the wound immediately and at monthly intervals. Skin atrophy is a side effect of steroid therapy. Consequently, only minimal amounts of steroids can be given with each injection, and the effects must be checked at monthly intervals.

The common wart, verrucus vulgaris, is ubiquitous and, contrary to the writings of Samuel Clemens, is not necessarily caused by the handling of frogs or toads—however, one must keep this theory in mind when taking the history. In my own personal experience, warts on the hands and fingers, as well as those on the plantar surface of the feet, thrive on surgical excision and electrocoagulation. These painful forms of treatment are essentially useless. There are several effective proprietary remedies, which consist of 15 to 20 percent salicylic acid in colloidion. The patient is advised to first soak the wart in warm water and then, while it is moist and soft, apply a drop or two of the salicylic acid–colloidion solution. The surrounding skin is protected with a thin film of petrolatum. Several applications usually are sufficient for a cure. The squamous papilloma is a larger, flat, warty-looking lesion that may appear on the extremities or the neck and is best excised for both diagnosis and treatment.

INGROWN TOENAILS

Occasionally, an infant will have a bit of skin grow up over the toenail that has been cut too short. These are rarely infected and do not require an operation. The mother is taught to place a bit of cotton under the nail to lift it away from the skin. When the nail grows out, the problem is solved. Older children develop typical ingrown toenails when a nail that was cut too short grows into the soft tissue that covers the nail edge. This results

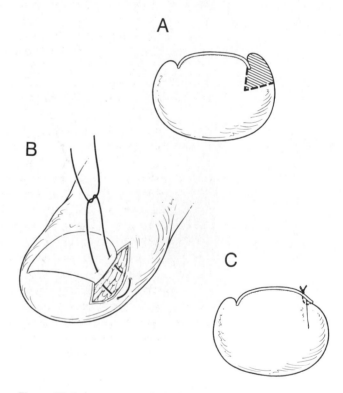

Figure 25–6. Ingrown toenail. **A.** A wedge excision is done of the hypertrophic skin and granulation tissue. **B.** A nylon suture is passed through the nail and skin, then back through the nail. **C.** The suture draws skin beneath the nail.

in granulation tissue that becomes infected. The nail is not at fault; the problem is the overgrown infected soft tissue. The removal of a part or the whole nail will more likely than not lead to recurrence. In early cases, the nail can be elevated with cotton. More cotton is pushed under the nail each day, until it is lifted away from the skin. This treatment may be combined with warm soaks initially. If this treatment is unsuccessful, rather than removing the nail, a wedge of the hypertrophied skin and granulation tissue is removed, and the skin is sutured beneath the nail with a single nylon mattress suture (Fig. 25–6).

REFERENCES

1. Sessions RB: Nasal dermal sinus—new concepts and explanations. Laryngosope 92:1, 1982
2. Naidich TP, Bauer BS, McLone DG, et al: Nasal dermal sinuses and cysts. Acta Radiol (Stockholm) (Suppl) 369:322, 1986
3. Thaller SR, Bauer BS: Cysts and cystlike lesions of the skin and subcutaneous tissue. Clin Plast Surg 14:327, 1987
4. Pensler JM, Bauer BS, Naidich, TP: Craniofacial dermoids. Plast Reconstr Surg 82:953–958, 1988
5. Kernahan DA: Cysts, sinuses and fistulae. In Kernahan DA, Thomson HG (eds): Symposium on Pediatric Plastic Surgery. St. Louis, Mosby, 1982, pp 31–36
6. Moelenbeck FW: Pilomatrixoma (calcifying epithelioma): A statistical study. Arch Dermatol 108:532, 1973
7. Castilla EE, Dutra MDG, Orioli-Parreiras IM: Epidemiology of congenital pigmented nevi: I. Incidence rates and relative frequencies. Br J Dermatol 104:307, 1981
8. Rhodes AR, Melski JW: Small congenital nevocellular nevi and risk of cutaneous melanoma. J Pediatr 100:219, 1982
9. Illig L, Weidner F, Hundeiker M, et al: Congenital nevi <10 cm as precursors to melanoma: 52 cases. A review and new conception. Arch Dermatol 121:1274, 1985
10. Quaba AA, Wallace AF: The incidence of malignant melanoma (0 to 15 years of age) arising in "large" congenital nevocellular nevi. Plast Reconstr Surg 78:174, 1986
11. Trozak DJ, Rowland DR, Hu F: Metastatic malignant melanoma in prepubertal children. Pediatric 55:191, 1975
12. Bauer BS, Vicari FA: An approach to excision of congenital giant nevi in infancy and early childhood. Plast Reconstr Surg 82:1012–1021, 1988
13. Kaplan E, Nickoloff BJ: Clinical and histological features of nevi with emphasis on treatment approaches. Clin Plast Surg 14:277, 1987
14. Rhodes AR, Wood WC, Sober AJ, Mihm MC: Nonepidermal origin of malignant melanoma associated with giant congenital nevocellular nevus. Plast Reconstr Surg 67:782, 1981

26
Pyloric Stenosis

Successful treatment of pyloric stenosis is one of the great surgical triumphs of this century.[1,2] Hirschsprung, a Danish pediatric surgeon, described the clinical findings of the disease and established pyloric stenosis as a diagnostic entity in 1888, but he was unable to suggest effective therapy.[3] In the early 1900s, a number of patients survived gastroenterostomy and various types of pyloroplasty. This seems an amazing achievement when we realize that these dehydrated, malnourished infants were operated on with no intravenous fluids and relatively crude anesthesia. In 1912, almost by accident, Conrad Ramstedt performed an operation that remains essentially the same today.[4] By 1922, the mortality rate of this disease had fallen to approximately 25 percent.[5] Earlier diagnosis, advances in fluid therapy, and anesthesia have reduced the mortality rate to practically zero. The Ramstedt pyloromyotomy remains as the standard operation.

PATHOLOGY

Two sphincteric loops of circular muscle fiber encircle the pylorus and converge at the lesser curvature. The most proximal of these, or the left canalis loop end (called Torgersen's muscle), blends with normal muscle on the antral side of the pylorus.[6] It is the thickening of these circular muscle fibers that obstructs the lumen by compressing the mucosa. There is no evidence of inflammation at first, but submucosal edema and round cell inflammation appear after prolonged vomiting. Histologic examination has demonstrated hypertrophy as well as an increase in number of the circular muscle fibers. Grossly, the pylorus is a hard, whitish mass 2 cm long and 1 cm in diameter. In autopsy specimens, the pylorus may barely admit a 1-mm probe. The distal end of the enlongated pylorus projects into the duodenum just as

the uterine cervix protrudes into the vagina. The stomach proximal to the pylorus is dilated, and its walls are thickened and edematous.

ETIOLOGY

There is no conclusive evidence for the etiology of pyloric stenosis. The fact that pyloric stenosis occurs with a higher frequency in some families and is rare in blacks suggests a genetic factor, but no specific inheritance pattern has been established.[7,8] It has occurred in both identical and nonidentical triplets, suggesting a single dominant gene as being responsible for the disease.[9] Previous studies relying on light microscopy were thought to show abnormal ganglion cells, but Jona examined the hypertrophied muscle with electron microscopy and could find no evidence of degenerative changes or failure of maturation of the ganglion cells.[10] Dodge produced typical pyloric tumors in puppies by the prolonged administration of pentagastrin.[11] Pentagastrin also can stimulate isolated strips of pyloric muscle to contract.[12] However, others have been unable to determine whether this elevation is a cause or an effect of the obstructed stomach.[13]

DIAGNOSIS

The typical baby with pyloric stenosis begins to vomit during the third week of life, and 15 percent of patients have a history of regurgitation, or spitting up, from birth. In a few, the vomiting is delayed until the fifth or sixth week. At first, there is only regurgitation, but the vomiting soon becomes more forceful and finally is projectile. Typically, emesis occurs after each feeding and contains only milk or curds. Specific inquiry should be made about the color—green vomitus brings up the possibility of a duodenal obstruction. A tinge of blood or a coffee-ground appearance may be caused by chronic gastritis, but this is more characteristic of a hiatus hernia with esophagitis or a duodenal ulcer. The forcefulness of vomiting, with projection of up to 2 or 3 feet from the infant, is the most typical symptom. Most babies are voraciously hungry and will take a feeding immediately after vomiting.

Changes in formula and various medications (such as antispasmodics) frequently are tried. The family history becomes important if pyloric stenosis has occurred in siblings or other relatives.

Weight loss indicates a serious problem that demands investigation. Weight should be determined at birth and at intermediate checkups for comparison. A vomiting baby whose weight is increasing is likely to be a victim of overfeeding.

The physical examination must commence with the baby completely exposed in a warm, comfortable position, preferably on his mother's lap. The infant's general appearance depends on the duration of symptoms. If he has vomited for several days, there will be obvious evidence of dehydration: a depressed fontanelle, dry mucous membranes in the mouth, and poor skin turgor. The lungs should be examined with care because of the possibility of aspiration pneumonia in any infant who has been vomiting. The abdominal examination must be unhurried and conducted with warm hands. The infant's abdomen should be carefully observed during a feeding of sugar water. Peristaltic waves begin with a bulge in the left upper quadrant and progress as hourglass

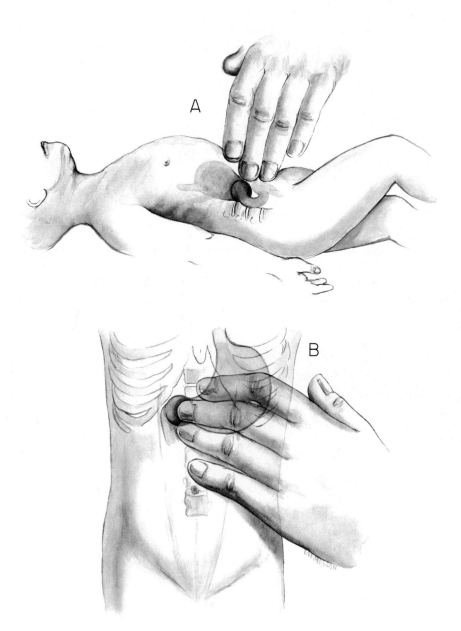

Figure 26–1. Palpation for pyloric tumor (Swenson).

constrictions across the abdomen to the left of the midline. A normal infant will develop a left upper quadrant bulge during feeding that does not move and disappears after a satisfactory burp. Palpation of a pyloric tumor is an art that requires great patience. The mass is oblong, smooth, and hard, and 1 or 2 cm in size. It is usually located in the epigastrium, just above the umbilicus and either in the midline or slightly to the right. Flexing the infant's knees and hips and giving him water or a honey-coated pacifier will relax the abdominal wall. It is helpful to sit on the baby's left side and palpate with the tip of the middle finger while the index and ring fingers depress the rectus muscle (Fig. 26–1). Occasionally, the mass appears to be superficial and is found with gentle palpation. More often, the tumor is deep and can be outlined only with steady pressure. When the firm mass is found, it is rolled under the fingers for positive identification. It is easy to mistake a tense rectus, the liver edge, or the right kidney for a pyloric mass. A pyloric olive should be unmistakably palpated on two separate occasions before recommending an operation. A tense, fussy baby will not relax long enough for the mass to be felt under the rectus, and an overdistended stomach will cover the mass. Spontaneous vomiting during feeding not only empties the stomach but also causes temporary complete relaxation of the abdominal muscles. If the baby does not vomit, a nasogastric tube is passed, and the stomach is emptied. The baby is then given a bottle of sugar water or a pacifier, and palpation is again performed. With persistence and experience, almost 100 percent of pyloric masses are palpable. The only thing more satisfying than actually palpating the tumor is helping a student feel the elusive mass for the first time!

Unfortunately, the diagnosis is in doubt more often than some clinicians would like to admit. I have been unable to palpate the olive only to have the infant continue to vomit, then return with obvious findings and a positive roentgenogram a week or more later. I reluctantly confess to recommending an operation on three occasions, based on palpating a mass, when at operation the pylorus was either normal or, at most, only slightly thickened. Whenever competent physicians disagree on the physical findings or if the history is atypical, other studies are indicated. Formerly, an upper gastrointestinal examination with barium was recommended. Now, however, an ultrasound study of the pylorus should be performed before a barium examination. Over the past 12 years, several studies have demonstrated the accuracy of this diagnostic tool.[14–16] Ultrasound observations that suggest pyloric stenosis include a bulls-eye appearance of the central or stellate echo, surrounded by a thickened pyloric muscle (Fig. 26–2). Pyloric canal length is more accurate in delineating the hypertrophic pylorus than are measurements of muscle mass thickness and pyloric diameter. Stunden et al. studied 200 consecutive infants, 112 with pyloric stenosis and 88 normal babies.[17] They achieved 100 percent accuracy by measuring canal length. The normal pyloric canal measured from 5 to 14 mm, whereas in pyloric stenosis, the canal length

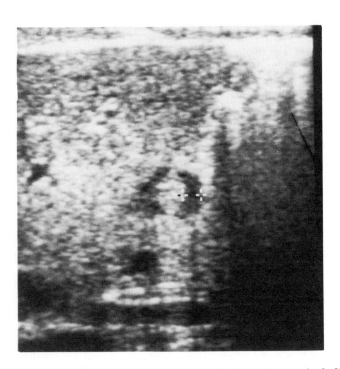 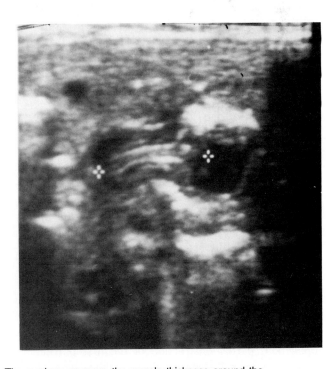

Figure 26–2. Ultrasound study of pyloric stenosis. **Left.** The markers measure the muscle thickness around the bulls-eye. **Right.** The markers measure the elongated pyloric canal.

varied from 18 to 28 mm. Thus, there was no overlap between normal and abnormal in this dimension as there was in both muscle thickness and overall diameter. The examination must be done by an experienced ultrasonographer, using a real-time scanner. Echogenic milk curds and barium impede transmission of the sound waves. Therefore, the infant's stomach should be emptied with a nasogastric tube and washed with normal saline. The infant is then allowed to take glucose water, or the stomach is distended with saline. Criteria for a positive study include a canal longer than 16 mm, diameter greater than 11 mm, and circular muscle more than 2.5 mm. Shouldering may be seen at each end of the canal, and there is little passage of liquid through the pylorus despite the visibly increased peristalsis.

Ultrasonography has confirmed the long-held clinical suspicion that a rare infant may have a mild degree of pyloric stenosis that resolves with time. Stunden's series included four older infants who had all the criteria for pyloric stenosis but without significant canal obstruction. Ultrasonography is most useful in those infants with doubtful findings on palpation. Ultrasonographic examination is as accurate as the clinical examination in making an early positive diagnosis. If the ultrasound study reveals a normal pylorus in an infant with significant vomiting, an upper gastrointestinal examination is mandatory to search for other diseases, such as gastroesophageal reflux or a partial upper intestinal obstruction.

Roentgenographic Studies

An upright film of the abdomen occasionally will reveal a single, long, air–fluid level in the distended stomach, with little or no gas distal to the pyloric canal. Always look for a double bubble sign indicating a partial duodenal obstruction, which might mimic a pyloric obstruction. The stomach must be emptied with a nasogastric tube before and after a barium swallow to minimize the dangers of aspiration. The esophagus is studied to rule out a hiatus hernia or stenosis. Gastroesophageal reflux may be produced with abdominal wall pressure and is accentuated when the infant lies flat on the back. The definitive roentgenographic finding is elongation and narrowing of the pyloric canal (Fig. 26–3). During fluoroscopy, strong gastric peristaltic activity is seen. As barium enters the duodenum, the cervixlike protrusion of the pylorus may be outlined. Repeated saline irrigations are necessary to remove the barium, which may otherwise remain in the stomach for several days.

Differential Diagnosis

Other obstructing lesions—such as an antral web, gastric duplication, partial obstruction of the first portion of the duodenum, and gastroesophageal reflux—should be demonstrated by a barium or ultrasound study. One

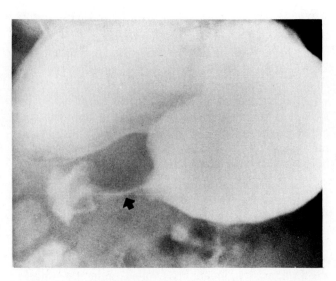

Figure 26–3. The string sign characteristic of pyloric stenosis.

should try keeping the infant in a prone position if gastroesophageal reflux is suspected.

Vomiting is a symptom of so many other diseases that may be confused with pyloric stenosis that only a few of the more important diseases can be listed here. A good general guide is that a baby with pyloric stenosis will continue to be hungry and active unless he is severely dehydrated. Babies with metabolic problems or central nervous system lesions are likely to be lethargic, to feed poorly, and to have other symptoms that are unusual in babies with pyloric obstruction. A subdural hematoma or hydrocephalus can cause projectile vomiting as well as irritability. The head circumference will be in the upper percentiles, and transillumination of the skull may suggest the diagnosis. Infants with the salt-losing adrenogenital syndrome vomit during the second or third week of life, but their degree of dehydration is out of proportion to their vomiting. The abnormal genitalia of girls with this disease aids in the diagnosis; afflicted boys have normal genitalia. These infants have a high serum potassium and low chloride and sodium, whereas babies with an obstruction will have hypokalemia. The diagnosis of adrenal insufficiency is made by measuring the serum and urine 17-ketosteroids.

Persistent vomiting in the neonatal period also is a prominent feature of a number of inborn metabolism problems, especially of those associated with protein intolerance. Early diagnosis of these diseases is essential to prevent mental retardation or death, as well as to give the family the benefit of genetic counseling. A history showing the unexplained death of a sibling is helpful. Physical findings of jaundice hepatomegaly, coarse facial features, hypotonia, and an abnormal urine odor are suggestive of a metabolic problem, but usually the history and physical examination provide little help in making a diagnosis. The classification and specific diagnosis of many of these disorders is extremely complex, but a few simple laboratory determinations—including the serum ammonia level, blood gases, and a test for reducing substances in the urine—are helpful in deciding which infants require expert evaluation and sophisticated biochemical study.[18] An elevated plasma ammonia level after protein feeding provides the clue that should lead to a study of enzyme deficiencies in the urea cycle. Disorders of organic acid metabolism, such as methylmalonic propionic or isovaleric acidemia, cause severe metabolic acidosis demonstrable by blood gas determination. A positive urine test for reducing substances will lead to the diagnosis of galactosemia. Phenylketonuria and a number of other diseases result in a positive urine reaction with ferric chloride. The problem with phenylketonuria is complicated by the fact that as many as 9 percent of infants with this problem also have a definite pyloric stenosis.[19]

PREOPERATIVE MANAGEMENT

The vomitus in babies with pyloric stenosis contains varying amounts of chloride, sodium, and potassium, but there is always an excess of chloride. Chloride losses measured via a nasogastric tube vary from 129 to as high as 162 mEq/L, with sodium concentrations of 71 to 112 mEq/L and potassium concentrations of 7.2 to 16 mEq/L. The volume of gastric juice lost through vomiting or tube drainage may be as high as 100 ml/day. This excessive chloride ion loss eventually results in extracellular chloride depletion and metabolic alkalosis. This is a unique situation, since almost all other abdominal surgical conditions, whether intestinal obstruction, peritonitis, or trauma, result in either isotonic electrolyte losses or sodium depletion.

The initial renal compensation to metabolic alkalosis involves the excretion of an alkaline urine, containing sodium from the extracellular space and potassium from the cell. This results in conservation of hydrogen ion and will maintain the blood pH. The renal loss of potassium combined with the loss in the vomitus will not be reflected in serum hypokalemia until cellular potassium is severely depleted. If vomiting continues, the kidney will commence to conserve sodium and will excrete an acid urine containing ammonia and acid anions. Thus, an acid urine and hypokalemia are late signs of metabolic alkalosis, at which point one also sees severe hypochloremia and a rise of the blood pH. At the same time, a rising BUN is indicative of prerenal azotemia secondary to severe dehydration. Clinically, these biochemical findings may be predicted from the duration of the baby's vomiting and the loss of 0.5 to 1 kg body weight.

Preoperative care is aimed at the restoration of these fluid and electrolyte losses. At the same time, the stomach is emptied and irrigated with saline through a nasogastric tube to obviate the danger of vomiting and aspiration while the baby is awaiting an operation. The diagnosis is made in the vast majority of infants shortly after the onset of symptoms. Many infants show no clinical signs of dehydration and have normal serum electrolytes. Such patients are given their normal maintenance volume of fluid as half-strength saline with additional potassium and are operated on within a few hours of admission to the hospital. When one finds a history of weight loss, clinical signs of dehydration, and an elevated urine specific gravity, the serum chloride will be in the range of 85 to 90 mEq/L. There will be minimal hyponatremia and a normal serum potassium. Initial therapy aimed at correcting the dehydration and mild hypovolemia consists of administering a bolus of normal saline at 20 ml/kg body weight. When the infant urinates, half-normal saline is administered, containing potassium chloride at 40 mEq/L. This solution contains 115 mEq chloride, 75 mEq sodium, and 40 mEq potassium per liter. The additional potassium is given primarily to increase the chloride, but it also is helpful in replenishing the cellular potassium losses. All solutions are given in either 5 or 10 percent dextrose. A volume of this solution equivalent to the measured recent weight loss is given during the first 6 to 12 hours after hospital admission. The serum electrolytes are then rechecked, and when the baby has a lusty cry, moist mucous membranes, and a urine excretion of 1 ml/kg, he is ready for surgery. The rare infant with severe dehydration and tissue loss from starvation will require hyperalimentation for several days with 20 percent dextrose and amino acids, in addition to the initial water and electrolyte replacement. An example of this form of management can be found in the treatment of a 3.5-week-old baby who was 1.5 kg under her birth weight on admission to the hospital. Her BUN was 143 mg/100 ml, the serum chloride was 54 mEq, the sodium 138 mEq, and the potassium 4.6 mEq/L. She was initially given normal saline and serum albumin to restore volume, followed by a potassium-containing solution. Her serum electrolytes returned to normal within 24 hours after admission to the hospital, but hyperalimentation and replacement of nasogastric losses were continued for 8 days before operation. As a result, she gained 1 kg, her BUN returned to normal, and she tolerated her pyloromyotomy without incident.

THE OPERATION

A carefully performed pyloromyotomy not only cures the baby overnight but is an esthetically pleasing and highly satisfying operation.

Few surgeons will agree on the choice of incision

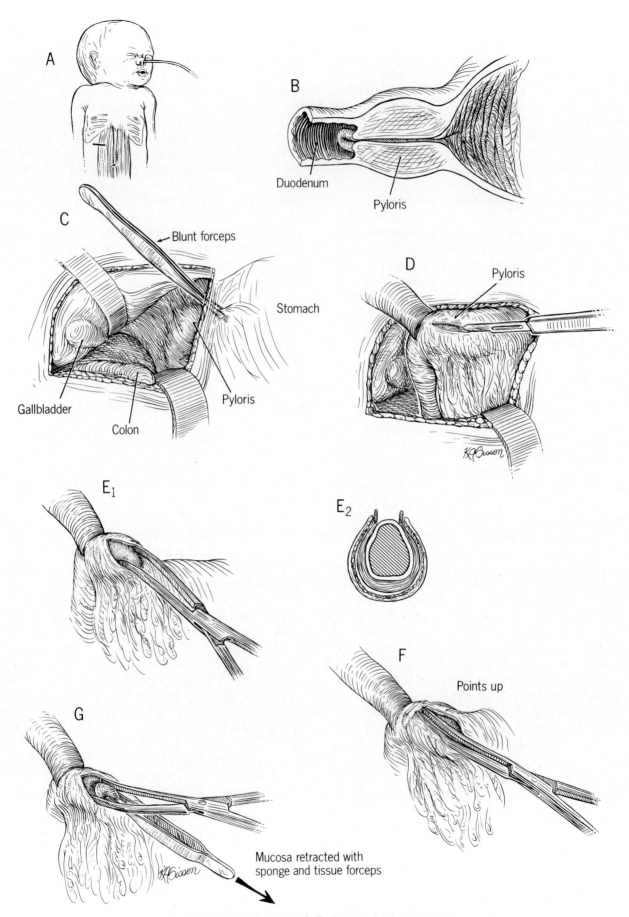

A

B

Duodenum

Pyloris

C

Blunt forceps

Stomach

Gallbladder

Colon

Pyloris

D

Pyloris

E₁

E₂

F

Points up

G

Mucosa retracted with
sponge and tissue forceps

Figure 26–4. A through **G.** Technique of pyloromyotomy.

and technique in the performance of this classic, simple operation. Vertical rectus-splitting or retracting operations were abandoned because of the higher incidence of wound evisceration. The Robertson muscle-splitting operation is so far lateral as to make it difficult to deliver the pyloric tumor into the wound.[20] Incisions that divide the skin and anterior rectus sheath transversely and the posterior rectus sheath and peritoneum vertically are unduly complex and require considerable retraction.[21,22] A simple transverse incision through all layers of the rectus sheath, muscle, and peritoneum directly over the liver provides direct access to the pylorus with minimal retraction. An incision placed over the liver has an additional advantage in that the small intestine never appears in the wound and, therefore, is not subjected to trauma, which could lead to adhesions.

The operation described here evolved from initial experiences with the muscle-splitting incision, modified with the help of colleagues, the surgical literature, and several generations of surgical residents.

Technique

The stomach is emptied once again with a size 14 french orogastric tube that is removed before the induction of anesthesia. The entire abdomen is prepared and draped with sterile towels, which intersect at the umbilicus and mark the oblique costal margin. These drapes are held in place with 0.5 inch Steristrips. A 3 cm transverse incision is made, extending from the lateral edge of the rectus sheath at the costal margin toward the midline (Fig. 26–4). The skin and anterior sheath are cut with the scalpel, and the muscle is divided with the electrocautery. Protecting the wound edges with moist sponges, the posterior sheath is elevated with two hemostats and opened in the line of the incision. The incision will be directly over the liver, which is elevated into the wound and retracted upward with a 1 cm malleable retractor (Fig. 26–4). A second retractor protected with a bit of moist gauze depresses the colon. The greater curvature of the stomach is then seen between these two retractors, and the anterior wall of the stomach can be grasped with a blunt tissue forceps and drawn into the wound. The stomach is held with a sponge, and the pylorus is brought into the wound by traction on the stomach to the left. The retractors are removed from the wound as soon as the stomach is grasped. With a large mass, it is sometimes necessary to depress the wound edges in order to deliver the pylorus. While the assistant continues to hold the stomach, the surgeon applies the left index finger to the duodenal end of the pylorus. With the mass stabilized, the pyloric vein and the bare avascular area between the blood vessels converging from the greater and lesser curvatures are identified. An incision in the pylorus is then made, commencing 2 mm proximal to the pyloric vein and extending onto normal stomach

muscle for 0.5 cm (Fig. 26–4D). This incision is never more than 1 mm deep. The firm pyloric muscle is then split to allow the mucosa to pout into the wound. A special instrument, such as the Benson spreader or a curved hemostat with the round outside edge ground down, is preferable to an ordinary hemostat.[23] The rounded outside edges of a hemostat tend to slip out of the wound, whereas a flat thin surface spreads the muscle in one tidy maneuver. The tips of the spreader are inserted into the center, or thickest, portion of the pylorus and spread until the muscle separates, exposing mucosa (Fig. 26–4E$_1$, E$_2$, F). The spreader is then moved proximally to completely separate Torgerson's muscle in the stomach. There are always a few muscle fibers remaining to be separated in the distal end of the incision adjacent to the duodenum (Fig. 26–4G). These final fibers are demonstrated by retracting backward on the gastric mucosa.[24] When separating these fibers, which actually protrude into the duodenum, the points of the spreader must be held up out of the wound rather than pointed downward to dig into the duodenum (Fig. 26–4F). An alternate method of separating these fibers is to grasp the muscle edge with blunt forceps and apply lateral traction. When the two edges of the pylorus muscle can be moved independently, the separation is complete (Fig. 26–5). Occasionally, it is necessary to ligate or coagulate a small vessel, but bleeding ceases when the pylorus is dropped back into the abdomen. With the liver immediately beneath the incision, the wound is easily closed. Continuous 4–0 monofilament polyglyco-

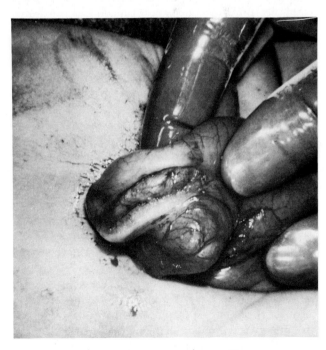

Figure 26–5. The completed pyloromyotomy. The mucosa pouts through the muscular incision, which extends well back onto the stomach.

late sutures may be used in both the posterior and anterior rectus sheath. The skin is approximated with Steri-strips.

POSTOPERATIVE CARE

Maintenance intravenous fluids are continued until the infant is taking at least half his or her required caloric intake by mouth. Most surgeons advise commencing oral feedings 4 to 6 hours after the operation. I prefer to start postoperative feedings the next morning. The first feeding is 15 ml of sugar water. If this is tolerated, the feedings are advanced to half-strength formula and then to increasing volumes of full-strength formula. Within 24 hours, most infants are taking their full formula and are ready for discharge from the hospital. In the event of postoperative vomiting, the volume is reduced to that tolerated and then slowly advanced again.

Complications

Duodenal perforation is the result of overzealous separation of fibers at the distal end of the pylorus with the pointed end of a hemostat. The duodenal mucosa pouts out, and a bit of bile leaks into the wound. The defect is easily closed with one or two interrupted nonabsorbable 5–0 sutures. A tab of omentum is brought up and tied over the wound with the suture ends. The stomach is kept empty with a nasogastric tube for 48 hours before feedings are commenced. There seems to be less postoperative vomiting when the duodenum has been perforated, perhaps because a more than adequate separation of the muscle was achieved.

Perforation of gastric mucosa occurs when the initial separation is too vigorous. The mucosa must be closed first, and then the pyloric muscle is sutured. The pyloromyotomy is then performed in a fresh area, away from the original incision.

Postoperative vomiting usually is the result of too-rapid advancement of the postoperative feedings. An increase from 1 ounce to 3 ounces often seems to be more than many babies will tolerate. Perhaps there is residual edema that causes a relative obstruction. Reduction of the volume usually will take care of the problem in a day or so. Vomiting that persists for 7 to 10 days raises the possibility of an incomplete pyloromyotomy. If the vomiting is forceful and follows every feeding, a barium meal is indicated. If there is still an obstruction, the infant is given intravenous fluids, and the stomach is irrigated. The baby is given nothing by mouth for 24 hours. Feedings are then resumed as in the postoperative period. If there is again persistent vomiting, another operation is advised. In such a case, one usually finds an incomplete incision on the stomach side of the pylorus.

Henderson et al. described cardiac and respiratory arrest caused by hypoglycemia when the intravenous fluids were discontinued in the postoperative period before resumption of an adequate oral intake.[25] They found evidence for depletion of glycogen in liver biopsies taken from malnourished babies at operation. This complication can be prevented by preoperative hyperalimentation as well as by continued administration of glucose-containing fluids in the postoperative period.

RESULTS

All infants operated on for pyloric stenosis now survive. Many long-term follow-up studies indicate that these infants have normal gastrointestinal function and no increased incidence of ulcer disease. However, radiographic studies sometimes indicate a narrowed pylorus for as long as 7 to 10 years after a successful pyloromyotomy.[26]

REFERENCES

1. Hayes MA, Goldenberg LS: Collective review, pyloric stenosis surgery. Surg Gynecol Obstet 104:105, 1957
2. Ravitch MD: The story of pyloric stenosis. Surgery 48:1117, 1960
3. Hirschsprung H, Von Angeborenor F: Pylorosstenosei; beobachtungen bei Sauglingen. Jabrb F Kinderklinek 28:61, 1888
4. Ramstedt C: Zr Operation der angeborenon Pylorostenosis. Med Klin 8:1702, 1912
5. Wollstein M: Healing of hypertrophic pyloric stenosis after the Fredet-Ramstedt operation. Am J Dis Child 23:511, 1922
6. Torgersen J: Muscular build and movements of the stomach and duodenum. Acta Radiol (Stock) [Suppl] 43:3, 1943
7. Shim W, Campbell A, Wright S: Pyloric stenosis in the racial groups of Hawaii. J Pediatr 76:89, 1970
8. Carter CO: Genetics of infantile pyloric stenosis. In Bergsma D (ed): Report on the Fourth Conference on the Clinical Delineation of Birth Defects. Baltimore, Williams & Wilkins, 1972
9. Janik J, Nagaraj H, Lehocky R: Pyloric stenosis in identical triplets. Pediatrics 70:282, 1982
10. Jona JZ: Electron microscopic observation in infantile hypertrophic pyloric stenosis (IHPS). J Pediatr Surg 13:17, 1978
11. Dodge JA: Production of duodenal ulcers and hypertrophic pyloric stenosis by administration of pentagastrin to pregnant and newborn dogs. Nature 225:284, 1970
12. Rogers IM, Macgillion F, Drainer IK: Congenital hypertrophic pyloric stenosis: a gastrin hypothesis pursued. J Pediatr Surg 11:173, 1976
13. Spitz L, Zail SS: Serum gastrin levels in congenital hypertrophic pyloric stenosis. J Pediatr Surg 11:33, 1976
14. Teele RL, Smith EH: Ultrasound in the diagnosis of idio-

pathic hypertrophic pyloric stenosis. N Engl J Med 296:1149, 1977

15. Khamapirad T, Athey P: Ultrasound in the diagnosis of hypertrophic pyloric stenosis. J Pediatr 102:23, 1983

16. Tunell WP, Wilson D: Pyloric stenosis: Diagnosis by real time sonography, the pyloric muscle length method. J Pediatr Surg 19:795, 1984

17. Stunden R, LeQuesne G, Little K: The improved ultrasound diagnosis of hypertrophic pyloric stenosis. Pediatr Radiol 16:200, 1986

18. Burton BK, Nadler HC: Clinical diagnosis of the inborn errors of metabolism in the neonatal period. Pediatrics 61:398–405, 1978

19. Partington MW: The early symptoms of phenylketonuria. Pediatrics 27:465, 1961

20. Robertson DE: Congenital pyloric stenosis. Ann Surg 112:687, 1940

21. Randolph JG: The evaluation of an ideal surgical incision for pyloric stenosis. Arch Surg 93:489, 1966

22. Scharli AF, Sieber WK: Surgical approach for the Ramstedt procedure in hypertrophic pyloric stenosis. Surg Gynecol Obstet 128:355, 1969

23. Benson CD: Infantile hypertrophic pyloric stenosis. In Pediatric Surgery, 2nd ed. Chicago, Year Book, 1969, vol 2, p 821

24. Quinby WC Jr: Complete pyloromyotomy without duodenal perforation. Surgery 59:627, 1966

25. Henderson BM, Schubert WK, Aug G, Martin LW: Hypoglycemia with hepatic glycogen depletion: A postoperative complication of pyloric stenosis. J Pediatr Surg 3:309, 1968

26. Steincke O, Roelsgaard M: Radiographic followup in hypertrophic pyloric stenosis. Acta Paediatr Scand 49:4, 1960

27
Intussusception

Intussusception, like pyloric stenosis, is another of those dramatic pediatric diseases that usually is easily recognized and treated. This disease has a long and fascinating medical history. The ancient Greeks, including Hippocrates, treated intestinal obstruction with enemas or insufflation of air into the anus. Perhaps the accidental reduction of an intussusception led to the centuries-old popularity of the enema as a medical and home remedy. Although intussusception was clearly recognized and on rare occasion successfully treated by the rectal injection of air, water, carbon dioxide, or hydrogen sulfide, the modern treatment was first implemented by Hirschsprung in 1876.[1] In 1905, he reported 107 cases treated with controlled hydrostatic reduction with only a 35 percent mortality rate.[2] The first successful operation for intussusception took place in Tennessee in 1835.[3] The controversy over the relative merits of operative versus hydrostatic reduction did not commence until the reports of Jonathan Hutchinson were published in 1873.[4] This controversy continued in this country until the late 1950s, when Dr. Paul Fox and the late Dr. Willis Potts of the Children's Memorial Hospital in Chicago were the last to advocate operative reduction for every child with intussusception.[5,6] All aspects of intussusception were reviewed in great detail by Dr. Mark Ravitch in a series of articles that culminates in his classic monograph of 1959.[7] This work continues to be the most valid authoritative source of information on this fascinating topic. Even though Chicago surgeons were the last to advocate operative therapy, we take some satisfaction in the fact that Ravitch's interest in intussusception was inspired by a paper given by Dr. E. H. Miller in 1933, in which the poor results of the operative treatment of intussusception at the Children's Memorial and Cook County Hospitals of Chicago were presented.

PATHOLOGY

An intussusception is the invagination of one segment of intestine into another. In most cases, this commences just proximal to the ileocecal valve. As it progresses, the ileum with its mesentery is drawn into the cecum and on into the colon. The lead point is termed the intussusceptum. The neck of the intussusception compresses the entrapped bowel—this, together with traction on the mesentery, produces lymphatic and mesenteric venous obstruction. One finds engorgement of the mucosa at the lead point and increasing edema up to the point of mesenteric arterial obstruction. The intussusceptum and varying portions of the invaginating bowel become gangrenous. Meanwhile, there is increasing proximal distention of the small bowel with sequestration of large volumes of intestinal secretions. In experimental intussusceptions created in dogs, Ravitch found vascular engorgement, mucosal sloughing, and bacterial penetration of the serosa within 38 hours. A similar process occurs in children.[8] There are exceptions to these usual findings, however. If the lesions commence in the ileum, a 2- or 5-layered intussusception occurs as the original ileoileal intussusception is drawn into the cecum. Other forms of intussusception include simple jejunal or ileal lesions, intussusception of the appendix, and gastroduodenal intussusception.[9–11]

ETIOLOGY

There is no specific etiology for the usual ileocolic intussusception. Gross found a lead point—such as Meckel's diverticulum, a polyp, intestinal duplication, or lymphoma—in only 43 of 702 children.[11] Direct observation

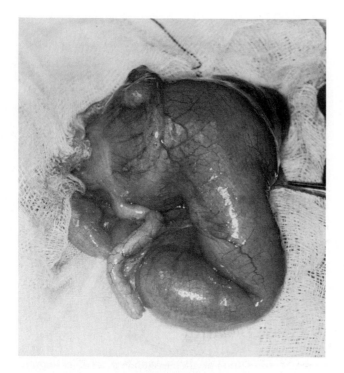

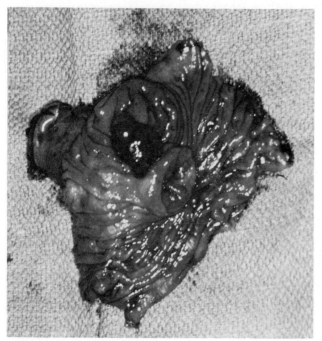

Figure 27–1. Specific lead points. **Top.** Duplication of the terminal ileum. **Bottom.** Polyp of the cecum.

acute gastroenteritis in infants. It was found in the stools of 37 percent of 30 children with intussusception.[12] Other studies have demonstrated an increased serologic response to adenoviruses in children who have had intussusception.[13,14] Viral gastroenteritis could increase peristalsis and thereby predispose to an intussusception or cause hypertrophy of lymphoid tissue in the terminal ileum. Segmental hyperperistalsis is the most probable explanation for intussusceptions that occur in the immediate postoperative period in children.

Specific Lead Points

Approximately 5 percent of all childhood intussusceptions have a specific lead point. In Ein's series and in our own experience, these children are older than the average, and a barium enema is less likely to achieve a reduction.[15] A Meckel's diverticulum is the most common lead point, followed by polyps and duplications of the bowel. Other specific lead points include ectopic gastric mucosa, eosinophilic granuloma of the ileum, papillary lymphoid hyperplasia of the ileum, hemangiomas, and submucosal hemorrhage secondary to hemophilia or Henoch's purpura (Fig. 27–1).[16–19] Lymphosarcoma of the intestine is the most common cause of intussusception in children over 6 years of age (Fig. 27–2).[20] The tumor arises from lymphoid follicles in the distal ileum. There may be either a large polypoid mass or infiltration of the submucosa, with involvement of the mesenteric lymph nodes. Intussusception also is a complication of the thick inspissated feces in the terminal ileum of a child with cystic fibrosis of the pancreas. In Shwachman's series, the average age was 9 years.[21] We saw one child with a recurrent intussusception who had both cystic fibrosis and colon polyps.

of the small intestine during any abdominal operation suggests that an intussusception may be initiated by a localized ring of intestinal spasm. Occasionally, one sees these localized areas of hyperperistalsis temporarily invaginate into the adjacent distal intestine. This phenomenon is frequently observed in dogs.

The human rotovirus is a major etiologic agent for

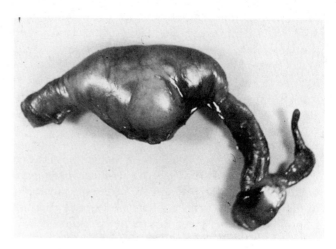

Figure 27–2. Lymphosarcoma of the terminal ileum that produced an intussusception. There had been chronic abdominal pain for 3 months.

CLINICAL FINDINGS

Typically, a baby with an intussusception pulls up his or her legs and screams with pain. When the attack is over, the baby is pale and limp. The child's mother is certain that this scream is no ordinary cry and that something serious has gone wrong. The onset is sudden, and the pains recur at intervals from 5 minutes to a half-hour until the baby is so exhausted and dehydrated that he can only lie still and moan. Victims of this ailment vomit their last feeding at the onset, and if the disease continues, the vomiting continues and becomes stained with bile. The passage of blood and mucus with the stool completes the classic picture: abdominal pain, vomiting, and the "currant jelly stool." These symptoms vary in their intensity, but pain, as indicated by rhythmic intense crying with vomiting, should never be dismissed as simple colic even though the baby does not appear to be ill. A coexisting illness—such as diarrhea, an upper respiratory infection, or (especially) otitis media, which causes pain and crying—may obscure the early symptoms. These babies are sometimes so sleepy between episodes of pain that they are admitted to the hospital with the diagnosis of meningitis or other central nervous system disorder.

PHYSICAL EXAMINATION

Early in the course of the disease, the vital signs are normal, but as abdominal distention and vomiting continue, there is fluid loss and bacteremia, which cause tachycardia, fever, and eventually hypovolemic shock. Potts paid particular attention to the infant's facial expression. During the spasm, the baby generally has an expression of pain or a sudden, startled, anxious look. Potts once cancelled an operation for intussusception because on the operating table the baby smiled at him. "Babies with intussusception don't smile," he remarked.[22] By simple observation, one can observe the rhythmic bouts in which the infant pulls up his or her legs, thrashes about, and cries. During these episodes, one may hear hyperperistaltic rushes by auscultation of the abdomen. Between episodes of pain, when the child relaxes, careful palpation may reveal the presence of a sausage-shaped mass. This will be in the upper midabdomen, tucked under the liver, where it is very difficult to find. It is helpful to palpate the abdomen while sitting or standing at the head of the baby. In this position, you can stabilize the mass between the posterior abdominal wall and the liver, where it will be less evasive. For a while, the child's abdomen remains scaphoid; it then commences to distend. When the diagnosis is delayed, one encounters severe abdominal distention with visible coils of bowel and peristaltic waves. Tenderness is an ominous sign of peritonitis, gangrene, or perforation. Dance's sign often is described—a sensation of emptiness in the right lower quadrant—but this is of little value in making the diagnosis. The rectal examination is most important. The tip of the intussusception may be felt, and even if the child has not passed blood in the stool, there should be some bloody mucus on the examiner's fingertip (Fig. 27–3).

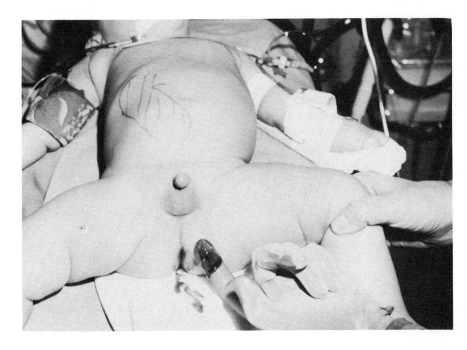

Figure 27–3. The classic findings of an intussusception. The sausage-shaped mass is outlined on the abdominal wall, and the examining finger covered with bloody mucus.

ATYPICAL INTUSSUSCEPTION

A case is termed "atypical" anytime one of us misses a straightforward diagnosis, even when the problem is the physician's ignorance rather than unusual symptoms in the patient. In spite of this inherent difficulty, there are a few children with intussusceptions that do not follow the classic pattern. The signs and symptoms of intussusception are remarkably similar throughout the world, except that in some areas of Africa, the average patient age is significantly higher, diarrhea is more common, and colic is less severe.[23] A preceding disease (most frequently dysentery) can mask the early symptoms of intussusception, particularly when there are bloody stools. There is, however, a less severe form of intussusception associated with minimal or no pain, no crying, and a delayed onset of vomiting. Rectal bleeding also is less frequent in this group of patients. This less acute entity, although more difficult to diagnose, is fortunately associated with minimal morbidity, mainly because of the absence of ischemia in the intussuscepted bowel. Children with this form of the disease are listless and have vague abdominal pain but no sign of a complete intestinal obstruction.[24-27] On careful examination of the records of 20 patients, Janik found some of the signs of intussusception in almost every case.[28] He proposed the term "nonischemic intussusception," rather than the terms "painless" and "atypical" that had been used previously. Janik found that these children had a 25 percent incidence of a specific lead point, and all of the intussusceptions were easily reduced either at operation or with a barium enema. Some of these children had undergone several hospitalizations and prolonged abdominal symptoms before a correct diagnosis was finally made.

POSTOPERATIVE INTUSSUSCEPTION

In our experience, bowel intussusception is the most common cause of intestinal obstruction during the first postoperative week.[29] This unique complication most often follows an intraabdominal or retroperitoneal operation, but has occurred after thoracic operations and even after biopsy of a cervical lymph node.[30] The incidence of this complication seems to be higher in children who are receiving postoperative irradiation and chemotherapy for malignancies.[31] Dammert and Votteler reviewed 81 cases collected from the literature and found that only 11 had a lead point, such as an inverted appendiceal stump, the resection site of a Meckel's diverticulum, or traumatized intestine.[32] Once you think of the diagnosis, the clinical picture becomes relatively straightforward. The child recovers as expected, the abdomen becomes flat, and he or she passes gas and may even tolerate liquids or food by mouth for several days after operation. The patient then vomits and becomes distended. At this point, we usually blame premature feeding and a continued postoperative ileus. Careful auscultation of the abdomen, however, reveals intestinal sounds, and supine and upright roentgenograms of the abdomen demonstrate a picture of obstruction rather than paralytic ileus. The problem is compounded by the fact that these children rarely have typical cramping abdominal pain and will improve with gastric drainage. A barium enema is of no help because these lesions occur in the ileum or jejunum. The diagnosis depends on the plain roentgenograms and a high index of suspicion. At operation, these intussusceptions generally are easily reducible, although we have observed gangrenous intestine requiring resection in two neglected patients.

MANAGEMENT

When a child with suspected intussusception is admitted to the emergency room of a hospital, a nasogastric tube is passed to decompress the stomach, and administration of intravenous fluids is started. If the symptoms have persisted for longer than 24 hours and if the child has a fever with an elevated white blood count, it is wise to administer antibiotics. A narcotic, such as Demerol (1 mg/kg body weight), may be given to relieve the pain. This medication also serves to sedate the child for a barium enema and is a suitable premedication in the event an operation is needed. If the child's condition is stable after the initiation of treatment, he or she is taken directly to the x-ray department. Supine and upright roentgenograms of the abdomen are obtained.

The barium enema was first used to diagnose an intussusception by William Ladd in 1913.[33] Currently, a controlled barium enema is the most reliable diagnostic technique for an ileocolic intussusception and is the accepted treatment for at least 75 percent of cases. Proper sedation is extremely helpful in preparing the child for this procedure. It is almost impossible to administer a satisfactory enema to an infant who is crying, moving, and periodically writhing in pain. Furthermore, several assistants are necessary. A lubricated straight catheter is inserted into the rectum and held in place with generous amounts of adhesive tape. The buttocks are taped together to further secure the catheter and to prevent leakage of barium. Many radiologists prefer a Foley balloon catheter, but there's danger of lacerating the rectum if the balloon is too large. The barium is administered from a container 3 feet above the table, and the flow is observed fluoroscopically until the meniscus of the intussusception is identified. This is usually in the transverse or proximal descending colon. At this time, a film is taken to outline the barium column between the intussusceptum and the colon. A coiled spring sign is diagnostic (Fig. 27–4). Occasionally, the intussusception is so rap-

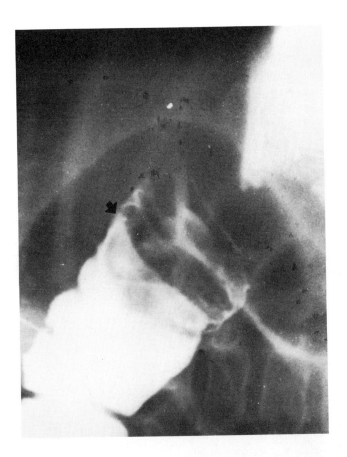

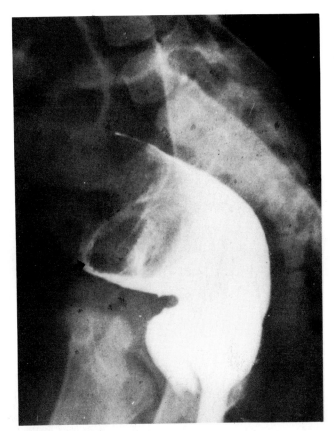

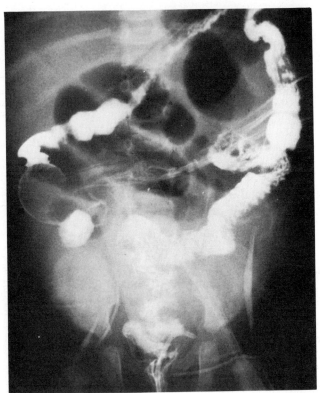

Figure 27–4. Barium enema findings in children with intussusception. **Top left.** The coiled spring sign, found here in the transverse colon. **Top right.** An intussusception in the rectum. **Bottom left.** The arrow points to a duplication of the cecum found during a barium enema reduction of the intussusception.

idly reduced that one wonders if it was really there! At other times, it is necessary to maintain pressure for several minutes. The reduction is followed by fluoroscopy. As long as the barium column advances, the attempt at reduction continues. A second or third attempt may be made after the child has evacuated the barium. A small injection of a rapid-acting tranquilizer is helpful if the child cries or is otherwise uncooperative. Our rate of success with barium enema reduction has improved with the addition of satisfactory sedation. In fact,

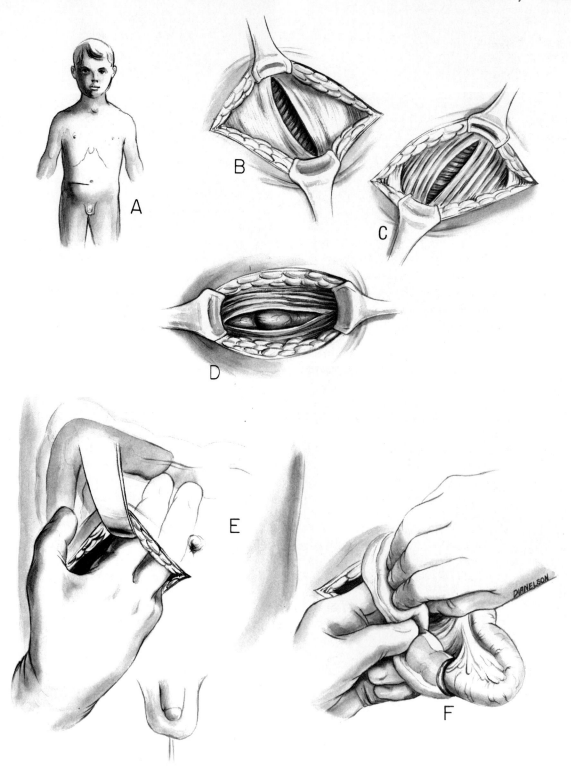

Figure 27–5. A through **F.** The surgical reduction of an intussusception.

nearly all the intussusceptions operated on in our hospital during the past 5 years have required resection for gangrenous bowel. The success rate of barium enema reduction has varied among several series of patients from 45 to 80 percent.[34–38] Glucagon will relax various portions of the gastrointestinal tract, including the colon. Hoy et al. took advantage of this property and administered glucagon to 25 children with intussusceptions just before the barium enema. Reduction was achieved in 21 patients (84 percent).[39] A barium enema reduction is considered successful when the contrast material freely refluxes into the terminal ileum. Following the procedure, all symptoms are relieved, and most children are able to take a liquid diet and are discharged from the hospital within 24 hours. When an intussusception is diagnosed very early, the entire process can be performed on an outpatient basis.

Surgical Management of Intussusception

A child who initially has prolonged symptoms, bloody stools, severe abdominal distention, and tenderness with signs of shock has gangrenous or at least severely compromised bowel. Plain films of the abdomen will clearly demonstrate a small intestinal obstruction. In this situation, a barium enema is not necessary to make the diagnosis, and the time spent in a fruitless attempt at a barium reduction is better used in preparing the child for operation. Antibiotics, blood transfusions, plasma, and intravenous fluids are required to treat septicemia and to replace lost fluid volume. When the child's vital signs have stabilized and he or she is excreting urine at 1 ml/kg per hour, the child is ready for surgery.

The lack of reflux of barium into the terminal ileum is sufficient evidence that an operation is indicated. Finally, because of the high incidence of lymphosarcoma of the bowel and other lead points in children over 6 years of age, we believe that these patients should also undergo surgery, even if the barium enema has successfully reduced the intussusception.

The skin incision is placed higher than the classic McBurney incision and is transverse, so that it can be extended medially if necessary. It is slightly below the umbilicus (Fig. 27–5). The oblique muscles are split in the direction of their fibers right to the edge of the rectus sheath. If more exposure is necessary, the anterior and posterior rectus sheath may be incised, but the muscle is merely retracted. The surgeon then inserts the index and third fingers into the incision and, with the opposite hand exerting counterpressure on the abdominal wall, traces the intussusception to its lead point. The index and third fingers then commence to exert pressure on the lead point until it has been reduced sufficiently to be delivered through the incision. If it is not possible to reduce the intussusception in this fashion,

the incision must be enlarged so that the entire mass can be delivered onto the abdominal wall. Then the entire hand encircles the mass and applies gentle pressure to reduce edema. The opposite hand then squeezes the bowel backward. Traction should never be used. Resection is indicated if the intussusception cannot be reduced manually or if, after reduction, the bowel is gangrenous or perforated. We prefer to cover the bowel with warm, moist laparotomy pads for at least 5 minutes to determine whether the purple, engorged bowel will become pink and obviously viable. If there is doubt, it is safer to resect and perform an end-to-end anastomosis. The presence of a specific lead point, such as a Meckel's diverticulum or a duplication, is also an indication for resection. Do not be fooled by an edematous engorged ileocecal valve, which on palpation feels like a polyp! We prefer an end-to-end anastomosis over exteriorization procedures, provided that the child has been adequately resuscitated before the operation. The choice of technique depends on the surgeon. An open, one-layer anastomosis is satisfactory. If the child is in good general condition, we perform an appendectomy after reduction of the intussusception.

Postoperative complications are directly related to the patient's pathology. A child who has had an easily reduced lesion is usually ready to go home in 3 or 4 days. On the other hand, when gangrenous intestine is resected, all of the potential complications of abdominal surgery can be anticipated.

RECURRENT INTUSSUSCEPTION

It is always wise to warn the parents that an intussusception may recur, with the average recurrence rate in several series at about 4 percent.[40] There is a greater recurrence rate following barium enema reduction than following surgery. Some early recurrences following barium enema reduction may actually have represented an incomplete reduction in the first place. Since parents are well aware of the symptoms of an intussusception, the duration of symptoms is considerably shorter in subsequent episodes. Ein reviewed 35 recurrent intussusceptions in 28 children; only 2 specific lead points were found.[41] Perhaps this is because 21 of the recurrences were again treated with barium enemas, and specific lead points that could have been found at operation were overlooked. The treatment of children with recurrent intussusceptions must be individualized. Perhaps because of the earlier diagnosis of recurrent intussusception, these are just as easily, if not more readily, reduced by barium enema. For this reason and because of the infrequency of a specific lead point, Ein has recommended continued barium enema reductions after as many as four or five episodes. In older children who

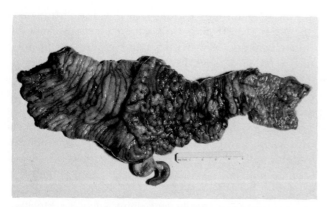

Figure 27–6. Resected specimen of the terminal ileum and cecum demonstrating hypertrophy of Peyer's patches in the ileum.

have a higher incidence of tumors (specifically lymphosarcoma), an operation should be performed at the first recurrence. In those under 1 to 2 years of age, repeated barium enema reductions are acceptable, although the family usually becomes alarmed at every minor episode of abdominal pain, and there is always the possibility that the child could have a specific lead point. In these children, we advise an operation at the second recurrence, with resection of a short segment of the terminal ileum and the cecum. One invariably finds marked hypertrophy of Peyer's patches in the terminal ileum (Fig. 27–6). Other local pathology includes duplications and polyps.

REFERENCES

1. Hirschsprung H: ET Tilfaelde of subakut Tarminsagination. Hosp Tid 3:321, 1876
2. Hirschsprung H: 107 Falle von Darminvagination bei Kindern, Behandelt in Konigen Louisey-Kinderhospital in Kopenhagen Wahrend der Jahre 1871–1904. Mitt Grenzgeb Med Chir 14:555, 1905
3. Thompson WW: A case of intussusception in which an operation was successfully resorted to by John RW Wilson, M.D. of Rutherford County, Tennessee, in December, 1831. Transylvania J Med 8:486, 1835
4. Hutchinson J: A succesful case of abdominal section for intussusception. Proc R Med Chir Soc 7:195, 1873
5. Fox PF: Intussusception: Surgical treatment. Surg Clin North Am 36:1501, 1956
6. Potts WJ: The Surgeon and the Child. Philadelphia, Saunders, 1959, pp 162–170
7. Ravitch MM: Intussusception in Infants and Children. Springfield, Ill, Thomas, 1959
8. Ravitch MM: Intussusception in Infants and Children. Springfield, Ill, Thomas, 1959, pp 46–48
9. Forshall I: Intussusception of the vermiform appendix with a report of seven cases in children. Br J Surg 40:305, 1953
10. Apfelberg DB, Glicklich M, Tang TT: Gastroduodenal intussusception in a child. Surgery 69:736, 1971
11. Gross RE: The Surgery of Infancy and Childhood. Philadelphia, Saunders, 1953, p 281
12. Konno T, Suzuki H, Kutsuzawa T, et al: Human rotovirus and intussusception. N Engl J Med 297:945, 1977
13. Gardner PS, Knox EG, Court SDM, et al: Virus infection and intussusception in childhood. Br Med J 2:697, 1962
14. Clarke EJ Jr, Phillips IA, Alexander ER: Adenovirus infection in intussusception in children in Taiwan. JAMA 208:1671, 1969
15. Ein SH: Leading points in childhood intussusception. J Pediatr Surg 11:209, 1976
16. Doberneck RC, Deane WM, Antoine JE: Albuquerque, NM: Ectopic gastric mucosa in the ileum: A cause of intussusception. J Pediatr Surg 11:99, 1976
17. McGreevy P, Doberneck RC, McLeay JM, Miller FA: Recurrent eosinophilic infiltrate (granuloma) of the ileum causing intussusception in a two-year-old child. Surgery 61:280, 1967
18. Schenken JR, Kruger RL, Schultz L: Papillary lymphoid hyperplasia of the terminal ileum: An unusual cause of intussusception and gastrointestinal bleeding in childhood. J Pediatr Surg 10:259, 1975
19. Bower RJ, Kiesewetter WB: Colo-colic intussusception due to a hemangioma. J Pediatr Surg 12:777, 1977
20. Wayne ER, Campbell JB, Kosloske AM, Burrington JD: Intussusception in the older child-suspect lymphosarcoma. J Pediatr Surg 11:789, 1976
21. Shwachman H: Gastrointestinal manifestations of cystic fibrosis. Pediatr Clin North Am 22:787, 1975
22. Fox P: Personal communication
23. Chapman JA: Intussusception in Rhodesian Africans: A contrast with the accepted clinical picture. J Pediatr Surg 8:43, 1973
24. Ravitch MM: Consideration of errors in the diagnosis of intussusception. Am J Dis Child 84:17, 1952
25. Ein SH, Stephens CA, Minor A: The painless intussusception. J Pediatr Surg 11:563, 1976
26. Geller RM, Hays DM: Subacute intussusception: A clinical entity in pediatric surgery. Am Surg 28:83, 1962
27. Bergdahl S, Hugosson C, Lauren T, Soderlung S: Atypical intussusception. J Pediatr Surg 7:700, 1972
28. Janik JS: Nonischemic intussusception. J Pediatr Surg 12:567, 1977
29. Raffensperger JG, Baker RJ: Postoperative intestinal obstruction in children. Arch Surg 94:450, 1967
30. McGovern JB, Gross RE: Intussusception as a postoperative complication. Surgery 63:507, 1968
31. Cox JA, Martin LW: Postoperative bowel obstruction: Ileus or intussusception? Arch Surg 106:263, 1973
32. Dammert G, Votteler TP: Postoperative intussusception in the pediatric patient. J Pediatr Surg 9:817, 1974
33. Ladd WE: Progress in the diagnosis and treatment of intussusception. Boston Med Surg J 168:542, 1913
34. Gierup J, Jorulf H, Livaditis A: Management of intussus-

ception in infants and children: A survey based on 288 consecutive cases. Pediatrics 50:535, 1972

35. Marks RM, Sieber WK, Girdany BR: Hydrostatic pressure in the treatment of ileocolic intussusception in infants and children. J Pediatr Surg 1:566, 1966

36. Wayne ER, Campbell JD, Burrington JD, et al: Management of 344 children with intussusception. Radiology 107:597, 1973

37. Ein SH, Stephens CA: Intussusception: 354 cases in 10 years. J Pediatr Surg 6:16, 1971

38. Minami A, Fujii K: Intussusception in children. Am J Dis Child 129:346, 1975

39. Hoy, GR, Dunbar D, Boles ET: The use of glucagon in the diagnosis and management of ileocolic intussusception. J Pediatr Surg 12:939, 1977

40. Herman BE, Becker J: Recurrent acute intussusception: A survey. Surg Clin North Am 40:1009, 1960

41. Ein SH: Recurrent intussusception in children. J Pediatr Surg 10:751, 1975

28
Disorders of the Spleen

Stephen E. Dolgin
John G. Raffensperger

Not so long ago, spleens were removed almost with abandon, causing, we thought, no harm to the patient. The observation by King and Shumacker that splenectomies in young children may be followed by overwhelming sepsis dispelled this notion and revived interest in the functions of the spleen.[1] It is a complex organ that filters undesirable material from the blood and has an important role in the immune system. Its rich blood supply and vascular anatomy favor its function as a filter. The central arteries branch from the segmental trabecular arteries at a right angle and pass through the white pulp, which consists of clusters of lymphatic tissue. Here, plasma and small particles are retained, a process that localizes foreign proteins within the germinal centers and is important in antibody formation. The blood continues with an increased hematocrit in the central arteries to the red pulp, where red cells contact phagocytic endothelial cells. The fast component of the spleen's circulation continues through endothelialized vessels as in any other organ. The blood that is in the slow circulation leaves the endothelialized vessels within the cords of Billroth.[2,3] The slow circulating blood next enters tortuous endothelium-lined sinuses, where there are clefts or slits measuring 1 by 3 μm. Here the cells become hypoxic, and old cells or those that cannot change shape are left behind and phagocytized. Encapsulated bacteria also are removed from the circulation in a similar manner. The filtration process can remove intracellular organisms, such as the malarial parasite.[4] The spleen also is a source of humoral antibodies, especially of IgM and IgG antibodies, in response to intravenous antigens. The spleen manufactures specific antibodies, opsonins, that are necessary for encapsulated organisms, such as the pneumococcus or *Haemophilus influenzae*, to become phagocytized. Thus, splenectomy in childhood, indeed at any age, or congenital absence of the spleen impairs the immune response to bacterial infections.

POSTSPLENECTOMY SEPSIS

The tremendous increased risk for sepsis after splenectomy in children must enter into any decision to remove the spleen. Furthermore, whenever splenectomy is advised, the parents must be warned of this risk. Most infections occur within 2 years after the splenectomy.[5] In a series of 1413 splenectomies reviewed by the Surgical Section of the American Academy of Pediatrics, the mortality rate due to sepsis depended on the original diagnosis. This varies from 0.51 percent after splenectomy for spherocytosis to 6.19 percent for portal hypertension or malignancy. It is most significant that there was an 0.9 percent mortality rate after splenectomy for trauma because of delayed sepsis.[6]

In most series, the risk of sepsis is greater when the splenectomy was performed before 5 years of age.[7,8] However, there is still a risk in older children and adults.[9–11] Postsplenectomy sepsis commences with a sudden onset of fever, nausea, and lethargy and may progress to coma and death within 24 to 48 hours. The sepsis is accompanied by shock and often disseminated intravascular coagulation. Even with prompt, massive antibiotic treatment, the mortality rate is still in the range of 50 percent.

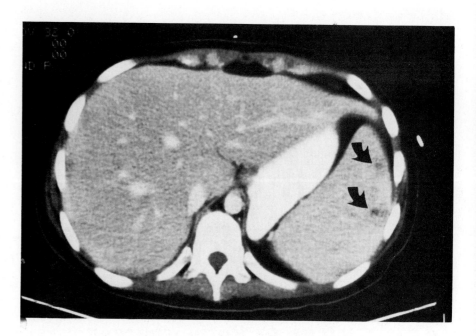

Figure 28–1. CT scan demonstrating multiple small abcesses in a teenage girl with acute lymphoblastic leukemia.

If possible, elective splenectomy is delayed until after the child is 5 years of age. The risk of postsplenectomy sepsis can be reduced further by vaccinating the child with a polyvalent pneumococcal vaccine a month before the operation. Recently, we have given *H. influenzae* type B vaccine. After the splenectomy, prophylactic oral penicillin is given, preferably for the lifetime of the patient, but at least for 5 years. If there is a penicillin allergy, trimethoprim-sulfamethoxazole is given. We also advise that all patients who have had a splenectomy wear a Medic-Alert bracelet and seek immediate medical attention for any febrile illness.

The evaluation of splenic function commences with a history that focuses on episodes of jaundice or purpura and a physical examination to determine the size of the spleen. Blood counts and an evaluation of the peripheral smear provide information on the shape of red blood cells and the numbers of platelets. Liver–spleen scans, which depend on the uptake of the reticuloendothelial system for radionuclides, provide information on the size and function of the spleen and will demonstrate filling defects, such as hemangiomas or abscesses. Computed tomography (CT) also will demonstrate small splenic defects, such as the abscesses seen in immunodeficient children (Fig. 28–1). Isotope-tagging techniques provide more specific information on the sequestration of blood cells within the spleen. The patient's own red cells may be tagged with chromium (^{51}Cr). Disappearance of the isotope from the circulation provides an index of hemolysis. Increased localization of the isotope within the spleen indicates sequestration of the tagged cells.

INDICATIONS FOR SPLENECTOMY

Splenectomy incidental to Hodgkin's disease and trauma is discussed in other chapters. The primary hematologic disorders cured or alleviated by splenectomy are congenital hemolytic anemia and idiopathic thrombocytopenic purpura. Other indications include hemangiomas, thalassemia, Gaucher's disease, and abscesses. Splenectomy occasionally is indicated for acquired hemolytic anemia and inborn errors of metabolism, but these patients must be studied with great care to be certain that operation is indicated. The indications for splenectomies in our hospital are listed in Table 28–1.

TABLE 28–1. INDICATIONS FOR SPLENECTOMY IN 151 CHILDREN, 1977–1987

Indication	Number
Spherocytosis	41
Idiopathic thrombocytopenic purpura	31
Hodgkin's disease (staging)	24
Incidental to renal transplantation	13
Leukemia	5
Thalassemia	7
Portal hypertension (splenorenal shunt)	4
Abscess	4
Autoimmune hemolytic anemia	4
Sickle cell disease	4
Wandering spleen	3
Miscellaneous	11

Hereditary Spherocytosis

Congenital hemolytic anemia can be inherited from either parent as a mendelian dominant trait. Consequently, there is usually a history of the disease in a parent as well as in other relatives. When the disease is found in one child, his or her siblings should be tested for the abnormality.[12] There is a membrane deficiency of spectrin, the most important structural protein in the red cell. The membrane skeleton determines the shape of the erythrocyte and allows the reversible deformability, so a normal cell can withstand its passage through the capillaries. When spectrin is deficient, the red cell is spherical and cannot traverse the spleen's microcirculation. Thus, it is trapped and destroyed in the red pulp.[13]

The disease is characterized by jaundice and anemia at birth, but thereafter its severity is variable. The hemoglobin stabilizes at 8 to 10 g, although recurrent episodes of anemia with jaundice do occur. On physical examination, there may be barely detectable scleral icterus, and the spleen is uniformly enlarged. Spherocytes of varying size are seen on the blood smear, and the reticulocyte count will vary from 7 to 20 percent. If the child is jaundiced, there will be a rise in the indirect bilirubin, with increased urobilinogen in the urine. The diagnosis is established by the osmotic fragility test, which demonstrates hemolysis of the cells in saline concentrations just below isotonicity. Although some patients with hemolytic anemia may live into adulthood with minimal symptoms, there is an increased risk of gallstones, and simple infectious diseases may precipitate hemolytic crises. Before operation, every child must have ultrasonography, since the presence or absence of gallstones decides the type of surgical incision. We recommend simultaneous cholecystectomy and splenectomy when there are gallstones. The splenectomy should be performed when the child is relatively well and never during a hemolytic crisis. After splenectomy, patients with spherocytosis are clinically well. They continue to have a slightly elevated bilirubin and the reticulocyte count is high, but the survival rate of their red blood cells is either normal or only very slightly impaired.[14]

Elliptocytosis follows a hereditary pattern similar to that of spherocytosis, but it is clinically milder. Occasionally, however, a child with elliptocytosis will have hemolytic crises and develop gallstones.

Idiopathic Thrombocytopenic Purpura

Thrombocytopenia commonly is found in children with sepsis, malignancy, or lupus erythematosus and sometimes occurs secondary to a drug hypersensitivity. The term idiopathic thrombocytopenic purpura (ITP) is reserved for those patients with normal bone marrow who show a marked reduction in platelet count but no associated systemic disease.

ITP most commonly develops in children between 2 and 4 years of age. With adults, the disease occurs primarily in women, but there is no such sexual distinction in children. The disease starts in children who were previously well or who had at most a mild infectious illness. The first symptoms are easy bruising in response to trauma, spontaneous ecchymoses, and petechiae. Approximately one third of affected children have nosebleeds, melena, or bleeding from oral mucous membranes. Intracranial hemorrhage is the most serious complication and has been reported in from 1 to 2 percent of children with ITP. This usually occurs within 6 weeks of the onset. One third of infants afflicted by neonatal ITP with extracutaneous bleeding develop intracranial hemorrhage.[15] On physical examination, the child rarely appears ill; he will have petechiae and ecchymoses. The tip of the spleen may be palpable, but an enlarged spleen or liver suggests another diagnosis. At the onset, platelet counts are often below 20,000/mm^3, anemia remains proportional to blood loss, and there may be slight eosinophilia. A bone marrow examination will demonstrate increased numbers of megakaryocytes.

ITP is no longer "idiopathic." The disease should now be termed "immune thrombocytopenic purpura." IgG, the most important host defense antibody, is a bridge between particle-bound antigens and the reticuloendothelial (RE) cells. The RE cells in the spleen clear sensitized cells or particles, such as platelets. Thus, the binding of IgG to platelets with their subsequent clearance by the spleen's RE cells is the major mechanism for platelet destruction in ITP. Measurement of platelet-associated IgG is a useful adjunct in diagnosis.

Therapy

About 80 percent of children with ITP recover without any form of therapy. Of these, 50 percent recover within 6 weeks of the onset, and the rest are well within a year. There is some controversy over the use of corticosteroids, since there is no real evidence that steroid therapy changes the natural course of the disease.[16,17] On the other hand, steroid therapy may temporarily increase the platelet count by blocking the removal of antibody-coated platelets from the circulation.[18] If steroid therapy is used, prednisone is given in a dose of 1 to 4 mg/kg per day. If there is no remission, administration of the drug is discontinued after 3 weeks. In the absence of overt bleeding, children with ITP are allowed to continue a normal life, although they must avoid activity that may result in trauma.

Spontaneous recovery or response to steroid therapy after the persistence of thrombocytopenia for 1 year is distinctly unusual. Formerly, the treatment of choice for chronic ITP was splenectomy. Some 70 to 90 percent of children who undergo splenectomy recover completely.[19,20] Before operation, a determined search should be made for an underlying disease that would contraindicate a splenectomy. In a series studied at the Cincinnati Children's Hospital, Zerella et al. found that splenectomies were performed in 30 of 183 children with ITP.[21] Of these splenectomies, 10 (30 percent) were performed as an emergency operation for persistent gastrointestinal hemorrhage or hematuria, and 7 patients showed evidence of intracranial hemorrhage. The platelet counts in these 10 patients ranged from 0 to 12,000/mm^3. Two patients died in the postoperative period from massive intracranial hemorrhage. The rest were alive and well at the time of the study.

Recurrence after splenectomy may be secondary to an overlooked accessory spleen, which may be located at a second operation by the use of intraoperative scanning with technetium-99m-labeled red cells and a sterile probe.[22]

There are now very few indications for splenectomy, since at least 75 percent of children with ITP will have an initial, rapid increase in their platelet counts after treatment with intravenous IgG.[23,24] The exogenous IgG is bound to the monocytes and macrophages of the spleen, thus competing with the platelets. The initial course of therapy consists of 2 g/kg of IgG given over 2 to 5 days. Although the response to IgG is more rapid than with steroid treatment, it is not as rapid as after splenectomy. Thus, an operation is still indicated in children recalcitrant to medical therapy and perhaps in emergency situations, such as intracranial hemorrhage.[25]

Thalassemia

The thalassemia syndromes are inherited disorders that result from defective synthesis of one or more of the polypeptide chains of hemoglobin. In these syndromes, the red blood cell has a low hemoglobin content. In addition, the cell membrane is deficient, and there is some destruction of the red cell in the spleen. Historically, the thalassemias have been found most often in patients of Mediterranean and African origin, and there is usually a family history. The child is anemic and requires regular transfusions. The spleen and liver are enlarged and bony changes develop, for example, prominent cheek bones, a protruding upper jaw, and frontal bossing of the skull. Roentgenograms demonstrate osteoporosis and marrow expansion. Afflicted children are chronically ill, with growth retardation and chronic infections, and are subject to hemolytic crises. They develop gallstones and are at risk to acquire hepatitis from frequent blood transfusions. Diagnosis of the specific hemoglobin pattern is made by electrophoresis. Supportive treatment consists of tranfusions to maintain the hemoglobin level and iron-chelating agents to remove the excess iron stores. Splenectomy is indicated when there is progressive splenomegaly, which results in secondary

hypersplenism. Splenectomy reduces the child's transfusion requirements and makes him or her more comfortable by eliminating the encroachment of the enlarged spleen on other organs. Partial splenic embolization has been recommended in thallasemia.[26] Unfortunately, the complications of embolization included fever, pleural effusion, and a convulsion. The morbidity was greater than that for splenectomy.

Miscellaneous

Children with sickle cell anemia usually autoinfarct their spleens by the age of 18 months. Thereafter, they are essentially asplenic and are susceptible to overwhelming infections. Occasionally, however, splenomegaly persists and red cells are sequestered in the spleen.[27] During crises, the child may become acutely anemic as a result of a precipitous fall in hemoglobin. Radioactive-tagged red blood cells are rapidly taken up in the spleen to prove the diagnosis. Splenectomy is helpful in preventing the sequestration crises and will decrease the child's transfusion requirements. Gaucher's disease is inherited as an autosomal recessive trait and is caused by a deficiency of the lysosomal enzyme, cerebroside—B glycoside. This leads to an accumulation of cerebroside in the reticuloendothelial cells of the spleen, liver and bone marrow.[28] This results in thrombocytopenia. The hematologic response to splenectomy is good and the patient may be improved by removal of the huge space occupying organ.[29,30] Partial splenic embolization has been advocated in lieu of splenectomy to partially ablate the spleen without the risk of surgery or postoperative sepsis.[31] I could not recommend this procedure because the risks of infarction, abscess and sepsis after embolization outweigh the minimal current risk of preoperative mortality.

Gaucher's disease is a metabolic disorder with autosomal recessive inheritance that involves a defect in the enzyme glucocerebrosidase, which allows the accumulation of glucosyl ceramide in the RE system. The spleen, liver, and bone marrow are the common sites of involvement. In the rarer types, II and III, the central nervous system also is affected. In the more common type I, or nonneuronopathic type, which affects Ashkenazi Jews, the central nervous system is spared. This disease has a variable clinical picture with a wide range of ages of onset, severity, and outcome.[28]

Splenomegaly is a common manifestation of Gaucher's disease and often has been treated by splenectomy. The indications are hypersplenism largely affecting the platelets and pressure symptoms from the enormity of the spleen. Splenectomy has been highly effective for these indications.

Some have argued that since the underlying disease is not affected by splenectomy and the rate of accumulation of glucosyl ceramide is not reduced, there can be rapid progression of bone and liver disease because of an increased accumulation in these sites after splenectomy.[29] In addition, Walker's review, which included nine cases of splenectomy for Gaucher's disease, suggested that these patients may be at especially high risk of sepsis after splenectomy.[30] For these reasons partial splenectomy has been advocated by some.[31–33]

At the Mount Sinai Medical Center in New York City, 12 children ages 15 months through 15 years have undergone spleen surgery for type I Gaucher's disease. Eight total splenectomies were performed. Four children underwent successful partial splenectomy. In 1 of the patients who underwent total splenectomy, partial splenectomy had been abandoned because of hilar bleeding. Another had been returned to the operating room from the recovery room to complete the splenectomy because of significant bleeding from the splenic remnant after partial splenectomy. There has been no evidence of sepsis in any of these 12 patients, and all were cured of hypersplenism. However, serious bone pathologic signs after splenectomy developed in 4 of the 8 patients who underwent total splenectomy. The youngest patient, a 15-month-old infant who underwent partial splenectomy, developed rapid regrowth of the splenic remnant and underwent completion splenectomy only 5 months after partial splenectomy in preparation for a bone marrow transplant.[34]

PARTIAL SPLENECTOMY

The spleen is completely mobilized and one pole that has a single artery and vein with surface lobulation is selected for preservation. Careful ligation of the individual arteries and veins to the remaining bulk of the spleen is performed, causing a line of ischemic demarcation that usually conforms to the lobulation on the surface. The large specimen is excised along this line of demarcation. Bleeding along the cut surface is controlled with a few silk ligatures to the occasional bleeding vessel and with a generous compress of microfibrillar collagen held on the surface under gentle pressure for a few minutes. A closed suction drain is left in place and is removed early postoperatively when there is no bleeding. Since it is possible that partial splenectomy may not be successful, it is wise to prepare all these patients with a polyvalent pneumococcal vaccine (Pneumovax) and to make sure that the family knows that splenectomy is likely. After partial splenectomy, we have performed a liver-spleen scan before discharge to document a well-perfused residual segment of spleen. Usually, this residual segment has been approximately the size of a normal spleen for the age of the child. We have not continued prophylactic antibiotics if the scan shows a well-perfused remnant.

The regrowth of the spleen remnant seen in our youngest patients is expected in at least 20 percent of the cases based on our experience plus the reported cases of partial splenectomy for Gaucher's disease. Since this is a logical consequence of leaving some spleen in this disease, the incidence may prove greater as the years pass, which would dampen the enthusiasm for this operation in this setting.

Tumors of the spleen include hemangiomas and hamartomas, which can cause severe thrombocytopenia and anemia even in the newborn period.[35,36] These lesions may be diagnosed by observing an enlarged spleen in a patient with thrombocytopenia. The specific diagnosis can be made by abdominal CT, ultrasonography, or radionuclide scans. Splenectomy is indicated regardless of the child's age. Lymphangiomas of the spleen may be associated with systemic lymphangiomatosis. There is a large, soft, spongy abdominal mass, which on ultrasound is contiguous with the spleen.

The wandering spleen is one that does not know it is supposed to be firmly attached to the greater curvature of the stomach and fixed securely in the left upper quadrant of the abdomen. The splenorenal, splenocolic ligaments and the peritoneal attachments to the diaphragm and lateral abdominal wall are completely absent. The freely movable spleen is associated with anomalies of intestinal fixation.[37,38] The wandering spleen also has been seen in association with the prune-belly syndrome.[39] The spleen, freed of all its attachments except its pedicle, is free to move about the abdominal cavity. It may appear in the pelvis on 1 day and the midabdomen the next. It may be asymptomatic and mistaken for an abdominal tumor. An astute examiner may palpate a notch in the spleen and make a brilliant guess about the diagnosis. More often, however, the child will have recurrent bouts of undiagnosed abdominal pain or will have an acute abdomen secondary to splenic torsion and infarction. We have observed three patients, all different. The first had abdominal pain and vomiting as an infant, for which he first had a pyloroplasty and then a gastric volvulus (reported in an earlier edition of this book). Finally, 14 years later, at age 19, he returned with an abdominal mass and thrombocytopenia. At operation, the spleen was on a long pedicle and was twisted. Another patient was a 7-year-old boy with a palpable abdominal mass and mild pain. An ultrasound examination demonstrated that the mass was the consistency of spleen, and there was no spleen in the usual location. At operation, there was a nonrotation of the midgut and a partial splenic infarction. The third patient was a 2-year-old girl with Le Jeune dwarfism, with an abdominal mass that also appeared to be spleen on an ultrasound examination. At operation, she had a nonrotation of the midgut, a preduodenal portal vein, and multiple small ectopic spleens in addition to the main mass. Necrosis of the spleen secondary to torsion has been associated with

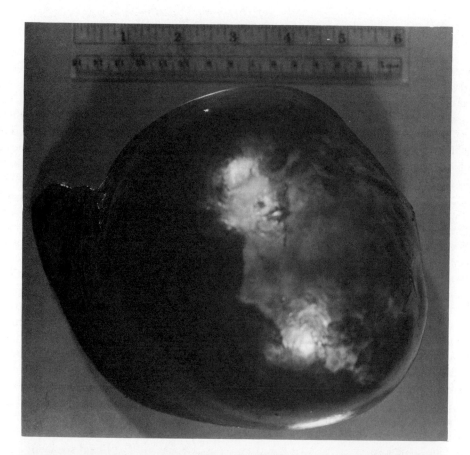

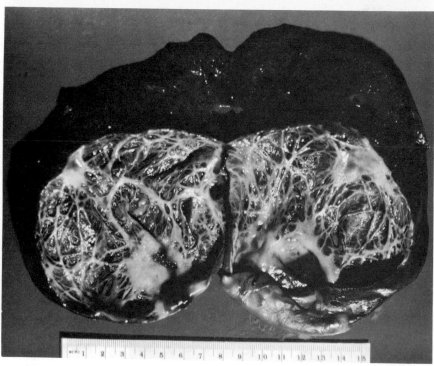

Figure 28–2. Epidermoid cyst of spleen. **Top.** This was a huge, smooth left upper-quadrant mass. **Bottom.** Cut surface showing trabeculations and the epithelial lining.

abscess formation and sepsis. Thus, the wandering spleen is life threatening and not just a curiosity.[40] The new imaging techniques have taken the guesswork (and the glory) out of the diagnosis, since the wandering spleen can be identified with certainty. At operation, if the spleen is infarcted, it must be removed. Otherwise, it can be fixed in the left upper quadrant by simple suture of the hilum to the posterior peritoneum, or a pocket of peritoneum could be created to immbolize the spleen.[41]

Most cysts seen in the United States are noninfectious, although echinococcal cysts may be seen in immigrant children. Since almost all cysts of the spleen are lined by squamous epithelium, it is possible that they are of congenital origin. It is far more likely, however, that they are really pseudocysts secondary to a previous traumatic intrasplenic hematoma. The hematoma is absorbed, leaving fluid in an irregularly septated cyst lined with flattened squamous epithelium. They are diagnosed by palpating a left upper quadrant mass, which on ultrasound or CT examination is cystic. They are filled with either straw-colored or greenish fluid, suggesting brokendown old blood. The wall is trabeculated and smooth (Fig. 28–2). In the past, splenectomy was the recommended treatment, but now a partial splenectomy is perfectly feasible.[42,43] Another, simpler way to preserve the spleen is merely to aspirate the fluid, then remove the outer wall of the cyst. The smooth lining is then approximated to the spleen's capsule with a running hemostatic lock stitch.[44]

Classically, splenic abscesses were due to endocarditis, sickle cell disease, trauma, or systemic sepsis.[45] The typical, solitary, large abscess is rarely seen in children. A totally different type of abscess is now seen in the hospital population of immunodeficient children. One of our children suffered with aplastic anemia and a necrotizing perianal infection and then developed splenic abscesses. Three others were children with acute lymphoblastic leukemia being treated with intensive chemotherapy. Each was persistently septic, one with *Candida* and the other with staphlococci, even with adequate intravenous antibiotics. Neither had specific abdominal symptoms, although on retrospective questioning, both had noted mild left shoulder pain. CT scans demonstrated small, multiple lesions in the spleen that were correctly interpreted as abscesses. The spleens were not particularly enlarged, but each child became afebrile after splenectomy. It was important to remove the focus of infection in preparation for a bone marrow transplant.

TECHNIQUE FOR SPLENECTOMY

If there are gallstones, a transverse incision that crosses both rectus muscles is used for combined splenectomy and cholecystectomy. Otherwise, for an elective splenectomy, the child is placed on the right side with the table broken to increase the space between the iliac crest and the ribs (Fig. 28–3). The patient is rolled back slightly so that more of the abdomen is exposed than the back. The incision is in the flank and extends into the oblique musculature of the abdomen, almost to the lateral border of the rectus sheath. Care is taken to prevent damage to the 10th and 11th intercostal nerves, which lie between the transversalis and internal oblique muscles. After incision of the skin, subcutaneous tissues, and fascia with a scalpel, the rest of the incision is made with the cutting current of the electrocoagulation unit. With this incision, the small intestine falls completely away from the operating field. In the course of the operation, it never requires manipulation or packing. This significantly reduces postoperative ileus and hastens recovery. When the peritoneum is opened, separate the caudal end of the spleen from the colon. When the lower pole of the spleen has been separated from the colon, it is grasped with a moist sponge and brought forward and inferiorly to expose its posterior peritoneal attachments. These attachments are divided with the cutting current, with great care taken to coagulate any small vessels. As these attachments of the spleen are divided, the spleen is withdrawn further into the incision until the diaphragmatic attachments also are divided under direct vision.

When removing a spleen for hematologic disease (especially for thrombocytopenia), one must be meticulous in controlling each small vessel to prevent postoperative hemorrhage. There is usually a short peritoneal fold between the upper pole of the spleen and the greater curvature of the stomach. This is divided between ligatures to include the uppermost short gastric vessels. These arteries may be only a few millimeters in length. It is consequently necessary to suture-ligate them on the stomach side in order to prevent postoperative hemorrhage. When all the short gastric vessels have been suture-ligated and divided, the spleen, with the tail of the pancreas, is delivered into the incision. The vessels in the splenic hilum are individually dissected and sutureligated. Lymph nodes often obscure the main artery and vein, so it is frequently safer to ligate the vessels after they bifurcate near the spleen. If the splenic artery is ligated first, the spleen contracts, providing an autotransfusion. When the spleen has been removed, a search for accessory spleens is made in the splenic hilum, along the dorsal surface of the pancreas, in the greater omentum, and along the mesocolon (Fig. 28–4). The bed of the spleen is packed with a warm moist pad, and then a search is made for bleeding vessels. Each must be ligated or coagulated to leave a completely dry field. Wound closure is accomplished with continuous polyglycolate sutures. When the lower intercostal nerves and

238

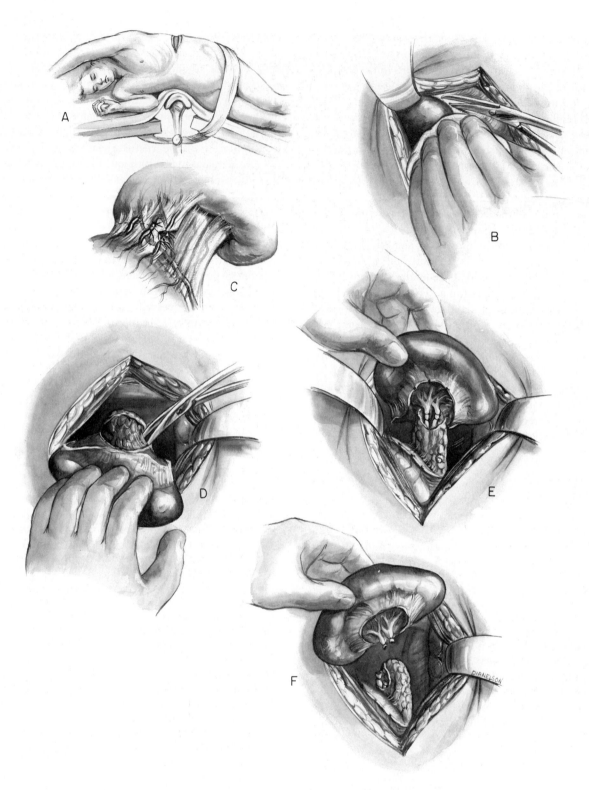

Figure 28–3. Technique for splenectomy with a lateral flank incision. This is appropriate when there are no gallstones and the operation is being performed for hematologic purposes. The child is placed on her side, and the operating table is broken to elevate the left flank. Hemostasis is obtained with the electrocautery and careful ligation of the short gastric and splenic vessels. Suture ligatures are used on the gastric side to prevent loosening of the ligature in the event of postoperative gastric distention.

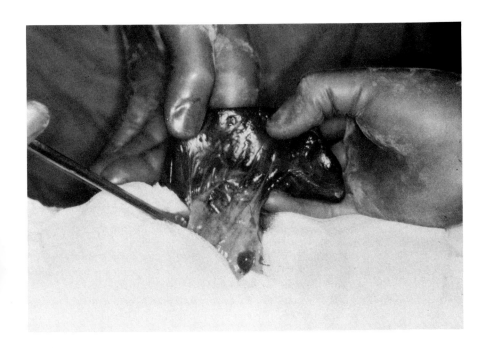

Figure 28–4. Ectopic spleens are most commonly found either in the hilum or, as shown here, along the pancreas.

the wound are infiltrated with bupivacaine, immediate postoperative pain is minimized, and the need for narcotics is greatly reduced. This allows immediate ambulation, eliminates ileus and the need for a gastric tube, and hastens recovery. Within the past 5 years, 80 percent of our patients have been discharged home on the third postoperative day.

REFERENCES

1. King H, Schumacker HB: Splenic studies: Increased susceptibility to infection after splenectomy performed in infancy. Ann Surg 136:239, 1952
2. Peters AM: Splenic blood flow and blood flow kinetics. Clin Haematol 12:422, 1983
3. Weiss L: The red pulp of the spleen: Structural basis of blood flow. Clin Haematol 12:375, 1983
4. Hooareesuwan S, Ho M, Wattanagoon Y: Dynamic alteration in splenic function during acute falciparum malaria. N Engl J Med 317:675, 1987
5. Horan M, Colebutch JH: Relation between splenectomy and subsequent infection: A clinical study. Arch Dis Child 37:398, 1962
6. Eraklis A, Filler R: Splenectomy in childhood: A review of 1413 cases. J Pediatr Surg 7:382, 1972
7. Walker W: Splenectomy in childhood: A review in England and Wales, 1960–64. Br J Surg 63:36, 1976
8. Singer DB: Postsplenectomy sepsis. Perspect Pediatr Pathol 1:285, 1973
9. Robinette CD, Fraumeni JF: Splenectomy and subsequent mortality in veterans of the 1939–45 war. Lancet 2:127, 1977
10. Balpanz JR, Nesbitt ME, Jarvis L, Krivit W: Overwhelm-

ing sepsis following splenectomy for trauma. J Pediatr 88:458, 1976
11. Chaikop E, McCabe C: Fatal overwhelming postsplenectomy infection. Am J Surg 149:534, 1985
12. MacKinney AA, Morton NE, Kosower NS, Schilling RF: Ascertaining genetic carriers of hereditary spherocytosis by statistical analysis of multiple laboratory tests. J Clin Invest 41:554, 1962
13. Croom R, McMillan C, Orringer E, Sheldon G: Hereditary spherocytosis: Recent experience and current concepts of pathophysiology. Ann Surg 203:34, 1986
14. Schilling RF: Hereditary spherocytosis, a study of splenectomized persons. Semin Hematol 13:169, 1976
15. Grosfeld JL, Naffis D, Boles T Jr, Newton WA Jr: The role of splenectomy in neonatal idiopathic thrombocytopenic purpura. J Pediatr Surg 5:166, 1970
16. McClure PD: Idiopathic thrombocytopenic purpura in children: Should corticosteroids by given? Am J Dis Child 131:357, 1977
17. Zuelzer WW, Lusher JM: Childhood idiopathic thrombocytopenic purpura: To treat or not to treat? Am J Dis Child 131:360, 1977
18. Shulman NR, Marder VJ, Weinrach RS: Similarities between known antiplatelet antibodies and the factor responsible for thrombocytopenia in idiopathic purpura—physiologic, serologic, and isotopic studies. Ann NY Acad Sci 124:499, 1965
19. Block GE, Evans R, Zatchuk R: Splenectomy for idiopathic thrombocytopenic purpura. Arch Surg 92:484, 1966
20. Charlesworth D, Torrance HB: Splenectomy in idiopathic thrombocytopenic purpura. Br J Surg 55:437, 1968
21. Zerella JT, Martin LW, Lampkin GC: Emergency splenectomy for idiopathic thrombocytopenic purpura in children. J Pediatr Surg 13:243, 1978
22. Wallace D, Fromm D, Thomas D: Accessory splenectomy

for idiopathic thrombocytopenic purpura. Surgery 9:134, 1982

23. Bussel JB, Schulman J: IV IgG in the treatment of chronic immune thrombocytopenia purpura as a means to defer splenectomy. J Pediatr 103:651, 1953

24. Warrier I, Lusher JM: IV IgG treatment for chronic ITP in children. Am J Med 76:193, 1984

25. Waerner S, Abildgaard C, French B: Intracranial hemorrhage in children with idiopathic thrombocytopenia purpura. Pediatrics 67:453, 1981

26. Pringle K, Spigos D, Tau W, Politis C: Partial splenic embolization in the management of thalassemia major. J Pediatr Surg 17:884, 1982

27. Topley JM, Rogers DW, Stevens MC: Acute splenic sequestration and hypersplenism in the first five years in homozygous sickle cell disease. Arch Dis Child 56:765, 1981

28. Brady RO, Barranger JA: Glucosylceramide lipidosis: Gaucher's disease. In Standbury JB, Wyngaarden J, Goldstein J, et al: The Metabolic Basis of Inherited Disease, 5th ed., New York, McGraw-Hill, 1983, pp 841–846

29. Rose JS, Grabowski GA, Barnett SH, Desnick RJ: Accelerated skeletal deterioration after splenectomy in Gaucher's type I disease. AJR 139:1202, 1982

30. Walker W: Splenectomy in childhood: A review in England and Wales, 1960–4. Br J Surg 63:36, 1976

31. Bar-Maor JA, Govrin-Yehudain J: Partial splenectomy in children with Gaucher's disease. Pediatrics 76:398, 1985

32. Rodgers BM, Tribble C, Joob A: Partial splenectomy for Gaucher's disease. Ann Surg 205:693, 1986

33. Rubin M, Yampolski I, Lambrozo R, et al: Partial splenectomy in Gaucher's disease. J Pediatr Surg 21:125, 1986

34. Hobbs JR, Jones KH, Shaw PJ, et al: Beneficial effect of pre-transplant splenectomy on displacement bone marrow transplantation for Gaucher's syndrome. Lancet 1:1111, 1987

35. Spencer S, Coulter-Knopp A, Day D, et al: Splenic hemangioma with thrombocytopenia in a newborn. Pediatrics 79:960, 1987

36. Symptomatic splenic hamartoma: Report of two cases and review of the literature. Pediatrics 66:261, 1980

37. Thompson J, Ross R, Pizzaro S: The wandering spleen in infancy and childhood. Clin Pediatr 19:222, 1980

38. Taha A, Bugonski R, El-Shapie M: Torsion of a wandering spleen: A rare cause of acute abdomen. Contemp Surg 31:16, 1987

39. Teramoto R, Opas LM, Andrassy R: Splenic torsion with prune-belly syndrome. J Pediatr 89:91, 1981

40. Kelly K, Chusid MJ, Camitta BM: Splenic torsion in an infant associated with secondary disseminated Haemophilus influenzae. Clin Pediatr 21:365, 1982

41. Stringel G, Sovey P, Mercer S: Torsion of wandering spleen: Splenectomy or splenopexy. J Pediatr Surg 74:373, 1982

42. Sink J, Filstom H, Kivks D, et al: Removal of a splenic cyst with salvage of functional splenic tissue. J Pediatr 100:412, 1982

43. Khan A, Bensoussan A, Blanchard H, et al: Partial splenectomy for benign cystic lesions of the spleen. J Pediatr Surg 21:749, 1986

44. Touloukian R, Seashore J: Partial splenic decapsulation: A simplified operation for splenic pseudocyst. J Pediatr Surg 22:135, 1987

45. Chum C, Ropp M: Splenic abscess. Medicine 59:50, 1980

29
Rectal Prolapse

Prolapse of the rectum is a troublesome but usually self-limiting problem affecting children from 1 to 3 years of age. During this period the rectal mucosa is loosely attached to the underlying muscularis.[1] In addition, the sacrum is somewhat flattened rather than curved posteriorly. This directs intraabdominal pressure toward the anus instead of into the hollow of the pelvis. Diarrhea, straining, and any condition that reduces pelvic tissue tone will predispose to prolapse. Such conditions include malnutrition, cystic fibrosis of the pancreas, exstrophy of the bladder, meningomyelocele, and repair of an imperforate anus.

The prolapse usually involves only 2 or 3 cm of mucosa, which appear only when the child strains at stool. There may be some bleeding along with the prolapse, but not before. This points to an important difference between prolapse of a rectal polyp and true prolapse. With a rectal polyp, the family will describe bleeding before the appearance of a "raspberry" at the anus. A true rectal prolapse looks like a rosette of red mucosal tissue. With sphincter paralysis, as with a meningomyelocele, the entire rectal wall may prolapse for several inches. If the bowel is not reduced promptly, the mucosa bleeds, becomes progressively edematous, and is more difficult to reduce.

The diagnosis is made easily if the child prolapses the rectum while straining in the office. This also may occur after a rectal examination. The evaluation must always include a careful digital examination for a polyp, and if there is a history of rectal bleeding, proctoscopy is indicated. The stools are examined for ova and parasites, and a sweat test for cystic fibrosis of the pancreas must always be performed.

TREATMENT

Treatment of obvious predisposing causes—such as intestinal parasites, infectious diarrhea, constipation, or cystic fibrosis—will cure the prolapse. There is a rarely specific etiology, but the usual prolapse is reduced easily by the parents, and the problem spontaneously disappears after a few months. The parents are often frightened and "want something done." They should be reassured and given gloves to aid in the reduction, and a diet should be prescribed that is designed to soften the stool. There is no benefit in the old practice of taping the child's buttocks together. This is messy and ineffective.

Several authors have recommended submucosal injection of such sclerosing solutions as 30 percent saline or 5 percent phenol in oil.[2,3] Injections produce considerable submucosal and perirectal fibrosis. We observed one child who had developed a rectal stricture following an injection at another institution. In addition, Kay and Zachary reported 3 perirectal abscesses in 51 patients injected with 30 percent saline.[3] This procedure does not appear to be indicated in the usual simple mucosal prolapse.

When there is prolapse of the entire rectal wall, particularly with a patulous anus, that recurs persistently over a period of several months, we prefer the presacral operation described by Ashcraft et al.[4] The child is anesthetized and placed in the prone position with his buttocks strapped apart. The rectum is liberally irrigated with povidone-iodine before the skin is prepared. A midline incision is then made over the coccyx, which is removed. This allows access to the rectum in the presacral space. The rectum is dissected along its posterior wall until the levator sling is identified. The sling is lifted away from the rectum, and when sufficiently mobilized, the sling is sutured from side to side so that the rectum is snug against either a size 8 Hegar dilator or the surgeon's fifth finger.

After the levator sling has been tightened, the posterior wall of the rectum is drawn up and sutured to the presacral fascia. Thus, the rectum is suspended from within the pelvis, and by tightening of the sling, it is curved forward in such a way that intraabdominal pressure is directed toward the sacrum. We originally used heavy silk sutures, as recommended by Ashcraft, but after one patient "spit out" her silk sutures, we decided on polyglycolic acid material. This problem was the only complication in nine patients, and we have had no recurrences. This appears to be a simple, reliable operation that will effectively cure a severe rectal prolapse.

Postoperatively, the child is given a clear liquid diet and mineral oil until there is a bowel movement.

REFERENCES

1. Herzog B: Rectal prolapse in childhood. Helvetica Chir Acta 37:575, 1970
2. Wyllie GG: The injection treatment of rectal prolapse. J Pediatr Surg 14:62, 1979
3. Kay N, Zachary R: The treatment of rectal prolapse in children with injections of 30 percent saline solutions. J Pediatr Surg 5:334, 1970
4. Ashcraft K, Amoury R, Holder T: Levator repair and posterior suspension for rectal prolapse. J Pediatr Surg 12:241, 1977

SECTION IV

Trauma

Accidental injury is the chief cause of death in children from 1 to 14 years of age. Most injuries in children, however, are simple contusions, lacerations, and fractures. Trauma of this magnitude, along with some one-system injuries, can be cared for by skilled surgeons in a well-equipped community hospital. Ideally, in the emergency rooms of general hospitals, there should be separate facilities for children so the child and his parents can be spared the sight of sick, injured, or drunk adults. The young patient with multiple or complex injuries, especially those with central nervous system damage, should be transferred to special pediatric trauma centers. The trauma center must have a transportation and communications system that includes trained paramedics, nurses, and surgeons to treat children at the accident scene or to aid in the treatment at local hospitals. This team expedites transportation of the child to a children's center.

In our hospital, the trauma team consists of an on-call pediatric surgeon, a pediatric surgical fellow, general surgery residents, and consultants from all the pediatric surgical specialties. A general surgery resident goes with the transport nurses to stabilize the child for transfer, which may be by either helicopter or ambulance.

Paramedics require special training to deal with children and must have guidelines as to when the injured child should be taken to a special center. It is essential for everyone concerned with traumatized patients to reflexively know, understand, and apply the ABCs of trauma. At the accident scene, airway management often requires the insertion of an oral airway or even an endotracheal tube. Initially, the cervical spine and long bones are immobilized, and, if possible, intravenous fluids are started. However, rapid transport to a hospital emergency room is preferable to sophisticated resuscitation efforts in the field.

Assessment of the child in the emergency room begins with a rapid total body survey, commencing with the airway and breathing. Again at this point, it may be necessary to ensure efficient ventilation by the use of an oral or endotracheal airway, needle thoracentesis, or chest tube placement. The circulation is quickly assessed by observation of skin color, capillary refill, and palpation of the pulses. Simultaneous with this initial evaluation, obvious external bleeding is controlled, and blood is drawn for type and crossmatch, hematocrit, and serum amylase. A large-bone intravenous line is inserted, and 20 ml/kg of warm lactated Ringer's solution is given if the vital signs are depressed. The level of consciousness is assessed, and the Glasgow coma score is determined.

Next, the spine, abdomen, and extremities are quickly evaluated, and cardiac monitoring is instituted. While the child is still in the emergency room, a gastric tube is passed to prevent vomiting and aspiration and to relieve acute gastric distention. If there is no blood at the urinary meatus, a catheter is passed into the bladder to determine the presence of hematuria and to measure urinary output. This initial resuscitation should be accomplished in no more than 10 to 20 minutes! Now, a more detailed physical examination is performed to search for overlooked or occult trauma, such as an unexpected bruise or bullet hole in the patient's back. The chest is again palpated and auscultated, and the tracheal position is examined. Carefully palpate and auscultate the abdomen looking for bruises, tenderness, and distention. Palpate and compress the pelvis and finally, run your hands up and down each extremity searching for an overlooked fracture and to palpate for each peripheral pulse. Also at this time, portable x-rays are obtained of the cervical spine and chest. These examinations will determine the need for further consultation, imaging studies, and treatment. A fractured femur is placed in a traction splint and immobilized. Other long bone fractures are splinted until there is time for proper radiographic evaluation. If there is no central nervous system injury, it is perfectly proper at this time to give intravenous analgesia to relieve the pain of fractures. While the child is in the emergency room and x-ray suite, particular attention must be paid to prevent hypothermia. All intravenous fluids are prewarmed in the emergency room, and while the child is exposed on the examining table, infra-red lights are used to prevent heat loss.

At our hospital, children with head and suspected abdominal injuries are taken for computed tomography (CT) as soon as they are resuscitated. In fact, the child in coma with a dilated pupil may have the intravenous line and other tubes inserted while the CT scan is in progress. If there is suspected abdominal injury or if the child cannot cooperate for an abdominal examination, a CT of the abdomen is taken at the same time as the head CT. Roentgenograms are obtained also of the chest and long bones. If there is a suggestion of urethral or bladder injury, the initial evaluation also includes a cystourethrogram.

There are few indications for an immediate operation in an injured child. Acute intracranial hematomas must be drained within minutes. Open fractures or major soft tissue wounds must be debrided and closed when the child is hemodynamically stable. Penetrating wounds of the abdomen will require an urgent laparotomy. On the other hand, children with blunt abdominal injuries are often stable, and even though they may have had an immediate episode of bleeding, their bleeding will stop, and they can be observed in an intensive care unit. If these children show signs of ongoing blood loss or unstable vital signs, they may still require an immediate operation.

When one surgeon plans and directs the child's overall care, there is less likelihood that occult injuries will be overlooked. In our hospital, the child with injuries in more than one organ system is admitted to the pediatric surgical service for evaluation and stabilization. It is sometimes necessary for the general surgeon to determine the relative importance of various injuries and the sequence of their treatment by the surgical specialists. Optimum care of the traumatized child includes immediate attention to his or her nutritional and psychologic support and includes long-range plans for full physical and psychologic rehabilitation.

30
Soft Tissue Trauma

There are several principles of trauma care that should be applied to children with even the most trivial injuries. A child's cry is often worse than his injury, and a trickle of blood frightens both the child and parents. Sincere, conscientious efforts to soothe the child and the parents pay large dividends, not only in making the job easier but in improved public relations. Insist that the parent stay with the child during treatment. Even if the mother is upset, she is more likely to calm down when she holds her child's hand and sees that the physician and nurses are doing good work. She will then have a better understanding of postoperative instructions.

The immediate application of an ice bag or a sterile towel soaked in iced saline will relieve the pain and swelling of ordinary contusions and burns. If the child is an unreasonable 2- or 3-year-old, one has the choice of using restraints or sedation. A full body restraint must be terrifying to an injured child, and there is the further danger that he or she will vomit and aspirate while restrained because of being unable to turn to the side. A mixture of 2 mg each of Demerol and Phenergan per kilogram of body weight, up to a maximum of 50 mg, will produce tranquility within 20 to 30 minutes. This combination provides pain relief with sedation and is superior to barbiturates and narcotics. It provides suitable sedation for suture of lacerations, painful dressing changes, debridement, and for the reduction of simple fractures. Any child who has been sedated for an outpatient procedure must have vital signs checked and must be observed in the emergency room until he or she is completely awake and responding appropriately.

ANESTHESIA

An unhurried approach and conversation to distract the child are important to every procedure performed under local anesthesia. One percent lidocaine may be sprayed on open lacerations or abrasions from a syringe without a needle, or it may be applied on a soaked sponge. This drug is also effective when sprayed on mucous membranes. A nearly painless injection through normal skin can be obtained with the following technique. As the skin is prepared with a cool antiseptic solution, the child is told that the cold will help make the skin numb. When the child is accustomed to the antiseptic, you then lightly touch the site with a fingertip. Gradually increase the finger pressure on the site of injection, and then slip a 27-gauge needle with the bevel down beneath your finger. Continued pressure on the needle tip while injecting the anesthetic agent raises a skin wheal without the usual jab. More anesthetic is then slowly injected through the skin wheal. Local infiltration usually is sufficient, although digital or other regional blocks are successful in a cooperative child.

Children with extensive soft tissue injuries or those with nerve or tendon involvement require admission to the hospital and general anesthesia.

LACERATIONS

The skin about any laceration is washed with soap and water, after which the wound is irrigated with a syringe and sterile saline. Bleeding from simple lacerations usually can be controlled with pressure. In rare cases a bleeding vessel will require ligation with fine catgut. Superficial wounds are closed with strips of sterile adhesive tape applied at right angles to the wound, with care to evert, rather than invert, the edges. In deeper wounds, fat and fascia are first closed with 5–0 or 4–0 chromic catgut placed so that the knot is inverted. Care must be taken to correctly match creases, edges of hairlines, and other skin landmarks and to avoid dog ears at the end of the laceration. Even in wounds, where sutures are required for deeper layers, every effort should be made to close the skin with sterile tape strips. Children often are more frightened of having sutures removed than of the original procedure. Furthermore, the tape strips can be left undisturbed for prolonged periods, thus providing the wound with continued support. More extensive wounds with ragged beveled edges require debridement with a scalpel in order to achieve improved healing and a straight-line scar. When skin sutures are necessary, only 6–0 or 5–0 nylon should be used, so as to minimize suture marks about the wound. These sutures are removed as soon as possible, and the wound is supported with sterile tapes for 10 to 14 days. Alternatively, 6–0 catgut placed through the skin will dissolve in a few days, leaving a nice scar without the need to remove sutures.

Minor skin losses over areas of fat and muscle may be treated by undermining adjacent tissue to develop local flaps that may be closed without tension. More extensive avulsions require skin grafting. Undermined wounds that produce a flap present a difficult problem. It is safe to suture a flap that is wider than it is long, but if the flap is long and narrow, it should be sequentially excised until there is active bleeding; otherwise the flap will necrose. Whenever there is a doubt about the viability of large skin flaps, the child should be admitted to the hospital, and repair should be carried out in the operating room with general anesthesia to achieve an optimum closure. A compression dressing and rest of the involved area are essential until healing has taken place.

After repair of traumatic wounds in the emergency room, the responsible surgeon must give the parents detailed instructions for care of the child and the dressings. Rest and elevation are recommended until the first dressing change. If there are complaints of fever, unusual discharge on the dressings, or pain that is not relieved by acetaminophen or aspirin, the child must be returned and the wound must be inspected.

Minimal dressings are used for elective abdominal and thoracic incisions in order to reduce respiratory restraint. However, traumatic wounds of the face and extremities require meticulous dressing techniques. A properly applied dressing will absorb exudate, control edema and bleeding, and, most importantly, immobilize the injured area. One layer of nonadherent material, such as lightly impregnated petrolatum gauze, is placed next to the wound. Absorbent gauze is then cut to fit the wound area and surrounding contours. On the face and scalp, small dressings may be held in place with elastic adhesive tape, but in general a Kerlix gauze bandage will serve to hold the dressing in place. On the hand, fingers are individually dressed. Then the entire hand and the forearm are encased in a voluminous dressing that is firmly secured with multiple strips of adhesive tape. A similar dressing is used for foot injuries. All extremity injuries, including small wounds of the digits, are dressed in this manner because active children will remove the bandage and soil the wound if anything less is applied.

PENETRATING WOUNDS

Puncture wounds produced by fragments of wood or shards of glass are more serious than they appear on the surface. These wounds frequently are deep, with severing of tendons and nerves, and there is always the possibility that a foreign body has broken off under the skin. The safest course to follow is to cover the wound with a sterile dressing and obtain an x-ray of the area. Large wood and glass splinters will be outlined against radiolucent fat, and even if negative, the x-ray may be helpful from a medicolegal standpoint if a foreign body is later found in the wound. Transillumination of an extremity against a bright light often will reveal the location of a foreign object. If the x-ray is negative, the wound must be explored to its depths, cleansed, and irrigated. Deep wounds may require drainage and a pressure dressing rather than suture of the superficial layers. Family members are warned about the possible presence of an overlooked foreign body and instructed to return if there is any wound drainage.

Bites

A mentally deranged sibling or parent may bite a child, but human bites are more common in fights between teenagers, when a clenched fist may strike an opponent's teeth. This often produces puncture wounds that are contaminated with anaerobic streptococci, fusiform bacilli, spirochetes, and other oral bacteria.[1] The result is a rapidly progressive synergistic infection. Human bite wounds are debrided, liberally irrigated with povidone-iodine solution, and left open. Broad-spectrum antibiotics, including penicillin, are administered in the hospital while the wound is treated with wet dressings. Small wounds will heal spontaneously, but a larger bite may require a delayed primary closure or a skin graft.

Dog bites are a common emergency room problem. Usually the animal is a family pet who has been teased by the child. German shepherds are the most common offenders and can inflict serious bites. Tooth abrasions and small wounds require only local cleansing and a nonadherent dressing. More extensive dog bites are usually parallel, crescent-shaped, deep lacerations with considerable surrounding contusion and hematoma (Fig. 30–1). They are contaminated with a variety of organisms, particularly *Pasturella multocida*, which is sensitive to penicillin.

Small children can be severely mauled by large dogs, and bites on the trunk may cause peritonitis or

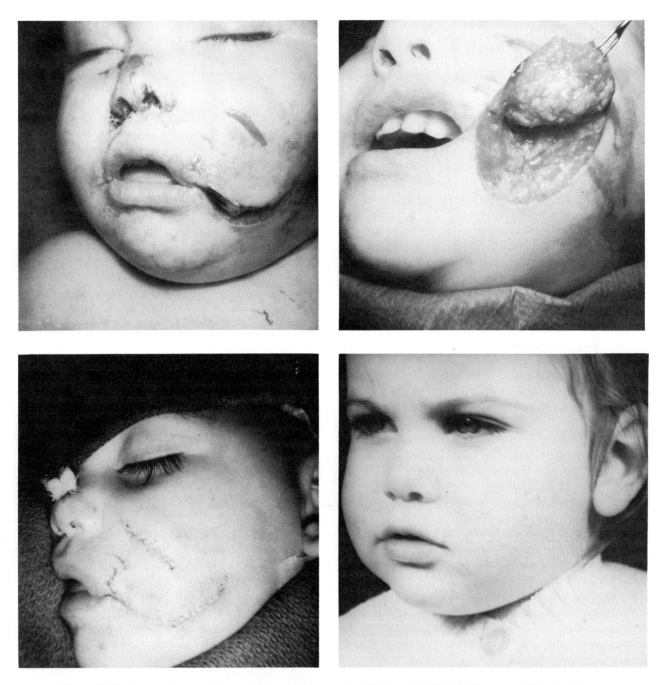

Figure 30–1. German shepherd bite to the face of a 1-year-old child. **Top left.** Multiple bites were inflicted by the closing jaws. **Top right.** Undermining by the lower teeth produced a flap. **Bottom left.** The wound was debrided and closed under general anesthesia. **Bottom right.** Result 6 months later. (*Courtesy of Dr. Richard Schultz*)

death.[2] Schultz and McMasters reviewed the results in 116 children under 10 years of age who had suffered severe dog bites, most of which were on the face.[3] They obtained successful primary closures of these wounds after extensive wound cleaning with soap and water, together with the excision of 1 to 2 mm of skin on either side of the wound to remove shelved edges of skin and to open deeper layers to further irrigation and debride-

ment. Of these patients, 30 percent required later scar revision, and interestingly, 32 percent became involved in personal litigation with the dogs' owners. Our own experience indicates that facial wounds usually can be closed after adequate debridement in the hospital. Although antibiotics should be given, their effectiveness in preventing infections is questionable.[4] Bites inflicted by other household pets and rodents are cleansed, irrigated, and left open. Bites by wild carnivores, especially skunk, fox, raccoon, bat, and wild dog bites, carry a significant threat of rabies. In the United States, 1 to 3 cases of human rabies have occurred yearly since 1960. The incidence in dogs has dropped from 8000 cases in 1946 to 129 in 1975. Unfortunately, the wild carnivores mentioned maintain an appreciable reservoir of rabies in this country.[5]

The two agents most commonly used to protect patients bitten by suspected animals are duck embryo vaccine, prepared from embryonated duck eggs infected with a fixed virus, and immune globulin, which is antirabies gamma globulin concentrated from the plasma of hyperimmunized human donors.

The US Public Health Service currently recommends the following approach to dog and wild animal bites. A bite by a domestic animal that has been vaccinated for rabies poses no threat, and only wound care is indicated. After a bite by a domestic dog, the animal is observed for 10 days by a veterinarian. If the dog remains well, nothing further must be done. If the bite was inflicted by a wild animal or a domestic dog whose behavior is suspicious, the animal is killed and the head is sent under refrigeration to the nearest state public health laboratory, where the brain is examined by fluorescent microscopy. In the meantime, the patient is given an immediate dose of 20 IU/kg of rabies immune globulin. Half the dose is injected around the wound, and the rest is given in the buttock. If the fluorescent test is positive or if the animal cannot be found, a series of 21 doses of duck embryo vaccine must be given. Two are given daily, subcutaneously, for the first 7 days, then one dose is given daily for another week. In addition, booster doses are given 10 and 20 days later. Most patients develop pain and erythema at the injection site, and 30 percent will develop a low-grade fever and malaise. The incidence of anaphylaxis is high enough that antihistamines and epinephrine should be available when each dose is given. The decision to administer rabies prophylaxis is difficult. Health departments are able to provide up-to-date information on the current incidence of rabies in the local animal population when doubtful situations arise.

Snakebite. The pit viper, rattlesnake, copperhead, and cottonmouth water moccasin are the most common poisonous snakes in North America. Bites by poisonous snakes cause severe immediate pain, with rapidly progressing local edema and tissue destruction. In addition, there are hemolysis and prolongation of the prothrombin and bleeding times. If there is not local pain within an hour after the bite, it is likely that the snake was nonpoisonous. First aid treatment consists of the application of a broad tourniquet just tight enough to occlude the lymphatics and veins. Local cooling may be of some benefit

but should not be prolonged. Immediate excision rather than incision of the fang marks will remove a larger concentration of venom than suction treatment. There is considerable morbidity associated with wound excision. Consequently, this treatment may be avoided if there is immediate access to antivenin. Wyeth laboratories produces a polyvalent antivenin that is effective against pit viper bites. Ten vials of the antivenin diluted in saline are given intravenously within the first hour of treatment. More is given as required. One child bitten by a rattlesnake required 75 vials to control her symptoms.[6] It is difficult to estimate the amount of antivenin required, and serum sickness due to horse serum is a common complication. Coral snake bites require a specific antivenin. In addition, coral snake venom causes paralysis of the cranial nerves and respiratory arrest. Thus, endotracheal intubation and ventilator support may be necessary.[7] Antibiotic administration, fluid therapy, blood transfusions, and local wound debridement or even fasciotomy may become necessary in the management of severe snake bite.

TETANUS PROPHYLAXIS

Tetanus is most likely to occur after puncture wounds, dirty lacerations, or crush injuries in children who have not had a full immunization series. A surprisingly large number of children are encountered in city emergency rooms for whom there is only a vague history of immunizations or about whom there is reason to believe that no immunizations have been given. The Infectious Disease Committee of the American Academy of Pediatrics has made the following recommendations for tetanus prophylaxis in children with injuries.[8] Children with clean minor wounds who have completed a primary series of tetanus toxoid or received a booster dose within 10 years require no further therapy. If the history is uncertain or more than 10 years have elapsed, they are given a booster dose of toxoid. For serious or contaminated wounds, a booster dose is given if one has not been given during the past 5 years. If the history is uncertain, the child with a contaminated or puncture wound is given a booster dose and, in addition, 250 to 500 units of tetanus immune globulin.

SOFT TISSUE INJURIES OF THE UPPER EXTREMITIES

Injuries of the hand and arm carry the potential threat of crippling nerve and tendon injuries. Further, deformities of fingers or the hand are cosmetically unattractive.

A careful functional examination of the hand is carried out before any disturbance of the wound. Simple

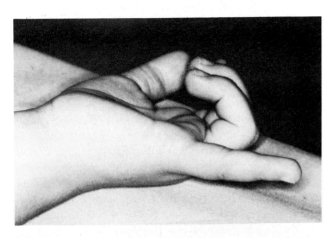

Figure 30–2. This child sustained a palmar laceration, with division of both the sublimus and profundus tendons to the fifth finger. The affected digit remains in extension when the hand is at rest.

observation of the child's hand during repose and in activity often will lead to a diagnosis of nerve or tendon damage (Fig. 30–2). Considerable patience is required, however, to distinguish between disuse of a part because of pain or because of anatomic injury. A cooperative patient can actively flex and extend the wrist and each digit. Specifically observe for flexion of the terminal phalanx to determine function of the profundus tendon. Adduction and abduction of the index and ring fingers to and from the middle finger constitute a test for ulnar nerve motor function. Next, have the child raise his or her thumb away from the palm and touch the tip of the little finger to determine median nerve activity. There is considerable overlap in sensory areas, but the lateral surface and tip of the little finger are wholly innervated by the ulnar nerve. The palmar surface and tip of the thumb are supplied by the median nerve. Commence the sensory examination with a wisp of cotton, then test with the tip of an intravenous needle. Radial nerve damage results in wristdrop and loss of sensation at the dorsal web space between the thumb and the second metacarpal. When there is any suggestion of nerve or tendon injury, examination of the wound itself must be carried out in the operating room with the child under anesthesia. Further, if there is bleeding from a small, deep hand wound, one must never blindly clamp with a hemostat. The bleeding is controlled with pressure, and when the wound is prepared, it may be extended until the bleeding point is clearly visible.

Fingertip Avulsions
Children frequently get fingertips caught in slammed doors. If the digit is hanging by a flap, it is gently washed and irrigated, and the remainder of the finger is painted with tincture of benzoin. The avulsed tissue is gently replaced and held with crisscross strips of sterile tape

(Fig. 30–3). A mitten pressure dressing is then applied, and the child's parents are instructed to keep the entire hand and arm elevated on pillows for 2 days. There is less trauma and equally good apposition of the tissue with tapes as there is with sutures. The tape strips are left in place for 10 days to 2 weeks. At that time, there may be a patch of black skin, but frequently there is complete healing. Partial avulsions that dislocate the nail require a digital block for anesthesia and careful replacement of the nail on its matrix beneath the dorsal skin. The fingertip is again held with sterile tapes. Even though the nail loosens, it will protect the sensitive underlying tissue until a new nail grows.

A variety of surgical treatments have been described for complete amputation of the fingertip. These include coverage of the defect with flaps of palmar skin and with advancement flaps from the lateral surface of the finger.[9] Douglas and Illingworth independently have described a treatment that consists of simple dressings and that results in regrowth and remodeling of the fingertip.[10,11] The wound is cleansed gently but not debrided, and the exposed bone is left intact. The wound is then covered with crisscross sterile tape strips and a bulky mitten dressing. The initial dressing is left in place for 2 weeks. Both Douglas and Illingworth observed healing within 11 to 12 weeks, with an excellent cosmetic result. This technique is satisfactory for infants, who heal relatively rapidly. We have observed the development of considerable excess granulation tissue in fingers

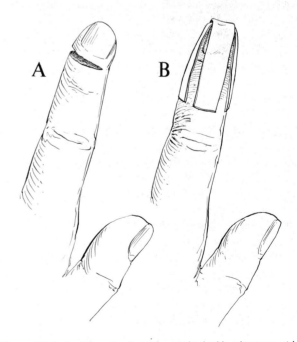

Figure 30–3. Avulsion of a fingertip repaired with crisscross strips of sterile tape. Occasionally, it is necessary to approximate the subcutaneous tissue with one or two catgut sutures. The hand is then encased in a large bulky dressing that extends to the elbow.

treated in this fashion, and the duration of healing seems excessive. The application of a small split-thickness skin graft achieves rapid healing, especially in older children. The fingertip is gently cleansed by soaking the finger in soap and water. After a digital block or the application of 1 percent lidocaine to the raw tissue, the hematoma is removed, and the digital arteries are ligated if they are still bleeding. Next, the inside of the upper arm is infiltrated with lidocaine, and a small split-thickness skin graft is cut with a razor blade held with a hemostat. This graft is held in place with crisscross strips of tape, and a bulky dressing is applied to the entire hand. With either the simple dressing treatment or a split-thickness skin graft, contraction of the wound pulls normally innervated volar skin up over the tip, and the finger is tapered rather than blunt as after a palmar flap graft.

Firecracker explosions and injuries from machinery often result in the amputation of one or more fingers and soft tissue loss from other portions of the hand. Every possible viable piece of tissue should be salvaged. If there is tissue of doubtful viability, it is sometimes best to cleanse and debride obviously dead tissue and then dress the wound and reassess it again in 24 or 48 hours for a delayed primary closure. Under no circumstance should the wound be closed under tension. Often, flaps of skin from a traumatically amputated finger may be used to resurface another, and split-thickness grafts or abdominal flaps are used to cover bone and tendons. With microsurgical techniques, cleanly amputated digits and limbs may be replanted, but frequently injuries of this type involve explosions or crushing wounds that result in extensive tissue damage.

Tendon Injuries

When an initial evaluation suggests that a tendon has been severed, the child is admitted to the hospital, and the wound is examined in the operating room. The entire hand is washed with soap and water, and the wound is irrigated. Then, if there is no concern about tissue viability, a tourniquet is inflated on the arm to provide a dry field in which to extend the incision, identify anatomic landmarks, and find the retracted ends of the severed tendon. Most lacerations must be extended to provide exposure of the involved tendon sheath. These incisions must follow transverse volar creases or extend laterally along the finger just volar to the neurovascular bundle. Under no circumstance should an incision cross a flexion crease or be extended vertically along a finger. When the wound is clean and the resulting repair can be covered with viable tissue, primary tendon repairs are indicated in children. Extensor tendons are thin and difficult to suture, but a satisfactory repair can be achieved by overlapping the tendon ends with 5–0 polypropylene or polyester sutures. The wrist is then splinted in extension, and the fingers are allowed minimal but

comfortable flexion. The healing is more rapid, and the results of primary flexor tendon repairs are better, in children than in adults.[12] Both the sublimus and profundus tendons are repaired in the palm and wrist—the profundus tendon distal to the sublimus insertion and the flexor of the thumb may both be repaired primarily. The decision for primary tendon repair becomes more difficult in no-man's-land, or the area between the distal palmar crease and the first interphalangeal joint. Both the profundus tendon and the sublimus tendon pass through a snug sheath from the palm to the fingers. Consequently, postoperative edema and scarring result in adherence of the tendon to the sheath. Since early normal finger function can be obtained with only the profundus tendon, the sublimus is resected in this area, and only the profundus is sutured. Unlike the experience with adults, excellent results are obtained with primary repair of the profundus tendon in this area.[13,14] Wide resection of the sheath, leaving only pulleys at the midportions of each phalanx, allows the tendon to glide in a bed of fat rather than becoming adherent to the sheath. If conditions are not ideal, however, or if the operator is not experienced in hand surgery, it is still wise to merely close the skin and defer tendon repair to a later date. Delayed direct tendon suture will still provide a good result.[15] If there is severe scarring in the hand, a better procedure is to first create a smooth tunnel to function as a gliding surface. This is effected by inserting a Silastic catheter between the proximal and distal outer end of the tendon. Either specially prepared rods or size 8 to 10 French Silastic catheters may be used. After a wait of 3 to 4 weeks to allow wound healing and joint mobilization with passive exercises, a tendon graft of palmaris longus is inserted in another procedure.[16] The pullout wire technique for flexor tendon repair leaves no irritating foreign body in the wound. However, direct suture of the tendon ends with nonreacting 5–0 polypropylene with a Bunnell weave is just as satisfactory. The initial splint and dressing are left in place for 10 days. At that time, the dressing is changed, and the skin sutures are removed with the child under anesthesia. Splinting is then continued for a total of 3 weeks.

PERIPHERAL NERVE REPAIR

Nerve injuries in children are detected only by meticulous clinical examination, combined with a high index of suspicion when the laceration is at the wrist or deep in the palm. Nerves also may be injured by fractures about the elbow and by direct contusions. Primary nerve repair is always indicated in clean wounds. Nerve regeneration is more rapid in children than in adults, and the accompanying perineural blood vessels are much easier to identify in fresh injuries than at delayed repair.

With magnification, even the branches of the median and ulnar nerves in the palm and digital nerves can be repaired with success. Extension of the original laceration with gentle proximal and distal dissection is necessary to correctly identify the injured nerve and to develop sufficient length for a tension-free anastomosis. Before nerve anastomosis, particularly near a joint such as the wrist, it is helpful to apply a sterile, padded metal splint to maintain immobility. The intrinsic nerve anatomy is carefully studied with magnifying loupes or with the operating microscope. Longitudinal superficial vessels and major nerve bundles provide landmarks for the accurate apposition of nerve ends. The epineurium from the distal end of the nerve is rolled back to expose the nerve fascicles, which are then cut back 1 to 2 mm. Two lateral stay sutures of 6–0 or 7–0 monofilament material are then inserted to appose the fascicles and the identifying blood vessels. The epineurium is then rolled and sutured to the proximal epineurium.[17] This epineurial cuff prevents the escape of axons from the sutured area. Nerve injuries must be splinted for at least 6 weeks.

WRINGER INJURIES

Injuries to the arm that are secondary to the limb being drawn between the rollers of a wringer-type clothes washer are becoming rare. The severity of the injury is determined by the distance between the rollers, the size of the child's arm, and the duration of time during which the rollers spin in one area. The most severe skin damage occurs at the elbow or axilla, where the rollers spin for prolonged periods of time, causing abrasions and exerting a shearing force that avulses skin from the fascia. The best initial treatment of wringer injuries consists of gently washing the arm with soap and water, then covering the skin with a nonadherent fine mesh gauze. The entire limb is then encased in a bulky compression dressing consisting of fluff and a bandage. The dressing should provide firm but moderate pressure from the fingertips to the axilla. The arm is elevated, and the dressing is changed after 2 or 3 days. An occasional child will lose some skin, which will require a graft. When healing has occurred, the child is encouraged to continue his or her usual activities. Soaking in warm water and washing the dishes provide excellent physiotherapy.

LOWER EXTREMITY SOFT TISSUE INJURIES

A barefoot child who cuts the sole of his or her foot on glass or a tin can has a grossly dirty foot and a badly contaminated wound. Further, the blood supply to the sole of the foot is poor. These are ideal conditions for a severe infection. For initial treatment, the entire foot is immersed in a basin of warm soapy water. Then gross dirt is removed with a surgical scrub brush and more soap. The wound edges are further washed, and the wound is liberally irrigated with sterile saline. Open wounds of the foot rarely should be sutured. Neglect of this advice results in deep wound infections from which the sutures must then be removed anyway. Even gaping wounds can be coapted with a properly applied dressing or one strip of sterile adhesive tape. The dressing for even a small laceration must be bulky enough to resist dirt and water and should extend to the knee to make sure it stays in place. During the first 48 hours after injury, the child must have bedrest with the foot elevated. The dressing is then changed, and if there is no infection, another bulky dressing is applied, and the child is allowed to walk with the aid of crutches. Since the adoption of this ironclad rule as an alternative to suturing plantar lacerations in our emergency room (over the protests of successive groups of residents), there have been few plantar infections caused by trauma.

Puncture wounds also are treated with prolonged soaking, after which the thick outer plantar skin around the puncture site is trimmed away with a number 11 blade to provide better drainage. Retained foreign bodies are removed only in the operating room under general anesthesia and x-ray control.

BICYCLE SPOKE INJURIES

The urge to get from one place to another as fast as possible sets in very early. Rather than being left behind to walk, younger siblings beg to be allowed to ride on the luggage racks of their elders' bicycles. This is a satisfactory arrangement until the passenger gets an ankle caught in the spokes. Usually, there is only a minor abrasion, but the lacerations that come to the attention of a surgeon are more likely to be serious skin avulsions over the medial malleolus of the ankle. There is a great urge to clean the wound and suture the flap in the optimistic hope that mangled tissue with no blood supply will heal. Children treated in this fashion, as seen in our surgical outpatient clinic, require up to 2 months to heal. Within a week, the flap becomes necrotic (Fig. 30–4) and requires debridement. The wound must then be dressed until it has granulated and will accept a split-thickness skin graft. The wound may appear to be minor to a surgeon, but the loss of a summer's play means a great deal to a child. Special carriers have been devised to prevent these injuries and should be standard equipment on bicycles in families with small passengers.[18]

The initial treatment for a bicycle spoke injury with a flap ideally should take place in the operating room

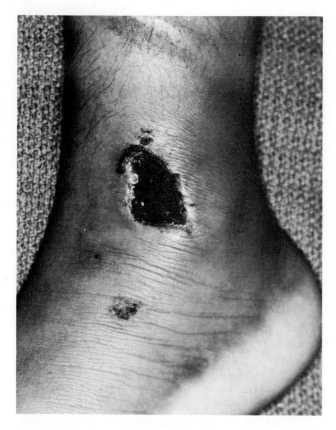

Figure 30–4. A 10-day-old bicycle spoke injury. The flap was sutured in the emergency room but became necrotic, requiring debridement and coverage with a split-thickness skin graft.

under either general or block anesthesia. After washing and irrigating the wound, all undermined skin and flaps of tissue are debrided until there is active bleeding. It is futile to suture flaps that have not only been devascularized but crushed and torn as well. If the resulting wound has exposed the malleolus, it is covered by rotating a full-thickness flap of skin forward from between the bone and the Achilles tendon. The defect over the soft tissue in this area is then covered with a split-thickness skin graft (Fig. 30–5). Even with less extensive injuries, a bulky compression dressing and a splint, together with bedrest and elevation of the foot, are essential to healing.

CRUSH INJURIES

In pediatric surgical practice, a crushed leg usually is the result of an automobile wheel passing completely over one or both limbs. There is severe shock due to blood and plasma loss, extensive contamination with street dirt, and devitalized tissue. There is also likely to be arterial and nerve damage. The initial management of these patients includes a search for injuries to the head, chest, and abdomen. A bulky sterile dressing is applied in the emergency room, and plasma is given

until whole blood is available. It is very difficult to assess arterial obstruction by palpating the pulses until shock has been corrected. Occasionally, edema and hematoma may obscure the dorsalis pedis pulse as well as the femoral and popliteal arteries. Resuscitation with fluids should commence in the emergency room and continue in the x-ray department, where films are taken of the long bones. An arteriogram should be obtained if there is any concern about a vascular injury. If the injury is below the femoral area, a percutaneous arteriogram is performed. Otherwise, it may be necessary to thread a catheter up one femoral artery and inject contrast material into the aorta. If neither of these techniques is feasible, arrangements should be made to perform arteriography in the operating room with the artery under direct vision. Examination with Doppler ultrasonography may give additional aid in evaluating arterial obstructions.

Degloving injuries occur when full-thickness skin is sheared away from the fascia. There is also underlying contusion and hematoma of the muscles. However, there are usually no fractures or arterial injuries. Treatment varies according to the condition of the avulsed skin. This skin is usually severely contaminated, abraded, and completely unsuitable for replacement on the limb. In the operating room, the leg is elevated, obvious bleeding is controlled, and the wound is extensively washed and irrigated with normal saline. Below the knee, all fascial compartments are opened to prevent postoperative vascular compression. The flaps of skin and devitalized muscle are excised until healthy bleeding tissue is found. Muscle that is blue and hemorrhagic and that does not contract is removed to decrease the possibility of gas gangrene. It may be possible to spread out the excised skin and, with a Brown dermatome, to cut split-thickness grafts, which are then applied to the denuded tissue. This procedure rarely is feasible because of abrasions and damage to the avulsed skin. Our procedure has been to dress the wound with saline-soaked, fine mesh gauze and a bulky dressing. The limb is then elevated, and the child is treated with antibiotics. It is necessary to continue plasma and blood transfusions because there are usually considerable ooze and exudate from the wound for 24 to 48 hours. At the end of 48 hours, the child's general condition has stabilized and oozing from the wound has diminished, and it is then possible to reevaluate tissue that was of borderline viability at the first operation. The wound is then covered with meshed skin grafts and redressed. At successive dressing changes, raw areas are again grafted until the wound is completely closed. Whirlpool treatments and physical therapy aid in achieving a functioning limb, but from a cosmetic point of view, the limb will be more slender than normal because of the loss of subcutaneous fat.

Open fractures in crush injuries are treated with meticulous debridement and fixation of the fracture with

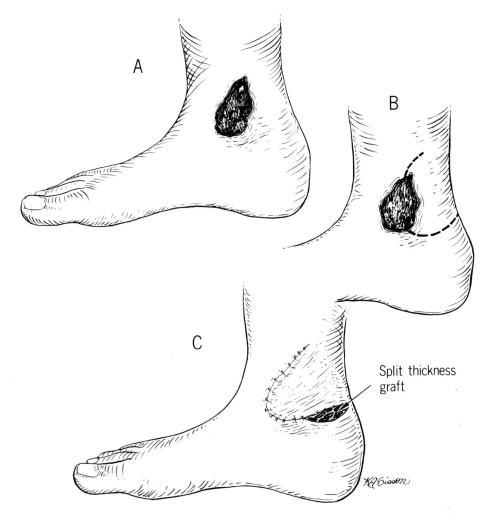

Figure 30–5. The flap created by the bicycle spoke is debrided until there is pink tissue that bleeds freely. The defect is closed by mobilizing a flap from the posterior portion of the ankle. Any defect left by the mobilized flap is covered with a split-thickness graft. This technique allows coverage of the malleolus with full-thickness skin.

either traction or external skeletal fixation. Internal fixation is avoided because of the increased risk of infection. The transfer of composite flaps of tissue with the aid of microvascular surgery has allowed soft tissue coverage of areas, such as a fractured tibia or the foot, where in the past it has been difficult to achieve satisfactory skin coverage.

TRAUMATIC AMPUTATION

Almost any extremity, fingers, legs, and arms may be successfully replanted with the aid of microvascular surgery. The extremity must be taken from the scene of the accident, placed in iced saline, and transported with the patient to a suitable center where microvascular surgery is available. While the child is being resuscitated in the operating room, the extremity is washed and debrided, and the nerves, arteries, and veins are isolated and identified. It is helpful to perform a fasciotomy on the limb before its replantation. The bone may be shortened and is then secured with internal fixation. Arterial flow is next established, either by direct anastomosis or with the aid of a vein graft. Blood is allowed to freely exit from the veins until they are repaired. The nerves are next anastomosed, and all repaired structures are covered with viable muscle. Open areas of skin may be grafted after several days. Prolonged physical therapy and rehabilitation are essential if the child is to obtain the most benefit from these prolonged, tedious procedures.

REFERENCES

1. Mason AL, Koch SL: Human bite infections of the hand. Surg Gynecol Obstet 51:591, 1930
2. Wiseman N, Chochinov Fraser V: Major dog attack injuries in children. J Pediatr Surg 18:533, 1983

3. Schultz RC, McMasters WC: The treatment of dog bite injuries, especially those of the face. Plast Reconstr Surg 49:494, 1972

4. Thomson HG, Svitek V: Small animal bites: The role of primary closure. J Trauma 13:20, 1973

5. US Public Health Service. MMWR 25 (51), 1972

6. Buntain W: Successful venomous snakebite neutralization with massive antivenin infusion in a child. J Trauma 23:1012, 1984

7. Kitchens C, Van Mierop L: Envenomation by the eastern coral snake (*Micrurus fulvius fulvius*). JAMA 258:1615, 1987

8. Report of the Committee on Infectious Diseases, 20th ed., Elk Grove Village, Ill. American Academy of Pediatrics, 1986, p 358

9. Kutler W: A new method for fingertip amputation. JAMA 133:29, 1947

10. Illingworth CM: Trapped fingers and amputated fingertips in children. J Pediatr Surg 9:853, 1974

11. Douglas BS: Conservative management of guillotine amputations of the finger in children. Aust Paediatr J 8:86, 1972

12. Rouk BK, Wakefield AR, Houston JT: Surgery of Repair as Applied to Hand Injuries. Baltimore, Williams & Wilkins, 1973

13. Weeks PM, Wray KC: Management of Acute Hand Injuries. St. Louis, Mosby, 1973, p 227

14. Palletta FX: Pediatric Plastic Surgery: Trauma. St. Louis, Mosby, 1967, vol 1, p 107

15. Arons MS: Purposeful delay of the primary repair of cut flexor tendons in "some-man's-land" in children. Plast Reconstr Surg 53:638, 1974

16. Hunter JM, Salisbury RE: Use of gliding artificial implants to produce tendon sheaths. Plast Reconstr Surg 45:564, 1970

17. Ducker TA, Garrison WB: Surgical aspects of peripheral nerve trauma. Curr Prob Surg 111:39, 1974

18. Berry T, Burg F, Kravitz H: The toddler as a bicycle passenger. Pediatrics 49:443, 1972

19. Zuker R, Stevenson J: Proximal upper limb replantation in children. J Trauma 28:544, 1988

31
Facial Injuries

Bruce S. Bauer
Jay M. Pensler

Facial injuries range from minor lacerations to large-scale avulsions with serious loss of tissue resulting from vehicular accidents and dog bites. Soft tissue trauma in combination with facial bone fractures is less common but typically occurs in motor vehicle accidents.

INITIAL ASSESSMENT OF INJURY

A detailed history includes the circumstances, the current status of immunizations, and the time elapsed since the injury. The physical examination will reveal accompanying trauma and will detail the extent and nature of the facial injuries. In addition to photographic documentation, the medical record should include a sketch of the injury, with reference to the vermilion border, the eyebrow, the lacrimal puncta, and the facial nerve. Examination for dental injuries is necessary when there is a perioral laceration. Periorbital injuries may suggest damage to the globe or entrapment of extraocular muscles and periorbita. The function of nerves of the face must be assessed before administration of anesthesia.

Simple lacerations of the face can be repaired in the emergency room, using local anesthesia with sedation. The choice of repair, in the emergency room or in the more controlled setting of the operating room, is based on the child's age and ability to cooperate, the complexity of the repair, the need for specialized equipment, and proper pediatric anesthesia.

Facial wounds are thoroughly cleansed. The removal of dirt and debris generally requires an anesthetic. Actual debridement in facial soft tissue injuries should be carried out very conservatively. The rich vascular supply of the face usually minimizes tissue loss and risk of infection. More radical debridement may necessitate complex reconstruction, which would be delayed till a later date.

A careful appraisal of the depth of the defect and the amount of tissue lost will help plan the reconstruction. Subcutaneous tissue planes should be closed to recontour the defect and to relieve distracting tension on the skin closure. Skin sutures should be placed equidistant from the edge of the wound, evenly spaced along the long axis of the wound, and tied with the proper amount of tension. A subcuticular pullout suture of 4–0 or 5–0 nylon omits direct cutaneous suture marks along the length of the laceration.[1] Mild 6–0 chromic catgut sutures placed through the skin will dissolve, obviating the necessity to remove skin sutures, yet they will leave no cross hatching.

In most simple lacerations, direct closure of the wound is possible. In some instances, however, tissue loss will be sufficient to require local flaps, Z-plasty, or a skin graft. The simplest closure is the best at the time of initial repair. An unfavorable orientation of the scar line may be revised later with a Z-plasty or a rotational flap. In some cases of obviously significant tissue loss, the method of choice is to close some areas directly and to resurface the remaining denuded area with a split-thickness skin graft. The graft may be applied at the time of initial repair if the recipient site is clean and viable or a few days later if subsequent debridement or intervening cleansing of the open wound seems to be indicated.[2,3] This technique allows for optimal healing of the initial wound without undue skin tension or compromising local flaps. Secondary revisions can be made as indicated after full scar maturation has taken place. The degree and direction of distortion can be assessed at that time.

FACIAL WOUNDS

Forehead lacerations frequently are associated with vehicular accidents in which the head strikes the dashboard or windshield. Special attention must, therefore, be paid to accompanying head or spinal injuries and to the removal of foreign material, such as glass. Routine x-ray or computed tomography (CT) scan (often needed in evaluation of the concomitant head injury) may be helpful in locating glass particles. The injury commonly extends through the full thickness of soft tissue down to the periosteum or bone. The underlying bone should be seen or felt to evaluate for a fracture. Function of the temporal branch of the facial nerve must always be assessed before injection of local anesthesia. The nerve courses along a line from a point 0.5 cm below the tragus of the ear, extending toward the eyebrow, and passing 1.5 cm above the lateral aspect of the eyebrow. Any lacerations in this region may involve the temporal branch of the facial nerve.

Eyebrow lacerations are particularly common in toddlers who fall and strike the edge of a piece of furniture. Eyebrows must never be shaved for the repair of wounds! Exact realignment of the browline is necessary to avoid a steplike defect as the scar forms. Debridement of the skin in the eyebrow should be performed with the cutting blade at an angle to the skin edge to parallel the plane of the eyebrow hairs.

Eyelid tissue is particularly delicate and expansile. Relatively minor injuries to the palpebral area can cause a significant amount of edema and dislocation. Patients and their families should be advised of this anticipated swelling and discoloration to spare them unnecessary apprehension. Assessment of the integrity of the lacrimal drainage system when the injury involves the medial portions of the lid may require probing or instillation of fluorescein. In addition, the status of the canthal ligaments must be evaluated carefully for an unsuspected rupture and subsequent traumatic telecanthus. Medial canthal ligament disruption should, if at all possible, be repaired at the time of injury. Repair usually requires transnasal wiring or wiring of bone fragments if a large enough piece remains attached to the avulsed ligament. Through-and-through lacerations of the lids should be closed in layers, using an absorbable suture (such as catgut) on the conjunctival layers and a nonabsorbable, nonreactive material (such as nylon) on the tarsal plate and skin. It is not necessary to repair septum orbitale and orbicularis oculi muscle in simple lacerations to the lids. Careful examination of the globe and evaluation of extraocular muscle function should accompany the repair of any lid laceration, and ophthalmologic consultation should be obtained.[4]

The course of Stensen's duct is deep to the middle third of a line drawn from the tragus of the ear to the midportion of the upper lip. This corresponds roughly to the anterior–posterior limits of the masseter muscle. The opening of the duct into the mouth is opposite the second maxillary molar. The buccal branch of the facial nerve is in close approximation to Stensen's duct. It is repaired by direct approximation over a fine plastic catheter placed within the duct, across the site of repair, and secured as a stent to aid healing and patency. A transected facial nerve should be repaired primarily under magnification with loops or microscope.

Lacerations of the lips can involve the skin, the mucosa, and the intervening orbicularis oris muscle. As a rule, mucosal defects should be realigned and their edges loosely approximated. Transected muscle is repaired with clear nylon sutures, and the skin is closed with very fine cutaneous sutures or a pullout subcuticular stitch. In through-and-through lacerations of the mouth, the skin and muscle should be reapproximated and the mucosa closed very loosely, if at all. Careful realignment of the vermilion border of the lip is of critical importance in preventing notching and visible mismatching. Lacerations at the oral commissure require detailed attention to the recreation of the commissural apex to prevent webbing and subsequent stricture formation. Significant disruption of the commissure may benefit from splinting for 6 to 9 months postrepair to avoid contracture. In general, loosened or avulsed teeth may be replaced in their sockets and held with dental wiring.

Intraoral soft tissue injuries usually are the result of a child falling on his or her face with a sharp object in the mouth, causing a mucosal puncture wound of the roof of the mouth. Lacerations of the palate rarely if ever need repair and will heal spontaneously. Similarly, lacerations of the tongue, though ragged or bifid at the tip, will heal without noticeable abnormality. If the lacerations are large enough to require suturing, general anesthesia is required.

The ear has a rich vascular supply, and tissue recuperation may proceed in a manner quite unlike that of other areas of the body. Thus, every possible bit of tissue is salvaged. Total or near-total amputations should be evaluated for replantation by microvascular technique if the amputated part was not crushed or shredded. Other techniques involving complex flap coverage of the cartilage may be of benefit. Burying the amputated part in a subcutaneous pocket on the chest or abdomen is a futile exercise, since the cartilage subsequently will melt away.

The soft tissue overlying the nasal skeleton is unique

and difficult to replace if it is destroyed or lost. For this reason, debridement of nasal injuries should avoid discarding irreplaceable tissue that might have survived. Avulsed skin flaps simply are replaced and held with a few peripheral sutures. If the success of this method seems unlikely, the avulsed flap may be amputated completely, defatted, and converted to a full-thickness skin graft. This is then laid in place over the defect and carefully sutured. When this available skin cover seems unsuitable or is missing, it often is advisable to simply leave the wound open and allow spontaneous reepithelialization. Local or distant flaps or full-thickness skin grafts for nasal reconstruction are better left to secondary repair.

Debris embedded in the skin and soft tissue of the face frequently is associated with blunt trauma and abrasion injuries. Unless removed completely, this debris will become permanently affixed to the tissues and will remain as an unsightly discoloration in the area of injury. Copious irrigation and vigorous cleansing of the wound will remove most of the foreign material. Isolated dirt particles are picked out with a scalpel, and entire areas of tattooed tissue may be treated by dermabrasion. The easiest time to extricate these disfiguring particles of foreign material is during the initial repair. This may be an indication for general anesthesia.

FACIAL FRACTURES

Facial fractures in children are much less common than they are in adults.[5] Fractures in children under the age of 5 years constitute no more than 1 percent of all facial fractures.[6]

The lower incidence of facial fractures in children is due to the relative prominence of the cranial skeleton as compared to the face, together with the elasticity of children's bones.

Favorable factors in the treatment of facial fractures in children are the capacity for rapid union by periosteal osteogenesis and the greater ability of a child's bones to remodel. Unfavorable factors arise from the nature of deciduous dentition, in which the shape and shallowness of the roots make their use as a means of immobilization difficult. The fact that the tooth buds of the permanent dentition fill much of the remainder of the bone makes it difficult to perform direct interosseous wiring without damage.

Certain facial bone trauma, especially to the mandibular condyles, may result in deformity because of interference with growth.

Some 45 percent of facial fractures in children result from traffic accidents, and 28 percent result from falls.[6] Some 57 percent of cases are associated with multiple trauma, and 41 percent show an associated cranial injury.

Observation will disclose nasal bleeding, blood-stained drooling, swelling, bruising, and ecchymosis. The presence of a laceration below the symphysis menti is always an indication for both a careful clinical examination for tenderness over the condylar region of the mandible and an x-ray. Physical examination should involve careful palpation of the bony facial skeleton to detect an underlying deformity. Always check for dental occlusion, loose teeth, and the range of mandibular movement and deviation. Look for paresthesia in the infraorbital and mental nerve distributions. If there is evidence of bruising around the eye, examine for range of movement of the extraocular muscles, diplopia, or evidence of ocular injury (such as hyphema).

The increasing availability and fine detail of CT scans and the frequent need for determination of associated head trauma make CT scan the optimal technique for evaluation of facial fractures. Although tomograms are useful, CT scan is the definitive study for evaluation of the nasal and ethmoin area and the orbit floor for blowout fractures. It also can be used to evaluate condylar head displacement. The waters, posteroanterior, submentovertical views may still be used effectively for evaluation where CT is unavailable.

If the fractures of the mandible are multiple or displaced (Fig. 31–1), reduction and immobilization should be implemented. If the teeth are too immature to support intermaxillary fixation, Gunning-type splints fabricated with quick-cure acrylic are secured to the body of the mandible by circumferential wiring and to the maxilla by wiring through the pyriform opening, thus avoiding the danger of tooth loss.

In children, immobilization for 3 weeks is sufficient for union of most mandibular fractures.

Extraction of teeth in the line of fracture is seldom indicated if there is good dental hygiene. Stabilization of loose or partially separated teeth associated with dentoalveolar injuries can be carried out by wiring them to adjacent stable teeth.

Fractures of the mandibular condyle may be bilateral or unilateral and frequently occur from indirect violence. A small laceration over the point of the chin frequently is present. Two types of injury occur. The more common is a fracture through the neck of the condyle with medial dislocation of the head. The second is a compression injury in which the head is flattened and may be driven through the thin bone of the temporal fossa. This compression injury is more likely to result in growth disturbance of the affected side of the mandible and possible ankylosis of the temporomandibular joint.

Treatment of condylar fractures remains controversial, with options ranging from aggressive open reduction to graduated diet and exercise only. In the unilateral case, the more conservative approach now seems to be

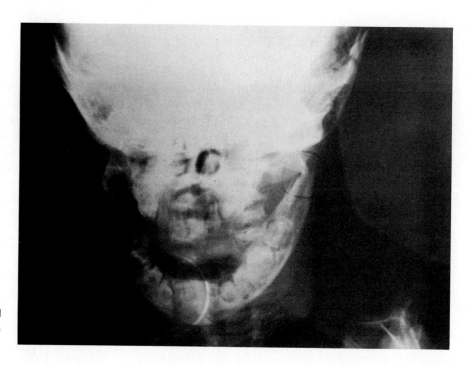

Figure 31–1. Bilateral condylar fracture and fracture of the right body of the mandible, requiring immobilization.

in favor, most certainly in children requiring remodeling of the condyle.

Fractures of the Nose

Unless seen early, deformity of the nasal bones frequently is masked by swelling so that doubt may remain as to the presence of a fracture. X-rays of the nasal bones in children are not particularly helpful. If in doubt, it is advisable to arrange for a further examination in a few days when swelling has subsided and the nasal skeleton can be more accurately palpated. If deformity is present, it is often more easily corrected at that time.

In young children, the nasal bones can be manipulated by a hemostat with the jaws wrapped in moistened cotton. The nose is packed gently with petrolatum gauze for 24 hours postoperatively, and a cast is applied for a period of 1 week (Fig. 31–2).

The development of a saddle nose may follow damage to the septal cartilage from either a hematoma or an abscess. Even when evacuated immediately in the postoperative period, some nasal deformity may occur.

Fractures of the middle third of the face are associated with severe trauma, blood-stained sputum, and malocclusion, and at times the entire middle third of the facial skeleton may be movable. If there is involvement of the zygomatic bones, open reduction of the fractures probably will be necessary, with direct interosseous wiring or by application of miniplates for rigid fixation to

a point on the unfractured facial skeleton. This reduction may be augmented by intermaxillary fixation with a Gunning-type splint, as for a fractured mandible, and suspension wiring (Fig. 31–3).

A forceful blow on the globe of the eye may cause fracturing or a blowout of the thin bony floor of the orbit, with prolapse of orbital contents into the antrum.

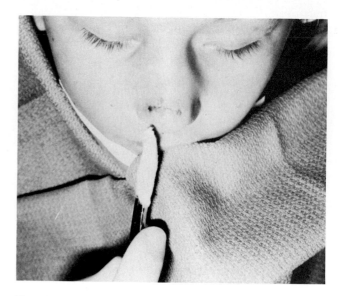

Figure 31–2. Cotton-wrapped hemostat used for manipulation and reduction.

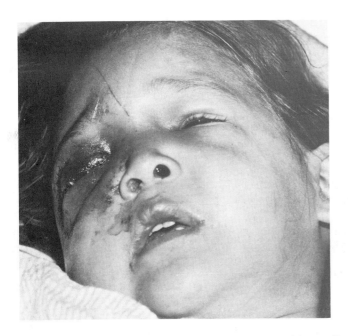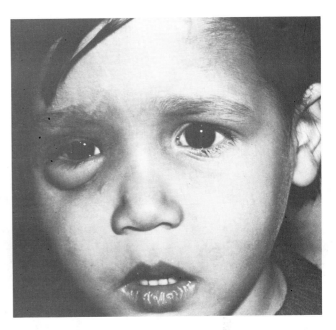

Figure 31–3. Left. A comminuted fracture of the maxillary–zygomatic complex. **Right.** The result a few days after reduction and direct wiring through infraorbital and frontozygomatic incisions.

As a result, movement of the globe is restricted, particularly on upward gaze, with diplopia, enophthalmus, and pseudoptosis. Tomograms of the orbital floor will reveal the defect and show the soft tissue shadow of the prolapsed orbital contents. At operation, the conjunctiva is grasped with forceps below the pupil, and an attempt is made to roll the eye upward. Upward rolling will be prevented by the entrapment of soft tissue in the orbital floor fracture.

Initial treatment of orbital floor defects of less than 7 mm consists of observation to determine if the diplopia will resolve spontaneously. If the diplopia does not correct itself, a direct surgical approach to the fracture site is performed through an incision over the infraorbital ridge. The periosteum of the floor of the orbit is elevated, the fracture is exposed, and the orbital contents are freed. The floor is then repaired with either autogenous bone graft (split cranial is ideal) or Silastic sheeting for small defects. The latter can be complicated by late implant extension.

Despite adequate surgical care, careful testing will show persistent muscle imbalance in about 45 percent of patients, although residual diplopia is seldom a problem.[7] Because of these results, there are some advocates of a nonoperative approach to this condition.[8,9] Along with muscle imbalance, some degree of enophthalmus is a common sequel of a blowout fracture.[10]

REFERENCES

1. Hartman LA: Intradermal sutures in facial lacerations: A comparative study of clear monofilament nylon and polyglycolic acid. Arch Otolaryngol 103:542, 1977
2. Schultz RC, Oldham RJ: An overview of facial injuries. Surg Clin North Am 57:987, 1977
3. Goldwyn RM, Rueckert F: The value of healing by secondary intention for sizeable defects of the face. Arch Surg 112:285, 1977
4. Whitaker LA, Schaffer DB: Severe traumatic oculoorbital displacement: Diagnosis and secondary treatment. Plast Reconstr Surg 59:352, 1977
5. Waite DE: Pediatric fractures of the jaw and facial bones. Pediatrics 51:551, 1973
6. Rowe NL: Fractures of the jaws in children. J Oral Surg 27:497, 1969
7. McCoy FJ, Chandler RA, Crow ML: Facial fractures in children. Plast Reconstr Surg 37:209, 1966
8. Emery JM, Van Noorden GK, Schlermitzaner DA: Orbital floor fractures: Long-term follow-up of cases with and without surgical repair. Trans Am Acad Ophthalmol Otolaryngol 75:802, 1971
9. Puttermann AM, Stevens T, Urist MJ: Nonsurgical management of blow-out fractures of the orbital floor. Am J Ophthalmol 77:232, 1974
10. Converse JM, Smith B, Obear MF, Wood-Smith D: Orbital blow-out fractures: A ten-year survey. Plast Reconstr Surg 39:20, 1967

32

Head and Spinal Cord Injuries in Children

David G. McLone
Yoon S. Hahn

HEAD INJURY

Impact to the skull is an inevitable part of childhood play. The automobile, high-rise buildings, increased participation in contact sports, and the apparent increase in the number of battered children have added to the frequency and severity of head injuries in children. In the vast majority of cases, the injury to the nervous system is insignificant.

Occasionally, the brain is the primary site of injury, or processes are set in motion that will secondarily injure the nervous system. Little can be done about the primary injury, but a great deal can now be done about the secondary damage. The secondary brain damage resulting from ischemia, raised intracranial pressure (ICP), or a mass lesion will compound the primary damage and initiate a process leading to irreversibility or mortality if intervention is not prompt.

Trauma accounts for about one third of all pediatric surgical admissions, and one half of these children have incurred a head injury. One child in 10 will suffer a significant head injury during school years, and one third of these children will be hospitalized.

Mortality figures for head injury in children vary widely. There are about 100,000 accidental deaths per year in North America, and approximately 25,000 are children. Studies at one time showed that of those children admitted in coma, one half to three quarters died. Recent studies paint a somewhat more optimistic picture, with a mortality rate of 20 to 40 percent.[1-4]

General Management

The fact that some children who eventually die from a head injury are awake when admitted to the hospital supports a more liberal criterion for admission. Of these deaths, 70 percent occur in the first 48 hours.[5] No perfect set of criteria exist for deciding who should be hospitalized for observation, which results in the admission for observation of a large number of children who recover completely without any treatment. This is done in the hope that the children who will deteriorate later are included in this larger group. This should place the child with an impending intracranial disaster in a situation where the diagnosis can be made promptly and the appropriate therapy can be administered swiftly.

Effective criteria for admission of a child with a head injury but not in coma include:

1. A history of loss of consciousness
2. A skull fracture
3. Labile physiologic response (vomiting, irritability, behavioral changes)
4. Convulsion
5. Cerebrospinal fluid leak
6. Caretakers who do not appear able to adequately observe the child at home

The lack of an adequate history should influence the decision in favor of admitting.

Admission to the hospital of a child with a head injury requires that the hospital have an area for constant observation, personnel conversant with the care of

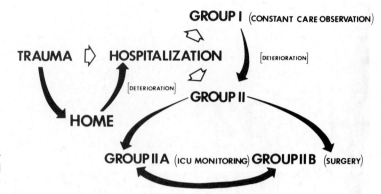

Figure 32–1. A flow chart showing the pathways for management of a child with a head injury. Criteria for admission and movement from group to group are described in the text.

trauma, emergency equipment available for pediatric patients, a computed tomography (CT) scanner, and a readily available neurosurgeon. Pediatric endotracheal tubes and volume respirators are essential for the care of some of these children. The absence of any of these capabilities precludes admission and demands transfer to another hospital.

Children not admitted should be watched closely at home, and their parents should be instructed to return to the hospital if the child's level of consciousness deteriorates or if one of the other criteria for admission is met.

Children can be divided into two groups after admission (Fig. 32–1). Group 1 includes children who are alert to lethargic and who have stable vital signs and no focal neurologic deficits. The second group includes children who show any of the following: stupor or coma, unstable vital signs, focal signs, an open or penetrating wound, a depressed skull fracture, or a cerebrospinal fluid leak.

Although controversial, we believe that all children admitted with the diagnosis of head injury should have skull films or a CT scan. It is prudent, where possible, to obtain CT scans on all head injuries that require admission to a hospital. Depressed fractures need repair, and linear fractures that cross major dural venous sinuses or the middle meningeal artery or that cross the cranial pneumatized sinuses require close observation and may require further diagnostic procedures. An occasional linear fracture will expand over the following weeks because of the herniation of intracranial contents through the fracture (Fig. 32–2). It is, therefore, important to follow all skull fractures for at least 6 weeks.

Awake Child. Group 1 patients should be admitted to areas of the hospital where frequent vital signs can be obtained and where nurse/patient ratios are such that close observation is possible. Observations should include:

1. Level of consciousness
2. Blood pressure and pulse

3. Pupils (size, equality, reactions)
4. Movement of the extremities

Until the child is determined to be stable, frequent observations should be recorded. A pulse monitor with an alarm is used between observations. Deterioration in any one of these categories moves the child into group 2.

A shocklike state with hypotension and tachycardia is almost never the result of intracranial events. Occasionally, very young children can loose enough blood intracranially or into the subgaleal space to produce shock. Other sources of blood loss should be sought when this occurs in older children. Conversely, hypertension and bradycardia are early indicators of an expanding intracranial mass. The changes in blood pressure and pulse usually are progressive (Fig. 32–3). Therefore, a decrease in pulse or an elevation in blood pressure should make one either increase the frequency of vital sign monitoring or move the patient to group 2.

Some children will require intravenous fluids because of persistent vomiting. The intake, output, and electrolytes of these children should be watched closely. Inappropriate antidiuretic hormone (ADH) syndrome is seen occasionally after a head injury in children. Confusion, alterations in levels of consciousness, and seizures can be precipitated by the ensuing hyponatremia. Profound hyponatremia with seizures can cause irreversible damage to the central nervous system. If profound hyponatremia exists and the child is symptomatic, 3 percent saline may be used to restore normal serum osmolality.

Occasionally diabetes insipidus occurs following a head injury. It is usually transient and seldom requires the use of antidiuretic hormones.

Group 2 patients include those children who have obvious or suspected surgical lesions and need immediate further diagnostic studies to determine whether a surgical lesion exists.

Little can be done to correct tissue destruction and cell death occurring as part of the primary event, but continued bleeding, advancing edema, ischemia, hypoxia, hypercarbia, open wounds, and depressed fractures can be controlled and corrected.

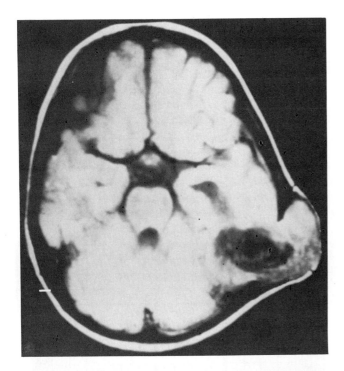

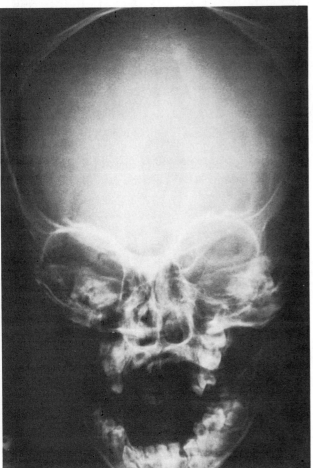

Figure 32–2. Top. An MRI demonstrates extrusion of traumatized brain tissue through a skull fracture. **Bottom.** Plain skull film of another child shows a growing skull fracture (arrows).

Comatose Child. The comatose child is a special subgroup in group 2. Many of these children will not have surgical lesions but diffuse brain injuries. Often, these are the children with multiple injuries involving other organ systems.

The initial management of these children is designed to resuscitate the child and prevent further damage. If one is going to be involved in care of these children, the following steps should be memorized and implemented immediately when confronted with the comatose child. Although these steps may be repeated elsewhere in this text, they are listed here to further emphasize their importance.

- Step 1: Establish an airway. Essentially all comatose children should have an intratracheal tube placed immediately. ASSUME THE CHILD HAS A SPINE INJURY! If the child is not breathing, ventilate the child and make sure the air is moving in both lungs.
- Step 2: Make sure the heart is beating. Assess peripheral pulses. If the heart is not beating or pulses are not adequate, begin closed chest massage.
- Step 3: Stop the bleeding.
  Step 4: Obtain venous access and begin fluid resuscitation and send blood for typing and crossmatching. Isotonic crystalloid should be given in amounts necessary to make the child euvolemic. Children with head injuries should not be kept dry.

The airway should be cleared and an endotracheal tube inserted immediately. Remember that there is always the possibility of an unstable cervical spine fracture. A tracheostomy usually is not acutely needed but often is desirable for long-term care. Serial blood gases should be determined to prove that ventilation and exchange are adequate.

Tissue hypoxia and hypercarbia compound any intracranial insult. Cerebral vasculature dilates in response to the fall in pH. As the P_{CO_2} increases so does intracranial pressure, and a previously delicate balance may shift toward rapid deterioration. Hyperventilation leads to a decline in the P_{CO_2}, an increase in the pH, and cerebral vascular constriction. Hyperventilation is an effective way to rapidly reduce intracranial pressure. Unlike the adult, the cerebral vasculature of children remains sensitive to hyperventilation for several days, and controlled ventilation may be used to reduce intracranial pressure for long periods of time.[6]

If the child is stable, that is, fractures are stabilized and chest tubes are placed, the next step should be a CT scan to determine if there is an intracranial mass. Remember through all of this we are assuming this child has a spine injury. Resuscitation should not be delayed to obtain a cervical spine x-ray, which may show alignment but give little information about stability. In fact,

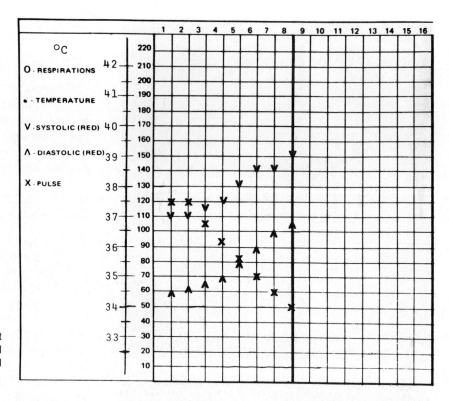

Figure 32–3. Patient observation sheet showing the changes in blood pressure and pulse of a child deteriorating from increased intracranial pressure.

if you have time for only one x-ray, get a chest x-ray.

Magnetic resonance imaging (MRI) is another valuable tool in the evaluation of traumatic lesions of the brain. In view of the precise anatomic and pathologic sensitivity, MRI is useful in patients with severe head injury in whom CT scans fails to demonstrate anatomic substrate for the degrees of coma or neurologic deficits. MRI can define a small subdural hematoma not detectable on CT scans or show axonal injury in the white matter of brain (Fig. 32–4). However, many of these lesions may not be of any clinical significance. MRI with its current prolonged scan time is unlikely to supplant the CT scan for the diagnosis of acute head injury or to improve the outcome of injured patients. Rather, it is of great prognostic value.

The Glasgow coma scale (GCS) has been widely accepted and used as an objective neurologic assessment of head injured patients (Table 32–1).[7] This scale has a limited usefulness for children under 3 years of age. The assessment on the "eye opening response" is applicable for patients of any age. However, in assessing a "best motor response," caution is required with infants to differentiate "withdraw" or "flexion" of all extremities from true "localizing to pain." A more obvious problem is the "verbal response" in neonates and infants. The subscoring system of the GCS "best verbal response" needs modification for use in children under 36 months of age.

GCS should be assessed at a reasonably early time after the injury or at the initial neurologic assessment.

The lack of cooperation by a child makes the neurologic examination difficult. The initial examination is most crucial. Be sure to watch for spontaneous reactions of the child. Make brief but repeated examinations rather than one long, perfect examination.

After the child has been resuscitated, and it is determined that the child does not have a surgical lesion, modern transducer technology makes it possible to continuously monitor ICP. This has potential benefit and little risk to the child. The signs and symptoms of deterioration because of ICP often occur late, and the effective-

TABLE 32–1. GLASGOW COMMA SCALE

Eye Opening
4   Spontaneous
3   Reaction to speech
2   Reaction to pain
1   No response

Best motor response
6   Spontaneous (obeys verbal command)
5   Localizes pain
4   Withdraws in response to pain
3   Abnormal flexion in response to pain (decorticate posture)
2   Abnormal extension in response to pain (decerebrate posture)
1   No response

Best verbal response
5   Oriented
4   Confused/disoriented
3   Inappropriate words
2   Incomprehensible sounds
1   No response

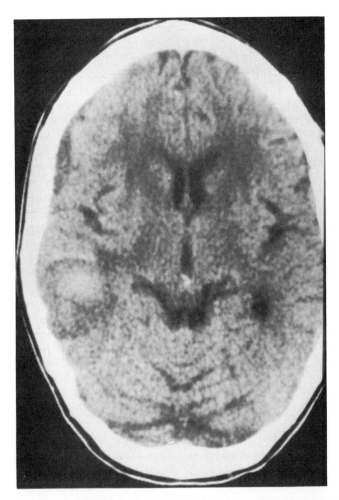 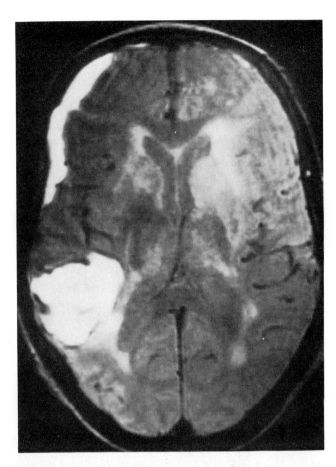

Figure 32–4. The difference between **Left.** A CT scan. **Right.** An MRI demonstrating intracranial lesions: subdural hematoma, intracerebral hematoma, and diffuse white matter injury.

ness of therapy may be impossible to evaluate without an intracranial monitor.

Indications for ICP monitoring include (1) GCS (or children's coma score [CCS]) of 8 or less, (2) no intracranial mass lesion after the mass is evacuated, and (3) patients who are pharmacologically paralyzed. Monitoring ICP has demonstrated that the clinical state of a patient does not always reflect the ICP. Although almost all patients who are developing midbrain dysfunction show a simultaneous elevation in ICP, many patients with elevated ICP, including plateau waves, do not show signs of neurologic deterioration.

As cerebral vasomotor tone begins to fail, systemic arterial pressure, which is usually elevated at this point, gains unimpeached entry into the intracranial compartment. If the resistance vessels are capable of response to a decrease in blood Pco_2, hyperventilation or osmotic agents may reduce ICP and retrieve the child. However, if resistance vessels are permanently damaged as a result of ischemia, vasoconstrictor tone is lost, vasomotor paralysis ensues, and vessels dilate passively. Ultimately,

mean systemic arterial pressure and ICP become equal, cerebral blood flow ceases, and the child dies.

The dose of Mannitol or the effect of hyperventilation can be determined only by monitoring ICP. An arterial line allows the monitoring of systemic arterial pressure so that cerebral perfusion pressure (the difference between ICP and systemic arterial pressure) can be maintained at a level sufficient to ensure brain perfusion. The number of patients requiring ICP monitoring is about the same as the number requiring surgery, which is a small minority of the head injuries admitted to the hospital.

The most important early factors are brain compression and distortion rather than changes in ICP per se. The speed or rate at which such changes in brain shape occur is a major factor in determining brain dysfunction. Brain shift causes distortion of the vasculature, with edema and decreased cerebral blood flow. Later, as ICP approaches systemic arterial pressure, cerebral perfusion pressure falls, and cerebral blood flow diminishes.

If the child is in status epilepticus, anticonvulsants,

phenobarbital, or diazepam is indicated in doses appropriate to stopping seizures. The physicians should be prepared to deal with the depressed respirations that frequently follow as a result of the postictal state and direct action of the medications. Phenytoin (Dilantin) is a better drug in the awake child but has a delayed effect if given orally and is absorbed poorly from intramuscular depots. Therefore, it is most useful given slowly intravenously. Seizure medication obviously is needed, but it would be a mistake to sedate a child to make the child more comfortable, thereby altering the child's level of consciousness and losing this useful vital sign to assess neurologic deterioration. Comatose patients and patients with open depressed skull fractures also should be started on anticonvulsants. Analgesics or narcotics that alter the child's state of consciousness should be used only when absolutely necessary.

The efficacy of barbiturates in doses to induce coma (barbiturate coma) to protect the brain is yet to be established. However, barbiturates can lower ICP in cases were hyperventilation and osmotic agents have failed.

Before determining if a patient has a surgical lesion, osmotic agents to reduce ICP are indicated only if the patient is deteriorating and is not responding to hyperventilation. A neurosurgeon must be available before giving the patient Mannitol. The administration of Mannitol to all patients with severe head injuries is definitely contraindicated. Hyperosmolar agents dehydrate the normal brain and may allow hematomas or edematous brain to expand. Unless prompt surgical decompression is carried out, the rebound associated with these agents makes the state of the child with a mass lesion even worse. In those children without surgical lesions and with ICP within normal limits, Mannitol is not indicated.

Children with evidence of dangerously increased intracranial pressure without a surgical lesion benefit from controlled ventilation and the prolonged use of hyperosmotic agents. Mannitol is usually only effective for about 72 hours because it leaks slowly across the blood–brain barrier and decreases the effective osmotic gradient. Monitoring of serial blood gases and ICP in an intensive care facility is an essential part of this management.

It is essential that the injured child receive adequate calories. All too often we focus on the injury and neglect the child's nutritional needs. The caloric requirements of the injured child are increased over the normal state. If these nutritional demands are met, the rate of recovery improves, and complications are fewer.

SPECIFIC MANAGEMENT

Scalp Lacerations

Lacerations of the scalp without evidence of underlying injury to the skull should be treated by shaving the area around the laceration, scrubbing the wound, and removing any foreign material. The skin edges may be bleeding profusely from multiple points, requiring rapid hemostasis. Rather than attempting to close off individual bleeding points, hemostats should be applied to the galea aponeurotica and everted over the skin edge. This maneuver is almost always successful in preventing further hemorrhage. No attempt should be made to determine depression of the skull fracture or a defect by probing the wound. A linear fracture needs no treatment, and a depressed fracture should be managed in the operating room. Both fractures should show on skull films or CT scans. Probing through a skull defect could result in unnecessary injury or contamination of the brain and its coverings. After the wound is debrided and cleansed, the skin edges are closed in a single layer with a monofilament suture.

Skull Fractures

Linear Fractures. Linear skull fractures indicate that there has been significant trauma and should alert one to the possibility of intracranial bleeding. Fractures that cross major dural sinuses or the middle meningeal artery or that pass into the foramen magnum are the most likely to involve delayed intracranial hematomas. Observation for 48 to 72 hours is needed for this group of children.

Fractures that extend into cranial sutures frequently will continue in the line of the suture, producing diastasis, especially if the squamous suture is involved. If the linear fracture is associated with a laceration of the underlying dura mater and the pia arachnoid enters this defect, the fracture may not heal and may grow wider with time. This growing fracture is produced by the pulsation of cerebrospinal fluid between the bone edges and is seen more frequently in younger children. A follow-up skull film taken 4 to 6 weeks after injury is indicated if a palpable mass is developing along the fracture line. It usually occurs within the first 6 weeks after the injury (Fig. 32–2).

Ping-Pong Fractures. Trauma to the skull at delivery or during the neonatal period may result in a dent in one of the cranial bones rather than a fracture. The depression may be small or may involve an entire cranial plate. We elevate all of these depressions through a small skin incision with introduction of a periosteal elevator beneath the bone. Pressure on the depressed segment elevates its level with the surrounding bone.

Depressed Fractures. Depressed skull fractures that are displaced more than the thickness of the skull should be surgically elevated. A conventional and coronal CT scan usually will make the diagnosis (Fig. 32–5). If there is a rent in the dura mater, it also should be repaired. The onset of epilepsy is correlated with the sever-

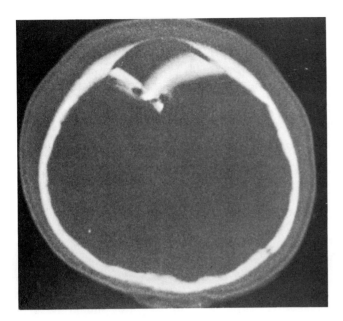
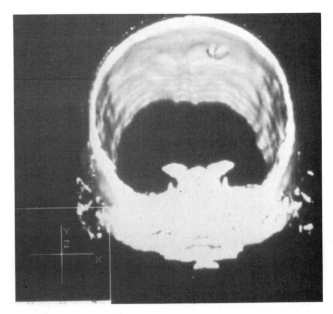

Figure 32–5. CT scan using different techniques to demonstrate depressed skull fractures in children. **Left.** Bone window shows depressed fragments and a large subgaleal hematoma. **Right.** Three-dimensional scan shows fragments protruding into the intracranial compartment.

ity of the injury.[8–10] Parenchymal injury with acute subdural hematoma or diffuse cerebral edema and a depressed skull fracture increase the possibility of seizures. We have not elevated minimally depressed fractures over major dural sinuses unless they have occluded the sinus. All children with a depressed fracture should have a CT scan before surgery to rule out other lesions.

Compound Depressed Fractures. All of these fractures should be repaired in the operating room. The hair and other debris should be removed from the wound. Debridement of the skin edges is important. Depressed or loose pieces of bone that are not grossly contaminated can simply be elevated and replaced. Any dural laceration or injury to the underlying brain is then addressed. The field is irrigated with large volumes of saline, and the wound is closed with monofilament suture.

Basal Skull Fracture. Fractures that pass into the basicranium are certainly more common than x-rays or clinical signs would indicate. As with linear fractures over the convexity of the skull, the vast majority are benign. Some of these fractures will traverse foramina of cranial nerves and interrupt their function. Surgical decompression of these nerves is, in most cases, not indicated. The presence of periorbital ecchymosis, raccoon eyes (bilateral black eyes), or contusion over the mastoid process (battle sign) should alert one to the possibility of a basilar skull fracture and the possibility of a cerebrospinal fluid (CSF) leak.

Fractures of the petrous, frontal, ethmoidal, and sphenoid bones can result in a direct communication between basal cerebrospinal cisterns and the ear, nose, or cranial air sinuses. Almost all traumatic CSF leaks will close spontaneously, usually within 14 days. Persistent or recurrent leaks, as with spontaneous leaks, require a craniotomy, closure of the fistula, and dural repair. Occasionally, air will enter the cranial cavity through the defect. The pneumoencephalus can be seen on plain skull roentgengrams.

The draining of CSF from an orifice should not be occluded by a dressing. We prefer keeping the patient lying flat in bed for 1 or 2 weeks until the CSF leakage ceases. This favors the flow of CSF from inside to out and decreases the possibility of contamination of CSF pathways. Other physicians advocate repeated lumbar puncture and maintaining the patient in the sitting position. This creates a negative ICP and prevents flow across the defect, allowing it to seal. Both methods are effective, but the former, keeping the child lying flat, seems less hazardous. The effectiveness of prophylactic antibiotics is debatable.

Hematomas of the Scalp and Cephalohematomas

A subgaleal hematoma results from bleeding into the space above the periosteum (Fig. 32–6). A cephalohematoma unlike a subgaleal hematoma is confined inside the boundaries of the cranial sutures. On palpation, many cephalohematomas feel like depressed skull fractures because the outer rim of clotted blood is firm and elevated, whereas the center is liquid and soft. Skull films show that the bone usually is not depressed but often has a linear fracture. Only rarely will either of the lesions in

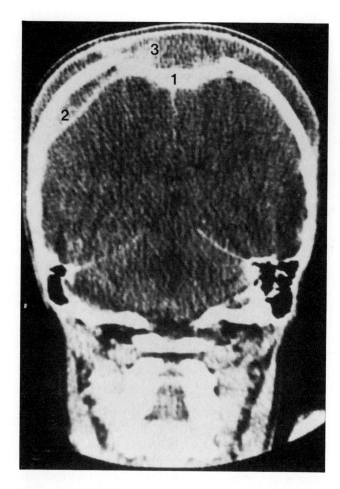

Figure 32–6. A coronal CT scan demonstrates (1) a depressed fracture, (2) epidural hematoma, and (3) a subgaleal hematoma.

themselves require treatment. In rare cases, the hematoma will calcify and require cosmetic surgery. One should resist the urge to drain these fluid cavities. Infection in this space leads to an open draining wound, a scalp defect, and prolonged hospitalization for the child.

All children with a significant scalp hematoma should have a CT scan. Some of these children are bleeding on both sides of the skull from open diploë in the fracture line. A significant epidural hematoma can develop.

Intracranial Hematomas

Acute Subdural Hematomas and Chronic Subdural Effusions.
The extravasation of blood between the dura mater and the pia arachnoid opens a potential space for an acute or chronic collection of fluid (Fig. 32–7). Subacute hematomas seen in adults and older children are rare in children under 2 years of age. These hematomas may be transient or occasionally followed by a relentlessly progressive effusion. Most of the chronic subdural effusions (hematomas) occur in chil-

dren under 2 years of age. Acute subdural hematoma of childhood is not necessarily associated with massive cerebral injury, as is the case in adults (Fig. 32–8). Subdural hematomas usually result from minor trauma or shaking of the child. They usually appear as thin laminar clots over the cerebral convexity. Occasionally, however, they are massive, and few children survive this type of injury.

We have documented the progression of acute laminar hematomas into expanding chronic subdural effusions. Early intervention prevents the development of membranes and the onset of relentless progression often seen with chronic effusions. The chronic subdural effusion of childhood remains an enigma. This lesion's relentless progression, producing a significant morbidity among the affected children, continues to puzzle pediatric neurosurgeons. The diagnosis of a subdural hematoma is made by CT scan or MRI. If a subdural hematoma is a possibility, a contrast-enhanced scan should be performed to reveal the occasional isodense hematoma. Diagnostic subdural taps often give erroneous results and are dangerous. Acute subdural hematomas cannot be aspirated, and the extent of chronic subdural hematomas cannot be determined by this method. We have seen CSF aspirated and interpreted as hygroma fluid, clear fluid converted to grossly hemorrhagic fluid by lacerating a cortical vein, and several cases of subdural hematomas converted to subdural empyemas.

Chronic subdural effusions can be difficult to differentiate clinically from hydrocephalus. They usually are associated with an increasing head circumference. Both have symptoms of increased ICP, lethargy, vomiting, and irritability. Biparietal enlargement, a sunken fontanelle, and a history of trauma favor a subdural hematoma.

In older children subdural hematomas are very much like those of the adult. Acute lesions are associated with significant cerebral damage. The subacute hematoma becomes clinically evident a few days or a couple of weeks later. The adult-type chronic subdural hematoma, a lenticuliform collection of xanthochromic fluid under the convexity of the skull, is rare. Acute and subacute adult-type hematomas require craniotomies, whereas chronic hematomas can be treated adequately through burr holes or subdural–peritoneal shunt. CT scanning and MRI remain the best diagnostic tools.

Epidural Hematoma.
Bleeding between the dura mater and the skull is either from meningeal arteries or venous bleeding from either meningeal veins, dural sinuses, or the diploe system of the skull. This lesion has a characteristic clinical picture. The trauma usually is not severe and may or may not be associated with loss of consciousness or skull fracture. The injury is followed by a period of apparent well-being. This lucid interval varies from hours to days and is then followed

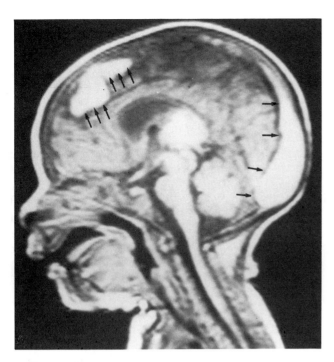

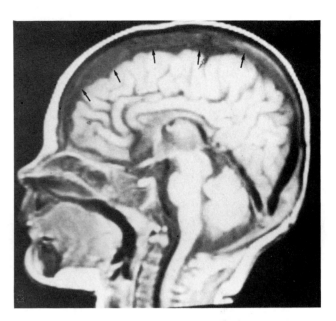

Figure 32–7. Sagittal MRIs of children with **Left.** an acute subdural hematoma (arrows). **Right.** a chronic subdural hematoma (arrows).

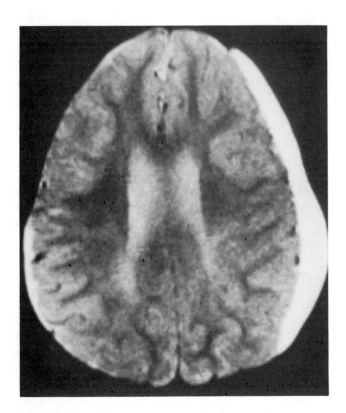

Figure 32–8. An MRI demonstrates clearly bilateral subdural hematomas.

by rapid deterioration. This is an emergent surgical lesion. The morbidity and mortality are low if the diagnosis is made early and the clot is evacuated. Unfortunately, too many of these children are sent home or admitted to inconstant observation areas of a hospital, where they deteriorate to an irretrievable state during sleep.

The diagnosis is made quickly by CT scanning (Fig. 32–9). Rapid surgical decompression by removing the blood clot through either a craniotomy or craniectomy is life-saving. If diagnostic studies are not available or the child has deteriorated and is not responding to hyperventilation, an attempt at diagnosis and decompression should be made, first on the side of the dilated pupil. Diagnostic burr holes are the least acceptable means of management and should be used only in extreme cases.

Lobar Edema. If the force resulting in injury was directed predominantly to one portion of the brain, the edema that develops often is focal. This commonly occurs in only one temporal lobe and often involves one of the frontal or occipital lobes. This focal edema expands rapidly and may act as a mass lesion, producing brain shift. It may also initiate a cycle of surrounded brain compression, decreased cerebral blood flow, edema, and compression. When this advancing edema does not respond to conservative measures or if the brain shift is significant, craniotomy and lobectomy are indicated. If the lobar edema is located in the parietal lobe—especially

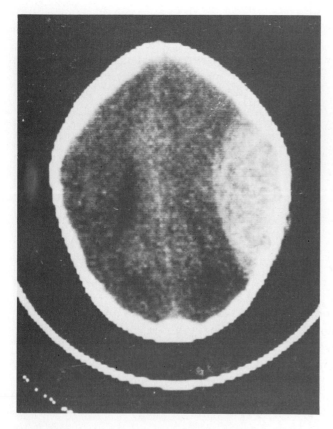

Figure 32–9. CT scan of an acute epidural hematoma. In spite of this huge hematoma, the child recovered completely.

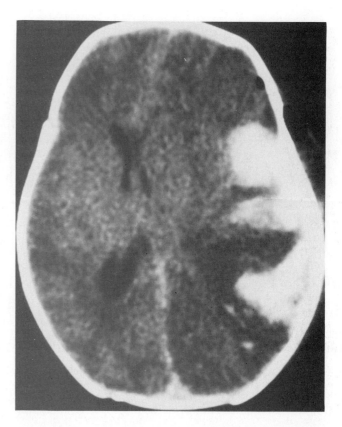

Figure 32–10. A CT scan shows diffuse injury to a hemisphere with contusion, an intracerebral hematoma, and marked shift of midline structures.

the left parietal lobe—surgical intervention is not indicated because of the profound neurologic deficit that follows removal of this lobe of the brain.

Intracerebral Hematomas

Extravasation of blood into brain parenchyma is not uncommon after a head injury. CT scanning or MRI will identify these previously unsuspected lesions. Most of them are small and do not require surgery. Surgery is indicated for those that act as mass lesions, with evidence of increased ICP or brain shift. The frontal, occipital, and temporal tips are the most common sites. Lesions under the motor cortex or left parietal lobe should be managed conservatively if possible (Fig. 32–10).

CT scanning or MRI is again the most effective diagnostic tool, with craniotomy and evacuation of the hematomas the most effective treatment. Removal of intracerebral hematoma through a burr hole usually is inadequate.

Intraventricular Hemorrhage

CT scans demonstrate bleeding into the ventricular system even in awake patients. Surgical therapy usually is not indicated, but posttraumatic hydrocephalus may develop later.

Penetrating Wounds

The size of the object, the location of entry, and the depth of penetration obviously are important, but the velocity also is important because the more rapid the projectile, the more force exerted against the surrounding nervous system, other things being equal (Fig. 32–11). Through-and-through low-velocity missiles do minimal damage to the brain, whereas a tangential wound from a high-velocity weapon may cause considerable brain damage. If the object is still projecting from the child's head, no attempt should be made to remove it until the child is prepared in the operating room. The projectile may be temporarily restraining a major bleeding source, such as a dural sinus. CT scan and occasionally an angiogram should be performed to rule out sinus injuries or intracerebral hematomas.

We debride the entrance wound and site of exit if it is a through-and-through wound. No attempt should be made to debride the tract through cerebral substance, since this only extends the injury. Readily accessible bone, hair, and clothing should be removed, the wound irrigated, the dura closed, and the skin sutured. If a dural graft is needed for closure of the dura mater, pericranium should be used. Postoperative antibiotics and anticonvulsants should be given.

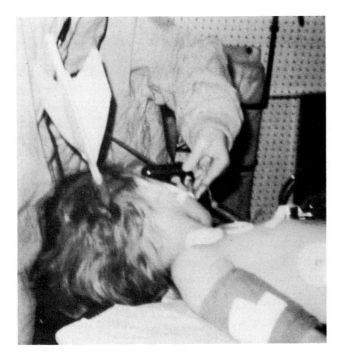

Figure 32–11. A lawn dart thrown over the garage embedded itself in the child's skull over the lateral sinus. The dart was removed in the operating room, and the child recovered completely.

Laceration of Dural Sinuses

Lacerated major dural sinuses hemorrhage massively. Several steps are important in the management of sinus lacerations. First, one must anticipate or entertain the possibility of sinus laceration. This enables one to make proper preparation for sinus bleeding. These lesions must be managed in the operating room with intravenous lines, and blood should be ready, with local coagulant materials available. Every attempt must be made to preserve the function of the dural sinuses. They should be ligated only when this is the only means available to stop the bleeding. Placing an absorbable gelatin sponge over the open sinus and turning the dural flaps (one from either side) over the sinus will control most lacerations.

Posttraumatic Hydrocephalus

Bleeding into the subarachnoid CSF pathways can produce obstruction to the circulation of CSF. This obstruction may be acute and transient. Occasionally, it results in permanent scarring in the arachnoid villi, leading to malabsorption of CSF and permanent hydrocephalus. Children who are making progress and then deteriorate should be investigated for the possibility of acute hydrocephalus. The diagnosis can be established by CT scan. Diversion of CSF to a body cavity or to an external drainage system will control the progression and, if performed early, will prevent brain damage.

Results

Little is known about the long-term effect of head injuries incurred during childhood. In severe head injuries, if coma exceeds 24 hours, a significant sequel can be expected in about half of the children.[1-4] Only now are psychologic studies bringing to light learning disabilities previously unsuspected in these children.[11,12]

A great deal of information is now available on acute problems associated with head injury in adults. Studies are being directed at the pediatric age group. Among the most striking findings of these investigations are the marked difference in physiologic response of the child's brain when compared to that of the adult and the much more optimistic prognosis for useful survival. It now appears that a child who reaches an emergency room in coma, breathing, and able to survive for 6 hours has a 60 percent chance of useful survival in spite of coma persisting beyond the initial 6 hours. The common occurrence in brain-injured children of weeks of coma, including decerebration, with the almost abrupt return to full function, constitutes one of the most striking events in medicine.

SPINAL CORD INJURIES

The child with a spinal cord injury presents similar management problems to the severe head-injured patient. Not only can anoxia and ischemia make the primary injury worse, but also failure of proper initial management can extend the level of irreversible damage.

Spinal cord injury in children comprises about 0.65 to 9.47 percent of spinal injuries of all ages. The incidence of spinal cord injury increases with age, particularly after the age of 12. Male children are slightly more frequent victims than females (1.6:1). Pedestrian-related motor vehicle accidents and falls are the most frequent causes of spinal cord injury in young children in contrast to passenger-related motor vehicle accidents in older children. High cervical injuries (C4 and above) in young children are more frequent, particularly atlantooccipital dislocation and odontoid fractures. A particular problem in children is the high frequency (36 to 66.7 percent) of spinal cord injury without radiographic abnormality (SCIWORA).[13,14] This again emphasizes the point that a normal lateral cervical spine x-ray does not rule out a spinal cord injury or an unstable spine in children. When no evidence of fracture or subluxation is found, dynamic flexion and extension x-rays should be obtained when the child is stable. Furthermore, delaying other resuscitative measures to obtain a cervical spine film makes little sense. Assume that the cervicle spine is unstable and proceed with resuscitation.

Anatomic and biomechanical differences certainly exist between children and adult spines.[15,16] The vertebral facets of children are shallowly angulated, and the vertebral bodies are wedge-shaped, predisposing to greater mobility. The child's head is disproportionately larger and, therefore, expose the spine to different inertial forces. The fulcrum of the neck motion occurs between C2 and C3 in children (C5 and C6 in adults). The maturation of the spine per se, its vasculature, paraspinal musculature, ligaments, and bony structure are important variables. Maturation of the vascular supply to the spine and radiographic complete fusion of the dens synchondrosis occur by the age of 13.

Birth injuries of the spinal cord are the result of excess traction during delivery. The spinal cord and meninges can be totally disrupted in the absence of bony injuries. In addition, brachial plexus and traumatic arachnoid cysts are common in traction injury during delivery.

Management of Spinal Cord Injuries

All children with a history of a neck injury or multiple trauma should be managed as if they have spine instability or a spinal cord injury until proven otherwise. Children with spinal cord injuries are treated like other patients with multiple trauma; airway and blood pressure are stabilized first. At times, the insertion of an appropriate airway into a patient with a spinal cord injury may require intubation. This should be done to prevent the onset of hypoxia and hypoxic brain damage. The techniques for inserting the airway are simple. The child's head should be held, and slight traction should be applied in line with the long axis of the body while intubation is occurring. Slight extension with a small roll under the shoulders is permissible in the young child, but flexion must be avoided. Appropriate intravenous lines are then inserted, and blood is sent for typing and cross-matching. The bladder is catheterized, and usually a nasogastric tube is inserted. During these manipulations, care is taken to prevent further injury to the already damaged spinal cord. Immobilization should be carried out at the scene of the accident. A firm collar should be applied, or the child should be placed on a board with sandbags on either side of the head and tape across the forehead to immobilize the head and neck.

Clinical Feature

The clinical features of spinal cord injuries in children are similar to those seen in adults. However, it is not uncommon to see some withdrawal reflex in the extremities within hours after a complete transection of the spinal cord, giving the false impression of an incomplete cord injury. The spinal cord injury can be classified into four discrete types:

1. Transection of cord. All modalities of function of the spinal cord are involved below the level of injury.

2. Anterior cord syndrome. Since the spinothalamic and corticospinal tracts are involved, one can demonstrate a loss of pain and temperature sensation with motor function loss below the level of involvement. However, the posterior column function (touch, position, and vibration) modalities are intact.

3. Brown-Sequard syndrome. Half of the spinal cord is transected. Therefore, the function of half of the spinal cord is lost: ipsilateral motor weakness (corticospinal tract) and loss of touch, position, and vibration sense (posterior column sign). Pain and temperature senses (spinothalamic tract) of the opposite side of the lesion are lost.

4. Central cord syndrome. The lesion is confined in the central zone of the cord, usually by ischemic necrosis, and is centripedal with decreasing effects toward the periphery of the cord. Fibers involving the arms are more involved than fibers to the legs. Therefore, one may see quadriparesis with more involvement of the arms than legs (corticospinal tract plus anterior horn cell involvement). Since the spinothalamic tract often is spared or partially involved, sensory changes are rather indefinite. This lesion commonly is caused by hypertension injury and usually associated with no overt fracture or dislocation of the cervical spine. This syndrome is more frequently observed in older children and young adults.

The posterior column may be selectively involved after trauma. However, a pure posterior cord syndrome is a rare occurrence. The key change after a cord injury, particularly of the cervical region, is a parasympathetic overflow through the vagus nerve, since the sympathetic outflow is lost due to cord injury. A systemic vascular resistance drops, and generalized vasodilatation occurs. With the loss of sympathetic innervation to the heart, parasympathetic function leads to varying degrees of bradycardia, and cardiac output increases. This effect is usually well tolerated in children and young adults. In most of the cases, sympathomimetics, such as alpha and beta receptors, for example, dopamine, are not necessary.

The neurologic examination requires accurate observation and recording in conjunction with a detailed neurologic history. The details of the accident and the evolution of symptoms often can provide a clue to the nature of the pathologic process. Children may remain in spinal shock for days, then may improve neurologically. Therefore, neurologic evaluation should be repeated to observe either deterioration or improvement. Localization of the spinal cord lesion often requires a thorough understanding of the horizontal and longitudinal sectional anatomy. In general, the higher the lesion in the cervical cord, the greater the loss of motor, sensory, and respiratory impairments.

Gastrointestinal function also is seriously impaired, particularly in the spinal shock stage. Ileus and fecal retention or impaction is common and gradually improves as the other reflexes return. The loss of sweating, due to an impaired sympathetic outflow, also is seen in the acute stage. Therefore, heat control is lost in the area of involvement, particularly with a higher cervical cord lesion. Late adaptation occurs with the return of local vasomotor responses.

Diagnostic Assessment

The radiographic investigation of children with a suspected spine injury poses special problems, since movement of a patient with an unstable spine may precipitate permanent damage of an already injured cord. Therefore, the examination should be performed without movement of the spine. The child should be lifted as one piece, retaining alignment. The initial basic lateral and anteroposterior cervical spine x-ray examination, once the child is stable, is sufficient. Later, a more detailed systematic evaluation of the spine can be carried out.

It is extremely important to see the whole seven cervical vertebrae. Failure to demonstrate particularly the lower cervical region in the lateral view will result in missing lesions in this area. Gentle traction on the arms may bring down the shoulder to visualize the lower cervical area, or the swimmer's technique is required (upward traction on one arm and downward traction on the other). For patients unconscious because of an associated head injury or multiple injuries, whole spine x-rays should be obtained.

Other views include anteroposterior open mouth to show the relationship of occiput to C1 and the odontoid process or the supine oblique views to evaluate facet injury. Tomography is useful when the fractures are dubious or not well seen on plain films, particularly an area between C7 and T1, where conventional technique fails to visualize fractures clearly. Demonstration of prevertebral soft tissue swelling on the lateral cervical spine x-ray is an extremely important clue of SCIWORA.

CT has the advantage of visualizing the relationship of the fracture to the spinal cord. CT with metrizamide myelography allows even more diagnostic evaluation of the spinal cord and surrounding structures. Two good reasons to perform myelography are (1) incomplete spinal cord injury and (2) progression of neurologic deficit.

MRI is useful to evaluate the extent of the parenchymal injury and the relationship of the cord to surrounding structures (Fig. 32–12). Again, because of the time required to complete this study, it is usually not useful in the acute stage of management.

Spinal cord dysfunction can be electrophysiologically quantitated by using somatosensory evoked potential (SSEP) and, more recently, motor evoked potential (MEP). SSEP is an indirect analysis of the integrity of sensory pathways. Average evoked potentials are re-

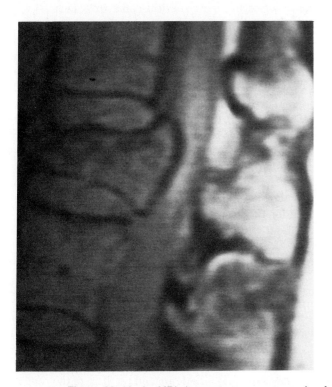 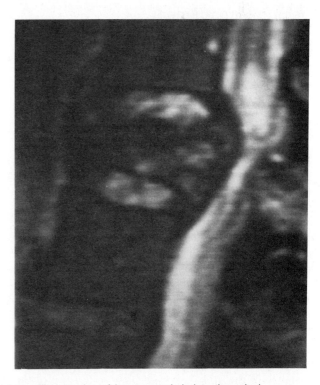

Figure 32–12. An MRI demonstrates a compression fracture with extrusion of bone posteriorly into the spinal canal, compressing neural elements. **Left.** T1 image. **Right.** T2 image.

corded from the scalp, brain, and spinal cord using various sites of remote peripheral stimulations. Neither the stimulation nor the recording method have been strictly standardized, but SSEP and MEP are reliable means of assessing neurologic function in children with spinal cord injuries. In general, acute injuries are manifested primarily by changes in the amplitude, whereas chronic injuries are associated with the appearance of bizarre long latency. The absence of cortical SSEP immediately after an acute spinal cord injury correlates with severe pathologic changes and poor prognosis for subsequent clinical recovery.

The ideal treatment is to accomplish an early restoration of the vertebral alignment and early rigid immobilization of the unstable cervical spine so that the child can be upright and mobilized as his or her general condition allows. The halo device offers an excellent alternative means of managing cervical spine instability in young children. Among numerous benefits of the halo device, one of its main advantages is that it obviates a need for confinement in bed. Early mobilization and ambulation can reduce medical complications from prolonged confinement. Under fluoroscopic control, it allows for external reduction of the bony offset with subsequent immobilization by adjusting the halo apparatus. In addition, it allows easy access for anterior or posterior cervical fusion without disruption of spinal alignment. The halo can be applied safely and is well tolerated by younger children. In selected patients, it provides an alternative to surgery.

Specific Management

Atlantooccipital Dislocation.
Atlantooccipital dislocation is not an uncommon spine injury (1 percent of all cervical cord injury) and is associated with extremely high mortality rates. Between 19 and 35 percent of patients dying of cervical spine injuries showed this type of injury in postmortem examination.

The craniocerebral junction of children is less stable than that of adults. The occipital condyles are small, and the articular plane is almost horizontal. With advancing age, the joint planes become more vertical and deeply, firmly seated in the articular facet of the atlas. Therefore, atlantooccipital dislocation is three times more common in children. The halo ring is an excellent device for the initial alignment of the craniospinal axis with minimal traction. Posterior craniocervical fusion is then performed. One can do this procedure with the halo device in place so that the craniocervical spine is kept well aligned.

Jefferson's Fracture.
This is a very rare type of burst fracture in young children and occurs with a squeezing injury of the atlas or with a blow to the top of the

head. Children usually refuse to move their necks because of nuchal rigidity and limitation of motion. Dysphagia is not uncommon. Cervicomedullary and spinal cord injury are absent in 50 percent of these patients.

Treatment involves immobilization in a halo device for about 12 weeks and then a hard cervical collar for another 4 to 6 weeks. In a facet injury, a posterior cranioatlantoaxis fusion is recommended.[16]

Atlantoaxial Dislocation.
Fracture–dislocation of the odontoid process with high cervical spine injury is the commonest form of spine injury in children. It has been estimated that fractures of the dens compose 75 percent of the cervical spine injuries in children, as contrasted with 10 to 15 percent in adults. Atlas and axis are firmly held by ligaments. Anteriorly, the anterior atlantooccipital membrane joins with the anterior longitudinal ligament binding the basilar portion of the occipital bone (clivus) to the anterior ring of C1 and the odontoid process of C2. The odontoid process is held in close approximation to the anterior atlantic arch (C1) by the alar ligaments, transverse ligament, and cruciform ligament and the tectorial membrane. The apical ligament (atlantodental ligament) is rather weak and, in most instances, simply provides a small vessel to the bone.

There are primarily three types of fractures in the odontoid process. A type I fracture goes through the tip of the odontoid process and probably represents an avulsion fracture where the alar ligament attaches. Usually, no treatment is necessary except for external immobilization with a hard cervical collar or halo for 3 or 4 months.

In contrast, when a type II fracture occurs at the base of the dens at the site of its union (neurocentral synchondrosis), there may be a disruption of the blood supply, and nonunion can occur in approximately 20 percent of the children. The posterior dislocation creates more nonunion problems than the anterior dislocation. If the distance between the posterior wall of the atlantic arch to the dens (atlantodental interval) is more than 4 mm in children, one should suspect a fracture–dislocation. We have achieved good union with the use of the halo device for many young children, eliminating the need for posterior cervical fusion.

Type III fractures of the body of C2 should heal with external immobilization for 8 to 12 weeks. This fracture usually runs through the superior articular facets of C2.

Os Odontoideum.
Os odontoideum is a round or oval piece of bone with a smooth border either in the position of the odontoid process or more proximal to the base of the occipital bone. Usually, there is a gap between the os odontoideum and the base of the remain-

ing odontoid process. Os odontoideum is now thought to be the result of previous trauma.

Hangman's Fracture. This type of fracture is an avulsion of the C2 pedicles, with some degree of dislocation of the C2 vertebral body on C3. This fracture is found both in a judicial hanging and in any hyperextension injury of the neck. In the case of a motor vehicle accident, the avulsed arches decompress the cervicomedullary junction, and therefore neurologic deficits are rare. This type of lesion seldom requires surgical intervention but requires external immobilization with a halo device for 8 to 12 weeks.

Mid and Lower Cervical Spine Injuries. These injuries occur most commonly because of C5–6 dislocation. Injuries to the anterior vertebrae usually are caused by axial loading and flexion forces in which compression and fracture occur. Similar to a burst fracture of the thoracic spine, osseous or extruded disc materials can be displaced posteriorly, compressing the spinal cord.

Treatment of mild compression fracture or axial loading fracture of the mid or lower cervical spine without paralysis is rigid orthosis for about 12 weeks. However, more severe form of injuries, such as unilateral facet dislocation, bilateral facet dislocation, and burst fractures, require immediate halo ring placement or skeletal traction and closed reduction. Later surgical intervention with fusion is indicated.

Injuries to the Thoracic and Lumbar Spine. Fracture–dislocations of this portion of the spine are relatively uncommon in children. However, once it occurs, permanent neurologic deficits are common.

Wedge fractures generally are stable, whereas those with greater than 50 percent wedging are potentially unstable because of damage to laminae, facets, and ligaments. Generally, surgical intervention is required. Otherwise, instability ensues, and a progressive kyphosis develops with the passage of time.

Burst fractures are caused by axial loading and often are associated with fractures of lamina, facets, and pedicles. The fragments can be displaced into the spinal canal, and dural lacerations are common. When rotation is added to the axial loading, the vertebral body is literally sliced through the bursting injury, and this is called a "slice fracture."

Thoracolumbar or upper lumbar spine injuries most often are associated with lap belt injuries. This type of fracture occurs when the lap belt is worn above the iliac crests or when the belt slides up during the accident.

Intraabdominal injuries are common with lap belt injuries and should not be overlooked in children with neurologic deficits.

The single most important factor determining the subsequent outcome of spinal cord injury is the initial extent of the injury. Unfortunately, there is very little evidence that any surgical, conservative, or pharmacologic treatment improves outcome.

REFERENCES

1. Hahn YS, McLone DG, Chyung CH, et al: Head injuries in children under 36 months of age. Childs Nervous System 4:1, 1988
2. Humphreys RP, Jamimovich R, Hendrick B, Hoffman H: Severe head injuries in children. Concepts Pediatr Neurosurg 4:230, 1983
3. Mahoney WJ, D'Souza BJ, Haller JA, et al: Long-term outcome of children with severe head trauma and prolonged coma. Pediatrics 71:75, 1983
4. Zuccarello M, Facco E, Zampieri P, et al: Severe head injury in children: Early prognosis and outcome. Childs Nervous System 1:158, 1985
5. Snoek JW, Minderhoud JM, Wilmink JT: Delayed deterioration following mild head injury in children. Brain 107:15, 1984
6. Bruce VA, Langfitt TW, Miller JD, et al: Regional cerebral blood flow, intracranial pressure and brain metabolism in comatose patients. J Neurosurg 38:131, 1973
7. Teasdale G, Jennett B: Assessment of coma and impaired consciousness: a practical scale. Lancet 2:81, 1974
8. Annegers JF, Grabow JD, Groover RV, et al: Seizures after head trauma: A population study. Neurology 30:683, 1980
9. Hahn YS, Fuchs S, Flannery AM, et al: Factors influencing posttraumatic seizures in children. Neurosurgery 22:864, 1988
10. Jennett B: Trauma as a cause of epilepsy in childhood. Dev Med Child Neurol 15:56, 1973
11. Chadwick O, Rutter M, Thompson J: Intellectual performance and reading skills after localized head injury in childhood. J Child Psychol 22:117, 1981
12. Levin HS, Eisenberg HM, Wigg NR: Memory and intellectual ability after head injury in children and adolescents. Neurosurgery 11:668, 1982
13. Cheshire DJE: The paediatric syndrome of traumatic myelopathy without demonstrable vertebral injury. Paraplegia 15:74, 1977
14. Pang D, Wilberger JE Jr: Spinal cord injury without radiographic abnormalities in children. J Neurosurg 57:114, 1982
15. Bailey DK: The normal cervical spine in infants and children. Radiology 59:712, 1952
16. Ruge JR, Sinson GP, McLone DG, Cerullo LJ: Pediatric spinal injury: The very young. J Neurosurg 68:25, 1988

33
Abdominal Trauma

_____ *William J. Pokorny*

Almost 90 percent of serious abdominal injuries in children less than 14 years of age are the result of blunt trauma. During the preschool years, falls are the predominant form of injury, whereas in elementary school, bicycle accidents and, increasingly, auto–pedestrian injuries predominate. As a child reaches the midteen years, high-speed motor vehicle accidents and penetrating wounds associated with violent crimes become the primary sources of trauma. The history of trauma usually is obvious. However, because of the thin abdominal wall and weak protecting musculature in the young child, even trivial trauma may result in visceral injury. Major lesions may result from a seemingly minor or forgotten incident, such as a belly-flopper on a sled. The costal margin of the young child does not extend down as far as that of an adult and provides less protection for the upper abdominal viscera. This accounts for the relatively higher incidence of splenic and hepatic injuries in children.

Children with abdominal injuries are more likely to suffer concomitant head, chest, or extremity injuries than adults, and these injuries generally are the result of an automobile accident or a bad fall. At Ben Taub General Hospital in Houston from July 1985 through June 1986, 3038 children under 14 years old were seen in the emergency center for trauma, and 394 were admitted. Although the majority of those admitted had skeletal and head injuries, only 10 required laparotomy.

Careful repeated clinical examination is essential to the early diagnosis and correct management of abdominal injuries. The surgeon may use a number of diagnostic aids, but these must be interpreted in light of the clinical findings. After the child's airway, ventilatory status, circulation, and level of conciousness have been evaluated and resuscitation has been begun, the abdomen is examined as part of a thorough overall examination. Observe first for obvious bruises or penetrating injuries. One should compress the lower chest and pelvis to check for tenderness or instability. The entire abdomen and flanks are gently and superficially palpated. Areas of localized tenderness about obvious sites of injury are marked with a pen for later comparison. The initial examination may be misleading. A child with an apparently nontender abdomen may have a ruptured spleen or liver. On the other hand, one who is frightened and crying but essentially unhurt may appear to have a rigid, tender abdomen. Pallor, poor capillary filling, and tachycardia are signs of hemorrhage, which may be intraperitoneal.

If there is any suggestion of an abdominal injury, blood should be drawn for a complete blood count, serum amylase, and typing and crossmatching. A plastic intravenous catheter should be placed securely in the upper extremity if possible, and lactated Ringer's solution should be started. An oral or nasogastric tube is inserted, and the aspirate is examined for blood. After any form of trauma, children are apt to cry and gulp air. The resulting acute gastric dilatation causes pain, tenderness, and abdominal distention. The abdomen that appears to be distended and tender may improve remarkably after emptying of the stomach.

Catheterization of the urinary bladder is performed in all children with abdominal trauma unless there is evidence of urethral or bladder neck injury. Indications of urethral or bladder neck injuries include blood from the meatus, pelvic fractures, perineal or scrotal hematomas, and a high floating prostate. If a urethral injury is suspected, a retrograde cystogram must be performed to rule out such injury before placing a urethral catheter. Blood in the urine is an indication for an intravenous pyelogram and cystogram or a contrast-enhanced abdominal computed tomography (CT) scan. These studies are important to demonstrate injury to the urinary tract and to alert the surgeon to congenital anomalies, particularly a solitary kidney, which will affect operative therapy. The urinary output is an important indication of tissue perfusion and is a guide for fluid and blood replacement. The rectal examination must not be forgotten, particularly with injuries to the pelvis and penetrating wounds. If the child's vital signs indicate hemorrhage, a second large intravenous line is placed, preferably in the superior vena cava, as a second portal for transfusion and to monitor central venous pressure.

Although it is rarely necessary to rush a child directly to the operating room for abdominal trauma, a gunshot wound or blunt trauma that injures the major vessels, fractures the liver, or tears the hepatic veins will result in severe shock and rapid distention of the abdomen because of massive hemorrhage. A needle paracentesis will quickly establish the diagnosis of intraperitoneal hemorrhage in this situation. Resuscitation may require the use of type-specific or, rarely, O-negative blood because these patients often exsanguinate before blood can be crossmatched. A minimum of 6 units of whole blood must be ready in the operating room. If possible, a cell-saver should be used to collect uncontaminated lost blood for reinfusion. When the incision is made, the tamponading effect of abdominal distention is released, and the hemorrhage can be torrential.

The condition of most children with abdominal trauma is not critical, and after the initial evaluation and resuscitation in the emergency room, other studies are indicated. All indicated roentgenograms are obtained in one visit to the x-ray department. These include an intravenous pyelogram if there is hematuria or flank tenderness, a cystogram if there has been lower abdominal trauma or pelvic fracture, and upright roentgenograms of the chest and abdomen that may demonstrate previously unrecognized thoracic trauma or a pelvic fracture. Furthermore, they may form a baseline for studying complications that may arise in the postoperative period. Films of the skull, spine, and long bones are obtained as indicated as long as the child's vital signs are stable. The responsible surgeon and a radiologist should review the films while the child is still on the x-ray table. If there is indication of free air or if the patient's condition remains unstable because of continuing hemorrhage, the patient should be taken directly to the operating room. On the other hand, if the patient remains stable but is suspected of having serious intraabdominal injury, one of three steps may be taken: (1) clinical observation and monitoring in a pediatric intensive care unit, (2) peritoneal lavage, or (3) abdominal CT scan. Clinical observation alone may be inadequate in that it may lead to a delay in diagnosis of the severely injured child. However, observation plus timely use of CT scanning may be in the best interest of the young patient if an unnecessary operation is to be avoided.

If the abdominal findings are equivocal in an awake, alert, and cooperative child, a CT scan and continued observation are indicated. Touloukian observed that the majority of children with insignificant injuries showed considerable improvement within 12 to 18 hours.[1] Once the child has settled down after the initial experience with tubes, needles, and x-rays, further careful palpation of the abdomen is performed. One must work to develop a good rapport with the child. Tenderness in the immediate vicinity of a contusion or penetrating wound is expected. Spreading tenderness or tenderness remote from the injured area indicates trouble. In Touloukian's experience, as in ours, there were neither fatalities nor an appreciable morbidity with the policy of continued observation in equivocal cases. If the child's abdominal findings are clearly worsening, particularly if blood transfusions or increased fluids are required to maintain the vital signs, an operation or further diagnostic tests are indicated.

Children under 3 years of age and those with concomitant head or thoracic injuries are difficult to evaluate on clinical grounds alone. With these children, special diagnostic techniques are most helpful.

PERITONEAL LAVAGE

Neither paracentesis nor lavage should be used routinely in children with blunt trauma. Either procedure will add to the child's apprehension and make it more difficult to evaluate abdominal tenderness that develops after the procedure.[2]

Although peritoneal lavage is a very sensitive tool to demonstrate intraperitoneal bleeding,[3–6] it is a major procedure in a small child. Care must be taken by the surgeon not to injure the intraperitoneal or retroperitoneal organs or vascular structures. This includes the bladder, which in an infant may extend to the umbilicus when distended. Likewise, the apprehensive, frightened child frequently has aerophasia, with marked gastric distention. For this reason, both the bladder and stomach must be decompressed with appropriate catheters before doing a peritoneal lavage. As in adults, the open technique is preferred, and the child must be adequately restrained. Buffered Ringer's lactate solution should be used in a dose of 10 ml/kg per 1000 ml.[7] The solution is run into the peritoneal cavity over a 10-minute period. The child is turned several times to mix the liquid, which is then allowed to run out by gravity. Grossly, bloody fluid is considered a positive result, and if the fluid is crystal clear, one may conclude definitely that there is no significant intraperitoneal injury.

Peritoneal lavage must be interpreted also in the light of the information gained from CT imaging. Lavage is so sensitive that children with insignificant splenic lacerations, who would have recovered without an operation, have been operated upon. Lavage should be reserved for the child with associated injuries that make clinical evaluation difficult and those children requiring immediate surgical intervention for extra-abdominal injuries when CT scanning is unavailable.

COMPUTED TOMOGRAPHY

CT scanning now is used routinely in our medical centers to evaluate the injured child. Its role in evaluating splenic, hepatic, and renal injuries is clear, and with the addition of oral contrast, it has been helpful in diagnosing gastric and duodenal injuries (Figs. 33–1 and 33–2).[8–10] Indications include (1) suspected intraabdominal injury, (2) stable vital signs, (3) slowly declining hematocrit, (4) a requirement for persistent fluid resuscitation, (5) neurologic injury, (6) a multiply injured patient requiring general anesthesia, (7) multiple bleeding sources, and (8) blood in the urine. The disadvantages associated with routine CT scanning include the amount of time required to do the study and the expense. CT scans have proven ineffective in demonstrating pancreatic and intestinal injuries when performed immediately after the injury,[11,12] although the next day these injuries are picked up on CT scan.

It is our policy to obtain an abdominal CT scan on all children with major blunt truncal injury who are hemodynamically stable and who do not have increasing peritoneal signs. Following this policy and observing patients with known and stable splenic and hepatic injuries, we and others have dramatically decreased the number of children undergoing laparotomy.[13,14] At Ben Taub General Hospital between July 1975 and June 1978, all patients sustaining significant blunt abdominal trauma underwent peritoneal lavage, and those with positive results underwent laparotomy. During this 3-year period, 59 patients had exploratory laparotomy. Although 9 had gastrointestinal injuries, 13 explorations were negative, 10 had splenectomies only, and 11 were found to have isolated hepatic injuries. During the more recent 3-year period, July 1983 through June 1986, routine abdominal CT scans were obtained, and hemodynamically stable patients with known splenic and hepatic injuries were observed in the pediatric intensive care unit. During this period, only 21 patients underwent laparotomy. Although a similar number, 10, had gastrointestinal injuries, only 3 required splenorrhaphies and 1 required hepatorrhaphy. None underwent splenectomy, and none had a negative laparotomy. Seventeen of these patients underwent immediate laparotomy based on clinical findings on arrival at the emergency center, and 4 underwent CT scan and were admitted for observation. All 4 were operated on within 24 hours of admission. Two were

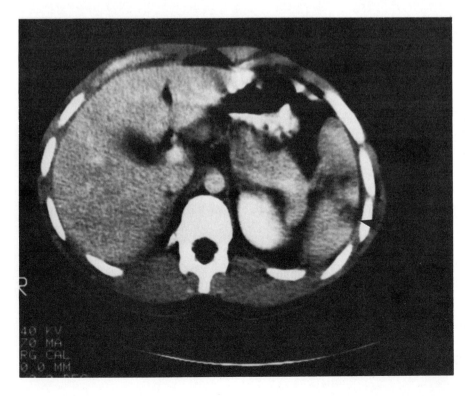

Figure 33–1. CT scan of the abdomen showing transection of the spleen through the hilum. This 17-year-old was treated nonoperatively.

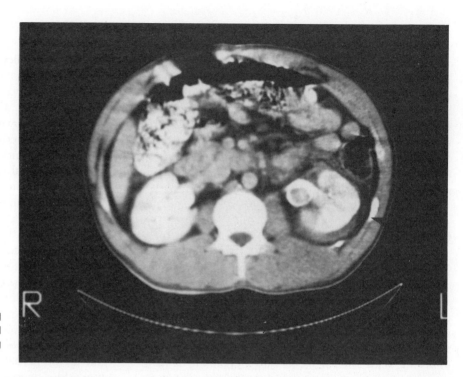

Figure 33–2. CT scan showing left perirenal hematoma, contusion of the upper pole, and a hematoma within the renal pelvis following blunt trauma.

taken to surgery based on evidence of continued hemorrhage, and 2 developed signs of peritoneal irritation.

PREEXISTING LESIONS

One must always keep in mind the possibility of a preexisting congenital defect or neoplasm when evaluating a child with abdominal trauma. The removal of a solitary kidney may be catastrophic. Hydronephrosis and renal tumors are the most common lesions brought to light by trauma. The injury itself is usually relatively minor, but pain and hematuria draw attention to the flank mass. Three mesenteric cysts have been seen at Children's Memorial Hospital that were asymptomatic until an episode of abdominal trauma caused hemorrhage within the cyst.

PENETRATING WOUNDS

Stab and gunshot wounds of the abdomen are seen more frequently these days in urban areas. In addition to street violence and other forms of assault, children may be the victims of stab wounds inflicted by a parent or babysitter. Children are also seen who have been impaled by automobile bumpers or who have wounds from shards of glass and sharp spikes of fences. Penetrating perineal wounds in small children caused by sexual abuse can lead to rectal and vaginal injuries, with secondary disruption of the rectal sphincter mechanism, peritoneal sepsis, and death.[15]

No more than two thirds of abdominal knife wounds penetrate the abdominal cavity.[16,17] Consequently a selective approach has evolved in determining the indications for surgery in these patients.[18] If the child's vital signs are stable and there is no abdominal tenderness, it is safe to merely observe him or her, with repeated abdominal examinations. During the period of observation, flat and upright roentgenograms of the abdomen are obtained, the stomach is kept empty with a nasogastric tube, and the child is given maintenance intravenous fluids. If no signs of peritoneal irritation develop within 48 hours, the patient may be discharged from the hospital. Wound sinogram and peritoneal lavage provide no more information than simple, frequent observation. Other penetrating wounds, as from shards of glass, require wound debridement under general anesthesia. If penetration of the abdominal cavity is found, a laparotomy may be performed at the same time.

When signs of peritonitis develop or if the vital signs suggest ongoing hemorrhage, an exploratory operation is indicated. The small intestine is the most commonly injured organ. Simple closure of small intestinal wounds with irrigation of the peritoneal cavity is all that is required. Small lacerations of the liver and spleen are repaired. There is some controversy over the proper management of left colon wounds. If there is minimal soilage of the peritoneal cavity and a small laceration, the wound may be safely sutured. On the other hand, impalement injuries of the descending colon or rectum should be repaired, and a proximal, completely diverting colostomy should be performed. Gunshot wounds, particularly those involving the colon or major vessels, carry a significantly increased risk of postoperative complications or death.[19,20]

A gunshot wound inflicted at close range results in multiple injuries to the intraabdominal organs. The greatest danger is in overlooking a small perforation of the intestine. Consequently, every inch of the intestine must be examined. Pancreatic and liver perforations are drained, but splenic injuries usually can be repaired. The missile track in a pistol or rifle wound may not always be estimated by observing the wounds of entrance and exit. The bullet trajectory may follow a curved tissue plain of least resistance. If there is no exit wound, the bullet must be localized by x-ray. If no bullet is found on roentgenograms of the chest and abdomen, a bullet embolus is possible, and x-rays must be taken of the extremities.

SURGERY

Some of the most difficult operations are those performed to treat abdominal trauma. If possible, blood volume deficits are corrected before the operation commences. In addition, the patient must be monitored with central venous or pulmonary artery pressure determinations, electrocardiogram, and arterial pressure, and oxygen saturation must be monitored with an arterial line and a Foley catheter appropriate for the child's size. The stomach must be emptied with a large-bore gastric tube. Both the surgeon and the anesthesiologist must have sufficient help to deal with major hemorrhage. The surgical setup must include vascular clamps, two functioning suction units, a sternal splitting saw, and a reliable electrosurgical unit. The entire abdomen, chest, and thighs are prepared and draped into the sterile field. This must include the flanks well around to the 11th rib, so that drains may be brought out through the posterior abdominal wall if necessary. A long, midline incision that can be extended into either pleural cavity or up the sternum provides the best exposure for a complete abdominal exploration and repair of any injury encountered.

After opening the abdomen, blood or fluid is removed with suction and sponges. Attention is first directed toward areas suspected of being injured. Massive hemorrhage, as from a lacerated major vessel, is controlled first with manual pressure. If it is possible to achieve proximal and distal control, the laceration is then repaired. Rarely, it is necessary to have an assistant control the bleeding point with pressure while the aorta is encircled at the diaphragmatic hiatus. At some point during the operation, a systematic inspection of the abdomen is carried out. First, the small intestine is eviscerated onto moist laparotomy pads; then, with retraction in the upper abdomen, the left lobe of the liver is inspected and palpated. The anterior wall of the stomach is in-

spected, after which the lesser sac is entered through the gastrocolic omentum, and the posterior wall of the stomach and the pancreas are observed. The retractor is then shifted to the right upper quadrant, and the right lobe of the liver, the superior vena cava, the right adrenal, and the kidney are observed and palpated. The liver is elevated with a retractor, and the duodenum is explored. If there is any hematoma in this area, the duodenum is mobilized to the left as far as the aorta. The right abdominal gutter and ureter are then observed, the retractor is moved to the pelvis, and the lower abdomen is inspected, particularly with a retroperitoneal hematoma in mind. The small intestine is then shifted to the right, and the exploration is carried up the left gutter to the left kidney, adrenal, and spleen. At this point, the left transverse colon is elevated, and the small intestine is inspected, commencing at the ligament of Treitz.

TRAUMA TO THE SPLEEN

The spleen is the most commonly injured intraperitoneal organ in blunt trauma to the abdomen in childhood. The symptoms of splenic injury are those of hemorrhage into the peritoneal cavity. However, shock is unusual in children with a ruptured spleen unless there are other injuries. Abdominal pain and pallor, with tenderness in the left upper quadrant, suggest the diagnosis. Fractured ribs in the left lower chest and abrasions on the left side also draw attention to the spleen. As the child is observed, tenderness spreads to other abdominal quadrants. He or she often will complain of pain in the left shoulder, particularly when lying down or during bimanual palpation of the flank (Kehr's sign).

The initial hematocrit may be within normal limits, but as the child is resuscitated, the hematocrit will drop during the first 6 to 12 hours of observation. All these signs may be obscured by associated injuries. Plain films of the abdomen may suggest the diagnosis when the greater curvature of the stomach is indented by a hematoma or ruptured spleen. The diagnosis is confirmed by CT scan of the abdomen. With our current program of observation and CT scanning, it is unusual to see the delayed rupture described by Zabinski and Harkins and later by Lorimer unless the original trauma was not brought to the attention of the physician.[21,22] The CT scan may be repeated 10 to 14 days after the injury and before discharge to rule out the possibility of an expanding subcapsular hematoma.[23]

For years, the standard management of a ruptured spleen was an immediate splenectomy. However, it is now known that children who have undergone a splenectomy are at increased risk of developing an overwhelming infection. It was initially believed that sepsis did not follow splenectomy performed for trauma, but Belfauz et al. found this to be false in their 12 cases.[24] Splenectomy results in several immunologic defects, including a poor response to intravenous particulate antigens, a deficiency in phagocytosis, and a decreased serum IgM and properidin.[25–27] No age range is exempt from postsplenectomy sepsis, and *Streptococcus pneumoniae* is the most common infecting organism.[28] Ein et al. found that splenectomy for thalassemia and portal hypertension gives the highest risk of infection. The difference in risk between splenectomies for trauma and hematologic problems, respectively, may very well represent the difference in the completeness of the splenectomy. When one operates for trauma, there is no search for accessory spleens. The accessory spleens, as well as fragments of traumatized spleen left behind after the operation, may be sufficient to protect the patient from sepsis. The majority of splenic injuries will respond to nonoperative management. Thirty-five of 56 children at the Toronto Children's Hospital and 37 of 42 at Children's Hospital National Medical Center with ruptured spleens were managed nonoperatively.[29,30] When operative intervention is required for associated injuries or to control bleeding, the spleen should be repaired.[31–33] In the 2-year period, 1975–1976, 21 patients less than 14 years of age underwent splenectomy at Ben Taub General Hospital. Since 1979, only 1 child has required splenectomy. In the last 2 years, only 1 child required a splenorrhaphy.[32] In the rare instance when this is not possible, autotransplantation of thin sections of the spleen into the omentum may provide some protection from sepsis.

The site and extent of injury must be defined by CT scan or isotope imaging. After the splenic injury is confirmed by CT scan, the child may be treated nonoperatively provided he or she can be monitored in an intensive care unit by a surgical–anesthesia team prepared to intervene at any time.[34] If this is lacking, it is safer to operate and repair or remove the damaged spleen. Patients who have massive bleeding should be operated on promptly.

The usual child with a ruptured spleen and no other injuries, and with a diagnosis confirmed by a CT scan, may be safely observed in the hospital until the pain and tenderness have subsided, usually in 7 to 10 days. The child is then sent home to continue limited activity for 1 month. Follow-up scans indicate that wedge-shaped defects or even complete separation of the spleen may persist for up to 3 months, but there have been no long-term sequelae in children treated in this manner.[35]

TRAUMA TO THE LIVER AND BILIARY TRACT

The liver is a large, richly vascularized organ enclosed in a thin, friable capsule. The hepatic veins are short

and inaccessible to the surgeon and empty into the suprarenal inferior vena cava. These anatomic facts explain the difficulties in treating major hepatic injuries. Fortunately, most liver injuries are either shallow lacerations on the dome of the right lobe or small penetrating wounds that stop bleeding spontaneously. Stone and Ausley found that 137 of 203 liver injuries reviewed at Emory University required only drainage because there was no active bleeding at the time of the laparotomy.[36] Such relatively minor lacerations following blunt trauma cause abdominal pain and tenderness, perhaps on the right side, but are difficult to distinguish from splenic injuries. Afflicted patients may experience tachycardia, but there are no signs of shock. The vital signs return to normal after initial resuscitation with a balanced salt solution, but over the first 6 to 12 hours of observation, the hematocrit falls.

In this group of patients the abdominal CT scan will confirm the diagnosis (Fig. 33–3). If the scan reveals a laceration with normal liver tissue on either side, continued observation without an operation is acceptable in that most children will respond to nonoperative management.[8] If a nonoperative approach is elected, the child must be constantly monitored in an intensive care unit, blood must be available for immediate transfusion, and the child must be given nothing by mouth. The surgical and anesthesia services must be prepared to take the child immediately to the operating room on a 24-hour basis. Indications for operation are similar to those described for splenic injuries and include associated injuries and persistent hemorrhage.[9] Evidence of decreased perfusion of the liver on the isotope study is an indication for operation. Before scans were routinely obtained at Children's Memorial Hospital in cases of suspected liver injuries, a 6-year-old girl with minimal abdominal findings developed septic shock and died 5 days after her injury. A pool table had fallen across her abdomen and crushed the left lobe of her liver. The necrotic lobe could have been detected with a scan. The appropriate treatment would have been a left hepatic lobectomy.[37]

At the other end of the spectrum of liver injury is the patient with major blunt trauma who has additional central nervous system, thoracic, or skeletal trauma. Kaufman and Burrington reported that 60 percent of their patients had additional major trauma.[38] In all series, there has been an overall 20 percent mortality rate; these are the children who die shortly after reaching the hospital from hemorrhagic shock.[39] Hemorrhagic shock and massive transfusion also account for most of the delayed complications, including respiratory failure, coagulation defects, metabolic acidosis, and renal failure, that are seen after operation in these patients.

For the child who continues to be in shock from hemorrhage despite resuscitation, there should be no

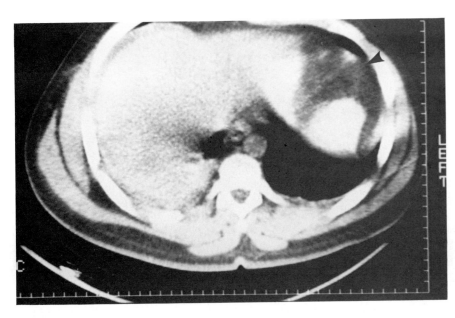

Figure 33–3. CT scan diagnostic of a subcapsular hematoma of the right lobe of the liver. This was treated nonoperatively.

delay in performing diagnostic tests to determine the exact site of hemorrhage, since the source will become all too apparent when the abdomen is opened. After initial resuscitation in the emergency room with rapid infusions of balanced salt solution, the child is taken directly to the operating room for continued shock therapy, monitoring, anesthesia, and laparotomy. We take the child to the x-ray department on the way to the operating room for a one-shot urogram only if there is hematuria.

In the operating room, the child is rapidly transfused, given oxygen and a relaxant, and intubated. This allows control of the airway and ensures better oxygenation than with the child's spontaneous respirations. Hypothermia has little to offer the child with a major hepatic injury because of the time required to lower the body temperature. In our hands, the combination of hypothermia and blood loss has led to irreversible cardiac arrest.

A generous midline incision, which can be converted into a sternum-splitting incision if necessary to control the suprarenal vena cava, provides the most rapid exposure of the liver. Initial hemostasis is obtained by packing the obviously hemorrhaging areas with moist pads. One may then remove blood with suction, and while the hemorrhage is being tamponaded with manual pressure, transfusions are given until the vital signs improve. When there is plenty of blood available, the packs are removed to evaluate the liver wound. In anterior lacerations, it frequently is possible to control bleeding points with direct suture ligature. Under no circumstances should the laceration be sutured closed or packed with absorbable hemastatic agents. This merely converts an open, easily drained wound into a closed pocket that invites continued hemorrhage into the liver substance, as well as infection and hematobilia.

If there is continued hemorrhage from deep within

the liver that does not appear to originate from a tear in the vena cava or hepatic veins, the wound is repacked, and the hepatic artery is dissected in the porta hepatis. Ligation of the hepatic artery that supplies the affected lobe appears to be safe and effective and has reduced the need for lobectomy. In addition to making this contribution to hepatic surgery, Mays warned against the traditional Pringle maneuver in which the entire porta hepatis is clamped.[40] Interruption of portal flow to each lobe only contributes to hypoxic tissue damage and decreased function in uninjured liver tissue. Canty and Aaron reported successful right hepatic arterial ligation as an alternative to liver resection in children.[41] Liver resection is indicated when arterial ligation fails to control the hemorrhage or when a segment of liver appears to be devascularized, in which case the resection is a debridement of necrotic liver tissue. Stone and Ausley reported an 18 percent mortality in 17 children requiring liver resection.[36] They proposed packing the liver wound with a pedicle graft of omentum as another alternative to liver resection. Only 1 of their 12 patients treated with an omental graft died.

Hepatic vein lacerations may be particularly difficult to control and are life threatening. The vein is first controlled with finger pressure. Then, when everything is ready, one attempt should be made to apply a vascular clamp to the torn vessel or to suture the laceration beneath the finger. These efforts are almost always hampered by poor exposure and the obscuring of the field with blood. Repeated attempts to control the hemorrhage in this fashion will fail and result in further injury to the hepatic veins and inferior vena cava. Consequently, the steps described by Mays should be undertaken without delay.[40] The wound is packed, the midline incision is extended to the suprasternal notch, and the sternum is split in the midline. The right pleural cavity is entered, and the diaphragm is split in the midline to the juncture of the inferior vena cava and the hepatic veins. Meanwhile, an assistant has cut extra holes in a size 20–26 French chest tube, which is filled with saline and then clamped. The pericardium is opened, the right atrial appendage is encircled with a pursestring suture and opened, and the tube filled with saline is passed down the cava. The tube is positioned in such a fashion that the distal end is just below the renal veins, and the extra hole is within the right atrium. The cava may then be encircled within the pericardium and around the catheter above the renal veins. Blood is shunted through the tube so that when the porta hepatis is crossclamped, there is a dry field for the repair of venous lacerations. The clamps on the porta hepatis must be opened every 15 minutes to avoid hypoxic damage to the liver.

Rarely, a patient is encountered with generalized bleeding from large liver injuries who remains in shock, with worsening hypothermia and coagulopathies. In these cases, it is prudent to pack the injury with gauze and rapidly close the abdomen so that the patient may be resuscitated and warmed. The patient can then be returned to the operating room in several days in a more controlled fashion. Regardless of what is done to the liver itself, drainage of the area is most important. Blood, bile, and serum accumulate under the diaphragm and cause infection unless there is adequate, dependent drainage of the suprahepatic and infrahepatic spaces. Drains to the anterior abdominal wall do not provide dependent drainage. Drainage of the common duct or gallbladder is not indicated unless these structures are injured.

Although there is controversy about administration of prophylactic antibiotics after liver surgery, we believe that broad-spectrum antibiotics should be given during surgery and for 3 days after a major resection or hepatic artery ligation. After that time, antibiotics are used only with clinical evidence of sepsis or positive cultures of the drainage. Pleural effusions often are the first sign of a subphrenic collection. The effusion is tapped and then drained with a chest tube. If a subphrenic abscess develops, the child should be returned to the operating room for drainage of the subphrenic space. If the original drains have been removed, the drainage tract may be reopened under sterile conditions. Adhesions are broken down, and loculated collections of fluid are drained.

There have been few reports of injury to the extrahepatic biliary system in children. Even complete division of the common bile duct may pass undetected until the child develops jaundice and bile ascites. Although end-to-end anastomosis of severed bile ducts in children has been performed successfully, when the distal bile duct is injured, choledochoduodenostomy is an alternate procedure.[42–44]

Hematobilia

When hematemesis follows recovery from abdominal trauma, hematobilia should be the first diagnostic consideration. The average interval between the trauma and the onset of the bleeding is 4 weeks, but the range is from 4 days to 5 months. In our cases, the hepatic injury went unnoticed until the hemorrhage commenced. However, hematobilia also has occurred after the suture of deep liver lacerations. Patients with hematobilia complain of a cramping right upper quadrant and are jaundiced or have an elevation of the serum bilirubin. Selective hepatic angiography confirms the diagnosis by demonstrating extravasation of contrast material (Fig. 33–4). Various techniques have been used in the management of hematobilia, from hepatic lobectomy to embolization and continued observation.[45–47] We have avoided hepatic lobectomy by securing control of the right hepatic artery in the hilum and then opening the cavity. On two occasions, it was possible to successfully suture-ligate the bleeding artery. The cavity was then left open and widely drained. However, since Hendren et al. have demonstrated successful healing of the traumatic aneurysm with serial angiograms, delay and observation of the child in the hospital seem to be worthwhile.[47]

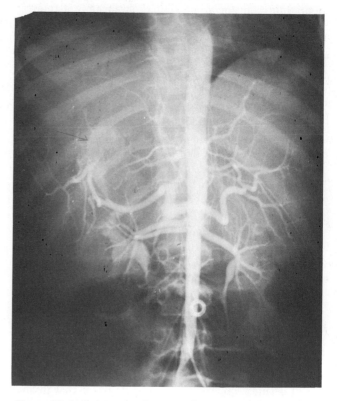

Figure 33–4. Aortography demonstrating extravasation of contrast material from the hepatic artery.

TRAUMA TO THE GASTROINTESTINAL TRACT

Rupture of the stomach secondary to blunt trauma is rare in children but does occur when severe upper abdominal trauma follows the ingestion of a large meal.[48,49] Typically, the child is hit in the epigastrium, and the stomach bursts along the greater curvature.[50] Older children complain of excruciating abdominal pain and develop a rigid abdominal wall as if an ulcer had perforated. If there is a delay in diagnosis, as may occur in the younger or abused child, peritonitis and shock may develop. We observed one 10-month-old infant who was kicked by his father soon after he had consumed a full bottle of milk. This infant did not arrive at the emergency room until he was in deep shock, and he subsequently died. Another child operated on at our hospital fell from a second story window immediately after supper. She too was in deep shock on arrival 6 hours after the injury but was successfully resuscitated. This child, as well as others mentioned in various reports, had a ruptured spleen in addition to a large rent on the anterior curvature of the stomach. The mechanism of injury in these cases is that of a bursting balloon. All have in common a painful, boardlike abdomen and large amounts of free air visible on upright roentogenograms if the diagnosis is delayed. Resuscitation and immediate laparotomy are required. At operation, the abdomen is completely irrigated with warm saline. Every nook and cranny of the abdominal cavity must be explored to remove food particles, which, if left, will become nidi for abscesses. Since the stomach has been ruptured by a bursting force, the edges of the wound are ragged and must be debrided until there is healthy tissue; then the wound is closed in two layers. Most recover uneventfully. However, one of our children and two reported in the literature developed postoperative gastric fistulas and subphrenic abscesses.

Trauma to the Duodenum

The duodenum is fixed against the posterior abdominal wall and is subject to shearing and crushing injuries by being forced against the vertebrae. The most common injury in childhood is the intramural hematoma. The trauma that produces a hematoma is of a lesser magnitude than that found in most abdominal injuries and is more likely to be a direct, pointed blow to the upper abdomen, as from a bicycle handlebar or a fist. The injury may have been so trivial that its history must be elicited by direct questioning. Indeed, child abuse is sufficiently common in these patients that the history of trauma often is never obtained. Pain with epigastric and right upper quadrant tenderness may occur immediately after the injury, but symptoms are likely to be delayed for 2 to 7 days. The most important symptom is persistent

bilious vomiting. Physical findings include dehydration, right upper quadrant tenderness, and the sensation of an ill-defined mass in the epigastrium.

Laboratory findings include an elevated white blood count and a dropping hemoglobin and hematocrit. If the diagnosis is delayed, hypochloremia, hypokalemia, and a high urine specific gravity may develop secondary to the persistent vomiting. An elevated amylase also is a common finding. However, clinically significant pancreatitis is unusual. Plain roentgenograms reveal a gasless abdomen except for a dilated stomach and sometimes a double bubble sign of duodenal obstruction. Felsen and Levin have described the characteristic coiled spring sign and the stacked coin sign seen on barium examination of the stomach and duodenum (Fig. 33–5).[51]

The physical findings in duodenal hematoma immediately after the injury often are ill-defined, and since there are no signs of peritonitis or rapid hemorrhage, an immediate operation is not indicated. In the past, most authors recommended surgical drainage of the hematoma, primarily because this would allow exploration to rule out other injuries. Some patients were operated on with the mistaken diagnosis of appendicitis.[52–54]

Associated injuries are extremely rare and may be

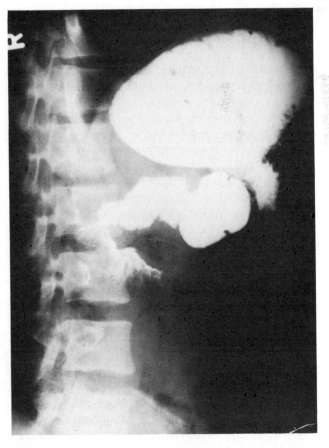

Figure 33–5. Duodenal obstruction due to traumatic hematoma.

ruled out by a careful clinical examination and abdominal CT scan. Current therapy consists of gastric drainage, replacement of lost fluids and electrolytes, and continued administration of intravenous fluids to provide the child's maintenance needs.[55–58]

Children with an incomplete obstruction study will be relieved of their symptoms within 3 to 5 days and will have no sequelae. Those with a complete obstruction are treated with nasogastric decompression and total parenteral nutrition. Although the majority of duodenal hematomas will resolve by 10 days postinjury, some may require 3 weeks.[59] If there is continued obstruction, which in our experience is rare, an operation is indicated. In a child requiring operation, the hematoma was extensive, including the entire duodenum and the first portion of the jejunum as well as the head and body of the pancreas. It is difficult to be sure at operation if the blood clot is submucosal or if the muscle layers have been separated. The hepatic flexure is mobilized to expose the second and third portions of the duodenum, where a longitudinal incision is made. Clot is removed by irrigation and with a sponge forceps. A second incision is then made at the ligament of Treitz to remove clot from the fourth portion of the duodenum and the jejunum. It is difficult to predict the length of time that these children will require intravenous fluids. Consequently, all those with complete obstruction should be supported with intravenous nutrition.[58]

Perforating Duodenal Injury. Perforations of the duodenum range from simple lacerations to complete disruption, with associated bile duct and pancreatic injury. Retroperitoneal perforations may show subtle signs. There may be only minimal upper abdominal and back pain without the tenderness usually associated with a gastrointestinal perforation. Peritoneal lavage is not helpful in the diagnosis of retroperitoneal perforations. The only way to make an early diagnosis in retroperitoneal duodenal injuries is to continually ask the question, "Does this child have a perforated duodenum?" and actively look for evidence of the diagnosis. Plain films of the abdomen must be searched carefully for scattered, small air bubbles in the right upper quadrant and transverse megacolon, as well as for obliteration of the right psoas muscle. Roentgenograms taken after injection of a water-soluble contrast agent through the gastric tube may demonstrate the perforation before it can be diagnosed clinically.[60] Contrast-enhanced CT scan of the abdomen is the diagnostic modality of choice and is very accurate, but the diagnosis must be considered and the study ordered. It is not unusual for a child with retroperitoneal duodenal injury to be sent home from the emergency center after what is thought to be a trivial abdominal injury only to return with abdominal pain.[61] Frequently, the pain localizes to the right lower quadrant

and may be confused with appendicitis.[61,62] An elevation of the serum amylase is seen with duodenal injuries because of reabsorption of pancreatic enzymes from the retroperitoneal space. At operation, the entire duodenum from the first portion to the ligament of Treitz must be mobilized and visualized if there is any evidence of hematoma, bile-stained material, or air bubbles in the retroperitoneal space. Operative management depends on the site and extent of the duodenal injury as well as associated injuries, particularly pancreatic and vascular injuries.[63,64] Treatment has ranged from simple suture to a Whipple resection of the duodenum and pancreas. The surgeon must be familiar with the various diverting and decompressing techniques, including primary repair with a jejunal patch, primary repair with tube gastrostomy and jejunostomy, pyloric exclusion and repair, diverticularization and repair, and pancreaticoduodenectomy.[65] In those situations when the patients involved are extremely ill, it is best to do as little as is necessary to achieve a safe closure and thorough, adequate drainage. Simple repair and drainage of a stab wound or small-caliber, low-velocity gunshot wound of the duodenum will be sufficient. However, simple repair of a duodenal injury resulting from blunt trauma or large-caliber gunshot wound is rarely sufficient, since there is a high incidence of leakage, with duodenal fistula formation. Corley and his colleagues at the Cook County Hospital saw a reduction in the mortality rate from duodenal injuries from 32 percent to 12 percent during a 7-year period, after the establishment of a uniform plan of treatment.[66] This reduction in mortality rate was achieved primarily by the addition of an effective internal decompression with an afferent jejunostomy tube. Leakage after simple suture of duodenal lacerations is the result of the extensive damage and devitalization of surrounding tissues, together with the high hydrostatic pressure developed in the poorly decompressed duodenum from the biliary and pancreatic secretions. Simple drainage with a nasogastric or gastrostomy tube may be ineffective in decompressing the edematous, partially obstructed duodenum. The duodenal repair may be reinforced with a jejunal patch,[67] and the severely injured duodenum may be protected by closure of the pylorus and the performance of a gastrojejunostomy or diverticularization.[65,68]

Our experience with 10 children on the pediatric surgery service at Ben Taub and Texas Children's Hospital suggests that the majority (7) of duodenal injuries in children may be treated by duodenorrhaphy and drainage, whereas those with massive injuries (3) require duodenorrhaphy and pyloric exclusion with gastrojejunostomy or pancreaticoduodenectomy.[61] Although 2 patients who underwent simple closure and drainage developed fistulae, all closed by the 22nd postoperative day. Two others developed pancreatic fistulae, which closed in

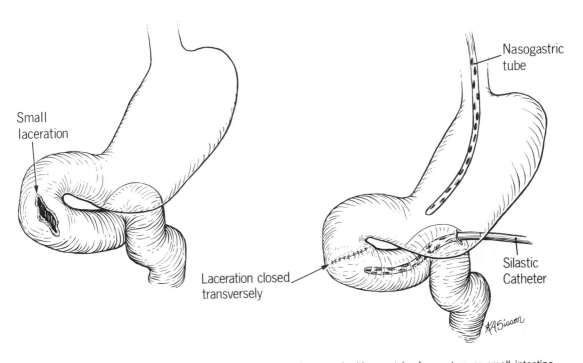

Figure 33–6. Small duodenal lacerations are closed and covered with a patch of omentum or small intestine. Then the duodenum is drained with a Silastic tube that exits at the ligament of Treitz.

the second postoperative week. Adequate intravenous or jejunal nutrition plays an important role in the care of these children.

Although each case must be individualized, the following would appear to be a rational approach to duodenal injuries. The ascending colon and hepatic flexure are reflected to the left for complete duodenal exposure. The ligament of Treitz is then taken down, and a Kocher maneuver is performed so that the entire duodenum is mobilized. Simple lacerations are sutured transversely with two layers of nonabsorbable sutures. Omentum or an adjacent loop of jejunum is placed over the repair as a patch, and the wound is adequately drained. In more extensive injuries, a soft Silastic tube may be inserted distal to the injury and threaded back into the duodenum for decompression. A second catheter may be placed distally for jejunal feedings (Fig. 33–6). For more severe injuries, we have mobilized the duodenum and jejunum in similar fashion, but instead of closing the duodenal wound, we debrided the edges and brought up an adjacent loop of jejunum for a side-to-side anastomosis. The entire area was then covered with a pedicle of omentum (Fig. 33–7). Children with combined duodenal and pancreatic wounds should have the repair protected by diverting the gastric flow with a pyloric exclusion and gastrojejunostomy or diverticulization. All children with duodenal injuries require long-term gastric and duodenal decompression. All should be started on jejunal or intravenous alimentation to provide for their

increased nutritional needs during their prolonged period of intense catabolism.

Intestinal Injuries

Direct force that compresses the small bowel against the spine results in avulsion of the intestine from the mesentery. There is antemesenteric rupture and sometimes complete transection of the bowel. These injuries occur just distal to the ligament of Treitz or proximal to the ileocecal valve, where the intestine is relatively fixed as it crosses the vertebrae.[69] Colon injuries secondary to blunt trauma are much less common, and the diagnosis may be delayed because of a lack of physical and radiographic findings despite a serious intestinal injury. Even with complete transection of the proximal jejunum, there may be very little spillage into the peritoneum of jejunal fluid and air because of the development of a paralytic ileus.[70] Contrast-enhanced CT scans of the abdomen may demonstrate only scant free fluid or blood, since the ileus prevents the contrast from reaching the perforation. In the Children's Memorial series, there were 20 perforations of the jejunum or ileum but only 1 of the cecum. All of these children had a history of major trauma, either an automobile accident, a fall, or a severe beating by a parent. They were in shock on admission to the emergency room, with rigid, severely tender abdomens. They required an immediate laparotomy. The typical injury is illustrated in Figure 33–8. These patients require rapid resuscitation with intrave-

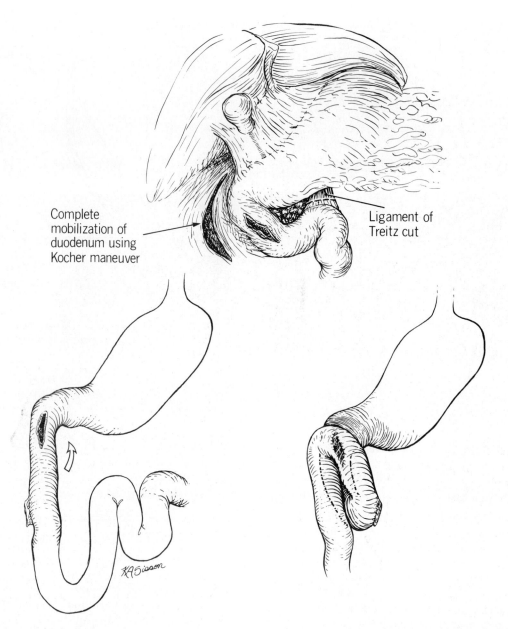

Complete
mobilization of
duodenum using
Kocher maneuver

Ligament of
Treitz cut

Figure 33–7. Extensive duodenal lacerations are closed and patched with small intestine, or a loop of small intestine is anastomosed to the laceration to achieve broad coverage of devitalized tissue and good internal drainage.

nous plasma, lactated Ringer's solution, antibiotics, and an immediate operation. When the site of injury is located, the involved intestine is wrapped in warm, moist pads while the abdominal cavity is generously lavaged with saline. Resection and anastomosis of the injured intestine are required if there is associated mesentery damage and surrounding hematoma. Otherwise, simple closure is warranted. The cecal injury was exteriorized because of severe fecal contamination resulting from a 6-hour delay in arriving at the hospital. All of these children survived.

Rectal Injuries

Since rectal injuries may be very painful and the child cannot cooperate, an examination under anesthesia is indicated.[15] Rectal injuries are treated in the standard fashion.[66] Mucosal or superficial anal injuries usually resolve with conservative treatment, as do full-thickness injuries below the internal sphincter following primary repair. Injury above the level of the internal sphincter is protected by a colostomy and drainage. Intraabdominal perforation is excluded at the time of colostomy or, if present, is repaired and protected by the colostomy.[71–73]

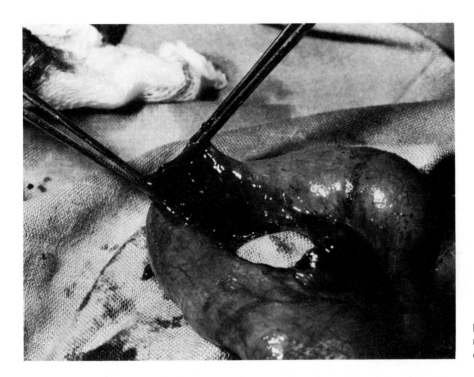

Figure 33–8. Avulsion of the ileum from its mesentery and perforation resulting from child abuse.

PANCREATIC INJURIES

In a review of injured children at Boston City Hospital, Welch found pancreatic injuries in 4 percent of the children admitted with blunt abdominal trauma.[62] When promptly diagnosed and surgically treated, pancreatic injuries rarely are fatal.[74,75] However, they frequently are associated with other life-threatening injuries and may be recognized only at laparotomy. In our own series of 51 children with pancreatic injuries treated operatively at Ben Taub General Hospital, 41 had significant associated injuries.[76] There were only 4 deaths, and none were directly due to the pancreatic injury. Mortality does correlate with the number of organs injured, particularly with major vessel injury.

The pancreas is a retroperitoneal organ lying transversely in the posterior epigastrium directly over the first and second lumbar vertebral bodies. The flat diaphragms and high costal margins of the young child leave the pancreas in a relatively unprotected position across the spine. The thin abdominal wall and weak abdominal musculature also leave the pancreas vulnerable to injuries as a result of what would be an insignificant blow in an adult. In the preadolescent, injuries to the pancreas are most often the result of blunt trauma to the abdomen that compresses the gland between the vertebral body and the offending object.[77,78] Most blunt injuries result in a contused gland, but in a third or more, the gland is transected. Although the classic injury involves bicycle handlebars, the vast majority result from accidents that involve motor vehicles. Because a large force is required to injure the pancreas, child abuse should be suspected in any case where no clear explanation for the injury can be established.[79] In adolescents as in adults, the penetrating injuries are common and often result from crimes of violence.[77,80,81] Penetrating injuries almost always result in perforation or laceration of the gland. The male predominance increases with age.

Children with blunt pancreatic injuries fall into three clinical groups. In the first are those who have mild to moderate epigastric and back pain, with tenderness over the epigastrium. Most, but not all, have an elevated serum amylase. Although a moderately elevated serum amylase is not in itself an indication for operation or even of pancreatic injury, an elevated amylase with associated persistent or increasing abdominal finding is a strong indication for operation.[82,83] The pain and physical findings of these children typically improve within 24 hours and abate within 72 hours. The amylase by then usually has returned to normal. The second group is made up of a small minority in whom the pain does not completely subside. These children usually are discharged and develop persistent abdominal pain and, weeks later, a pancreatic pseudocyst. To detect the development of pseudocysts, all children with pancreatic injuries should be followed for several weeks after injury with urinary amylase determinations and sonography or CT scan.[84] In the third group are the children with immediate severe pain, tenderness, and paralytic ileus. In this group, the clinical indications for surgery usually are clear. An elevated serum amylase or peritoneal fluid amylase obtained by paracentesis may be helpful in diagnosing these injuries.

Diagnostic Tests

Amylase. The serum amylase will be elevated in approximately 10 percent of those patients with a penetrating injury of the pancreas. When the serum amylase is drawn immediately after the injury, it is elevated in only approximately 60 percent of patients with blunt trauma. Although the serum amylase determination should be made in patients with blunt abdominal trauma, a single elevated amylase in a recently injured patient with no evidence of intraabdominal injury is of little significance.[82] In addition, the level of hyperamylasemia does not correlate with pancreatic injury. Therefore, the decision to operate on a child with suspected acute pancreatic injury should be based on factors other than the serum amylase level.[83] However, if the diagnosis is delayed, the serum amylase will become elevated, and a persistent hyperamylasemia is an indication of pancreatic injury.[85]

Computed Tomography. Although there was initially enthusiasm for the use of CT scans in all intraabdominal injuries, more recent experience has shown an unacceptably high number of false negative and false positive studies in patients with pancreatic injuries who were studied within a few hours of injury from blunt trauma.[11,12] The diagnostic errors have been attributed to the following: (1) lacerations of the pancreas may produce little immediate change in density, (2) there may be minimal separation of the injured fragments, and (3) immediately after the injury, there may be little evidence of posttraumatic pancreatitis. However, 24 hours after the pancreas is injured, the CT scan will demonstrate changes in density, separation of fragments, and posttraumatic pancreatitis[11] (Fig. 33–9).

Treatment

The majority of children with pancreatic injuries have contused glands and will respond to nasogastric decompression, sedation, and intravenous fluids. Sonography is valuable in detecting resolution of the inflammatory mass or the development of a pseudocyst.[86] The urinary amylase nearly always is elevated in those patients who develop complications of their pancreatic injury, such as pseudocyst or fistula.[85]

Children with severe pancreatic injuries have significant peritoneal findings and are operated on immediately, following necessary resuscitation. At laparotomy, the first priority is control of hemorrhage, the second priority is control of contamination of the peritoneal cavity by gastrointestinal perforations, and the third priority is treatment of the pancreatic injury.[86] In most cases, associated injuries are present that may be life threatening and must take priority in treatment. Any pancreatic injury may be treated with thorough and adequate drainage in the presence of other life-threatening injuries.[87] Definitive operative care of the drained pancreas may be delayed to a later date.

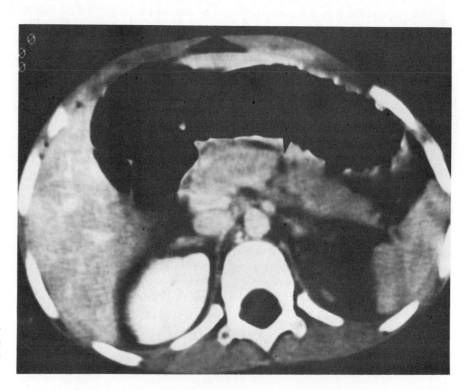

Figure 33–9. CT scan of the abdomen showing transection of the pancreas. The scan was taken 24 hours after a horse had fallen across the patient's abdomen.

Operative management of pancreatic injuries must include (1) careful definition of the injury, (2) control of hemorrhage, (3) control of pancreatic secretions, and (4) conservation of pancreatic function.[76,77] Determinants of selection of operative repair and the ultimate outcome include extent of glandular injury, including ductal injury,[88] site of ductal injury,[89] and associated injuries, particularly duodenal injuries. These factors have been incorporated into the grading system shown in Table 33–1.[90]

The operative treatment for contusion of the pancreas is drainage of the injury and lesser sac. Drainage should be dependent, with the drains brought out through the flank. The drain exit through the abdominal wall should be loose to allow free egress of the pancreatic fluid. Larger lacerations should be closed with monofilament nonabsorbable sutures and drained. The treatment of a transection depends on the location of the injury and the viability of the distal segment.[91,92] Primary repair of the pancreatic ducts has been accomplished, but this is difficult, time consuming, usually unsuccessful, and seldom indicated.[93] If a significant portion of viable pancreas is present distal to the transection, this segment of pancreas may be preserved. The proximal transection is suture closed, and a Roux-en-Y jejunal loop is used to drain the distal pancreas.[94] If transection is through the tail, the small distal segment is simply excised, and the proximal portion is closed and drained. Whereas experimental animals will grow normally after 75 to 90 percent pancreatectomies,[95,96] insulin deficiency has been reported in patients after extensive resections to the right of the superior mesenteric vessels.[86,89,97] It is prudent to preserve significant portions of the pancreas whenever possible.

Whipple procedures are reserved for those patients who, in addition to extensive injuries of the head or neck of the pancreas, have a nonreconstructable duodenal injury.[98,99] Lesser injuries to the head and neck of the pancreas can be treated by suture and drainage, and when necessary for major ductal injury, a Roux-en-Y loop may be used to drain the distal segment or proximal

ductal injury.[100] Lesser duodenal injuries can be treated by repair and drainage or by pyloric exclusion and gastrojejunostomy.[80]

Postoperative complications directly attributable to pancreatic injury include fistulae, pancreatic pseudocysts, and pancreatic abscess formation. In reviewing 27 children operated on immediately after injury, Stone found that complications included 1 fistula, 1 pseudocyst, and 1 abscess.[101] In reviewing 47 children operated on immediately after injury at Ben Taub Hospital, Graham et al. reported 1 pseudocyst and 11 fistulae, all of which closed spontaneously within 4 weeks.[76]

Pseudocysts of the pancreas usually are the result of a blunt traumatic injury to the pancreas. A history of trauma may be difficult to obtain in the case of a toddler, but a high degree of suspicion must be maintained in children with abdominal pain and epigastric mass. Nearly all have had persistent symptoms of intermittent vomiting, anorexia, and abdominal pain since the time of injury. However, the interval between injury and primary operation for pseudocyst drainage varies from several days to months and averages 4 to 6 weeks. Nearly all of these patients have an elevated amylase level. Contrast studies of the gastrointestinal tract are helpful, but sonography has become the most useful means of localizing the mass and of differentiating a solid inflammatory mass from a pseudocyst of the pancreas.

Pancreatic pseudocysts in adults are complications of a chronic disease process (usually alcoholism or biliary disease) that causes scarring and permanent distortion of the ductal system.[102,103] The high incidence of recurrence and chronic fistula formation following operative drainage, particularly external drainage of a pancreatic pseudocyst in adults, reflects the progression of the underlying disease process.[104] In contrast, pancreatic pseudocysts in children are a complication of an acute traumatic or viral illness superimposed on a normal gland.[105–108] The process is not progressive, and with resolution of the inflammatory changes of the acute injury, the ductal system usually opens.

Therefore, the response to treatment and prognosis differs between children and adults. In children, recurrence of pancreatic pseudocysts and persistent external fistulae are quite uncommon even after external drainage.[107] For this reason as well as the significant rate of spontaneous intraabdominal rupture, bowel obstruction, and inanition, large or symptomatic pseudocysts should be drained when diagnosed rather than awaiting maturation of the cyst wall.[103,109] Most pancreatic pseudocysts that are present for more than 6 weeks can be drained internally either by a cystogastrostomy or with a Roux-en-Y loop.[107,110] If the time since injury is less than 6 weeks, the cyst wall may not be sufficiently developed to support an anastomosis. In this case, adequate external drainage is accomplished with

TABLE 33–1. CLASSIFICATION OF PANCREATIC INJURY

Grade	Injury
I	Contusion/hematoma (minimal parenchymal damage)
II	Capsular/parenchymal disruption without major ductal injury
IIIa	Capsular/parenchymal disruption with ductal involvement distal to the superior mesenteric vessels; the duodenum is intact
IIIb	Capsular/parenchymal disruption with ductal involvement to the right of the superior mesenteric vessels; the duodenum is intact
IV	Combined extensive pancreatic/duodenal crush injuries

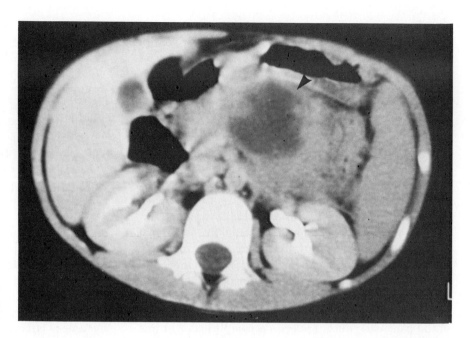

Figure 33–10. CT scan of pancreatic pseudocyst. The child remained asymptomatic, and the pseudocyst resolved without surgery.

catheters and Penrose drains placed in a dependent position.

Spontaneous resolution of pancreatic pseudocysts that have been followed by ultrasound studies have been reported[84,111,112] (Fig. 33–10). However, these patients must be followed closely, since untreated pseudocysts may develop serious complications. In our experience, nearly all children with pancreatic pseudocysts have one or more of the triad of symptoms of pain, vomiting, and fever. Therefore, operative delay is unwarranted in children with large or symptomatic pancreatic pseudocysts.[12,113,114]

REFERENCES

1. Touloukian RJ: Abdominal trauma in children. Surg Gynecol Obstet 127:561, 1968
2. Hendren WH, Kim SH: Trauma of the spleen and liver in children. Pediatr Clin North Am 22:349, 1975
3. Powell RW, Smith DE, Zarina CD, et al: Peritoneal lavage in children with blunt abdominal trauma. J Pediatr Surg 11:973, 1976
4. Drew R, Perry JF, Fischer RP: The expedience of peritoneal lavage for blunt trauma in children. Surg Gynecol Obstet 145:885, 1977
5. DuPriest RW, Rodriguez A, Shatney CH: Peritoneal lavage in children and adolescents with blunt abdominal trauma. Am Surg 48:460, 1982
6. Beaver BL, Colombani PM, Fal A, et al: The efficacy of computed tomography in evaluating abdominal injuries in children with major head trauma. J Pediatr Surg 22:1117–1122, 1987
7. American College of Surgeons Committee on Trauma, Collicott PR (chairman) (ed): Pediatric Trauma in Advanced Trauma Life Support Courses, Instructor Manual. Chicago, American College of Surgeons, 1984, pp 293–301
8. Cooney DR: Splenic and hepatic trauma in children. Surg Clin North Am 61:1165, 1981
9. Karp MP, Cooney DR, Berger PE, et al: The role of computed tomography in the evaluation of blunt abdominal trauma in children. J Pediatr Surg 16:316, 1981
10. Kane NM, Cronan JJ, Dorfman GS, DeLuca F: Pediatric abdominal truma: Evaluation by computed tomography. Pediatrics 82:11, 1988
11. Jeffrey R, Federle M, Crass R: Computed tomography of pancreatic trauma. Radiology 147:491, 1983
12. Smith S, Nakayama D, Gantt N: Pancreatic injuries in childhood due to blunt trauma. J Pediatr Surg 23:610–614, 1988
13. Oldham KT, Guice KS, Ryckman F, et al: Blunt liver injury in childhood: Evolution of therapy and current perspective. Surgery 100:542, 1986
14. Moore TC: Nonoperative management of blunt abdominal trauma in childhood (Letter). Surgery 101:380, 1987
15. Pokorny WJ, Pokorny SF, Gonzales ET, Black CT: Perineal injuries in infants and children. In Brooks BJ (ed): The Injured Child. Austin, University of Texas Press, 1985
16. Freeark RJ: Penetrating wounds of the abdomen. N Engl J Med 291:185–188, 1974
17. Stein A, Lissoos I: Selective management of penetrating wounds of the abdomen. Trauma 8:1014, 1968
18. Thompson SJ, Moore EE, Van Duzer-Moore S, et al: The evolution of abdominal stab wound management. J Trauma 20:478, 1980
19. Sinclair MC, Moore T, Morris JA: Penetrating abdominal injuries in children and adolescents. Am Surg 41:342, 1975
20. Tunnell WP, Knost J, Nance FC: Penetrating abdominal injuries in children and adolescents. J Trauma 15:720, 1975

21. Zabinski EJ, Harkins AN: Delayed splenic rupture—a clinical syndrome following trauma. Arch Surg 46:186, 1943
22. Lorimer WS: Occult rupture of the spleen. Arch Surg 89:434, 1964
23. Touloukian RJ: Abdominal injuries in children: A perspective for the 1980s. In Brooks BF (ed): The Injured Child. Austin, University of Texas Press, 1985, pp 53–60
24. Belfauz JR, Nesbit ME, Jarvis C, Kririt N: Overwhelming sepsis following splenectomy for trauma. J Pediatr 88:458, 1976
25. Rowley DA: The formation of circulatory antibody in the splenectomized human being following intravenous injection of heterologous erythrocytes. J Immunol 65:515, 1950
26. Carlisle HN, Saslow S: Proper levels in splenectomized persons. Proc Soc Exp Biol Med 102:150, 1959
27. Morales IC, Montaner A: Immunological studies in the postsplenectomy syndrome. J Pediatr Surg 10:159, 1975
28. Ein SH, Shandling B, Simpson JS, et al: The morbidity and mortality of splenectomy in childhood. Ann Surg 185:307, 1977
29. Ein SH, Shandling B, Simpson JS, et al: Nonoperative management of traumatized spleen in children. How and why. J Pediatr Surg 13:117, 1978
30. Eichelberger MR, Randolph JG: Abdominal trauma. In Welch KJ, Randolph JG, Ravitch MM, et al (eds): Pediatric Surgery, 6th ed. Chicago, Year Book, 1986, pp 154–174
31. LaMura J, Chung-Fat SP, SanFilippo JA: Splenorrhaphy for the treatment of splenic rupture in infants and children. Surgery 81:497, 1977
32. Upadhyaya P, Nayak NC, Moitra S: Experimental study of splenic trauma in monkeys. J Pediatr Surg 6:767, 1971
33. Wesson DE, Filler RM, Ein SH, et al: Ruptured spleen—when to operate. J Pediatr Surg 16:324, 1981
34. Haller JA, Pokorny WJ: Pediatric trauma. In Mattox KL, Moore EE, Feliciano DV (eds): Trauma. E. Norwalk, CT, Appleton & Lange, 1988, pp 629–644
35. Fischer KC, Russello P, Eraklis A, Treres S: Nonoperative treatment of children with splenic rupture. Extended follow-up with scintigraphic assessment of healing. J Nucl Med 18:596, 1977
36. Stone HH, Ausley JD: Management of liver trauma in children. J Pediatr Surg 12:3, 1977
37. Jona JZ, Goldstein R: Compression hepatic necrosis in a child. J Trauma 17:402, 1977
38. Kaufman JM, Burrington JD: Liver trauma in children. J Pediatr Surg 6:585, 1971
39. Susan EM, Klotz D Jr, Kottmeier PK: Liver trauma in children. Pediatr Surg 10:411, 1975
40. Mays T: Hepatic trauma. Curr Probl Surg 13:10, 1976
41. Canty TG, Aaron WS: Hepatic artery ligation for exsanguinating liver injuries in children. J Pediatr Surg 10:693, 1975
42. Hartman SW, Greaney EM Jr: Traumatic injuries to the biliary system in children. Am J Surg 108:150, 1964
43. Noone RB, Mackie JA, Stoner R: Liver and bile duct laceration from blunt abdominal trauma in children. Ann Surg 166:824, 1967
44. Caro AM, Ocana Losa JM: Complete avulsion of the common bile duct as a result of blunt abdominal trauma—case report of a child. Pediatr Surg 5:60, 1970
45. Bismuth H: Hemobilia. N Engl J Med 288:617, 1973
46. Guillen J, Elliot DP: Traumatic hemobilia—a case report. J Trauma 11:886, 1971
47. Hendren WH, Warshaw AL, Fleischili DJ, Barlett MK: Traumatic hemobilia: Nonoperative management with healing documented by serial angiography. Ann Surg 17:991, 1971
48. Vassy LE, Klecker RL, Koch E, Morse TS: Traumatic gastric perforation in children from blunt trauma. J Trauma 15:184, 1975
49. Asch MJ, Coran AG, Johnston PW: Gastric perforation secondary to blunt trauma in children. J Trauma 15:187, 1975
50. Siemens RA, Fulton RL: Gastric rupture as a result of blunt trauma. Am Surg 43:229, 1977
51. Felsen B, Levin EJ: Intramural hematoma of the duodenum: diagnostic roentgen sign. Radiology 63:823, 1954
52. Wiot JF, Weinstein AS, Felsen B: Duodenal hematoma induced by coumadin. AJR 86:70, 1961
53. Freeark RJ, Corley RD, Norcross WJ, Strohl EC: Intramural hematoma of the duodenum. Arch Surg 92:463, 1966
54. Steward DR, Byrd CL, Schuster SR: Intramural hematoma of the alimentary tract in children. Surgery 68:550, 1970
55. Webb AJ, Taylor JJ: Traumatic intramural hematoma of the duodenum. Br J Surg 54:50, 1967
56. Mahour GH, Woolley MD, Gans SL, Payne VC Jr: Duodenal hematoma in infancy and childhood. J Pediatr Surg 6:153, 1971
57. Fullen WD, Selle JG, Whitley DJ, et al: Intramural duodenal hematoma. Ann Surg 179:549, 1974
58. Holgerson LO, Bishop HC: Non-operative treatment of duodenal hematoma in children. J Pediatr Surg 12:11, 1977
59. Touloukian RJ: Protocol for the nonoperative treatment of obstructing, intramural duodenal hematoma during childhood. Am J Surg 145:330, 1983
60. Karnaze GC, Sheedy PF, Stephens DH, McLeod RA: Computed tomography in duodenal rupture due to blunt abdominal trauma. J Comput Assist Tomogr 5:267, 1981
61. Pokorny WJ, Brandt ML, Harberg FJ: Major duodenal injuries in children: diagnosis, operative management and outcome. J Pediatr Surg 21:613, 1986
62. Welch KJ: Abdominal trauma. In Ravitch MM (ed): Pediatric Surgery, 3rd ed. Chicago, Year Book, 1979, pp 125–149
63. Deadhar MC, Duleep KS, Gill SS, Eggleston FC: Retroperitoneal rupture of the duodenum following blunt trauma. Arch Surg 96:263, 1968
64. Stone HH: Pancreatic and duodenal trauma in children. J Pediatr Surg 7:670, 1972
65. Martin TD, Feliciano DV, Mattox KL, Jordan GL: Severe duodenal injuries: treatment with pyloric exclusion and gastrojejunostomy. Arch Surg 118:631, 1983
66. Corley RD, Norcross WJ, Shoemaker WC: Traumatic injuries to the duodenum. Ann Surg 181:95, 1975
67. McInnis WD, Aust JB, Cruz AB, Root HD: Traumatic

injuries of the duodenum: A comparison of 1 closure and the jejunal patch. J Trauma 15:847, 1975

68. Jordan GC, Beall AC: Diagnosis and management of abdominal trauma. Curr Probl Surg 8:23, 1971

69. Schenk WG, Lolnchyna V, Moylan JA: Perforation of the jejunum from blunt abdominal trauma. J Trauma 23:54, 1983

70. Kakos GS, Grosfeld JL, Morse TS: Small bowel injuries in children after blunt abdominal trauma. Ann Surg 174:238, 1971

71. Black CT, Pokorny WJ, McGill CW, et al: Ano-rectal trauma in children. J Pediatr Surg 17:501, 1982

72. Robertson HD, Ray JE, Ferrari BT, et al: Management of rectal trauma. Surg Gynecol Obstet 154:161, 1982

73. Slim MS, Makaroun M, Shammai AR: Primary repair of colo-rectal injuries in childhood. J Pediatr Surg 16:1008, 1981

74. Jones R, Shires G: The management of pancreatic injuries. Arch Surg 90:502–508, 1965

75. Thompson RJ, Hinshaw DB: Pancreatic trauma: Review of 87 cases. Ann Surg 163:153, 1966

76. Graham J, Pokorny W, Mattox K, et al: Surgical management of acute pancreatic injuries in children. J Pediatr Surg 13:693, 1978

77. Stone HH, Stowers KB, Shippey SH: Injuries to the pancreas. Arch Surg 85:525, 1962

78. Othersen H, Moore F, Boles E: Traumatic pancreatitis and pseudocyst in childhood. J Trauma 8:535, 1968

79. Pena S, Medovy H: Child abuse and traumatic pseudocyst of the pancreas. J Pediatr 83:1026, 1973

80. Graham J, Mattox K, Jordan GL, et al: Traumatic injuries of the pancreas. Am J Surg 136:744, 1978

81. Sims E, Mandal A, Schlater T, et al: Factors affecting outcome in pancreatic trauma. J Trauma 24:125, 1984

82. Olsen W: The serum amylase in blunt abdominal trauma. J Trauma 13:200, 1973

83. Moretz J, Campbell D, Parker D, et al: Significance of serum amylase level in evaluating pancreatic trauma. Am J Surg 130:739, 1975

84. Bradley E, Clements L: Spontaneous resolution of pancreatic pseudocysts: Implications for timing of operative intervention. Am J Surg 129:23, 1975

85. Cogbill T, Moore E, Kashuk J: Changing trends in the management of pancreatic trauma. Arch Surg 117:722, 1982

86. Stuber JL, Templeton AW, Bishop K: Sonographic diagnosis of pancreatic lesions. Am J Roentgenol Radium Ther Nucl Med 116:406, 1972

87. Jordan GL Jr: Injury to pancreas and duodenum. In Mattox KL, Moore EE, Feliciano DV (eds): Trauma. Norwalk, CT, Appleton & Lange, 1988, pp 473–494

88. Levine R, Glauser F, Berk J: Enhancement of the amylase-creatinine clearance ratio in disorders other than acute pancreatitis. N Engl J Med 292:329, 1975

89. Robey E, Mullen J, Schwab C: Blunt transection of the pancreas treated by distal pancreatectomy, splenic salvage and hyperalimentation. Ann Surg 196:695, 1982

90. Pokorny WJ: Pancreatic injuries in children. In Buntain WL (ed): Management of Pediatric Trauma. New York, Grune & Stratton, 1989

91. Weitzman J, Rothschild P: The surgical management of

92. Weitzman J, Swenson O: Traumatic rupture of the pancreas in a toddler. Surgery 57:309, 1965

93. Martin L, Henderson B, Welsh N: Disruption of the head of the pancreas caused by blunt trauma in children: A report of two cases treated with primary repair of the pancreatic duct. Surgery 63:697, 1968

94. Letton D, Wilson J: Traumatic severance of pancreas treated by Roux-Y anastomosis. Surg Gynecol Obstet 109:473, 1959

95. Hallman GL, Jordan GL: Subtotal pancreatectomy and growth of young mice. JAMA 191:167, 1965

96. Dragstedt LR: Some physiological problems in surgery of the pancreas. Ann Surg 118:576, 1943

97. Northrup W, Simmons R: Pancreatic trauma: A review. Surgery 71:27, 1972

98. Cameron A, Southcott R, Blake J, et al: Successful Whipple's operation for pancreatic injury. Injury 16:233, 1985

99. Halgrimson C, Trimble C, Gale S, et al: Pancreaticoduodenectomy for traumatic lesions. Am J Surg 118:877, 1969

100. Bozymski E, Orlando R, Holt J: Traumatic disruption of the pancreatic duct demonstrated by endoscopic retrograde pancreatography. J Trauma 21:244, 1981

101. Stone H: Pancreatic and duodenal trauma in children. J Pediatr Surg 7:670, 1972

102. Jordan G, Howard J: Pancreatic pseudocysts. Am J Gastroenterol 45:444, 1966

103. Becker W, Pratt H: Pseudocysts of the pancreas. Surg Gynecol Obstet 127:744, 1968

104. Warren W, Marsh W, Sandusky W: An appraisal of surgical procedures for pancreatic pseudocyst. Ann Surg 147:903, 1958

105. Cooney D, Grosfeld J: Operative management of pancreatic pseudocysts in infants and children: A review of 75 cases. Ann Surg 182:590, 1975

106. Leistyna J, Macaulay J: Traumatic pancreatitis in childhood. Am J Dis Child 107:644, 1964

107. Pokorny W, Raffensperger J, Harberg F: Pancreatic pseudocysts in children. Surg Gynecol Obstet 151:182, 1980

108. Pollard P, Chavrier Y: Pseudocyst of the pancreas in a child aged 13 years. Ann Chir Infant 13:395, 1972

109. Wool G, Goldring D: Pseudocyst of the pancreas: Report of five cases and review of literature. J Pediatr 70:586, 1967

110. Stone H, Whitehurst J: Pseudocysts of the pancreas in children. Am J Surg 114:448, 1967

111. Dahman B, Stephens C: Pseudocysts of the pancreas after blunt abdominal trauma in children. J Pediatr Surg 16:17, 1981

112. Gorenstein A, O'Halpin D, Wesson D, et al: Blunt injury to the pancreas in children: Selective management with ultrasound. J Pediatr Surg 22:1110–1116, 1987

113. Eisebaum S, Grant RN, Cohen A: Hemorrhagic pseudocyst and pancreatitis in a ten-year-old boy. Am Surg 36:387, 1970

114. Moazzenzadah A, Fernandez L, Zamora B: Intraperitoneal rupture of pancreatic pseudocyst: Report of a case and review of the literature. Am Surg 42:589, 1976

traumatic rupture of the pancreas due to blunt trauma. Surg Clin North Am 48:1347, 1968

34
Genitourinary Trauma

Any child who has suffered major trauma must have a urine examination for blood. The first voided urine specimen represents only bladder urine and may not accurately reflect bleeding from the kidneys. A urinary catheter should be inserted as a part of the initial emergency room evaluation because this is the only certain way to obtain a satisfactory sample, and the catheter will allow accurate measurement of the urine volume as the child is resuscitated. The only contraindication to immediate catheterization is the possibility of a urethral injury. If there is gross blood at the meatus and perineal tenderness after either direct perineal trauma or a pelvic fracture, a urethrogram is performed before insertion of the catheter. Obvious flank abrasions, ecchymosis, and tenderness are further clues to renal injury, whereas lower abdominal pain and tenderness or clinical evidence of a pelvic fracture are signs of a bladder perforation. The abdominal findings after injury of the urinary tract are nonspecific. Retroperitoneal hematomas will leak bloody fluid into the peritoneal cavity, causing tenderness. In addition, nerve irritation from a lower thoracic or flank injury will cause muscle spasm.

Children with suspected abdominal injuries and all those with serious trauma should have computed tomography (CT) scanning of the abdomen. This single study will demonstrate renal injuries with great accuracy, as well as damage to other solid organs. The intravenous pyelogram (IVP) is still a useful tool in evaluating renal trauma. It will demonstrate bilateral renal function and extravasation. If the IVP is normal, one may be confident that there is no major renal injury. The IVP may be performed rapidly in the emergency or operating room with portable x-ray equipment. If a child is in shock with rapid intraabdominal hemorrhage, the one-shot IVP is the most useful test one can obtain before operation. In the initial evaluation, a CT scan with contrast material will demonstrate renal lacerations, fractures, and avascular segments that eventually may require an operation.

An arteriogram will rarely provide more information unless a pedicle injury is suspected because of severe trauma and a nonvisualizing kidney. Figure 34–1 compares the IVP, CT scan, and an arteriogram in a boy with a solitary kidney in whom the lacerated upper pole was avascular.

When there is hematuria with only mild flank tenderness and when either an IVP or CT scan is normal or at most demonstrates mild distortion of the calyces, one may diagnose a renal contusion. There is no correlation between the amount of hematuria and renal injury, but in most cases, the hematuria clears after several days of bedrest. There are no long-term sequelae, such as hypertension, after a simple renal contusion, and the child may return to normal activities after 2 weeks.

RENAL PEDICLE INJURY

Severe blunt trauma, especially in sudden deceleration injuries, may completely avulse the renal pedicle. The mobile kidney is forcefully displaced away from the fixed aorta; this stretches the renal artery and disrupts the intima. Thrombosis then occurs distal to the intimal tear (Fig. 34–2). In these injuries, there may be only microscopic hematuria. The CT or IVP will reveal nonvisualization on the affected side (Fig. 34–3).

If the child's condition is sufficiently stable, an immediate transfemoral arteriogram must be performed. If the patient is in shock and requires a laparotomy for other injuries, the surgeon must keep in mind a renal pedicle injury and explore the renal artery from the aorta to the kidney.

Most cases of renal pedicle injury have been diagnosed too late to salvage the kidney. Consequently, the usual treatment has been nephrectomy.[1-3] Skinner, however, salvaged the kidney in a 37-year-old man after making the diagnosis of right renal artery thrombosis by aortogram within 10 hours of the injury.[4] The injured

296

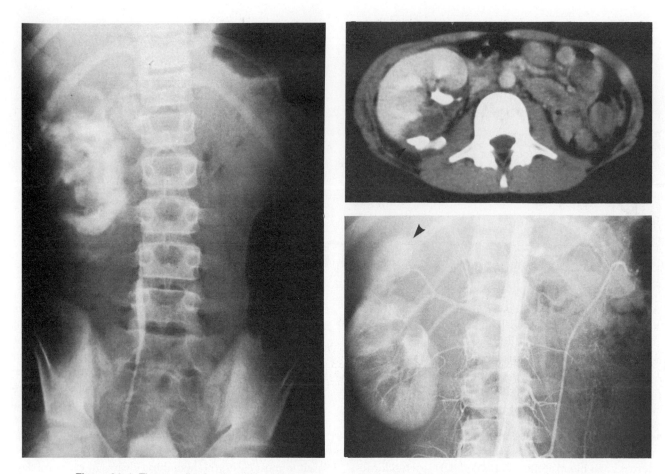

Figure 34–1. Three studies in a boy with major trauma to a solitary kidney. He required drainage of the hematoma and extravasation and had hypertension for several months. **Left.** The IVP demonstrates extravasation of contrast material, indicating a major renal injury. **Top right.** The CT demonstrates the laceration and a separated segment. **Bottom right.** The arteriogram shows the separated segment.

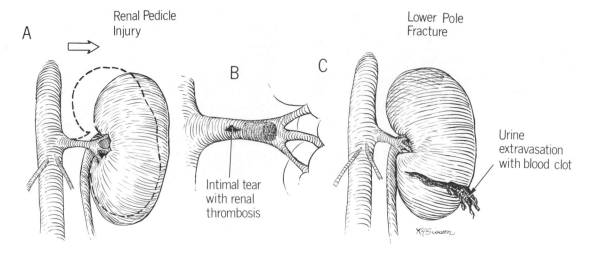

Figure 34–2. A. The mechanism of this renal pedicle injury was a deceleration force that stretched the renal artery. **B.** An intimal tear resulted, with renal artery thrombosis. **C.** A typical pole injury with hemorrhage and urinary extravasation.

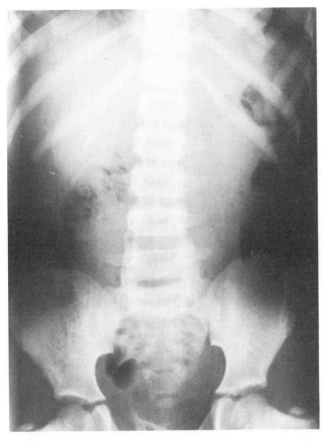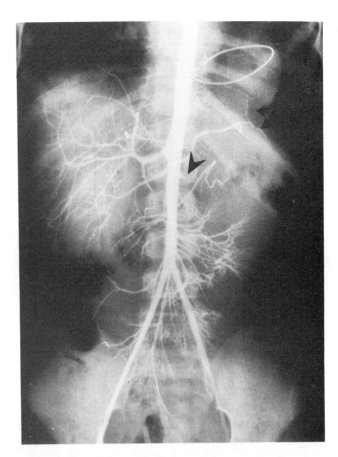

Figure 34–3. Left. Intravenous pyelogram demonstrating absence of renal function on the left. **Right.** An immediate transfemoral arteriogram was performed. There was only a short stub of a renal artery. There was also a ruptured diaphragm with the spleen in the left chest.

vessel was resected, and a Fogarty catheter was used to remove a distal clot. The kidney was then perfused with 1000 ml cold Ringer's solution containing mannitol and heparin. Guttman et al. made the diagnosis at laparotomy in a child with a torn vena cava as well as several other injuries.[5] They removed the kidney and repaired a hole in the pelvis, as well as the intimal tear, and then reimplanted the kidney after irrigating it with Sack's solution at 4C. At 6 months, the child had a normal IVP.

RENAL FRACTURE

The kidney is nestled within a soft bed of perirenal fat and is protected by the vertebrae and the rib cage. Thus, severe trauma is necessary to fracture the kidney. In most cases, major renal trauma is secondary to a motor vehicle accident or a severe fall. Almost half of children with these severe renal injuries will have trauma of other organ systems. Fortunately, hemorrhage is contained within Gerota's fascia and rarely requires an immediate operation for control. In Karp and associates' series of

44 patients, 66 percent of those with initial hematuria had associated injuries, but only 4 required an immediate operation on a kidney.[6] The CT scan allowed excellent definition of the injury but tended to exaggerate the amount of extravasation of urine, which in itself was not an indication for surgery. Either a CT scan with contrast or an IVP will identify a severely injured kidney, which will visualize poorly and will demonstrate extravasation of contrast material outside the kidney. It is most important to identify an avascular upper or lower pole, which may be resected, with salvage of the remaining kidney if an operation is indicated. Also, if the poles are separated but still have a blood supply, the entire kidney may either heal spontaneously or be repaired and salvaged.

Treatment

No more than 20 percent of children with injuries to the parenchyma and renal collecting system require an operation.[7–10] The usual child with hematuria, flank tenderness, and minimal findings on radiologic studies requires only bedrest, observation of the vital signs, and the volume of blood lost in the urine. In most cases, the urine becomes clear within 3 or 4 days. Repeated urinalyses are obtained for several more days, and another CT scan is obtained a month after the injury. The indications for operation are controversial, since even severely lacerated kidneys with major urinary extravasation will heal with normal function. On the other hand, the potential morbidity from infection and secondary hemorrhage must be weighed against the minimal risk of an earlier operation. An operation is indicated when there is hemorrhage with an expanding flank mass associated with urinary extravasation. An arteriogram or scan that demonstrates a major avascular area supports the decision to operate.

Technique

The injured kidney must be approached from the peritoneal cavity. The aorta, vena cava, and renal artery and vein are exposed by an incision in the posterior parietal peritoneum medial to the inferior mesenteric vein. Once the renal pedicle is encircled with tapes, the colon may be reflected and Gerota's fascia opened. A retroperitoneal hematoma about the kidney must never be opened until the renal pedicle is definitely secured. When the vessels are controlled, Gerota's fascia is opened, the clot is removed, and the kidney is inspected. Totally avulsed segments or avascular portions of the kidney are removed, and pelvocalyceal tears are sutured with 4–0 chromic catgut. Bleeding is controlled first by the application of vascular clamps to the renal artery, after which individual bleeding vessels are suture-ligated. If one pole is devitalized, the renal capsule is stripped back, and a partial nephrectomy is performed (Fig. 34–4). After closure of the pelvis and control of hemorrhage, either

the capsule or adjacent renal fat and fascia may be used to cover the raw surface. Generous drainage with large Penrose drains out the flank completes the procedure. Deep lacerations may be controlled by suture-ligation of individual vessels and closure of the renal parenchyma with chromic catgut.

The management of retroperitoneal hematomas found at laparotomy for other injuries is still controversial. This is obviously the situation where a preoperative IVP or CT is most helpful. If the hematoma is found during abdominal exploration, a pyelogram is performed on the operating table. If this x-ray does not demonstrate extravasation of contrast and if the hematoma remains stable during the rest of the operation, the hematoma is left alone. If, however, there is evidence of renal injury, the problem is best solved by controlling the renal pedicle (as described) and exploring the damaged kidney. Devitalized tissue is debrided, hemostasis is attained, and the area is liberally drained. If this is not done, one is faced with the prospect of delayed hemorrhage in a patient who has already been through a major operation. In addition, the combination of hematoma and urine is more likely to become contaminated and infected once the abdominal cavity has been opened.

The plan of therapy outlined has resulted in maximal salvage of renal tissue. At the Children's Memorial Hospital, only 3 nephrectomies and 1 heminephrectomy were necessary for trauma during the 16-year period 1971 through 1987. One other operation was required to control hemorrhage from renal laceration in a child with crossed renal ectopia. One of the nephrectomies might have been avoided if a retroperitoneal hematoma had been opened during an operation to remove a rup-

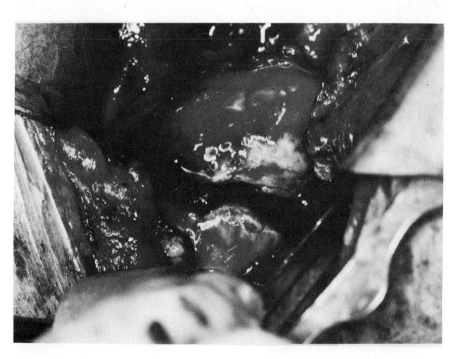

Figure 34–4. The lower pole of the kidney was completely avulsed. This pole was removed, and the remaining kidney was sutured and salvaged.

tured spleen. The child had his spleen removed, and 3 days later a heminephrectomy was performed. Infection was then followed by a secondary hemorrhage, which necessitated completion of the nephrectomy.

PREEXISTING LESIONS

Tumors and congenital defects, particularly hydronephrosis and horseshoe kidneys, are susceptible to minor injury. During the past 12 years, there have been 4 children at our hospital with Wilms' tumors, 3 with hydronephrosis, and 1 with crossed renal ectopia referred after trauma. In such patients, treatment is directed to the underlying disease.

URETERAL AVULSION

Ureteral avulsion may occur with severe trauma in which there is a sudden hyperextension of the spine that imposes tension on the ureter. The avulsion takes place at the pelvoureteral junction and is almost always bilateral.[11,12] In the reported cases there were extensive associated injuries that delayed the diagnosis. IVPs, however, demonstrated extravasation of all contrast material, with no visualization of the ureters. The diagnosis is confirmed with retrograde pyelography. It is helpful to leave the retrograde catheter in place to aid in identification of the distal ureter, which is embedded in hematoma and edema. Treatment consists of primary ureteral anastomosis performed with interrupted 5–0 chromic catgut over a Silastic stent tube. The ureteral anastomosis is spatulated, and the splinting catheter is brought out as a nephrostomy. Delay in diagnosis results in anuria, urinary ascites, infection, fibrosis, and possible loss of a kidney.

TRAUMA TO THE BLADDER AND URETHRA

Even a minimal blow to the dome of a distended bladder results in an intraperitoneal perforation, since a child's bladder extends well up into the peritoneal cavity. An improperly applied seat belt is sufficient to rupture the bladder in a deceleration accident. During the first 48 hours, urine in the peritoneal cavity causes little reaction. There may be mild distention and some pain, but there are no really significant peritoneal signs. Only the most careful examiner will remember to examine the child for free fluid. The diagnosis of a bladder injury will unfold when contrast leaks out of the bladder during the IVP or cystogram. Small tears in the dome of the bladder are obvious because the contrast material will leak out

into the abdominal gutters (Fig. 34–5). There rarely are any other injuries in such cases, and treatment consists of an exploratory laparotomy, closure of the bladder in two layers with an absorbable suture, and liberal perivesical drainage. A cystotomy tube is left in place to decompress the bladder for 10 to 14 days, and two Penrose drains are placed adjacent to the bladder and brought out through lateral stab wounds.

Extraperitoneal ruptures of the bladder and urethra are quite a different matter. These injuries are secondary to major pelvic fractures. Fractures of the femurs and laceration of the rectum are the most commonly associated injuries. We also saw a transected vagina together with a urethral–vaginal fistula after a school bus had run over a 5-year-old girl. In the usual case, the pelvic ring is compressed, and the pubic rami are fractured on either side. The broken bones shear through the urethra at the fixed triangular ligament. The puboprostatic ligament is ruptured. Blood clot and extravasated urine force the bladder and prostate up and out the pelvis.

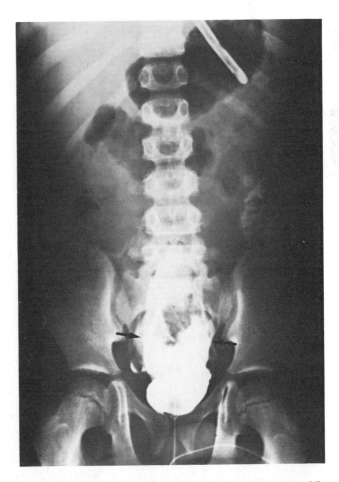

Figure 34–5. This 5-year-old child was a passenger in an automobile that struck a tree. There was no pelvic fracture, but he had lower abdominal tenderness and hematuria. Contrast material escaped from the bladder up both gutters of the peritoneal cavity.

Pelvic fractures are massive injuries in themselves. Quinby reviewed 19 children; 9 required an operation for visceral injuries and 5 more were operated on to control massive hemorrhage.[13] These children are in shock because of blood loss, and they have intense pain, with suprapubic fullness. The first step in their management is resuscitation with lactated Ringer's solution, which is followed by whole blood transfusions. The evaluation must include an examination of the rectum for perforation. In older boys, the prostate may be freely movable high above a fluctuant blood clot. When the child is stabilized, roentgenograms are obtained of the pelvis, abdomen, chest, and any other possible fractures. A catheter is passed 2 to 3 cm into the anterior urethra, and contrast material is injected (Fig. 34–6). If there is no urethral injury, the catheter is passed into the bladder, and a cystogram is performed. Posterioanterior and lateral views are important because a filled bladder could obscure a posterior leak. A perivesical hematoma will compress and elevate the bladder. It is important to carefully examine the x-rays because contrast material that extravasates from a ruptured urethra into a hematoma may be contained and thus appear to be within the bladder. If there is no injury of the bladder, urethra, or rectum and the child is hemorrhaging severely, angiography should be considered in order to localize the bleeding point.[14] The femoral artery opposite the obvious injury is catheterized. A flush aortogram is performed

to rule out other visceral injuries, after which the catheter is advanced just proximal to the opposite obturator artery and injections are made to determine the exact site of bleeding. When this is accomplished, 2 to 4 mm fragments of Gelfoam mixed with contrast material are injected under fluoroscopic control. Most often, the hemorrhage originates from the branches of the obturator artery supplying the pubic rami.

When a bladder or urethral injury is diagnosed, an operation is indicated as soon as the child's vital signs are stable. Sufficient blood for transfusion to replace two or three times the child's blood volume must be at hand. Two large-bore upper extremity cannulas for transfusion, with central venous pressure and arterial monitoring, are essential. Two working suction tips, an electrocautery, bone wax, and an assortment of urethral catheters are also necessary. It is probably wise that a general surgeon and urologist work together because there is controversy over the management of these patients, complications are frequent, and the long-term results are less than satisfactory.

The entire abdomen, perineum, and upper thighs are prepared and draped into the operative field, so that one has access to the urethra as well as to the abdomen. Lacerated arteries adjacent to the pubis can usually be electrocoagulated, and bone ooze is controlled with wax.

Ligation of the hypogastric arteries may be indicated

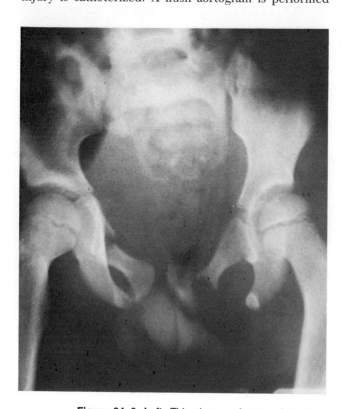 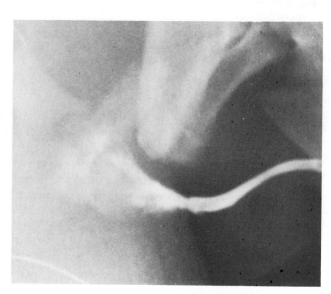

Figure 34–6. Left. This shows a fracture through the pubic ramus caused when an automobile ran over this boy's pelvis. **Right.** The urethrogram demonstrated extravasation of contrast material from the posterior urethra.

when other techniques fail. Once hemorrhage is controlled and the child is stabilized, attention is directed to the urinary tract. Perforations of the bladder are closed, and the bladder is drained with a suprapubic catheter. The torn end of the distal urethra may have retracted below the urogenital diaphragm and the prostatic urethra may be held up by edema and hematoma. The obvious goal of the operation is to save the child's life. Consequently, control of hemorrhage, drainage of the extravasated urine, and suprapubic diversion of urine are the first considerations.

These are rare lesions, particularly in children, and we must rely somewhat on experience obtained with adult patients. Morehouse is of the opinion that attempts to realign the stricture, particularly with metal sounds, does more damage to the injured urethra and increases the incidence of incontinence and impotence.[15] He simply drains the bladder with a suprapubic tube and even avoids perivesical drains. If there is only an incomplete tear of the urethra, healing with spontaneous voiding will occur within 10 days. On the other hand, with complete tears, he believes that simple bladder drainage results in less fibrosis, which must be dealt with at a secondary repair after a delay of 3 to 4 months. Forty-one of his patients were treated by this technique. Of these, 40 became continent without stricture, and 36 had satisfactory potency after the deliberate secondary repair. However, most other surgeons think that unless the patient's general condition is too poor to continue with the operation, an attempt should be made to realign the disrupted urethra. My own limited experience with urethral rupture, which is supported by a report on a series of 7 children in the Mayo Clinic,[16] seems to indicate that excellent results can be obtained with immediate urethral realignment.

Technique
Interlocking metallic sounds and even the usual rubber catheters should be avoided because in all probability these will increase the injury. Rather, a soft, straight Silastic tube with additional fenestrations that will lie within the urethra is passed into the meatus and through the urethra (Fig. 34–7). The bladder itself is then widely opened at the dome. Further dissection about the bladder neck or prostate is contraindicated to minimize further damage to the pelvic nerves. It is particularly important not to convert a partial tear into a complete transection. If the Silastic catheter appears in the bladder, one can assume that the urethra is partially intact. If there is complete separation, a second catheter may be passed through the bladder and out through the bladder neck and torn urethra, where it is sutured to the first catheter, which may then be drawn into the bladder. The Silastic stent is then brought to the outside and securely sutured to itself, so that there is a continuous

tube that is not likely to be pulled out. Three to four catgut sutures can be inserted between the prostate and the urogenital diaphragm to maintain satisfactory approximation. Further, as edema and hemorrhage subside, the bladder and prostate descend, and the torn urethra will come into apposition if it is aligned with a catheter. A suprapubic tube drains the bladder, and the fenestrated Silastic catheter allows for drainage of exudate from the urethra.[17]

During the postoperative period, blood and intravenous fluids are given as is necessary to stabilize the vital signs and to maintain a urinary output of 1 ml/kg. Broad-spectrum antibiotics are administered, pending culture results, after which an agent, such as gantrisin, is used until all urinary drains have been removed and the urine is sterile. With the fenestrated tube, a cystogram may be performed through the cystotomy tube to detect continued leakage. Long-term follow-up is necessary to detect and to dilate urethral strictures.

PERINEAL INJURIES

Genital, urethral, and rectal trauma fortunately are uncommon in children. Blunt trauma most often is the result of a straddle-type injury in which the child falls on the crossbar of a bicycle or a similar hard object.[18] Penetrating injuries also may be accidental as a result of a fall, but these are more often the result of rape or child abuse. There are often long-term sequelae with this group of injuries, which must be treated as early as possible.

Blunt Trauma
Most straddle injuries involve only contusions, which require bed rest and an ice bag. In girls, there may be periurethral lacerations that bleed profusely. These require careful examination in the operating room under general anesthesia, ligation of bleeding points, and loose approximation of the tissues with absorbable sutures. Since there will be considerable edema, a Foley catheter is indicated for a day or two. After the acute injury has subsided, warm sitz baths are indicated. Since the penile urethra is mobile, it is practically never injured by blunt trauma, but the bulbous region is fixed beneath the symphysis pubis and is vulnerable to contusion or laceration. A tear in the urethral mucosa results in the appearance of blood at the urethral meatus. Rapid swelling of the perineum indicates a severe injury with urinary extravasation and hematoma.

The appearance of blood or bloody urine at the meatus is an indication for a urethrogram. A small catheter is inserted into the meatus for several centimeters, and 10 to 15 ml of dilute contrast material is injected and observed fluoroscopically. In most cases there is

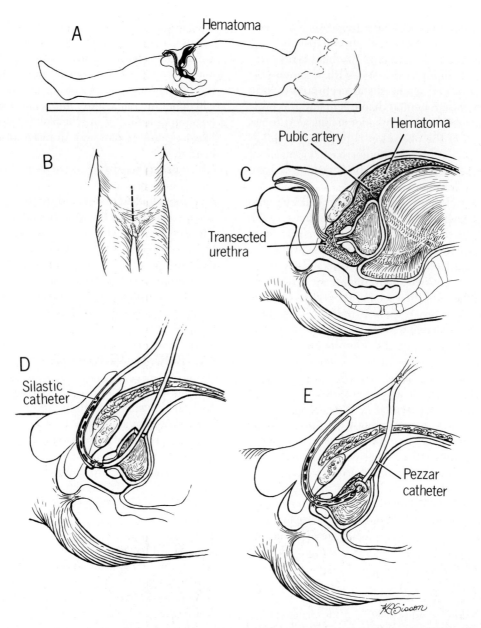

Figure 34–7. A, B, and **C.** Perivesical hematoma associated with a severe pelvic fracture. A midline incision is used to expose the bladder. **D.** In such a case, the bladder is widely opened, and a fenestrated Silastic catheter is passed through the urethra. If this appears in the bladder, it is sutured to a pezzar catheter. Otherwise, a second catheter is passed out the bladder neck and the urethral catheter is found in the laceration. The two catheters are sutured together, and the urethral catheter is brought into the bladder, where it remains as a stent for the transected urethra (**E**).

only a partial transection, and it is possible to advance the catheter on into the bladder, where it must remain for at least 10 days until the urethra has healed.

Surgical Treatment. When a catheter cannot be advanced into the bladder, an operation is indicated. Just as in urethral injuries associated with fractures of the pelvis, the principles of treatment are drainage of the extravasation and urinary diversion with a suprapubic cystotomy. When the diagnosis has been delayed, this

may be all that can be accomplished. However, it is desirable to repair the urethra at the same time.[19] The child must be placed in an exaggerated lithotomy position. The skin preparation and draping include the lower abdomen, perineum, and thighs. The urethra is approached through the midline perineal incision extending through the superficial fascia of the perineum (Colles' fascia). Blood and urine encountered beneath this layer are drained. At this point, another attempt can be made to pass a suction Silastic catheter into the bladder. If this is not possible, it is necessary to incise through Buck's fascia, which envelops the corpora spongiosum and urethra. The proximal urethra is identified by passing a catheter from the opened bladder until it appears in the field. Once identified, the urethra is mobilized sufficiently for anastomosis with fine catgut sutures over a Silastic catheter, with multiple holes cut to lie in the injured urethra. The wound must be closed very loosely over several Penrose drains. If the extravasation has extended beneath the superficial fascia onto the abdominal wall, the involved areas also must be drained.

Penetrating Injuries

Every child in whom there is a suspicion of penetrating vaginal injury, either by rape or by accidental impalement, must be examined under general anesthesia. In either situation, the history often is vague, and the little girl is brought to the emergency room because of vaginal bleeding. Rape must be strongly considered if the child has been left alone with an older male babysitter or if there are contradictory statements. Attempts to examine an acutely disturbed child with a painful genital injury in the emergency room are futile, and serious damage could be overlooked. The usual injury is a periurethral laceration that extends up the vault of the vagina, but we have seen one traumatic rectovaginal fistula and a traumatic evisceration of small intestine through a posterior vaginal tear. The child is placed on the operating table in the lithotomy position with the abdomen ex-

posed. Vaginal aspirates or swabs are taken to study for sperm in any case of suspected rape. The usual lacerations are loosely closed, and a Foley catheter is inserted for 2 days. If there is a high vaginal laceration, it is necessary to explore the abdomen. A colostomy must be performed when there is a laceration through the vagina into the rectum and for third degree rectal tears. A perineal repair is performed several months later.

Male Genital Injuries

A foreskin that gets caught in a zipper causes embarrassment and pain but only minor damage to the penis. Usually, the zipper can be opened after the injection of a bit of local anesthesia. Otherwise, the zipper may be cut away from the pants and a circumcision performed in the operating room that removes the foreskin along with the zipper.

More serious genital injuries result from burns and avulsions. Debridement of genital burns should be accomplished with dressing changes rather than surgical excision in order to save every scrap of viable epithelium. Skin grafts take well to the shaft of the penis for initial coverage, but secondary repairs usually are necessary to release scar tissue, which shortens the apparent penile length (Fig. 34–8).

Avulsions of the scrotum and penile skin are bizarre injuries that usually result from the patient becoming entangled in machinery. The skin separates superficial to Buck's fascia, and the glands are left intact, since

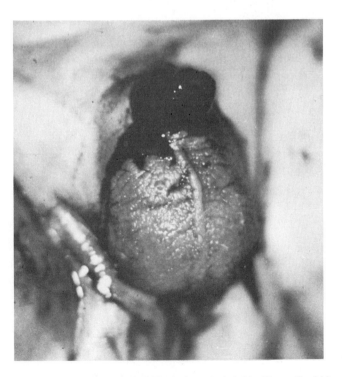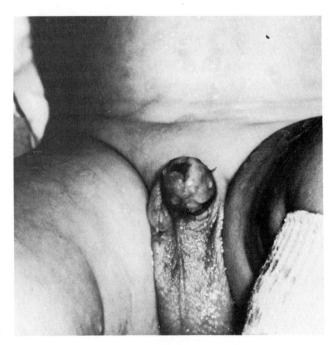

Figure 34–8. Left. A dog mauled this 10-month-old boy, inflicting bites on the lower abdomen and avulsing the skin from his penis. Right. The same boy 4 months after coverage of the wound with a split-thickness skin graft.

the skin is more adherent in this area. The injured area is cleaned and debrided, although there is a strong temptation to suture back the avulsed skin. The denuded penis is best covered with a single sheet of split-thickness skin taken from the adjacent thigh. This is sutured in place and held with a stent dressing.[20] The testicles can be placed in subcutaneous pockets on the medial aspect of the thigh after avulsion of the scrotum.

REFERENCES

1. Nelson RP, Sullivan MJ, Richter J, Russo M: Complete avulsion of the renal pedicle with survival: Case reports and literature review. J Trauma 16:2, 157, 1976
2. Grablowsky OM, Weichert RF III, Goff JB, Schlegel JU: Renal artery thrombosis following blunt trauma: Report of four cases. Surgery 67:895, 1970
3. Levine EF, Hessl JM: Renal artery occlusion following blunt abdominal trauma. J Urol 112:553, 1974
4. Skinner DC: Traumatic renal artery thrombosis: A successful thrombectomy and revascularization. Ann Surg 177:214, 1973
5. Guttman FM, Homsy Y, Schmidt E: Avulsion injury to the renal pedicle following blunt trauma: Survival of the patient and the kidney. Paper presented at the American Pediatric Surgical Association Meeting, Acapulco, April 20, 1977
6. Karp M, Jewett T, Kuhn T, et al: The impact of computed tomography scanning on the child with renal trauma. J Pediatr Surg 21:617, 1986
7. Cass A: Blunt renal trauma in children. J Trauma 23:123, 1983
8. Mandour W, Lai M, Linke C, Frank I: Blunt renal truma in the pediatric patient. J Pediatr Surg 16:669, 1981
9. Javadpour N, Guinan P, Bush IM: Renal trauma in children. Surg Gynecol Obstet 136:237, 1973
10. Reid IS: Renal trauma in children: A ten-year review. NZ J Surg 42:260, 1973
11. Johnson JM, Chernov MS, Cloud DT, et al: Bilateral ureteral avulsion. J Pediatr Surg 7:723, 1972
12. Boston VE, Smyth BT: Bilateral pelvicureteric avulsion following closed trauma. Br J Urol 47:149, 1975
13. Quinby WC: Fractures of the pelvis and associated injuries in children. J Pediatr Surg 1:353, 1968
14. Barlow B, Rottenberg RW, Santulli TV: Angiographic diagnosis and treatment of bleeding by selective embolization following pelvic fracture in children. J Pediatr Surg 10:939, 1975
15. Morehouse PD: Posterior urethral injury etiology, diagnosis, initial management. Symposium on Genitourinary Trauma. Urol Clin North Am 4:69, 1977
16. DeWeerd JH: Immediate realignment of posterior urethral injury. Symposium on Genitourinary Trauma. Urol Clin North Am 4:75, 1977
17. Warwick RT: A personal view of the immediate management of pelvic fractures and urethral injuries. Symposium on Genitourinary Trauma. Urol Clin North Am 4:81, 1977
18. Ezell WW, McCarthey RP: Mechanical traumatic injury to the genitalia in children. J Urol 102:788, 1969
19. Devine CJ, Devine PC, Horton CE: Anterior urethral injury. Urol Clin North Am 4:25, 1977
20. Culp DA: Genital injuries: etiology and management. Urol Clin North Am 4:143, 1977

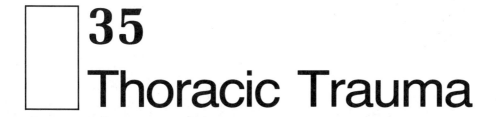

35
Thoracic Trauma

Marleta Reynolds

Major thoracic injuries are a serious threat to life, particularly when associated with cranial or abdominal trauma. Of 51 children with blunt thoracic trauma reported by Levy, 16 children had concomitant skull fractures, 9 had ruptured spleens, and 38 had long bone fractures.[1] There was an overall mortality rate of 30 percent in this series, primarily due to associated head injuries. Since our designation as a pediatric trauma center (2½ years ago), we have admitted 1118 injured children. Thoracic trauma occurred in only 4 percent and did not contribute to the death of any patient. At Children's Memorial Hospital, 97 percent of all chest injuries were from blunt trauma.

In the newborn period, chest injuries are associated with delivery. Between 3 and 5 years of age, there is a peak in the incidence of foreign body aspiration. At the end of the first decade of life, when children are small and difficult for a driver to see, there is a high incidence of blunt injuries to the chest from automobile accidents. In teenagers, there is a significant increase in the incidence of penetrating wounds to the chest. Most of these injuries occur in the brutal environment of the ghetto, where stab and gunshot wounds occur frequently.

Compression injuries to the vertebral column occur when the child engages in vigorous sports. We deal with three categories in this chapter: (1) birth injuries, (2) injuries associated with blunt trauma, and (3) penetrating wounds.

GENERAL MANAGEMENT

Accurate assessment of thoracic injuries in the emergency room is critical because a child with impaired ventilation can deteriorate rapidly. First, determine if there is airway obstruction, pneumothorax or hemothorax, or evidence of cardiac tamponade. Noisy respirations with retraction of the thorax, particularly in a comatose child, should lead to immediate examination of the oropharynx. Laryngoscopy, with insertion of an endotracheal tube, is the safest and most rapid way to ensure an open upper airway. If this cannot be accomplished, immediate tracheostomy should be performed. In an infant, needle cricothyrotomy can provide adequate ventilation. Diminution of breath sounds or shift of the trachea and apical cardiac impulse, with cyanosis or tachypnea, is an indication for diagnostic thoracentesis. If there is a return of air or blood, a chest tube should be inserted without waiting for an x-ray of the chest. Obviously, prior roentgenograms of the chest are desirable if the patient's condition permits.

TECHNIQUE FOR CHEST TUBE INSERTION

Air, blood, chyle, or pus may be evacuated from the chest through a tube inserted through an intercostal space and connected to a waterseal drainage bottle. If the pleural cavity is not obliterated by adhesions, the tube is always inserted at the midaxillary line through the fifth to the seventh intercostal spaces. The child rests in a supine position, with the affected chest slightly elevated on a folded towel. The chest is at the edge of the examining table or bed. An assistant holds the child's arm over his head so that the entire axilla is exposed; in addition, the child's body is bent away from the affected side to open the interspaces. The entire chest is painted with povidone-iodine and draped with sterile towels. One percent lidocaine is infiltrated into the skin and subcutaneous tissues. The needle is directed to the next highest rib, and the periosteum is injected. During injection of the local anesthetic, the needle is slid into the

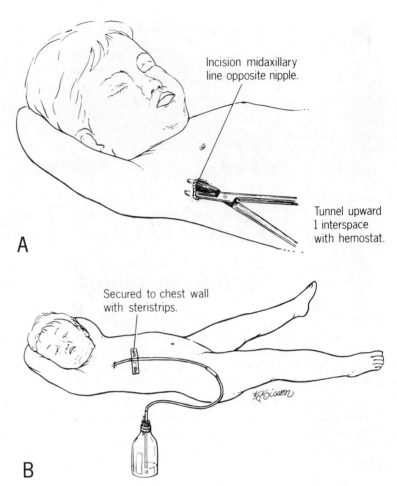

Incision midaxillary
line opposite nipple.

Tunnel upward
1 interspace
with hemostat.

Secured to chest wall
with steristrips.

A

B

Figure 35–1. Chest tubes in children should be inserted through the midaxillary line opposite the nipple. **A.** Tunnel subcutaneously to insert the tube one interspace higher than the incision. **B.** Use a lot of tape and a suture to secure the tube.

pleura over the rib. In this manner, the intercostal vessels are avoided. A 1 cm skin incision is made, and with a curved hemostat the subcutaneous tissues are dissected and undermined so that the course of the tube is tunneled upward to pass over the next highest rib. The chest tube may be inserted with a pair of curved forceps and secured to the skin with a suture ligature (Fig. 35–1). When the tube is properly placed, there will be a rush of air into the waterseal bottle with each breath if there is a pneumothorax.

A properly inserted tube should be directed toward the apex. In this location both air and fluid are drained from the pleural cavity (Fig. 35–2). A tube never should be inserted into the second intercostal space anteriorly in a child, and if a lower interspace is used, there is danger that either the liver or the spleen will be injured.

A patient who arrives at the emergency room in extremis with a penetrating chest wound may require immediate endotracheal intubation and an open thoracotomy to relieve pericardial tamponade or to control massive hemorrhage. If the patient's condition can be improved with these measures, he or she is taken directly to the operating room for completion of the operation.

THORACIC INJURIES ASSOCIATED WITH BIRTH

Respiratory efforts by the newborn at birth, vigorous attempts to resuscitate obtunded newborns, coughing paroxysms or inhalation therapy, and obstetric manipulation all can lead to thoracic injury. In many instances, all that is required is conservative management and supportive therapy. In other cases, the underlying pulmonary or congenital lesion is so severe that it, rather than the incidental thoracic trauma, is responsible for the ultimate outcome of therapy. A fractured clavicle is the most common injury. Aside from the obvious deformity from malalignment of the clavicular fragments, there is no distress.

Barotrauma from aggressive ventilatory support can result in pneumothorax, pneumomediastinum, subcutaneous emphysema, or interstitial emphysema. In most of these birth injuries, it is only necessary to give supportive care, and the entrapped air is eventually reabsorbed. In cases of significant pneumothorax, chest tubes with waterseal drainage are inserted to remove the intrapleural air and to facilitate reexpansion of the lung.

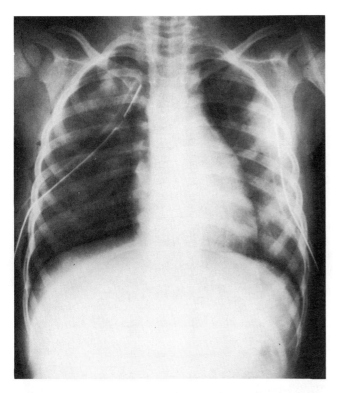

Figure 35–2. Properly placed chest tubes inserted to drain air from bilateral pneumothoraces. This child was struck by a car and brought to the emergency room in severe respiratory distress. The air has been evacuated, but one can see evidence of bilateral pulmonary contusion.

PENETRATING WOUNDS TO THE CHEST

Gunshot and stab wounds of the chest are seen with increasing frequency in young teenagers as a result of urban street fights. The location of the wound is important in assessing the injury to underlying vital organs. Usually, there is damage only to the lung parenchyma with pneumothorax, which can be managed with a tube thoracostomy connected to a waterseal drainage system. Prompt reexpansion of the lung occurs unless there is an organized blood clot that prevents drainage of the accumulated blood and maintains collapse of the lung. It is occasionally necessary to surgically decorticate an organized or infected blood clot in a hemothorax that was initially inadequately drained.

The compelling danger of penetrating wounds is the possibility of injury to mediastinal structures (e.g., heart, great vessels, or esophagus) or penetration into the upper abdomen. If the direction of the missile or knife crossed the midline or entered the mediastinal area, a barium swallow is indicated to determine if the esophagus is injured. The patient must be observed for evidence of cardiac tamponade. Mediastinal emphysema

suggests injury to either the tracheobronchial tree or the esophagus. Neck vein distention, pulsus paradoxus, shock, and distant cardiac sounds are indications for pericardial aspiration. Definite findings may occur late in acute cardiac tamponade, so one must be prepared to perform diagnostic pericardial tap if there is any question of cardiac injury.

Aspiration of the pericardium formerly was considered therapeutic, but today, if cardiac tamponade occurs, open thoracotomy or median sternotomy is considered preferable because of the danger of continued bleeding.[2] Continuing or uncontrolled pneumothorax, as well as severe or continuing hemorrhage into the pleural space, is an indication for open thoracotomy.

Many stab wounds of the chest are delivered with a downward thrust, resulting in penetration of the diaphragm and injuries to structures or organs in the upper abdomen. In such circumstances, surgery is mandatory. In one of our patients, the wound of entry penetrated the thorax in the right fifth intercostal space. The knife blade penetrated the diaphragm and injured the left lobe of the liver and stomach. In addition, the right phrenic nerve was injured, resulting in continued respiratory distress and gastroesophageal reflux because of paralysis of the right diaphragmatic crus.

BLUNT TRAUMA TO THE CHEST

Multiple rib fractures with a flail segment are rare in young children because their elastic thoracic cages absorb considerable bending force. In older children, however, multiple rib fractures and flail chest occur more frequently. The paradoxic movement of the chest wall with respiration decreases the efficiency of ventilation and may lead to respiratory failure.[3] Younger patients subjected to severe compression injuries of the thorax may develop a syndrome known as "traumatic asphyxia," which occurs when the chest wall is severely compressed while the glottis is closed.[4] This results in increased pulmonary and systemic venous pressure, extravasation of blood into the lung parenchyma, and petechial hemorrhages over the face and upper chest. The full extent of pulmonary damage may not be immediately apparent. Clinically, the child may appear to be well, and the chest roentgenogram on admission may demonstrate clear lung fields. Progressive asphyxia occurs within the next 2 or 3 days, and repeated chest roentgenograms show fluffy or linear densities in the lung fields, indicative of perivascular and peribronchial hemorrhages.[5] Earlier signs of pulmonary contusion or traumatic wet lung may occur in the form of increased respiratory effort combined with clinical signs of hypoxemia. Arterial blood gases should be checked at frequent intervals to determine the need for ventilatory support and endotracheal intuba-

308

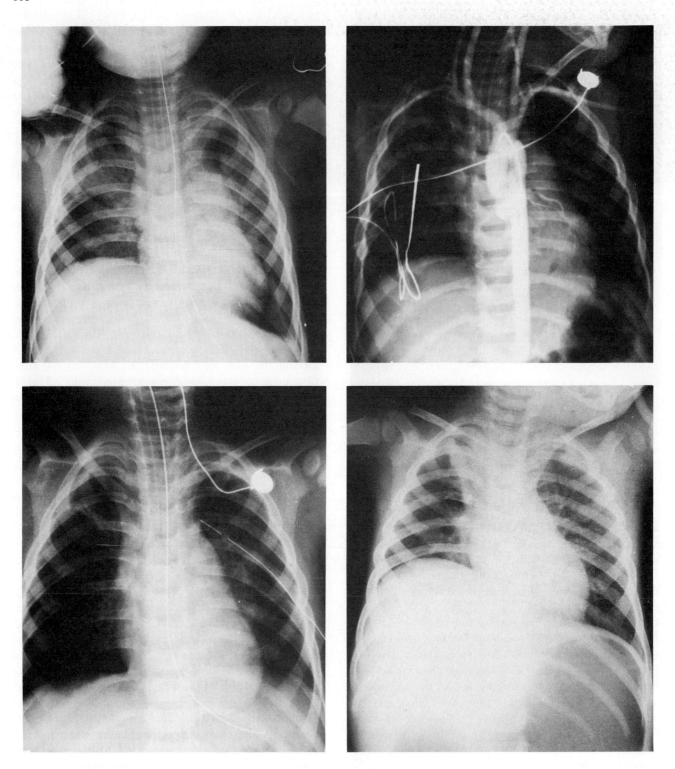

Figure 35–3. Multiple rib fractures, including a fracture of the right first rib. This 2-year-old boy was struck by an automobile and sustained a cerebral concussion and fractures of the humerus and femur in addition to his severe chest injury. **Top left.** On admission to the hospital, the boy was cyanotic, with shallow respirations. He was intubated and placed on a respirator. Note the early pneumothorax on the left. **Top right.** Concern over his widened mediastinum led to the performance of an aortogram to rule out an aortic transection. **Bottom left.** Five days later, he is still on ventilator support with an endotracheal tube, but his lungs had markedly cleared. **Bottom right.** The patient required 20 days of intubation with ventilatory support. After positive pressure ventilation was withdrawn, the elevation of the right diaphragm secondary to phrenic nerve injury became apparent. This boy spontaneously recovered over the following year. He now has no posttraumatic sequelae.

tion. Humidity, the removal of secretions, and positive inotropic drugs may all be required to support the child until the lung injury subsides.

After blunt chest trauma, the child may have little initial respiratory distress. The common complication of blunt chest trauma is a localized pulmonary contusion, with hemorrhage and edema of the lung underlying the injury. The degree of respiratory distress is in direct relation to the amount of involved lung. A bloody pleural effusion may develop several days later. These children must be observed closely, with serial roentgenograms and blood gas determinations. Treatment consists of pain relief, high humidity, increased oxygen concentration, and respiratory support in the case of severe hypoxemia with carbon dioxide retention. An intercostal nerve block may relieve pain and prevent atelectasis. A chest tube with waterseal drainage is indicated for a pleural effusion. Long-term respiratory support occasionally is indicated. Figure 35–3 illustrates serial roentgenograms of a 2-year-old boy who was struck by an automobile. He was unconscious on admission to the emergency room with cyanosis, tachycardia and shallow respirations. An endotracheal tube was inserted, and he was placed on positive pressure ventilation. His initial roentgenograms demonstrated patchy infiltrates and a minimal pneumothorax. The widened mediastinum led to concern about a ruptured aorta, and consequently an aortogram was performed. This child required a chest tube to drain the left pneumothorax and 20 days of endotracheal intubation. Part of his problem was paralysis of the left diaphragm secondary to the fracture of his right first rib.

A persistent pneumothorax that does not respond to tube drainage or extensive mediastinal or subcutaneous emphysema suggests rupture of the bronchus or trachea. Air also may dissect into the peritoneal cavity or the pericardium. However, these findings are not always present, and the diagnosis of ruptured bronchus may be difficult to make. The loose peribronchial tissues may maintain continuity of the bronchial wall and limit air leak even though the integrity of the bronchial lumen is impaired by separation of the ends of the ruptured bronchus. Often, the primary finding is persistent atelectasis of the lung distal to the site of rupture.[6] Occasionally, the only significant finding immediately after trauma is hemoptysis.

The most dependable method for establishing a diagnosis of rupture of the bronchus is immediate bronchoscopy. Successful repair has been reported from 3 months to 8 years after initial injury.[7–9] Leape reported a 6 cm separation of the left mainstem bronchus that was successfully diagnosed by bronchoscopy and repaired immediately after the trauma.[10] The right mainstem bronchus is easily accessible through a right posterolateral thoracotomy. Exposure of the left mainstem bronchus may require mobilization of the aorta and division of the liga-

mentum arteriosum. Repair is accomplished by end-to-end anastomosis. It is necessary for the anesthesiologist to intubate selectively the uninjured contralateral bronchus in order to maintain adequate ventilation during the operation. Postoperatively, periodic follow-up bronchoscopy is indicated to evaluate and, if necessary, to dilate strictures at the site of repair.

Rupture of a leaf of the diaphragm has been reported in association with blunt trauma to the thorax.[11–13] In this situation, roentgenograms of the chest may demonstrate stomach or loops of bowel above the level of the diaphragm. Because of the severity of the trauma required to produce rupture of the diaphragm, this event usually is associated with concomitant injury to upper abdominal organs, especially the stomach, liver, spleen, and bowel. Acute diaphragmatic rupture should, therefore, be repaired through a laparotomy incision, so that the abdominal organs also may be inspected thoroughly and repaired. Pulmonary injury usually can be managed by closed thoracostomy.

REFERENCES

1. Levy JL: Management of crushing chest injuries in children. South Med J 65:1040, 1972
2. Mattox KL, Beall AC, Jordan GL, DeBakey ME: Cardiorrhaphy in the emergency center. J Thorac Cardiovasc Surg 68:886, 1974
3. Eichelberger MR, Randolph JG: Thoracic trauma in children. Surg Clin North Am 61:1181, 1981
4. Haller JA Jr, Donahoo JS: Traumatic asphyxia in children: Pathophysiology and management. J Trauma 11:453, 1971
5. Kilman JW, Charnock E: Thoracic trauma in infancy and childhood. J Trauma 9:863, 1969
6. Urschel HC Jr, Razzuk MA: Management of acute traumatic injuries of tracheo-bronchial tree. Surg Gynecol Obstet 136:113, 1973
7. Al-Omeni MW: Traumatic rupture of left mainstem bronchus. Arch Surg 99:346, 1969
8. Logeais Y, Florent GD, Danrigal A, et al: Traumatic rupture of the right main bronchus in an eight-year-old child successfully repaired eight years after injury. Ann Surg 172:1039, 1970
9. Danis RK, Schweiss JF: Late repair of bronchial rupture in a child by bronchial replantation. J Pediatr Surg 11:235, 1976
10. Leape LL: Bronchial avulsion: Successful repair after bilateral pneumothorax. J Thorac Cardiovasc Surg 62:470, 1971
11. Estrera AS, Landay MJ, McClelland RN: Blunt traumatic rupture of the right hemidiaphragm: Experience in 12 patients. Ann Thorac Surg 39:525, 1985
12. Radhakrishna C, Dickinson SJ, Shaw A: Acute diaphragmatic hernia from blunt trauma in children. J Pediatr Surg 4:553, 1969
13. Melzig EP, Swank M, Scaleberg AM: Blunt traumatic rupture of diaphragm in children. Arch Surg 11:1009, 1976

36
Vascular Injuries and Limb Gangrene

VASCULAR INJURIES

A normal child will tolerate ligation or thrombotic obstruction of major arteries without loss of limb. In years past, the subclavian artery was used for the Blalock-Taussig subclavian–pulmonary artery anastomosis, and the brachial artery often was ligated after angiography without immediate sequelae. The femoral artery may thrombose after cardiac catheterization, without loss of limb. I have removed the common iliac artery for a fibrosarcoma with only minimal temporary pallor and coolness of the leg. This is possible because children have no arteriosclerosis, and there are excellent collateral vessels around major arteries. Even though collateral flow is satisfactory for immediate limb salvage, obstruction of major vessels is associated with long-term retarded limb growth. These changes may not become obvious until the child is 4 to 6 years old and are most prominent after 10 years of age.

Unfortunately, in children, especially infants under 1 year of age, underlying disease can cause spontaneous gangrene. Children with these diseases require vascular access. An arterial puncture or venous cutdown is then blamed for the gangrene and limb loss. The tragedy is compounded when legal action is taken against the physician when the disease and not the procedure is at fault.

In older children, vascular trauma is most often the result of penetrating injuries with gunshots, stabs, and impalement on broken shards of glass. This penetrating trauma results in immediate hemorrhage or a large hematoma and loss of peripheral pulses.

When there is a wound in the vicinity of a major vessel, exploration is indicated on clinical grounds alone. A preoperative angiogram seldom is indicated.[1] Treatment consists of wide surgical exposure with proximal and distal control of the injured vessel. One leg, in addition to the injured area, is prepared and draped into the sterile field in case it is necessary to take a saphenous vein graft. In most injuries, simple arterial repair with interrupted monofilament sutures is all that is indicated. With gunshot wounds, it is necessary to debride the artery, and a vein graft may be indicated to relieve tension. With magnification and fine suture material, it is possible to suture vessels as small as 1 to 2 mm in diameter. Thus, major arteries in small infants can be repaired. The long-term results may be improved by repair of associated injured veins. The most important cause of death with penetrating vascular injuries is immediate, massive hemorrhage, but Moore and Peter have reported survival of a 4-year-old child with a gunshot wound of the abdominal aorta.[2] Direct blunt trauma may result in intimal disruption and gradual thrombosis of major arteries. The symptoms of pallor, weakness, and temperature changes in the extremity may develop over several days. The diagnosis is suspected by absent or diminished arterial pulsations beyond the injury and is confirmed by Doppler examination and an arteriogram.[3] In most cases, it is necessary to resect a segment of artery, which is replaced with a graft.[4] Blunt extremity injury that results in fractures or dislocation may cause intimal disruption or transection of major vessels. The presence or absence of pulses must be noted and recorded in every single injured extremity. If there are signs of diminished circulation, a Doppler study is performed. If there is not prompt improvement, an angiogram is indicated. Crush injuries that fracture the femur and the femoral artery often are associated with other serious trauma that may take precedence. If at all possible, however, the fracture must be stabilized with internal fixation and the artery repaired. Most often, a fasciotomy will be indicated. The combination of a crush injury, fracture, and vascular obstruction often results in such severe tissue damage that an amputation becomes necessary.

Supracondylar fractures of the humerus result from a fall on the outstretched hand. When there is severe displacement of bone fragments, the brachial artery may become trapped, lacerated, or contused. Even if there is no direct arterial damage, severe soft tissue edema can interfere with circulation. The end result of vascular insufficiency is ischemic necrosis of forearm muscles, with fibrosis of the nerves, and a deformed anesthetic hand, a Volkman's ischemic contracture. This tragic sequence is avoided by prompt reduction of the fracture under general anesthesia and skeletal traction with a Kirschner wire drilled through the ulna 3 cm from the tip of the olecranon. The arm is then held in traction with the shoulder abducted and the arm elevated.

There must be no encircling cast or dressing. In most cases, the radial pulse will return after reduction of the fracture. The hand is evaluated at hourly intervals for pulse, capillary refill, and tissue perfusion. Documentation of the pulse with Doppler ultrasonography will enhance the clinical findings. If the pulse does not return but there is good capillary refill and a warm, pink hand, nothing further is done. In most cases, the pulse will reappear. In a review of supracondylar fractures, loss of pulsation was found in the brachial artery in only 25 of 1919 patients, and the incidence of Volkman's contracture is only 1.1 per 1000 cases.[5]

There is no reason for complacency, however, and the limb must be closely observed. If there is poor capillary refill, pallor, or coolness of the hand after reduction of the fracture, an arteriogram is indicated.[6] If the brachial artery is obstructed, the arm is explored. A longitudinal incision is made from the flexor crease of the elbow, medial to the biceps tendon, and extending along the middle of the volar surface of the forearm to the flexor crease of the wrist.[7] The brachial artery is exposed and decompressed, and the fascia overlying the muscle compartments is opened, allowing the muscle bellies to bulge. A local anesthetic or papaverine is applied to the adventia of the artery to relieve spasm, but in most cases, a segment of contused artery must be resected and replaced with a vein graft. A Fogarty catheter will aid in removing clots and in dilating the artery for anastomosis. The wound is left open, and the arm is replaced in traction, with a loose sterile dressing. After the edema has subsided, the wound is closed secondarily.

Vascular injury from cardiac catheterization, angiography, and intraarterial monitoring lines accounts for most arterial obstructions in children under 1 year of age. O'Neill et al. reviewed 41 thromboembolic complications in 4000 infants with umbilical artery catheters.[8] Signs of vascular obstruction included pallor or cyanosis of the feet, legs, or buttocks. In O'Neill's series, the catheter was removed at the first sign of trouble. Fifteen infants with obstruction distal to the femoral artery had limb survival without an operation, but the authors rec-

ommended aortic thrombectomy for aortic or iliac clots. Complications included intestinal gangrene secondary to mesenteric artery obstruction and renal infarcts or hypertension. The incidence of aortic thrombosis secondary to umbilical artery catheters is reduced by the addition of heparin and by avoiding hyperosmolar fluids. In our nursery, abdominal ultrasonography performed at the cribside accurately diagnoses aortic clots. Treatment with urokinase and heparin is instituted immediately and has been successful in early cases. If this fails, aortic thrombectomy is indicated provided the infant is in satisfactory general condition.

With increased experience, femoral artery thrombosis has become an infrequent sequela of cardiac catheterization. There were only 35 arterial injuries at the Toronto Children's Hospital in 12,000 catheterizations from 1966 to 1981.[9] In this series, when pulses disappeared after the procedure, the child was given heparin and observed for 4 to 8 hours. Arterial exploration was performed if the pulse remained nonpalpable. Simple thrombectomy restored the pulse in 70 percent of 17 patients, whereas a vein patch angioplasty was performed in 8 children with restoration of all pulses. There was only 1 amputation, and this was in a 1.74 kg infant with heart failure. Leblanc et al. now give heparin to children weighing less than 7.5 kg and do not operate. Others are divided on the indications for surgery in catheter-related femoral artery thrombosis when there is an absent pulse but good capillary filling and a warm, pink leg.[10–12] In otherwise healthy children, it is perfectly satisfactory to give heparin and observe the limb. When the circulation remains intact, an operation is not absolutely necessary, but one can anticipate a leg length discrepancy and perhaps claudication. Delayed vascular reconstruction has allowed resumption of normal leg length when performed before the adolescent growth spurt. However, when there is pain, pallor, and poor perfusion, a thrombectomy is indicated.

Most iatrogenic vascular injuries, such as ligation of the brachial artery during an attempted venous cutdown, occur during the emergency resuscitation of very ill children. Often the child's underlying disease caused hypovolemia and vasospasm, which make venous access difficult. If the accidental arterial injury results in limb ischemia and the child's general condition will permit an operation, repair of the artery is indicated. Obviously, this is a difficult decision that must be individualized.

LIMB ISCHEMIA AND GANGRENE

It is worthwhile to discuss diseases that may result in limb ischemia and gangrene in the context of vascular injury. Limb gangrene often is blamed on an essential vascular access procedure that is alleged to have caused an arterial injury.

Gross reviewed the literature on childhood embolism and thrombosis in 1945.[13] There have been other reports of spontaneous limb gangrene in newborn and older infants.[14,15] A review article on this topic, which also documents an extensive personal experience, appeared in the August 1985 *Current Problems in Surgery*.[16] Thrombosis of major arteries in the newborn infant is associated with a wide variety of infectious and metabolic disease.[17-21] Infants of diabetic mothers are particularly at risk for spontaneous arterial thrombosis, and blood hyperviscosity may be an underlying factor in infants with spontaneous gangrene.[22] Hyperviscosity is determined by the hematocrit, the deformability of the red blood cell, and the plasma viscosity. When the venous hematocrit is over 65, most newborns will have hyperviscous blood. This is seen in babies who are born to diabetic mothers and in those with chromosomal abnormalities. Placental insufficiency with intrauterine hypoxia accounts for the polycythemia found in many babies with these conditions. They may have seizures, irritability, hypotonia, or congestive heart failure as well as peripheral cyanosis and limb gangrene. When symptomatic, these infants are treated with partial exchange transfusions using fresh frozen plasma or albumin instead of blood.[23]

Upper extremity thrombosis has been reported in a considerable number of neonates with arterial insufficiency, regardless of etiology. Birth trauma may account for this, since a number of reported patients have had an above average birth weight. Wiseman et al. attempted an axillary artery thrombectomy in an infant born to a prediabetic mother, but the thrombus recurred, and an amputation was necessary.[24] It is unlikely that an operation will succeed unless the underlying disease is corrected.

Severe diarrhea with hypernatremic dehydration is one of the most prominent causes for limb gangrene in infants under 1 year of age.[25,26] These infants often are premature and are malnourished before the acute illness. The diarrhea leads to hypovolemia, hemoconcentration, and intense vasospasm, and often the serum sodium is over 160 mEq/liter. There is severe metabolic acidosis, and sepsis causes endotoxin damage to vascular endothelium. These infants often are brought to the hospital in extremis and require the rapid administration of intravenous fluids. Venous or arterial sampling is necessary to determine serum electrolytes and blood gases for optimum therapy. This is the situation in which a vascular access procedure is most often blamed for extremity gangrene.[27] An arterial or venous puncture may contribute to the limb ischemia by further damage to vascular endothelium or by locally increasing vasospasm. When signs of extremity ischemia appear in this clinical

setting, heparin should be administered through all vascular lines, and topical nitroglycerin paste is applied to the extremity. At the same time, the underlying disease is treated with fluids and antibiotics. Unfortunately, cerebral edema and convulsions may complicate rapid fluid therapy. The physician and his patient are between a rock and a hard place. Changing the venipuncture site may result in gangrene of another limb (Fig. 36–1). Intraosseous fluid therapy may be the best way around this no-win situation.

Purpura fulminans complicates a number of infectious diseases. The most serious are septicemia due to the meningococci or streptococci.[28,29] These children arrive at the hospital in overwhelming septic shock. There is poor peripheral perfusion, and ischemic changes develop at areas of skin pressure. Gangrene may be limited to patchy areas on the skin, or entire extremities may be involved (Fig. 36–2). They may require vascular

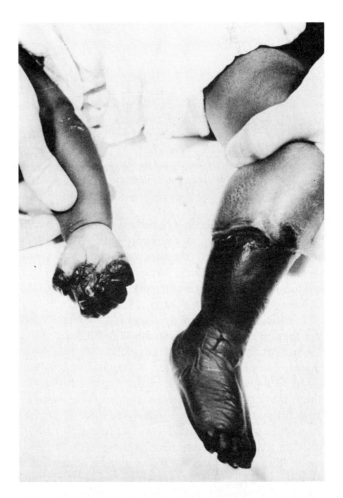

Figure 36–1. This 6-month-old infant with severe diarrhea and dehydration first had a venous cutdown performed at the saphenous vein in the ankle. When the foreleg became ischemic, the IV was switched to a needle venipuncture on the back of the hand. This too became ischemic. Both the distal portion of the hand and the foreleg were amputated.

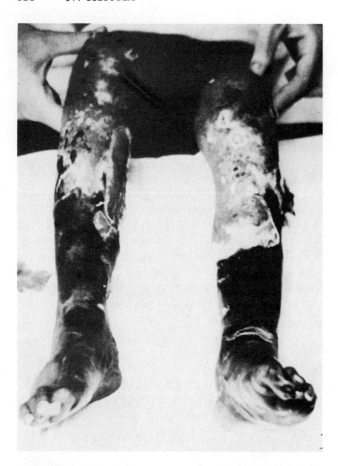

Figure 36–2. A 4-year-old boy with streptococcal sepsis that resulted in purpura fulminans and lower extremity gangrene. Note the patchy areas of skin gangrene above the demarcated areas.

access, which again may contribute to limb ischemia. In one reported case, an extremity with a heparinized posterior tibial arterial cutdown was spared.[30] This suggests the value of heparin, particularly the usefulness of administering heparin through all catheters used for vascular access.

When ischemic changes appear in an extremity during therapy for any overwhelming illness, the status of the patient and the peripheral circulation must be meticulously examined and recorded. A Doppler study is indicated to determine patency of the major arteries, but there is no place for an arteriogram in these patients. In addition to treating the underlying disease, heparin is useful, and topical nitroglycerin ointment may be applied for its vasodilating effect. If there is no improvement, the site of vascular access should be moved to another location, even though ischemic changes may occur there as well. When gangrene becomes obvious, the skin is treated with silver sulfadiazine and loose fluffy bandages. Collateral flow may improve the vascularity. Consequently, debridement or amputation is delayed until the eschar commences to separate in order to salvage as much tissue as possible.

REFERENCES

1. Meagher D, Defore W, Mattox K, et al: Vascular trauma in infants and children. Trauma 19:532, 1979
2. Moore T, Peter M: Thru and thru gunshot penetration of distal abdominal aorta in a 4 year old child managed by aortic transection, debridement, and reanastomosis with survival. J Trauma 19:537, 1979
3. Richardson J, Fallot M, Nagaraj A, et al: Arterial injuries in children. Arch Surg 116:685, 1981
4. Stanton PE Jr, Brown R, Rosenthal D: External iliac artery occlusion by bicycle handle injury. J Cardiovasc Surg 27:728, 1986
5. Walle A: Supracondylar fracture of the humerus in children. Br J Accident Surg 16:296, 1985
6. Broudy A, Jupiter J, May J: Management of supracondylar fracture with brachial artery thrombosis in a child: case report and literature review. J Trauma 19:540, 1979
7. Eaton R, Green W: Epimysiotomy and fasciotomy in the treatment of Volkman's ischemia contracture. Orthop Clin North Am 3:175, 1972
8. O'Neill J, Neblett W, Born M: Management of major thromboembolic complication of umbilical artery catheters. J Pediatr Surg 16:972, 1981
9. Leblanc J, Wood AE, O'Shea MA, et al: Peripheral arterial trauma in children. A fifteen year review. J Cardiovasc Surg 26:325, 1985
10. Flinigan D, Keifer T, Schuler J, et al: Experience with iatrogenic pediatric vascular injuries. Ann Surg 198:430, 1983
11. Klein M, Coran A, Whitehouse W, et al: Management of iatrogenic arterial injuries in infants and children. J Pediatr Surg 17:933, 1972
12. Smith C, Green R: Pediatric vascular injuries. Surgery 90:20, 1981
13. Gross R: Arterial embolism and thrombosis in infancy. Am J Dis Child 70:61, 1945
14. Strokes G, Shumacker H: Spontaneous gangrene in infancy. Angiology 3:226, 1952
15. Smith J, Currarino G, Goldberg H, et al: Gangrene of the extremities in the newborn and infant. Am J Surg 109:306, 1965
16. Villavicencio J, Gonzalez-Cerna J, Velasco P: Acute vascular problems of children. Curr Probl Surg, 22, 1985
17. Hsi AC, Davis DJ, Sherman FC: Neonatal gangrene in the newborn infant of a diabetic mother. J Pediatr Orthop 5:358, 1985
18. Oppenheimer E, Esterly J: Thrombosis in the newborn: comparison between the infants of diabetic and non diabetic mothers. J Pediatr 159:549, 1965
19. Hunter AG, Jimenez CL, Carpenter BF, MacDonald I: Neuroaxonal dystrophy presenting with neonatal dysmorphic features. Early onset of peripheral gangrene, and a rapidly lethal course. Am J Med Genet 28:171, 1987
20. Shaffer WO, Aulicino PL, DuPuv TE: Upper extremity gangrene of the newborn infant. J Hand Surg [Am] 9A:88, 1984
21. Rayner CR, Lloyd DJ, Ward K: Neonatal upper limb ischaemia. The case for conservative management. J Hand Surg [Am] 9:57, 1984

22. Papageorgiov A, Stern L: Polycythemia and gangrene of an extremity in an infant. J Pediatr 81:985, 1972
23. Oski F, Naiman J (eds): Hematological Problems in the Newborn, 3rd ed. Philadelphia, Saunders, 1982, pp 87–96
24. Wiseman N, Briggs J, Bolton V: Neonatal arterial occlusion with ischemic limb gangrene. J Pediatr Surg 12:707, 1977
25. Comoy S, Karabus C: Peripheral gangrene in hypernatremia dehydration of infancy. Arch Dis Child 50:616, 1975
26. Amitai I, Goder K, Husseini N, Rousso M: Hypernatrimia dehydration complicated by peripheral gangrene in infancy. Isr J Med Sci 19:538, 1983
27. Nabseth D, Jones J: Gangrene of the lower extremities after femoral venipuncture. N Engl J Med 268:1003, 1963
28. Schaller RT Jr, Schaller JF: Surgical management of life-threatening and disfiguring sequelae of fulminant meningococcemia. Am J Surg 151:553, 1986
29. Jacobsen ST, Crawford AH: Amputation following meningococcemia. A sequela to purpura fulminans. Clin Orthop 185:214, 1984
30. Issacman SH, Heroman WM, Liohtsev AL: Purpura fulminans following late-onset group B beta-hemolytic streptococcal sepsis. Am J Dis Child 138:915, 1984

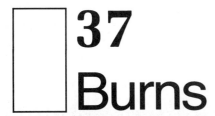

37
Burns

_____ *David P. Meagher, Jr.*

Burn wounds are a common cause of injury, disability, and permanent disfigurement in childhood. No other form of trauma causes such physiologic and psychologic injury because every organ system is affected. Fears about pain, disfigurement, length of hospitalization, cost, quality of future life, and even death arise in the process of dealing with extensive thermal trauma. Even a small burn, managed on an outpatient basis, can result in significant functional impairment if not dealt with appropriately. Burns are second only to automobile accidents as cause of death during childhood. An estimated 1500 to 2500 children die from thermal injury in the United States each year. Over the last 10 to 20 years, changes in treatment protocols, the development of new medications and skin substitutes, and the establishment of burn centers have resulted in tremendous improvements in all forms of burn care.

ETIOLOGY

The majority of thermal injuries in childhood result from an accident in the home. Toddlers are naturally inquisitive and tend to be burned when they pull over a container of hot liquid on themselves. The resultant scald affects the head, face, shoulders, and upper extremities. These often are spotty, deep, partial-thickness wounds. Young children also suffer scalds from immersion in hot water. There is a characteristic distribution of the burn with symmetrical injury to the lower extremities coupled with sparing of the soles or a small area on each buttock.[1] Child abuse should be strongly suspected in these cases (Fig. 37–1). In a recent 5-year review of patients admitted

to our Burn Center, 68 percent were 4 years of age or under, and 64 percent were scalded. Boys are injured by scalding 2 to 2.5 times as often as girls.[2,3] Older children are fascinated by matches and often have easy access to flammable liquids, such as gasoline. These wounds commonly are full thickness in depth, involving much of the body surface area. The majority of fatal burns come from this group of injuries.

In our recent experience, child abuse or parental neglect was suspected in 15 percent of the cases. Similar findings have been noted by others.[4,5] Burned children come disproportionately from economicallly disadvantaged and single-parent families. There is a tendency toward large families having a prior history of stresss.[2] Often, the burned child has been left under the supervision of other young children. A self-inflicted burn may be the result of either preexisting emotional instability or inadequate supervision. Children of all ages may become trapped in a burning room where they are exposed to smoke inhalation or airway burns.

CLASSIFICATION

Burns may be classified by etiology as scald, flame, contact, electrical, or chemical. Further, the severity of a burn is determined by its depth as well as the percentage of body surface involved. Initially, the etiology and the percentage of body surface burned are easily determined, but the depth can only be estimated. Scald burns, in particular, may not declare their actual depth for 5 to 8 days after injury. A partial-thickness burn is one that spares the deeper skin appendages and can heal sponta-

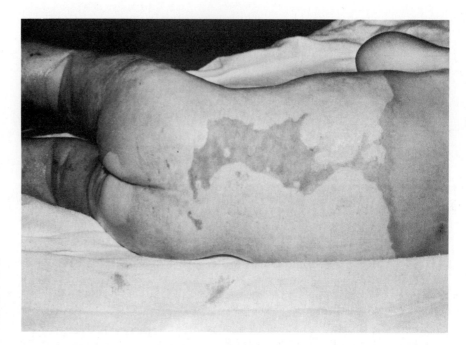

Figure 37–1. Deep partial- and full-thickness burns on a 13-month-old child subjected to nonaccidental trauma. Note the bandlike distribution on the trunk coupled with unburned areas on the buttocks where the skin was in contact with the cooler tub.

neously. Skin grafts may or may not be indicated. A full-thickness burn requires skin grafting for wound closure. These definitions can be compared to the original classification of first-, second-, and third-degree wounds (Fig. 37–2).

A first-degree burn implies a superifical injury of the epidermis, with the basal layers left intact. The skin is red, edematous, and painful. Rapid healing takes place by regeneration of the epithelium from the basal layers, with desquamation of the superficial corneum. The second-degree burn is best subclassified as either a superficial or deep partial-thickness wound. It characteristically involves the epidermis and upper dermis but spares the dermal appendages. There are blistering and erythema of the skin immediately after the burn, but healing usually takes place by regeneration of skin from deeper epidermal cells and dermal appendages. In the case of a deep partial-thickness burn, the epithelium after such healing is thin and unstable. Later, these wounds have a distinct tendency to develop leathery hypertrophic scars. Because of these problems, most burn centers now advise skin grafting or overgrafting the deep partial-thickness burn. We currently define these burns as those that require 14 to 21 days for spontaneous healing. Clinically, it is often very difficult to decide whether a burn is a deep partial-thickness or full-

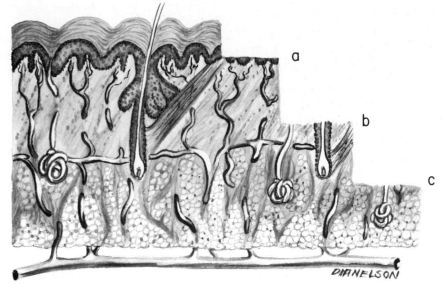

Figure 37–2. A first-degree burn involves only the superficial epithelium, resulting in redness of the skin with an occasional blister. A burn down to **(a)** injures the superficial epithelium and is considered a superficial partial-thickness injury. When the skin is damaged to **(b)**, there is a deep partial-thickness burn. Spontaneous healing frequently results in hypertrophic scarring. Skin grafts frequently are used to improve the ultimate result. A burn down to **(c)** or deeper is a full-thickness injury that requires a skin graft.

thickness injury. This is particularly true of scalds and at the edge of flame burns. The tissue may be bright red or white after the initial blisters are broken.

A full-thickness or third-degree burn is one in which the entire skin has been destroyed. The tissues are dry, charred, or dark brown after a full-thickness flame burn (Fig. 37–3). Thrombosed veins may be seen through the translucent skin and are clearly indicative of the depth of the injury. The full-thickness burn will weep little fluid from its surface and is anesthetic. Although a number of techniques have been described for early determination of the depth of a burn, few have withstood the test of time. Unfortunately, a child's skin is thinner than that of an adult, and a burn that would be partial-thickness in an adult often is full-thickness in a child. Some authorities have added a fourth category of thermal injury. When underlying tendons, muscles, or bone are severely injured, the wound is said to be a fourth-degree burn. These wounds obviously have a significant impact on the survival or future function of the area involved.

Burns are further classified according to the extent of the burn on the body. In order to determine the overall severity of a burn, the age of the child, the location and depth of the burn, and the percent total body surface area (TBSA) involved are considered. Thus, a minor burn involves less than 10 percent of the body surface, is partial-thickness and does not involve the face, hands, perineum, or feet. Also excluded from the minor category are electrical or inhalation injuries. A 10 to 20 percent TBSA burn is considered moderate if less than 10 percent of the total area is full-thickness. Any burn of 20 percent or more TBSA in children is severe, especially if half of the area is full-thickness injury. Any burn in a child under 2 years of age is more serious because of the thin skin and the difficulties in preventing infection and

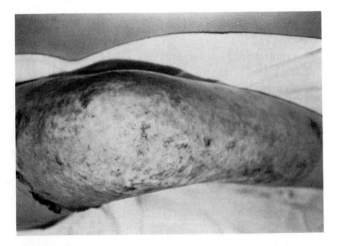

Figure 37–3. A localized full-thickness flame burn on the lower extremity of an 8-year-old boy. Most of the wound is whitish, insensitive, and leathery.

maintaining adequate nutrition. A full-thickness burn of more than 30 percent TBSA is a real threat to life. However, with optimum care in a burn center, survival with 80 to 90 percent burns is not uncommon.

PATHOLOGY OF THE BURN WOUND

Jackson, in 1953, described three concentric zones of significant thermal injury in the burn wound.[6] On contact with thermal or chemical energy, there is immediate coagulation necrosis of the skin's superficial layers. In this zone of coagulation, temperatures exceeding 45C (113F) result in denaturation of protein exceeding the capacity for cellular repair. The depth of tissue damage is determined by the temperature and duration of contact with the source of heat. Beneath the top layer of coagulation necrosis, there is a zone of stasis containing damaged but still viable tissue. There is reduction of capillary blood flow to this zone because of injury to the microcirculation. Prevention of additional injury and dehydration can allow survival of this layer.[7,8] Venous thrombosis leads to infarction in this zone and can convert the wound from a deep partial-thickness burn to one with full-thickness loss.[9] In a deeper zone of hyperemia, there is vasodilatation with the ability of cells to heal within 1 week. Although necrotic tissue may release toxins into the circulation and is the site of immediate red cell hemolysis, it is no longer metabolically active but remains as a culture medium until it is debrided or sloughed. The deeper, viable, injured zones are of greatest importance in the first hours after injury. It is here that appropriate therapy can have an impact on the ultimate result.

With thermal injury, capillary permeability is increased, resulting in free loss of plasma proteins and electrolytes into the extravascular space. This injury to the capillary membrane is such that the colloid oncotic pressure is no longer able to keep plasma proteins within the blood vessels. In extensive partial-thickness burns, about one half of the lost fluid and protein remains in the extravascular tissues, whereas the remainder is lost to evaporation from superficial weeping and blister fluid.[10] In severe burns, these fluid losses take place primarily during the first 12 hours after injury. Furthermore, with the onset of burn shock, there is loss of endothelial vascular integrity in unburned areas, resulting in further exudation of fluid and protein from the vascular space.[11,12] A phase of protein and fluid reabsorption from the injured zones usually commences within 48 hours postinjury.

In the last 20 years, particular attention has been given to the effects of prostaglandins in thermal injury.[13] These studies have revealed markedly increased levels of prostinoids, mainly PGE_2, in burned skin and blister fluid. Attempts at therapeutic manipulation of the zone of stasis with prostinoid inhibitors, however, have been largely unsuccessful. In 1980, thromboxane was isolated from burn blister fluid.[14] Preservation of dermal microcirculation using specific thromboxane synthetase inhibitors, such as dipyridamole and imidazole, has been demonstrated.[15,16] Thromboxane synthetase inhibition reduces platelet adherence and prevents erythrocytes and leukocytes from sticking to the wall of blood vessels. The end result is vasodilatation. Confirmation of similar effects in humans is under investigation. If they are confirmed, specific antithromboxane agents may prevent progressive dermal ischemia and increase the survival of damaged skin. Robson and Heggers have summarized the advances in this area.[17]

Further derangements in the skin's normal function include a loss of regulation of body temperature because of injury to the sweat glands, as well as an increase in evaporative water losses through the wound. In terms of patient survival, the loss of skin as a barrier against bacterial invasion also is important. Not only are the usual bacteriostatic properties of normal skin destroyed, but dead tissue becomes a perfect culture medium for the proliferation of bacteria. For years, it has been thought that the major source of serious burn wound infection was the environment in which the patient was cared for. Elaborate precautions, including strict isolation of major burn patients in laminar flow rooms, have been followed. Support for this environmental concept comes from clinical evaluation of epidemic infections of a single organism within a burn unit. Within the last few years, increased attention has been given to evidence that the patient may be the major source of infection.[18,19] Increasing knowledge of immunology has stimulated interest in failure of local immunity as a potential cause of burn wound sepsis.[20] Deitch and Smith have presented evidence that there is a substance (or substances) present in the blister fluid of burned patients that suppresses the normal lymphocyte response to mitogens.[21] It is not yet known whether this factor is locally produced or generated in the serum.

An extensive thermal injury exerts pathophysiologic responses far beyond the burn wound itself. Evidence in both humans and experimental animals has demonstrated depression in cardiac output in excess of that expected from plasma loss.[22,23] Cross-perfusion studies have shown a similar effect on unburned animals. The hypovolemic state, even when transient, is reflected in diminished urinary output and increases in circulating norepinephrine, cortisol, aldosterone, antidiuretic hormone, and renin angiotensin. The 17-ketosteroid levels remain elevated as long as the burn wound is open. The hypermetabolism associated with burns is associated with heat loss through evaporation of water from the burn wound, as well as through chronic catecholamine stimulation.[24] The tremendous stress reaction of a major burn, unlike the reaction to a single surgical insult, is

prolonged for weeks or months after injury. The patient's endogenous nutritional supplies are rapidly depleted unless sufficient supplemental calories, vitamins, and protein are supplied to meet the increased needs. The metabolic response to the burn wound is in proportion to its severity. Curreri has shown in adults that a dietary program that supplies 25 kcal/kg body weight plus 40 kcal/percent burn can circumvent the effects of the metabolic response.[25] Since 1982, we have preferred to use the Galveston formula advocated by Carvajal et al.[26] The daily caloric requirements of the burned child are as follows:

$$1800 \text{ kcal/m}^2 \text{ body surface area}$$
$$\text{plus}$$
$$2200 \text{ kcal/m}^2 \text{ burn surface area}$$

In our hands, this has proven to be an excellent means of estimating the caloric needs of the burned child.

EVALUATION AND INITIAL MANAGEMENT OF MINOR BURNS

Burns involving less than 10 percent TBSA in children over 1 year of age usually can be managed on an outpatient basis. Exceptions are made for cases involving the face, hands, perineum, or feet.

Except for trivial burns, infants are admitted to the burn center. If there is any question of child abuse or the ability of the family to follow instructions, the child is admitted until social services evaluates the family situation. There is no harm in initiating treatment on an outpatient basis, then later admitting the child for debridement and grafting if necessary. The family should be advised from the outset that a partial-thickness burn may be deep enough to require surgical intervention.

After initial assessment of the child, the burn, and the family, the child is medicated with a narcotic analgesic as long as the vital signs are stable. The burn and surrounding skin are gently washed with dilute povidone-iodine (Betadine) soap or sodium hypochlorite (Chlorox) solution. Subsequent wound care is administered avoiding the use of povidone-iodine in order to limit excessive iodine absorption. Sterile gloves are worn whenever touching the wound. Currently, we advise the debridement of all blisters at the time of initial evaluation. Though somewhat controversial, this advice is based on experimental data mentioned earlier as well as on the need for a clean, moist surface to which a biosynthetic dressing can be applied.[14–17,21] After debridement, an assessment of the wound is made. If the surface is moist and light pink in color, the wound probably is superficial to mid-partial-thickness in depth. For the past several years we have used Biobrane biosynthetic dressing on these wounds with significant success (Fig. 37–4). The material must be applied in complete contact with the wound using a gentle stretch. There should be ample

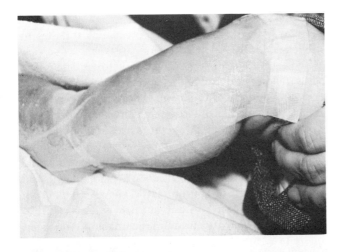

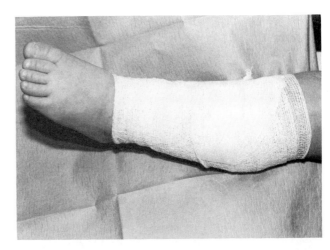

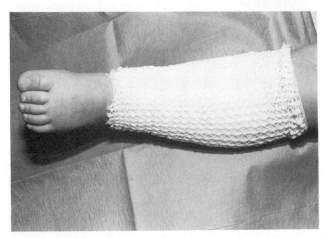

Figure 37–4. Dressing technique for outpatient scald burns. **Top left.** Thin porous Biobrane is stretched to cover the debrided moist burn. The biosynthetic is held in place with adhesive strips. **Top right.** Gauze bandages are applied to help hold the Biobrane in contact with the wound and absorb exudate. **Left.** Elastic mesh is used to secure the gauze.

overlap on the surrounding unburned skin to allow the Biobrane to be secured with adhesive strips. A bulky gauze dressing is then applied and covered with an elastic mesh. The wound is reexamined 36 to 48 hours later. If the biosynthetic has adhered, it can be either left open or protected with a few layers of gauze. The burn is then inspected every 3 to 5 days until healed. The wound becomes pain-free within 12 hours after application of the biosynthetic. Should the Biobrane fail to adhere, a new piece can be applied if the wound remains clean and moist. Biobrane should *not* be applied over eschar. If at any point eschar is present, silver sulfadiazine cream on fine mesh gauze is used, then covered with a layer of absorbent gauze. Should the burn fail to heal by 14 days postinjury, indicating a deep partial-thickness wound, consideration can be given to admission for application of split-thickness skin grafts.

EVALUATION AND INITIAL MANAGEMENT OF SEVERE BURNS

Treatment of the severely burned child begins with an evaluation of the airway, circulation, and burn wound on admission to the emergency room or burn center.

In addition to the usual equipment for airway management and resuscitation, sterile sheets should be available to cover the child. Treatment must be carried out in a warm room where there is minimal traffic and where all personnel are masked and wearing sterile gowns.

Burns of the Airway

The mouth, nose, and pharynx may be burned by hot gases or actual flames. Fortunately, direct inhalation rarely causes damage to the trachea or lungs because of reflex laryngeal spasm. These patients may be cyanotic and apneic at the scene of the accident, often requiring resuscitation by firemen. The direct thermal injury is obvious because of facial edema and singed nasal hairs. Prophylactic nasotracheal intubation to forestall acute upper airway obstruction is indicated in any patient with significant facial burns (Fig. 37–5). Most patients with inhalation injury do not wheeze or produce carbonaceous sputum for 24 to 48 hours after injury.[27] The endotracheal tube usually can be removed within 48 hours after the edema has subsided. Tracheostomy is now rarely indicated in the care of the acute burn. Humidification and supplemental oxygen therapy are provided to any patient suspected of having an inhalation injury whether intubation is necessary or not.

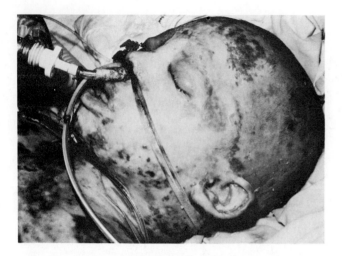

Figure 37–5. This 7-year-old boy sustained massive flame burns to 96 percent of his body. Prompt nasotracheal intubation, fluid resuscitation, and treatment of his inhalation injury allowed him to survive, permitting subsequent wound coverage using autologous cultured epithelium at another institution.[83] Note the use of umbilical tape in securing the tubes.

Children trapped in a closed space not only are subjected to direct thermal injury but also are at risk for developing carbon monoxide poisoning as well as pulmonary injury due to inhalation of chemicals in smoke. The type of gases produced in a fire depends on the material being burned, the temperature of the fire, and the amount of oxygen present. Burning plastics cause particularly severe pulmonary damage. The polyvinyl-

chloride used in plastics decomposes to yield high temperatures, thick smoke, and high concentrations of hydrogen chloride gas.[28] In many cases, smoke particles are coated with irritating aldehydes, ketones, and organic acids. The majority of these particles are large and are deposited in the upper airway, where mucosal irritation occurs, with the risk of subsequent airway compromise.[29] Volatile gases, as well as chemicals adsorbed onto particles, may gain entry into the lower respiratory tract where, within minutes, cilia cease functioning, resulting in impaired mucous clearance.[30] Chemotactic substances, such as histamine, are then released. Oxides of nitrogen and sulfur as well as phosgene gas can result in severe injury, the clinical appearance of which may be delayed for hours.

There are no good early criteria for diagnosis of a pulmonary burn. Wheezing with respiratory distress may not become obvious for 24 to 48 hours. Early x-ray changes consist only of a fine infiltrate or hyperinflation (Fig. 37–6). Unfortunately, respiratory complications have emerged as the dominant killer of patients with major thermal injury. In a review of patients over 15 years of age, Herndon et al. found that 21 percent of all patients and 61 percent of patients who died had an inhalation injury.[31] In younger children, the incidence of inhalation injury is much lower, but the mortality remains high. In a series of 500 patients 14 years of age or younger, there was a 6 percent incidence of inhalation injury with a 40 percent mortality.[30] In our own experience over the past 5 years, the incidence of significant pulmonary injury has been 2.5 percent with a 12

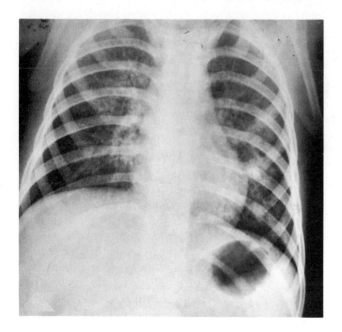
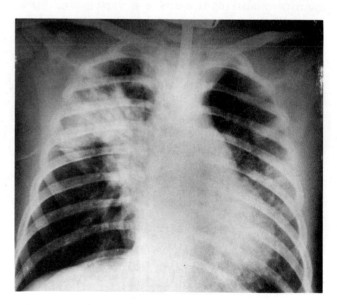

Figure 37–6. Left. A chest x-ray immediately after this inhalation injury revealed only minimal infiltrates. **Right.** The same patient 24 hours later, with consolidation in both lung fields and such severe respiratory distress that a tracheostomy was necessary. Tracheostomy currently is rarely indicated in the treatment of pulmonary burns.

percent mortality. Techniques for earlier diagnosis of lower airway damage include xenon lung scanning and fiberoptic bronchoscopy.[32,33] The first stage of inhalation injury is acute pulmonary insufficiency, the second is pulmonary edema, and the last is bronchopneumonia.[34]

Carbon monoxide poisoning is suggested by cherry-red skin and is confirmed by finding a minimum of 20 percent carboxyhemoglobin in the blood.[35] The clinical effects of carbon monoxide are secondary to the combination of carbon monoxide with hemoglobin, the displacement of oxygen, and the interruption of the oxygen transport system. Carbon monoxide also shifts the oxyhemoglobin curve to the left, increasing the affinity of oxygen for hemoglobin and, thereby, further reducing oxygen delivery to the tissues. Symptoms rarely develop until the carboxyhemoglobin is greater than 10 percent. Early symptoms include headache, fatigue, weakness, nausea, vomiting, and impaired judgment. With higher levels, tachycardia and hyperventilation lead to seizures and coma. Levels greater than 60 percent usually are fatal.[29] The mainstay of treatment remains supplemental oxygen (100 percent F_iO_2).

Smoke inhalation can produce a variety of findings, ranging from congestion and edema of the mucosa to complete necrosis and sloughing of the respiratory epithelium. Deep to the mucosa there is peribronchiolar and perivascular edema. This elevation of extravascular lung water appears to be directly related to the toxic effect of smoke inhalation and not to the burn itself.[36] The edema fluid weeps into the bronchi and, together with sloughed epithelial cells, results in bronchial obstruction. Initial treatment of any child suspected of having an airway burn consists of supplemental humidified oxygen, postural drainage, and endotracheal suction. Moylan and Chan, in a double-blind prospective study, demonstrated a fourfold greater mortality for inhalation injury treated with steroids when compared to controls with comparable injury treated without steroids.[37] Perhaps of greatest importance to the survival of a patient with inhalation injury is the markedly decreased pulmonary compliance. This has been demonstrated in both animals and humans.[31,38]

Resuscitation

After evaluation of the airway, the child's clothing is completely removed, and he or she is placed on sterile sheets. IV access is established expeditiously; with massive burns, a central venous line may be of great benefit in fluid management. If necessary, these lines may be established through burned tissue as long as they are removed as soon as practical. Blood is drawn for complete blood count, electrolytes, urea nitrogen, total protein, and albumin levels. Patients with very large burns may need a typing and crossmatching of blood shortly after arrival. A throat culture for Group A streptococci is obtained. In the Denver area, streptococcal infection is endemic, so we administer prophylactic penicillin until the culture is negative. Fluid resuscitation is instituted with an initial bolus of 20 ml/kg of Ringer's lactate. An accurate baseline body weight and height are quickly obtained for use in subsequent calculations. In burns of 20 percent TBSA or greater, a Silastic Foley catheter is inserted for urinary monitoring. A nasogastric tube is passed to prevent the gastric dilatation frequently seen with major burns. Tetanus prophylaxis is given if indicated.

Using a modified Lund-Browder diagram, the percentage of body surface area burned is estimated and drawn on the diagram (Fig. 37–7). This diagram illustrates the changes in relative body surface area in children of different ages. Because the head is larger and the lower extremities smaller in children than in adults, the standard rule of nines can misrepresent the magnitude of the injury. If they are defined, relative areas of partial- and full-thickness burns are drawn, and the diagram is then placed in the child's hospital record.

Burn shock has been recognized and treated for almost 40 years by a variety of fluids and recipes. Accurate observations of urinary output, pulse rate, sensorium, and hematocrit have been used to assess therapy. Cope and Moore, in 1947, first popularized a surface area formula for burn resuscitation and proposed that fluids be given in relationship to the size of the burn.[39] The formula of Evans et al., which uses 1 ml each of plasma and isotonic saline per kilogram per percent body surface area burned, was formulated because the losses into the burn wound consist primarily of plasma and extracellular fluid.[40] In addition to plasma and saline calculated on the basis of burned area, the child's maintenance fluids were given as well. A maximum of 50 percent burn surface area was used. One half of the first day's requirement was given during the first 8 hours postburn, with the other half being given over the remaining 16 hours. This formula has been used in some institutions for years with success. However, in a review of 100 patients treated with the Evans formula, Hutcher and Haynes noted that the predicted quantities of fluid fell short by as much as 50 to 100 percent in children weighing less than 20 kg.[41] The Brooke army formula was similar in volume of fluid but cut the amount of colloid by one half.[42] The maximum burn size and maintenance fluids were unchanged. Although some clinicians continued to prefer resuscitation using plasma and blood, Baxter and Shires demonstrated that patients with extensive burns responded well to electrolyte solutions without colloid.[43,44] Moncrief concluded that since the capillary membrane is permeable to protein as well as electrolytes and water, colloid solutions given during the first 24 postburn hours would leak out into the tissue.[45] Based on research such as this, the modified Brooke and Park-

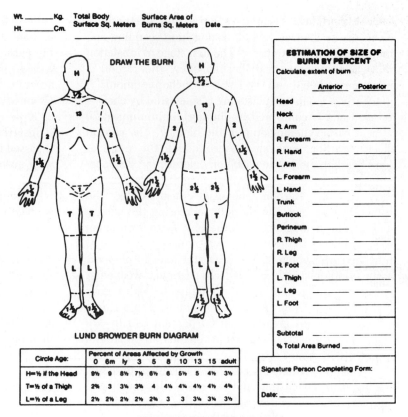

Wt. _____ Kg.   Total Body   Surface Area of
Ht. _____ Cm.   Surface Sq. Meters   Burns Sq. Meters   Date _____

DRAW THE BURN

LUND BROWDER BURN DIAGRAM

Circle Age:	Percent of Areas Affected by Growth								
	0	6m	1y	3	5	8	10	13	15	adult
H=½ if the Head	9½	9	8½	7½	6½	6	5½	5	4½	3½
T=½ of a Thigh	2¾	3	3¼	3½	4	4¼	4½	4½	4½	4¾
L=½ of a Leg	2½	2½	2½	2¾	2¾	3	3	3¼	3¼	3½

ESTIMATION OF SIZE OF BURN BY PERCENT

Calculate extent of burn

	Anterior	Posterior
Head		
Neck		
R. Arm		
R. Forearm		
R. Hand		
L. Arm		
L. Forearm		
L. Hand		
Trunk		
Buttock		
Perineum		
R. Thigh		
R. Leg		
R. Foot		
L. Thigh		
L. Leg		
L. Foot		
Subtotal		
% Total Area Burned		

Signature Person Completing Form:

Date: _____

Figure 37–7. Body surface area in infants and older children.

LUND-BROWDER BURN DIAGRAM

land formulas have become very popular throughout the world.[44,46] These entirely crystalloid formulas mandate the administration of 3 and 4 ml/kg per percent body surface area burned during the first 24 hours, respectively. Administration of supplemental protein is not considered until the second day postburn.

The use of colloid for burn resuscitation in the form of blood, plasma, or albumin has been advocated by some for years. The main objection has been the increase in vascular permeability postburn, with subsequent extravasation of protein into the interstitial space.[45] Carvajal et al., using radioiodinated serum albumin in a rat model, have shown that effective transcapillary sieving of albumin molecules into burned skin essentially stops by 8 hours postinjury.[47] In further studies using a more extensive scald burn model requiring fluid resuscitation, Carvajal et al. showed that edema in the burned tissue was greatest at 3 hours postburn.[48] Neither albumin extravasation nor water accumulation was seen in the unburned tissue. These same investigators have demonstrated a minimal effect of burn depth on the microvascular sieving of albumin.[49] Burn edema developed rapidly and with equal severity in superficial as well as deeper burns.

Burn resuscitation based on the use of hypertonic lactated saline has been popularized by Monafo et al.[50,51]

Proponents of this form of resuscitation claim that the volume of fluid required for resuscitation is less, that sustained hypernatremia with consequent increase in serum osmolality develops, that the sodium load counteracts the effect of antidiuretic hormone, and that hypertonic saline is more cost effective.[52,53] Little mention is made that patients resuscitated using hypertonic saline are quite thirsty and, when allowed to take unlimited fluids orally, tend to convert their resuscitation to a more isotonic one. Carvajal recently has compared, in a thorough fashion, resuscitation with hypertonic lactated saline to more conventional techniques on both theoretical and practical grounds and found no therapeutic advantage of the former for the burned child.[54]

In our experience, pediatric burn patients having greater than 30 percent TBSA injuries are more easily resuscitated with fewer complications with the early use of colloid. A major problem with adult burn formulas is that the child's maintenance fluid requirements are not directly proportional to the weight of the child. The estimate of burn-related losses is determined primarily by the extent of tissue injury and not the child's weight.[55] Thus, most adult formulas tend to underhydrate the small child or the child with a small burn and overhydrate the older child with extensive burns. For the last 7 years we have used successfully the Ringer's lactate–colloid

(Galveston) formula first proposed by Carvajal in 1975.[56,57] The total fluid requirements for the first day are estimated as follows:

$$2000 \text{ ml/m}^2 \text{ body surface area}$$
$$\text{plus}$$
$$5000 \text{ ml/m}^2 \text{ burn surface area}$$

One half of the calculated fluid volume is administered during the first 8 hours postburn, with the remainder given over the following 16 hours. We begin resuscitation using Ringer's lactate to which is added 12.5 g of 25 percent albumin (50 ml) at 4 to 6 hours postinjury. Initially, we avoid supplemental dextrose because of the reactive hyperglycemia related to stress. The child's Dextrostix is followed closely, and at the first sign of a drop, 5 percent dextrose is added to the fluid infusion. This usually occurs between 12 and 24 hours postburn. In the practical management of the burned patient, it must be recalled that none of the formulas are entirely accurate for each situation. Unusual losses may result in an increased need for fluid.

Circumferential burns of an extremity or the thorax present another hazard. Eschar can have the consistency of leather and become unyielding to the underlying edema. This is most commonly seen with flame burns but also can come into play with electrical and scald burns. The effect is the same as that of a skintight cast over a swollen fracture. Venous obstruction results in further edema and potential loss of distal circulation. This situation in the thorax can significantly restrict movement and thereby effect respiration. Longitudinal incisions should be made through the eschar down to viable tissue. The eschar separates, resulting in prompt restoration of circulation (Fig. 37–8). Escharotomies also may be necessary on the dorsum of the hands and feet as well as on each digit. Incisions on the chest should be longitudinal, starting at each midaxillary line. A transverse incision across the junction of the chest and abdomen helps provide further relief. Because the areas are anesthetic, these procedures can be performed at the bedside. Blood for possible transfusion should be available, since blood loss occasionally is significant. The incisions are dressed using silver sulfadiazine cream as on the remainder of the burns.

The initial care of a burned child can be summarized as follows:

1. Evaluate airway—intubate if indicated.
2. Draw blood for CBC, electrolytes, BUN, Dextrostix, total protein, and albumin levels—type and crossmatch if necessary.
3. Insert IV line and infuse Ringer's lactate—calculate first day's fluid needs per Galveston formula after height, weight, and body surface area are available.
4. Insert Silastic Foley catheter if greater than 20 percent TBSA burned or there are genital burns present.
5. Insert nasogastric tube for major burn.
6. Give tetanus prophylaxis as indicated.
7. Obtain throat culture—start penicillin if streptococcol infections are endemic to the region (discontinue if culture negative).
8. Before tubbing or wound debridement, administer morphine sulfate intravenously if vital signs are stable.
9. Begin an intensive care flow sheet.

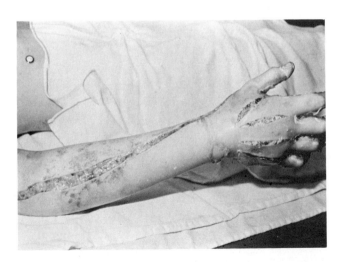 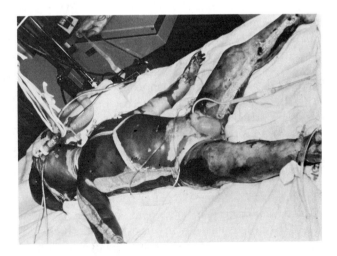

Figure 37–8. Left. In the case of full-thickness extremity burns, escharotomies frequently are required to preserve circulation distally. **Right.** In the case of major burns, full-thickness wounds on the thorax can result in marked ventilatory restriction. Note the placement of escharotomies and the separation of eschar achieved.

TREATMENT OF THE BURN WOUND

The principles of burn wound therapy are simple yet somewhat difficult to achieve. Since many partial-thickness burns will heal spontaneously, the wound must be protected from mechanical trauma and bacterial contamination. On the other hand, the eschar of a deep partial- or full-thickness burn must be not only protected from bacterial invasion but also excised so that the wound can be closed with skin grafts. Before the era of topical antimicrobials, burns were dressed with moist, bulky dressings. With these techniques, about one fourth of the wounds would heal within 2 weeks postinjury. The occlusive dressing technique was associated with a high incidence of wound infection and sepsis during the second and third postburn weeks. Topical therapy with 0.5 percent silver nitrate in bulky wet dressings significantly reduced the incidence of burn wound sepsis.[58] Although silver nitrate is still used in some centers, this solution is messy and hypoosmolar. It leaches out sodium, chloride, and potassium ions and may cause water toxicity. Hyponatremia can develop very rapidly, particularly in infants with extensive burns. Supplemental electrolyte therapy frequently is required, with careful monitoring of serum and urinary sodium and potassium levels.

Mafenide acetate (Sulfamylon) was the next topical antimicrobial to be introduced. This is the only topical agent that has definitely been shown to diffuse rapidly through full-thickness eschar to the burn wound–blood interface.[59] For maximum benefit, it should be reapplied every 12 hours. Unfortunately, mafenide is a potent carbonic anhydrase inhibitor that impairs the renal tubular buffering mechanism, which can result in severe metabolic acidosis.[60] The severity of this problem is related to the surface area being treated. Patients with respiratory insufficiency, including inhalation injury, should be monitored closely. When less than 20 percent TBSA is treated for a brief period, the drug is relatively safe. We have found it to be particularly useful on burned ears and localized areas of burn wound infection.

Silver sulfadiazine, synthesized by Fox by substituting silver for the ionized sulfonamide hydrogen of sulfadiazine, is effective against *Pseudomonas, Staphylococcus aureus,* and a variety of other organisms that colonize burn wounds.[61] This agent currently is the most widely used topical antimicrobial drug. Transient leukopenia sometimes is seen a few days after beginning treatment. Whether this is a primary effect of the burn or a complication of the drug is unclear. In our experience, the white blood cell count usually will return to normal despite the continued use of silver sulfadiazine. In children, the use of a closed dressing technique is preferable. Silver sulfadiazine can be applied directly from a jar onto fine mesh gauze. This gauze is then placed on the

burn wound in a single layer and covered with absorbent dressing held in place by stretchable net. Except in unusual circumstances, the dressings are changed daily. At the time of the daily dressing change, the child is placed in a hydrotherapy tub. A sample of the bath water can then be obtained and submitted to the microbiology laboratory for identification and quantification of the bacteria present. This allows us to monitor the predominant wound flora and helps anticipate potential burn wound sepsis. The bath water culture is routinely done every 2 to 3 days when treating a major burn. Sodium hypochlorite solution is added to the bath water, resulting in a final dilution of 1:120. If evidence of infection is present, the concentration can be doubled to 1:60.

Other topical agents, such as nitrofurazone (Furacin), povidone-iodine, gentamicin, and cerium nitrate, have been advocated in the past. Each has advantages and disadvantages, but none has withstood the test of time. All of the topical antimicrobials will, when properly used, decrease the incidence of bacterial invasion of the wound and subsequent sepsis. Unfortunately, these agents delay the separation of eschar and, if relied on exclusively for wound management, will delay the ultimate closure of full-thickness injuries. Consequently, there has been a return to earlier surgical debridement of wounds. Primary excision and grafting of small, deep, nonlife-threatening burns during the first few postburn days is a highly acceptable and desirable practice (Fig. 37–9). Such areas as hands, where early skin coverage leads to improved function, are particularly suitable for early excision and grafting.[62,63]

Surgical procedures for excision of the burn wound basically fall into three categories, namely, tangential

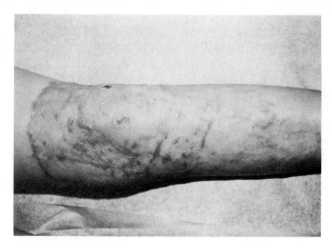

Figure 37–9. The localized full-thickness burn illustrated in Figure 37–3 underwent tangential debridement with application of a minimally expanded meshed autograft within 24 hours of admission to the burn center. The child was discharged 1 day later. The appearance is acceptable at 4 months postburn.

excision, tangential debridement, or excision to fascia. The concept of tangential excision was first described by Janzekovic in 1970 and further refined by Jackson and Stone in 1972 in classic articles.[64,65] With this procedure, the burn wound is excised down to healthy appearing deep dermal tissue, which is classically covered immediately with split-thickness autograft. The procedure usually is carried out within the first week postburn, before bacterial colonizaton of the eschar. Failure to cover the wound bed immediately with skin graft or a physiologic biosynthetic covering will result in desiccation of the wound, with further necrosis and loss of the remaining dermal elements. This technique has decreased hypertrophic scarring, achieved earlier wound healing, and shortened hospital stays.[66] Disadvantages include increased operative blood loss and need for considerable experience for successful use of the technique.

Tangential debridement is used in the care of full-thickness wounds. The eschar is sharply excised until viable subcutaneous tissue is exposed. At this point, the wound can be covered with skin grafts as available or, alternatively, xenograft, homograft, or a biosynthetic dressing. This probably is the most common surgical technique in use today. Following excision, the wound must be inspected frequently and not allowed to desiccate. The application of a temporary wound covering, such as pigskin or Biobrane, provides an excellent test of the recipient bed vis-a-vis future acceptance of autograft. The major advantage of this technique is preservation of subcutaneous tissue, allowing retention of normal body contours.

Excision to fascia can be used in the care of the massively burned child (>60 percent TBSA), burn wound sepsis, and localized full-thickness wounds. In the last case, excision can be used to accelerate wound closure but, in our experience, is rarely indicated because of the poor cosmetic result. Burn wound sepsis is defined as bacteria exceeding 10^5 organisms per gram of burned tissue, with active invasion of underlying unburned tissue. Parks et al. have demonstrated a definite role for aggressive excision of the burn wound in the control of established burn wound sepsis in children.[67] Their mortality rate of 14 percent represents a significant improval in survival. A major factor in the survival of children with massive thermal injury appears to be early aggressive excision of eschar with wound closure using autograft or biosynthetics. Massive early excision of the burn wound to fascia within 72 hours of admission, followed by coverage using cadaver allograft, has been compared to serial debridement and grafting.[68] There was no significant difference in survival noted. It was postulated that long-term morbidity would be greater in the group excised to fascia. The same authors now believe that application of this early aggressive approach may not be appropriate in the care of scald burns.[69] We concur with this

assessment. Currently, we reserve the technique of excision to fascia for cases of established burn wound sepsis. In our hands, massive thermal burns in children are best handled by early serial tangential excision with autografting as available.

Over the last 5 years, improved survival in adult and pediatric victims of major thermal injury has been documented.[70] Much of this improvement appears to be related to increasing emphasis on early excision of the burn wound.[71,72] There remains controversy on exactly how early is early enough, but most agree that excision of the wound should begin within 1 week postinjury. These impressive results with major burns can be further confirmed by the experience of our burn center over the last 8 years. The overall mortality for burns greater than 50 percent TBSA was 6.3 percent. The single death occurred in 1983 in a child burned over 100 percent of his body. For burns greater than 80 percent TBSA, the mortality was 17 percent. In general, this reflects our attention to prompt excision of the burn wound, coupled with aggressive nutritional support starting within 48 hours postinjury. Within the past 2 years, Herndon et al. have shown that the primary early determinants of survival in children with massive thermal injury are no longer the size and severity of the burn wound.[73] The presence of preadmission shock and inhalation injury were the primary factors determining mortality. Multiple organ failure usually related to sepsis remain the primary late determinants of mortality.

Wound Coverage

Burns of less than 20 percent TBSA usually can be grafted completely with the patient's own skin in one operative procedure. We attempt to graft the face, hands, and areas of functional significance with sheets of skin unless the child is massively burned. In that case, the idea is to cover as much as possible using mesh autograft. Smaller burns also can be grafted with either sheet graft or unexpanded meshed skin. The thighs and buttocks are our first choice for donor sites. Currently, our dermatome of choice is the Padgett electric instrument, although on occasion, we still use the air-driven Brown dermatome. For harvesting sheet grafts of uniform thickness, the Reese drum dermatome has distinct advantages. The depth of graft harvested varies with the age of the patient as well as donor and recipient sites. In general, we use grafts varying from 0.008 to 0.012 inch in thickness. In the case of massive burns where the same donor sites may need to be reharvested up to 10 times, we use grafts of 0.005 to 0.006 inch.

The Meshgraft dermatome allows one to cut slits into a strip of skin up to 3 inches wide, allowing expansion ratios from 1.5:1 to 12:1. In practice, we routinely use 1.5:1 except for the massively burned child, where 3:1 expansion is more practical. In our climate, expansion greater than 3:1 results in frequent desiccation of the wound as well as a worse functional and cosmetic result. An advantage of the mesh graft is the ease with which it can be applied to irregular surfaces. Mesh grafting is also preferable when skin is applied immediately after excision. The improved drainage via the interstices allows better take of the skin on graft beds that would be unsuitable for sheet grafts. Mesh grafting is one of the most important factors in the survival of children with massive burns.

The successful take of a skin graft requires that the recipient site be free from gross infection and necrotic tissue and that it have an adequate blood supply. The graft must be protected from shearing forces by immobilization for 4 to 5 days. With larger burns, it is advantageous to have enough surgical personnel to allow the simultaneous harvesting and application of skin grafts. The tendency of sheet grafts to curl is overcome by stabilizing the skin at its center, then rubbing toward the edge with the back of a tissue forceps. On the face and other delicate areas, the graft is sutured in place with 5–0 chromic sutures, grafts in other areas are secured using surgical staples. Donor sites are covered with either Biobrane, Xeroform, or Scarlet Red after hemostasis has been obtained. When used properly, we have found the biosynthetic to have distinct advantages. At the end of the procedure, the grafts are covered with Neosporin ointment on Adaptic, followed by gauze bandages and elastic net dressing. The donor sites are covered with an absorbent gauze, such as Kerlix. Grafted extremities are immobilized in plaster casts, which along with the gauze dressings, help prevent desiccation in a semi-arid climate. The interstices of the mesh usually will fill in within 1 week if desiccation and infection are prevented. For uninfected wounds, prophylactic cephalosporin is administered for one dose preoperatively and 48 hours postoperatively. Support for antibiotic prophylaxis has been provided by Alexander et al.[74]

Wound Dressings

Homograft and Amnion.
Skin grafts taken from cadavers have been used to cover burn wounds for many years. Homograft skin is the proverbial gold standard to which all other wound dressings are compared.[75] Ideally, skin is harvested from a cadaver within 18 hours of death in the morgue or operating room under aseptic conditions. The skin is taken at a depth of 0.012 to 0.015 inch thickness. It is then stored in a balanced salt solution containing human plasma and an aminoglycoside antibiotic. When stored at 4C, the viability can be routinely maintained for 14 days and occasionally for up to 30 days. Modern skin banks can further cryopreserve cadaveric skin with storage at −196C for an indefinite period. The homograft must be ABO-matched with the recipient.

The prime indication for cadaveric homograft is as a temporary physiologic skin substitute for massively burned patients with large areas of full-thickness loss until autografts are available for wound coverage. Homograft skin can be maintained on the burn wound for prolonged periods of time, probably secondary to the natural immunosuppression of the burned patient.[76] The major disadvantages to the routine use of homograft are limited supply, the need for specialized skin banks to process and store the product, the relatively high cost ($300 to $600 per square foot), and potential transmission of disease. Anecdotal reports of the transmission of acquired immune deficiency syndrome (AIDS) by homograft skin brings its further usage into question.

The use of amnion as a skin substitute was first suggested in 1910. The techniques of its preparation and clinical use have been described by Thomson and Parks.[77] It was found in this study to be a cost-effective biologic dressing for immediate placement on superficial partial-thickness burns. An additional use includes application as a temporary dressing on excised wounds before autografting. In a series of pediatric patients having both partial- and full-thickness burns, Walker et al. found that the amnion-treated group was more comfortable and more mobile, required fewer dressing changes, and had a shorter hospital stay.[78] We have no experience with this biologic dressing, having found that many of these same advantages are available off the shelf in a biosynthetic product.

Xenograft and Biosynthetics.
Pigskin xenograft, when used on fully debrided uncontaminated wounds, will adhere to the wound surface, reduce bacterial colony counts, limit fluid and protein loss, reduce pain, and increase the rate of epithelialization.[69] Pigskin is commercially available in frozen or lyophilized forms. A product impregnated with silver nitrate for help in controlling bacterial colonization has been introduced. When pigskin is allowed to adhere to a partial-thickness wound, there is proliferation and spread of epithelial cells under the biologic dressing. Once keratinization has occurred, the pigskin detaches, leaving a healed epidermal layer.[69] After application, the wound must be protected from shear forces and inspected frequently for infection. Pigskin also can be applied as a protective barrier on granulating and excised wounds.

A number of synthetic and biosynthetic products have been developed and recommended for use on the burn wound (e.g., Opsite, Epi-Lock, and Biobrane). We have had extensive experience with Biobrane over the last 6 years. It has been found to be particularly useful on superficial and middepth partial-thickness wounds, donor sites, clean granulating, and fully excised full-thickness burns. A secondary, though less cost-effective, use is as a protective covering for mesh autografts. Con-

TABLE 37–1. MAJOR CLINICAL BENEFITS OF BIOBRANE

Pain reduction

Reduced dressing changes

Flexible dressing allows joint movement and promotes ambulation

Can observe wound healing through Biobrane or detect purulence
  if present

comitant use of topical antimicrobials has not been necessary in the case of partial-thickness burns.[79] Biobrane is a bilaminate biosynthetic dressing consisting of a thin flexible silicon membrane bonded to a layer of nylon fabric mesh. Both layers are coated with a layer of type I porcine collagen, which stimulates fibrin ingrowth. Water vapor transmission is only slightly higher than that of normal skin. The elasticity and flexibility allow excellent conformance to the wound. The translucent nature allows inspection of the wound (Table 37–1). The product is now available in multiple forms, each having its own advantages and indications. A multicenter study has shown that Biobrane is as effective as frozen human cadaver homograft for temporary coverage of freshly excised full-thickness burn wounds before autografting.[80]

PERMANENT SKIN REPLACEMENT: THE FUTURE OF BURN CARE

Ultimately, the ideal burn wound covering will be a biosynthetic material that is immediately available and that, when placed on an excised burn wound, will be incorporated rapidly and permanently replace the basic functions of skin.[81] Remensnyder has provided us with a composite list of desirable characteristics of a permanent skin substitute (Table 37–2).[81] In the last 5 to 10 years,

TABLE 37–2. DESIRABLE CHARACTERISTICS OF A PERMANENT SKIN SUBSTITUTE

Rapid adherence

Appropriate water vapor transfer

Intact bacterial barrier

Nonantigenic

Nontoxic

Hemostatic

Bacterial suppressant

Encourages fibrous ingrowth and bond

Flexible and elastic

Durable

Ease of handling

No wound contraction

Compatible surface change

Low cost

Long shelf life

(Data from *Remensnyder*.[81])

considerable progress has been made toward recognizing this goal. The artificial skin of Burke and Yannas is a bilaminate consisting of a collagen matrix bound to a thin silicone membrane, which serves as a vapor and bacterial barrier. Host tissue uses the collagen matrix as a scaffolding in which a neodermis is made. When this process is complete, the silicone layer is removed, and thin autografts are applied to the surface. This forms an epidermal layer. The details of development, as well as the results of early clinical trials, were provided by Burke in his Presidential Address to the American Burn Association in 1982.[82] Commercial production of this product will soon begin.

In recent years, following the pioneering research of Green, Gallico et al. have grown sheets of cultured epidermal cells rapidly and began to evaluate their clinical application.[83] The current status of this work as well as the background of its development have been presented by these researchers.[84] The future of this technique, particularly if it can be coupled with a neodermis, such as that developed by Burke, looks very promising. The use of cultured allogeneic epidermis has been evaluated on partial- and full-thickness wounds.[85] Successful application on partial-thickness wounds was noted, but the cells failed to grow well on full-thickness wounds. The success of this technique is based on the fact that epidermal cells apparently fail to stimulate a rejection response in the host. This system, if perfected, has obvious advantages over the autologous techniques. Particularly if a neodermal product can be combined with the allogeneic cells, the potential for a readily available permanent skin replacement exists.

SUMMARY OF BURN WOUND CARE

Rapid advances have been made in burn wound care since the introduction of effective topical antimicrobial agents. It is difficult to know whether the excellent results obtained with a particular agent or technique are the result of the method itself or the enthusiasm with which it is applied. In our experience, topical silver sulfadiazine is superior to other antimicrobials. It is well tolerated by patients and has greatly reduced the risk of burn wound sepsis. We prefer early surgical excision and grafting for deep burns small enough to be covered by the child's own skin. If complete coverage is not feasible because of the size of the burn, the eschar is surgically debrided and Biobrane is applied until adequate autografts are available. Deep partial-thickness wounds should be covered with thin autografts to improve both the functional and cosmetic results. Much of this overgraft may slough with time, leaving a better result underneath. Waiting for good granulation tissue is no longer acceptable. The wound should be closed with autograft or biosynthetic as soon as it is free from necrotic tissue.

Nutrition

In the total care of the burned child, nothing is more important than maintaining adequate nutrition. This can be difficult when the child initially has a paralytic ileus and is then depressed, in constant pain, and subjected to frequent operative procedures. As long as the burn wound is open, the degree of catabolism in a major thermal injury (>50 percent TBSA) may demonstrate resting metabolic rates that can reach twice basal levels. The child frequently develops and maintains a temperature 1 to 2C above normal. This represents an upward set of the thermoregulatory mechanism in the brain. The hypermetabolism appears to be a generalized systemic response involving the entire body.[86] Without intensive nutritional support, in addition to what the child will eat, there can be excessive weight loss, increased risk of infection, wound conversion to full-thickness, and loss of skin grafts.

The impressions of nurses and parents are not sufficient in evaluating the burned child's caloric intake. The statement "He took his lunch well" is meaningless. An accurate daily calorie count with a determination of protein intake is essential. Each of our burn patients undergoes a nutritional evaluation by the burn team nutritionist. For burns of 15 percent TBSA or greater, a soft Silastic catheter is passed via the nose into the stomach shortly after admission. Enteric feedings usually can be instituted in even massive burns within 48 hours. For smaller wounds, feedings are begun within 24 hours. After calculation of caloric goals using the Galveston formula, feedings are begun using cow's milk (20 kcal/ounce). This provides a palatable, well-tolerated formula having the recommended 20 percent of the calories as protein. The volume is advanced as tolerated over 24 to 48 hours. For children less than 1 year of age, one of the standard infant formulas is used. In order to boost the protein content from 9 to 11 percent to the desired level, a modular protein supplement can be added when dealing with larger burns. The child is allowed to take a high-calorie high-protein diet ad libitum when ready.

In addition to the milk feedings, vitamin supplements containing trace metals are provided in near physiologic doses. Children with massive burns occasionally will require increased supplementation. Research into the normal daily requirements, as well as the effect of excessive supplements, has provided somewhat conflicting data. Until further data are available about vitamin and mineral supplements in the burned child, supplementation should not greatly exceed the established guidelines for healthy children, unless a deficiency has been documented.[87]

We attempt to minimize the length of time burned children are npo before operative procedures. Solid food is withheld for the usual interval while milk feedings are continued until 3 to 4 hours preoperatively. With care, this has not resulted in an increase in the anesthetic complication rate. Postoperatively, milk feedings are resumed on return from the recovery room and rapidly advanced in volume back to preoperative levels. If possible, an attempt is made to catch up the missed feedings. Bolus feedings, initially on an hourly basis and then every 2 to 3 hours, are preferred. This tends to better simulate the physiologic state while allowing neutralization of excess gastric acidity. On occasion, with massive burns, the volume of milk required may be better tolerated if it is provided as a continuous drip. We have attempted to circumvent this problem with volume by adding a calorie–protein supplement to the milk. Without a significant change in osmolality, the caloric density can be increased to 1.2 kcal/ml at a reasonable cost.

We, like most burn centers, prefer to avoid the use of central hyperalimentation. There are instances, such as early in the course of a massive burn with inhalation injury or when an infant develops severe diarrhea from rotovirus, when transient central hyperalimentation is necessary. It must be realized, however, that the risk of catheter-related complications is significant. Some situations also warrant an attempt at using an enteric elemental diet. There are numerous commercial products on the market, usually having approximately 1 to 2 kcal/ml. Unfortunately, many of these are hyperosmolar, resulting in impressive diarrhea themselves when used near full strength. The percentage of protein in most of these preparations is below the recommended 20 to 25 percent. Finally, when compared to the cost of milk plus or minus a modular protein supplement, these commercial preparations are more expensive.

For years, the optimal means of assessing the nutritional status of the burned patient has been debated. A daily calorie count and documentation of protein intake is only a starting point. Measurement of daily weight provides a crude assessment of nutritional status. In our center, a nutritional flow sheet is used to record the various parameters in the assessment. Concentrations of serum proteins can be used as indicators of visceral protein status. Visceral proteins are necessary for wound healing, oncotic pressure, host defense mechanisms, substrate transport, and enzyme functions. Protein levels commonly used to indicate visceral protein status include serum albumin, transferrin, retinol-binding protein, and prealbumin.[86] Though they do not monitor acute changes, we follow total serum protein and albumin levels at least 3 times a week. For more severe injuries, we recently have begun to obtain serum transferrin and prealbumin levels on a weekly basis. Serum transferrin may be the most reliable indicator of current protein status because of its short half-life of 8 to 10 days. The mainstay of our nutritional assessment program is the urinary urea nitrogen method of determining nitrogen (N_2) balance:

Nitrogen balance = (protein intake/6.25) − (UUN + X)

where:

UUN = urine urea nitrogen (g/24 hr)
X = 2 (0–4 years)
    3 (4–10 years)
    4 (>10 years)

In the case of a major thermal injury, the patient's remaining unhealed burn surface area is recalculated weekly. The nutritional needs are then reassessed by formula. A 24-hour UUN level is obtained, and N_2 balance is calculated. A value of plus 3 to 5 is believed to be adequate. For smaller children, because of lack of cooperation in obtaining a 24-hour urine collection, the temporary insertion of a Silastic Foley catheter unfortunately is required. The same evaluation is performed at any time there is a marked change in the patient's overall status. We have found the UUN method of determining N_2 balance to be quite helpful in assessing the nutritional needs of the burned child. A number of burn centers have tried to perfect indirect calorimetry as a more accurate means of assessing nutritional status.[87,88] They have believed this to be an excellent technique providing very accurate results. Others, including ourselves, have found it very difficult to obtain uniformly reliable data. The ultimate role of indirect calorimetry in the routine clinical assessment of nutritional status has yet to be determined.

Sepsis

Delayed closure of the burn wound, poor nutrition, and sepsis continue to pose a major threat to children with thermal injury. During the first few days after the burn, the most likely source of contaminating bacteria is the patient. Previously, it was thought that the major source of infection after this was colonization of the eschar from the hospital environment. This concept resulted in the application of rigid reverse isolation techniques. These techniques continue is vogue in some centers. Recently, however, there has been increasing attention directed at the patient being the most important source of infecting organisms.[18,19,89] As with many problems, both mechanisms probably are operative. Until further data are available, we continue to place children with greater than 40 percent TBSA burned in reverse isolation until sufficient wound closure has occurred.

Antibiotic prophylaxis has limited effectiveness in burn therapy. Because streptococci are endemic to the Rocky Mountains, it has been our policy to routinely administer penicillin to new burn patients until their throat culture is negative. This policy recently has come into question in our unit. MacMillan, in a 10-year study of burn sepsis, found that septic complications occurred twice as frequently in patients treated with penicillin.[90] It has been questioned whether penicillin can alter the wound flora sufficiently to allow the emergence of antibiotic-resistant organisms, particularly methicillin-resistant *Staphylococcus aureus* and *Candida albicans*.[91] These two organisms are now the predominant pathogens in our unit. Enteric gram-negative organisms, particularly *Pseudomonas*, have become much less common. Because of this fact, we continue to administer cephalosporin prophylaxis against *S. aureus* around grafting procedures.

Suppurative thrombophlebitis is truly an iatrogenic complication. There is a natural tendency to leave intravenous catheters in place longer when venous access is limited by the burn wound. This is obviously a poor practice. Considerable planning is required to make the most of each vein. In our experience, the infected vein usually is the site of the intravenous line on admission. Saphenous veins at the groin are used only as a last resort, and the intravenous line should be left in place for less than 48 hours. If suppurative thrombophlebitis is suspected, the catheterization site is opened, and the contents of the vein are cultured. Aggressive excision of the vein is required when gross pus is present.

Unfortunately, all progress brings new problems. We have noted an increasing incidence of fungi in burn wounds. *C. albicans* and *Aspergillus* are the most common fungi found in burn wound cultures. As the effectiveness of antimicrobial agents increases, fungal infections may well become more prevalent. In hopes of decreasing this risk, we attempt to remove all indwelling lines and urinary catheters as soon as practical. All patients with large burns (>40 percent TBSA) are begun on enteric nystatin antifungal prophylaxis. The use of broad-spectrum antibiotics is limited. Appropriate cultures are monitored, and, with the first indication of fungus, topical nystatin cream is added to the silver sulfadiazine dressings. This has proven to be an effective means of keeping wound colony counts under control. If invasive fungal infection is suspected, quantitative wound biopsies are obtained, and systemic antifungal therapy is instituted.

We have found repeatedly that a simple bath water culture obtained before the addition of the sodium hypochlorite provides excellent insight into the type and degree of colonization of the burn wound. This is routinely performed every 3 days for larger burns. A culture obtained 2 days before grafting can be useful in dictating the perioperative antibiotic prophylaxis. If impending sepsis is suspected, the bath water culture can help identify the presumptive organism and allow accurate sensitivities to be available at the time sepsis actually develops. Hypothermia, deterioration of the wound, loss of grafts, disorientation, and intolerance of enteric feedings are all clinical signs of invasive sepsis. Feeding intolerance is one of the earliest signs. Fever and white blood cell counts are difficult to interpret.[92] Blood cultures and quantitative burn wound biopsies document invasive burn wound sepsis. Broad-spectrum parenteral antibiotics providing coverage for gram-negative organisms and *S. aureus* are begun until culture results are obtained.[93] The antibiotic coverage is then narrowed to treat the specific organism isolated. As mentioned earlier, aggressive surgical excision or debridement of eschar has been shown to have a prominent place in the prevention and treatment of burn wound sepsis.

Burn Wound Scars

Rehabilitation of the burned child may require many years. However, if thought is given to predictable patterns of burn scarring at the outset, joint contractures can be minimized. Burns involving flexion creases are at risk for producing future limitation of motion. Areas of particular concern include the neck, axillae, antecubital and popliteal fossae, hips, and, of course, the hands and feet. As soon as practical after admission to the burn center, the patient is evaluated by occupational and physical therapists. Knees and elbows are splinted in extension. The shoulders can be widely abducted with bulky gauze dressings or splints. The hand presents particular problems in that flexion of the interphalangeal joints may dislocate the extensor tendon slip so that it becomes a flexor. Skeletal traction with pins drilled vertically through the distal phalanx and nail, then attached by rubber bands to a hayrake or banjo traction device, will help prevent contractures and allows excellent positioning of the hand and fingers for grafting. This technique, originally described by Larson et al., has been evaluated in a prospective manner and found to be safe and effective.[94,95] For over 10 years, we have used suspension on a majority of severely burned hands and feet. The neck must be splinted in extension as early as possible to prevent dense scarring and contracture, which can be severe enough to interfere with endotracheal intubation.

In addition to early splinting, the child must be encouraged to use his or her joints as often as possible. Active and passive range of motion exercises are taught to the child, parents, and caregivers, with daily monitoring by the therapist. Children will use their hands and upper extremities to play with bathtub toys. Splinting is continued after the child is discharged from the hospital until the range of motion has stabilized. Progressive improvement may take place for up to 1 year after the injury. Established contractures can be improved with serial casts in some patients, whereas many require reconstruction by dividing the band of scar tissue and inserting additional skin. Z-plasties are useful in many locations. Recently, silicone tissue expanders have been

perfected and can prove to be very helpful in selected areas.

Deep dermal burns, as well as interstices in mesh autografts, can heal by epithelialization, resulting in thick hypertrophic scars. This is seen commonly along the edges or between skin grafts. During this phase of healing, the child may complain of severe itching. Scratching results in loss of epithelium and further scar formation. Enteric preparations, such as Benedryl and Atarax, can be helpful for varying time intervals, but, unfortunately, tolerance develops fairly soon. Keeping the healed burns moisturized with a cream, such as cocoa butter, seems to provide considerable relief. McDonald and Deitch have identified a number of variables in the development of hypertrophic scars and grafts.[96] Children and blacks have a significantly higher incidence than adults and whites, respectively. The presence of dermal elements in a graft bed resulted in decreased skin graft hypertrophy. Skin grafts performed within 14 days of injury looked better than those performed after 2 weeks. Hypertrophic scars may be prevented or improved by the application of custom-fitted pressure garments for 6 to 15 months after injury. While awaiting the arrival of the custom-fitted product, tubular compression bandages can be of assistance. These have definite advantages over the classic elastic bandage. For increased pressure in selected areas, an elastomere insert can be fashioned and placed under the pressure garment. Facial masks made of elastic cloth or clear plastic can apply pressure to burn scars and result in significant improvement in the child's appearance (Fig. 37–10).

ELECTRICAL BURNS

The most common electrical burn in childhood occurs when a toddler chews on a defective or exposed electrical cord. Saliva is an excellent electrolyte solution for conduction of electricity. The lower lip and corner of the mouth are most frequently involved, although the tongue and tooth buds also may be injured. Initially, the child has severe pain that interferes with eating. He or she may not be able to swallow saliva. Within a few hours after the injury, there is severe edema of the skin and buccal mucosa. The injured area then turns white, with a surrounding area of erythema. The necrotic tissue gradually demarcates, turns into black eschar, and eventually sloughs. The natural course of the injury is then one of healing by contracture and epithelialization (Fig. 37–11). The end result is scarring of the lips and varying degrees of obliteration of the angles of the mouth. In extreme cases, this results in microstomia. During separation of the eschar, there is considerable danger of hemorrhage from an eroded labial artery. Parents should

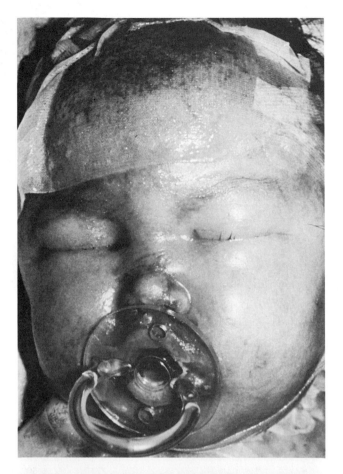

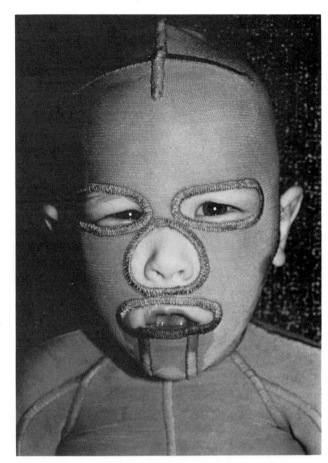

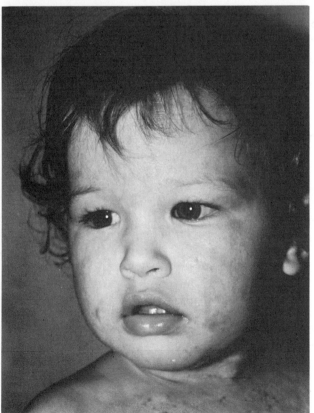

Figure 37–10. Pressure therapy for hypertrophic scarring. **Top left.** An 8-month-old female 2 days postscald burn. The entire face was bright red and edematous secondary to deep partial-thickness burns. **Top right.** A custom-fitted elastic compression mask was used on hypertrophic scars. **Left.** Same child at 9 months postburn.

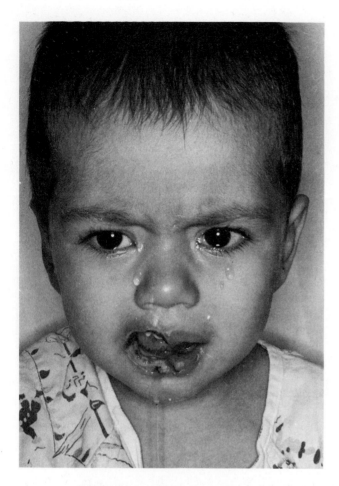 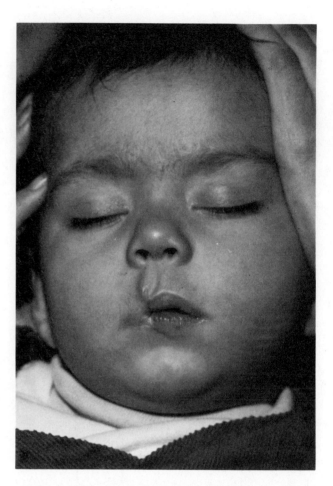

Figure 37–11. Left. A severe electrical burn of the angle of the mouth after slough of necrotic tissue. **Right.** Healing by scar contracture requiring future reconstructive surgery. This type of contracture can be avoided in selected patients by use of microstomia splints.

be advised of this possibility and instructed in techniques to control bleeding. The injury also may interfere with nutrition, growth, and speech. The proper treatment for these injuries has been debated for years. Although still recommended by some surgeons, early excision and repair are not carried out mostly because of the difficulty in assessing the degree of injury. Most surgeons have adopted the policy of allowing spontaneous slough of the eschar, with attempts at preventing contracture using intraoral splints.[97,98] Secondary operative procedures may then be performed to correct residual deformity as needed. The intraoral splint, when worn continuously for 6 to 8 months, prevents microstomia. The device is custom-made in one of several forms for the patient as soon as his condition permits. An expansile appliance consisting of acrylic sections that fit into the commissures of the mouth, connected with adjustable steel bars, allows regulation of the pressure with a set screw. The cosmetic result using these simple devices is superior to that obtained with surgical reconstruction of the lip.[99]

Older children occasionally sustain electrical burns

when accidentally coming into contact with high tension wires. The extent of the injury is determined by the sites of entrance and exit of the current, the amount of thermal energy generated by the arc of the spark, and the length of time the patient is in contact with the source of electricity. Since the electrical current preferentially travels along blood vessels, there is not only the initial effect of heat and electricity but also the possibility of delayed thrombosis of major vessels.[100] There can also be damage to major peripheral nerves. A significant possibility of electrical injury to the heart exists, with resulting cardiac arrhythmia. It is, unfortunately, impossible to determine the full extent of the injury at the initial examination. The skin may appear to be intact except for wounds at the entrance and exit sites. Vascular trauma may result in progressive necrosis of muscles and subcutaneous tissues, with delayed skin changes. Initially, these patients require large volumes of Ringer's lactate solution and sodium bicarbonate to correct fluid losses and acidosis. Escharotomy and fasciotomy must be urgently considered if evidence of a compartment syndrome develops. A compartment syndrome is seen in severely swollen extremities when secondary vascular compromise develops from the constriction of edematous tissue. Operative debridement is begun as soon as devitalized tissue is recognized. This may require multiple trips to the operating room. There is often a temptation to amputate an extremity that appears to contain large amounts of necrotic tissue because of potential sepsis. Aggressive local care, with frequent dressing changes to hasten the separation of small pockets of necrotic material in preparation for grafting, will improve the patient's overall condition. A surprising level of function may be salvaged, especially in highly motivated youngsters.

REFERENCES

1. Lenoski EF, Hunter KA: Specific patterns of inflicted burn injuries. J Trauma 17:842, 1977
2. Libber SM, Slayton DJ: Childhood burns reconsidered: The child, the family, and the burn injury. J Trauma 24:245, 1984
3. Smith RW, O'Neill TJ: An analysis into childhood burns. Burns 11:117, 1984
4. Deitch EA, Staats M: Child abuse through burning. J Burn Care Res 13:373, 1982
5. Harmel RP Jr, Vane DW, King DR: Burn care in children: Special considerations. Clin Plast Surg 13:95, 1986
6. Jackson DM: The diagnosis of the depth of burning. Br J Surg 40:588, 1953
7. Zawacki BE: The natural history of reversible burn injury. Surg Gynecol Obstet 139:867, 1974
8. Zawacki BE: Reversal of capillary stasis and prevention of necrosis in burns. Ann Surg 180:98, 1974
9. Massiha H, Monafo WW: Dermal ischemia in thermal injury: the importance of venous occlusion. J Trauma 14:705, 1974
10. Birke G, Liljedahl SO, Plantin LO, et al: Studies on burns, IX: The distribution and losses through the wound of I-131-albumin measured by whole body counting. Acta Chir Scand 134:27, 1968
11. Arturson G: Pathophysiological aspects of the burn syndrome with special reference to liver injury and alterations of capillary permeability. Acta Chir Scand (suppl) 274:1, 1961
12. Jelenko C III, Jennings WD Jr, O'Kelley WR III, et al: Threshold burning effects on distant microcirculation, II: The relationship of area burnt to microvascular size. Arch Surg 106:317, 1973
13. Anggard E, Artursson G, Jonsson CE: Effect of prostaglandins in lymph from scalded tissues. Acta Physiol Scand 80:46, 1979
14. Arturson G: Arachidonic acid metabolism and prostaglandin activity following burn injury. In Ninneman J (ed): Traumatic Injury: Infection and Other Immunologic Sequelae. Baltimore, University Park Press, 1983, pp 55–78
15. Heggers JP, Ko J, Robson MC, et al: Evaluation of burn blister fluid. Plast Reconstr Surg 65:798, 1980
16. DelBeccaro EJ, Robson MC, Heggers JP, et al: The use of specific thromboxane inhibitors to preserve the dermal microcirculation after burning. Surgery 87:137, 1980
17. Robson MC, Heggers JP: Pathophysiology of the burn wound. In Carvajal HF, Parks DH (eds): Burns in Children: Pediatric Burn Management. Chicago, Year Book, 1988, pp 27–32
18. Deitch EA, Maijima K, Berg R: Effect of oral antibiotics and bacterial overgrowth on the translocation of the GI tract microflora in burned rats. J Trauma 25:385, 1985
19. Robson MC: The effect of admitting skin bacteria and burn treatment on burn wound sepsis. Presented at the 6th Annual Meeting of the North American Burn Society, Snowbird, Utah, January 24–30, 1988
20. Deitch EA, Dobke M, Baxter CR: Failure of local immunity: A potential cause of burn wound sepsis. Arch Surg 120:78, 1985
21. Deitch EA, Smith BJ: The effect of blister fluid from thermally injured patients on normal lymphocyte transformation. J Trauma 23:106, 1983
22. Moncrief JA: Effect of various fluid regimens and pharmacologic agents on the circulatory hemodynamics of the immediate post-burn period. Ann Surg 164:723, 1966
23. Baxter CB: Crystalloid resuscitation of burn shock. In Polk HC Jr, Stone HH (eds): Contemporary Burn Managements. Boston, Little, Brown 1971, pp 7–32
24. Wilmore DW, Long JM, Mason AD Jr, et al: Catecholamines: Mediators of the hypermetabolic response to thermal injury. Ann Surg 180:653, 1974
25. Curreri PW: Metabolic and nutritional aspects of thermal injury. Burns 2:16, 1976
26. Hildreth M, Carvajal HF: Caloric requirements in burned children: A simple formula to estimate daily caloric requirements. J Burn Care Rehabil 3:78, 1982
27. Moylan JA: Smoke inhalation and burn injury. Surg Clin North Am 60:1533, 1980
28. Dyer RF, Esch VH: Polyvinyl chloride toxicity in fires. JAMA 235:393, 1976
29. Charnock EL, Mechon JJ: Postburn respiratory injuries in children. Pediatr Clin North Am 27:661, 1980
30. Herndon DN, Langner F, Thompson P, et al: Pulmonary injury in burned patients. Surg Clin North Am 67:31, 1987
31. Herndon DN, Thompson PB, Traber DL: Pulmonary injury in burned patients. Crit Care Clin 1:79, 1985
32. Pruitt BA, Erickson DR, Morris A: Progressive pulmonary insufficiency and other pulmonary complications of thermal injury. J Trauma 15:369, 1975
33. Hunt JL, Agee RN, Pruitt BA: Fiberoptic bronchoscopy in acute inhalation injury. J Trauma 15:641, 1975
34. Stone HH, Martin JD: Pulmonary injury associated with thermal burns. Surg Gynecol Obstet 129:1242, 1969
35. Trunkey D, Parks S: Burns in children. Curr Probl Pediatr 6:36, 1976
36. Herndon DN, Barrow RE, Traber DL, et al: Extravascular lung water changes following smoke inhalation and massive burn injury. Surgery 102:341, 1987

37. Moylan JA, Chan CK: Inhalation injury: An increasing problem. Ann Surg 188:34, 1978

38. Head JM: Inhalation injury in burns. Am J Surg 139:508, 1980

39. Cope O, Moore FD: The redistribution of body water and the fluid therapy of the burned patient. Ann Surg 125:1010, 1947

40. Evans EI, Pennel OJ, Robinette PW, et al: Fluid and electrolyte requirements in severe burns. Am J Surg 135:804, 1952

41. Hutcher N, Haynes BW: The Evans formula revisited. J Trauma 2:453, 1962

42. Reiss E, Stirman JA, Artz CP, et al: Fluid and electrolyte balance in burns. JAMA 152:1309, 1953

43. Batchelor ADR, Kirk J, Sutherland AB: Treatment of shock in the burned child. Lancet 1:123, 1961

44. Baxter CR, Shires T: Physiological response to crystalloid resuscitation of severe burns. Ann NY Acad Sci 150:874, 1968

45. Moncrief JA: Burns. N Engl J Med 288:444, 1973

46. Pruitt BA Jr: Fluid and electrolyte replacement in the burned patient. Surg Clin North Am 58:1291, 1978

47. Brouhard BH, Carvajal HF, Linares HA: Burn edema and protein leakage in the rat. I. Relationship to time of injury. Microvasc Res 15:221, 1978

48. Carvajal HF, Linares HA, Brouhard BH: Relationship of burn size to vascular permeability changes in rats. Surg Gynecol Obstet 149:193, 1979

49. Carvajal HF, Linares HA: Effect of burn depth upon edema formation and albumin extravasation in rats. Burns 7:79, 1980

50. Monafo W, Chuntrasakul C, Ayrazian VH: Hypertonic sodium solutions in the treatment of burn shock. Am J Surg 125:778, 1973

51. Monafo WW, Halverson JD, Schechtman K: The role of concentrated sodium solutions in the resuscitation of patients with severe burns. Surgery 95:129, 1984

52. Bowser BH, Caldwell FT Jr: The effects of resuscitation with hypertonic vs. hypotonic vs. colloid on wound and urine fluid and electrolyte losses in severely burned children. J Trauma 23:916, 1983

53. Bowser-Wallace BH, Caldwell FT Jr: A prospective analysis of hypertonic lactated saline v. Ringer's lactate-colloid for the resuscitation of severely burned children. Burns 12:402, 1986

54. Carvajal HF: Controversies in fluid resuscitation. In Carvajal HF, Parks DH (eds): Burns in Children: Pediatric Burn Management. Chicago, Year Book, 1988, pp 51–77

55. Carvajal HF: A physiologic approach to fluid therapy in severely burned children. Surg Gynecol Obstet 150:379, 1980

56. Carvajal HF: Acute management of burns in children. South Med J 68:129, 1975

57. Carvajal HF: Resuscitation of the burned child. In Carvajal HF, Parks DH (eds): Burns in Children: Pediatric Burn Management. Chicago, Year Book, 1988, pp 78–98

58. Moyer CA, Brentano L, Cravens D: Treatment of large human burns with 0.5% silver nitrate solution. Arch Surg 90:812, 1965

59. Harrison HN, Bales H, Jacoby F: The behavior of mafenide acetate as a basis for its clinical use. Arch Surg 103:449, 1971

60. White, NG, Asch MJ: Acid-base effects of topical mafenide acetate in the burned patient. N Engl J Med 284:1281, 1971

61. Fox CL Jr: Silver sulfadiazine: A new topical therapy for *Pseudomonas* in burns. Arch Surg 96:184, 1968

62. Bondoc CC, Quinby WC, Burke JF: Primary surgical management of the deeply burned hand in children. J Pediatr Surg 11:355, 1976

63. Mahler D, Benmeir P, BenYakar Y, et al: Treatment of the burned hand: early surgical treatment (1975–85) vs. conservative treatment (1964–74). A comparative study. Burns 13:45, 1987

64. Janzekovic Z: A new concept in the early excision and immediate grafting of burns. J Trauma 10:103, 1970

65. Jackson DM, Stone PA: Tangential excision and grafting of burns: The method and a report of 50 consecutive cases. Br J Plast Surg 25:416, 1972

66. Engrav LH, Heimbach DM, Reus JL, et al: Early excision and grafting vs. nonoperative treatment of burns of indeterminant depth: A randomized prospective study. J Trauma 23:1001, 1983

67. Parks DH, Linares HA, Thomson PD: Surgical management of burn wound sepsis. Surg Gynecol Obstet 153:374, 1981

68. Herndon DN, Parks DH: Comparison of serial debridement and autografting and early massive excision with cadaver skin overlay in the treatment of large burns in children. J Trauma 26:149, 1986

69. Herndon DN, Curreri PW, Abston S, et al: Treatment of burns. Curr Probl Surg 24:341, 1987

70. Demling RH: Improved survival after massive burns. J Trauma 23:179, 1983

71. Pietsch JB, Netscher DT, Nagaraj HS, et al: Early excision of major burns in children: Effect on morbidity and mortality. J Pediatr Surg 20:754, 1985

72. Tompkins RG, Burke JF, Schoenfeld DA, et al: Prompt eschar excision: A treatment system contributing to reduced burn mortality. Ann Surg 204:272, 1986

73. Herndon DN, Gore D, Cole M, et al: Determinants of mortality in pediatric patients with greater than 70% full-thickness total body surface area thermal injury treated by early total excision and grafting. J Trauma 27:208, 1987

74. Alexander JW, MacMillan BG, Law EJ, et al: Prophylactic antibiotics as an adjunct for skin grafting in clean reconstructive surgery following burn injury. J Trauma 22:687, 1982

75. Pruitt BA, Levine NS: Characteristics and uses of biologic dressings and skin substitutes. Arch Surg 119:312, 1984

76. Ninnemann JL, Fisher JC, Frank HA: Prolonged survival of human skin allografts following thermal injury. Transplantation 25:69, 1978

77. Thomson PD, Parks DH: Monitoring, banking and clinical use of amnion as a burn wound dressing. Ann Plast Surg 7:354, 1981

78. Walker AB, Cooney DR, Allen JE: Use of fresh amnion as a burn dressing. J Pediatr Surg 12:391, 1977
79. Hansbrough JF, Zapata-Sirvent R, Carroll WJ, et al: Clinical experience with Biobrane biosynthetic dressing in the treatment of partial thickness burns. Burns 10:415, 1984
80. Purdue GF, Hunt JL, Gillespie RW, et al: Biosynthetic skin substitute versus frozen human cadaver allograft for temporary coverage of excised burn wounds. J Trauma 27:155, 1987
81. Remensnyder JP: Burn wound coverings and biologic dressings. In Carvajal HF, Parks DH (eds): Burns in Children: Pediatric Burn Management. Chicago, Year Book, 1988, pp 182–192
82. Burke JF: Observations on the development of an artificial skin: Presidential address, 1982 American Burn Association Meeting. J Trauma 23:543, 1983
83. Gallico GG, O'Connor NE, Compton CC, et al: Permanent coverage of large burn wounds with autologous cultured human epithelium. N Engl J Med 311:448, 1984
84. Gallico GG, O'Connor NE: Cultured epithelium as a skin substitute. Clin Plast Surg 12:149, 1985
85. Madden MR, Finkelstein JL, Staiano-Coico L, et al: Grafting of cultured allogeneic epidermis on second- and third-degree burn wounds on 26 patients. J Trauma 26:955, 1986
86. Souba WW, Schindler BA, Carvajal HF: Nutrition and metabolism. In Carvajal HF, Parks DH (eds): Burns in Children: Pediatric Burn Management. Chicago, Year Book, 1988, 119–144
87. Turner WW, Ireton CS, Hunt JL, et al: Predicting energy expenditures in burned patients. J Trauma 25:11, 1985
88. Saffle JR, Medina E, Raymond J, et al: Use of indirect calorimetry in the nutritional management of burned patients. J Trauma 25:32, 1985
89. Deitch EA, Winterton J, Li M, et al: The gut as a portal of entry for bacteremia: Role of protein malnutrition. Ann Surg 205:681, 1987
90. MacMillan BG: Burn wound sepsis: A ten-year experience. Burns 2:1, 1987
91. Durtschi MB, Orgain C, Counta GW, et al: A prospective study of prophylactic penicillin in acutely burned hospitalized patients. J Trauma 22:11, 1982
92. Parrish RA, Novak AH, Heimbach DM, et al: Fever as a predictor of infection in burned children. J Trauma 27:69, 1987
93. Dacso CC, Leuterman A, Curreri PW: Systemic antibiotic treatment in burned patients. Surg Clin North Am 67:57, 1987
94. Larson DL, Evans EB, Abston S, et al: Skeletal suspension and the treatment of burns. Ann Surg 168:981, 1963
95. Harnar T, Engrav L, Heimbach D, et al: Experience with skeletal immobilization after excision and grafting of severely burned hands. J Trauma 25:299, 1985
96. McDonald WS, Deitch EA: Hypertrophic skin grafts in burned patients: A prospective analysis of variables. J Trauma 27:147, 1987
97. Leake JE, Curtin JW: Electrical burns of the mouth in children. Clin Plast Surg 11:669, 1984
98. Palin WE, Sadove AM, Jones JE, et al: Oral electrical burns in a pediatric population. J Oral Med 42:17, 1987
99. Hartford CE, Kealey GP, Lavelle WE, et al: An appliance to prevent and treat microstomia from burns. J Trauma 17:356, 1977
100. Haberal M: Electrical burns: A five-year experience—1985 Evans lecture. J Trauma 26:103, 1986

38
Trauma in the Neonate

An infant is likely to be injured during birth if the labor is prolonged or difficult and if there is a forceps or breech delivery. Trauma accounts for 2 percent of neonatal deaths, and there are an estimated 20 infants injured at birth for every 1 who dies.[1,2]

CEPHALOHEMATOMA

Difficult deliveries frequently result in rupture of a blood vessel under the infant's scalp. Cephalohematomas occur beneath the periosteum and are limited anteriorly by the attachment of the periosteum to the coronal suture. Subgaleal accumulations of blood are not limited by the soft, loosely adherent galea. The soft central portion of the blood clot may feel like a depressed skull fracture, and indeed scalp hematomas may be associated with skull fracture or intracranial hemorrhage. X-rays of the skull and a careful neurologic evaluation are indicated. It is best to await spontaneous reabsorption of the clot. If the hematoma is very large or if it appears that ulceration of the overlying scalp is imminent, aspiration with a syringe and needle under absolutely sterile conditions may be performed. When needling is insufficient, an open drainage through a curvilinear incision is indicated. If this is not accomplished in larger, persisting hematomas, disfiguring calcification with alteration of skull growth may occur. Sufficient blood may be lost into a scalp hematoma to require transfusion. The other serious complication is infection.

SPINAL CORD INJURIES

A breech injury together with traction or extreme flexion of the head can cause hemorrhage and laceration of the cervical cord without fracture or dislocation of the spine.[3]

The child with a high spinal cord injury may die in respiratory failure immediately after birth or may have varying degrees of flaccid paralysis. Absence of sweating below the lesion may cause thermoregulatory difficulties. If the baby does survive, he or she is likely to be hyperreflexic and spastic. Since there is no satisfactory therapy, every effort should be made to identify those at risk before delivery. Babies with hyperextended heads in the breech presentation should be delivered by Cesarean section.[4]

PERIPHERAL NERVE INJURY

Birth paralysis of the seventh nerve is unilateral and associated with edema and hemorrhage. Pressure during birth causes constriction of the nerve within the bony canal. Examination reveals edema and ecchymosis, with unilateral weakness of the face. The baby is unable to close the eye on the affected side, and when he or she cries, there is a definite asymmetry of the face. Treatment consists of careful eye hygiene and taping the lid shut to prevent corneal abrasions. Recovery generally begins by the second week after birth and continues over a period of several months. Patches of necrosed fat may be left in subcutaneous tissue of the face after an injury of this sort.

Traction of the head, trunk, or arm during birth may result in varying degrees of damage to the brachial plexus. Associated defects include fractures of the clavicle or humerus and facial palsy. The electromyelogram is helpful in delineating the pathology.[5] Three types of such damage have been described. The upper arm, or Erb–Duchenne, is the most common type, in which injury at the junction of the anterior primary divisions of the fifth and sixth cervical roots results in paralysis, primarily of the deltoid, supraspinatus, infraspinatus, brachiaradialis, and supinator brevis muscles. The lower arm, or Klumpke, type involves the eighth cervical and first dorsal roots, with paralysis of the intrinsic muscles of the hand and of the flexors of the wrist and fingers. Sympathetic nerve fibers may be damaged, causing Horner's syndrome. In the third type, the entire arm is involved, with flaccid paralysis and sensory loss. Clinically, in the newborn period, the affected extremity hangs lifeless at the side, with the elbow straight and with loss of active movement. The differential diagnosis includes fracture of the clavicle or humerus. A chest x-ray should be obtained because an associated phrenic nerve palsy results in elevation of the diaphragm with respiratory distress.

Gradual recovery during the first few months of life is the rule, although recovery is rarely complete. The paralyzed extremity should be supported with the shoulder in 70° to 90° of abduction and 90° of external rotation. In the newborn, this may be implemented by securing the arm to the sheets with bandages and pins. Later, a light brace is applied that also will hold the forearm in full supination and the hand in the functional position. Several times a day, a full range of passive motion of all joints is carried out to help prevent contractures.

SKELETAL TRAUMA

Fractures of the clavicle result in obvious pain and limitation of motion on the injured side. There also will be a bump or swelling over the injured bone. The diagnosis is confirmed with an x-ray; treatment consists of a figure-eight bandage of stockinette partially filled with sheet wadding. The bandage is pinned in place and tightened every day by the mother. Fractures of the midshaft of the humerus result in pain and failure to move the affected arm. The diagnosis is confirmed with an x-ray, and treatment consists of merely strapping the arm to the chest with a soft Velpeau's bandage. Healing is complete within 3 weeks.

PNEUMOTHORAX

Pneumothorax usually results from overzealous attempts to artificially inflate the lungs immediately after birth. However, it also has occurred secondary to chest compression when no attempts at artificial ventilation have been made (Fig. 38–1). When there is significant respiratory distress, a chest tube is inserted in the midaxillary line opposite the nipple and connected to an underwater seal. This results in prompt expansion of the lung and eliminates pulmonary compression as a factor in the infant's respiratory distress. Occasionally, a pneumothorax of less than 25 percent is observed in an infant showing minimal distress. Most of these small collections of air will reabsorb within 24 hours. On the other hand, if artificial ventilation is necessary, pneumothorax of any degree may be aggravated by positive pressure. Consequently, a chest tube is indicated. Simple aspiration will only make matters worse because as the lung expands it will be lacerated by the needle.

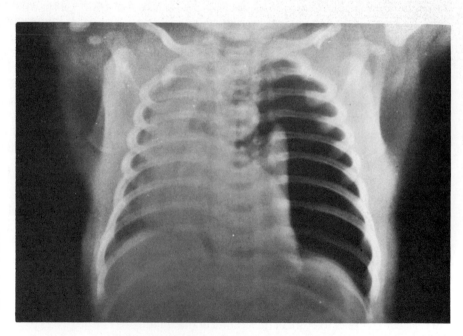

Figure 38–1. A 9-pound infant born after a long, difficult delivery. At birth, he was noted to have a fracture of the left clavicle, after which he developed severe respiratory distress secondary to tension pneumothorax. There was a prompt expansion of the lung after insertion of a chest tube.

ABDOMINAL INJURIES

Until recently, most reports on intraabdominal visceral injuries in neonates were from autopsy series.[6] Closer observation of the neonate, prompt transfusion, correction of coagulation abnormalities, and surgery have resulted in survivors of liver and spleen injuries.[7–10] A review of our own experience as well as of the cases reported in the literature has resulted in a fairly clear clinical picture of the infant with intraperitoneal bleeding. The typical victim is larger than average and was born in a forceps or breech delivery. One of our patients with a ruptured spleen also had an incompatibility requiring an exchange transfusion. The onset of lethargy with refusal to take feedings occurs during the first 48 hours after birth. Such infants are pale, have tachypnea, and after 24 hours develop abdominal distention. Ecchymosis of the abdominal wall, bluish discoloration about the umbilicus (Cullen's sign), and a blue scrotum are more specific signs of intraperitoneal hemorrhage.

The hemoglobin and hematocrit levels are reduced, and there may be bleeding at venipuncture sites because of a coagulation defect. Abdominal x-rays demonstrate loops of intestine floating in a fluid-filled abdomen, and there may be displacement of the stomach from a blood clot around the spleen. Ultrasonography performed at the cribside will demonstrate reliably fluid within the abdominal cavity, and often lacerations of the liver or spleen. Computed tomography (CT) scans will demonstrate liver or spleen injury.

The liver and kidneys usually opacified, whereas the spleen did not. In our own cases, the diagnosis of hemoperitoneum was proven with a single abdominal paracentesis. Although several authors have reported suture repair of the neonatal liver, in our experience, newborn liver is too fragile to hold sutures. Our patient did not stop bleeding until he was given fresh whole blood.[11] Rickham and Johnston successfully treated two infants with hemoperitoneum solely by transfusion.[12] Splenectomy has been performed in most infants with rupture of the spleen, but concern over postoperative infections led Matsuyama et al. to successfully repair a lacerated spleen with catgut sutures.[13] We attempted nonoperative treatment of hemoperitoneum in a newborn, but the infant continued to bleed and not only required 600 ml of blood but had respiratory distress secondary to abdominal distention. At operation, the spleen was completely fragmented, and there was hemorrhage from branches of the splenic artery. Every effort should be made to save the spleen, but with rupture of either the liver or spleen in the newborn, correction of coagulation defects with fresh whole blood and platelets will be necessary to control bleeding.

ADRENAL HEMORRHAGE

Some 75 percent of babies who develop adrenal hemorrhage have had a breech or traumatic delivery.[14] They have a retroperitoneal hematoma, easily observed with either an ultrasound or CT study. Later, when the hematoma calcifies, there may be concern about a neuroblastoma. An operation is not indicated if the diagnosis of adrenal hemorrhage can be made.

REFERENCES

1. Valdes-Sapena MA, Arey JB: The causes of neonatal mortality: An analysis of 501 autopsies on newborn infants. J Pediatr 77:366, 1970
2. Gresham EL: Birth trauma. Pediatr Clin North Am 22:317, 1975
3. Towbin A: Spinal cord and brain stem injuries at birth. Arch Pathol 77:620, 1964
4. Bresnan MJ, Abrams IE: Neonatal spinal cord transection secondary to intrauterine hyperextension of the neck in breech presentation. J Pediatr 84:734, 1974
5. Eng GD: Brachial plexus palsy in newborn infants. Pediatrics 48:18, 1971
6. Potter EL: Pathology of the Fetus and Newborn. Chicago, Year Book, 1952, p 96
7. Eraklis AJ: Abdominal injury related to the trauma of birth. Pediatrics 39:421, 1967
8. Leape LL, Bordy MD: Neonatal rupture of the spleen: Report of a case successfully treated after spontaneous cessation of hemorrhage. Pediatrics 47:101, 1971
9. Srouji MN, Williams ML, Werner JN: Neonatal rupture of the liver: Use of exchange transfusion to correct associated coagulation defects. J Pediatr Surg 6:56, 1971
10. Sokol DM, Tompkins D, Izant RJ Jr: Rupture of the spleen and liver in the newborn: A report of the first survivor and a review of the literature. J Pediatr Surg 9:227, 1974
11. Monson D, Raffensperger J: Intraperitoneal hemorrhage secondary to liver laceration in a newborn. J Pediatr Surg 2:464, 1967
12. Rickham PP, Johnston JH: Neonatal Surgery. New York, Appleton-Century-Crofts, 1969, p 245
13. Matsuyama S, Suzuki N, Nagamachi Y: Rupture of the spleen in the newborn: Treatment with splenectomy. J Pediatr Surg 11:115, 1976
14. Tank WS, David R, Holt JF, Morley GW: Mechanisms of trauma during breech delivery. Obstet Gynecol 38:761, 1971
15. Gross M, Kottmeier PK, Waterhouse K: Diagnosis and treatment of neonatal adrenal hemorrhage. J Pediatr Surg 2:308, 1967

39
Child Abuse

Kempe described the battered child syndrome in 1961, but various forms of child abuse have been noted for centuries and were well described in Dickens' novels.[1] There are many facets to the child abuse syndrome, varying from simple neglect to overt major trauma. Physicians who care for children have a moral and legal responsibility to not only treat the medical and surgical problems but also to obtain help from the proper child protection agencies.[2]

The first step is to suspect child abuse when there are unexplained or repeated injuries or when the magnitude of the trauma is out of proportion to the parent's explanation. An apparent prolonged interval between the injury and bringing the child for medical help, together with little apparent concern for the child, are meaningful observations. Frequently, grandparents or other relatives are sufficiently concerned about the child and the family situation to volunteer information that contradicts the parent's history. On physical examination, there are often signs of malnutrition, bruises, and old burns. Sexual abuse and injuries to the genitalia, in either sex, provide strong evidence of intentional injury. Since many of these victims have learned that a cry brings only another blow, they will submit to painful medical procedures without a whimper. Roentgenograms or radionuclide scans of long bones and the skull should be obtained any time there is a suspicion of child abuse, since fractures in various stages of healing are typical and are often accepted by a court as evidence.[3] An ophthalmologic examination also is useful in detecting child abuse that includes vigorous shaking of the child. There are petechial hemorrhages on the retina, which are an indication of similar injuries in the brain.[4] Although subdural hematomas, spinal injuries, and fractures are common in this group of patients, pediatric surgeons are more likely to treat abused children for burns and visceral and genital injuries.[5,6]

BURNS

Cigarette burns, a stocking distribution of scalds on the feet and legs, and hot plate burns of the buttocks are all characteristic. The Cook County Burn Unit reported 26 cases in which burning was the primary form of abuse and 17 others in which burns were subordinate to another form of intentional trauma over a 4-year period.[7]

From 1970 to 1986 at the Children's Memorial Hospital, child abuse was suspected in nearly 10 percent of burned children under 2 years of age, and many more children were admitted to the hospital with burn wounds due to neglect, if not outright intentional burning. The burns in these children are likely to be infected when seen in the emergency room. The poor nutrition and associated injuries make treatment more difficult. In the Cook County Hospital series, there was a 19 percent mortality rate in burns from child abuse.[7]

VISCERAL INJURIES

Delay and a poor history contribute to the high mortality rate seen with intraabdominal injuries.[8,9] The child with a ruptured intestine, the most common injury secondary to intentional trauma, will have unexplained abdominal distention, shock, and sepsis. With no history of obvious trauma, the diagnosis depends on eliciting abdominal tenderness and reliance on roentgen findings. Unexplained duodenal hematomas and pseudocysts of the pancreas are often the result of abuse, and a history will be obtained only after repeated questioning.

SEXUAL ABUSE

Both the male and female genitalia are targets of the most vicious abuse that one sees in pediatric practice.[10]

Boys may sustain rectal tears, bruising, lacerations of the penis and scrotum, or burns at the hands of baby sitters. More often than not, the mother's boyfriend is the perpetrator. This usually seems to be the result of mental imbalance, perhaps aggravated by jealousy of the child's real parent. Little girls may have varying degrees of bruising or lacerations of the vagina or rectum. Many times, these children are so hysterical that they cannot be examined properly in the emergency room. They must be examined under anesthesia, so that whatever repair is necessary may be performed. We have observed penetration of the vagina into the peritoneal cavity and several instances of third-degree lacerations from the vagina into the rectum. In these instances, we have performed a colostomy and then an elective repair of the rectovaginal fistula at a later date. Photographic evidence of the extent of injury, together with specimens of vaginal fluid, should always be obtained for evidence in these tragic cases.

Condyloma acuminata about the genitalia or rectum are also signs of sexual child abuse.[11] These are viral lesions transmitted like any other venereal disease. They may be removed by coagulation with the electrocautery or by freezing with liquefied nitrogen applied with a cotton swab.

The extent of child abuse and neglect is staggering. In the State of Illinois from July to December, 1976, 3856 cases were reported to the Central Child Abuse Registry.[12] Of these children, 55 percent were white, and 85 percent were from families with an annual income below $6000. Thus it would appear that poverty is at least one important factor. The child's mother is the most common offender, although the father, babysitters, and the mother's boyfriend are also offenders.

In Illinois, as in many other states, medical personnel must report cases of suspected child abuse to the Department of Children and Family Services. At the Children's Memorial Hospital, a Protective Services Team consisting of social workers, nurses, and physicians was formed in 1970. After a referral is made to this group, further consultation frequently is obtained from psychiatric personnel, the hospital's legal department, and law enforcement agencies. Approximately 150 children are referred to this team each year. A team approach is helpful, indeed necessary, if the child is to be restored to emotional as well as physical health. The natural tendency of a physician is to become angry with the family. This only makes the parents more hostile to and resentful of therapeutic attempts. Our attitudes are softened somewhat when we realize that in these cases the mother herself was often an abused child who attempted to escape a bad family situation by an early, unwise marriage.

Alcoholism, divorce, and poverty contribute to a continually deteriorating situation. The child becomes the target of a lifetime of unhappiness and suppressed hostility. Although the process of counseling and rehabilitation of the family must be carried out by skilled social workers in a variety of facilities, the physician will be called on to describe the injury and to provide evidence that it could, indeed, have been intentionally inflicted. For this reason, accurate descriptions of all injuries, including old bruises, cuts, and fractures, must be entered into the chart along with details of the current trauma. The history as related by the family is recorded, and supplementary data are added later. Photographs of the child's external wounds, as well as findings at operation, have been extremely helpful, particularly if the surgeon is called on to testify in court, which may happen if the child is to be placed in the state's custody. The importance of the physician's role in child abuse is emphasized by a report of one suit against a doctor for failing to make the diagnosis.[13]

Unfortunately, in spite of recent laws and awareness of the problem, children known to be injured by their parents are too frequently returned to the same home environment by responsible authorities, only to be injured again, sometimes fatally.

REFERENCES

1. Kempe CH, Silverman N, Steele BF: The battered child syndrome. JAMA 181:17, 1962
2. Kottmeier, P: The battered child. Pediatr Ann 16:343, 1987
3. Haase G, Ortiz V, Sfakianakis G, et al: The value of radionuclide bone scanning in the early recognition of deliberate child abuse. J Trauma 20:873, 1980
4. Harley R: Ocular manifestations of child abuse. J Pediatr Ophthalmol Strabismus 16:5, 1980
5. O'Neill JA, Meacham WR, Griffin P, Sawyers JL: Patterns of injury in the battered child syndrome. J Trauma 13:4, 322, 1973
6. Cullen JC: Spinal lesions in battered babies. J Bone Joint Surg 57B:264, 1975
7. Stone NH, Rinaldo L, Humphrey CR, Brown RH: Child abuse by burning. Surg Clin North Am 50:6, 1970
8. Garnall P, Ahlmed S, Jolleys A, Cohen SJ: Intraabdominal injuries in the battered baby syndrome. Arch Dis Child 47:211, 1972
9. Touloukian RJ: Abdominal visceral injuries in battered children. Pediatrics 42:642, 1968
10. Black C, Pokorny W, McGill C, et al: Anorectal trauma in children. J Pediatr Surg 17:501, 1983
11. McCoy C, Applebaum H, Besser A: Condyloma acuminata: An unusual presentation of child abuse. J Pediatr Surg 17:505, 1982
12. State Administrative Offices, 623 East Adams, Springfield, Ill., Child Abuse Registry: Memorandum of Feb. 3, 1977
13. Curran WJ: Failure to diagnose battered child syndrome. N Engl J Med 296:795, 1975

SECTION V

Tumors

Elaine R. Morgan
Edward S. Baum

Cancer is second only to trauma as the leading cause of death in children. In 1973, 2961 children from 1 to 14 years of age died from malignancy. This comprised 11 percent of the deaths in this age group, with a mortality of 5.6/100,000 population.[1]

The incidence of major malignant neoplasms is 124.5/1,000,000 in Caucasian children under 15 years of age. In black children, it is 97.8/1,000,000.[2] Leukemia accounted for 25 to 30 percent, and the central nervous system for 20 to 25 percent of these tumors. The next most common category is the lymphomas, which comprise 10 to 15 percent of childhood cancers. Neuroblastoma and Wilms' tumors each account for 7 percent of all childhood malignancies. In descending order of frequency are the rhabdomyosarcomas, liver tumors, and Ewing's sarcoma. Other soft tissue tumors, teratomas and miscellaneous histologic types, constitute the remainder.[2,3]

Relatively few malignant tumors in children currently are treated solely by surgical excision. Most are treated by a combination of surgical resection, chemotherapy, and radiation. Thus, the successful treatment of a child with a malignant tumor requires the cooperative approach of surgeons, pediatric oncologists, and radiation therapists.[4] A member from each of these disciplines should be involved from the onset so that the extent of the lesion is clearly understood by all who eventually will be involved in the child's management.

In some situations, notably osteosarcoma and some cases of retinoblastoma, ablative surgery may be indicated.[5,6] In others, particularly the rhabdomysarcomas, chemotherapy and radiation are sufficiently successful that mutilative operations are contraindicated.[7] It is, therefore, important that a surgeon understand the limitations as well as the successes of other modes of therapy. In other situations, notably with lymphomas and advanced neuroblastomas, the surgeon's role is primarily to assist in making the diagnosis with biopsy or staging procedures.[8,9] Furthermore, the surgical removal of a large portion of the tumor may enhance the effectiveness of chemotherapy, even if the entire tumor cannot be removed.[10]

The surgeon must continue to be involved with the child's care long after the operative procedure. Suspicious lumps may require biopsy to rule out recurrent tumor. A second-look operation may be indicated to determine if it is safe to discontinue chemotherapy. In addition, such procedures as the insertion of a central venous catheter may be helpful in maintaining the child's nutrition and will facilitate chemotherapy.

Surgical assistance also may be required to manage the complications of chemotherapy. In particular, a lung biopsy frequently is indicated to determine whether a pulmonary infiltrate is caused by *Pneumocystis carinii*. Close cooperation is indicated to determine the proper timing of additional treatment following an operation because radiotherapy and several of the chemotherapeutic agents retard wound healing.

Although chemotherapy has dramatically improved the prognosis of many pediatric neoplasms (particularly Wilms' tumor and the rhabdomyosarcomas), these drugs have significant side effects. Not only must the importance of these drugs be stressed to the family at the onset of treatment, but one must also warn of their possible side effects. Older children must be included in the discussion of long-term chemotherapy and radiation so they will know what to expect when side effects do occur. The commonly used drugs, with their indications and side effects, are listed in Table 40–2.

REFERENCES

1. Public Health Service: Vital Statistics of the United States, 1973. Rockville, MD, HEW, 1975, vol 2, part B
2. Young JL, Miller RW: Incidence of malignant tumors in U.S. children. J Pediatr 86:254, 1975
3. Miller RW, Dalager NA: U.S. childhood cancer deaths by cell type, 1960–68. J Pediatr 85:664, 1974
4. Farber S: The control of cancer in children. Neoplasia in childhood. In Farber S (ed): Proceedings of the University of Texas M.D. Anderson Hospital and Tumor Institute Twelfth Annual Clinical Conference on Cancer, 1967. Chicago, Year Book, 1969, pp 321–27
5. Chang P: Progress in the treatment of osteosarcoma. Med Clin North Am 61:1027, 1977
6. Reese AB: Tumors of the Eye, 2nd ed. New York, Hoeber, 1963
7. Johnson DG: Trends in surgery for childhood rhabdomyosarcoma. Cancer 35:916, 1975
8. Exelby PR: Solid tumors in children: Wilms' tumor, neuroblastoma and soft tissue sarcomas. CA 28:146, 1978
9. Sullivan MP, Fuller LM, Butler JJ: Hodgkin's disease in children. In Sutow WW, Vietti TJ, Fernbach DJ (eds): Clinical Pediatric Oncology. St Louis, Mosby, 1977, pp 408–443
10. Schabel FM: Concepts for systemic treatment of micrometastases. Cancer 35:15, 1975

40
Renal Masses

John G. Raffensperger
Elaine R. Morgan

Flank masses are a clinical problem throughout the pediatric age range. They are usually asymptomatic and are discovered by either the child's mother or a physician during a routine examination. Abdominal pain is unusual even when the mass is very large. Furthermore, urinary symptoms are rare. The usual signs of malignancy (such as anorexia, malaise, and weight loss) are seen only with the largest malignant tumors. Fever is more common with urinary tract obstructions, such as hydronephrosis, than with tumors. In addition, the presence of white blood cells in the urine suggests hydronephrosis or a duplication of the kidney rather than a tumor. The diagnosis of any abdominal mass commences with careful palpation. Renal masses are localized to the flank and are less mobile than intraperitoneal lesions, such as mesenteric or ovarian cysts. Cystic lesions and small Wilms' tumors will move with respiration, but larger Wilms' tumors are relatively fixed.

During the neonatal period, unilateral multicystic kidneys and congenital hydronephrosis due to a ureteropelvic junction obstruction are the most commonly encountered flank masses. The multicystic kidney is knobby to palpation and transilluminates easily (Fig. 40–1). Radiologic studies demonstrate absent function on the affected side, and ultrasonography shows the cysts with an absence of renal parenchyma. Careful evaluation of the opposite side is helpful, since approximately one fifth of multicystic kidneys are associated with other urinary abnormalities.

The treatment for a multicystic kidney is excision because of the danger of infection and the increased incidence of Wilms' tumors in dysplastic kidneys. An extraperitoneal flank incision is used. The ureter is atretic, the renal artery is absent, and the kidney is easily shelled out with blunt dissection. Bilateral polycystic kidneys must not be confused with the unilateral multicystic kidney. With multicystic kidneys, there is usually a strong family history of renal disease, and both kidneys are palpable. The infantile form of the disease is incompatible with life, since the kidneys are studded with literally thousands of 1 to 2 mm cysts. Pyelograms demonstrate poor function, with enlargement of both kidneys. There is no treatment for this condition short of renal transplantation. The adult type of polycystic renal disease may also be present in infancy. Often both kidneys are palpable, and radiologic study demonstrates bilateral distortion. The physical findings and the pyelogram may suggest bilateral Wilms' tumor because of pelvicalyceal distortion, but transillumination and echography demonstrate the cystic nature of the lesion. Renal function may be preserved by the removal of larger cysts and by unroofing smaller ones.

Hydronephrosis secondary to ureteropelvic stricture is equal in frequency to the congenital multicystic kidney as a cause of flank mass in the neonatal period. Hydronephrosis is seen in later childhood secondary to ureteral reflux and lower ureteral obstructions as well as to ureteropelvic abnormalities. Consequently, a cystogram, cystoscopy, and a retrograde pyelogram are indicated. Most hydronephrotic kidneys in childhood can be reconstructed and salvaged. Nephrectomy is indicated only if there is a nonfunctioning shell. Particularly in the neonatal period, the pelvis may be hugely dilated, but after decompression, there is sufficient cortex for satisfac-

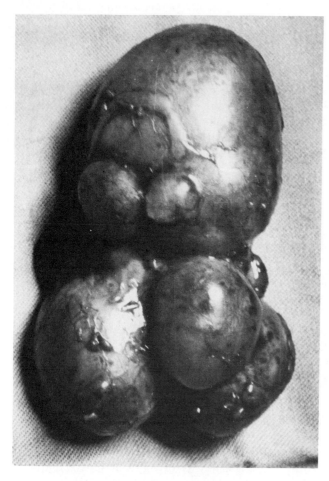

Figure 40–1. Unilateral multicystic kidney.

tory function even when the hydronephrotic kidney is solitary.

Duplication of the renal pelvis and ureter are common but usually asymptomatic. Occasionally, the upper obstructed duplication is tense and hard. It may then mimic a renal tumor or, more likely, a neuroblastoma because the inferior, functioning renal segment will be displaced downward.

Duplications become symptomatic when the upper ureter drains into the vagina or urethra to produce continuous urinary dribbling. When the upper segment is large enough to minic a tumor, it is usually a functionless shell. The treatment for this condition is heminephrectomy.

WILMS' TUMOR

Wilms' tumor (nephroblastoma) and neuroblastoma are the two most common solid intraabdominal malignant tumors in childhood. Neuroblastoma is more common than Wilms' tumor, particularly in younger children. The incidence of Wilms' tumor is 1 in every 13,500

live births, or approximately 450 new cases per year in the United States.[1,2] In 1961, Ravitch and Thomasson published an extensive review of Wilms' tumors, from the first published case in 1814 to the era of nephrectomy and postoperative radiation.[3] After Wilms published his extensive monograph on kidney tumors in 1899, almost all kidney tumors of childhood were grouped together and given his name. The lumping together of all embryomas as Wilms' tumors was recommended by Gross and Neuhauser in 1950.[4]

Some kidney tumors, especially those detected in early infancy, are benign. At the other end of the spectrum, there is a small group of tumors that are clinically more aggressive, are histologically distinct, and do not respond to the usual treatment. The surgeon must be aware of these variations so that the patient is not given radiation and chemotherapy needlessly on the one hand or treated with inappropriate drug regimens on the other.

Pathology

Wilms' tumors vary in size from a small mass limited to the renal fossa to huge lesions that extend from the diaphragm to the pelvis and cross the midline, displacing the aorta and inferior vena cava. The colon is lifted, and in larger tumors, there are thin-walled veins coursing over the surface. These are enlarged, along with the gonadal veins, when the renal vein is obstructed with tumor. There is a pseudocapsule that separates the tumor from normal kidney tissue and a fibrous capsule around the surface of the tumor. The cut surface is gray, lobular, and firm, but in larger tumors, there are hemorrhage, necrosis, and cystic degeneration. (Fig. 40–2) The renal pelvis is distorted but is invaded by tumor only in the end-stages of the disease. The gross pathology explains the usual radiographic findings of calyceal distortion without displacement of the kidney. Microscopically, the Wilms' tumor reveals its embryologic origins. There are three cell types, epithelial, stromal, and blastemal, which give the classic Wilms' tumor a triphasic appearance.[5] The stromal elements may consist of any type of connective tissue, including muscle, osteoid, or cartilage. The epithelial elements may resemble renal tubules, whereas the blastema consists of sheets of darkly staining cells.

Attempts have been made to grade the histologic appearance of Wilms' tumors to determine prognosis.[6] There are three unfavorable histology types that account for only 10 percent of cases but 60 percent of deaths. In anaplastic tumors, the nuclear diameter in any of the elements is three times larger than normal and is hyperchromatic with abnormal mitotic figures.[7] The rhabdoid form of Wilms' tumor contains large uniform cells with clear nuclei.[8] These lesions occur in younger children who have a high mortality, with metastases to brain, lung, and liver.[9] The third unfavorable type is the clear cell sarcoma, also called a "bone-metastasizing"

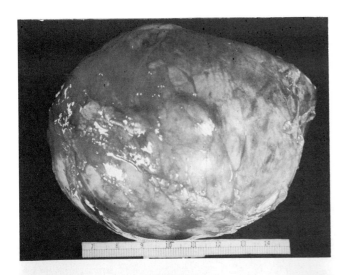

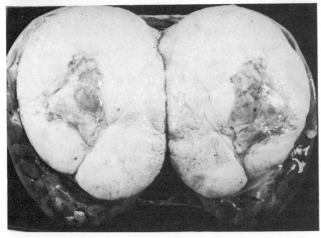

Figure 40–2 Top. Wilms' tumor removed from a 3-year-old child. **Bottom.** Cut surface demonstrating calyceal distortion.

Wilms' tumor.[10–12] There is a male predominance, and most tumors appear before 3 years of age. Microscopically, the tumor consists of a monotonous pattern of clear cells arranged in cords or trabeculae. This tumor metastasizes to the pelvis, spine, and ribs and has a particularly poor prognosis.

Classic Wilms' tumors invade blood vessels and can extend to the right atrium through the inferior vena cava. They metastasize to the lung and regional lymph nodes and, occasionally, to the liver. They may occur in extrarenal locations, most notably in the inguinal canal.[13] The pathology may be changed by therapy; in particular, lung metastases appear microscopically to be a more benign form of muscle tissue after chemotherapy.

There are several benign relatives of the classic Wilms' tumor that may be differentiated by a preoperative computed tomography (CT) scan and require a more limited operation. The cystic nephroma may occupy a part or all of the kidney, with cystic spaces interspersed

with immature mesenchyme. There may be islands of immature blastema or tubules reminiscent of a typical Wilms' tumor, although these lesions are clinically benign.[14] They are recognized on CT scan by their large cystic spaces[15] (Fig. 40–3). Nephroblastomatosis is defined as the presence of tumorlike lesions that consist of immature metanephric elements persisting beyond the 36th week of gestation.[16] These may be only subcapsular, flat, whitish plaques or microscopic nodules in the cortex (Fig. 40–4). Nephroblastomatosis may be a precursor to Wilms' tumor, is often found in bilateral Wilms' tumors, and may coexist with a classic tumor in the same kidney.[17] It is still unclear whether nephroblastomatosis exists as an independent tumor or is always a precursor to Wilms' tumor.[18]

The lesion usually is diffuse in one kidney, and since it usually follows a benign course, our policy has been to perform multiple biopsies, treat with chemotherapy, and follow up with CT scans and second-look operations for repeat biopsy and, if possible, excision of the lesion. A nephrectomy is not advised for nephroblastomatosis.

Bolande et al. have applied the term "congenital mesoblastic nephroma" to a group of neoplasms that would appear to fall within the spectrum of lesions previously considered to be Wilms' tumors.[19] This type of tumor, described as a leiomyoma, hamartoma, or fibroma, appears in newborn infants or during early infancy.[20–26] Grossly, the lesion is whorled and pale. Microscopically, there are woven bundles of spindle-shaped cells. A characteristic feature is the presence of thin-walled vascular channels interwoven among the spindle cells and most prominent near the periphery. Mitotic figures are rare, but islands of renal parenchyma

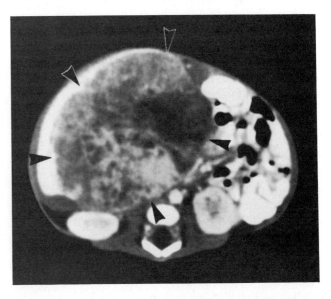

Figure 40–3. CT scan of a large cystic nephroma that was hanging off the lower pole of the kidney. This was removed with a wedge resection of the lower pole.

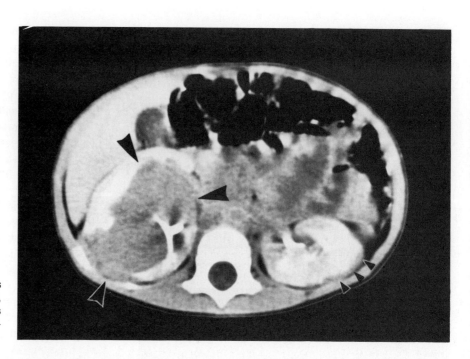

Figure 40–4. On the left, the large arrows point to a Wilms' tumor distorting the calyces, while on the right, the three small arrows point out surface plaques of nephroblastomatosis.

containing immature glomerular structures and tubules are seen more frequently. It is not clear whether these tumors are simple benign mesenchymal lesions (a benign form of Wilms' tumor) or a precursor of the malignant tumor. There does seem to be a spectrum even within this group of tumors, from the uniformly benign lesion to the malignant sarcoma. There have been two reported cases of mesoblastic nephroma that recurred, each in black females; one caused the child's death 4 months after its original removal.[27,28] After reviewing these two cases, Beckwith concluded that infants with congenital mesoblastic nephroma usually are curable with nephrectomy alone when the margins of the resected specimen are free from tumor.[29]

The surgeon must be alert to the variations in pathology found in the renal tumors of childhood. Postoperative treatment depends on an exact diagnosis, which requires close cooperation between the surgeon and pathologist. The pathologist should inspect the kidney in the operating room and study frozen sections to establish a preliminary diagnosis. This will then determine the need to carry out electron microscopic studies, special stains, or study with monoclonal antibodies. We now freeze a specimen of tumor for future studies as new diagnostic modalities are developed. Whenever there is doubt about the diagnosis, the pathologist should consult with the National Wilms' Tumor Registry.

Pathogenesis

Wilms' tumors are in the borderland between embryology and pathology in that they are associated with other congenital anomalies and some are potentially inheritable.[30] Fourteen of our 122 patients treated from 1975

to 1987 had associated congenital abnormalities (Table 40–1). There is an association between aniridia, Wilms' tumor, and deletion of the short arm of chromosome 11, band 13.[31–34] Children with the Beckwith-Weideman syndrome have a high incidence of abdominal tumors, particularly Wilms'.[35] These children, as well as those with hemihypertrophy, must be followed closely for the development of tumors.[36–38]

Congenital defects of the kidney, especially fused or horseshoe kidney, are associated with Wilms' tumors. In one retrospective series of children with Wilms' tumors, 27 percent with bilateral lesions had associated external genital anomalies, whereas only 2.3 percent of those with unilateral tumors had anomalies.[39] There also is a specific syndrome (Drash) consisting of male pseudohermaphroditism, glomerulonephritis, and mental retardation.[40,41] The tumor has appeared in siblings, cousins, and successive generations of the same family.[42–44] The heritable form of the disease is more likely to

TABLE 40–1. ASSOCIATED DEFECTS IN 122 PATIENTS WITH WILMS' TUMORS

Defect	Number
Beckwith-Weideman syndrome	2
Hemihypertrophy	3
Horseshoe kidney with extra ureter	1
Pelvoureteral stricture	1
Undescended testes	3
Soto's syndrome	1
DES exposure	1
Varicocele	1
Aniridia and mental retardation	1
Total	14

be bilateral and multicentric and will have a higher incidence of associated nephroblastomatosis as well as other congenital defects. Fortunately, at least 90 percent of unilateral Wilms' tumors appear to be sporadic without a genetic relationship. Surviving patients have a less than 2 percent risk of having offspring with the tumor.[45] Wilms' tumors are derived from the metanephric blastema cells, which normally disappear 4 to 6 weeks before term in normal gestations. Thus, nephroblastomatosis that develops from this metanephric precursor becomes malignant after a second hit from some unknown carcinogen.[46,47]

Clinical Features

Wilms' tumors usually appear as an asymptomatic abdominal mass. Pain occurs only if there is spontaneous hemorrhage or after trauma. Large tumors will rupture spontaneously, causing peritonitis that may be mistaken for appendicitis. Fever caused by tumor breakdown sometimes occurs, and hypertension is found in about 50 percent of patients.[48,49] On palpation, the tumor is smooth and slightly mobile and arises from the flank.

Large tumors not only extend across the midline but also seem to fill the abdomen. Always look for a varicocele in a boy with a left-sided tumor; this is a sign of renal vein occlusion.

Diagnostic Studies

The urinalysis rarely demonstrates hematuria unless there has been trauma to the kidney. After admission to the hospital, blood is drawn for typing and crossmatching, CBC, BUN, creatinine and coagulation studies. Intravenous fluids should be started promptly in anticipation of radiologic studies and an operation within 24 hours.

An intravenous pyelogram was formerly the primary diagnostic tool and, with the clinical examination, provided a correct diagnosis in 95 percent of patients. Ultrasonography is now the easiest and most rapid diagnostic test. This single study is a screening tool to be used when a tumor is suspected and to follow up those children who have congenital abnormalities known to be associated with Wilms' tumor. The ultrasound study will provide us with a presumptive diagnosis. It will detect tumor

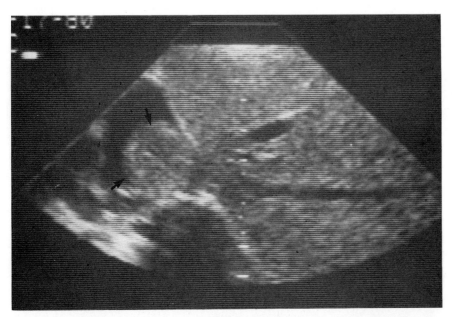

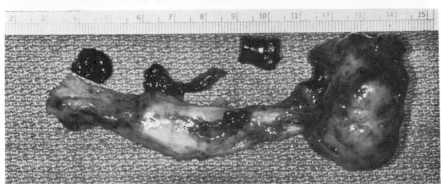

Figure 40–5. Top. Ultrasound study demonstrating Wilms' tumor bulging into the right atrium from extension up the inferior vena cava. The arrows indicate a tumor in the atrium. **Bottom.** Wilms' tumor specimen demonstrating the bulbous mass within the right atrium, with the long intracaval extension. Removed by cardiopulmonary bypass simultaneous with nephrectomy.

in the vena cava or right atrium as well as contralateral tumors. It is important to study the vena cava and atrium in every child with a Wilms' tumor because the removal of these extensions may require cardiopulmonary bypass[50-52] (Fig. 40–5). CT of the abdomen and chest always are performed, since this study often will differentiate between benign variants and the classic Wilms' tumor. Cystic nephroma in particular may be diagnosed. CT also provides information about extension of the tumor to adjacent organs and will demonstrate enlarged lymph nodes (Fig. 40–6). CT of the chest before operation detects metastases that, after the operation, may be difficult to differentiate from atelectasis or patchy pneumonia. With careful clinical and imaging studies, there should be little difficulty in differentiating Wilms' tumors from cystic lesions, hydronephrosis, renal abscess, and neuroblastoma, all lesions that may occur as a flank mass.

The diagnostic studies and preoperative preparation, consisting of blood transfusion when indicated, and the correction of fluid and electrolyte abnormalities, should take place simultaneously so the child is ready for an operation within 24 hours. There is no evidence that preoperative radiation or chemotherapy improves survival or makes a complete resection any easier by shrinking the tumor. If anything, the surrounding tissue becomes more vascular, the tumor is more friable, and healing is impaired. At the time of operation, intravenous lines are inserted in the upper extremities, and if the tumor is large, a central line is placed in the external jugular vein.

Surgical Technique

The removal of a Wilms' tumor requires a carefully planned anatomic dissection of the retroperitoneal great vessels. Gentleness in handling the tumor to prevent intraoperative spillage of the tumor from the rupture of the capsule is the single most important technical detail influencing survival.[53] Early ligation of the renal vein does not seem to be a critical factor in preventing relapse, and the role of lymph node dissection is still undetermined. However, unless all available lymph nodes are removed with the specimen, it is difficult to assess accurately the intraperitoneal spread of the tumor. The following description of the operation, illustrated in Figure 40–7, outlines the various steps in the operation.

A transverse incision from the flank across the mid-

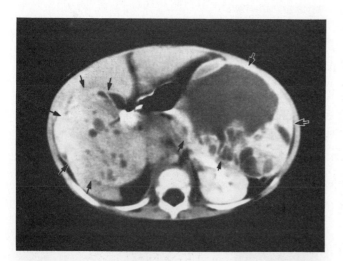

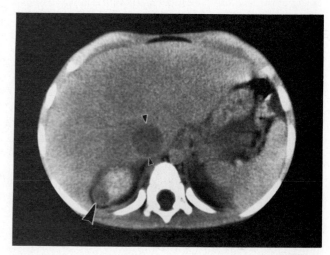

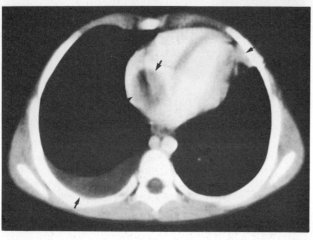

Figure 40–6. This study illustrates the value of CT study in abdominal tumors. **Top left.** The large primary tumor with a hydronephrosis secondary to a uteropelvic junction (UPJ) obstruction on the opposite side. **Top right.** This is a cut through the liver, which demonstrates tumor in the inferior vena cava (arrows). **Left.** A cut through the chest, which demonstrates a pleural effusion, tumor in the right atrium, and a metastasis to the left atrium. All gross tumor was removed at a single operation.

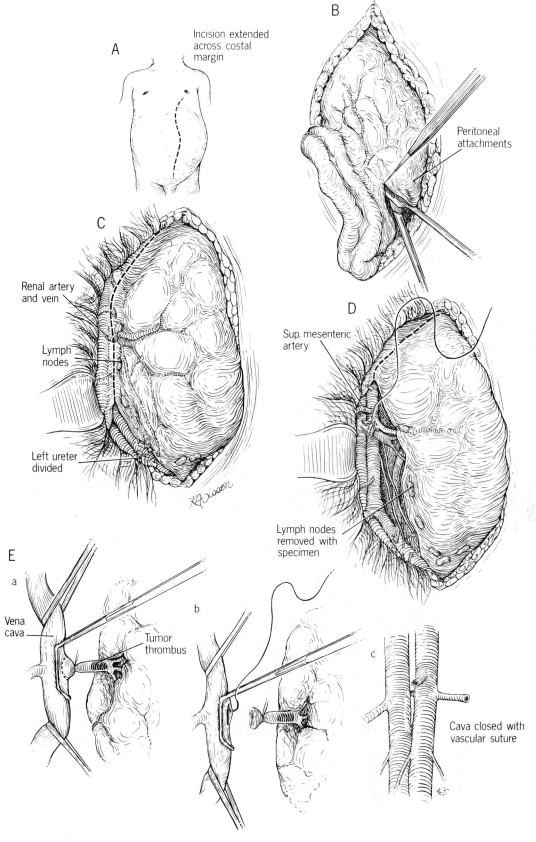

A

Incision extended
across costal
margin

B

Peritoneal
attachments

C

Renal artery
and vein

Lymph
nodes

Left ureter
divided

D

Sup. mesenteric
artery

Lymph nodes
removed with
specimen

E

a

Vena
cava

Tumor
thrombus

b

c

Cava closed with
vascular suture

Figure 40–7. A through H. Kidney resection for Wilms' tumor. (Continued)

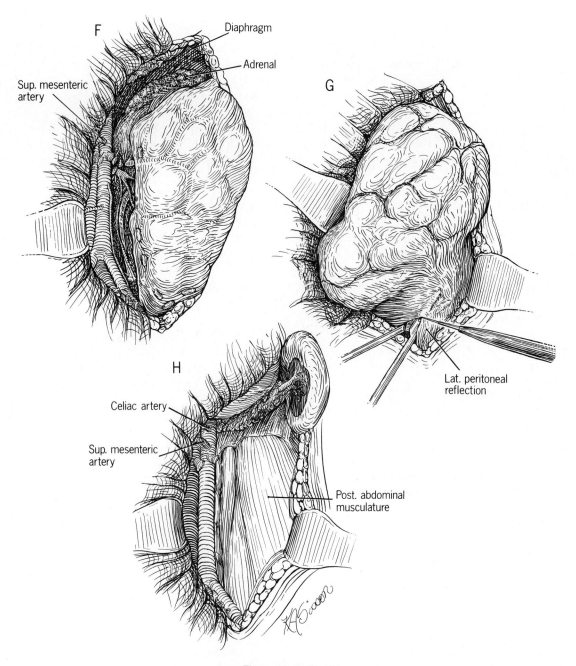

Figure 40–7. (Cont.)

line is satisfactory for small tumors. However, a paramedian incision from the pubis to the costal margin affords optimum exposure for large masses (Fig. 40–7A). We almost routinely divide the costal cartilages to allow for easier retraction of the chest wall that overhangs the kidney in the upper abdomen. The vertical incision provides excellent exposure of the vena cava and the aorta and, when extended across the costal margin, allows freeing of the upper pole from the diaphragm under direct vision. An oblique thoracoabdominal incision is satisfactory, but exposure of the vena cava, aorta, and other structures medial to the tumor has not been as satisfactory as a vertical incision.

The small intestine is eviscerated from the abdomen, and the liver is examined for metastases. The colon overlying the tumor is then held up by an assistant, and with a combination of a sharp scissors dissection and electrocoagulation, the peritoneum lateral to the colon is incised from the pelvis to the flexure (Fig. 40–7B). Electrocoagulation at this point is essential. Otherwise, the many small vessels in the peritoneum will ooze throughout the procedure. If the intestine or mesentery is adherent to the tumor, these structures are resected en bloc with the kidney. On the right side, the lateral attachments of the liver to the abdominal wall are divided to improve exposure at the upper pole. Although most authors recommend ligation of the renal vein at this point, we prefer to expose completely the inferior vena cava and the aorta in order to identify all of the major vessels. Commencing in the pelvis, the iliac vessels are identified and cleared of nodes and overlying tissue (Fig. 40–7C). The gonadal vessels between the aorta and inferior pole are ligated and divided. As the dissection proceeds up the aorta and vena cava, all tissue is freed medially and left attached to the specimen (Fig. 40–7D). On the left side, the inferior mesenteric vein is identified and mobilized to the right with the colon. Also on the left, the renal vein must be dissected free from the superior mesenteric artery. When the vena cava has been dissected above and below the renal vein, both vessels are palpated for tumors. If there is no tumor within the renal vein, it may be doubly ligated and divided (Fig. 40–7E). A 4–0 suture ligature also is applied to the caval side. If there is tumor within the vein but not in the vena cava, a Satinsky clamp is applied across the cava. The renal vein is then divided with a cuff of cava. Next, the intima is inspected for adherent tumor and the vessel closed with a continuous vascular suture. Tumor that extends up the vena cava for a short distance often can be removed by isolating the vena cava above and below with tapes. However, if the vein is solid to the diaphragm, it will be necessary to split the sternum and open the right atrium with cardiopulmonary bypass to remove intracaval or intraatrial tumor. After the aorta has been completely cleared and immediately after the vein has been divided, the renal artery may be ligated. This prevents distention of the tumor with blood. After the renal vein and artery have been controlled, the dissection commences again inferiorly. The previously opened plane on the iliac vessels is continued up the posterolateral abdominal wall directly on the fascia of the lumbar muscles. All lumbar fat is left attached to the specimen. This entire procedure is performed under direct vision with scissors and the electrocautery. The abdominal wall is retracted away rather than forcibly mobilizing the tumor (Fig. 40–7F). As the mobilization is continued superiorly, the diaphragm is encountered (Fig. 40–7G). The chest cage is retracted up and away from the mass so that the dissection may continue under direct vision. At this point, it usually is necessary to again dissect up along the aorta. Above the renal artery, between the aorta and the tumor, there are a number of small vessels and nerve fibers. In this area, great care must be taken to identify the superior mesenteric artery and to ligate every strand of tissue between the aorta and the tumor. If this is not done carefully, bleeding will obscure the anatomy. The dissection anteriorly on the aorta is then carried posteriorly until the plane of dissection on the diaphragm is encountered. The adrenal is removed along with the kidney unless the lesion is small and in the lower pole. The removed specimen should include the kidney, Gerota's fascia, fat from the lumbar fossa, and aortic lymph nodes from the iliac vessels to the superior mesenteric artery (Fig. 40–7H). Any areas in which the tumor may have gone outside the limits of this resection should be biopsied for a frozen section examination. If necessary, portions of the liver or pancreas may be resected. Bleeding from the renal fossa is then controlled with coagulation or suture ligatures, and the bed of the tumor is outlined with metal clips. We irrigate the tumor bed with half-strength Dakin's solution, change gloves and the wound towels, and then expose the contralateral kidney to search for another tumor. Gerota's fascia is opened, and the kidney is mobilized for complete visual inspection and palpation.

Postoperative Care

Following surgery, the stomach is decompressed until peristalsis returns, the urinary output is monitored, and extra whole blood or plasma is given as needed to replace oozing into the tumor bed. The immediate postoperative recovery usually is prompt, and we have observed minimal wound problems despite the extended incision. Perhaps this is because the abdomen is quite relaxed after the resection of a large tumor.

Staging

Further therapy awaits microscopic confirmation of the diagnosis and clinical pathologic staging of the disease. Close cooperation between the surgeon and the pathologist and radiologist is necessary to determine the extent of the disease. The National Wilms' Tumor Registry group staging is as follows:

Stage I: The tumor is limited to the kidney and is completely resected with an intact renal capsule. There is no residual tumor beyond the margins of the resection.

Stage II: The tumor extends beyond the kidney, but it is completely resected. There may be local extension with penetration through the renal capsule into the perirenal fat or beyond, or periaortic lymph nodes may be involved.

Stage III: The residual tumor is confined to the abdomen. The tumor was either biopsied or ruptured during the removal. Implants are on the peritoneal surface and involve lymph nodes beyond the limits of the resection.

Stage IV: Hematogenous metastases to the liver, lung, bone, or brain.

Stage V: Bilateral renal tumors, either initially or subsequently.

TABLE 40–2. CHEMOTHERAPY DRUGS

Name, Form, and Size	Storage	Stability	Administration	Principal Toxicities	Indication
Dactinomysin	Room temp.	Stable 2 weeks in solution	IV	Nausea, vomiting, myelosuppression, diarrhea, alopecia	Wilms' tumor, sarcoma
Doxorubicin, 10 mg vial	Room temp.	Stable 2 weeks in solution	IV	Myelosuppression, nausea, vomiting, stomatitis, fever, cardiomyopathy, alopecia	Wilms' tumor, sarcoma, Hodgkin leukemia
L-Asparaginase, 10,000 µg vial	Refrigerate	Stable 48 hours in solution	IV IM	Hypersensitivity reaction, hyperglycemia, hepatitis (reversible), convulsions	Lymphocytic leukemia, lymphoma
BCNU, 100 mg vial	Refrigerate	Use immediately after mixing	IV	Nausea, vomiting, myelosuppression	CNS tumors, lymphoma
Bleomycin, 15 µg vial	Room temp.	Stable 4 weeks	IV IM	Hypotension, pulmonary fibrosis	Lymphoma, testicular tumors
Cyclophosphamide, 25 to 50 mg tabs, 100, 200, or 500 mg vials	Room temp.	Tabs or stable solution—stable 24 hours	IV IM	Myelosuppression, hemorrhagic cystitis, nausea, vomiting, alopecia	Leukemia, neuroblastoma, lymphoma, sarcoma
Cytosine arabinoside	Refrigerate	Stable 2 weeks in solution	IV IM IT	Myelosuppression, nausea, vomiting, oral ulceration, CNS toxicity associated with its administration	Leukemia, lymphoma
Daunomycin, 20 mg vial	Room temp.	Stable 2 weeks	IV	Myelosuppression, nausea, vomiting, alopecia, cardiomyopathy	Leukemia, lymphoma, Wilms' tumor, neuroblastoma
5-Fluorouracil 500 mg/ 10 ml ampules	Room temp.	Discard opened ampule after using	IV PO	Myelosuppression, nausea, vomiting, diarrhea, stomatitis, cerebellar signs	GI tumors, hepatoma
Imidazole, carboxamide, 100 to 200 mg vials	Refrigerate	Stable for 12 hours after mixing	IV	Myelosuppression, nausea, vomiting, stomatitis	Sarcoma, lymphoma, neuroblastoma
Chlorambucil	Room temp.	Stable indefinitely	PO	Myelosuppression, nausea, vomiting, hepatotoxicity, dermatitis	Sarcoma
Methotrexate, 2 to 5 mg tabs, 5 to 50 mg vials	Room temp.	Tabs and solution stable	PO IV IM IT	Oral ulceration, myelosuppression, hepatitis osteoporosis, CNS toxicity associated with administration	Leukemia, osteogenic sarcoma, lymphoma
Nitrogen mustard, 10 mg vial	Room temp.	Use immediately after mixing	IV	Nausea, vomiting, myelosuppression, diarrhea, alopecia	Hodgkin's disease
Cisplatinum	Refrigerate	Use immediately after mixing	IV	Audio toxicity, nausea, vomiting, renal toxicity	Neuroblastoma, osteogenic sarcoma
Prednisone, 5 mg tabs	Room temp.	Stable	PO	Cushinoid appearance, euphoria, polyphagia	Leukemia, CNS tumor, lymphoma
Vincristine, 1 to 5 mg vials	Refrigerate	Stable for 2 weeks after mixing	IV	Peripheral neuropathy, obstipation, jaw pain, bone marrow depression	Leukemia, Wilms' tumor, neuroblastoma, lymphoma

Each year brings new advances in the care of children with Wilms' tumor, which historically has evolved from a combination of radiation therapy and one course of dactinomycin. National studies have identified those children who benefit from combinations of drugs, primarily vincristine, dactinomycin, and doxorubicin (Table 40–2). The survival rate has improved dramatically, but the toxic effects of radiation with chemotherapy are significant. Radiation causes atrophy of lumbar musculature and inhibits epiphyseal growth. Chemotherapy potentiates radiation, to result in hepatitis, pulmonary fibrosis, bone marrow depression, intestinal disturbances, and skin reactions. Over the years, treatment has been refined to minimize or eliminate these problems. Children with advanced disease do require radiation and multiple-drug therapy. They benefit immensely from the insertion of a central venous catheter that is used both for drug administration and for intravenous nutrition during bouts of anorexia or vomiting. Doxorubicin and cardiac irradiation can result in cardiomyopathy. Consequently, heart function must be monitored with echocardiography and radionuclide gated-pool flow (MUGA). Follow-up chest x-rays are obtained initially at 6-week intervals and then every 3 months. An abdominal ultrasound study is performed every 6 months. Patients with clear cell tumors should also have CT scans of the brain as well as nuclear bone scans searching for metastases. Abdominal ultrasonography is an excellent screening tool for more frequent follow-up because no radiation is required. The Fourth National Wilms' Tumor Study currently is in progress to determine the optimum modes of therapy based on findings from the prior studies. We can anticipate that children with Wilms' tumors diagnosed in 1988 will have an excellent opportunity for disease-free survival, but they will require medical supervision for the duration of their lives because secondary tumors are emerging as a long-term problem.

National Wilms' Tumor Study Results

The first nationwide cooperative study of Wilms' tumors commenced in 1969; eventually 349 of 606 patients were randomized.[54] This study demonstrated that children under 2 years of age with stage I tumors fared well without radiation therapy to the tumor fossa. Children over 2 years of age had a better survival rate when given radiation, and the study also demonstrated that children with advanced stage tumors survived better with a combination of dactinomycin and vincristine than with either drug alone. The second study, from 1974 to 1978, registered 755 children, and in the third national study there were 1164 patients.

The results of the three NWTS have shown the following[55–58]:

1. Patients with unfavorable histology, that is, anaplastic clear cell sarcoma and rhabdoid sarcoma,

have a significantly worse survival than patients with classic Wilms' tumors.
2. Postoperative radiation is unnecessary in patients with stage I favorable histology or anaplastic tumors and patients with stage II favorable histology tumors who receive two-drug therapy with vincristine and dactinomycin.
3. Patients with stage III favorable histology have a better outcome when they receive dactinomycin plus vincristine and either (a) doxorubicin plus 1000 rads to the tumor bed or (b) 2000 rads to the tumor bed.
4. The addition of cyclophosphamide to dactinomycin plus vincristine plus doxorubicin and radiation did not improve the outlook for patients with stage IV disease or tumors with unfavorable histology.
5. The best current 2-year relapse-free survival rates for patients on NWTS 3, by stage and histology are:

Stage I	90–93 percent
Stage II, favorable histology	90–91 percent
Stage III, favorable histology	83–88 percent
Stage IV or unfavorable histology	63–69 percent

NWTS IV currently is underway and is looking at (1) epidemiologic risk factors for Wilms' tumor, (2) correlation of gross and histologic morphology with outcome, and (3) late effects of treatment in the hopes of simplifying drug administration while shortening and intensifying drug delivery schedules. The current therapeutic recommendations are summarized in Figure 40–8.

We have now treated 215 children with Wilms' tumors at the Children's Memorial Hospital in Chicago from 1964 to June of 1987. There has been a steady improvement in survival rates. Since the formation of the National Wilms' Tumor Study groups, our patients have been treated according to protocol. In the 5-year period before 1969, there was only a 50 percent overall survival rate. Since 1975, we have treated 122 patients with 100 percent survival in stages I, II, and III (Table 40–3). There is still room for improvement because the survival rate in the 17 patients with stage IV tumors was only 47 percent overall. For patients operated on at our hospital, the survival rate was 63 percent.

BILATERAL TUMORS

Improved imaging techniques and the practice of exposing and carefully examining the contralateral kidney have resulted in an increased detection of bilateral tumors (Fig. 40–9). Seventeen of our most recent 122 patients had bilateral lesions, an incidence of 13 percent. In these patients, we must not only make every effort to cure the disease, but we must preserve kidney tissue. In

SCHEMA

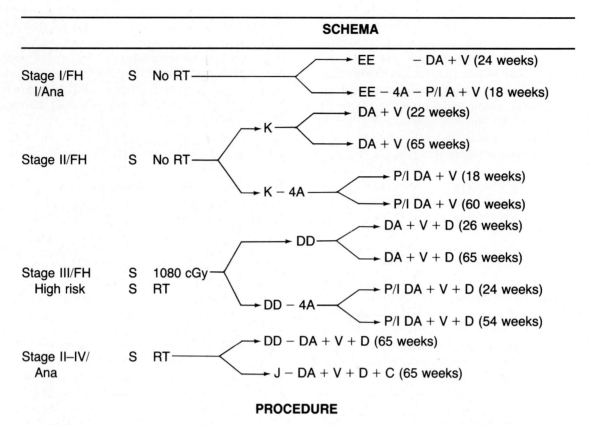

PROCEDURE

1. All patients should have an excretory urogram or opacified CT scan of the abdomen for accurate placement of radiation therapy portals.

2. The initial randomization to standard or pulsed, intensive chemotherapy is to take place within 72 hours of nephrectomy, which is day zero, but not later than 5 days thereafter.

3. The radiation therapist should be alerted and a simulation appointment requested for not later than day 9.

Figure 40–8. Fourth National Wilms' Tumor Study. Procedures and study design at a glance. S, surgery; RT, radiation therapy; FH, favorable histology; DA, dactinomycin; D, doxorubicin; V, vincristine; C, cyclophosphamide; Ana, anaplastic tumors; P/I, pulsed, intensive; High risk, clear cell sarcoma of kidney (CCSK, all stages), and stage IV/FH. CCSK patients and stage IV/FH patients receive XRT (1080 cGy) if the primary tumor would qualify as stage III were there no metastases.

the past, the kidney with the largest tumor was resected, and the tumor in the contralateral kidney was treated with either radiation or a heminephrectomy. Chemotherapy was then added to the treatment regimens. With these various modes of treatment, 8 of 14 patients treated at our hospital from 1956 to 1978 survived.[59] At least 3 of these deaths were caused by the vigorous radiation and chemotherapy programs in use at that time.

Bilateral nephrectomy and transplantation were attempted in several centers, but this procedure is no longer recommended except in a last-ditch effort to cure residual tumor.[60,61] In an effort to salvage as much renal tissue as possible, the recommendation has been made to biopsy, then administer chemotherapy, and then operate 3 to 6 months later to resect residual tumor.[62–64] It

is too early to evaluate the role of chemotherapy with delayed excision, and as yet, there is no completely satisfactory protocol for bilateral tumors because there is so much variability in their size, mode of presentation, and histology.

In 1976, Weiner recommended bilateral partial nephrectomies for large tumors.[65] This has been our choice of treatment since his report. When the diagnosis of bilateral tumors is made on preoperative studies, we plan on bilateral tumorectomy. This operation differs somewhat from a standard heminephrectomy because we follow the plane of the tumor pseudocapsule, with minimal effort to remove a rim of normal kidney with the tumor. It is necessary to completely mobilize the kidney after opening Gerota's fascia. The renal artery

TABLE 40–3. SURVIVAL RATES BY STAGE AND PATHOLOGY IN 122 PATIENTS 1975–1987, CHILDREN'S MEMORIAL HOSPITAL

Stage	Number	Survival Rate (%)
I	32	100
II	34	100
III	22	100
IV	17	47 of those treated overall
		63 of those whose entire treatment was at CMH
V	17	76
Sarcoma	13	38
Renal cell carcinoma	3	33
Benign variant	4	100

and vein are looped for control. The dissection is commenced, however, without clamping the renal vessels. By dissecting with the coagulation current on the surface of the kidney, a plane is started that can be continued with blunt dissection. Bleeding is controlled with coagulation, suture ligatures, and occasionally Gelfoam. It usually is possible to leave from one half to three fourths of each kidney after resecting the tumors (Fig. 40–10). When a contralateral small lesion is found after completing a nephrectomy, it is merely wedged out, leaving almost all the kidney. Multicentric small tumors also may be removed by wedge excisions or tumorectomy. When a biopsy of the contralateral kidney reveals nephroblastomatosis, the lesion is removed if possible, but most often this lesion is either multiple or diffuse

throughout the kidney. A biopsy is performed, chemotherapy is given, and the lesion is followed with CT scans. A second-look operation with rebiopsy is carried out at a later date. Thirteen of our most recent 17 patients treated for bilateral Wilms' tumor have survived (76 percent).

METASTATIC DISEASE

There were no lung metastases in our 32 stage I patients and they developed in only 3 of 56 stage II and III patients. All were cured by chemotherapy, radiation, and surgical resection. One child developed a second tumor, a chondromyxoid fibroma, 8 years after treatment for his Wilms' tumor. Eight of 17 patients with stage IV disease had lung metastases when first diagnosed. Four appear to be cured with surgical resection when the lung lesions persisted after drug and radiation therapy. Four patients died with lung and liver metastases unresponsive to therapy. The current NWTS protocol treats lung metastases that are present at onset with chemotherapy and total lung radiation. If the lesions fail to respond or recur after an initial response, they are removed surgically. Lung metastases that appear while the child is on therapy also are removed. Most lesions are on the surface of the lung and are removed easily by wedge resection. Only deeper or larger metastases require a lobectomy.

We have operated for multiple, recurrent metastases, with ultimate control of the disease. Aggressive surgical excision is preferable to repeated therapy with radiation, since pneumonitis and fibrosis with pulmonary

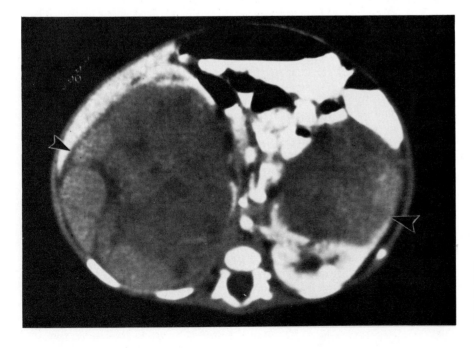

Figure 40–9. Bilateral, large Wilms' tumors. On the left, there is a rim of normal kidney around the darker tumor tissue. On the right, the arrow indicates tumor partly enveloped by a rim of normal kidney.

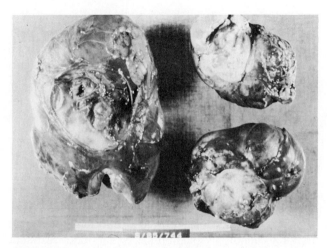

Figure 40–10. This child had a large focus of Wilms' tumor in the left kidney and two smaller lesions in the right. All were removed by tumorectomy, leaving more than 75 percent of her normal functioning kidneys.

failure are long-term complications of intense radiation to the lung.

Intracardiac extension of tumor from the vena cava is an invitation to tumor embolization. Consequently, these patients require a combined radical nephrectomy with simultaneous removal of the atrial tumor with the aid of cardiopulmonary bypass. All 4 of our patients have recovered from this combined approach and are alive and free of disease from 2 to 8 years. As an example of our aggressive surgical approach to Wilms' tumor, one of these children had a simultaneous resection of a lung metastasis and a wedge resection of a tumor from the contralateral kidney.

Involved portions of the liver should be resected at the time of the original operation for Wilms' tumor when there is either direct tumor invasion or a metastasis. Hepatic lobectomy rather than further radiation therapy is indicated for liver metastases. Chemotherapy must be delayed for at least 3 weeks after surgery to allow the liver to regenerate.[66–68]

Brain metastases, although rare, must be considered when a child develops central nervous system signs after the removal of a Wilms' tumor. These lesions may respond to radiotherapy and to excision.[69,70]

There are still problems to be solved in the management of children with Wilms' tumors. We hope that more children will survive as better and perhaps less toxic chemotherapeutic agents are developed. The problem is not over when the tumor has apparently been cured. Schwartz et al. found five cases of leukemia in children who were apparently cured of the original tumor.[71] Obviously, a child who has been treated for Wilms' tumor must be followed throughout his or her lifetime for new tumors and for complications of therapy.[72]

REFERENCES

1. Miller RW: Deaths from childhood cancer in sibs. N Engl J Med 279:122, 1968
2. Young JL, Miller R: Incidence of malignant tumors in U.S. children. J Pediatr 86:254, 1975
3. Ravitch MM, Thomasson B: Wilms' tumor. Urol Surv 11:83, 1961
4. Gross RE, Neuhauser EBD: Treatment of mixed tumors of the kidney in childhood. Pediatrics 6:843, 1950
5. Beckwith J: Wilms' tumors of childhood: A selective review from the NWTS pathology center. Hum Pathol 14:481, 1983
6. Beckwith J, Palmer N: Histopathology and prognosis of Wilms' tumor: Results from the First National Wilms' Tumor Study. Cancer 41:1937, 1978
7. Bonadio J, Storer B, Norkool P, et al: Anaplastic Wilms' tumors: A clinical and pathological study. J Clin Oncol 3:513, 1985
8. Haas J, Palmer N, Weinberg H, Beckwith J: Ultrastructure of malignant rhabdoid tumor of the kidney. A distinctive renal tumor of children. Hum Pathol 12:646, 1981
9. Palmer N, Sutow W: Clinical aspects of the rhabdoid tumor of the kidney: A report of the National Wilms' Tumor Study group. Med Pediatr Oncol 11:242, 1983
10. Morgan E, Kidd J: Undifferentiated sarcoma of the kidney: A tumor of childhood with histopathologic and clinical characteristics distinct from Wilms' tumor. Cancer 42:1916, 1978
11. Ugarte N, Gonzalez-Crussi F, Hsueh W: Wilms' tumor: Its morphology under one year of age. Cancer 48:346, 1981
12. Marsden HB, Lawler W: Bone metastasizing renal tumor of childhood: Histopathological and clinical review of 38 cases. Virchows Arch Pathol Anat 387:341, 1980
13. Thompson MR, Emmanuel IG, Campbell MS, Zachary RB: Extrarenal Wilms' tumor. J Pediatr Surg 8:37, 1973
14. Andrews M, Askin F, Fried F, et al: Cystic partially differentiated nephroblastoma and polycystic Wilms' tumor: A spectrum of related clinical and pathologic entities. J Urol 129:577, 1983
15. Madewell J, Goldman S, Davis C, et al: Multilocular cystic nephroma: A radiologic–pathologic correlation of 58 patients. Radiology 146:309, 1983
16. Machin G: Nephroblastomatosis and multiple bilateral nephroblastomatosis. Arch Pathol Lab Med 102:639, 1978
17. Bove K, McAdams A: The nephroblastomatosis complex and relationship to Wilms' tumor: A clinicopathologic treatise. Pediatr Pathol 3:185, 1976
18. Machin G: Persistent renal blastema (nephroblastomatosis) as a frequent precursor of Wilms' tumor: A pathological and clinical review. Part 3. Clinical aspects of nephroblastomatosis. Am J Pediatr Hematol Oncol 2:353, 1980
19. Bolande RP, Brough AJ, Izant RJ: Congenital mesoblastic nephroma of infancy. Pediatrics 40:272, 1967
20. Beckwith JB: Mesenchymal renal neoplasms of infancy. J Pediatr Surg 5:405, 1970
21. Waisman J, Cooper PH: Renal neoplasms of the newborn. J Pediatr Surg 5:407, 1970

22. Richmond H, Dougall AJ: Neonatal renal tumors. J Pediatr Surg 5:413, 1970

23. Smith TW, Allen MS, Gillenwater JY: Benign renal tumors in children: Report of a case. J Urol 110:470, 1973

24. Burkholder GV, Beach PD, Hall R: Tumors. J Urol 104:330, 1970

25. Reeder F, Morse TS: Renal leiomyoma in a newborn infant. Am J Surg 104:788, 1962

26. Bogdan R, Taylor DEM, Mostofi FK: Leiomyomatous hamartoma of the kidney. Cancer 31:462, 1973

27. Walker D, Richard GA: Fetal hamartoma of the kidney: recurrence and death of patient. J Urol 110:352, 1973

28. Joshi VV, Kay S, Milsten R, et al: Congenital mesoblastic report of a case with unusual clinical behavior. Am J Clin Pathol 60:811, 1973

29. Beckwith JB: Mesenchymal renal neoplasms of infancy revisited. J Pediatr Surg 9:803, 1974

30. Willis RA: The Borderland of Embryology and Pathology. London, Butterworth, 1962, chap 11

31. Pulling GP: Wilms' tumor in seven children with congenital aniridia. J Pediatr Surg 10:87, 1975

32. Fraumeni JF Jr, Glass AG: Wilms' tumor and congenital aniridia. JAMA 206:825, 1968

33. Riccardi V, Sujanski E, Smith A, et al: Chromosomal imbalance in the Aniridia-Wilms' tumor association: 11p interstitial deletion. Pediatrics 61:604, 1978

34. Vunis J, Ramsay N: Familial occurrence of the aniridian Wilms' tumor syndrome with deletion: 11p 13–14.1. J Pediatr 96:1027, 1980

35. Sotelo-Avila C, Gonzalez-Crussi F, Fowler J: Complete or incomplete forms of Beckwith-Weideman syndrome: Their oncogenic potential. J Pediatr 96:47, 1980

36. Fraumeni JF Jr, Geiser CF, Manning MD: Wilms' tumor and congenital hemihypertrophy: Report of five new cases and review of literature. Pediatrics 40:886, 1967

37. Pendergrass T: Congenital anomalies in children with Wilms' tumor. Cancer 37:403, 1976

38. Breslow N, Beckwith J: Epidemiological features of Wilms' tumor: Results of the National Wilms' Tumor Study. J Natl Cancer Inst 68:429, 1982

39. Behleshti M, Mancer J, Hardy B, et al: External genital abnormalities associated with Wilms' tumor. Urology 24:130, 1984

40. Goldman S, Garfinkel D, Dorst J: The Drash syndrome: Male pseudohermaphroditism, nephritis and Wilms' tumor. Radiology 141:87, 1981

41. McCoy F, Franklin W, Aronson A, Spargo B: Glomerulonephritis associated with male pseudohermaphroditism and nephroblastoma. Am J Pathol 7:387, 1983

42. Brown WT, Puranik SR, Altman DH, et al: Wilms' tumor in three successive generations. Surgery 72:756, 1972

43. Meadows AT, Lichtenfeld JL, Koop CE: Wilms' tumor in three children of a woman with congenital hemihypertrophy. N Engl J Med 291:23, 1974

44. Cordero J, Li F, Holmes L, et al: Wilms' tumor in five cousins. Pediatrics 66:716, 1980

45. Li F, Williams W, Gimbrere K, et al: Heritable fraction of unilateral Wilms' tumor. Pediatrics 81:147, 1988

46. Knudson A, Strong L: Mutation and cancer: A model for Wilms' tumor of the kidney. J Natl Cancer Inst 48:313, 1972

47. Bove KE, McAdams AJ: The nephroblastomatosis complex and its relationship to Wilms' tumor: A clinicopathologic treatise. In HS Rosenberg, RP Bolande (eds): Perspectives in Pediatric Pathology. Chicago, Year Book, 1976, pp 185–223

48. Mitchell JD, Baxter TJ, Blair-West JR, et al: Renin levels in nephroblastoma (Wilms' tumor). Arch Dis Child 45:376, 1970

49. Sukarchana K, Kieswetter WB, Tolentino W: Wilms' tumor and hypertension. J Pediatr Surg 7:573, 1972

50. Utley JR, Mobin-Uddin K, Segnitz RH, et al: Acute obstruction of tricuspid valve by Wilms' tumor. J Thorac Cardiovasc Surg 66:626, 1973

51. Schullinger JN, Santulli TV, Casarella WJ, et al: The role of right heart angiography in the management of selected cases. Ann Surg 185:451, 1977

52. Luck S, DeLeon S, Shkolnik A, et al: Intracardiac Wilms' tumor: Diagnosis and management. J Pediatr Surg 17:551, 1982

53. Leape LL, Breslow NE, Bishop HC: The surgical treatment of Wilms' tumor: results of the National Wilms' Tumor Study. Ann Surg 187:351, 1976

54. D'Angio GJ, Evans A, Breslow N, et al: The treatment of Wilms' tumor: Results of the National Wilms' Tumor Study. Cancer 38:633, 1976

55. D'Angio GJ, Evans A, Breslow N, et al: The treatment of Wilms' tumor: Results of the second National Wilms' tumor study. Cancer 47:2302, 1981

56. Bonadio J, Storer B, Norkool P, et al: Anaplastic Wilms' tumor: clinical and pathological studies. J Clin Oncol 3:513, 1985

57. Breslow N, Churchill G, Beckwith JB, et al: Prognosis for Wilms' tumor patients with metastatic disease at diagnosis. Results of the second National Wilms' tumor study. J Clin Oncol 3:521, 1985

58. D'Angio GJ, Evans A, Breslow N, et al: Results of the third National Wilms' tumor study (NWTS3): A preliminary report [Abstract]. Proc AACR 25:183, 1984

59. Wasiljew B, Besser A, Raffensperger J: Treatment of bilateral Wilms' tumors—A 22-year experience. J Pediatr Surg 17:265, 1982

60. DeMaria J, Hardy B, Brzezinski , et al: Renal transplantation in patients with bilateral Wilms' tumors. J Pediatr Surg 14:577, 1979

61. Penn I: Renal transplantation for Wilms' tumors: Report of 20 cases. J Urol 122:193, 1979

62. Ducos R, Falterman K: Needle biopsy and preoperative chemotherapy for massive unilateral and bilateral Wilms' tumor [Group minutes, March]. Pediatr Oncol 24:65, 1985

63. Kelalis P: Surgical treatment: NWTS recommendations. Dial Pediatr Urol 8:6, 1985

64. Tucker O, McGill C, Pokorny W, et al: Bilateral Wilms' tumors. J Pediatr Surg 21:1110, 1986

65. Weiner E: Bilateral partial nephrectomies for large bilateral Wilms' tumors. J Pediatr Surg 11:867, 1976

66. Wedemeyer PP, White JG, Nesbit ME, et al: Resection of metastases in Wilms' tumor: A report of three cases

cured of pulmonary and hepatic metastases. Pediatrics 41:446, 1968

67. Smith WB, Wara WM, Margolis LW, et al: Partial hepatectomy in metastatic Wilms' tumor. J Pediatr 84:259, 1974

68. Filler RM, Tefft M, Vauter GF, et al: Hepatic lobectomy in childhood: Effects of x-ray and chemotherapy. J Pediatr Surg 4:31, 1969

69. Traggis D, Jaffe N, Tefft M, et al: Successful treatment of Wilms' tumor with intracranial metastases. Pediatrics 56:472, 1975

70. Morgan SK, Buse MG: Survial following brain metastases in Wilms' tumor. Pediatrics 58:130, 1976

71. Schwartz AD, Lee H, Baum ES: Leukemia in children with Wilms' tumor. J Pediatr 87:374, 1975

72. Li F, Sellan S, et al: Second neoplasms after Wilms' tumor in childhood. J Natl Cancer Inst 71:1205, 1983

41
Neuroblastoma and Ganglioneuroma

John G. Raffensperger
Edward S. Baum

Neuroblastomas and related tumors are among the most baffling, interesting, and frustrating malignancies in childhood. Some well-advanced lesions may completely regress spontaneously or mature into benign ganglioneuromas. Others with similar histology relentlessly invade, metastasize, and cause death in spite of intensive therapy. Neuroblastomas have unique immune and biochemical properties that aid in their diagnosis and may someday provide answers to their mysterious behavior. Perhaps the riddles posed by neuroblastoma hold the key to understanding the behavior of other malignancies.

Neuroblastomas and ganglioneuromas are derived from cells that originate in the embryonic neural crest. These parent cells give rise to the sympathetic nervous system and adrenal medulla. Tumors may develop anywhere from the base of the skull to the presacral area. Most are found in the retroperitoneal space, where it is not always possible to determine whether a large lesion arose from the adrenal gland or from the adjacent sympathetic ganglia. Presumably, if the kidney is displaced inferiorly, the tumor arose from the adrenal. Approximately 25 percent of neuroblastomas originate in the mediastinum, pelvis, or neck.

PATHOLOGY

Grossly, the typical abdominal neuroblastoma is unencapsulated and is insinuated about the aorta and the renal and mesenteric vessels. It is densely adherent to adjacent structures and grows through tissue planes to invade the mesentery and intraabdominal organs. On cut section, there may be a rim of highly vascular tissue surrounding a semiliquid necrotic center. Solid portions are red to yellow, soft, and friable. Paravertebral neuroblastomas also may invade the vertebral foramina and compress the spinal cord. Metastases are common in adjacent lymph nodes but also occur in bone, liver, and skin. Ganglioneuromas and ganglioneuroblastomas, on the other hand, often are encapsulated and do not invade adjoining tissues, have smooth surfaces and are firm in consistency, and the cut surface is yellow.

Microscopically, a neuroblastoma varies from diffuse sheets of undifferentiated small round cells to recognizable neuroblasts (Fig. 41–1). Rosettes can be seen in about a third of these tumors, and with special stains, nerve processes may be observed. Calcification is seen in about 50 percent of neuroblastomas. Ganglioneuromas contain fully differentiated ganglion cells in a connective tissue stroma. Careful examination of ganglioneuromas often will demonstrate scattered islands of neuroblasts. These tumors must be termed "ganglioneuroblastomas" because the islands of malignancy may metastasize. It is possible that these tumors represent the maturation of a neuroblastoma into a ganglioneuroma. It is often difficult to differentiate neuroblastomas from other small, blue, round cell tumors, such as Ewing's sarcoma or lymphoma.[1] For this reason, tissue always must be obtained for electron microscopy to identify neurofilaments and neurosecretory granules.[2] Immunohistologic detection of a nerve-specific enzyme, neuronospecific enolase, and antibody studies for specific tumor antigens also are helpful.[3,4] All of these studies should be done in

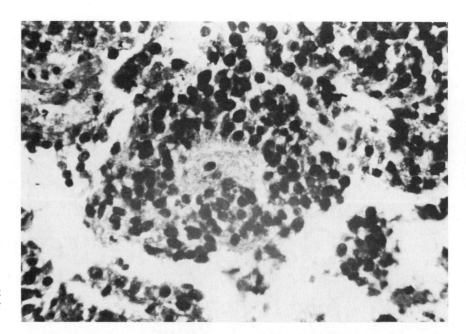

Figure 41–1. Neuroblastoma. The small dark cells are difficult to differentiate from other small cell malignant tumors.

every case, in the hope of further elucidating some of the mysteries of these tumors.

There are ongoing attempts to relate the histology of neuroblastoma to prognosis in individual patients. The Shimada classification takes into account the degree of tumor cell maturation, age, karyorrhexis index, and presence or absence of a neurofibromatous stroma.[5] The more fibrous the stroma and the more cells that have differentiated into ganglion cells, the better the prognosis.

BIOCHEMISTRY

There is an increased synthesis of dopa, dopamine, norepinephrine, and other catecholamines in neural crest tumors. Clinically, the most important metabolic pathways include the degradation of norepinephrine to vanilmandelic acid (VMA) and dopamine to homovanillic acid (HVA). The biochemistry by which these compounds are secreted and broken down has been described in detail by many authors.[6–8]

Levels of the norepinephrine derivative VMA are elevated in 80 percent of children with neuroblastoma, and when determinations of VMA, HVA, and total catecholamines are performed with 24-hour urine specimens, the diagnostic accuracy approaches 100 percent.[9,10] If the VMA level is elevated beyond 7 mg after 24 hours, the test is considered positive. If the VMA is not elevated, the total catecholamines in a 24-hour specimen are measured. Serial determinations of urinary catecholamine levels can be helpful in determining recurrences as well as the need for another operation or more chemotherapy. Neurospecific enolase and serum ferritin produced by neuroblasts may be useful tumor markers to indicate

prognosis and to follow the course of the disease.[11–13] Human neuroblastoma cell lines have multiple copies of a DNA sequence that is related to the Y-MYC and C-MYC oncogenes, termed N-MYC oncogene. Untreated primary neuroblastomas, especially those with widespread disease, have multiple copies of the N-MYC oncogene. Patients with amplification of the N-MYC oncogene have a worse prognosis; consequently, N-MYC amplification is an important prognostic indicator.[14–16]

IMMUNE ASPECTS, SPONTANEOUS REGRESSION, AND MATURATION

Neuroblastoma undergoes spontaneous regression more frequently than does any other human malignancy.[17] Furthermore, small neuroblastomas are incidental findings in 1 percent of infants at birth who die from other causes.[18] This spontaneous regression of both the primary tumor and metastases, leading to complete disappearance of the tumor, occurs almost exclusively in children under 1 year of age.

Maturation to a benign ganglioneuroma also may limit the course of the disease. The presence of ganglioneuroma in lymph nodes adjacent to the primary tumor provides indirect evidence that the tumor evolved from a malignant lesion.[19] Even more conclusive are patients in whom biopsies at successive operations have demonstrated the evolution from a highly cellular malignant lesion to one that has fewer mature cells with more stroma.[20,21]

There may be immunologic differences between patients who survived the disease and those who died.[22] Lymphocytes appear to be of some importance, since the mean pretreatment lymphocyte count of survivors was 7600, whereas the mean count in children who died was 5300. Furthermore, some correlation was found between survival and increased lymphocytic infiltration of the tumor. Lymphocytes from both surviving patients and those dying of their tumors demonstrated in vitro cytotoxic activity. A blocking antibody acts against the activity of the cytotoxic lymphocytes in children with active disease. There is also cytotoxic activity in the serum against tumor cells in patients with neuroblastoma, but unfortunately one also finds a blocking antibody against the serum cytotoxic activity. The blocking antibodies were not found in the serum of children cured of the disease.[23] More recent studies have failed to confirm any consistent relationship between prognosis and degree of lymphocytic infiltration of the tumor. In addition, the lower lymphocyte counts in children who die from the disease may reflect bone marrow displacement by tumor cells.[24] Attempts are now being made to direct the immune mechanism against neuroblastoma. Murine IgG$_3$ antibodies activate human complement and affect in vitro antibody-dependent cellular cytotoxicity.[25]

CLINICAL FINDINGS

More than half of the children with a neuroblastoma have an abdominal mass. Irritability, anorexia, weight loss, and fever are more common in children with neuroblastoma than in those with Wilms' tumors. Older children, in particular, are likely to have symptoms such as bone pain (which unfortunately is caused by metastases), fever of undetermined origin, or other vague and misleading symptoms. Skin metastases, proptosis, and lumps about the skull are other metastatic signs that may be present before the primary tumor is discovered. Chronic and occasionally severe intractable diarrhea may be associated with neural crest tumors, particularly ganglioneuromas and ganglioneuroblastomas. In these cases, in which catecholamine excretion is increased, other vasoactive intestinal hormones also have been isolated.[26] Neurologic symptoms consisting of paralysis and sensory changes may result from spinal cord pressure, dumbbell tumors, or cerebral metastases.[27] Even more unusual neurologic symptoms, consisting of ataxia speech impairment and rapid, flickering eye movements, have been described in children with neuroblastoma.[28] As yet, there is no explanation for this syndrome, termed "myoclonic encephalopathy," although it appears to be more commonly associated with mediastinal neuroblastomas. Attempts to explain the central nervous system damage as a toxic effect of elevated catecholamines would seem to be dispelled by the report of a patient in whom the myoclonus developed 19 months

after successful treatment, when the urinary catecholamine excretion was normal.[29]

On physical examination, the retroperitoneal neuroblastoma is hard and irregular, crosses the midline, and is fixed to surrounding tissues. In babies, the liver is more likely to be palpable than is the primary tumor. Indeed, the liver may be diffusely infiltrated with tumor, and a primary lesion may never be found. The liver will be hard and irregular and may fill almost the entire abdominal cavity. Mediastinal tumors are found on chest roentgenograms, which are often obtained for symptoms unrelated to the tumor. Pelvic neuroblastomas cause urinary, bowel, or rectal symptoms and are discovered on rectal examination.

An obvious abdominal mass is investigated with a computed tomography (CT) scan, which will demonstrate downward displacement of the kidney if the tumor originates in the adrenal, or medial displacement of the ureter with paravertebral masses. The CT scan also will demonstrate the relationship of the tumor to the celiac axis and mesenteric arteries or extension through the diaphragm, which will aid in determining the operability of the tumor (Fig. 41–2). CT scans are valuable in mediastinal or other paravertebral tumors to determine involvement of the spinal cord by extension through vertebral foramina (Fig. 41–3). Magnetic resonance imaging (MRI) may be superior in determining the extent of disease and operability. A 24-hour urine sample is obtained for catecholamines, and a test for serum neurospecific enolase and ferritin is carried out. It is essential to determine bone marrow involvement to define the extent of disease. Consequently, both bone scans and bone marrow aspiration are indicated. In some centers, radiolabeled meta-iodobenzyl guanidine allow imaging of bone as well as the primary tumor, since it is taken up by adrenergic tissue.[30]

Solitary neuroblasts may be mistaken for leukemia on bone marrow aspirates if rosettes are not present. Thus, it is essential to use biochemical tumor markers and monoclonal antibodies to be certain of the diagnosis, especially in the absence of a mass.[31] If the bone marrow is normal or nondiagnostic, an operation is indicated for either biopsy or tumor excision. Tissue must be preserved for routine and electron microscopy and a full battery of histochemical and immune studies.

While diagnostic studies are in progress, anemia, dehydration, or intercurrent infections are treated to prepare the child for an operation.

TREATMENT

Therapy for neuroblastomas depends on the child's age, the tumor's location, and clinical staging. Complete surgical removal, the treatment of choice, is more likely

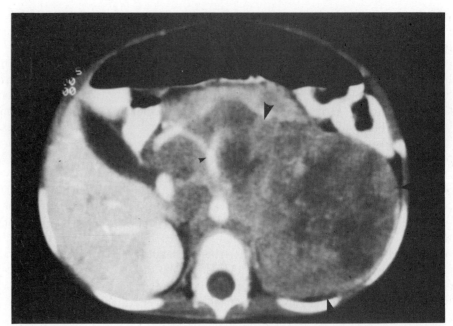

Figure 41–2. The large retroperitoneal neuroblastoma (large arrows) surrounds the celiac axis (small arrows). The hepatic and splenic arteries have the appearance of a seagull's wings.

to be possible in tumors located in the neck, mediastinum, or pelvis than with retroperitoneal lesions.

ABDOMINAL NEUROBLASTOMA

Abdominal neuroblastomas in infants and children under 1 year of age, especially when there is extensive liver involvement, have a unique prognosis. If a tissue diagnosis can be made on the basis of a bone marrow aspiration or by needle biopsy of the liver, an operation is not indicated. These are the children whose tumors are most likely to undergo spontaneous regression with little or no therapy.[32,33] Schnaufer and Koop studied 11 infants with stage IV-S lesions, 8 of whom survived.[34] Two of their patients died with respiratory distress and inferior vena cava compression because of a rapidly enlarging liver. In 2 children, they created a large ventral hernia with a Silastic patch as a temporary measure to decompress the abdomen. One of these patients survived; the other died with sepsis. One of our patients also died with sepsis after application of a Silastic patch. We now prefer to create a skin-covered ventral hernia by undermining the skin through a small upper abdominal incision. Then the fascia and peritoneum are divided in the midline.

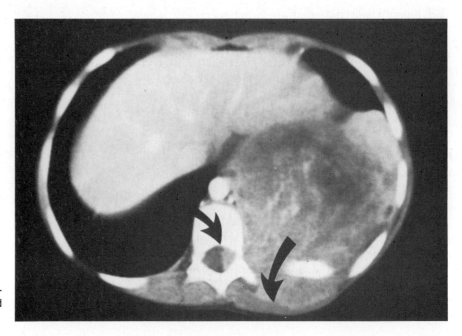

Figure 41–3. The arrows indicate a neuroblastoma extending into the spinal cord and the paravertebral muscles.

Surgical Technique

Preoperative imaging studies may indicate the extent of disease and operability, but what appears to be the primary tumor surrounding major vessels may actually be lymph nodes. Therefore, surgical exploration is indicated to remove the tumor if possible or at least to obtain a generous biopsy. To completely evaluate and remove the tumor, a long thoracoabdominal incision, as described for Wilms' tumor, is indicated. The entire chest and abdomen are prepared, and large-bore intravenous lines are placed in upper extremity or jugular veins. If a preliminary dissection indicates tumor invading adjacent organs or surrounding major vessels, it should only be biopsied, treated with chemotherapy, and reoperated when the tumor is smaller.

The aorta and inferior vena cava are identified, usually at the inferior edge of the tumor. With careful, persistent dissection, a plane may be found between the tumor and major vessels. It is often possible to separate lymph nodes from the tumor to preserve the mesenteric and celiac arteries. There should be no hesitation to remove one involved kidney, but if other organs are involved, the tumor should be left alone. All lymph nodes along the aorta and vena cava should be removed for complete surgical staging.

Paraspinal masses with extension through vertebral foramina or spinal cord involvement require a different approach. These patients are positioned on their side, and an incision is made that extends from the vertebra, transversely across the abdomen. In these lateral tumors, there is less involvement with the major vessels, and they can be freed from their intraabdominal attachments and dissected to the vertebra. Then, by removing bone from about the foramina, extensions into the spinal canal may be removed by a neurosurgical team. This simultaneous approach, which allows a complete one-stage tumor removal, is better than the usual approach via a posterior laminectomy and a separate anterior abdominal incision.

PELVIC NEUROBLASTOMA

Approximately 5 percent of neuroblastomas in children arise in the pelvis. The symptoms of urinary retention, constipation, and frequently edema and vascular engorgement of the legs draw attention to the tumor earlier than do abdominal masses. Rectal examination will reveal a firm mass posterior to the rectum in the presacral space that is indistinguishable from a presacral teratoma. A CT scan will demonstrate displacement of the bladder forward with ureteral obstruction. The diagnosis can be made if the usual tumor markers are elevated. Treatment consists of surgical excision by the presacral route, if possible, or, if necessary, by a combined sacral and ab-

dominal approach. In two series involving a total of 9 patients, all were under 2 years of age and most were very young infants.[35,36] All except 1 had survived from 3 to 22 years after the diagnosis had been made, even though complete excision was performed in only 2. The 1 child who died had an intestinal obstruction and no tumor at autopsy. The excellent survival rate with pelvic neuroblastomas once again appears to be related more to the young age of the patient at the time of diagnosis than to therapy.

MEDIASTINAL NEUROBLASTOMA

Posterior mediastinal tumors are of neurogenic origin. They may be completely asymptomatic and found incidentally on a chest roentgenogram. On the other hand, large thoracic neuroblastomas may cause severe respiratory distress in the neonatal period.[37] Other clinical findings may include Horner's syndrome and neurologic symptoms from spinal cord compression. The chest x-ray demonstrates a paravertebral soft tissue mass in the posterior mediastinum. Separation and erosion of the ribs are findings that help differentiate neuroblastomas from ganglioneuromas.[38] CT scans are most helpful in evaluating extension of the tumor through the foramina. The usual thoracic neuroblastoma is removed easily through a posterolateral thoracotomy. The pleura medial to the tumor is opened, and the mass is dissected free from the aorta and esophagus. Intercostal arteries are ligated as necessary, and occasionally it is necessary to remove portions of ribs with the mass. If preoperative studies suggest intraspinal extension, a combined neurosurgical–thoracic approach is planned. The patient is placed in a prone lateral position to provide access to the posterior mediastinum as well as the vertebral canal. After the mediastinal portion of the tumor has been mobilized, the foramina are opened by removing the lateral portion of the vertebral pedicle and arch. This provides excellent exposure of the intraspinal portion of the tumor and allows en bloc removal in one stage.

STAGING

Tumor staging is important to determine therapy and prognosis. A preliminary idea of the tumor stage is based on preoperative studies. Final staging must await the gross operative findings, combined with microscopic examination of lymph nodes and adjacent tissue. The staging system proposed by Evans et al. is used by most institutions. The stages are as follows[39]:

Stage I: Tumor confined to the organ or structure of origin.

Stage II: Tumors extending in continuity beyond the organ or structure of origin, but not beyond the midline. Regional lymph nodes on the ipsilateral side may be involved.*

Stage III: Tumors extending in continuity beyond the midline. Regional lymph nodes may be involved bilaterally.

Stage IV: Remote disease involving the skeleton, organs, soft tissue, or distant lymph node groups, etc.

Stage IV-S: This includes patients who would otherwise be in stage I or stage II, but who have remote metastases confined to one or more of the following sites: the liver, the skin, or the bone marrow, without radiologic evidence of bone metastases.

O'Neill et al. have refined the classification and prognosis of neuroblastoma in a retrospective study that took into account the child's age, the tumor stage, the Shimada histologic classification, and lymph node disease as well as the extent of surgical resection.[40] The Shimada subtypes 1, 2, and 4 had a good prognosis, whereas types 3 and 5 carried a poor prognosis. Sex, race, and site of disease did not influence outcome. Their survival rates, based on these criteria, are as follows:

	5-Year Survival
1. Favorable histology, stage I or II, lymph nodes either positive or negative	98%
2. Favorable histology, stage III, lymph nodes positive or negative	83%
3. Unfavorable histology, stage II, III, negative nodes	53%
4. Unfavorable histology, stage II, III, positive nodes	17%

In this study, complete tumor resection was associated with better survival rates in all groups, and the authors also noted a better prognosis when serum ferritin was low and when the neurospecific enolase was below 100 ng/ml at the time of diagnosis.

A series of 133 patients reported from France indicated an overall survival rate of 72 percent in children under 1 year of age and 32 percent in older children.[41] In this study, total resection of the tumor without metastases resulted in a 100 percent survival rate, and if metastases could be controlled, resection of the primary tumor improved survival.

There is some doubt if radiation or chemotherapy improves the outcome of patients with stage I or II tu-

mors. Evans et al. attempted to answer this question with a series of 49 patients treated between 1972 and 1981.[42] Thirteen patients under 1 year of age survived regardless of therapy. Surgery alone cured 91 percent of patients with stage I tumors. There was an 83 percent survival rate in stage II patients treated with surgical excision and a 62 percent survival rate when radiation with or without chemotherapy was added. Adjunctive therapy resulted in no improvement in stage II patients.

Members of the Children's Cancer Group reviewed 75 patients with stage II neuroblastomas treated with surgery alone and 66 who had surgery plus radiation.[43] Each group had similar survival rates. The size of the tumor and the extent of resection did not influence the outcome, and, in fact, there was evidence that residual tumor regressed spontaneously. The data identified a group of neuroblastomas whose growth is biologically limited.

The role of surgery in children with advanced neuroblastoma is less well defined. There is no advantage in attempted resection of a primary tumor unless the metastases can be controlled with chemotherapy. Grosfeld and Bachner obtained long-term survival in children with stage IV tumors when the primary lesion could be excised primarily or at a second-look operation, after treatment with chemotherapy.[44] These results have not been borne out by the Children's Cancer Group review.[45]

Intensive drug therapy with repeated courses of multiple drugs will induce remission of advanced disease, but as yet there are no cures. Treatment with high-dose chemotherapy or total body radiation together with bone marrow transplantation is being attempted in pilot studies.[46,47]

GANGLIONEUROMA

Ganglioneuromas represent the benign end of the spectrum of tumors that arise from the sympathetic ganglia. They occur most commonly in the posterior mediastinum but can arise from an abdominal parasympathetic ganglion. Radiographically, they are rounded densities that may contain calcifications. In the retroperitoneal area, they displace the ureter laterally.

Treatment

Surgical excision alone is sufficient treatment for a benign ganglioneuroma. Many microscopic sections of the tumor must be studied because there may be islands of neuroblastoma within the tumor.

REFERENCES

1. Triche T, Askin F: Neuroblastoma and the differential diagnosis of small, round blue cell tumors. Hum Pathol 14:569, 1983

---

*Tumors arising in midline structures (such as the pelvis), showing penetration of the capsule, or involving lymph nodes on the same side would be considered stage II. Bilateral extension is considered stage III.

2. Taxy J: Electron microscopy in the diagnosis of neuroblastoma. Arch Pathol Lab Med 104:355, 1980

3. Thiele C, McKeon C, Triche T, et al: Differential proto-oncogene expression characterizes histopathologically indistinguishable tumors of the peripheral nervous system. J Clin Invest 80:804, 1987

4. Oppedal B, Brandtzaeg W, Kemshead T: Immunohistochemical differentiation of neuroblastomas from other small round cell neoplasms of childhood using a panel of mono and polyclonal antibodies. Histopathology 11:363, 1987

5. Shimada H, Chatten J, Newton W, et al: Histopathological prognostic factors in neuroblastic tumors: Definition of subtypes of ganglioneuroblastoma and an age-linked classification of neuroblastomas. J Natl Cancer Inst 73:405 1984

6. Bohoun C: Catecholamine metabolism in neuroblastomas. J Pediatr Surg 3:114, 1968

7. Hinterberger H, Bartholomew RS: The chemical diagnosis of ganglioneuroma and neuroblastoma using random specimens of urine. Aust Paediatr J 6:222, 1970

8. Kaser H: Catecholamine-producing neural tumors other than pheochromocytoma. Pharm Rev 18:659, 1966

9. Williams CM, Greer M: Homovanillic acid and vanilmandelic acid in diagnosis of neuroblastoma. JAMA 183:836, 1963

10. Bell M: Neuroblastoma: Newer chemical diagnostic tests. JAMA 205:155, 1968

11. Zeltzer P, Marangos P, Evans A, et al: Serum neuron-specific enolase in children with neuroblastoma: Relationship to stage and disease course. Cancer 57:1230, 1986

12. Tsuchida Y, Hanna T, Iwanaka T, et al: Serial detrmination of serum neuron-specific enolase in patients with neuroblastoma and other pediatric tumors. J Pediatr Surg 22:419, 1981

13. Hann HWL, Evans A, Siegel S, et al: Prognostic importance of serum ferritin in patients with stages III and IV neuroblastoma. The Children's Cancer Study Group Experience. Cancer Res 45:2843, 1985

14. Cohn S, Herst C, Maurer H, Rosen S: N-MYC amplification in an infant with stage IV-S neuroblastoma. J Clin Oncol 5:1441, 1987

15. Nakagawara A, Ikeda K, Tsuda T, Higashi K: N-MYC oncogene amplification and prognostic factors of neuroblastoma in children. J Pediatr Surg 22:895, 1987

16. Brodeur G, Hayes A, Green A: Consistent N-MYC copy number in simultaneous or consecutive neuroblastoma samples from sixty individual patients. Cancer Res 47:4248, 1987

17. Everson T, Cole W: Spontaneous regression of cancer. Prog Clin Cancer 3:79, 1967

18. Beckwith J, Perrin E: In situ neuroblastomas: A contribution to the natural history of neural crest tumors. Am J Pathol 43:1089, 1963

19. Macmillan RW, Blanc WB, Santulli TV: Maturation of neuroblastoma to ganglioneuroma in lymph nodes. J Pediatr Surg 11:461, 1976

20. Koop CE: The Neuroblastoma Progress in Pediatric Surgery. Baltimore, University Park, 1972, vol 2, pp 1–28

21. Sitarz AL, Santulli TV, Wigger HJ, et al: Complete maturation of neuroblastoma with bone metastases in documented stages. J Pediatr Surg 10:533, 1975

22. Bill AH: Immune aspects of neuroblastoma. Am J Surg 122:143, 1971

23. Hughes M, Marsden HB, Palmer H: Histologic patterns of neuroblastoma related to prognosis and clinical staging. Cancer 34:1706, 1974

24. Chung HS, Higgins GR, Siegel SE, et al: Abnormalities of the immune system in children with neuroblastoma related to the neoplasm and chemotherapy. J Pediatr 90:548, 1977

25. Chueng N-KU, Lazarus H, et al: Ganglioside GD_2-specific monoclonal antibody 3F8: A phase I study in patients with neuroblastoma and malignant melanoma. J Clin Oncol 5:1430, 1987

26. Goemans-Jansen A, Engelhardt J: Intractable diarrhea in a boy with vasoactive intestinal peptide-producing ganglioneuroblastoma. Pediatrics 59:710, 1977

27. Bond JV: Unusual presenting symptoms in neuroblastoma. Br Med J 2:327, 1972

28. Senelick RC, Bray PF, Lahey ME, et al: Neuroblastoma and myoclonic encephalopathy: Two cases and a review of the literature. J Pediatr Surg 8:623, 1973

29. Detalieux C, Ebinger G, Maurus R: Myoclonic encephalopathy and neuroblastoma [Letter]. N Engl J Med 292:46, 1975

30. Feine U, Muller-Schauenburg W, Trevner J, et al: Meta-iodobenzyl guanidine (MIBG) labeled with I^{123}/I^{123} in neuroblastoma diagnosis and follow-up treatment with a review of the diagnostic results of the International Workshop of Pediatric Oncology held in Rome. Med Pediatr Oncol 15:181, 1984

31. Cheung N-KU, Von Hoff D, Strandjord S, et al: Detection of neuroblastoma cells in bone marrow using GD_2-specific monoclonal antibodies. J Clin Oncol 4:363, 1986

32. Schwartz AD, Dadash-Zedeh M, Lee H, et al: Spontaneous regression of disseminated neuroblastoma. J Pediatr Surg 85:760, 1974

33. Bond JV: Neuroblastoma metastatic to the liver in infants. Arch Dis Child 51:879, 1976

34. Schnaufer L, Koop CE: Silastic abdominal patch for temporary hepatomegaly in stage IV-S neuroblastoma. J Pediatr Surg 10:73, 1975

35. Bensahel H, Boureau M: Neoplasm. Ann Chir Infant 13:37, 1972

36. Ghazali S: Pelvic neuroblastoma: A better prognosis. Ann Surg 179:115, 1974

37. Haller JA Jr, Shermeta DW, Donahoo JS, et al: Life-threatening respiratory distress from mediastinal masses in infants. Ann Thorac Surg 19:364, 1975

38. Bar-Ziv J, Nogrady MB: Mediastinal neuroblastoma and ganglioneuroma. Am J Roentgenol Radium Ther Nucl Med 125:380, 1975

39. Evans AE, D'Angio GJ, Randolph J: A proposed staging for children with neuroblastoma. Cancer 27:374, 1971

40. O'Neill J, Littman P, Blitzer P: The role of surgery in localized neuroblastoma. J Pediatr Surg 20:708, 1985

41. LeTourneau J, Bernard W, Hendren W: Evaluation of the role of surgery in 130 patients with neuroblastoma. J Pediatr Surg 20:244, 1985

42. Evans A, D'Angio G, Koop L: The role of multimodel

therapy in patients with local and regional neuroblastoma. J Pediatr Surg 19:77, 1984

43. Matthay K, Sather H, Haase G: Excellent outcome of stage II neuroblastoma is independent of residual disease and adjuvant therapy. Children's Cancer Study Group, Operations Office, 199 Northlake, 3rd Floor, Pasadena, CA 91101

44. Grosfeld J, Baehner R: Neuroblastoma: An analysis of 160 cases. World J Surg 4:29, 1980

45. Sitarz D, Finkelstein J, Grosfeld J, et al: An evaluation of the role of surgery in disseminated neuroblastoma: A report from the Children's Cancer Study Group. J Pediatr Surg 18:147, 1983

46. August C, Serota F, Koch P, et al: Treatment of advanced neuroblastoma with supralethal chemotherapy, radiation and allogenic or autologous marrow reconstitution. J Clin Oncol 2:609, 1984

47. Hartman O, Kalifa C, Beaujeau F, et al: Treatment of advanced neuroblastoma with two consecutive high dose chemotherapy regimens and ABMT. Adv Neuroblastoma Res 175:565, 1985

42
Liver Tumors

Edward S. Baum
John G. Raffensperger

Primary liver neoplasms are third after Wilms' tumors and neuroblastomas as a cause of a malignant abdominal mass in infancy and childhood. Hepatic lesions are so uncommon that the experience of any one surgeon or hospital is severely limited. However, there is now sufficient shared information to establish guidelines for the diagnosis and management of these relatively rare tumors.

There is a wide variety of benign and malignant tumors of the liver. The most common discrete hepatic mass in childhood is the hepatoblastoma. Table 42–1 lists the diagnosis of 1237 liver tumors collected from the literature by Weinberg and Finegold.[1] Table 42–2 lists the benign and malignant liver tumors seen at the Children's Memorial Hospital in Chicago from 1952 to 1987.

The most common presenting symptom of liver tumor is an abdominal mass or swelling. Other symptoms include pain, loss of appetite, weight loss, and occasionally jaundice or fever. Vascular malformations may coexist with heart failure or coagulation disorders. On physical examination, there is a readily palpable abdominal mass connected to the liver. It is sometimes difficult, however, to differentiate a large retroperitoneal or renal mass from a liver tumor. An ultrasound examination is an excellent screening modality to determine the tumor's location and whether it is cystic, solid, or multiple. The computed tomography (CT) scan provides the most specific information about the tumor's location, size, blood vessel invasion, and operability (Fig. 42–1). These studies have supplanted the intravenous pyelogram (IVP) and aortogram in the study of solitary lesions. Suspected hemangiomas are well demonstrated with nuclear liver–spleen scans, and aortography is most useful in the study of hemangiomas as a preliminary to embolization. When the lesion is suspected of being malignant, chest roentgenograms and CT scans of the lung are indicated because of the high incidence of lung metastases.

Liver enzymes and the alpha-fetoprotein determination usually are within normal limits with benign tumors but are elevated in approximately 50 percent of children with malignancies.

TABLE 42–1. DIAGNOSES IN 1237 PEDIATRIC LIVER TUMORS FROM THE LITERATURE

Tumor	Number	%
Hepatoblastoma	532	43
Hepatocellular carcinoma	284	23
Benign vascular tumor	166	13
Mesenchymal hamartoma	75	6
Sarcoma	79	6
Adenoma	22	2
Focal nodular hyperplasia	22	2
Other	57	5

Data from Weinberg and Finegold.[1]

VASCULAR MALFORMATIONS

Infantile hemangioendothelioma and cavernous hemangiomas are the two principal vascular lesions encountered in the liver. They are benign but potentially lethal be-

TABLE 42–2. LIVER TUMORS TREATED AT CHILDREN'S MEMORIAL HOSPITAL, CHICAGO, 1952–1987

Malignant Liver Tumors		Benign Liver Tumors	
Type	Number	Type	Number
Hepatoblastoma	17	Hemangioma	12
Carcinoma	17	Hemangioendothelioma	5
Mesenchymal sarcoma	2	Hepatoma	6
Undifferentiated sarcoma	1	Hamartoma	7
Hemangiosarcoma	2	Teratoma	1
		Focal nodular hyperplasia	1
Total	39	Total	32

cause of the possibility of congestive heart failure secondary to arteriovenous shunting, thrombocytopenia, and rupture with intraperitoneal hemorrhage. One of our patients died with respiratory distress secondary to diffuse hemangioendotheliomas that caused enormous growth of the liver. Hepatomegaly is a consistent finding in children with hemangiomas, and often a bruit will be heard over the liver. Half the children with hepatic hemangiomas also have cutaneous lesions (Fig. 42–2). Petechiae and ecchymosis also may be present secondary to thrombocytopenia. Cavernous hemangiomas are usually solitary and confined to one lobe of the liver, which is grossly soft, with large vessels coursing over the surface.

Histologically, there are large dilated vascular spaces lined with vascular endothelium. Hemangioendotheliomas are pale, red-gray lesions 1 to 2 cm in diameter and are distributed throughout the liver. The vascular spaces are lined by budding, branching structures, are more cellular than a cavernous hemangioma, and may appear to be malignant.[2]

The appearance of the liver scan in hemangioendotheliomas is sufficiently characteristic that an accurate diagnosis may be made (Fig. 42–3). When a liver hemangioma is associated with cardiac failure, an arteriogram should be obtained to identify accurately the hepatic artery and the location of the shunt. In addition, a cardiac catheterization may demonstrate an increase in oxygen concentration at the hepatic veins, which will rule out congenital heart disease.

Treatment

Liver hemangiomas have the same tendency to regress as do cutaneous lesions.[3] Thus, for asymptomatic lesions, observation with serial liver scans is all that is necessary. Although radiation has been recommended for liver hem-

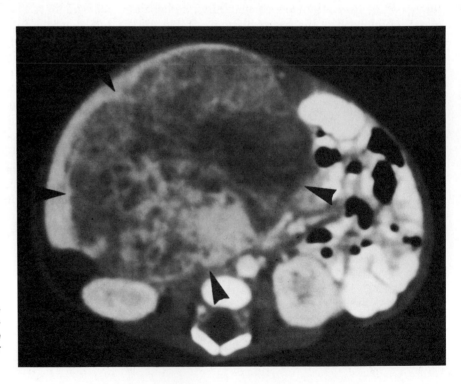

Figure 42–1. CT scan of a large hepatoblastoma of the right lobe of the liver in a 1-month-old child. This was resectable, but the main portal vein was adherent to a tumor in the hilum of the liver.

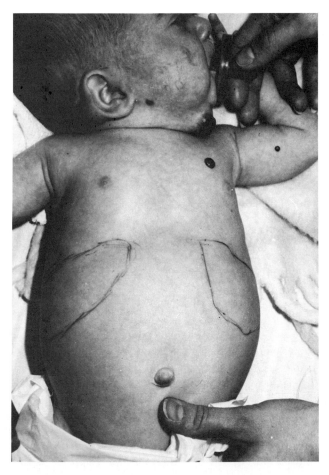

Figure 42–2. Cutaneous hemangiomas in an infant with hepatic hemangiomas who was in congestive heart failure. She responded to steroid therapy.

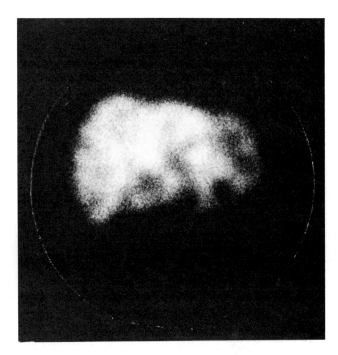

Figure 42–3. Liver scan demonstrating the multiple filling defects characteristic of hemangioendotheliomas.

angiomas, the good results attributed to this therapy are probably the result of spontaneous regression.[4] Steroid therapy, supplemented when necessary with hepatic artery embolization, is the mainstay of therapy.[5,6] Infants with cardiac failure secondary to a demonstrable intrahepatic shunt are helped with hepatic artery ligation.[7,8] In reported cases, the response has been dramatic, with immediate postoperative improvement and resolution of the hemangioma. There has been no ischemia of the liver parenchyma, demonstrable by changes in the liver enzymes. In one of our patients, hepatic artery ligation was of no help because there was an associated intracardiac defect. Multiple hemangiomas grew so rapidly, despite steroid therapy, in another patient that he suffered respiratory failure because of the huge liver. While he was on mechanical ventilation, we performed a ventral fasciotomy, by undermining the abdominal skin and dividing the fascia and peritoneum in the midline through a small upper abdominal incision. The liver herniated out into the subcutaneous space. After 4 months and no improvement with steroids and hepatic artery emboli-

zation, the patient was given 600 rads in four doses to the liver. He gradually improved, and the ventral hernia was closed when he was 2 years old. He is now 10 years old and has an apparently normal liver.[9] Hepatic lobectomy is technically feasible and reportedly successful, even in newborn infants.[10–13] In our series, there were five successful lobectomies for hemangiomas, and one infant died following surgery because of blood loss due to thrombocytopenia.

Ein and Stephens reported three neonates who died from uncontrollable hemorrhage during attempted resection.[14] Since both hepatic artery ligation and steroids have demonstrably hastened the natural resolution of diffuse hemangiomatosis, it seems logical to use these measures first. If the lesion fails to regress, it can be resected.

BENIGN LIVER TUMORS

Benign, solid liver tumors are less common than malignant lesions but may become sufficiently large to cause symptoms by compression of other intraabdominal structures.[15] Although there is no certain technique for differentiating benign from malignant lesions short of a biopsy, a child who has normal liver enzymes, a normal alpha-fetoprotein determination, and a CT scan that demonstrates a circumscribed avascular lesion may have a benign tumor.

The hepatic adenoma is a well-circumscribed, firm,

TABLE 42–3. CLINICAL DATA ON PATIENTS WITH MESENCHYMAL HAMARTOMA

Age	Sex	Symptoms	Pathology	Follow-up
5 years	F	Movable mass	14.5 × 13 × 6 cm mass attached by a broad pedicle	Well at 11 years
11 months	F	Abdominal distention, palpable mass	17 × 12 × 12 cm mass, 910 g	Well at 10 years
14 months	F	Hard abdomen, mass	Pedunculated 10 × 15 cm mass	Well at 14 years
5½ months	F	Irritable, large mass	6.5 × 5.5 × 5 cm mass	Well at 14 years
15 months	M	Smooth, nontender mass	13 × 17 cm mass	Well at 8 years
4 years	F	Smooth, nontender mass	15 × 14 × 8 cm mass	Well at 6 months

homogeneous, yellow-brown mass. Histologically, it is composed of hepatocytes that appear normal but show no lobular differentiation. Focal nodular hyperplasia is more common in girls and has been seen in teenagers who have taken oral contraceptives.[16] This is a solitary nodular mass that is seen most frequently on the inferior surface of the right lobe. Microscopically, nodules of hepatocytes are separated by bands of connective tissue and nests of ducts.

Mesenchymal hamartoma is a benign, cystic developmental anomaly that affects children under 5 years of age. The clinical data of our six patients with this lesion are listed in Table 42–3.[17] These were all asymptomatic children who had large, smooth, nontender masses, inseparable from the liver by palpation. These tumors can become extremely large but are always resectable. Ultrasonography demonstrates cystic spaces with septae. Nuclear scans or CT with contrast demonstrate a decreased blood supply, an important point in differentiating these lesions from malignant tumors or hemangiomas. At operation, these lesions are tense but cystic and smooth. There is no evidence for invasion of adjacent organs or the opposite lobe. A frozen section is done to definitely rule out malignancy because, in many cases, these lesions may be shelled out of the liver or simply removed by transecting a pedicle. Three of our patients required a formal lobectomy, however.

Solitary cysts of the liver either are caused by echinococcal infection or are termed "nonparasitic." The latter lesions are congenital malformations consisting of a simple cyst lined with cuboidal or squamous epithelium. They are asymptomatic and may be found during a routine examination. Ultrasonography demonstrates a solitary cyst with no septa. These lesions may be left alone, or if there is concern about the diagnosis, they are simply enucleated from the liver. Hydatid cysts occur in children from areas endemic for *Echinoccocus*, such as the southwestern part of the United States. We missed the diagnosis in a boy from Peru. Surgical excision is used for cysts that are easily accessible, but most are deep within the liver, and surgical removal can be hazardous. Currently, albendazole has proven useful in eliminating the

organism. A combination of drug therapy with aspiration of the cyst under ultrasound control may become the treatment of choice.[18]

MALIGNANT LIVER TUMORS

Hepatoblastoma and hepatocarcinoma are the two most common primary malignant tumors of the liver in childhood. The hepatoblastoma is rare beyond 3 years of age and is most common in children under 1 year. It is twice as frequent in boys and is usually present as a solitary mass arising from one lobe in an otherwise normal liver. The mass is encompassed by a layer of fibrous tissue that separates it from the liver substance (Fig. 42–4). On cut surface, the color varies from green to yellow depending on the amount of bile and fat in the tissue. There are also areas of hemorrhage and necrosis. Microscopically, epithelial cells arranged in cords are separated from the sinusoids. Kasai and Watanabe studied 70 cases of liver carcinoma and found that hepatoblastomas may be further differentiated into fetal and embry-

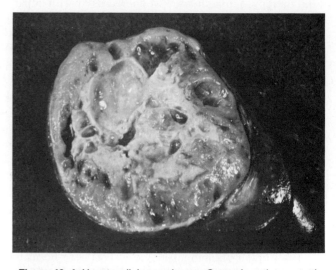

Figure 42–4. Hepatocellular carcinoma. Cut surface demonstrating areas of degeneration and cyst formation.

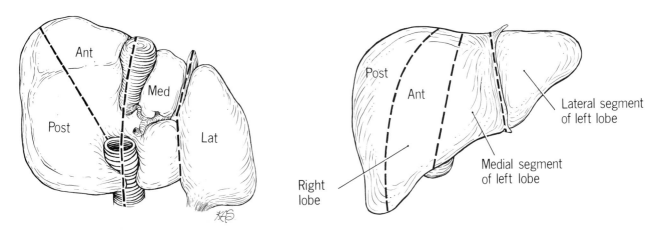

Figure 42–5. Anatomy of liver showing division into right and left lobes and segments.

onal tumors.[19] Half of the hepatoblastomas studied were of the better-differentiated fetal cell type, which appear to have a better prognosis. Hepatoblastoma may produce gonadotropin and precocious puberty in boys.[20]

Hepatocarcinoma also occurs more frequently in boys but in a wider age range than hepatoblastoma. It appears in children under 3 years old, with another peak incidence in children from 12 to 13 years of age. This tumor is similar to the adult form of liver cancer and, like the adult tumors, is more likely to be found in previously cirrhotic livers.[21] The hepatocarcinoma tends to be multicentric and more invasive than the hepatoblastoma. Microscopically, the cells are more polygonal, bizarre, and irregular. In addition, mitoses are common. We have observed liver carcinoma develop in two siblings with familial cholestatic disease, one with biliary atresia and one with hepatitis.

Treatment

Complete surgical excision is the treatment of choice for solid liver tumors. Before operation, the child should have a complete workup to exclude metastases to the lungs and bone. Coagulation studies should be performed and abnormalities corrected. Sufficient blood must be typed and crossmatched to transfuse the child with at least double the estimated blood volume. In addition, we have the family donate 2 fresh units of blood on the day of surgery and have fresh-frozen plasma and platelets ready in order to diminish coagulation disorders brought about by massive transfusions. Intravenous lines are inserted into the upper extremities or jugular veins, and all vital signs, including direct arterial venous pressures, are monitored. Although hypothermia and hypotensive anesthesia have been recommended for liver resections, we have not found these measures helpful in controlling hemorrhage.

Surgical Anatomy

Only benign tumors that have a narrow pedicle of liver tissue are amenable to local excision. Malignant lesions and large benign lesions require a hepatic lobectomy for cure. Furthermore, liver resections that follow anatomic segmental planes result in less blood loss than wedge resections. A line running from the gallbladder fossa to the inferior vena cava at the diaphragm divides the liver anatomically into the right and left lobes (Fig. 42–5). The medial segment of the left lobe lies between this line and the falciform ligament. The left lateral segment lies to the left of the falciform ligament. Most liver resections for cancer require an extended right lobectomy, which includes the medial segment of the left lobe.

The hepatic artery and bile ducts follow a segmental distribution within the liver. However, estimates of anomalies of the hepatic artery vary from 25 to 50 percent. Either a lobar hepatic artery or a superior mesenteric artery may arise from the left gastric. Furthermore, a segmental artery may arise from the opposite main hepatic branch. Although preoperative arteriography may aid in mapping anomalous vessels, it is difficult to distinguish anomalies from distortions caused by the tumor. Thus, it is necessary to trace the arterial supply from the main hepatic artery before any ligation. Accessory hepatic ducts also may be found, especially on the right side. The portal vein lies beneath the bile duct and the artery. The right branch is much shorter than the left and, of course, larger. The left portal vein sharply recurves just beneath the falciform ligament to supply the medial segment of the left lobe (Fig. 42–6). Therefore, in resecting only the left lateral lobe, the main left portal vein must not be ligated.

There are three major hepatic veins, plus a variable number of small veins that drain directly from the right lobe into the inferior vena cava. The middle hepatic

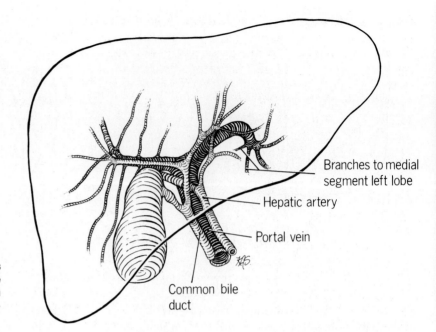

Figure 42–6. The left portal vein recurves beneath the falciform ligament to supply the medial segment of the left lobe. The main left portal vein must be protected when resecting only the left lateral lobe.

vein is in the plane between the right lobe and the medial segment of the left lobe. Care must be taken to leave this vein behind when resecting either lobe. The three main veins may empty into the vena cava separately, or the medial vein may join with either the right or left to empty into the cava as a common trunk (Fig. 42–7). In more than 60 percent of cases, the middle vein joins the left. The liver is attached to the diaphragm by the right and left triangular ligaments. These peritoneal folds are continuous with the coronary ligament, which separates so that a large portion of the liver is directly opposed to the diaphragm. The hepatic veins join the inferior vena cava within this bare area of the liver. Care must be taken to prevent injury to the veins when the peritoneal reflection commences to separate. The right coronary ligament is reflected down the right lateral abdominal wall as the hepatorenal ligament, which must be divided in order to roll the right lobe to the right to expose the retrohepatic inferior vena cava. Glisson's capsule, which envelops the liver in a fibrous cap-

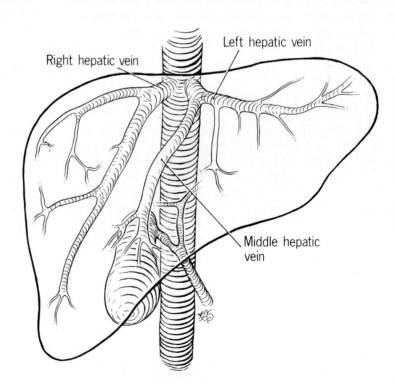

Figure 42–7. The hepatic veins. In 60 percent of cases, the left hepatic vein joins the medial vein to form a common trunk.

sule, also envelops the bile ducts and vessels in the porta hepatis and continues with these structures into the liver substance. This connective tissue provides substance to vessels and bile ducts within the liver tissue, so that when blunt dissection is employed while transversing the liver substance, these structures may be identified and individually clamped and ligated.

The monograph by Fortner et al. provides an excellent additional summary of the segmental anatomy of the liver and problems associated with resection.[22]

Surgical Technique

The entire chest, abdomen, and flank are prepared and draped into the sterile field. This will allow adequate room for extension of the incision into the chest and will allow a drainage incision to be made through the bed of the 11th rib. A transverse subcostal incision is adequate for left lobe lesions and for biopsy and evaluation of right lobe tumors.

When it is evident that a right lobectomy is indicated, the right subcostal incision may be extended across an interspace into the chest or, depending on the surgeon's preference, up the midline by splitting the sternum (Fig. 42–8A). With either approach, it is necessary to open the chest to gain access to the intrapericardial cava. Although there is some risk of spreading tumor cells, the histologic nature of the tumor should be determined by biopsy and frozen section. A needle biopsy will provide sufficient tissue with minimal danger of spilling malignant cells. While the frozen section is being processed, the extent of the tumor is determined by a preliminary dissection to expose the hepatic veins and porta hepatis. Extension of tumor into these areas or into the opposite lobe precludes a safe resection. Since chemotherapy and radiation may convert an inoperable mass into one that may be safely resected, it is wiser to make a tissue diagnosis and close the abdomen than to embark on an impossible resection for an inoperable tumor.

Left Hepatic Lobectomy. After the initial biopsy and exploration, the round and falciform ligaments are divided close to the abdominal wall and diaphragm (Fig. 42–8B). The left costal margin is then retracted upward, and the stomach is held down. The surgeon then grasps the left lobe and under direct vision divides the left triangular and coronary ligaments until the left hepatic vein is seen. This dissection may be commenced with the electrocautery, but as the peritoneal reflections widen, scissors dissection is employed in order to avoid the vein.

The tumor and left lobe are elevated and retracted to the right. This exposes the portal vein in the portal fissure. The portal veins, hepatic artery, and bile ducts are carefully dissected free from Glisson's capsule, fat,

lymphatics, and nerve fibers. The right branches should be encircled with colored tapes so that they are constantly in direct vision during the dissection, since it is very important that the blood supply to the right lobe be left alone. After carefully identifying, ligating, and dividing the structures in the portal fissures, the liver is allowed to fall back into the abdomen, and the left hepatic vein is dissected from Glisson's capsule back into the liver substance until it can be safely isolated and suture-ligated. Care must be taken at this point to avoid damage to the middle hepatic vein. The lobe is then removed by outlining the course of the resection with the electrocautery. Most of the dissection is performed bluntly by crushing liver tissue between the thumb and fingers. This technique leaves the vessels and ducts, which may then be clamped and ligated with a figure-eight suture. Hemostasis of the cut liver edge is obtained with additional sutures and with the electrocautery. Interlocking mattress sutures are likely to cut through the liver tissue, which is more friable in children, than to control bleeding.

Right Hepatic Lobectomy. An extended resection of the right lobe of the liver for tumor is a formidable surgical procedure. However, such operations have been carried out in children since 1952 with technical success.[23]

Unexpected massive hemorrhage is most likely to occur at the junction of the hepatic veins and the inferior vena cava. When the liver is retracted up and away from the cava, small vessels between the right lobe and the vein are stretched until they resemble strands of connective tissue (Fig. 42–8C). When these strands are cut, blood obscures the field, and attempts to clamp the vessels may injure the cava. Each vessel must be carefully suture-ligated (Fig. 42–8D). Attempts to blindly pass a clamp around one of the main hepatic veins when there is poor exposure also are likely to result in a torn vena cava.

Torrential bleeding from the cava cannot always be prevented, since tumor growth may make it difficult to dissect an adequate length of hepatic vein. For this reason, it is wise to encircle the infrahepatic cava and the intrapericardial cava with tapes before dissection of the hepatic veins. Then if the cava is torn, bleeding may be momentarily controlled by tightening the tapes while a vascular clamp is accurately placed across the tear.

After the cava has been encircled and the hepatorenal peritoneal reflections have been severed, dissection is commenced in the hepatoduodenal ligament. All fat and lymphatic tissue is removed to expose the hepatic artery, the common bile duct, and the portal vein. The cystic artery and duct are identified, ligated, and divided in order to expose the right branches high in the porta

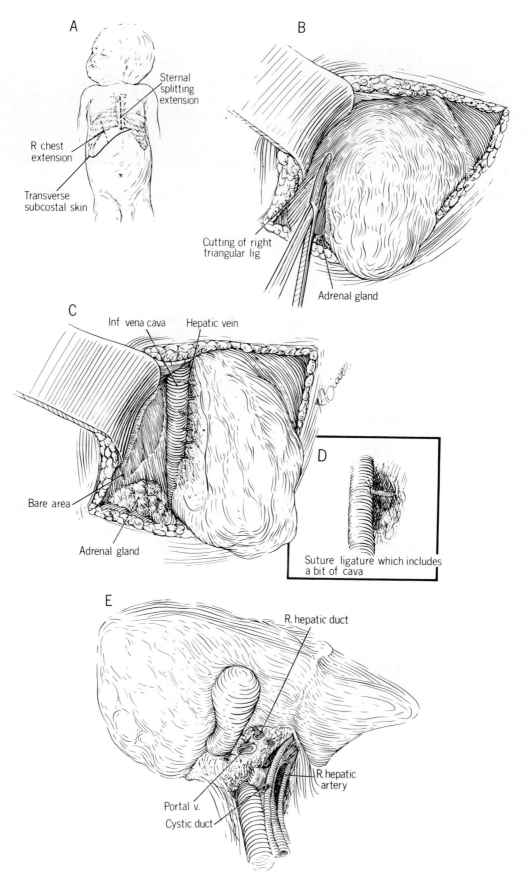

A

Sternal
splitting
extension

R chest
extension

Transverse
subcostal skin

B

Cutting of right
triangular lig

Adrenal gland

C

Inf vena cava   Hepatic vein

Bare area

Adrenal gland

D

Suture ligature which includes
a bit of cava

E

R. hepatic duct

R. hepatic
artery

Portal v.

Cystic duct

Figure 42–8A through I. Technique for right hepatic resection. (Continued)

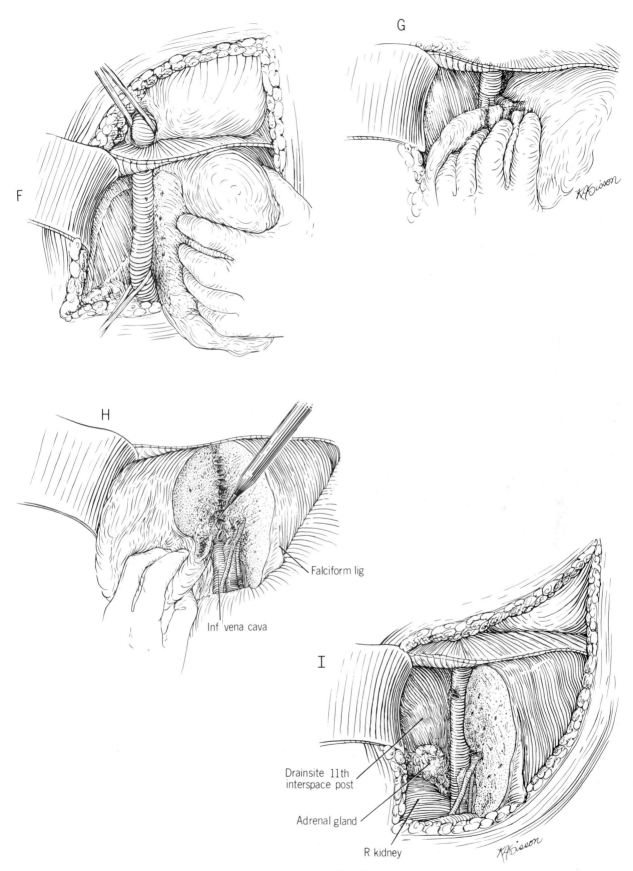

F

G

H

Falciform lig

Inf vena cava

I

Drainsite 11th
interspace post

Adrenal gland

R kidney

Figure 42–8. (Cont.)

hepatis (Fig. 42–8E). This dissection must proceed carefully, with the knowledge that congenital defects and distortion by the tumor make identification difficult. The vessels and ducts of the left lobe must be clearly visualized and left undisturbed.

The right duct is divided first to expose the artery and then the short right portal vein. The tumor and right lobe are then wrapped in moist laparotomy pads, and an assistant elevates the mass with the hand to expose the retrohepatic inferior vena cava (Fig. 42–8F). This dissection is best performed by opening and closing either a delicate forceps or a Metzenbaum scissors. All tissue that does not separate easily is suture-ligated with 5–0 vascular material flush with the cava. Metal clips are unreliable when applied on the cava side of these small vessels. This dissection must not be hurried. The right hepatic vein may be embedded in liver tissue, in which case it must be exposed by opening Glisson's capsule. A length of vein is then bluntly dissected until enough is exposed for safe suture-ligation (Fig. 42–8G). This entire process must be performed under direct vision, and it is best to suture-ligate the vessel in continuity. The final line of resection will be determined by the left lateral limits of the tumor but will be somewhere just to the right of the falciform ligament and will be directed to the left of the right hepatic vein. This will preserve the left hepatic vein and perhaps a portion of the middle vein. After marking the line of resection with the electrocautery, liver tissue is squeezed between the fingers, leaving the vascular structures to be clamped and suture-ligated (Fig. 42–8H,I).

After resection of either lobe, biopsies are taken at the margins of resection to determine if there is residual tumor. The raw liver surface may be covered with the falciform ligament that was left attached to the remaining liver substance. Several large Penrose drains containing a gauze wick are brought out of the flank so that the liver bed has dependent drainage.

During the procedure, a meticulous record is kept of ongoing blood loss. Fresh blood should be used when available. Otherwise fresh-frozen plasma is given at intervals along with whole blood. If oozing develops during the operation, blood is drawn for coagulation studies. Then, if necessary, platelets or other components are given as required. During the immediate postoperative period, continued oozing from the large wound will require either more whole blood or more plasma. The amount will depend on serial observations of the venous pressure, hematocrit, and urinary output.

Approximately 20 percent of the liver remains after an extended right hepatectomy. When this remaining liver is normal, overt hepatic insufficiency is unlikely. However, hypoproteinemia and hypoglycemia are hazards in the immediate postoperative period.[24] For this reason, 10 to 20 percent glucose should be administered through a central venous line, and fresh-frozen plasma or serum albumin should be given until the child has a normal diet. Vitamin K is given for a week or until the prothrombin time returns to normal levels. Postoperative complications include subphrenic collections of bile and blood, prolonged fever, pleural effusion, and prolonged ileus. Adequate drainage (as described) will help prevent local complications. We have observed serious postoperative gastrointestinal bleeding in two patients following hepatic lobectomy. The source of the hemorrhage was never discovered but was thought to be hematobilia.

Liver regeneration proceeds rapidly after resection, so that within a few weeks, liver function tests will have returned to normal and a scan will show return of liver substance. Dactinomycin and, presumably, other chemotherapeutic agents impair liver regeneration in patients and experimental animals after liver surgery.[25] Consequently, therapy must not be commenced until there is evidence of normal liver function in the postoperative period.

Results

Data on 252 malignant liver tumors were obtained from questionnaires sent to the Surgical Section of the Academy of Pediatrics in 1974. Of 78 children with hepatoblastomas who were treated with resection of their tumors, 45 (or 60 percent) survived. Of 33 children with hepatocellular carcinoma who were treated with resection, 12 survived. In this group, there were no survivors among patients who did not have a complete excision of tumor, although 3 hepatoblastomas that were initially unresectable became operable following radiation and multiple drug therapy.[26]

Children who have had a completely resected fetal type of hepatoblastoma will survive with no further therapy. All others require chemotherapy. A combination of vincristine, cyclophosphamide, doxorubicin, and 5-fluorouracil resulted in 17 of 18 patients surviving disease free for periods of 8 to 42 months, whereas 7 patients who were not given chemotherapy all died.[27] In another series, 19 of 29 children given chemotherapy survived, 14 of them for periods of 2 to 11 years after treatment.[28] Tumors judged to be unresectable on either the preoperative workup or at laparotomy may become resectable after chemotherapy or other treatment modalities, such as radiolabeled antiferritin antibodies.[29–31] Antitumor drugs dispersed in Lipiodol and given in the hepatic artery have caused rapid shrinkage of unresectable hepatoblastomas.[32]

REFERENCES

1. Weinberg A, Finegold M: Primary hepatic tumors of childhood. Hum Pathol 14:512, 1983

2. Dehner LP: Pediatric Surgical Pathology. St. Louis, Mosby, 1975, p 368

3. Braun P, Ducharme JC, Riopelle JL, et al: Hemangiomatosis of the liver in infants. J Pediatr Surg 10:121, 1975

4. Park WC, Phillips R: The role of radiation therapy in the management of hemangiomas of the liver. JAMA 212:1496, 1970

5. Holcomb G, O'Neill J, Mahoubi S, Bishop H: Experience with hepatic hemangioendothelioma in infancy and childhood. J Pediatr Surg 23:661, 1988

6. Brown SH Jr, Neerhout RC, Fonkalsrud EW: Prednisone therapy in the management of large hemangiomas in infants and children. Surgery 71:168, 1972

7. Delurimer AA, Simpson EB, Baum RS, et al: Hepatic artery ligation for hepatic hemangiomatosis. N Engl J Med 277:333, 1967

8. Mattiolli L, Lee KP, Holder TM: Hepatic artery ligation for cardiac failure due to hepatic hemangioma in the newborn. J Pediatr Surg 9:859, 1974

9. Ricketts R, Stryker S, Raffensperger J: Ventral fasciotomy in the management of hepatic hemangioendothelioma. J Pediatr Surg 17:187, 1982

10. Sompi E, Niemio K, Rouskamen O, et al: Cavernous hepatic hemangioma in the newborn infant: Case report. J Pediatr Surg 9:239, 1974

11. Graivier L, Votteler TP, Dorman GW: Hepatic hemangiomas in newborn infants. J Pediatr Surg 2:299, 1967

12. Tawes RL, Nelson JA, Hyde CA: Hepatic hemangiomas: successful resection in a neonate. Surgery 70:782, 1971

13. Matolo NM, Johnson DG: Surgical treatment of hepatic hemangioma in the newborn. Arch Surg 106:725, 1973

14. Ein SH, Stephens CA: Benign liver tumors and cysts in childhood. J Pediatr Surg 9:847, 1974

15. Vandza T, Valayer J: Benign tumors of the liver in children: Analysis of 20 cases. J Pediatr Surg 21:419, 1986

16. Mays ET, Christopherson WM, Barrows GH: Focal nodular hyperplasia of the liver: Possible relationship to oral contraceptives. Am J Clin Pathol 61:735, 1974

17. Raffensperger JG, Gonzalez-Crussi F, Skeehan T: Mesenchymal hamartoma of the liver. J Pediatr Surg 18:585, 1983

18. Morris D, Dyke S, Mariner S: Albendazole—objective response in human hydatid cysts. JAMA 253:2053, 1985

19. Kasai M, Watanabe I: Histologic classification of liver-cell carcinoma in infancy and childhood and its clinical evaluation. Cancer 23:551, 1970

20. Watanabe I, Yomagochi M, Kasai M: Histologic characteristics of gonadotropin producing hepatoblastoma: A survey of seven cases from Japan. J Pediatr Surg 22:406, 1987

21. Sinniah D, Campbell PE, Colebatch JH: Primary hepatic cancer in infancy and childhood: A survey of twenty cases. In Rickham PP, Hecker WC, Prevot J (eds): Progress in Pediatric Surgery. Baltimore, University Park, 1974, pp 141–70

22. Fortner JG, et al: Surgery in liver tumors. In Current Problems in Surgery. Chicago, Year Book, 1972, pp 1–56

23. Clatworthy HW Jr, Boles ET Jr: Right lobectomy of the liver in children. Surgery 39:850, 1956

24. Pinkerton JA, Sawyers JL, Foster JH: A study of the postoperative course after hepatic lobectomy. Ann Surg 173:800, 1971

25. Filler RM, Tefft M, Vawter GF, et al: Hepatic lobectomy in childhood: Effects of x-ray and chemotherapy. J Pediatr Surg 4:31, 1969

26. Exelby PR, Filler RM, Grosfeld JL: Liver tumors in children in the particular reference to hepatoblastoma and hepatocellular carcinoma. J Pediatr Surg 10:329, 1975

27. Evans A, Land V, Newton W, et al: Combination chemotherapy (vincristine, adriamycin, cyclophosphamide and 5-fluorouracil) in the treatment of children with malignant hepatoma. Cancer 50:821, 1982

28. Gauthier F, Valoyer J, Thai B, et al: Hepatoblastoma and hepatocarcinoma in children: Analysis of a series of 29 cases. J Pediatr Surg 21:424, 1985

29. Weinblatt M, Siegel S, Siegel M, et al: Preoperative chemotherapy for unresectable primary hepatic malignancies in children. Cancer 50:1061, 1982

30. Quinn J, Altman A, Robinson T, et al: Adriamycin and cisplatin for hepatoblastoma. Cancer 56:1926, 1985

31. Sitzman J, Order S, Klein J: Conversion by new treatment modalities of nonresectable to resectable hepatocellular cancer. J Clin Oncol 5:1566, 1987

32. Ogita S, Tokiwa K, Toniguchi H: Intra-arterial chemotherapy with lipid contrast medium for hepatic malignancies in children. Cancer 60:2886, 1987

43
Teratomas

Teratomas are rare, puzzling neoplasms containing a diversity of tissue not ordinarily found at the tumor's site. The term "teratoma" is derived from the Greek word meaning monster and accurately suggests the dichotomy of these lesions, that is, a combination of developmental anomaly and tumor. They are almost always found in children and frequently arise in the gonads. Extragonadal teratomas tend to occur near the midline of the body, indicating their possible origin from disorganized cells in the germinal layers of the primitive streak or notochord. The sites of origin of extragonadal teratomas are those often seen as common points of connection between conjoined twins. Despite considerable experimental work, the exact cellular origin of teratomas remains unknown. The two oldest schools of thought suggest either germ cells or undifferentiated embryonic cells.[1] The tissue is highly variable within a single tumor. There may be derivatives from only two germ layers, such as skin, skin appendages, and connective tissue. However, in most sacrococcygeal tumors, there is tissue from all three germ layers, including skin, teeth, nervous system, intestine, endocrine glands, cartilage, and bone (Fig. 43–1). There are also varying degrees of differentiation in individual tissues. The more differentiated tumors may contain well-developed extremities or a partially formed fetus (Fig. 43–2). The most immature component resembles undifferentiated embryonic cells. In general, teratomas containing well-differentiated tissue are benign. The more immature or poorly differentiated tissue is most often malignant. Unfortunately, a small nest of immature cells in an otherwise well differentiated teratoma may metastasize or lead to local recurrence.

SACROCOCCYGEAL TERATOMA

Data from 405 children with sacrococcygeal teratomas were collected by the Surgical Section of the American Academy of Pediatrics in 1973.[2] Seventy-four percent of these patients were female. The diagnosis was made on the first day of life in 205 patients. Seventy-four infants (18 percent) had associated congenital anomalies, most involving the musculoskeletal system. This large group of tumors was subdivided and classified according to the size of the intrapelvic portion of the tumor. In 186 patients, the bulk of the mass extended outside the pelvis and was readily visible. Only 39 patients had presacral lesions without external presentation. Intrapelvic or presacral tumors had a higher incidence of malignancy. As would be expected, there was considerable delay in diagnosis of the presacral lesions that were invisible to exterior observation. Thus, there is considerable clinical importance in defining sacrococcygeal teratomas as "presacral" or "postsacral."

There may be a genetic influence in their origin, since Ashcraft and his associates have described a familial syndrome of presacral teratomas, sacral defects, and anal stenosis.[3] The familial distribution in their series suggests an autosomal dominant transmission. Several other authors have described both a familial occurrence and associated birth defects.[4–6] Sacral tumors rarely occur in older children and adults. Usually, there has been a history of neglected draining sinuses or a long-standing mass lesion, suggesting onset at a much earlier time.[7]

Pathology

Benign teratomas are well encapsulated and contain varying degrees of solid and cystic components. Even well-encapsulated benign lesions often are intimately adherent to the coccyx. The cystic fluid may be serous, mucoid, or bloody, and the cyst lining often consists of recognizable squamous epithelium with sebaceous material and teeth. Limb buds and male genitalia also may protrude into the cyst cavity. Predominantly cystic tumors are more likely benign, and the incidence of malignancy rises in proportion to the amount of solid tissue. The variety of tissues within a single teratoma is apparent only on careful microscopic examination, which reveals

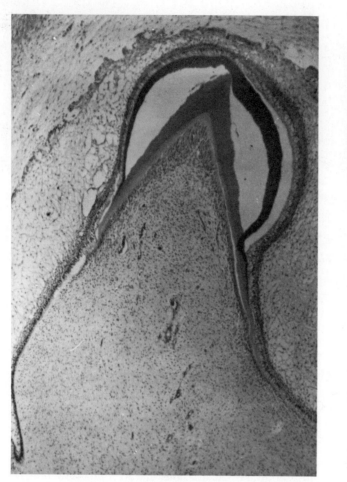

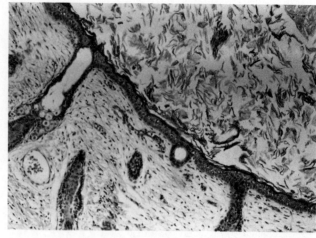

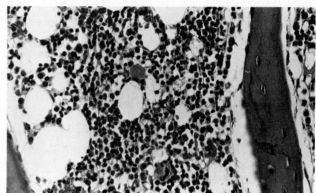

Figure 43–1. Microscopic sections of teratoma demonstrating tissues arising from all three germ layers. **Left.** Tooth bud. **Top right.** Skin and appendages. **Bottom right.** Bone marrow.

varying degrees of differentiation of almost every organ system.

In spite of the heterogeneity of tissues found in these tumors, the malignant component, when present,

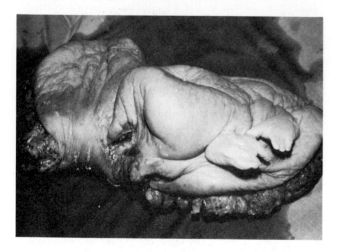

Figure 43–2. Sacrococcygeal teratoma with well-developed limb buds.

is almost always the yolk sac or endodermal sinus tumor.[8] This tumor is microscopically similar to the rat endodermal sinus, a yolk sac structure not found in humans but present in the early development of the fetal rat.[9] Epithelial structures predominate, with a papillary and tuboalveolar pattern of cystic spaces lined by columnar and cuboidal epithelium. Crussi and Roth have supported this origin of the endodermal sinus tumor with electron microscopic studies.[10] In our own series of 7 malignant sacrococcygeal teratomas, the malignant component was always of endodermal sinus origin.[11] Malignant sacral tumors infiltrate into the pelvic organs and metastasize to lymph nodes, liver, and lungs.

Diagnosis

Sacrococcygeal teratomas have been diagnosed before birth by fetal ultrasonographic examination.[12,13] The mass contains more solid elements and is more caudal than the usual meningomyelocele. Prenatal diagnosis is important because these tumors may be large enough to cause dystocia. Rupture of the tumor with massive hemorrhage may occur during birth. Thus, it is important to have the mother delivered by cesarean section in a center where the infant can receive immediate surgical treatment.

Unfortunately, sacrococcygeal teratomas that appear before 30 weeks gestation are associated with polyhydramnios and placentomegaly. All seven fetuses with this presentation died in utero, but diagnosis after 30 weeks was associated with survival.[14]

In well over half of the reported cases, a sacrococcygeal teratoma appears as an obvious caudal, skin-covered, firm or cystic mass. The mass may weigh more than the infant or be no more than a barely noticeable lump. The larger masses often distort and push the anus anteriorly (Fig. 43–3). A large presacral extension may compress pelvic veins, causing leg edema. In addition, we have observed an infant whose presacral tumor obstructed the bladder, causing renal failure and vesical rupture. The skin over large tumors is thin and may be discolored with hematoma and a network of blood vessels. Rarely, a teratoma is off to one side in a buttock. In older children, presacral teratomas can occur with constipation or nonspecific pelvic pain. There may be no obvious external mass, but rectal examination will reveal a firm tumor, often fixed to the sacrum. Draining sinus tracts or repeated episodes of abscess formation posterior to the anus also suggest an undiagnosed teratoma.

Other tumors, such as neuroblastoma, hemangioma, hamartoma, and chordoma, could be confused with a teratoma. However, all of these require excision for diagnosis and therapy. A cystic duplication of the rectum is palpable as a smooth, rounded lesion in the presacral space; imaging studies would clearly indicate its cystic nature. It is most important to differentiate a lipome-

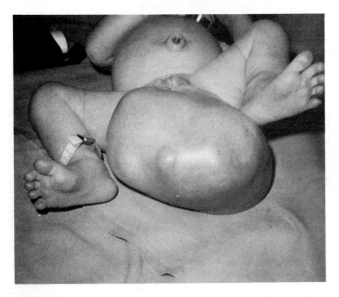

Figure 43–3. Large benign sacrococcygeal teratoma in a newborn infant.

ningocele from a teratoma. Clinically, the lipomeningocele is higher up the back and overlies the spinal canal. Roentgenograms demonstrate a spina bifida. Naidich et al. found it difficult to differentiate teratomas from lipomeningoceles with B-mode sonography because the teratoma was homogeneous and echogenic.[15] These authors observed that the lipomeningoceles were above the intergluteal cleft and extended through a spina bifida into the canal. Teratomas, on the other hand, were below the intergluteal cleft and extended anterior to the sacrum rather than into the canal. Presacral meningoceles are much softer and more fluctuant than a teratoma. Any imaging study, such as ultrasonography, computed tomography (CT), or myelogram, should easily differentiate a presacral meningocele from a teratoma.

Plain roentgenograms often demonstrate teeth or calcification in a teratoma. CT demonstrates septae and solid components in otherwise difficult to diagnose lesions. Either a lateral CT scan or magnetic resonance imaging (MRI) will demonstrate intrapelvic or intraspinal extensions of sacral lesions with great detail. The serum alpha-fetoprotein (AFP) is a useful test to differentiate between benign and malignant teratomas. In one series, the AFP was elevated in 31 of 32 malignant teratomas.[16] AFP also has been found to be elevated in the amniotic fluid when the infant has a teratoma.[17]

Surgery

When the child has been anesthetized, the rectum is irrigated with either 1 percent neomycin or a solution of povidone-iodine, after which an indwelling catheter is placed in the bladder, and the entire abdomen, back, perineum, and legs to the knees are prepared and draped (Fig. 43–4). If the lesion is primarily perineal with minimal extension into the pelvis or abdomen, the mass may be removed through a presacral incision. The infant is placed on the abdomen over a roll to elevate the hips. A sterile sheet should be under the abdomen and buttocks, and the entire lower back, perineum, and thighs should be draped into the sterile field. A curved transverse or inverted V incision is made over the mass, with the apex of the V overlying the coccyx. If the skin is thinned out over a large mass, some is left adherent to the tumor and excised with the specimen. The blood supply of a sacrococcygeal teratoma comes almost entirely from the middle sacral vessels. Consequently, the dissection is extended superior to the mass into the subcutaneous tissues overlying the sacrum. When the upper and lateral margins of the tumor and the sacrum have been exposed, the coccyx and the lowest sacral segment are transected. This allows exposure of the sacral vessels, which are ligated and divided. Further, the coccyx must be removed in order to prevent tumor recurrence. The fascia over the gluteus muscle is divided, and the tumor is sharply dissected away from the muscle. With malignant tumors, there may be no clear demarcation of the tumor's edge. Consequently, normal muscle should be transected with the electrocautery to provide a tumor-free margin. As the dissection proceeds about the mass, either an instrument or a finger must be inserted into the rectum at intervals to aid in identifying a safe plane of dissection that will not injure the bowel. Finally, the mass is removed with any excess skin, and the wound is irrigated with saline solution. Reconstruction is then carried out by suturing the levator ani muscle in the midline around the rectum. The gluteal muscles are then resutured to the sacrum, and an attempt is made to restore the normal intergluteal fold by attaching the skin to the tissues in the midline. The skin is closed over Penrose drains, and a pressure dressing is applied.

When the tumor extends into the pelvis higher than

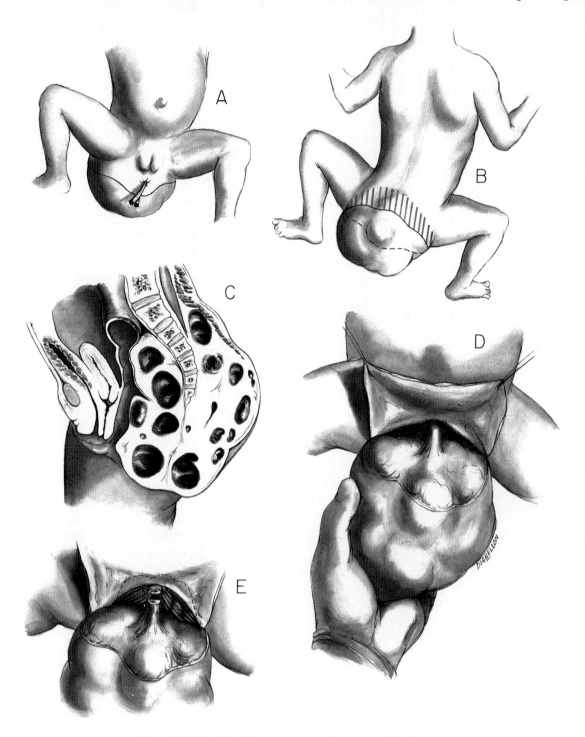

Figure 43–4. Excision of a sacrococcygeal teratoma. (Continued)

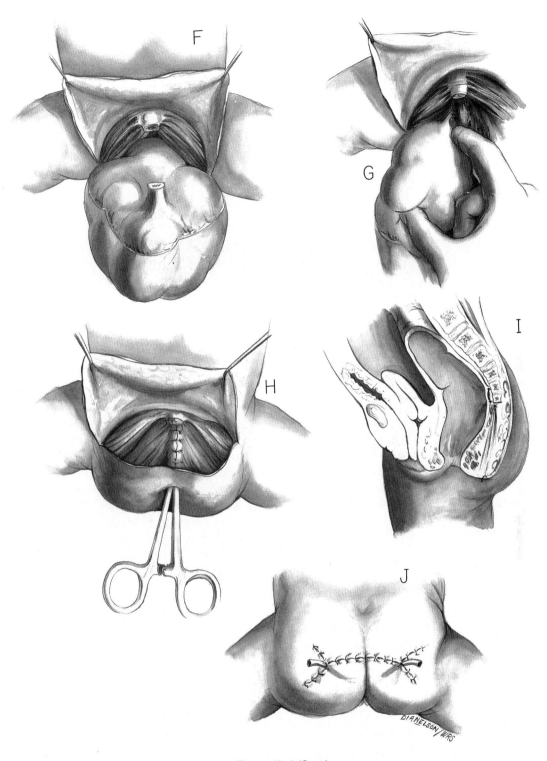

Figure 43–4 (Cont.)

the examining finger can reach from the rectum or if tumor is palpable in the abdomen, a laparotomy must be performed to free the tumor from intraabdominal attachments. In older children, the tumor is more likely to be malignant. Consequently, a preliminary abdominal exploration to free the tumor and to excise iliac and

aortic lymph nodes is indicated. A low transverse incision will provide excellent exposure of the intrapelvic tumor and allow one to separate the ureters, bladder, and rectum from the mass. If the dissection stays close to the tumor, danger to the pelvic nerves will be minimized. Although segments of the rectum or other pelvic organs

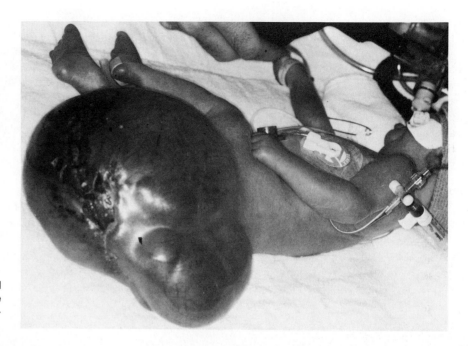

Figure 43–5. Large bleeding sacrococcygeal teratoma. In a case such as this, open the abdomen and clamp the aorta before attempting removal of the tumor.

may be removed in order to excise a malignant lesion, it is preferable to rely on chemotherapy to destroy residual tumor rather than performing a pelvic exenteration. A colostomy is indicated to protect a rectal suture line after excision of part of the bowel. After the tumor has been freed down to the sacrum from the abdominal approach, the child is turned on the side, and the sacral portion is removed. The lower two thirds of the sacrum can be removed safely with an invasive mass, since bladder control will be satisfactory if the third sacral nerve is preserved on one side.

We have observed three newborn infants with huge, bleeding sacrococcygeal teratomas. Two of these infants died from shock and hypothermia. The third infant was saved because we first opened the abdomen to obtain control of the aorta (Fig. 43–5). All of these infants went into shock very rapidly; they can be saved only with rapid blood transfusions through large-bore catheters and an immediate operation. The entire body below the nipples is prepared and draped into a sterile field. The abdomen is rapidly opened, and the aorta is compressed until it can be encircled with a tape and temporarily occluded. Blood is then replaced until the vital signs are stable and the infant is turned on the abdomen for excision of the teratoma.

Tumor recurrence is almost inevitable unless the coccyx is removed along with the mass.[18] In one of my patients, the mass did not involve the coccyx, which was left behind. Five years later, malignant endodermal sinus tumor developed even though the original teratoma was well differentiated. In an extended review of 254 teratomas of all types, Tapper and Lack found that the most important single prognostic sign of malignant recurrence was the incomplete removal of the tumor at the first operation.[19] There is a definitely higher incidence of malignancy when the diagnosis is made after 3 months of age. This observation correlates with the increased incidence of hidden, or presacral, tumors.

In every location, the malignant component of teratomas is the endodermal sinus tumor (Fig. 43–6). These were universally fatal until the advent of modern chemotherapy, introduced in the 1970s. In a series from Melbourne, 3 of 5 patients treated between 1976 and 1980 survived disease free, and the initial responses in 6 more patients are encouraging.[20] The best results are obtained when the primary malignant tumor is completely resected, either primarily or after its size has been reduced with chemotherapy.[21] The importance of

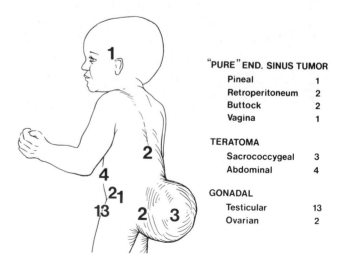

"PURE" END. SINUS TUMOR	
Pineal	1
Retroperitoneum	2
Buttock	2
Vagina	1
TERATOMA	
Sacrococcygeal	3
Abdominal	4
GONADAL	
Testicular	13
Ovarian	2

Figure 43–6. The endodermal sinus tumor may arise de novo from several sites, including the glands. It is also the malignant component of teratomas.

surgical resection has been borne out in our own experience with 9 children between 4 months and 7 years of age with endodermal sinus tumors. Two had benign tumors resected in the newborn period, but the recurrence was malignant. Radiation with multiple drug therapy and resection of residual tumor has resulted in apparent cure of 5 of these 9 patients. The serum AFP has been a valuable tumor marker in the follow-up of these patients. Serial CT scans will demonstrate reduction in tumor size during therapy but will not distinguish between residual scar or tumor. Surgical excision is essential to determine tumor activity as well as for cure.

The current chemotherapy regimen in use at our hospital for endodermal sinus tumors, regardless of location or organ, consists of vinblastine, bleomycin, cisplatin, and etoposide administered over a 6-day period. These drugs are then repeated every 3 weeks for six cycles. The child is completely reevaluated with tumor markers and CT scans to detect residual tumor.

TERATOMAS AT OTHER SITES

Although the pathology of teratomas is similar, their biologic behavior and symptoms depend on their location and the organ involved. Aside from their involvement with the gonads, teratomas are largely midline tumors, which may occur from the brain to the tail. The locations of teratomas encountered at our hospital are listed in Table 43–1.

Facial Teratoma

The epignathus is a rare congenital malformation. The infant is born with a mass of tissue protruding from the mouth. Although several different pathologic types of tumor have been reported, all are related to teratoma in that they contain derivatives of two or more germ layers that grow irregularly as a mixture of solid and cystic elements. Teeth and hair may be present in the

TABLE 43–1. BENIGN AND MALIGNANT TERATOMAS, 1952–1977

Benign		Malignant	
Location	Number	Location	Number
Sacrococcygeal area	25	Sacrococcygeal area	20
Ovary	5	Ovary	7
Anterior mediastinum	5	Testicle	3
Retroperitoneum	4	Retroperitoneum	2
Testicle	3		
Face	3		
Cervix	2		
Stomach	1		
Liver	1		

larger of the cysts, but the gross structure and the histologic picture usually are more like those of the fleshy teratomas that occur elsewhere.

Most epignathi are attached to the base of the skull in the posterior nasopharynx, near the site of Rathke's pouch and the closed craniopharyngeal canal. The tumor in one reported case was associated with an open Rathke's pouch, which in turn was associated with the cranial vault.[22] The origin of these tumors is thought to be similar to that of the sacrococcygeal teratomas, since they lie in an area that remains active in embryologic differentiation until well along in fetal life. In some of the cases, there is an intracranial extension of the tumor, with bony changes in the sella turcica and abnormalities of one or both parts of the hypophysis.

Associated congenital anomalies are frequent, and most infants with these tumors are stillborn. If the airway is compromised, a tracheotomy must be performed as a preliminary to x-ray studies and surgical attempts to remove the mass.

Cervical Teratoma

Teratomas in the neck may be sufficiently large to cause respiratory obstruction in the neonate, necessitating immediate surgical excision.[23] The mass is usually so large that endotracheal intubation, rather than a tracheotomy, is indicated. Occasionally the mass is smaller and occurs as an asymptomatic lesion in the anterior portion of the neck. The great majority of reported cases have been intimately associated with the thyroid gland, and only 1 in 67 of the tumors in children reported by Keynes was malignant.[24] Wide exposure through a transverse incision is necessary so that the recurrent laryngeal nerves may be identified and the thyroid vessels isolated in order to control the tumor's blood supply. Following surgery, the trachea, which has been distorted and flattened by the tumor, may require long-term support by means of either an endotracheal tube or a tracheostomy.

Mediastinal Teratoma

Teratomas arising in the anterior mediastinum cause respiratory distress in early infancy by compression of the trachea and the heart. On physical examination, the infant is cyanotic and tachypneic and may breathe better when lying on the abdomen. The anterior-posterior diameter of the chest may be increased, and the heart tones are muffled by the mass. Roentgenograms demonstrate a large mass that may be indistinguishable from the cardiac shadow. Indeed, the initial diagnosis may be congenital heart disease. A lateral roentgenogram, however, will demonstrate posterior displacement of the trachea. Smaller mediastinal teratomas may exist until adult life, when they may be discovered on an incidental roentgenogram. One dramatic symptom in adults has been the expectoration of hair. Most mediastinal teratomas are benign and well encapsulated. Only 12.9 percent of tumors in a series of 251 patients were malignant.[25] Surgical excision is best carried out through an anterior thoracotomy, which may be extended across the sternum into the opposite pleural cavity if more exposure is required. Intrapericardial teratomas cause cardiac tamponade in addition to respiratory distress. The tumor may be attached to the root of the aorta—3 operative deaths from aortic bleeding have been reported.[26]

We have had one teratoma in the left posterior mediastinum involving the esophagus. It was necessary to resect the esophagus with the tumor and eventually interpose a segment of transverse colon. The CT scan in our case made the diagnosis and demonstrated the esophageal involvement. Eight other cases of posterior mediastinal teratoma have been reported.[27]

Retroperitoneal Teratoma

Teratomas can arise either in the retroperitoneal space independent of the kidney or in an intrarenal location.[28,29] In either case, the tumor occurs as an abdominal mass with displacement or intrinsic distortion of the kidney, depending on the tumor's location. Intrarenal teratomas mimic Wilms' tumors and can be diagnosed only after nephrectomy. An unusual tumor that has been distinguished from teratomas is fetus in fetu, which represents an attempt at monozygotic twinning in the retroperitoneal space.[30] Most cases are diagnosed in infants who have an abdominal mass. The distinguishing feature is a well-formed vertebral column visible on an abdominal roentgenogram. The blood supply to the lesion arises from the host's superior mesenteric artery. Consequently, care must be taken in securing the blood supply to the mass.

Teratoma of the Stomach

The origin of gastric teratomas is difficult to fit into any of the current hypotheses. Approximately 50 cases have been reported in the literature, but only 2 have been in girls.[31–33] The presenting symptoms consist of abdominal enlargement, hematemesis, and a palpable upper abdominal mass. Roentgenograms demonstrate a mass that distorts the stomach, and at operation the lesion may either be in the stomach or arise from the stomach surface. Treatment consists of excision of the lesion with a small rim of the attached stomach wall. There are usually dense adhesions to the adjacent liver and colon, which make freeing the mass difficult. On the basis of reported cases, one may conclude that gastric teratomas are benign and that there are no recurrences after excision.

Teratoma of the Testicle

The various types of germ cell tumors, including benign teratoma, embryonal cell carcinoma, and endodermal sinus tumor, are the most common testicular tumors in childhood.[34] Embryonal carcinoma or endodermal sinus tumor usually occurs as an asymptomatic enlargement of the testicle in children under 2 years of age. Orchiectomy combined with chemotherapy has produced survival rates of over 80 percent.

The teratoma typically occurs as an asymptomatic scrotal mass in a boy between 3 and 4 years of age. Unfortunately, most testicular tumors are first thought to be hydroceles, and the diagnosis is thus delayed. This error can be avoided by noting the sensation of heaviness imparted by a testicular tumor as well as the absence of transillumination. Unfortunately, testicular teratomas may be bilateral.[35]

Teratoma of the Ovary

Benign cystic teratomas account for 30 to 40 percent of all ovarian cysts and tumors found in children.[36–38] Just as with all other teratomas, the malignant component most often is an endodermal sinus tumor that metastasizes to lymph nodes, the peritoneal surface, omentum, and liver.

Ovarian teratomas may occur in infancy but are most common in girls between 8 and 12 years of age. The symptoms are abdominal pain or a sense of fullness. Examination reveals a movable pelvic mass. There is no way to differentiate a teratoma from the other ovarian tumors unless a roentgenogram demonstrates a tooth or other calcium deposit within the mass.

There is one unusual pathologic entity associated with ovarian teratomas, gliomatosis peritonei.[39] Either after or at the time of laparotomy, the peritoneum becomes studded with small white nodules resembling tuberculous peritonitis, but which is actually glial tissue. This tissue is well differentiated and benign. Most patients can expect long-term survival after removal of the original tumor. It would appear that the patients with immature teratomas of the ovary with peritoneal metastases reported on by Kosloske et al. actually were afflicted with this benign form of gliomatosis.[40] An obvious cystic teratoma is removed by simply ligating the ovarian vessels and the fallopian tumor close to the mass. A complete exploration is made of the peritoneal cavity in order to find and remove any metastatic deposits or enlarged lymph nodes. However, since teratomas are bilateral in up to 25 percent of women during their reproductive years, it is necessary to carefully palpate and, if necessary, biopsy the opposite ovary.

REFERENCES

1. Crussi FG (ed): Extragonadal Teratomas. Series 2, Fascicle 18 Atlas of Tumor Pathology. Washington, DC, Armed Forces Institute of Pathology, 1982
2. Altman RP, Randolph JG, Lilly JR: Sacrococcygeal tera-

toma: American Academy of Pediatrics Surgical Section Survey—1973. J Pediatr Surg 9:389, 1973

3. Ashcraft KW, Holder TM, Harris DJ: Familial presacral teratomas. Birth Defects 11:143, 1975

4. Kenefick JS: Hereditary sacral agenesis associated with presacral tumors. Br J Surg 60:271, 1973

5. Smith J, Wixon D, Watson RC: Giant cell tumor of the sacrum: clinical and radiologic features in 13 patients. J Can Assoc Radiol 30:34, 1979

6. Izant RJ, Filston HC: Sacrococcygeal teratomas. Am J Surg 130:617, 1975

7. Miles RM, Stewart GS: Sacrococcygeal teratomas in adults. Ann Surg 179:676, 1974

8. Ein S, Mancer K, Adeyemi S: Malignant sacrococcygeal teratoma, endodermal sinus, yolk sac tumor in infants and children: a 32 year review. J Pediatr Surg 20:473, 1985

9. Teilum G: Endodermal sinus tumors of the ovary and testis: comparative morphogenesis of the so-called mesonephroma ovarii (Schiller) and extraembryonic (yolk sac–allantoic) structures of rat's placenta. Cancer 12:1092, 1959

10. Crussi FG, Roth LM: The yolk sac and yolk sac carcinoma: An ultrastructural study. Hum Pathol 7:675, 1976

11. Olsen MM, Raffensperger JG, Crussi FG, et al: Endodermal sinus tumor: A clinical and pathological correlation. J Pediatr Surg 17:832, 1982

12. Sherowsky RC, Williams CH, Nichols VB, et al: Prenatal ultrasonographic diagnosis of a sacrococcygeal teratoma in twin pregnancy. J Ultrasound Med 4:159, 1985

13. Seeds JW, Mittelstaedt CA, Cefalo RC, et al: Prenatal diagnosis of sacrococcygeal teratoma: An anechoic caudal mass. JCU 10:193, 1982

14. Flake A, Harrison M, Adzick N, et al: Fetal sacrococcygeal teratoma. J Pediatr Surg 21:563, 1986

15. Naidich TP, Fernbach SK, McLone DG, Shkolnik A: Sonography of the caudal spine and back: Congenital anomalies in children. AJR 142:1229, 1984

16. Tsuchida Y, Hasegawa H: The diagnostic value of alpha-fetoprotein in infants and children with teratomas: A questionnaire survey in Japan. J Pediatr Surg 18:152, 1983

17. Hecht F, Hecht BK, O'Keefe D: Sacrococcygeal teratoma: Prenatal diagnosis with elevated alpha-fetoprotein and acetylcholinesterase in amniotic fluid. Prenat Diagn 2:229, 1982

18. Donnellan WA, Swenson O: Benign and malignant sacrococcygeal teratomas. Surgery 64:834, 1968

19. Tapper D, Lack EE: Teratomas in infancy and childhood: A 54-year experience at the Children's Hospital Medical Center. Ann Surg 198:398, 1983

20. Dewan P, Davidson P, Campbell P, et al: Sacrococcygeal teratoma: Has chemotherapy improved survival? J Pediatr Surg 22:274, 1987

21. Billmire D, Grosfeld J: Teratomas in childhood: Analysis of 142 cases. J Pediatr Surg 21:548, 1986

22. Wilson JW, Gehweiler JA: Teratoma of the face associated with a patent canal extending into the cranial cavity (Rathke's pouch) in a three-week-old child. J Pediatr Surg 5:349, 1970

23. Jordan R, Gauderer M: Cervical teratomas: An analysis, literature review and proposed classification. J Pediatr Surg 23:583, 1988

24. Keynes WM: Teratoma of the neck in relationship to the thyroid gland. Br J Surg 46:466, 1959

25. Rusby NL: Dermoid cysts and teratoma of the mediastinum: A review. J Thorac Surg 13:169, 1944

26. Deeadayalu RP, Tuuri D, Dewall RA, et al: Intrapericardial teratoma and bronchogenic cyst: Review of literature and report of successful surgery in infant with intrapericardial teratoma. J Thorac Cardiovasc Surg 67:945, 1974

27. Karl S, Dunn J: Posterior mediastinal teratomas. J Pediatr Surg 20:508, 1985

28. Palumbo LT, Cross KR, Smith AN, et al: Primary teratomas of the lateral retroperitoneal spaces. Surgery 26:149, 1949

29. Dehner LP: Intrarenal teratoma occurring in infancy: Case report. J Pediatr Surg 8:369, 1973

30. Grosfeld JD, Stepita DS, Nance WE, et al: Fetus-in-fetu: Case report. Ann Surg 180:80, 1974

31. Azpiroz JAC, Valle EM, Herberth AF, et al: Gastric teratoma in infants: Case report. Am J Surg 128:429, 1974

32. Nandy AD, Sengupta, Chatterjee SK, et al: Teratoma of the stomach. J Pediatr Surg 9:563, 1974

33. Cairo M, Grosfeld J, Weetman R: Gastric teratoma: unusual cause for bleeding of the upper gastrointestinal tract in the newborn. Pediatrics 67:721, 1981

34. Giebink GS, Ruymann FB: Testicular tumors in children: Review and report of three cases. Am J Dis Child 127:433, 1974

35. Carney JA, Kelalis PP, Lynn HB: Bilateral teratoma of testis in an infant. J Pediatr Surg 8:49, 1973

36. Ein SH, Sarte MM, Stephens CA: Cystic and solid ovarian tumors in children: A 44-year review. J Pediatr Surg 5:148, 1970

37. Towne BH, Mahour GH, Woolley MM, et al: Ovarian cysts and tumors in infancy and childhood. J Pediatr Surg 10:311, 1975

38. Breen J, Maxon W: Ovarian tumors in children and adolescents. Clin Obstet Gynecol 20:607, 1977

39. Fortt RW, Mathie IK: Gliomatosis peritonei caused by ovarian teratoma. J Clin Pathol 22:348, 1969

40. Kosloske AM, Favara BE, Hays T, et al: Management of immature teratoma of the ovary in children by conservative resection and chemotherapy. J Pediatr Surg 22:839, 1976

44
Ovarian Tumors

An ovarian cyst or tumor must be considered in any girl with unexplained lower abdominal pain, an abdominal mass, or sexual precocity. The diagnoses of 350 ovarian cysts and tumors from five series of cases is listed in Table 44–1.[1–5] The most common lesions are the simple cysts, either follicular or lutein, and the benign cystic teratomas. Solid tumors are much less common and are more likely to be malignant.

DIAGNOSIS

A simple cyst may appear in the newborn infant as a mobile abdominal mass anterior to the rectum. It will transilluminate and often cannot be differentiated from a mesenteric cyst or intestinal duplication. An ultrasound examination will differentiate ovarian cysts from kidney lesions. An intrauterine torsion of an ovarian cyst results in toxicity, fever, and thrombocytopenia.

Ovarian torsion in an older child simulates appendicitis (Fig. 44–1). The history, however, will reveal a more acute onset of pain with radiation down the inner side of the child's thigh. Often the girl will remember the exact time of the onset of her pain, whereas the onset of appendiceal pain is less dramatic.

Normal uterine adnexa can undergo torsion that simulates a twisted ovarian cyst. There often is a history of lower abdominal pain, and the other side is subject to future torsion. Thus, contralateral adnexal fixation should be performed to prevent future problems.[6] When a girl has lower abdominal pain with equivocal physical findings, the question of an ovarian cyst is always raised, particularly if the rectal or pelvic examinations are not definitive. An ultrasound examination will accurately detect an ovarian mass as small as 2 cm in diameter. Furthermore, ultrasonography will reliably distinguish a solid from a cystic lesion. Roentgenograms are of value only in detecting lesions large enough to displace other organs or those containing calcifications.

TREATMENT

A ruptured corpus luteum cyst may cause acute lower abdominal pain and even a shocklike state in teenage girls. Unlike ovarian torsion, the symptoms rapidly subside. Often, by the time the patient reaches the hospital, there is only mild residual discomfort. If an ultrasound examination reveals a small cyst, the lesion may be observed safely through several menstrual cycles. If symptoms and the mass persist, an exploration with removal of the cyst is indicated. All other cysts and solid tumors require an operation. If the tumor is solid, the preoperative studies should include the usual metastatic workup and a computed tomography (CT) scan of the abdomen.

At operation, the bladder is catheterized, and the abdomen is opened with a low transverse incision. Simple cysts are removed by clamping and dividing the ovarian vessels, together with the suspensory ligament and the uteroovarian ligament. There is no need to remove the fallopian tube. All cysts must be opened and inspected in the operating room because there is a strong possibility of bilateral lesions if the cyst is a teratoma. Although some surgeons advocate routine bivalving and biopsy of the contralateral ovary, inspection with biopsy of any suspicious lesion is sufficient in children. An incidental appendectomy is then performed, and the wound is closed.

SOLID TUMORS

The most common ovarian tumor in childhood is the mature cystic teratoma.[7,8] At operation, the tumor is smooth and not attached to adjacent viscera. It should

TABLE 44–1. COLLECTED SERIES OF 350 OVARIAN CYSTS AND TUMORS[a]

Benign		Malignant	
Type	*Number*	*Type*	*Number*
Simple cysts	159	Malignant teratoma (includes embryonal carcinoma and endodermal sinus tumors)	13
Cystic teratomas	129	Papillary adenocarcinoma	6
Granulosa cell tumors	11	Dysgerminoma	7
Cystic adenomas	6	Granulosa cell carcinoma	5
Arrhenoblastoma	1	Lymphoma	2
Fibroma	2	Reticulum cell sarcoma	1
Hemangioma	2	Cystic sarcoma	1
Thecoma	1	Choriocarcinoma	3
Total	311	Fibrosarcoma	1
		Total	39

[a] In this combined series, there were 56 solid tumors, of which 39 were malignant.

be removed and submitted for immediate pathologic examination. Frozen sections are taken from solid portions of the tumor, and if there is only mature tissue from the three germ layers, nothing more needs to be done. When there is a large amount of solid or necrotic tissue on the cut surface of the tumor, one must suspect an immature or grossly malignant lesion. There are varying degrees of malignancy in immature teratomas, but the endodermal sinus tumor represents the malignant end of the spectrum. Clinically, these tumors grow rap-

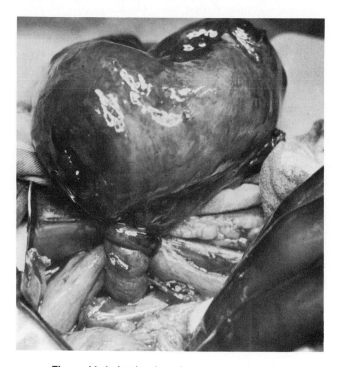

Figure 44–1. A twisted ovarian cyst in a teenage girl.

idly, and often there is ascites at the time of diagnosis. When an ovarian mass is attached to the omentum or intestine, it must be considered malignant at the outset. The incision must be enlarged to allow complete exploration of the liver, peritoneal surfaces, and the periaortic lymph nodes. All ascitic fluid is removed and saved to study for malignant cells. The tumor is handled gently to avoid spillage, the omentum is removed from the colon and stomach, and any adherent bowel is resected with the tumor. The ovarian vessels are ligated at their origin, and all lymph nodes along the vessels are removed. The fallopian tube is clamped and suture-ligated flush with the uterus. There is no advantage to removal of the uterus or opposite ovary. If a frozen section confirms the suspicion of malignancy, the iliac and periaortic nodes are removed.

Further treatment depends on the pathology. Children with granulosa cell tumors have all survived with no further therapy, but germ cell tumors, dysgerminoma, immature teratomas, and endodermal sinus tumors demonstrate varying degrees of malignancy. A review of tumors previously termed "embryonal carcinoma" or "malignant teratoma" has demonstrated that most of these are actually endodermal sinus tumors (Chapter 47).

The alpha-fetoprotein is elevated in endodermal sinus tumors but returns to normal levels with successful treatment. Formerly, the median survival for patients with these lesions was only 6 to 12 months.[9] There has been a high relapse rate, even when the original tumor appeared to be confined to the ovary. Consequently, all these lesions require postoperative chemotherapy.[10] In our hospital, a four-drug protocol of vinblastine, bleomycin, cisplatin, and etoposide is given to these patients, depending on the stage of their disease.

REFERENCES

1. Harris BH, Boles TE Jr: Rational surgery for tumors of the ovary in children. J Pediatr Surg 9:289, 1974
2. Adelman S, Benson CD, Hertzler JH: Surgical lesions of the ovary in infancy and childhood. Surg Gynecol Obstet 141:210, 1975
3. Thatcher DS: Ovarian cysts and tumors in children. Surg Gynecol Obstet 117:477, 1963
4. Towne BH, Mahour GH, Woolley MM, et al: Ovarian cysts and tumors in infancy and childhood. J Pediatr Surg 10:311, 1975
5. Ein SH, Darte JMM, Stephens CA: Cystic and ovarian tumors in children: A 44-year review. J Pediatr Surg 5:148, 1970
6. Russ J: Sequential torsion of the uterine adnexa. Mayo Clin Proc 62:623, 1987
7. Breen J, Maxson W: Ovarian tumors in children and adolescents. Clin Obstet Gynecol 20:607, 1977
8. Russell P, Painter D: The pathological assessment of ovarian neoplasms. V: The germ cell tumors. Pathology 14:47, 1982
9. Sikorowa L, Morcwski A, Pietkowski Z: Endodermal sinus tumors of the ovary. Clinicopathologic study of 6 cases. Oncology 36:187, 1979
10. Ehren I, Mahove G, Isaacs H: Benign and malignant ovarian tumors in childhood and adolescence. Am J Surg 147:339, 1984

45
Tumors of the Testicle

Testicular tumors represent only 1.5 percent of all childhood neoplasms. There is a peak age incidence at 2 years and a second period of increasing frequency during puberty. There are definite racial differences, with the highest incidence in Japanese boys and the lowest in blacks.[1,2]

Although etiologic factors in testicular tumors are no better understood than in other pediatric malignancies, there is a clear association of malignancy with the dysplastic undescended testicle. Gehring et al. found cryptorchid-associated malignant tumors in 37 of 529 adult patients with testicular tumors.[3] It is of great interest that 24 percent of these tumors occurred in the contralateral descended testicle. In this study, orchidopexy failed to prevent malignant degeneration, but it was noted that all the tumor patients had undergone the operation after the age of 6 years. An earlier orchidopexy may protect against malignant degeneration.

PATHOLOGY

Most childhood testicular tumors are of germ cell origin. Table 45–1 lists the more common testicular tumors, based on a collected series of 609 cases.[4] To this list may be added such miscellaneous tumors as the rhabdomyosarcomas, involving the paratesticular tissues, and leukemic infiltrates, which secondarily involve the testicle. Germ cell tumors formerly termed "embryonal carcinoma," "malignant teratoma," or "infantile orchioblastoma" are now recognized to be yolk sac or endodermal sinus tumors.[5] These account for 35 to 45 percent of all testicular tumors in childhood. The typical tumor is a homogeneous, yellow-gray mass with foci of hemorrhage. This tumor has a varying microscopic appearance but is characterized by a small group of epithelial cells

surrounding a central blood vessel, the Schiller-Duval body. The cells are clear and cuboidal.

Seminomas in children are exceedingly rare but appear more frequently in pubertal boys. They are essentially identical in appearance and behavior to the same tumors in adults. The nongerminal cell tumors include the Sertoli cell and Leydig cell lesions. Both of these tumors are associated with precocious sexual development, and about 10 percent are malignant.[6,7]

Rhabdomyosarcomas are the most common paratesticular neoplasms. Grossly, when these tumors are first seen, there is infiltration of the paratesticular tissues, the spermatic cord, and the skin. There are also likely to be grossly enlarged lymph nodes in the groin.

TABLE 45–1. TESTICULAR TUMORS IN CHILDREN: 609 CASES

Cell Type	Number of Cases	Percent
Germ cell origin (69.1% of all cases)		
Embryonal carcinoma	167	39.7
Teratoma	113	26.8
Teratocarcinoma	90	21.4
Mixed germ cell	40	9.5
Seminoma	11	2.6
Total	421	100.0
Nongerm cell origin (30.9% of all cases)		
Sarcoma	62	33.0
Interstitial cell	51	27.1
Lymphoma	38	20.2
Sertoli cell	29	15.4
Other	8	4.3
Total	188	100.0

Data from Giebink and Ruymann.[4]

DIAGNOSIS

Even though tumors are rare, as a matter of discipline, one must consider a testicular malignancy in every child who exhibits a scrotal mass. In almost every case of testicular tumor, a mistaken diagnosis of hydrocele has been made, often months previously. A testicular tumor is painless, heavy, and firm.

The most important function of scrotal transillumination is not to distinguish hernia from a hydrocele but to determine the presence of a testicular mass. Even minimal degrees of asymmetry between the two testicles should raise the suspicion of a tumor, particularly if there is a firm or indurated area in the larger organ. The differential diagnosis includes such benign conditions as orchitis, torsion, or contusion due to trauma. In the neonate, meconium peritonitis may be associated with a hard scrotal mass, but x-ray evidence of calcification in the peritoneal cavity and scrotum should make the diagnosis. Splenogonadal fusion also may resemble a tumor.[8]

Preoperative studies include routine blood counts and a chest x-ray. An ultrasound study of the abdomen is helpful in detecting other genitourinary anomalies or retroperitoneal lymph nodes. Complete studies for metastases are time-consuming and are not necessary if the lesion should turn out to be benign. It makes more sense to biopsy the tumor and if it is malignant to carry out further studies.

SURGICAL EXPLORATION

An exploration for a possible testicular tumor commences with an oblique groin incision that extends to the upper portion of the scrotum. The use of an oblique incision is contrary to the usual practice in pediatric surgery but allows wide exposure of the inguinal canal, from the scrotum to the internal ring. The cremaster muscle fibers are then encircled and clamped with a noncrushing vascular clamp. The testicle with its enveloping fascia, including the cremasteric muscle and the gubernaculum, is then delivered into the surgical field and is brought through a small slit in a plastic drape sheet, which is placed over the wound with the sticky side facing outward. A wedge biopsy is then taken from the mass. The instruments, sponges, and gloves are immediately discarded after the biopsy site is closed, and the testicle is wrapped in the plastic drape to avoid spilling tumor cells.

If the frozen section reveals malignant tissue, a radical orchiectomy is performed. The incision is extended so that the testicular vessels can be followed to their origin. The vessels are removed with all surrounding lymph nodes. Simple orchiectomy is sufficient treatment for a benign teratoma, but the endodermal sinus or other malignant germ cell tumors require further therapy. This is an aggressive tumor, which metastasizes to lymph nodes, brain, and bones. Kaplan and Firlit found nodal metastases in 4 of 10 boys with yolk sac tumors and originally recommended a radical retroperitoneal lymph node dissection.[9] In other series in which lymph node dissections were performed, no tumor was found.[10–12] Current recommendations are to do follow-up serum alpha-fetoprotein (AFP) level determinations. When there is no metastatic disease, this tumor marker falls to normal levels. Abdominal computed tomography (CT) scans are performed for evidence of periaortic lymph node enlargement.

Children with stage I tumors who have no nodal involvement or metastases have a 3-year disease-free rate of 84 percent whether they are treated with chemotherapy or not.[13] Children with advanced disease or those who develop metastases after initial surgery require systemic chemotherapy. An increasing level of AFP is regarded as a sign of relapse and an indication for adjuvant treatment. Various drug protocols are evolving, but in our hospital, a four-drug regimen using vinblastine, bleomycin, cisplatin, and etoposide is used.

The paratesticular rhabdomyosarcoma is the most common tumor of the spermatic cord or testicular supporting tissues. These are aggressive lesions that occur in boys of 9 to 10 years of age.[14] These children require node dissection, chemotherapy, and radiation appropriate to the stage of their disease, but disease-free survival is now better than 80 percent.[15]

TECHNIQUE OF NODAL DISSECTION

A long, vertical incision that will expose the aorta from the renal arteries to the iliac vessels is necessary. The small intestine is eviscerated to the right, and the posterior peritoneum is opened from the duodenum to the pelvis. After exposure of the renal arteries and veins, all lymphatic and areolar tissue is removed from the aorta and from between the aorta and inferior vena cava. If they have not previously been removed, the testicular vessels are taken with surrounding nodes and areolar tissue from their origin. At the end of the dissection, the aorta, iliac arteries, inferior mesenteric artery, and renal vessels should be cleared of all surrounding tissue. If nodes are palpable above the limits of this dissection, they should be removed separately for microscopic examination.

REFERENCES

1. Li FP, Fraumeni JF Jr: Testicular cancers in children: Epidemiologic characteristics. J Natl Cancer Inst 48:1515, 1972
2. Mostofi FK: Testicular tumors. Cancer 32:1186, 1973
3. Gehring GG, Rodriguez FR, Woodhead DM: Malignant degeneration of cryptorchid testes following orchiopexy. J Urol 112:354, 1974
4. Giebink GS, Ruymann FB: Testicular tumors in childhood. Am J Dis Child 127:433, 1974
5. Dehner L: Pediatric Surgical Pathology, 2nd ed. Baltimore, Williams & Wilkins, 1987, p 722
6. Talerman A: Malignant sertoli cell tumor of the testis. Cancer 28:446, 1971
7. Tamoney HJ, Noriega A: Malignant interstitial cell tumor of the testis. Cancer 24:547, 1979
8. Tsingoglov S, Wilkinson AW: Splenogonadal fusion. Br J Surg 63:297, 1976
9. Kaplan W, Firlit C: Treatment of testicular yolk sac carcinoma in the young child. J Urol 126:663, 1981
10. Tefft M, Vawter CF, Mistus A: Radiotherapeutic management of testicular neoplasms in children. Radiology 88:457, 1967
11. Gangai MP: Testicular neoplasms in an infant. Cancer 22:658, 1968
12. Sabio H, Bergert EO Jr, Farrow GM, et al: Embryonal carcinoma of the testis in childhood. Cancer 34:2118, 1974
13. Flamant F, Nihoul-Fekete C, Patte C, et al: Optimal treatment of clinical stage I yolk sac tumor of the testis in children. J Pediatr Surg 21:108, 1986
14. Cromie W, Rainey R, Duckett J: Paratesticular rhabdomyosarcoma in children. J Urol 80:122, 1979
15. Ghavimi F, Herr H, Jereb B, Flexby P: Treatment of genitourinary rhabdomyosarcoma in children. J Urol 132:313, 1984

46

Benign and Malignant Neoplasms of the Gastrointestinal Tract

Randall W. Powell

Neoplasms of the gastrointestinal tract occur rarely in infants and children and often progress to advanced stages because the diagnosis is delayed. The rarity of these neoplasms and their early nonspecific symptoms do not prompt diagnostic tests that would lead to early diagnosis and treatment.

NEOPLASMS OF THE MOUTH AND PHARYNX

The neoplastic lesions developing in the oral cavity and pharynx may be detected early due to symptoms of difficulty in feeding or respiratory obstruction. In the newborn, the large lymphangioma involving the tongue and floor of the mouth can cause severe upper airway obstruction requiring emergency control of the airway. Large teratomas originating from the oral cavity can cause respiratory embarrassment or feeding difficulties. These tumors should be totally excised. Other benign lesions of the oral cavity, tongue, and pharynx include hemangiomas, fibromas, hamartomas, congenital epulis, and various tumors related to dentition.

Malignant tumors are rare, representing 5 to 10 percent of all oral cavity tumors in children.[1] The most common of these are malignant lymphomas and rhabdomyosarcomas. The lymphomas involve the tonsils or other lymphatic tissue in the posterior pharynx and frequently occur with enlarged cervical lymph nodes. The role of surgery is for diagnosis. Rhabdomyosarcomas may involve the lips, tongue, palate, nasopharynx, and oropharynx. Surgical extirpation is the goal, with subsequent chemotherapy and possible radiation therapy in advanced stages. The nasopharyngeal rhabdomyosarcomas, be-cause of their parameningeal location, also require CNS prophylaxis (irradiation and intrathecal chemotherapy) to prevent the frequent meningeal spread.

Epithelial malignancies of the oral cavity and pharynx are extremely rare, but the incidence may increase with the popularity of oral tobacco products in the adolescent age group. These tumors may be recognized at advanced stages because of reluctance to seek medical attention.

NEOPLASMS OF THE ESOPHAGUS

The esophagus is a rare site for neoplasms in childhood. The most common solid tumor is the leiomyoma of the wall of the esophagus, which may appear as an abnormal shadow on a chest radiograph or may cause obstructive symptoms. A barium swallow reveals a smooth indentation into the lumen of the esophagus. An esophageal duplication often occurs in the same fashion and cannot be differentiated from the leiomyoma except by computed tomography (CT). At thoracotomy, the tumor usually can be separated readily from the esophagus without violating the esophageal lumen. With extensive tumor, resection with subsequent esophageal replacement may be necessary.[2]

Mucosal lesions of the esophagus are rarely reported. Aberrant gastric mucosa has caused obstructive symptoms in children and has been implicated in the development of adenocarcinoma of the esophagus in adults.[3] The aberrant mucosa can mimic a neoplastic lesion. Barrett's esophagus, a metaplastic change of the squamous epithelium of the esophagus to a columnar epithelium, can occur in children in the setting of chronic irritation by gastroesophageal reflux and is associated with an increased risk of carcinoma in adults. Lye ingestion can result in a long-term risk for the development of squamous carcinoma of the esophagus. Appelquist and Salmo reported 3 cases of squamous carcinoma developing after lye ingestion.[4] The mean age at the time of ingestion was 6.2 years, with an interval from ingestion to diagnosis of carcinoma from 13 to 71 years.

NEOPLASMS OF THE STOMACH

The stomach is another rare site for neoplasms in infants and children. Benign neoplasms predominate and include mucosal and gastric wall tumors. Leiomyomas and leiomyosarcomas frequently occur with bleeding, and because of the difficulty in determining the diagnosis at the time of surgery, a wide excision is recommended.[5] Gastric teratomas, though rare, appear as large epigastric or left upper quadrant masses, or with bleeding from ulceration of the gastric mucosa overlying the tumor (Fig. 46–1). A generous excision of the attachment site is curative in this benign lesion. Gastric teratomas usually occur in infants and almost exclusively in males.[6,7]

Gastric mucosal tumors are rare. Gastric polyps may occur in syndromes with diffuse polyposis, such as Peutz-Jeghers syndrome and generalized juvenile polyposis.

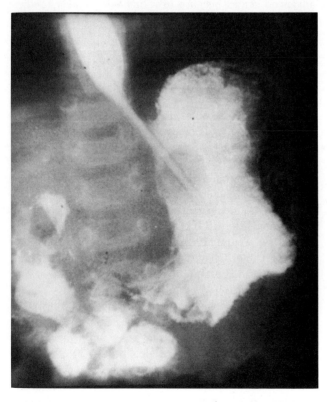

Figure 46–1. Upper gastrointestinal x-ray of a gastric teratoma of the greater curvature of the stomach. Note filling defect.

With increasing use of upper gastrointestinal flexible endoscopy, the pancreatic rest may represent the most frequent mucosal lesion. Adenocarcinoma is quite rare in children. McNeer reported 19 cases occurring in the 15 years or less age group of 501 total cases.[8] Since gastric adenocarcinoma occurs in children much as it does in adults, aggressive evaluation of a gastric ulcer in a child or adolescent is mandatory.[9]

NEOPLASMS OF THE SMALL INTESTINE

Non-Hodgkin's lymphomas predominate as the malignant tumor of the small intestine. These tumors usually occur in school-age children, and delays in diagnosis are common because of nonspecific symptoms. Acute symptoms in the form of colicky abdominal pain and blood in the stool occur when the lymphoma acts as a lead point for an intussusception.[10] The surgical treatment for this tumor is resection of the involved intestine with adjacent involved mesenteric nodes in patients with limited disease, followed by chemotherapy. In patients with extensive disease with large abdominal masses, a simple biopsy for diagnosis followed by intensive chemotherapy can result in salvage. Second-look operations if CT or contrast studies reveal residual disease can aid in salvage. In North America, Burkitt's lymphoma frequently involves the intestine and may cause ascites, abdominal or pelvic masses, or intestinal obstruction.[11] The lymphomas tend to occur in the distal ileum and can be demonstrated by contrast studies (Fig. 46–2). The tumor may appear grossly as a large mass, an infiltrating constricting lesion, or as ulcer or polyp.

Other malignant tumors of the small intestine include leiomyosarcoma, angiosarcoma, and carcinoid tumor. All of these neoplasms are extremely rare. Lesions that may mimic malignant tumors include hypertrophied Peyer's patches in the distal ileum, inflammatory bowel disease, and infections such as tuberculosis. Crohn's disease has been reported to be associated with an increased risk of adenocarcinoma of the small bowel (28 of 579 patients),[12] but none of the patients was younger than 21 years of age.

Benign neoplasms of the small intestine include polyps (Peutz-Jeghers and other polypoid syndromes), hemangiomas, lymphangiomas, leiomyomas, and neurofibromas. The multiple endocrine neoplasia (MEN) type 2b syndrome is characterized by mucosal neuromas throughout the gastrointestinal tract.[13] These patients tend to have typical facial features and develop medullary carcinoma of the thyroid and pheochromocytoma early in life.

Hemangiomas may cause acute or chronic blood loss, obstruction, pain, or rarely a mass lesion. Abraham-

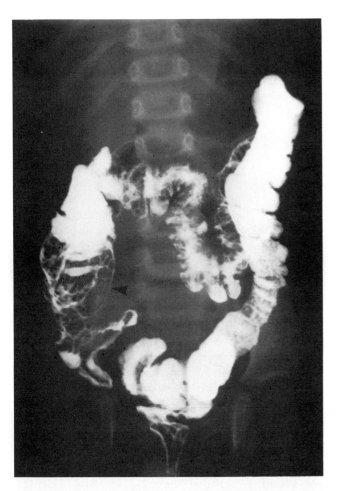

Figure 46–2. A 5-year-old boy with a 6-week history of vomiting and recurrent abdominal pain. Barium enema shows a normal colon, but reflux through the ileocecal valve reveals a mass within the distal ileum invaginating into the cecum.

son and Shandling reported 7 cases of their own and reviewed 58 other cases.[14] They classified the hemangiomas and discussed each type fully. They emphasized the frequent difficulty in demonstrating these neoplasms as the source of the patient's symptoms.

NEOPLASMS OF THE LARGE INTESTINE

Malignant neoplasms of the large intestine include lymphoma, adenocarcinoma, leiomyosarcoma, and carcinoid tumors. The carcinoid tumors in children occur most often in the appendix and are more frequent in females (3:1).[15] The tumor may cause obstruction of the appendiceal lumen, resulting in appendicitis or appendicitis symptoms. Ryden et al. reviewed 30 cases, and 29 had symptoms of appendicitis, with 25 having histologic evidence of acute appendicitis.[15] The tumors ranged from 0.1 to 2.5 cm, with tumor invasion into the muscularis

in 27 of the 30 cases, and 14 cases showed perineural involvement. Of the 27 patients available for follow-up, all were alive without evidence of disease 2 to 24 years after appendectomy. The recommended treatment for this tumor is simple appendectomy. The large tumor (>2 cm) at the base of the appendix or obvious nodal involvement may be best treated by right colectomy.

The colon is the most common site for adenocarcinoma in the gastrointestinal tract in children, but this tumor in children represents less than 1 percent of all malignant tumors of the large intestine.[16] The sex ratio, equal in adults, is a 2:1 ratio of male/female in pediatric age patients.[16] Middelkamp and Haffner in their review found that 95 percent of these tumors occur in the over 10 year age group.[17] Common symptoms include abdominal pain (90 percent), vomiting (40 percent), constipation (25 percent), weight loss (20 percent), blood in the stools (18 percent), and abdominal distention (13 percent).[17] These symptoms are often vague and, because of the rarity of the diagnosis, are not completely evaluated until late in the course of the disease. Occasionally, children with colon carcinoma will have signs and symptoms of acute appendicitis, and some authors recommend a thorough palpation of the colon when a normal appendix is found.[16,17] The locations of adenocarcinoma of the colon in children are similar to those in adults and are depicted in Figure 46–3.[18]

In the last 7 years at the University of South Alabama Medical Center, two children with adenocarcinoma of the colon have been treated. One was a 2-year-old female who had abdominal distention and evidence of intestinal obstruction. At celiotomy, an adenocarcinoma of the de-

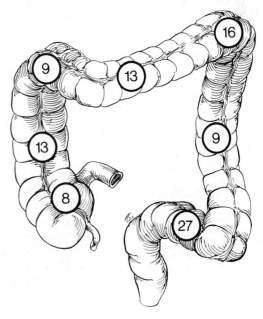

Figure 46–3. Distribution of 95 cases of carcinoma of the colon. (*Cain and Longino.*[18])

scending sigmoid colon area with lymph node metastases and peritoneal implants was found. The patient succumbed to diffuse abdominal carcinomatosis within a year after her initial operation. The second patient, an 11-year-old male, had abdominal distention and vague abdominal pain. On physical examination, significant ascites was present and CT was normal. A paracentesis yielded straw-colored fluid with a positive cytologic examination. Colonoscopy and barium enema revealed a constricting lesion near the hepatic flexure (Fig. 46–4), and biopsies revealed adenocarcinoma. At celiotomy, the entire omentum was replaced with tumor, and numerous peritoneal implants were seen. A palliative resection included the right and transverse colon and the omentum. The lesion near the hepatic flexure had constricted the colon lumen to approximately 0.5 cm. At present, this child is undergoing chemotherapy under an experimental protocol. Both of our patients had mucin-producing tumors, seen in at least 50 percent of colon carcinomas reported in children but in only 5 percent of adult patients.[16] The prognosis for children with adeno-

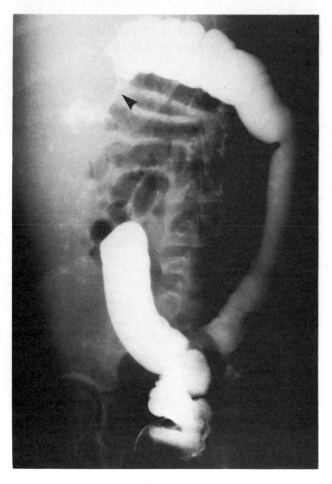

Figure 46–4. Annular constricting carcinoma of the transverse colon in an 11-year-old boy.

carcinoma of the colon is poor, with long-term survival reported as 2.5 percent.[16] The two factors that seem to produce the high mortality rate in children are delay in diagnosis so that the tumor is discovered in an advanced stage and the higher incidence of more aggressive, mucin-producing tumors. Aggressive use of the barium enema and colonoscopy in children with prolonged abdominal complaints may decrease the delay factor. Chemotherapy can be used in advanced cases with varying success.[19,20]

A number of conditions may predispose to the development of adenocarcinoma of the colon occurring in childhood, but usually malignancy develops after the second decade. These conditions include ulcerative colitis, Crohn's disease, polyposis syndromes (familial polyposis, Gardner's syndrome, Turcot's syndrome), nodular lymphoid hyperplasia, retinitis pigmentosa, ureterosigmoidostomy, and familial cancer syndrome.[1]

Benign tumors of the rectum include leiomyomas, adenomatous and juvenile polyps, villous adenomas, and hemangiomas. The mixed or predominantly cavernous hemangioma involving the rectum can be especially troublesome. These lesions frequently extend from hemangiomas of the lower extremity or buttock and can cause significant bleeding.[14] Patients may require a temporary diverting colostomy because of ulceration and bleeding. After the typical involution of this type of hemangioma, the colostomy can be closed. This method avoids perianal scarring and sphincter injury, which can occur with surgical excision or radiation therapy.

NEOPLASMS OF THE PANCREAS AND BILE DUCTS

Pancreatic neoplasms may appear as functional tumors arising from the islet cells or nonfunctional tumors of acinar or ductal origin. The functional tumors can occur early in life with symptoms of hypoglycemia (insulinoma) or severe diarrhea with electrolyte abnormalities (vasoactive intestinal peptide-secreting tumor). Symptoms of active or unusual ulcer disease should alert one to the possibilities of a gastrinoma (Zollinger-Ellison syndrome). Diagnosis of these tumors can be made by measurements of the active hormone and localization of the tumor by ultrasonography, CT, or surgical exploration. Excellent results can be obtained by removing the tumor or target organ.[21]

Nonfunctional tumors arising from acinar or ductal elements of the pancreas can be benign (cystadenoma) or malignant (adenocarcinoma).[21,22] These tumors usually occur as an abdominal mass with vague associated symptoms. The benign cystadenoma requires complete resection to prevent recurrence or recurrence with malignant

TABLE 46–1. CONDITIONS PREDISPOSING TO GASTROINTESTINAL TRACT MALIGNANCY

Condition	Site of Malignancy
Polyposis coli	
Familial polyposis	Colon
Gardner's syndrome	Colon
Turcot's syndrome	Colon
Peutz-Jeghers syndrome	Colon
Inflammatory bowel disease	
Ulcerative colitis	Colon
Crohn's disease	Small intestine and colon
Ureterosigmoidostomy	Colon
Ataxia telangiectasia	Stomach
IgA deficiency	Colon, stomach
Retinitis pigmentosa	Colon
Tylosis (palmar–plantar keratosis)	Esophagus
Glioma	Colon
Familial atypical mole–malignant melanoma syndrome	Colon
Lye ingestion	Esophagus

changes.[21,22] Adenocarcinomas appear in a similar fashion but rarely cause jaundice as in the adult. Many patients have metastatic disease. Resectable tumors of the head of the pancreas require pancreaticoduodenectomy, with a reasonable outlook for survival (5 of 22) and normal growth and development.[21]

Rhabdomyosarcoma represents the most common of the rare tumors arising in the bile ducts. The occurrence of cholangiocarcinoma in unresected choledochal cysts has led to the universal recommendation for complete excision of the cyst when first diagnosed.

CONDITIONS PREDISPOSING TO MALIGNANCY IN THE GASTROINTESTINAL TRACT

There are diseases and syndromes that predispose to the development of malignancy of the gastrointestinal tract (Table 46–1), and there are conditions in the gastrointestinal tract that may herald an increased risk of malignancies in other organ systems (Table 46–2).[23] In

TABLE 46–2. GASTROINTESTINAL TRACT CONDITIONS ASSOCIATED WITH OTHER MALIGNANCY

Condition	Site
Multiple endocrine neoplasia type 2b	Medullary carcinoma of thyroid
Gastrointestinal tract neuromas	Pheochromocytoma
Turcot's syndrome	
Colon polyposis	Brain

certain conditions, such as ulcerative colitis or polyposis syndromes, the risk of developing a malignancy can be eliminated by removing the target organ. Other conditions require knowledge of the risk and early diagnosis and treatment of the malignancy when it develops.

REFERENCES

1. Toomey JM: Tumors of the mouth and pharynx. In Bluestone CD, Stool SE (eds): Pediatric Otolaryngology. Philadelphia, Saunders, 1983, chap 52, pp 1038–1052
2. Nahmad M, Clatworthy HW Jr: Leiomyoma of the entire esophagus. J Pediatr Surg 8:829, 1973
3. Powell RW, Luck SR: Cervical esophageal obstruction by ectopic gastric mucosa. J Pediatr Surg 23:632, 1988
4. Appelquist P, Salmo M: Lye corrosion carcinoma of the esophagus. Cancer 45:2655, 1980
5. Wurlitzer FP, Mares AJ, Isaacs H Jr, et al: Smooth muscle tumors of the stomach in childhood and adolescence. J Pediatr Surg 8:421, 1973
6. Matias IC, Huang YC: Gastric teratoma in infancy: Report of a case and review of world literature. Ann Surg 178:631, 1973
7. Purvis JM, Miller RC, Blumenthal BI: Gastric teratoma: First reported case in a female. J Pediatr Surg 14:86, 1979
8. McNeer G: Cancer of the stomach in the young. Am J Roentgenol Radium Ther Nucl Med 45:537, 1941
9. Dixon WL, Fazzari PG: Carcinoma of the stomach in a child. JAMA 235:2414, 1976
10. Wayne ER, Campbell JB, Kosloske AM, Burrington JD: Intussusception in the older child—suspect lymphosarcoma. J Pediatr Surg 11:789, 1976
11. Dunnick NR, Reaman GH, Head GL, et al: Radiographic manifestations of Burkitt's lymphoma in American patients. AJR 132:1, 1979
12. Greenstein AJ, Sachar DB, Smith H, et al: Patterns of neoplasia in Crohn's disease and ulcerative colitis. Cancer 46:403, 1980
13. Carney JA, Go VLW, Sizemore GW, Hayles AB: Alimentary tract ganglioneuromatosis: A major component of the syndrome of multiple endocrine neoplasia, type 2b. N Engl J Med 295:1287, 1976
14. Abrahamson J, Shandling B: Intestinal hemangiomata in childhood and a syndrome for diagnosis: A collective review. J Pediatr Surg 8:487, 1973
15. Ryden SE, Drake RM, Franciose RA: Carcinoid tumors of the appendix in children. Cancer 36:1538, 1975
16. Andersson A, Bergdahl L: Carcinoma of the colon in children: A report of six new cases and a review of the literature. J Pediatr Surg 11:967, 1976
17. Middelkamp JN, Haffner H: Carcinoma of the colon in children. Pediatrics 32:558, 1963
18. Cain AJ, Longino LA: Carcinoma of the colon in children. J Pediatr Surg 5:527, 1970
19. Donaldson MH, Taylor P, Rawitscher R, Sewell JB Jr: Colon carcinoma in childhood. Pediatrics 48:307, 1971

20. Pratt CB, Rivera G, Shanks E, et al: Colorectal carcinoma in adolescents: Implications regarding etiology. Cancer 40:2464, 1977
21. Grosfeld JL, Clatworthy HW Jr, Hamoudi AB: Pancreatic malignancy in children. Arch Surg 101:370, 1970
22. Taxy JB: Adenocarcinoma of the pancreas in childhood: Report of a case and a review of the English language literature. Cancer 37:1508, 1976
23. Altman AJ, Schwartz AD: Malignant Diseases of Infancy, Childhood and Adolescence, 2nd ed. Philadelphia, Saunders, 1983, pp 1–21, 510–523

47
Mediastinal Masses

Mediastinal masses comprise a fascinating, heterogeneous group of tumors, congenital defects, and infections that are considered together only because of their common location. By arbitrarily dividing the mediastinum into anatomic areas, a lesion that appears on a roentgenogram of the chest may be classified with considerable accuracy. The space between the anterior pericardium and the sternum is the anterior mediastinum, which normally contains only loose areolar tissue and the thymus gland. The middle mediastinum includes the heart, pericardium, ascending aorta, trachea, mainstem bronchi, and peribronchial lymph nodes. The posterior mediastinum is traversed by the descending aorta, esophagus, vagus nerve, and the sympathetic chain. Figure 47–1 illustrates the various lesions that are most likely to occupy these anatomic divisions. There is some overlap because teratomas do occur within the pericardium and rarely in the posterior mediastinum. Lymphatic tumors may arise or perhaps extend into the anterior mediastinum. It is fairly safe to say, however, that enteric cysts and the neurogenic tumors are confined to the posterior mediastinum. The relative frequency of the various tumor types compiled from four hospital series is shown in Table 47–1.[1–3] The miscellaneous lesions included undifferentiated sarcomas, pericardial cysts, lipomas, and heterotropic lung, but unlike series including adults, there was only one substernal thyroid. Table 47–1 includes 355 mediastinal lesions seen at Children's Memorial Hospital from 1952 to 1986.

NEUROGENIC TUMORS

The pathology and treatment of the most common posterior mediastinal tumors, neuroblastoma and ganglioneuroma, are discussed in Chapter 41. Ganglioneuromas are more common in older children, where they are discovered on routine chest x-rays. Neuroblastomas occur in younger children and may become large enough in infants to cause respiratory distress.[4] The most important symptoms caused by these tumors result from spinal cord compression. There may be a gradual onset of weakness in the lower extremities or sudden neurologic decompensation with paralysis. Plain x-ray films demonstrate smooth rounded lesions in the posterior mediastinum and may show rib separation or bone erosion (Fig. 47–2). The computed tomography (CT) scan is most important in evaluating these lesions because it will reliably demonstrate intraspinal extension (Fig. 47–3). Formerly, it was often necessary to carry out a laminectomy to decompress the spinal cord before transthoracic excision of the primary tumor. For the past 5 years, with CT guidance, we have been able to plan combined thoracic and neurosurgical excision of these lesions in one stage. A myelogram may be necessary for complete evaluation of the intraspinal extension. At operation, the patient is placed in a prone lateral position. The chest is opened, and the tumor is mobilized from the aorta and vertebral body, removing segments of rib when necessary. The incision is extended to the spinous

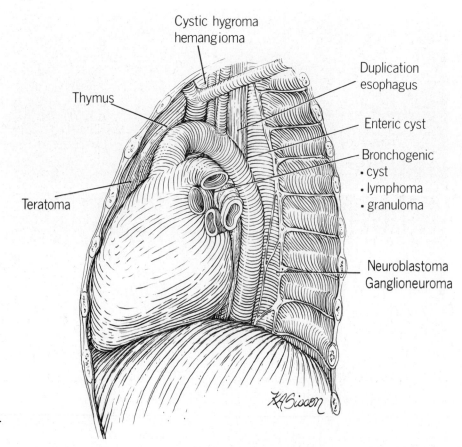

Figure 47–1. Sites of the most common mediastinal tumors in children.

processes of the vertebrae, and the neurosurgeon exposes the intraspinal extension by removing the lateral portions of the foramina and arch of the vertebrae. This technique has allowed complete one-stage removal of extensive tumors.

Neurofibromas, often in patients with von Recklinghausen's disease, also involve the posterior mediastinum, usually at the apex of the chest, in association with the brachial plexus.

Mediastinal neuroblastomas are more likely to be

TABLE 47–1. RELATIVE FREQUENCY OF TUMORS IN FOUR SERIES

Tumor Type	Series 1[a]	Series 2[b]	Series 3[c]	Series 4[d]
Neuroblastoma	9	13	28	52
Ganglioneuroma	6	16	11	16
Neurofibroma	3	7		7
Teratoma	8	21	5	10
Vascular lesions	4	9	5	15
Granuloma	9	3	1	7
Bronchogenic cysts	2	5	6	26
Duplication	6	7	11	11
Lymphoma	8	9	14	45
Thymus	8	4	7	10
Miscellaneous	17	11[e]	5	13
Total	80	105	93	355

[a] Haller et al.[1]
[b] Whittaker and Lynn.[2]
[c] Bower and Kiesewetter.[3]
[d] Data compiled at Children's Memorial Hospital, Chicago, 1954–1986.
[e] This includes only one thyroid tumor.

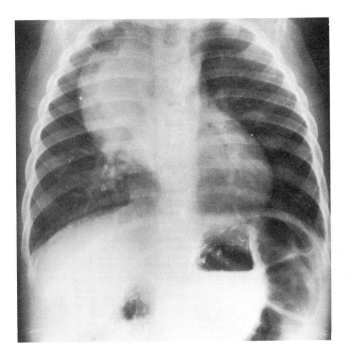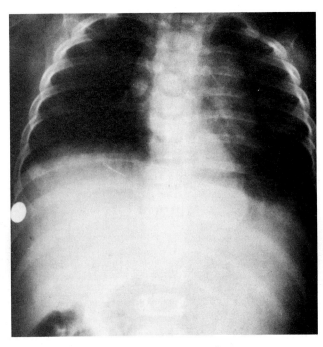

Figure 47–2. Left. Neuroblastoma involving the posterior mediastinum in a 10-month-old infant. **Right.** Neuroblastoma in left lower posterior mediastinum.

stage I or II lesions and have a better prognosis even without radiation and chemotherapy than abdominal lesions.

TERATOMAS

Teratomas produce symptoms when they are large enough to compress the trachea. We observed one newborn infant who was thought to have cyanotic congenital

heart disease, but his cyanosis was relieved when he lay in a prone position (Fig. 47–4).

A teratoma may be sufficiently large to fill one hemithorax and may be confused with a pleural effusion.[5,6] On physical examination, the chest may bulge forward, while the cardiac sounds are made distant or obscured by the mass. A lateral roentgenogram will demonstrate posterior displacement of the tracheal air column, and if an angiocardiogram is obtained, it will show that the

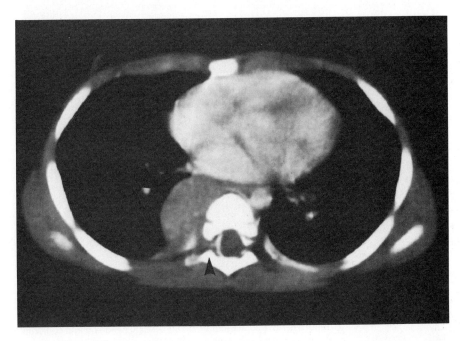

Figure 47–3. CT scan demonstrating a posterior neuroblastoma with spinal canal invasion.

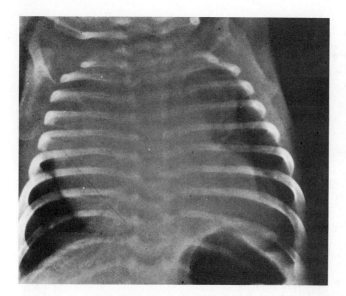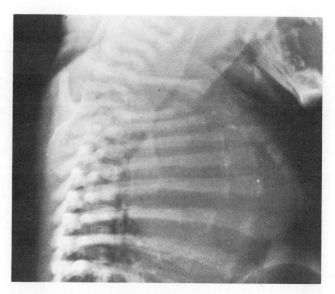

Figure 47–4. Anterior mediastinal teratoma that compressed the trachea, causing severe respiratory distress and cyanosis. **Left.** Posteroanterior view. **Right.** Lateral view.

heart is also displaced posteriorly. A teratoma may occur within the pericardium.[7] Infants with teratomas have shown symptoms of cardiac tamponade. Angiography demonstrates pressure on the heart and the great vessels. These tumors either densely adhere to the adventitia of the aorta or derive blood directly from the root of the aorta. Hemorrhage from an aortic tear may occur during their removal.

There are exceptions to every rule. Figure 47–5 illustrates the esophagogram of a 6-month-old boy with a teratoma in his posterior mediastinum that was inseparable from his esophagus. In a series of 21 mediastinal germ cell tumors at the Boston Children's Hospital, 12 were benign teratomas, and the remaining 9 had malignant components.[8] The malignant tumors were treated with excision and, when possible, with adjuvant chemotherapy. Only 2 patients were long-term survivors.

BRONCHOGENIC CYSTS

Bronchogenic cysts are almost always adjacent to the trachea or mainstem bronchi, usually at the carina. They are lined with respiratory epithelium and have cartilage and smooth muscle in their wall. A cyst only 2 to 3 cm in diameter causes wheezing, stridor, cough, and recurrent pneumonia. Cysts with identical histologic findings are found peripheral to or even completely separate from the lung.[9] These lesions are more properly termed "lung cysts" as a means of distinguishing them from cysts that are adherent to the main airway. The histologic similarity of these cysts is not surprising, since all of them are derived from the ventral or anterior primitive foregut.

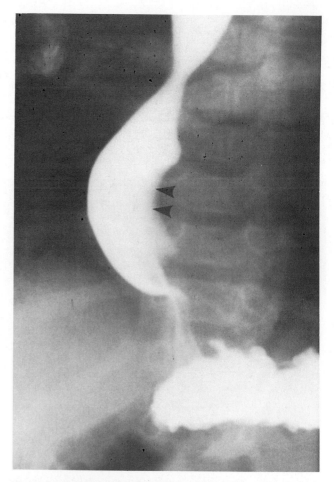

Figure 47–5. Esophagogram demonstrating distortion and compression by a posterior mediastinal teratoma.

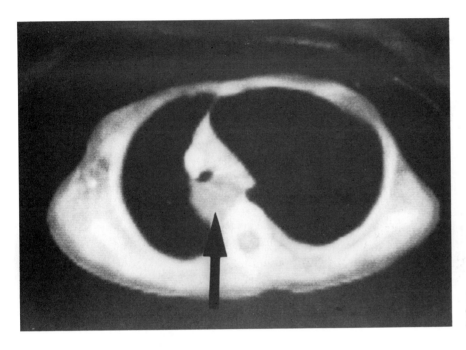

Figure 47–6. CT scan of a carinal broncho-genic cyst that caused left lung emphysema and mediastinal shift.

A bronchogenic cyst always must be considered in infants with respiratory distress, even in the newborn period.

When bronchogenic cysts are in the subcarinal or perihilar region, they are easily overlooked on plain radiographs. There may be signs of obstructive emphysema, indentation on the esophagus or cardiac silhouette, or other nonspecific findings.[10–13] Since 1979, we have used CT scans for every child suspected of having a bronchogenic cyst or unexplained airway obstruction[14] (Fig. 47–6). This study has brought to light previously undiagnosed cysts. Bronchoscopy is indicated only if there is some suspicion of a bronchial foreign body.

Treatment

Since a bronchogenic cyst may cause life-threatening respiratory distress, an emergency operation may be required. A right posterolateral thoracotomy provides excellent exposure of lesions at the carina and the right mainstem bronchus. The proximal left mainstem bronchus also is approached from the right side. Lesions that are more than 2 or 3 cm distal to the carina on the left mainstem bronchus must be approached from the left. Access to this area requires mobilization of the aorta, division of the ligamentum arteriosus, and retraction of the left main pulmonary artery. The vagus and the recurrent laryngeal nerve must be identified and protected. Most cysts are only loosely connected to the surrounding mediastinal areolar tissue and are easily dissected down to the point where they are intimately connected with the trachea or bronchus. At this point, sharp dissection with the thin blades of tenotomy scissors is indicated. One may want to remove the entire cyst in order to admire the resected specimen, but if necessary, a bit of the cyst wall should be left attached to the airway

as a safeguard against perforation of the bronchus. Any remaining bits of epithelium may be destroyed with the electrocautery. If the tracheal wall is entered, it may be repaired with a patch of pericardium or a bit of Gelfoam held in place with a flap of pleura.[15]

DUPLICATIONS OR ENTERIC CYSTS

Duplications may occur anywhere in the gastrointestinal tract, from the mouth to the anus. Duplications within the mediastinum must be included in the differential diagnosis of mediastinal masses. They present unique complications because of their location.

The most common enteric duplication within the mediastinum is an epithelium-lined cyst enclosed within the muscular wall of the esophagus (Fig. 47–7). There is controversy over the embryologic origin of such cystic duplications.[16]

Ciliated respiratory-type epithelium, gastric mucosa, and squamous epithelium can all be found within an esophageal duplication, since the esophagus is derived from multipotential foregut tissue. The best explanation for these cysts is that the esophagus initially has a lumen that during early growth becomes partially solid. The final lumen is then established by the formation of vacuoles that coalesce. One of several vacuoles may fail to become connected with the esophageal lumen and remain as an isolated cyst adjacent to the esophagus, sharing with it a common muscular wall. Small cystic esophageal duplications may remain asymptomatic, to be found on incidental chest roentgenograms. Others may be sufficiently large to compress the bronchus, causing either acute respiratory obstruction or repeated bouts of pneu-

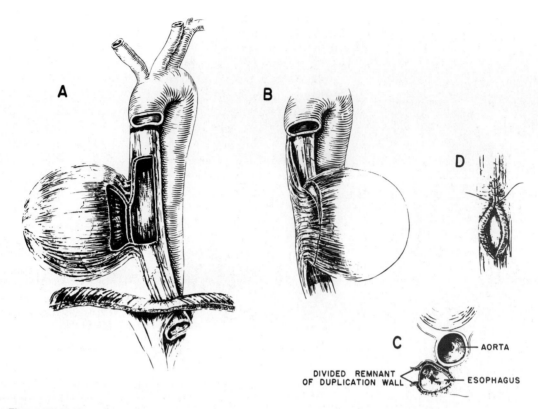

Figure 47–7. The most common form of enteric duplication within the mediastinum is this type of cystic lesion encompassed within the muscle layers of the esophagus. Only the mucosa is removed in the portion of the cyst adjacent to the esophagus. Enough muscle is left to close over the esophageal mucosa.

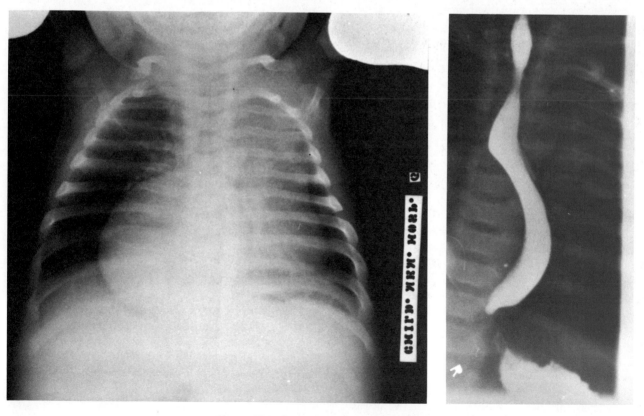

Figure 47–8. Cystic duplication of the esophagus.

monitis. One of our patients had been diagnosed as having asthma because of her repeated bouts of wheezing. Dysphagia is an unusual symptom because the esophageal lumen, though sometimes displaced, rarely is obstructed. Chest roentgenograms demonstrate a smooth, rounded mass projecting from the posterior mediastinum into the lung field (Fig. 47–8). Esophagograms demonstrate a smooth displacement of the lumen. When the lining mucosa consists of gastric epithelium, complications may occur, e.g., ulceration with perforation into the esophagus or lung. The child may then cough or vomit blood.[17]

Treatment

An intercostal incision should be made over the cyst. Those cysts in the upper third of the esophagus are best approached from the right side, but lower lesions may be approached through the left chest. There is usually little inflammatory reaction and no adhesion of the duplication to the lung.

The pleura over the cyst is opened, and the duplication is mobilized by sharply dissecting it from the surrounding areolar tissue and vagus nerve until a point is reached where the muscle layers of the cyst blend with those of the esophagus. An incision is then made 1 or 2 cm from the esophagus on the cyst wall through the muscular coat to the mucosa of the duplication. The mucosa of the duplication is not opened but is separated from the esophageal mucosa with sharp dissection. Thus the duplication is removed without disturbing the esophagus itself. The excess muscle that had splayed out over the base of the duplication is then sutured over the mucosa.

Tubular rather than cystic duplications within the esophagus are rare. In such cases, there is a tube lined with squamous epithelium that connects at each end within the esophagus.[18] Recurrent dysphagia was the only symptom in one of our patients. Roentgenograms demonstrated the double lumen. At operation, the esophagus was opened, and the septum that separated the duplication from the esophageal lumen was divided.

Enteric cysts or posterior mediastinal duplications of the intestine frequently are extensions of duplications that originate in the stomach or intestine (Fig. 47–9). They are most likely to be tubular and distinct from the esophagus but are densely attached to the vertebrae and may extend into the neck. The wall consists of smooth muscle, and the endothelium may be either intestinal or gastric. It is interesting, from both a clinical and an embryologic point of view, that these lesions often are associated with vertebral anomalies, especially hemivertebrae.[19,20]

There are at least five theories for the embryologic origin of these anomalies. The most probable assumes that early in embryonic life an adhesion forms between the ectoderm and endoderm that prevents proper cover-

ing of the notochord. This neurenteric band prevents medial migration of the paraxial mesoderm, which leads to the vertebral deformities. This same band adheres to a portion of the developing foregut and causes a traction diverticulum, which eventually results in the lengthy tubular duplication.[21]

Bleeding, perforation, infection, and pain are all caused by peptic ulceration within the duplication. The symptoms are usually chronic and baffling, since plain roentgenograms frequently demonstrate only inconclusive shadows. One of our patients was admitted to the hospital several times for unexplained anemia and occasional vomiting of brown material. Several chest roentgenograms and endoscopic studies were negative. Finally, an ill-defined mass appeared on the chest roentgenogram, which proved to be a tubular duplication extending from the stomach to the neck. Technetium scans to demonstrate gastric mucosa and CT should assist in making a correct diagnosis.

Since these lesions extend the length of the thorax, wide exposure is indicated. If the duplication extends through the diaphragm, one may suture the duplication

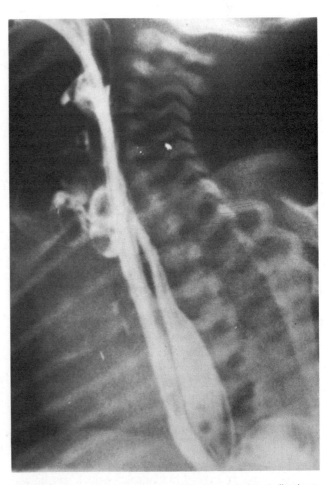

Figure 47–9. An enteric duplication within the posterior mediastinum that originated in the stomach. The child had recurrent bouts of chest pain and upper gastrointestinal bleeding secondary to peptic ulceration within the duplication.

closed and leave the abdominal portion for a second procedure. However, one of our patients developed a massive gastrointestinal hemorrhage 3 days after the thoracotomy. An emergency operation was required to remove the abdominal end of his duplication.

THYMUS

The thymus is often prominent in children as a sail-like shadow in the upper mediastinum. This thymic enlargement never causes symptoms, but if there is doubt about a tumor, a CT scan should settle the issue. An ectopic thymus can cause an abnormal shadow in the posterior mediastinum, which may require a biopsy for diagnosis. Thymic cysts are unusual, and malignant thymomas have been seen in children. These require a biopsy to differentiate them from lymphomas. The thymus has long been thought to play a role in myasthenia gravis.[22] The operation should be considered in patients of any age whose symptoms are refractory to medical treatment, but it seems most beneficial to those with early, mild symptoms.

Eventual recovery from myasthenia gravis was observed in 6 of 8 children, aged 10 to 16 years, in one series.[23] We have used a transcervical approach to thymectomy to reduce postoperative pain and the need for respiratory support. The best results are obtained when the maximum amount of thymic tissue is removed.[24] Thus, both transternal and cervical approaches may be important to remove thymic tissue from the diaphragm to the neck and laterally from one phrenic nerve to another.

MEDIASTINAL LYMPH NODE DISEASE

Although Hodgkin's disease and lymphoma usually occur as a neck mass, they can develop in the mediastinum, causing respiratory distress. If a diagnosis cannot be made on the basis of cervical node biopsy, bone marrow aspiration, or cells in pleural fluid, a mediastinal biopsy is indicated. Although mediastinoscopy is technically feasible in children, we have not been able to obtain sufficient tissue. For this reason, an anterior mediastinal exploration through a small submammary incision is preferable.

Granulomatous disease of the mediastinum deserves special mention. The enlarged lymph nodes encountered in tuberculosis and histoplasmosis may simulate lymphoma, and on one occasion, we made the mistaken diagnosis of a bronchogenic cyst in a 6-month-old infant who had a large tuberculous lymph node. Aside from the occasional difficulties in diagnosis, which can be resolved by a thorough history and skin tests, granulomatous involvement of mediastinal nodes may cause airway obstruction and the superior vena cava syndrome.[25–28]

Children who have had histoplasmosis frequently have a mild systemic disease diagnosed as flu weeks or months before the time they have airway compression symptoms secondary to a hilar mass. In such cases, an operation is indicated, both to confirm the diagnosis and to relieve the obstruction. There is evidence that surgical excision or drainage of involved lymph nodes will prevent the late development of a fibrosing mediastinitis, which entraps the superior vena cava and the airways.[29,30]

We once successfully drained an anterior mediastinal abscess at mediastinoscopy, but in the usual case, a thoracotomy is indicated. There is such dense fibrosis and reaction about the nodes that complete excision is hazardous. Consequently, it is safer to resect as much as possible and then open the node to clean out purulent and granulomatous material.

MISCELLANEOUS MEDIASTINAL MASSES

Cystic hygromas that occur in the lower cervical region are likely to have extensions in the upper mediastinum that require thoracotomy for complete removal. Rarely, a large mediastinal cystic hygroma may cause respiratory distress without a cervical component.[31,32] In one of our patients, a posterior mediastinal cystic hygroma caused a chronic chylothorax. Removal of the lesion, together with pleural stripping and long-term pleural drainage, prevented recurrence of the chylothorax.

CT scans are superior to plain chest x-rays in demonstrating the extent of cervicothoracic hygromas and allow one to plan an incision to remove the tumor in one stage.[33] Cystic hygromas insinuate themselves around the major vessels and nerves of the chest. In 6 of our patients, the jugular vein has been dilated and thin walled, making its dissection difficult. It is better to leave a few bits of hygroma wall behind than to risk damage to the recurrent nerve or a major vessel. Chest tube drainage is apt to be prolonged, and these children should be kept on intravenous alimentation and a no-fat diet until all drainage has ceased to avoid a chronic chylothorax.

The reported cases of mediastinal lipomas and liposarcomas in children are most likely examples of benign lipoblastomatosis.[34–36] These lesions, which may be quite large, cause respiratory distress through compression of the lung and the airways. The diagnosis can be made only by exploration and removal of the mass.

REFERENCES

1. Haller AJ, Mazur DO, Morgan WW: Diagnosis and management of mediastinal masses in children. J Thorac Cardiovasc Surg 58:385, 1969

2. Whittaker LD, Lynn HB: Mediastinal tumors and cysts in the pediatric patient. Surg Clin North Am 53:893, 1973

3. Bower RJ, Kiesewetter WB: Mediastinal masses in infants and children. Arch Surg 112:1003, 1977

4. Haller JA, Shermeta DW, Donahoo JS, et al: Life-threatening respiratory distress from mediastinal masses in infants. Ann Thorac Surg 19:364, 1975

5. Pate JW, Buker R, Korones SB: Mediastinal teratoma in the newborn. Surgery 54:533, 1963

6. Shackelford GD, McAlister WH: Mediastinal teratoma confused with loculated pleural fluid: Case report. Pediatr Radiol 5:118, 1976

7. Deenadayalu PR, Tuuri D, Dewall RA, et al: Intrapericardial teratoma and bronchogenic cyst. J Thorac Cardiovasc Surg 67:945, 1974

8. Lack E, Weinstein H, Welch K: Mediastinal germ cell tumors in childhood: A clinical and pathological study of 21 cases. J Thorac Cardiovasc Surg 89:826, 1985

9. Maier HC: Bronchogenic cysts of the mediastinum. Ann Surg 127:476, 1948

10. Gerami S, Richardson R, Harrington B, et al: Obstructive emphysema due to mediastinal bronchogenic cysts in infancy. J Thorac Cardiovasc Surg 58:432, 1969

11. Weichert RF, Lindsey ES, Pearce CW, et al: Bronchogenic cyst with unilateral obstructive emphysema. J Thorac Cardiovasc Surg 59:287, 1970

12. Delany DJ, Harned HS, Wright WE: Neonatal congestive heart failure due to mediastinal cyst: Case report. Pediatr Radiol 2:259, 1974

13. Grafe WR, Goldsmith EI, Redd, SF: Bronchogenic cysts of the mediastinum in children. J Pediatr Surg 1:384, 1966

14. Snyder M, Luck S, Hernandez R, et al: Diagnostic dilemmas of mediastinal cysts. J Pediatr Surg 20:810, 1985

15. Potts W: The Surgeon and the Child. Philadelphia, Saunders, 1972, pp 80–81

16. Skandakalis JE, Grey SW: Embryology for Surgeons. Philadelphia, Saunders, 1972, p 72

17. Chang SH, Morrison L, Shaffner L, et al: Intrathoracic gastrogenic cysts and hemoptysis. J Pediatr 88:594, 1976

18. Frank RC, Paul LW: Congenital reduplication of the esophagus. Radiology 53:417, 1949

19. Beardmore HE, Wiglesworth FW: Vertebral anomalies and alimentary duplications. Pediatr Clin North Am 5:451, 1958

20. Bentley JFR, Smith JR: Developmental posterior enteric remnants and spinal malformations. Arch Dis Child 35:76, 1960

21. Elwood SJ: Mediastinal duplication of the gut. Arch Dis Child 34:474, 1959

22. Wekerle H, Muller-Hermelink H: The thymus in myasthenia gravis. Clin Top Pathol 75:179, 1986

23. Youssef S: Thymectomy for myasthenia gravis in children. J Pediatr Surg 18:537, 1983

24. Jaretzki A, Penn A, Younger D, et al: "Maximal" thymectomy for myasthenia gravis: Results. J Thorac Cardiovasc Surg 95:747, 1988

25. Greenwood MF, Holland P: Tracheal obstruction secondary to histoplasma mediastinal granuloma. Chest 62:642, 1972

26. Woods, LP: Mediastinal histoplasma granuloma causing tracheal compression in a 4-year-old child. Surgery 58:448, 1965

27. Pate JW, Hammon J: Superior vena cava syndrome due to histoplasmosis in children. Ann Surg 161:778, 1965

28. Goodwin RA, Nickell JA, Des Prez RM: Mediastinal fibrosis complicating healed primary histoplasmosis and tuberculosis. Medicine 51:227, 1972

29. Zajtchuk R, Strevey TE, Heydorn WH, Treasure RL: Mediastinal histoplasmosis. J Thorac Cardiovasc Surg 66:300, 1973

30. Williams KR, Burford TH: Surgical treatment of granulomatous paratracheal lymphadenopathy. J Thorac Cardiovasc Surg 48:13, 1964

31. Bratu M, Brown M, Carter M, Lawson JP: Cystic hygroma of the mediastinum in children. Arch Dis Child 119:348, 1970

32. Moore T, Cobo J: Massive symptomatic cystic hygroma confined to the thorax in early childhood. J Thorac Cardiovasc Surg 89:459, 1985

33. Grosfeld J, Weber T, Vane D: One-stage resection for massive cervicomediastinal hygroma. Surgery 92:693, 1982

34. Kleinhaus S, Ducharme JC: Mediastinal lipoma in children: Case report. Surgery 66:490, 1969

35. Tabrisky J, Rowe JH, Christie S, et al: Benign mediastinal lipoblastomatosis: Case report. J Pediatr Surg 9:399, 1974

36. Wilson JR, Bartley TD: Liposarcoma of the mediastinum. J Thorac Cardiovasc Surg 48:486, 1964

48
Tumors of the Lung

C. Thomas Black
Richard J. Andrassy

The majority of pulmonary neoplasms in children are distant metastases from primary tumors in extrapulmonary locations. They comprise more than 80 percent of all lung masses in children. A variety of benign and malignant primary lung tumors also occurs in children. The scarcity of each tumor type makes it difficult to assess accurately the natural histories and optimal methods of treatment.

METASTATIC TUMORS

Most pediatric tumors, such as nephroblastoma (Wilms' tumor), osteosarcoma, hepatoblastoma, and rhabdomyosarcoma, metastasize preferentially to the lungs, whereas pulmonary involvement by central nervous system tumors and neuroblastoma is usually rare until the final stages of the disease. Although management of pulmonary metastases from specific tumor types is discussed in chapters relating to those primary tumors, some principles may be generalized.[1] Chemotherapy, and radiotherapy when appropriate, should be administered before surgery to eliminate micrometastases and to shrink the tumor, thus minimizing the volume of lung parenchyma that must be sacrificed for adequate resection. If or when tumor nodules become responsive to non-surgical measures, resection should be considered if enough lung parenchyma can be spared to avoid respiratory insufficiency. Because metastases frequently are multiple and may be both synchronous and metachronous, conserva-

tive excision is important. Multiple wedge resections usually are sufficient, but occasionally lobectomy or rarely pneumonectomy is necessary for complete removal of the tumor. Staged thoracotomies usually are employed when bilateral tumor nodules are present. Median sternotomy may allow simultaneous access to both hemithoraces, but posteriorly situated nodules are difficult to reach through this approach. Recurrent tumor does not contraindicate repeat thoracotomy and resection if adequate functional tissue will remain.

Wilms' tumor and osteosarcoma are the most common but not the only pulmonary metastases to be resected for childhood cancer. Combining cases from the Children's Memorial Hospital of Chicago and the University of Texas—M. D. Anderson Cancer Center in Houston, five children with metastatic hepatoblastoma underwent 19 thoracotomies for the resection of a total of 33 pulmonary metastases.[2] Four of these five children are alive an average of 30 months after their last thoracotomy. The only nonsurvivor had undergone resection of her primary tumor 15 months earlier and was free of intraabdominal recurrence. She had undergone two previous thoracotomies for resection of metastases but had developed several more tumor nodules, the largest of which had invaded pulmonary veins. She died shortly after resection of these metastases of a tumor embolism to the cerebrum. Resection of pulmonary metastases is indicated, since unresectable nodules that have become unresponsive to chemotherapy or radiotherapy are inevitably fatal.

PRIMARY TUMORS

Distinctions between benign and malignant forms of pediatric primary lung tumors often are subtle. Many histologic types have been identified, and classification is difficult.

Treatment of both benign and malignant primary tumors consists of a thorough bronchoscopic examination and biopsy, followed by thoracotomy. Bronchial sleeve resection or resection of the bronchus and lobectomy with bronchoplasty may be possible in selected patients for maximal tissue salvage. Five children aged 12 months to 12 years with bronchial tumors or malformations were managed successfully in this fashion at the Children's Memorial Hospital in Chicago.[3]

The following diagnostic considerations are listed in approximate order of frequency of occurrence.

A. Bronchial adenomas
   1. Carcinoids
   2. Adenoid cystic carcinomas (cylindromas)
   3. Mucoepidermoid carcinomas
B. Bronchogenic carcinomas
C. Inflammatory pseudotumors
D. Hamartomas and teratomas
E. Pulmonary blastomas
F. Other benign tumors
   1. Papillomas
   2. Chondromas
   3. Leiomyomas
   4. Hemangiomas
   5. Granular cell tumors (myoblastomas)
G. Sarcomas
H. Lymphomas

Bronchial Adenomas

Bronchial adenomas include carcinoid tumors, adenoid cystic carcinomas (cylindromas), and mucoepidermoid carcinomas. As a group, they comprise about 35 percent of all primary pulmonary neoplasms in children. Even so, there are less than 50 cases reported in the literature.[4] They are not, as their name erroneously implies, always benign tumors.

Bronchial carcinoid tumors are the most common bronchial adenomas and comprise approximately 60 percent of the reported cases. In a review of 21 patients under the age of 20 years with histologically proven bronchial carcinoids,[5] the most frequent presenting complaints were hemoptysis, cough, and pneumonia. The duration of symptoms ranged from 1 month to 12 years, with the mean duration of symptoms slightly over 1 year, excluding the patient who had symptoms for 12 years. These tumors generally involve major bronchi, which explains the fact that the symptoms and physical

signs are those of bronchial obstruction. The right lung is affected approximately twice as often as the left. Bronchoscopic biopsy is diagnostic in the majority of cases. However, these tumors are quite vascular and may hemorrhage.

Carcinoid tumors generally occur in one of two group patterns: (1) as endobronchial polypoid masses that produce segmental bronchial obstruction followed by atelectasis and infection or (2) as iceberg lesions with predominantly extrabronchial growth, the small intrabronchial extent of which gives rise to mucosal ulceration and hemoptysis. In routine histologic preparations, bronchial and intestinal carcinoids usually are indistinguishable.

Carcinoid tumors of the lung consist histologically of festoons and ribbons of small polyhedral cells with central nuclei and eosinophilic cytoplasm, arranged in a plexiform or organoid pattern that resembles the pattern of carcinoid tumors (argentaffinomas) of the gastrointestinal tract (Fig. 48–1).[6] Distant metastases are extremely rare, and no documented cases of carcinoid syndrome have been reported, although one patient was found to have an elevated serum 5-hydroxyindolacetic acid level.

Adenoid cystic carcinomas (cylindromas) represent the second group of bronchial adenomas, comprising about 10 percent of the total. These are most commonly found in the trachea and are made up of cuboidal or flattened epithelial cells, arranged in two layers. Histologically, they resemble mixed tumors of the salivary glands and basal cell carcinomas of the skin. Clinical presentation, physical signs, and diagnostic approach are all similar to those in patients with carcinoids. There is

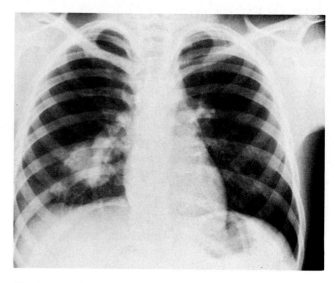

Figure 48–1. Chest film demonstrating a right lower lobe squamous cell carcinoma in a 10-year-old boy. (*LaSalle et al.*[6] *Used with permission.*)

a 40 percent chance of malignancy in adults with this tumor.

Mucoepidermoid carcinomas represent approximately 30 percent of bronchial adenomas. These pedunculated endobronchial tumors generally arise from the trachea or major bronchi. The epithelial component has somewhat of an epidermoid appearance, and the glandular lumen shows abundant mucus. The incidence of malignancy reported for children with this tumor appears to be extremely low, and survival should be at least 90 percent.

Primary Bronchogenic Carcinomas
Malignant bronchogenic tumors of the lung are rare in childhood; there are fewer than 50 cases reported in the literature. Adenocarcinoma is the most common type; squamous cell carcinoma of the bronchus occurs much less frequently than in adults. The average life expectancy for patients with such tumors is approximately 6 months after the onset of symptoms. Other histologic cell types include oat cell carcinomas, small cell carcinomas, and anaplastic carcinomas. Diagnosis usually is delayed, and metastases frequently are present at the time of diagnosis.

Inflammatory Pseudotumors
The term "inflammatory pseudotumor" includes a number of benign and presumably nonneoplastic lesions. Among these is a group of tumors variously designated as plasma cell granulomas, xanthofibromas, fibrous xanthomas, sclerosing hemangiomas, histiocytomas, and xanthogranulomas. Approximately 60 children with these

tumors are reported in the literature.[4,7] These lesions are characterized by an antecedent respiratory infection with mild or absent symptoms and a radiographic pattern showing a single, sharply circumscribed mass. Any lobe of the lungs may be affected, although the right lower lobe is the most common site. Approximately 50 percent of afflicted patients have an asymptomatic solitary peripheral mass on the roentgenogram. The rest have signs and symptoms of pulmonary infection, including fever, cough, and hemoptysis. A chest roentgenogram may show calcification in the mass. The cause is unknown, although experimental evidence suggests a viral etiology. The lesions may be as large as 12 cm in diameter, although they are usually between 2 and 5 cm. The histologic picture is chiefly one of chronic inflammation with fibrosis. Treatment consists of thoracotomy with wedge or segmental resection and frozen section histopathologic correlation.

Hamartomas and Teratomas
The term "hamartoma" was coined to describe benign tumors of an organ comprised of tissue normally occurring in that organ but arranged in an abnormal fashion. This rare diagnosis may be suspected when there is a persistent smooth round density on a chest x-ray or computed tomography (CT) scan. Some contain calcium, and skin tests are performed to rule out tuberculosis and fungal infections. (Fig. 48–2). Diagnosis often is made following thoracotomy and surgical resection. An interesting association of a smooth muscle tumor of the stomach and an extraadrenal paraganglioma occurring in conjunction

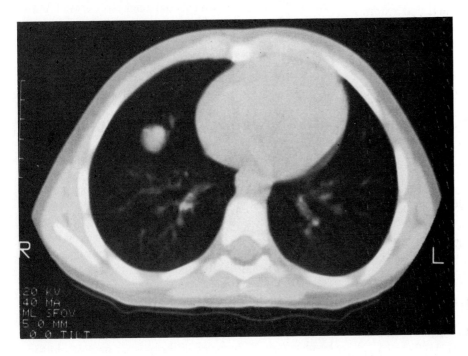

Figure 48–2. A hamartoma of the right lung. It is smooth and rounded and contains calcium.

with a pulmonary hamartoma has been twice reported in young girls.

Teratomas of the lung are malignant and extremely rare. Only one has been reported in an infant and one in an older child.[8]

Pulmonary Blastomas

Pulmonary blastomas are rare malignant neoplasms that histologically resemble fetal lung tissue. They generally arise in the peripheral portion of the lung and demonstrate variable clinical behavior. There have been 14 reported instances of pulmonary blastoma in the pediatric age group; the majority appear in adulthood.[4] Identification of the tumor generally is made at thoracotomy or autopsy. Operable lesions should be treated by lobectomy or pneumonectomy. The long-term survival of patients with this tumor has been under 50 percent.

Other Benign Tumors

Benign tumors of the tracheobronchial tree may arise from any of the tissue layers, but they are generally considered pathologic curiosities. Papillomatosis is a common laryngeal tumor of infancy and childhood that occasionally spreads distally, but generally only as far as the trachea. However, a squamous papilloma may drop into a peripheral bronchus as a solitary lesion (Fig. 48–3), requiring pulmonary resection.

Leiomyomas, chondromas, fibromas, neurogenic tumors, hemangiomas, and granular cell tumors (myoblastomas) all have been reported in the pediatric age group. In general, these benign tumors usually occur in the trachea or mainstem bronchus, with symptoms of distal obstruction. Preoperative bronchoscopy and CT scan are valuable in the assessment of the location and extent of bronchial tumors. As with other endobronchial tumors,

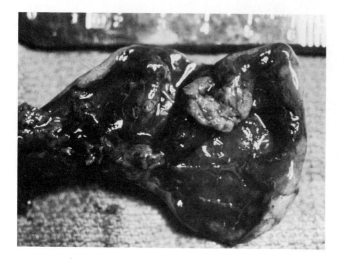

Figure 48–3. Laryngeal papillomatosis with a drop metastasis to the left lower lobe. It was removed by segmental resection.

sleeve resection or resection of a damaged lobe with limited bronchial excision and bronchoplasty may prevent unnecessary resection of normal lung.

Sarcomas of the Lung

Fibrosarcomas occur as pedunculated intrabronchial masses of fibrous tissue, although one child was reported to have a fibrosarcoma of the lung parenchyma.[9] Fever with signs of distal infection secondary to obstruction is the most common presenting symptom. Diagnosis should be established by bronchoscopy. Although these tumors may be removed bronchoscopically, there is a high incidence of local recurrence, and resection is the treatment of choice. These tumors are primarily locally invasive tumors and should be resected even when extensive. In 1986, Jimenez et al., in a review of the literature, found 10 cases of primary pulmonary leiomyosarcoma in patients under 8 years of age.[10] Interestingly, there have been no patients reported with this disease between the ages of 8 and 19 years. Cough, dyspnea, and signs of obstructive pneumonitis are usually present in such patients. A good outcome usually followed complete surgical resection. Primary rhabdomyosarcoma of the lung has been reported in six children aged 2 to 13 years.[4]

Lymphomas

Lymphomas involving the lung may include lymphosarcomas, reticulum cell sarcomas, and Hodgkin's disease. The lung generally is involved by direct spread from the mediastinal lymph nodes or thymus or by disseminated lymphoma. A few cases of primary pulmonary lymphoma have been reported in the pediatric age group, but one must make a differential diagnosis between pseudolymphoma and lymphocytic interstitial pneumonitis. The lung rarely provides the primary sign of Hodgkin's disease. Nonsurgical treatment of this disorder is the rule.[11]

PULMONARY COIN LESIONS

Spherical intrapulmonary masses that appear on a chest roentgenogram during or following an upper respiratory infection may be localized inflammatory lesions. Rose and Ward described 21 of these lesions that occurred during a 10-year period at the Children's Medical Center in Seattle.[12] These acute inflammatory processes resolve with antibiotic therapy, but small coin lesions may persist for several months. These may be pulmonary lesions associated with atypical measles. If there is a history of partial immunization to measles with an atypical skin rash that commences on the extremities and spreads toward the trunk with a febrile illness, the lesion should be observed.[13] However, if there is no previous history that suggests measles or other upper respiratory infection, any coin lesion that persists for 6 to 8 weeks should be biopsied by wedge resection.

DISCUSSION

The great majority of neoplastic lesions in infants and children prove to be metastatic, since primary pulmonary tumors in this age group are rare medical curiosities. Children who have persistent or recurrent pulmonary symptoms that do not clear with the usual expectorants and antibiotics should be suspected of having a space-occupying lesion. The child with these symptoms frequently is subjected to early diagnostic bronchoscopy to evaluate the possibility of a foreign body, whereas diagnostic procedures frequently are delayed in the older child or adolescent with a similar complex. Chest roentgenograms followed by early diagnostic bronchoscopy prove to be valuable in the majority of cases. Sputum collection and diagnostic cytology are rarely of benefit in this age group with these expected tumor types. Since the majority of lung tumors in the pediatric age group occur in the trachea or in the main bronchi, bronchoscopic biopsy facilitates early diagnosis and treatment. If this is unsuccessful or contraindicated, early diagnostic thoracotomy can prove of value in inflammatory, infectious, or neoplastic lesions. Limited bronchial and pulmonary resection may salvage normal lung tissue when the tumor is benign. Awareness of the possible occurrence of both benign and malignant lesions in infants, children, and adolescents is vital to early recognition and treatment.

REFERENCES

1. Baldeyrou GL, Lemoine G, Zucker JM, et al: Pulmonary metastases in children: the place of surgery. A study of 134 patients. J Pediatr Surg 19:121, 1984
2. Black CT, Luck SR: Resection of pulmonary metastases in hepatoblastoma. (in preparation)
3. Black CT, Luck SR, Raffensperger JG: Bronchoplastic techniques for pediatric lung salvage. J Pediatr Surg 23:653, 1988
4. Hartman GE, Shochat SJ: Primary pulmonary neoplasms of childhood: A review. Ann Thorac Surg 36:108, 1983
5. Andrassy RJ, Feldtman RW, Stanford W: Bronchial carcinoid tumors in children and adolescents. J Pediatr Surg 12:513, 1977
6. LaSalle AJ, Andrassy RJ, Stanford W: Bronchogenic squamous cell carcinoma in childhood: A case report. J Pediatr Surg 12:520, 1977
7. Berardi RS, Lee SS, Hammond PC, et al: Inflammatory pseudotumors of the lung. Surg Gynecol Obstet 156:89, 1983
8. Pound AW, Willis RA: A malignant teratoma of the lung in an infant. J Pathol 98:111, 1969
9. Holinger PH, Johnston KC, Gossweiler N, et al: Primary fibrosarcoma of the bronchus. Dis Chest 37:137, 1960
10. Jimenez JF, Uthman EO, Townsend JW: Primary pulmonary leiomyosarcoma in childhood. Arch Pathol Lab Med 110:348, 1986
11. Weiss LM, Yousem SA, Warnke RA: Non-Hodgkin's lymphomas of the lung. Am J Surg Pathol 9:480, 1985
12. Rose RW, Ward BH: Spherical pneumonias in children simulating pulmonary and mediastinal masses. Radiology 106:179, 1973
13. Laptook A, Wind E, Nussbaum M, et al: Pulmonary lesions in atypical measles. Pediatrics 62:42, 1975

49
Chest Wall Tumors

Any of the soft tissue tumors may involve the chest wall. The benign lesions, such as hemangiomas and cystic hygromas, are easily recognized and require only excision for cure. The skin incision should follow natural skin creases, and when the tumor involves or is adjacent to the breast, great care must be taken to avoid injury to the developing ductal tissue.

Malignant tumors may require full-thickness excision of the chest wall, including muscle, ribs, and pleura. The resulting defect may be closed with a prosthesis, or if the defect is posterior, it is usually possible to use adjacent muscle and the scapula for coverage.

Congenital deformities of the costal cartilages (such as fusion or unilateral overgrowth) frequently are misdiagnosed as tumors. They are limited to the costal cartilages and occur as a diffuse swelling rather than a discrete mass. Chest roentgenograms may demonstrate fusion or bifid ribs, but more often the ribs are entirely normal. To make certain there is no tumor, one must inspect oblique roentgenograms, which expose the costal cartilages in profile. Some of these defects may progress to a pectus carinatum or other more obvious chest wall defect. With infants, however, only reassurance and observation are required. If there is a discrete mass or any suspicion of a tumor on x-ray, of course a biopsy is indicated. Osteomyelitis may cause bone destruction sufficient to simulate a tumor.

Computed tomography (CT) scans have contributed to our ability to diagnose specific lesions, as well as to accurately determine the tumor's extent along ribs as well as pleural or lung involvement. Bone scans often will not differentiate among inflammatory lesions, healing fractures, or tumors but will indicate lesions in other bones that may suggest a metastatic tumor.

Osteochondromas are smooth, localized lesions with a cortex continuous with the adjacent rib. Although primary malignant tumors of the ribs are rare in children, they are more common than benign tumors.[1] Formerly, it was thought that Ewing's sarcoma was the most common rib tumor in childhood.[2] A Ewing's sarcoma will have periosteal new bone formation and a soft tissue mass (Fig. 49–1). In advanced cases, there may be pleural effusion or invasion of the underlying lung. Retrospective studies of patients thought to have Ewing's sarcoma have revealed that some were a primitive neuroectodermal tumor.[3] On routine microscopy, they are made up of small blue cells, not unlike the picture seen with lymphoma or neuroblastoma.

Primitive neuroectodermal tumors may arise anywhere in the body but are most commonly found in the chest wall, where they may originate from intercostal nerves. Electron microscopy and histochemical studies for neurospecific enolase have demonstrated the neural origin of these tumors. They may occur at any age and are most prevalent in teenage girls. They vary in size, but become large, extend along the ribs in both directions, and invade the pleural cavity, mediastinum, and lung. They are highly malignant, recur locally, and metastasize.[4] The chest x-ray and CT scan (Fig. 49–2) illustrate a primitive neuroectodermal tumor in a 14-year-old girl.

When the clinical and radiologic signs suggest a benign lesion, simple excisional biopsy of the rib along with adjacent intercostal muscle and pleura is adequate treatment. When a malignant lesion is suspected, we prefer to perform biopsy through a small incision. If a diagnosis of malignancy can be made with a frozen section, the operation may proceed. Otherwise, the incision is closed, and the permanent sections are reviewed. The operation for Ewing's sarcoma or a neuroectodermal tumor involves removal of one rib above and one rib below the tumor, with a margin of 4 to 5 cm in a longitudinal

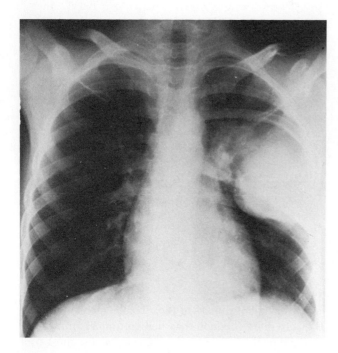

Figure 49–1. Ewing's sarcoma of the rib. Chest x-ray demonstrating a smooth mass.

lesion until the interspace below a normal rib has been reached. The portion of the chest wall containing the tumor is then removed. Any adherent lung is removed with the specimen. This usually involves only a simple wedge resection, but we have removed a lobe and, in one recurrent tumor, have performed a pneumonectomy. The tumor margins must be examined using frozen sections so that further tissue may be excised to ensure tumor-free margins.

The operated area should be irradiated with 4000 to 6000 rads over a period of 4 to 6 weeks. Intensive chemotherapy also is indicated. With this regimen, Rosen et al. reported survival of 12 consecutive patients with Ewing's sarcoma with no evidence of disease for anywhere from 10 to 37 months.[5]

Biopsy with radiation and chemotherapy is indicated for unresectable lesions. In the series of chest wall tumors reported on by Kumar et al., the lesions of 2 children became resectable after therapy. These patients were still alive at the time of the report. However, of the 8 children with unresectable tumors, only 2 survived.[6]

The Intergroup Ewing's Sarcoma Study also concluded that optimum treatment consisted of complete surgical resection, local radiation, and multimodal chemotherapy. With this aggressive approach, even patients who had an incomplete resection have survived for prolonged periods of time.[7]

It is still too soon to evaluate the results of treatment in children who have been diagnosed as having the primitive neuroectodermal tumor, but we have 3 children who have survived from 2 to 6 years after surgical resection, radiation, and three-drug chemotherapy.

direction. The initial incision must include a generous excision of a previous biopsy site. Skin flaps are elevated so that all muscle overlying the ribs is removed en bloc. An interspace is entered above or below the tumor, and the thoracic cavity is explored. Ribs and intercostal bundles are then transected proximal and distal to the

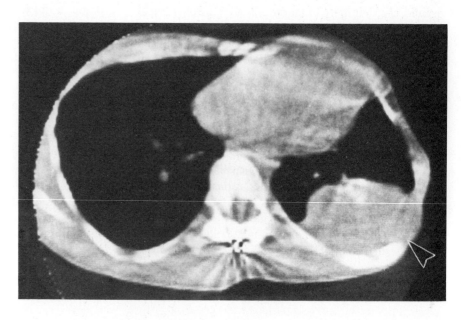

Figure 49–2. Primitive neuroectodermal tumor in a 14-year-old girl resected and treated by chemotherapy and radiotherapy. The patient was tumor free after 3 years.

REFERENCES

1. Joseph WL, Fonkalsrud WE: Primary rib tumors in children. Am Surg 38:388, 1972
2. Franken EA Jr, Smith JA, Smith WL: Tumors of the chest wall in infants and children. Pediatr Radiol 6:13, 1977
3. Askin F, Rosai J, Sibley R, et al: Malignant small cell tumor of the thoracopulmonary region in childhood: A distinctive clinicopathologic entity of uncertain histogenesis. Cancer 43:2438, 1979
4. Linnoilo R, Tsokos M, Triche T, et al: Evidence for the neural origin and PAS-positive variants of the malignant small cell tumor of thoraco pulmonary region (Askin tumor). Am J Surg Pathol 10:124, 1986
5. Rosen R, Wollner N, Tan C, et al: Disease-free survival in children with Ewing's sarcoma treated wtih radiation therapy and adjustment for drug sequential chemotherapy. Cancer 33:384, 1974
6. Kumar AP, Green A, Smith JW, et al: Combined therapy for malignant tumors of the chest wall in children. J Pediatr Surg 12:991, 1977
7. Thomas P, Foulkes L, Gilula L, et al: Primary Ewing's sarcoma of the ribs: A report from the Intergroup Ewing's Sarcoma Study. Cancer 51:1021, 1983

50
Breast Lesions

Symmetrical enlargement of the breasts is common in neonates. Often there is a secretion of cloudy fluid, which has been referred to as "witches' milk." This change is attributed to estrogen and prolactin from the maternal circulation. The swelling is soft and diffuse, but in some infants there is local tenderness with hyperemia. This may proceed to a pyogenic infection and an abscess that requires drainage.

PREMATURE THELARCHE

Enlargement of one or both breasts without other signs of precocious puberty is relatively common (Fig. 50–1). Unfortunately, the national publicity concerning can-

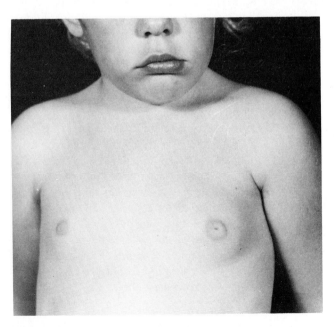

Figure 50–1. Premature thelarche. This is normal breast tissue that develops for no apparent reason in prepubertal girls.

cer of the breast often causes the child's mother to be tremendously concerned about this perfectly benign, self-limiting lesion. A small subareolar mass usually develops at the age of 1.5 to 4 years. On palpation, the mass is a slightly nodular subareolar disc of tissue. This may persist until the girl reaches puberty, but often it regresses and then reappears. Precocious puberty can be ruled out by observing a normal labia with no pubic hair. If desired, a vaginal swab may be used to determine if the vaginal cells display any estrogenic effect.[1] The surgeon must steadfastly refuse to biopsy this small breast tissue, since biopsy will cause a small, underdeveloped breast. Breast enlargement associated with genital development and growth acceleration is a manifestation of precocious puberty. A history should be obtained to rule out the ingestion of corticosteroids, contraceptives, or other hormones. Other drugs, such as digoxin and anticonvulsants, also may cause breast enlargement. Functionally active ovarian and adrenal tumors also may cause precocious puberty. Frequently, even exhaustive study will fail to give a definite etiology.

BREAST TUMORS

Hemangiomas, lymphangiomas, and other soft tissue tumors may involve the breast at any age. If excision is required, great care must be taken not to disturb the subareolar tissue so that the breast will not eventually be deformed. A galactocele is a soft, fluctuant cystic mass that may appear in boys as well as girls during the first months of life. Excision is the treatment of choice. True breast masses are rare in children. At our hospital, from 1975 to 1985, there were 19 teenage girls with fibroadenoma, 5 with virginal hypertrophy, 1 with cystosarcoma phylloides, 2 with neurofibromas, and only 1 with infiltrating ductal carcinoma in a child who had a previous history of radiotherapy.[2]

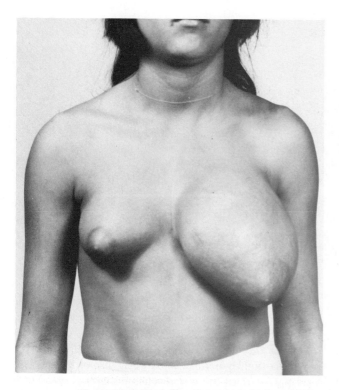
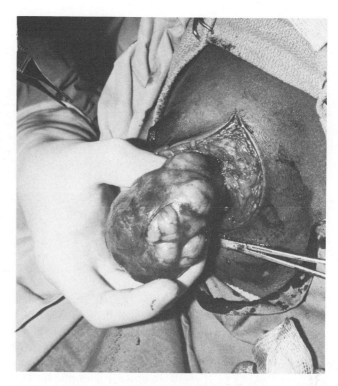

Figure 50–2. Giant fibroadenoma. **Left.** Firm nodular masses, which may involve almost the entire breast. **Right.** An excised mass.

The most common breast mass in teenage girls is the fibroadenoma. The peak age incidence is between 14 and 15 years, but younger girls also may have this lesion. It is more common in black girls.[3] The fibroadenoma appears as a firm, discrete, movable mass, which may become from 10 to 15 cm in diameter (Fig. 50–2). Grossly, the fibroadenoma is firm, gray to white, and well circumscribed. It may be dissected free from normal breast tissue by keeping instruments directly on the tumor capsule. The usual histologic pattern is similar to that of the adult intracanalicular fibroadenoma.

Cystosarcoma phylloides is even more unusual in teenage girls. These grow rapidly and become very large. Unlike the same lesion in older women, most are benign, although there have been reports of local recurrence or metastasis.[4,5] Local excision is the treatment of choice.[6]

Virginal hypertrophy also resembles fibroademona, except that both breasts may be involved, with rapid growth. The breast may be huge, firm, diffusely enlarged, and pendulous, with prominent superficial veins. There may be an ill-defined discrete mass. A reduction mammoplasty through a submammary incision is indicated to reduce the size of the breast and relieve the girl of the excessive weight.

Intraductal papilloma has been described in children. This lesion may be confused with carcinoma. Simple excision is all that is indicated.[7]

Carcinoma of the Breast

Fortunately, cancer of the breast is extremely rare in children under 20 years of age. In the age group between 10 and 15 years, the incidence of cancer of the breast is almost the same in boys as in girls. Carcinoma of the breast in prepubertal girls seems to be of a lower grade of malignancy than is encountered in older children and adults. The case reported by Lippitt et al. of a ductal carcinoma cured by a simple mastectomy appears to be typical for this age group.[8] On the other hand, carcinoma of the breast does develop in older teenagers, following the same clinical course of lymphatic and distant metastases as seen in adults.[9,10]

Juvenile secretory carcinoma has occurred in both boys and girls, from 3 to 17 years of age.[11] It has coexisted with juvenile papillomatosis and has been shown not to be a hormone-dependent tumor.[12] This appears to be a slowly growing, locally recurring malignancy, which metastasizes to axillary lymph nodes. It occurs as an asymptomatic breast mass, which should be biopsied and studied, and if the diagnosis is confirmed, a simple mastectomy with adequate margins is recommended along with axillary node sampling. Sufficient tissue should be left to allow breast reconstruction.

Gynecomastia

Pubertal boys frequently find a small, tender breast bud during self-examination. Usually, several months pass by before they tell their parents, who then take the boy to a physician. On physical examination, there is discernible enlargement of the breast. On palpation, the lesion varies in size but is usually no more than 2 to 3 cm in diameter and is slightly tender. It usually disappears within 6 months.

True sexual abnormalities, such as hermaphroditism or Klinefelter's syndrome, can be ruled out by physical examination or endocrine studies, if indicated. On rare occasion, gynecomastia will increase and persist, causing the boy considerable embarrassment. In such cases, excision is performed for cosmetic purposes. We prefer a submammary incision because circumareolar incisions frequently do not provide sufficient exposure. A skin flap is elevated with the areola until the extent of the breast tissue is demonstrated. Excision is then carried down to the pectoral fascia. The wound must be absolutely dry before it is closed. As an added protection against hematoma formation, suction drains and a pressure dressing are routinely used.

REFERENCES

1. Altcher A: Premature thelarche. Pediatr Clin North Am 19:543, 1972

2. Bauer B, Jones K, Talbot C: Mammary masses in the adolescent female. Surg Gynecol Obstet 165:63, 1987

3. Bower R, Bell MJ, Ternberg JL: Management of breast lesions in children and adolescents. J Pediatr Surg 11:337, 1976

4. Amerson RJ: Cystosarcoma phylloides in adolescent females: A report of seven patients. Ann Surg 171:849, 1976

5. Hoover HC, Trestioranu A, Ketcham AS: Metastatic cystosarcoma phylloides in an adolescent girl: An unusually malignant tumor. Ann Surg 181:279, 1975

6. Molit D, Golladay E, Gloster E, Jiminez J: Cystosarcoma phylloides in the adolescent female. J Pediatr Surg 22:907, 1987

7. Bloem JJ, Misere JF: Giant form of intraductal papilloma of the breast. J Pediatr Surg 6:65, 1971

8. Lippitt WH, Medart WS, Ramsey SN: Breast cancer in a 10-year-old girl. Surgery 68:395, 1970

9. Nichini FM, Goldman L, Lapayowker MS, et al: Inflammatory carcinoma of the breast in a 12-year-old girl. Arch Surg 105:505, 1972

10. Byrne MP, Fahey MM: Gooselaw breast cancer with axillary metastases in an 8½-year-old girl. Cancer 31:726, 1973

11. Karl S, Ballantine T, Zaino R: Juvenile secretory carcinoma of the breast. J Pediatr Surg 20:368, 1985

12. Ferguson T, McCarty K, Filstom H: Juvenile secretory carcinoma and juvenile papillomatosis: Diagnosis and treatment. J Pediatr Surg 22:637, 1987

51
Malignant Lymphomas

John G. Raffensperger
Elaine R. Morgan

Tumors arising from lymphoid tissue account for 10 to 15 percent of childhood malignancies in the Western world and up to 50 percent of tumors in African children. The malignant lymphomas are divided into two groups, Hodgkin's disease and the non-Hodgkin's lymphomas. Each of these groups is further subdivided on the basis of cell type. Any may involve the liver, spleen, bone, bone marrow, lung, or skin as well as lymphatic tissue.

The surgeon's primary involvement is in obtaining tissue for the initial diagnosis. During the past 20 years, the staging laparotomy has been used to aid the oncologist in determining the extent of the disease. Surgical resection is rarely feasible except when a lymphosarcoma is localized to the gastrointestinal tract.

HODGKIN'S DISEASE

One of the patients originally described by Hodgkin was a 10-year-old child.[1] Perhaps by coincidence, 10 years is the mean age of diagnosis of Hodgkin's disease in all patients up to 15 years of age. Although Strum and Rappaport were unable to document the diagnosis of Hodgkin's disease in children under 3 years of age, the youngest patient among three other reviews was 2 years old.[2–4] In these three series, covering a total of 223 patients, there was a 90 percent preponderance in boys in the under-10 age group. By the midteen years, the male:female ratio is 1.4:1, or the same as in adults.

Pathology

Histologic examination is required both to make the diagnosis and for classification according to the system devised by Lukes and Butler (the Rye modification).[5,6] This classification recognizes the following types of Hodgkin's disease: (1) lymphocytic predominance, (2) nodular sclerosis, (3) mixed cellularity, and (4) lymphocytic depletion. The nodular sclerosing form is most common in children. Lymphocyte predominance carries the best prognosis but is rare.[7] Survival in nodular sclerosis and mixed cellularity types is approximately the same.[8]

The multinucleated giant cell, or the Sternberg-Reed cell, has been considered essential to the diagnosis of Hodgkin's disease. Variants of this cell type, such as lacunar cells, sometimes are seen. On the other hand, Sternberg-Reed cells also are found in other conditions, such as cat-scratch fever, measles, and infectious mononucleosis.[9,10]

Clinical Findings

The most common presenting symptom of children with Hodgkin's disease is an enlarged, nontender cervical lymph node. Fever, anorexia, loss of weight, and night sweats are not common in children, except in advanced disease. Adenopathy in other areas, such as the axilla or groin, is much less frequent, and few children will have a palpable liver or spleen.

Early in the disease, the cervical adenopathy of lymphomas seems no different from the usual shotty

TABLE 51–1. MICROSCOPIC FINDINGS IN 50 CONSECUTIVE CERVICAL LYMPH NODE BIOPSIES

Reactive hyperplasia	23
Hodgkin's disease	10
Non-Hodgkin's lymphoma	6
Undifferentiated sarcoma	2
Metastatic rhabdomyosarcoma	2
Metastatic neuroblastoma	1
Papillary carcinoma of the thyroid	1

lymph nodes found in any child. A persistent nontender node that appears in the absence of a respiratory or dental infection must be seriously considered for biopsy. The pathology of 50 consecutive cervical lymph nodes biopsied at the Children's Memorial Hospital is shown in Table 51–1.

A suspicious lymph node must be totally removed under general anesthesia. It is important to obtain the largest node available, since smaller, more accessible nodes may merely show reactive hyperplasia when an adjacent node contains Hodgkin's disease. On rare occasions, Hodgkin's disease may occur with only mediastinal adenopathy. A small anterior thoracotomy incision is necessary to obtain adequate tissue for diagnosis in these children.

Clinical Staging

Hodgkin's disease is believed to commence in a single group of lymph nodes and then involve other adjacent areas in an orderly progression. The frequency with which the mediastinal nodes are skipped by disease that involves the left cervical area and the abdomen is explained by the direct communication of the thoracic duct. It is more important with children than with adults to make every effort to limit therapy because extensive irradiation can lead to serious long-term side effects in the growing child. For this reason, various methods have been devised for the staging of Hodgkin's disease. The Ann Arbor classification is currently the most widely used.[11–13] This system recognizes that all current clinical methods of evaluation—including the physical examination, bone marrow aspiration, liver function tests, and lymphangiography—are unreliable in determining the full extent of disease.

The staging classification of Hodgkin's disease according to symptoms involves two main categories: (A) no systemic symptoms, (B) systemic symptoms. Classification of a patient as symptomatic (category B) requires the presence of one or more of the following features: unexplained loss of more than 10 percent of the body weight in the 6 months before admission, unexplained fever with temperature above 38C, and night sweats. Further classification by extent of involvement can be made as follows.

I: A single lymph node region or a single organ or site (I_e).

II: Two or more lymph node regions on the same side of the diaphragm (II) or localized involvement of an extralymphatic organ or site and one or more lymph node regions on the same side of the diaphragm (II_e).

III: Lymph node regions on both sides of the diaphragm (III), which may also be accompanied by localized involvement of an extralymphatic organ or site (III_e), involvement of the spleen (III_s), or both (III_{es}).

IV: Diffuse or disseminated involvement of one or more extralymphatic organs or tissues, with or without lymph node enlargement. The classification of a patient as stage IV should be further classified by defining the site by symbols.[11]

Staging is carried out by clinical and radiologic examinations and, in selected patients, by the staging laparotomy. The gallium-67 citrate scanning technique allows a general survey of bone, lymph node, and abdominal organ involvement but is accurate in no more than 70 to 80 percent of cases. The computed tomography (CT) scan provides little more accuracy because enlarged nodes may represent hypertrophy due to infection and small tumor nodules will be overlooked. Lymphangiography is difficult to perform in small children and at best fails to demonstrate periportal or splenic nodal groups. The lymphangiogram was erroneous in one third of 55 patients studied at the Boston Children's Hospital, and in the series of Dudgeon et al., there was a 69 percent false positive rate and a 10 percent false negative rate.[14,15] Lymphangiograms are easier to obtain in older children but must be interpreted with caution. When combined with CT and gallium scans, radiologic staging may provide useful information.[16,17]

The Staging Laparotomy. Studies at Stanford University on the progression of Hodgkin's disease from one area to another led to the use of an exploratory laparotomy to determine the need for extended radiation to organs and lymph nodes below the diaphragm.[18,19] Hays applied these studies to children and found that a laparotomy changed the stage of disease in approximately 40 percent of patients.[20] Accurate staging as determined by laparotomy was considered important so therapy could be directed to involved tissue with great accuracy, thus limiting the complications of therapy while not missing involved areas that were not demonstrated by other studies. During the 1970s, many institutions, including our own, performed staging laparotomies on every child in whom the diagnosis of Hodgkin's disease was made. Table 51–2 illustrates our results. The laparotomy changed the stage in 12 patients; the spleen and splenic hilar nodes were found to be positive in 10.

In recent years, the necessity for the staging laparot-

TABLE 51–2. HODGKIN'S DISEASE: RESULTS OF LAPAROTOMY

Total patients with Hodgkin's disease	37
Patients who did not undergo laparotomy	7
Misdiagnosis	3
Clinical stage IV	4
Patients who underwent laparotomy	30
No. positive	13
No. negative	17
Diagnosis made at laparotomy	2
Change in stage by laparotomy	12
Lower stage (I or II)	2
Higher stage (III or IV)	10

omy has been questioned. It is not indicated when the child has stage IV disease, as evidenced by a positive bone marrow or biopsy evidence of organ disease. Extensive mediastinal involvement often is treated with chemotherapy, so the findings at laparotomy would not alter the treatment. The risk of abdominal involvement is almost nil in children with lymphocyte-predominant disease apparently limited to the right neck. Others believe that a laparotomy is not required in stages I and II disease if treatment is to be with chemotherapy or if relapses can be treated effectively with chemotherapy after initial radiation.[21] Institutions, such as the Mayo Clinic, continue to perform staging laparotomies in order to avoid the undertreatment of occult disease as well as the toxicity and complications of overtreatment.[22] The Children's Hospital of Los Angeles also recommends a staging laparotomy in all patients with stage I and II disease. If the subdiaphragmatic area is negative, radiation may be localized to the exact area of disease.[23] The oncologists in our hospital have adopted a selective approach to staging laparotomy. If a satisfactory lymphangiogram cannot be obtained, a laparotomy is performed. In most older children, the lymphangiogram provides excellent visualization of the iliac and lower abdominal periaortic nodes. If there is no suspicion of disease on the lymphangiogram, CT scan, or gallium scan, we do not perform a laparotomy. Since these studies cannot evaluate the spleen and splenic hilar nodes, our radiotherapists include these areas in the field of radiation. If there is any discrepancy among the various diagnostic techniques, a laparotomy is performed.

The technique of performing a staging laparotomy is as follows. The entire abdomen, including one iliac crest, must be prepared and draped into the field. We prefer a transverse incision, which is curved downward from the left costal margin to just above and to the right of the umbilicus. Alternatively, a paramedian incision may be used. The spleen is removed in all patients over 4 years of age. In younger children, either needle biopsy of the spleen or a hemisplenectomy is performed. All lymph nodes must be removed from the splenic hilum

and from the superior surface of the splenic vein. A wedge biopsy and three needle biopsies are then performed on each lobe of the liver. While warm, moist laparotomy pads are placed over the liver biopsy sites and in the splenic bed, the intestine is eviscerated from the abdomen to the right. The posterior peritoneum is then opened from the renal artery inferiorly to the bifurcation of the iliac arteries. Lymph nodes are removed from the paraaortic and iliac chain regardless of their size, although special attention must be given to obviously enlarged nodes. Several large nodes are selected for removal from the mesentery, and the posterior peritoneum is closed with a running suture.

The intestine is then returned to the abdominal cavity, and by retracting the liver superiorly, more nodes are removed from the porta hepatis. Finally, by retracting the stomach anteriorly, the aortic nodes at the diaphragm are visualized, and several are removed. Nodes may be removed with minimal blood loss by opening the overlying peritoneum and dissecting the loose areolar tissue away with scissors. The node is then elevated, and a metal clip is applied to the remaining tissue. All specimens must be properly labeled and placed in separate jars. The hemostatic clips are also markers for future reference. While the abdomen is being closed, one member of the surgical team makes an incision over the iliac crest. This must be sufficiently large to allow a 3 cm elevation of periosteum from the bone. A small chisel and hammer are then used to remove a wedge of bone and marrow. The marrow cavity is packed with bone wax, and the incision is closed. In small children, the iliac crest may be composed mostly of cartilage. Consequently, one must be sure to go deeply enough to obtain marrow.

Previously, postsplenectomy sepsis was a major complication of this operation. For that reason, hemisplenectomy has been suggested as a means of sampling the spleen while leaving enough tissue in place to avoid sepsis.[24,25] Since the advent of effective vaccines and the use of prophylactic antibiotics, the risk of postsplenectomy sepsis has almost disappeared.[26] We continue to perform a complete splenectomy because of the risk of overlooking disease, except in the occasional child younger than 4 years of age.

Therapy

Radiation therapy is the treatment of choice for stage I or II disease and in older children with stage III disease limited to the spleen or upper paraaortic nodes.[27] Patients with stage III disease with involvement of lower abdominal or iliac nodes, those with stage IIIB disease, and those with massive mediastinal disease probably benefit from a combination of chemotherapy and low-dose radiation.[28] Some very young children with stage II disease may be similarly treated in order to use a lower dose of radiation. Those with stage IV disease usually are treated with more extensive chemotherapy consisting of two noncross-resistant regimens. The chemotherapy regimens commonly used today are MOPP (mechlorethamine, vincristine, procarbazine, and prednisone) and ABVD (doxorubicin, bleomycin, vinblastine, and dacarbazine) or other combinations of these drugs.

Results

The current 2-year disease-free survival rates are as high as 80 percent in stage IV disease and up to 95 percent in stage I disease. The 5-year survival rates are only slightly lower. As the results of treatment improve, there is greater concern over the side effects of radiation and chemotherapy. Radiation affects the growing skeleton and damages the heart, and the MOPP regimen results in male sterility. Secondary malignant tumors will develop in some of the survivors. Thus, the optimum approach to children with Hodgkin's disease has not been fully determined.

NON-HODGKIN'S LYMPHOMA

The non-Hodgkin's lymphomas are more common in childhood than Hodgkin's disease, and there is an even greater preponderance of males. There is one age peak at 4 to 5 years and another at 10 to 11 years.[29] These rapidly growing, aggressive tumors occur in the abdomen, the anterior mediastinum, and lymph nodes of the head and neck, as well as peripheral sites. The distinction between lymphoma and leukemia is often difficult, but, in general, with leukemia at least 25 percent of the bone marrow is replaced by malignant cells. Historically, as lymphoma progressed, many children developed lymphocytic leukemia. Fortunately, with modern therapy, this progression is seen with less frequency.

Pathology

This group of lymphomas is categorized as follows: lymphoblastic, undifferentiated Burkitt's, undifferentiated non-Burkitt's, and large cell or histiocytic types.[30] Other systems of classification also are used.

The lymphocytic, poorly differentiated type is most common in children in the United States and the Western world, whereas the undifferentiated Burkitt's lymphoma is most common in Central Africa. In the United States, Burkitt's lymphoma is more likely to occur as a large abdominal mass than as the typical jaw tumor seen in Africa. Recently, immunologic techniques have been used in the further classification of the non-Hodgkin's lymphomas. Tumors may now be described as T cell, B cell, or null cell. The mediastinal tumors are more commonly T cell, and abdominal tumors are more often B cell.

The poorly differentiated lymphocytic lymphoma is most likely to involve extranodal sites as well as the mediastinum and subsequently undergo leukemic transformation. Histologically, lymph nodes are diffusely replaced by uniform lymphoid cells with round to oval nuclei. Mitoses are abundant, and the starry sky appearance of histocytes is often noted, as in Burkitt's lymphoma.

Clinical Findings

Since non-Hodgkin's lymphomas grow so rapidly, children are likely to have advanced disease. Although the first sign may be only an asymptomatic, enlarged lymph node, more children have rapidly progressing dyspnea and cough due to mediastinal nodes or pleural effusion. In this situation, it is necessary to establish an exact diagnosis rapidly. Enlarged peripheral lymph nodes should be biopsied, and an emergency bone marrow examination is indicated. When there is severe tracheal or superior vena cava obstruction and no easily obtainable lesion for biopsy, it may be necessary to remove a mediastinal node. In this situation, a general anesthetic may be hazardous, but a biopsy under local anesthesia also is dangerous. We prefer to take the child to the operating room and perform all required biopsies and the insertion of a central venous catheter under general endotracheal anesthesia. The endotracheal tube allows a more tranquil, exact operation. It is left in place, and the child is placed on a ventilator and kept in the intensive care area during the induction of therapy. The child is ventilated, and the endotracheal tube is left in place until the tumor has shrunk and the tracheal obstruction is relieved.

Abdominal lymphomas may cause chronic abdominal pain, a mass, or ascites and can mimic appendicitis or cause an intussusception. Three of our patients initially had a gangrenous intussusception. In Ein et al.'s series of 1200 children with intussusceptions, only 11 had a lymphoma.[31] They noted a high incidence of preexisting abdominal symptoms and weight loss before the acute episode. In addition, only 1 of the 11 intussusceptions could be reduced with a barium enema, and in that case a filling defect was seen on barium enema. The symptoms of lymphoma can mimic inflammatory bowel disease. When there is only abdominal pain, intestinal roentgenograms may demonstrate nonspecific thickening of the wall or effacement of the mucosa. Abdominal ultrasonography, CT scans, and gallium scans all aid in the diagnosis by demonstrating enlarged lymph nodes or a mass in the mesentery and bowel wall. Patients with disseminated disease often will have a positive bone marrow, and this examination is indicated in all cases. An exploratory laparotomy is not indicated when the diagnosis can be established by other means. Staging systems are not indicated, since therapy is based only on whether the disease is localized or disseminated.

Therapy

Lymphomas, especially of the Burkitt's type, are the most rapidly growing tumors in the human body. Not only do they grow rapidly, but with therapy and even before the initiation of treatment, tumor cells become necrotic and release metabolites that result in the tumor lysis syndrome. Nucleic acid purines are converted to uric acid, which may precipitate in the kidney, causing renal failure. Children with widespread lymphomas are at the greatest risk of developing this problem. It must be anticipated and, hopefully, prevented by pretreatment with allopurinol (10 mg/kg per day), alkalinization of the urine, and administration of one and one half to two times the usual daily intake of fluid to promote a brisk diuresis.

Surgical treatment of the lymphomas is limited to resection of tumors of the bowel and mesentery. Many of these occur as an acute abdomen, and the tumor is found during an exploration for intestinal obstruction or suspected appendicitis. Often, the mass is localized to the ileum or cecum, and a right hemicolectomy with ileal and mesenteric resection is indicated. Adjacent mesenteric or enlarged periaortic nodes should be removed for biopsy, and the margins of resection are studied with frozen section at the time of operation. These patients can expect a 90 to 100 percent disease-free survival rate when treated with adjuvant chemotherapy.[32,33] In the past, debulking operations of large, unresectable tumors were thought to be beneficial. This is no longer true, since chemotherapy results in rapid debulking, and an extensive operation may delay chemotherapy.[34] These patients must be followed carefully by a surgeon, however, because intestinal perforation through an area of necrotic tumor is a potential hazard. There are a number of chemotherapy regimens designed for lymphoma, depending on cell type and extent of disease. Patients with lymphoblastic lymphoma respond to a 10-drug regimen, whereas those with nonlymphoblastic lymphoma are given 4 drugs.[35] Multiinstitutional studies are continuing to improve the results in these patients.

REFERENCES

1. Hodgkin T: On some morbid appearances of the absorbent glands and spleen. Medical Clinical Transactions. London, Medical Chir. Soc., 1832, p 56
2. Strum SB, Rappaport H: Hodgkin's disease in the first decade of life. Pediatrics 46:748, 1970
3. Teillet F, Schweisguth O: Hodgkin's disease in children. Clin Pediatr 8:698, 1969
4. Norris DG, Burgert EO Jr, Cooper HA, et al: Hodgkin's disease in childhood. Cancer 36:2109, 1975
5. Lukes RJ, Butler JJ: The pathology and nomenclature of Hodgkin's disease. Cancer Res 26:1063, 1966
6. Lukes RJ, Craver LF, Hall TC, et al: Report of the nomenclature committee. Cancer Res 26:1311, 1966
7. Russell K, Donaldson S, Cox R, Kaplan H: Childhood Hodgkin's disease: patterns of relapse. J Clin Oncol 2:80, 1984
8. Dearth J, Gilchrist G, Burgert E, et al: Management of stage I to III Hodgkin's disease in children. J Pediatr 5:829, 1980
9. Strum SB, Park JK, Rappaport H: Observation of cells resembling Sternberg-Reed cells in conditions other than Hodgkin's disease. Cancer 26:176, 1970
10. Lukes RJ, Tindle BH, Parker JW: Reed–Sternberg-like cells in infectious mononucleosis. Lancet 2:1003, 1969
11. Carbone PP, Kaplan HS, Musshoff K, et al: Report of the committee on Hodgkin's disease staging classification. Cancer Res 31:1860, 1971
12. Rosenberg SA, Boiron M, DeVita VT, et al: Report of the committee on Hodgkin's disease staging procedure. Cancer Res 31:1862, 1971
13. Rappaport H, Berard CW, Butler JJ, et al: Report of the committee on histopathological criteria contributing to staging of Hodgkin's disease. Cancer Res 31:1864, 1971
14. Filler RM, Jaffe N, Cassady JR, et al: Experience with clinical and operative staging of Hodgkin's disease in children. J Pediatr Surg 10:321, 1975
15. Dudgeon D, Kelly R, Ghory M, et al: The efficacy of lymphangiography in the staging of pediatric Hodgkin's disease. J Pediatr Surg 21:233, 1986
16. Castellino R: Imaging techniques for staging abdominal Hodgkin's disease. Ca Treat Rep 66:697, 1982
17. Lang B, Littman P: Management of Hodgkin's disease in children and adolescents. Cancer 51:1371, 1983
18. Rosenberg SA, Kaplan HS: Evidence for an orderly progression in the spread of Hodgkin's disease. Cancer Res 26:1225, 1966
19. Glatstein E, Guernsey JM, Rosenberg SA, et al: The value of laparotomy and splenectomy in the staging of Hodgkin's disease. Cancer 24:709, 1969
20. Hays DM: The staging of Hodgkin's disease in children reviewed. Cancer 35:973, 1975
21. Irving M: Hodgkin's disease: Is staging laparotomy necessary? Br J Surg 72:589, 1985
22. Windebank K, Gilchrist G: Hodgkin's disease. Pediatr Ann 17:204, 1988
23. Lally K, Arnskin M, Siegel S, et al: A comparison of staging methods for Hodgkin's disease in children. Arch Surg 121:1125, 1986
24. Boles E, Haase G, Hamoudi A: Partial splenectomy in staging laparotomy for Hodgkin's disease: An alternate approach. J Pediatr Surg 13:581, 1978
25. Tubbs R, Thomas F, Norris D, Firor H: Is hemisplenectomy a satisfactory option to total splenectomy in abdominal staging of Hodgkin's disease? J Pediatr Surg 22:727, 1987
26. Hays D, Ternberg J, Chen T, et al: Postsplenectomy sepsis and other complications following staging laparotomy for Hodgkin's disease in childhood. J Pediatr Surg 21:628, 1986
27. Sweet D, Kinneally A, Ullmann J: Hodgkin's disease: Problems of staging. Cancer 42:957, 1978
28. Lange B, Littman P: Management of Hodgkin's disease in children and adolescents. Cancer 51:1371, 1983
29. Murphy SB, Davis LW: Hodgkin's disease and the non-

Hodgkin's lymphomas in childhood. Semin Oncol 1:17, 1974

30. Murphy S: Childhood non-Hodgkin's lymphoma. N Engl J Med 299:1466, 1978

31. Ein S, Stephens C, Shandling B, Filler R: Intussusception due to a lymphoma. J Pediatr Surg 21:786, 1986

32. Murphy S, Hustu H, Rivera G, et al: End results of treating children with localized non-Hodgkin's lymphoma with a combined modality approach of lessened intensity. J Clin Oncol 1:326, 1983

33. Jenkin R, Anderson J, Chilcote R, et al: The treatment of localized non-Hodgkin's lymphoma in children: A report from the Children's Cancer Study Group. J Clin Oncol 2:88097, 1984

34. Kaufman B, Burgert E, Banks P: Abdominal Burkitt's lymphoma: Role of early aggressive surgery. J Pediatr Surg 22:671, 1987

35. Anderson J, Wilson J, Jenkin D, et al: Childhood non-Hodgkin's lymphoma: The results of a randomized therapeutic trial comparing a 4 drug regimen (LOMP) with a 10 drug regimen LSA$_2$-L$_2$. N Engl J Med 30:559, 1983

52
Soft Tissue Tumors

Muscle, fat fascia, blood vessels, and other connective tissues are the source of a wide variety of childhood tumors, varying from hemangioma to highly malignant killers. Most are readily palpable. Others, such as the sarcomas of the genitourinary tract, produce early, distinctive symptoms. Any lump or mass lesion in a child must be considered potentially malignant and should be biopsied. After making this dogmatic statement, it must be admitted that there are some exceptions. One of the most important is the small bud of developing breast tissue that may be present as a tender subareolar lump in a young girl. Immunizations, or baby shots, when given into the anterolateral part of the thigh may leave an indurated mass that consists of fat necrosis and may resemble a tumor. The history is most important. If in doubt, aspiration sometimes returns a bit of yellow cloudy fluid. Obvious hemangiomas or cystic hygromas are easy to diagnose clinically. Benign conditions are much more common than malignant tumors, and we must excise a number of "lumps and bumps" if we are to diagnose the early sarcomas.

There are some clinical signs that may aid the surgeon in arriving at a preoperative guess about the nature of the lesion. Small, circumscribed, subcutaneous lumps adjacent to the orbit of or at the suprasternal notch usually are epidermoid cysts. Subcutaneous lesions, particularly those that follow the course of a nerve and are associated with café au lait spots, often are nerve sheath tumors. A small mass that on palpation seems to be intradermal often will turn out to be a dermatofibroma. Masses that are deep to the subcutaneous tissue and those that have undergone a rapid increase in size or are associated with pain or edema are the most likely to be malignant. Computed tomography (CT) scans have proven to be extremely helpful in evaluating soft tissue tumors, especially those on the extremities. Often, an experienced radiologist can differentiate benign from malignant lesions, and scans will determine the extent of the lesions.

BIOPSY

It is inappropriate to perform a wide excision that needlessly sacrifices normal tissue to remove a benign lesion. On the other hand, when a tumor that has been simply shelled out is found to be a highly malignant sarcoma, we can be certain that tumor was left in the wound.

A 2 to 3 cm mass that may be circumscribed with a margin of tissue but leaves an easily closed wound with no cosmetic or functional impairment is completely excised. This accounts for the majority of common skin and subcutaneous lesions. The admonishment to take a margin of normal tissue around the tumor usually indicates the excision of an overlying ellipse of skin and dissection through fat rather than on the surface of the tumor. This type of excision is designed primarily for those lesions that turn out to be fibromas. A specimen of larger tumors may be obtained with a needle biopsy, under local anesthesia, to make a definitive diagnosis by permanent microscopic section before surgical excision. Alternatively, a small incisional biopsy may be performed. If the pathologist can make a satisfactory diagnosis with a frozen section, the definitive excision may proceed under the same anesthetic. Regardless of which technique is chosen, one will spill tumor cells. However, if the tumor is malignant, the biopsy site will be liberally resected with the tumor.

When the lesion is clearly malignant, there is no hesitation to perform a wide radical excision that encompasses the tumor with a safe margin of normal tissue, even if this excision requires the mobilization of skin flaps or grafting. The management of soft tissue tumors requires the cooperation of the surgeon, the pathologist, and the oncologist.

Many of these lesions are extremely rare in the pediatric age group. Some (particularly fibrous lesions) are peculiar to childhood and are quite cellular, with mitotic figures, yet are benign. Furthermore, there has been a radical change in the management of the most common malignant tumors, the rhabdomyosarcomas. Mutilating surgical procedures, such as amputation and pelvic exenteration, are rarely indicated, since chemotherapy has proven to be highly successful.

LIPOMATOUS TUMORS

The usual adult form of lipoma is exceedingly rare in childhood. When one palpates a soft, subcutaneous mass and thinks it is a lipoma, the diagnosis usually is cystic hygroma. We have encountered 7 cases of lipoma, of which 2 occurred on the lower extremity, 1 on the abdominal wall, 3 on the back, and 1 in the axilla. These tumors were soft to palpation, and roentgenograms demonstrated a sunburst effect of radiolucencies that radiated from the tumor into muscle bundles. These were poorly defined lipomatous masses that diffusely infiltrated the muscle bundles. When these tumors are encapsulated, they are termed "lipoblastoma." When they are not encapsulated, the proper term is "lipoblastomatosis." They consist of embryonal fat, and although they may grow rapidly and will recur if incompletely excised, they are benign.

In an analysis of 35 cases, 88 percent occurred in infants under 1 year of age.[1] The lesions occurred most commonly on the trunk and extremities, and although some were encapsulated, most infiltrated the surrounding fibromuscular tissue planes. There were no deaths due to tumor in this series, but there was a 14.3 percent incidence of recurrence, apparently because of incomplete original excision.

The CT scan in Figure 52–1 is of a 1-year-old child whose original tumor was palpable in the paravertebral region. The superficial portion was removed, but there was a prompt recurrence, and the CT scan demonstrated not only the posterior mediastinal tumor but extradural extension. The tumor was removed with a combined thoracic–neurosurgical approach, and her spine was stabilized with a bone graft. We have observed 1 recurrence after incomplete excision, and Stringel et al also reported that 1 of their 4 cases recurred but was cured after a second excision.[2] There is no evidence that this tumor progresses to liposarcoma. In fact, the fat cells tend to mature with age.

LIPOSARCOMAS

Liposarcoma appears to be extremely rare in childhood, with essentially no unequivocal cases recorded in patients below the age of 5 years. There are 4 liposarcomas in our tumor records. One liposarcoma on the shoulder of a 10-year-old boy did not recur during 3 years of follow-up after a radical local excision. A huge retroperitoneal mass in a 12-year-old girl was resected along with the right ureter. She was then treated with radiation and chemotherapy. No tumor was found at a second look 2 years later, and she is still alive and tumor free 13 years after her original operation. One other child survived excision of a retroperitoneal liposarcoma, and another died.

FIBROMA, FIBROMATOSIS, FIBROSARCOMA

The fibromatoses are poorly understood, unpredictable lesions because there is so little correlation with their microscopic appearance and their biologic behavior. There are a large number of descriptive terms applied to these tumors.[3]

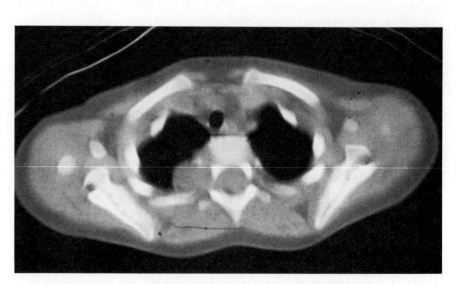

Figure 52–1. CT scan of a child with a lipoblastoma of the posterior mediastinum with intraspinal extension.

Classification of Fibrous Tissue Tumors of Childhood

  I. Fibromatosis colli (torticollis, sternomastoid tumor)
 II. Hereditary gingival fibromatosis
III. Congenital fibromatosis
     A. Solitary
     B. Generalized
 IV. Congenital fibrosarcoma-like fibromatosis (congenital or infantile fibrosarcoma)
  V. Digital fibrous tumor of Reye (infantile dermal fibromatosis)
 VI. Diffuse (muscular) infantile fibromatosis (infantile myofibromatosis)
VII. Fibrous hamartoma of infancy
VIII. Juvenile aponeurotic fibroma
 IX. Juvenile hyaline fibromatosis
  X. Fibromatosis (infantile, juvenile, not otherwise classified)
 XI. Nasopharyngeal angiofibroma (?)

From a clinical standpoint, regardless of histologic classification, age, or location of the tumor, all the fibrous tumors have a tendency to recur locally if they are not completely excised with a margin of normal tissue. Thus, close cooperation with the pathologist is essential. After removing the tumor, the surgeon should excise additional tissue from various locations in the wound for frozen section. The pathologist should mark the surface of the tumor with India ink and examine every area where it approaches the margins of resection. To make matters more complicated, some of these lesions have a tendency to regress spontaneously.

The most common fibromatosis is the sternocleidomastoid tumor, which occurs as a mass in the muscle, with tortocollis. The proper term for this lesion is "fibromatosis colli." At one time, this was thought to result from birth trauma, but it has its onset before birth, and it is the position of the infant's head that necessitates a breech delivery. The tumor will resolve with warm soaks, massage, and gentle stretching exercises.

Digital fibrous tumors that appear in children under 1 year of age also form a recognizable type of fibromatosis.[4] Typically, there is a smooth nodule that first appears on the lateral or distal extensor surface of the digit. If growth occurs, it is usually longitudinally along the finger or toe. Digital fibrous tumors are very cellular lesions that tend to recur promptly after excision. Since there is always a feeling of uncertainty about the prognosis of any individual lesion, the first recurrence should be treated with a wide local excision, taking all the overlying skin and stripping periosteum from the bone. When the pathologist clearly can make the diagnosis of digital fibroma, further recurrences are observed. These tumors tend to undergo spontaneous regression. We also have seen recurrent small nodules in the incision

regress after injection of triamcinolone acetonide (Kenalog).

The fibrous hamartoma of infancy occurs in the axillary region or upper arm, usually during the first few months of life. This lesion is localized to the subcutaneous tissues and shows little tendency to recurrence after excision.[5] Nodular fasciitis is a reactive lesion involving the fascia of the back, which is not truly a tumor but occurs as a mass lesion. It also shows little tendency to recur. Juvenile hyaline fibromatosis is a descriptive term for multiple subcutaneous tumor nodules that contain a large amount of ground substance. They grow steadily, are multiple, and produce deformity of the hands and face and hypertrophy of the gums and nailbeds. They do not recur after excision, but multiple new tumors appear over the course of the patient's life.[6]

Congenital fibromatosis, or myofibromatosis, may appear as a solitary mass in the skin, muscle, or viscera, or there may be multiple lesions with visceral involvement.[7] Isolated fibromatosis may be excised if the lesion is cosmetically unacceptable or in a location where it interferes with function.[8] Wiswell et al. collected 170 patients with infantile myofibromatosis from the literature, most from 1980 to 1988.[9] They had solitary lesions, often at birth, with discrete nodules in the skin or muscle, most of which regressed spontaneously. Ninety infants had multiple lesions, and 33 of them had visceral involvement. Twenty-five patients died because of multiple cardiopulmonary or gastrointestinal tumors. When the diagnosis is made on a biopsy of a subcutaneous mass, the child should have CT scans performed of the lung and abdomen, searching for additional lesions. We have had 2 children with skin and visceral involvement. One with splenic nodules recovered with spontaneous regression. The second child had skin lesions over her shoulder and arm and jaundice secondary to common bile duct obstruction. Her jaundice was relieved with a portojejunoduodenostomy. All of her lesions are regressing 3 years after the diagnosis was made.

Fibromatosis or Aggressive Fibromatosis

These terms describe a lesion that has a tendency to recur after excision, may require radical surgery including amputation for cure, and for which both radiation and chemotherapy have been suggested as adjuvant treatment. In one series, 2 of 10 children died of progressive disease.[10] Despite behavior that, by any criteria, would be considered malignant, this lesion has a very benign appearance. Histologically, it consists of a monotonous spindle cell tumor with a large amount of collagen between the cells. An occasional mitosis is seen, but significant nuclear atypia are absent. Despite this soothing histologic picture, the tumor tends to infiltrate into muscle, along fascial planes, and into periosteum and bone. More important, there may be extensions at a distance from the tumor or in a proximal direction, or there may be multicentric foci.[11] They occur with equal frequency on the head and neck, trunk, or extremities and occur as firm, deep tumor masses.

Treatment. A small tumor no more than 2 to 3 cm in diameter should be excised with a margin of normal tissue. When the diagnosis is established, the child should be studied carefully with either CT or magnetic resonance imaging (MRI), searching for multicentric foci. If the lesion is in an extremity, the entire limb must be studied because we have observed secondary lesions 10 cm proximal from the primary lesion, with normal intervening tissue. Unless one can be certain that the original margin of normal tissue was at least 2 cm, the child should be reoperated on to obtain more extensive margins. If the initial tumor is large, an incisional biopsy would perhaps be the best first step. Then, with information from permanent histologic sections and radiologic studies, a proper operation may be planned.

Wide surgical excision that does not interfere with function is the accepted mode of therapy for this lesion. Unfortunately, wide surgical excisions often are limited by essential bones, nerves, and vessels. Ideally, there should be a minimum of 2 cm of normal tissue on either side, with more both proximally and distally, in order to remove extensions along fascial planes. Multiple frozen sections are obtained during the operation to be absolutely certain of tumor-free margins. If the tumor abuts against bone, the periosteum should be removed. Individual major arteries and nerves are dissected on their sheath, and frozen sections are taken of adjacent tissue. Thus, a wide surgical excision is a carefully planned, anatomically executed operation. When the tumor is adjacent to major vital structures, we cannot claim to have performed a wide excision unless these are taken also. This becomes a problem with tumors that are on the foot or adjacent to the tibia, where the tumor must be skimmed off.

Although radiotherapy has been recommended when excision is impossible, high doses are required.[12] Chemotherapy certainly should be used at the first recurrence, especially if further excision would compromise function.[13]

Raney et al. have summarized the current status of chemotherapy for these lesions and reported on 3 patients treated with vincristine, dactinomycin, and cyclophosphamide in whom there was either complete disappearance or greater than 75 percent shrinkage of the tumor.[14]

Congenital Fibrosarcoma

Congenital fibrosarcomas appear at birth or during the first 3 months of life. Otherwise, from a clinical stand-

point, they are no different than any other fibrosarcoma in that they will recur locally and metastasize. The ambivalence of this lesion can best be summed up by quoting from Dehner:[3] "The histology of the lesion in terms of cellularity, mitotic activity and even necrosis is similar in most respects to that of a conventional fibrosarcoma in the adult." And: "In order to reduce the possibility of unnecessary radical surgery, the authors prefer the term 'congenital fibrosarcoma-like fibromatosis.'" Microscopically, however, these tumors differ from the fibromatoses by having a herringbone appearance, and on electron microscopic study, there are immature fibroblasts and histiocytic cells.[15]

Blocker et al. reviewed 52 cases of congenital fibrosarcoma and found that 37, or 71 percent, were on the extremities, where there was a local recurrence rate of 32 percent and a mortality rate of 5 percent.[16] There were 15 tumors on the trunk or head and neck, with a recurrence rate of 33 percent, but the metastatic and mortality rates were 26 percent, indicating a more aggressive behavior for axial tumors. This pattern of behavior certainly warrants treating congenital fibrosarcomas with the same degree of surgical aggressiveness as those at an older age. Wide local excision should be carried out at the first operation. This is not possible with some tumors of the extremities, where the tumor involves adjacent bone and nerves. Fibrosarcomas require diligent pathologic and radiologic study to determine if all margins of the tumor have been excised and the presence of proximal or metastatic lesions. Reexcision or amputation must be carried out if the tumor margins are not clear. Carroll, at our institution, successfully salvaged the leg of a child with a fibrosarcoma by removing a tumor of the thigh that had invaded the femoral vessels by complete excision, with microvascular replacement of the artery with a vein graft. Also, we have a 5-year cure in a child who, at 3 months of age, had a tumor that surrounded the iliac artery and vein as well as the femoral nerve. She has a functioning leg 5 years after resection of the tumor along with these structures. A third child, who had a neck tumor removed in the neonatal period that recurred within 2 months, is now tumor free 3 years after complete excision of the tumor with a portion of the mandible. In these 3 patients, multiple frozen sections were taken until adjacent tissue was found in all dimensions that was free from tumor. In the case of the neck tumor, this required 50 frozen section examinations. Fourteen of the 37 extremity lesions found by Blocker et al. in the literature required an amputation at some point in their treatment.

Although the efficacy of adjuvant chemotherapy has not been established, treatment with vincristine, dactinomycin, and cyclophosphamide has resulted in tumor shrinkage with subsequent surgical resection in 2 children.[17] This treatment may, in the future, allow less extensive operations, with improved survival rates. The same principles outlined here apply to older children with fibrosarcoma.

RHABDOMYOSARCOMAS

Rhabdomyosarcomas follow Wilms' tumors and neuroblastomas as the most frequent malignancies in childhood. The peak age of incidence is between 3 and 5 years, but these tumors of striated muscle may be seen at any age, from birth on. The typical sites are the head and neck, the genitourinary tract, the extremities, and the trunk. These tumors have also been found in the bile duct and the perianal region.[18,19]

Pathology

There are three subtypes of rhabdomyosarcoma: the pleomorphic, which is unusual in childhood, the alveolar cell, which primarily affects the extremities of older children, and the embryonal cell rhabdomyosarcoma, which is most frequent in the pediatric age group. The benign counterpart of rhabdomyosarcoma, the rhabdomyoma, occurs in younger children and may be located either superficially in the soft tissues or in the myocardium.[20-22]

The embryonal rhabdomyosarcoma has individual characteristics depending on its site of origin. When it occurs in the bladder, vagina, or nasopharynx, it bulges outward beneath the mucous membrane to grossly resemble a bunch of grapes. Thus the term "sarcoma botryoides" is applied to these soft, myxomatous, protruding, grapelike masses. Microscopically, there is a chaotic, highly cellular pattern, with hyperchromatic, variegated nuclei. Striations may be found in the cytoplasm, especially with electron microscopy. Histologically, it may be difficult to distinguish this lesion from the other small cell tumors of childhood, such as Ewing's sarcoma and neuroblastoma. The tumor's site of origin is helpful in determining its definitive pathology.

Rhabdomyosarcomas grow rapidly, infiltrating adjacent tissues and organs. Before the introduction of chemotherapy, widespread metastases with local recurrence was the rule following surgical excision. These lesions metastasize to bone and bone marrow as well as to the lung. Lymphatic metastases vary according to the site of origin of the tumor and must be considered when planning surgical therapy. A compilation of 264 patients in the Intergroup Rhabdomyosarcoma Study revealed the following incidence of lymphatic metastases regardless of cellular type.[23]

Site of Origin	Percent Metastatic
Genitourinary tract	19
Extremities	17
Trunk	10
Head and neck	3
Orbit	0

From these data, one may surmise that lymph node dissection is important in the staging and treatment of rhabdomyosarcomas that involve the genitourinary tract, extremities, and trunk.

Staging

The Intergroup Rhabdomyosarcoma Study recommended the following grouping system, which is similar to that used for Wilms' tumors, based on available clinical, laboratory, and surgical findings. This staging system not only is helpful in determining the prognosis and treatment for an individual child but also allows comparison of various treatment modalities among large groups of patients.[24]

- GROUP I. Localized disease, completely resected
  A. Tumor confined to muscle or organ
  B. Infiltration beyond origin, but microscopic confirmation of complete resection
- GROUP II. Regional disease, grossly resected with:
  A. Microscopic residual tumor
  B. Nodal involvement or extension into adjacent organs
- GROUP III. Incomplete resection, or biopsy only
- GROUP IV. Distant metastases present at the onset of treatment

Recently, efforts have been made to improve on this system of staging by taking into account the site of the tumor and its natural history.[25,26]

Rhabdomyosarcoma of the Head and Neck. Tumors that develop from the nasopharynx or auditory canal have bloody or purulent drainage, and on examination one may find a red, globular mass that is easily biopsied. Lesions that develop from the muscles of the head and neck appear as mere asymptomatic, deep-seated swellings. These must be differentiated from lymph nodes, metastatic neuroblastomas, and the various benign cysts that involve the head and neck. A biopsy is indicated for any firm mass that cannot be explained readily by its location or other symptoms. Orbital lesions may cause pain and swelling about the eye, with proptosis and diplopia.

Rhabdomyosarcoma of the Genitourinary Tract. Any vaginal discharge, particularly if it is bloody, requires an examination under anesthesia, with biopsy of suspicious lesions (Fig. 52–2). Chronic vaginal foreign bodies and urethral prolapse may simulate a tumor. We have observed endodermal sinus tumors originating from the vagina as well as simple benign fibromatous polyps in newborn infants, which resemble sarcoma botryoides.

Lesions of the bladder are more difficult to diagnose because at first one finds only increased difficulty in

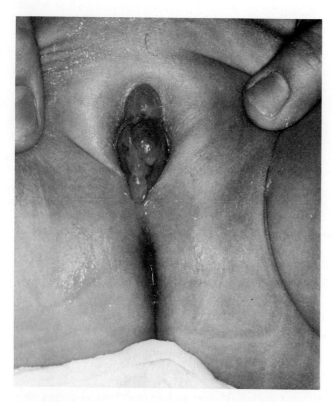

Figure 52–2. Sarcoma botryoides of the vagina. This is a red, polypoid, friable lesion.

urination, which may simulate an infection. Prostatic lesions often are not diagnosed until there is complete urinary obstruction. Following catheterization, a suprapubic mass may still be felt, and on rectal examination, a prostatic lesion bulges into the rectum and is easily palpable.

Rhabdomyosarcoma of the Trunk and Extremities.
Subcutaneous mass lesions are common complaints in children. Only by continually thinking of malignancy will early lesions be diagnosed. Firm, fixed masses deep within a muscle must be biopsied. A deep-seated hematoma following trauma is almost impossible to differentiate from a tumor. However, since most active children have frequent falls, a history of trauma should not lead one to procrastinate in advising a biopsy.

Preoperative Studies
Lesions about the head and neck are best studied with CT scans, which will assess intracranial extension and bone invasion. Cystoscopy or examination of the vagina and uterus under anesthesia will allow biopsy of obvious lesions. CT scans allow evaluation of the extent of the lesion and retroperitoneal lymph node involvement. Ultrasonography is useful in follow-up after baseline studies. MRI and CT scans are necessary for adequate evaluation of the trunk. Gallium and bone scans may be helpful

in detecting nodal and bone lesions in all locations. Bone marrow examination also is indicated in the search for metastatic disease. As yet, there are no biologic markers of any value in rhabdomyosarcoma.

Treatment
Formerly, surgery with radiotherapy was the only effective treatment for rhabdomyosarcoma. Often these operations involved radical pelvic exenterations or amputations. Even with these operations, the cure rate was dismal. Fortunately, chemotherapy has tremendously improved survival rates in all locations with far less aggressive operations.

Genitourinary Tract.
Surgical excision is no longer the primary mode of therapy in tumors of the vagina, uterus, bladder, or prostate.[27] When first diagnosed, these lesions are merely biopsied. We have removed exophytic vaginal lesions with electrocautery without sacrifice of the vaginal wall. Treatment is then commenced with "pulse VAC" (vincristine, dactinomycin, and cyclophosphamide) at monthly intervals. Repeat CT scans and examinations under anesthesia with biopsies are then carried out from 6 to 8 weeks after the initiation of therapy. Residual tumor in the vulva or vagina may be resected with salvage of a functioning vagina. We have resected one half or more of the vagina with reconstruction of an adequate organ, and in one child, the vagina was removed from the cervix to the urethra and immediately replaced with a segment of colon. Lesions of the cervix may require a hysterectomy, but the ovaries and other pelvic organs are left alone. At the time of operation for these lesions, the iliac and paraaortic nodes should be removed for staging. Often, continued chemotherapy without radiation is all that is required for cure; survival rates of better than 90 percent are being achieved. Chemotherapy has not been as successful in boys with tumors of the prostate or trigone of the bladder. At this time, radiation therapy is recommended commencing 6 weeks after the initiation of chemotherapy. Over the course of 5 weeks, 4500 rads are delivered to the local area. Previous studies demonstrated that radiation that was started at a later date was less effective.[28]

When repeated studies and biopsy show continued disease, surgical resection is indicated. At our hospital, from 1974 to 1983, 10 children were treated with chemotherapy, radiation, and local tumor excision. Eight children were alive and well, without evidence of disease, from 3 to 8 years after their original diagnosis. Only 1 child, who had pulmonary metastases at the time of diagnosis, died.[29] There may be occasional patients who do not respond to this regimen and will require pelvic exenteration. Paratesticular rhabdomyosarcomas metastasize to regional lymph nodes. Thus, treatment consists of a radical orchiectomy with hemiscrotectomy, retroperitoneal lymph node dissection, and chemotherapy.

Head and Neck. Tumors that originate from the nasopharynx, the sinuses, and the middle ear extend directly into the meninges in 35 percent of patients.[30] Consequently, these patients are given cranial radiation along with intrathecal chemotherapy.[31] Other head and neck tumors have a better prognosis, with approximately 90 percent being relapse free 2 years after treatment with radiation and chemotherapy.[32]

Trunk and Extremities. Rhabdomyosarcomas arising in the trunk and extremities of children have a poorer prognosis than those involving the head and neck or genitourinary tract.[33,34] The main reason for this difference is the predominance of the alveolar histologic type of tumor in the trunk and extremities. There is also a 17 percent incidence of regional lymph node involvement in extremity lesions at the time of diagnosis.[35] Local excision of the tumor is the mainstay of therapy. Ideally, the tumor should be removed along with its entire muscle group from origin to insertion. When fascial planes are crossed, it is necessary to remove more than one muscle group, but essential nerves and vessels should not be sacrificed because microscopic residual tumor is controlled with postoperative radiation and chemotherapy.

Unfortunately, the initial excision often is performed without a diagnosis, and the margins of the resection are inadequate. In this situation, a second, more extensive wound excision is indicated. Regional lymph nodes should also be removed for complete tumor staging. Postoperative chemotherapy and radiation are given depending on the stage of disease. Stage II tumors with microscopic residual fare as well as stage I lesions, since local radiation and chemotherapy are effective in this situation. Amputation adds little to a wide local resection. Surgical excision of recurrent or metastatic tumor along with more radiation and more intensive chemotherapy has saved a few children.[36]

Results

There were 897 patients in the Intergroup Rhabdomyosarcoma Study from 1972 to 1978. The long-term survival rates are listed below according to their clinical stage and histologic type.[37]

Clinical Group	Alveolar Histology		All Other Types	
	Number	Mortality (%)	Number	Mortality (%)
I	13	38.5	63	4.8
II	35	45.7	102	22.5
III	33	60.6	195	44.6
IV	32	90.6	78	74.4
Total	113		438	

The alveolar histologic type has a higher mortality rate in each stage. In addition, this study demonstrated that tumors, regardless of cell type, that were in a site precluding complete surgical excision also had a worse prognosis.

THE INTERGROUP STUDY

From 1972 to 1984, the intergroup study included 47 children with embryonal type tumors of the female genital tract.[38] The survival in this group was superior to that of sarcomas in other locations. Twenty-one of 28 patients with vaginal tumors were treated initially with chemotherapy only or with drugs plus radiation. Thirteen then had a hysterectomy with partial vaginectomy, and all survived. Four others had only a partial vaginectomy, and these patients also survived. Three of 6 children who had only biopsy plus chemotherapy and radiation died. Recurrent disease developed in 7 children, 5 of whom survived with radical surgery and more intense therapy. There were 10 children with uterine tumors, 6 of whom survived after various combinations of surgery, chemotherapy, and radiation. Seven of 9 children with vulvar tumors were alive and free of disease after surgical excision and chemotherapy.

This study demonstrated the value of conservative surgery with combined chemotherapy in curing these tumors while preserving function.

CONGENITAL SARCOMA

Congenital sarcoma of an extremity noted at birth usually is classified as embryonal sarcoma. Grossly, these lesions

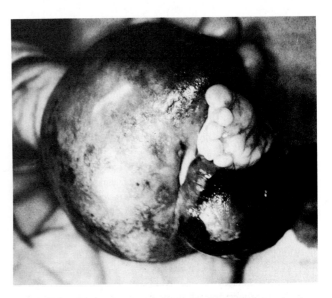

Figure 52–3. An embryonal sarcoma involving the lower leg in a newborn infant. The child has been tumor free for 3 years since amputation.

are huge masses that infiltrate all layers of the extremity (Fig. 52–3). Microscopically, there is diffuse invasion of muscle, nerves, and fascial planes by small, poorly defined cells. Most reported cases have required amputation.[39] Shafer, however, was able to locally excise a 4 by 5 cm, poorly demarcated lesion and thus salvage the limb.[40] Despite the malignant histologic picture, these tumors have an excellent prognosis and require neither radiation nor chemotherapy following surgical excision.

REFERENCES

1. Chung EB, Enzinger FM: Benign lipoblastomatosis. Cancer 32:482, 1973
2. Stringel G, Shandling B, Mancer K, Ein S: Lipoblastoma in infants and children. J Pediatr Surg 17:277, 1982
3. Dehner P: Pediatric Surgical Pathology, 2nd ed. Baltimore, Williams & Wilkins, 1987, p 886
4. Beckett JH, Jacobs AH: Recurring digital fibrous tumors of childhood: A review. Pediatrics 59:401, 1977
5. Enzinger F: Fibrous hamartoma of infancy. Cancer 18:241, 1965
6. Woyke S, Domagala W, Markiewicz C: A 19-year follow-up of multiple juvenile hyaline fibromatosis. J Pediatr Surg 19:302, 1984
7. Chung E, Enzinger F: Infantile myofibromatosis. Cancer 48:1807, 1981
8. Fraser G, Dimmick J, Maysmith D: Solitary congenital fibromatosis of the scalp: A case report. J Pediatr Surg 20:221, 1985
9. Wiswell T, Davis J, Cunningham B, et al: Infantile myofibromatosis: The most common fibrous tumor of infancy. J Pediatr Surg 23:314, 1988
10. Rao B, Horowitz M, Parham D, et al: Challenges in the treatment of childhood fibromatosis. Arch Surg 122:1296, 1987
11. Rock M, Pritchard D, Reiman H, et al: Extra-abdominal desmoid tumors. J Bone Joint Surg 66:1369, 1984
12. Greenberg H, Goebel R, Weisrelbaum R, et al: Radiation therapy in the treatment of aggressive fibromatosis. Int J Radiat Oncol Biol Phys 7:305, 1981
13. Stein R: Chemotherapeutic response in fibromatosis of the neck. J Pediatr 90:482, 1977
14. Raney B, Evans A, Granowetter L, et al: Nonsurgical management of children with recurrent or unresectable fibromatosis. Pediatrics 79:394, 1987
15. Gonzales-Crussi F, Wiederhold M, Sotelo-Avila C: Congenital fibrosarcoma: Presence of a histiocytic component. Cancer 46:77, 1980
16. Blocker S, Koenig J, Ternberg J: Congenital fibrosarcoma. J Pediatr Surg 22:665, 1987
17. Ninane J, Gosseye S, Panteon E, et al: Congenital fibrosarcoma: Preoperative chemotherapy and conservative surgery. Cancer 58:1400, 1986
18. Akers DR, Needham ME: Sarcoma botryoides (rhabdomyosarcoma) of the bile ducts with survival. J. Pediatr Surg 6:474, 1971
19. Srouji MN, Donaldson MH, Chatten J, et al: Perianal rhabdomyosarcoma in childhood. Cancer 38:1008, 1976
20. Kilman JW, Craenen J, Hosier DM: Replacement of entire right atrial wall in an infant with a cardiac rhabdomyoma. J Pediatr Surg 8:317, 1973
21. Shaher RM, Farina M, Alley R, et al: Congenital subaortic stenosis in infancy caused by rhabdomyoma of the left ventricle. J Thorac Cardiovasc Surg 63:157, 1972
22. Dehner LP, Enzinger FM, Fout RL: Fetal rhabdomyoma: An analysis of 9 cases. Cancer 30:160, 1972
23. Lawrence W Jr, Hays DM, Moon TE: Lymphatic metastasis with childhood rhabdomyosarcoma. Cancer 39:556, 1977
24. Maurer HM: The intergroup rhabdomyosarcoma study (NIH): Objectives and clinical staging classification. J Pediatr Surg 10:977, 1975
25. Donaldson S, Belli J: A rational clinical staging system for childhood rhabdomyosarcoma. J Clin Oncol 2:135, 1981
26. Lawrence W, Gehan E, Hays D, et al: Prognostic significance of staging factors of the UICC staging system in childhood rhabdomyosarcomas: A report from the Intergroup Rhabdomyosarcoma Study (IRS 111). J Clin Oncol 5:46, 1987
27. Kumar A, Wrenn E, Fleming I, et al. Combined therapy to prevent pelvic exenteration for rhabdomyosarcoma of the vagina or uterus. Cancer 37:118, 1979
28. Raney G, Hays D, Maurer H, et al: Primary chemotherapy plus radiation therapy (RI) and/or surgery for children with sarcoma of the prostate, bladder or vagina: Preliminary results of the Intergroup Rhabdomyosarcoma Study (IRS 11) 1978–82. Abstracted Proc ASCO, 1983, p 243
29. Kaplan W, Firlit C, Berger R: Genitourinary rhabdomyosarcoma. J Urol 130:116, 1983
30. Teft M, Fernandez C, Donaldson M, et al: Evidence of meningeal involvement by rhabdomyosarcoma of the head and neck in children. Cancer 42:253, 1978
31. Raney R, Tefft M, Maurer H, et al: Results of intensive treatment of children with cranial para-meningeal sarcoma: A report from the Intergroup Rhabdomyosarcoma Study. Proc Am Assoc Cancer Res 23:120, 1982
32. Wharan M, Foulkes M, Lawrence W, et al: Soft tissue sarcoma of the head and neck in childhood: Nonorbital and nonparameningeal sites. Abstracted Proc ASCO, 1983, p 160
33. Raney R, Ragab A, Ruymann F, et al: Soft tissue sarcoma of the trunk in childhood: Results of the Intergroup Rhabdomyosarcoma Study. Cancer 49:2612, 1982
34. Hays D, Soule E, Lawrence W, et al., for the IRS Committee: Extremity lesions in the Intergroup Rhabdomyosarcoma Study (IRS 1 Preliminary Report). Cancer 48:1, 1982
35. Heyn R, Hays D, Lawrence W, for the IRS Committee: Alveolar rhabdomyosarcoma and lymph node spread: A preliminary report from the Intergroup Rhabdomyosarcoma Study (IRS II). Abstracted Proc ASCO 3:80, 1984
36. Raney R, Crist W, Maurer H, et al: Prognosis of children

with soft tissue sarcoma who relapse after achieving a complete response. Cancer 52:44, 1983

37. Hays D, Newton W, Soule M, et al: Mortality among children with rhabdomyosarcomas of the alveolar histologic subtype. J Pediatr Surg 18:412, 1983
38. Hays D, Shimada H, Raney B, et al: Clinical staging and treatment results in rhabdomyosarcoma of the female genital tract among children and adolescents. Cancer 61:1893, 1988
39. Chamberlain JW, Lawrence K: Congenital sarcoma of extremities: Report of two cases. Am J Dis Child 62:1, 1941
40. Shafer A: Sarcoma of the leg in a newborn infant. J Pediatr 56:97, 1960

53
Peripheral Nerve Tumors

Tumors of the peripheral or cranial nerves that arise from the nerve sheath or Schwann cells are usually benign, and symptoms depend on the tumor location. Diagnosis and treatment consist of local excision, with preservation of any involved major nerve.

Single, benign neurofibromas that are not associated with von Recklinghausen's disease may be simply excised with expectation of cure. More extensive neurofibromas in peripheral nerves may still be resected and the nerve anastomosed after a period of nerve lengthening with an implantable tissue expander. At the initial operation, the tumor is assessed and biopsied. The tissue expander is placed beneath the nerve at a distance from the tumor. It is then gradually inflated, and the nerve is lengthened until the tumor can be removed and the nerve sutured with the aid of an operating microscope.

Unfortunately, neurofibromas in children with von Recklinghausen's disease are extensive, may involve visceral organs, and are more likely to become malignant during the first two decades of the child's life.

The plexiform neurofibroma is the most difficult peripheral nerve tumor in childhood. Thirteen of 22 children with this lesion treated at our hospital had definite café au lait spots.

Grossly, the plexiform neurofibroma is a poorly defined mass consisting of enlarged nerve trunks with extension along adjacent nerves and into tissue planes. Some individual nerve trunks may be up to 1 cm or more in diameter, whereas others may taper in the form of a carrot or radish (Fig. 53–1). In following individual nerves, one may also find beadlike enlargements. These frequently are palpable along superficial nerves remote from the main mass. Cervicothoracic lesions infiltrate into the adventitia of major blood vessels and involve the trachea and tongue. Scalp and facial lesions infiltrate the skin, particularly the eyelid, so that all of the tissue from the periosteum to the epidermis is diffusely involved with tumor.

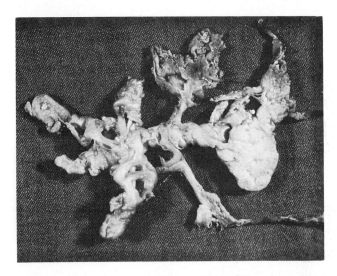

Figure 53–1. Plexiform neurofibroma dissected from the brachial plexus.

DIAGNOSIS AND CLINICAL COURSE

Even though plexiform neurofibromas are microscopically benign, many of these lesions pursue a relentless course, causing airway and esophageal obstruction, grotesque deformity requiring amputation of extremities, and severe cosmetic problems when they involve the face. Plexiform neurofibromas in the submucosa of the colon or small intestine may simulate Hirschprung's disease.[1-3]

The usual presenting complaint is that of a mass lesion that on palpation feels like a bag of worms. The diagnosis is made easily if there are associated café au lait spots or a familial history of von Recklinghausen's disease. There is a slight male preponderance. Six of our patients were mildly mentally retarded, and 2 had progressive central nervous system deficits. Of 85 pa-

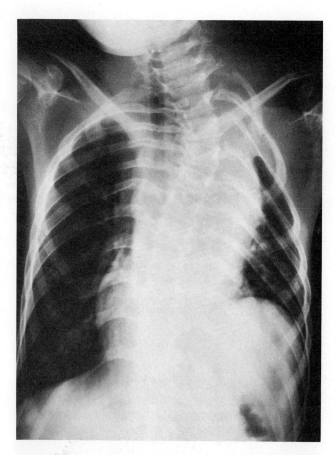

Figure 53–2. Extensive plexiform neurofibroma involving the brachial plexus and mediastinum.

tients reviewed by Adkins and Ravitch during a 25-year period, 36 percent had orthopedic problems, such as kyphoscoliosis, and 22 percent had neck or head masses.[4] Diagnostic studies vary from simple excision biopsy of peripheral tumors to extensive radiologic studies of cervicothoracic lesions (Fig. 53–2). Vertebral abnormalities with or without central nervous system signs are indications for a myelogram. Computed tomography (CT) has been helpful in evaluating involvement of cranial nerves at the base of the skull and mediastinal extension.

THERAPY

Plexiform neurofibromas, although usually benign, progress relentlessly through the fascial planes to surround blood vessels and major nerve trunks. These lesions should be excised as completely as possible during the first operation whenever the child has a mass. Complete excision is often feasible when the tumor is on the trunk or an extremity. One patient in our series required a below-the-knee amputation when three previous procedures failed to halt the tumor's growth. The cosmetic appearance of children with lesions of the face and scalp can be improved by excising gross tumor, but usually a complete excision is impossible because the dermis is infiltrated over wide areas. In the neck, the bulk of the tumor with most of its extensions can be removed through a radical neck dissection. It may be necessary to remove the vagus nerve and jugular vein along with the tumor, but the main nerve trunks are identified with a bipolar nerve stimulator and spared. Diffuse involvement of the brachial plexus may defeat the goal of complete removal, since it will leave the child with a semiparalyzed arm. Diffuse involvement of the upper mediastinum may require a combined approach to the neck and chest. Splitting the sternum, with resection of the clavicle, was necessary in 2 patients who had extensive recurrent plexiform neurofibromas extending from the base of the skull to within the pericardium.

NEUROFIBROSARCOMA

Ten percent of malignant nerve sheath tumors develop during the first two decades of life. At least 40 percent of these are in children with von Recklinghausen's disease.[5,6] Patients with central tumors, particularly cervicomediastinal lesions, will develop malignancies at an earlier age than those with peripheral tumors. These patients also are more likely to have von Recklinghausen's disease and have a poorer survival rate after the malignancy develops.

In 1972, we reported on 9 patients with cervicomediastinal plexiform neurofibromas.[7] Since then, 4 have developed either a malignant schwannoma or a neurofibrosarcoma. One boy died at age 9 and the other at 18 years of age with rapidly growing extensive lesions. Both families refused chemotherapy. One girl developed a malignant supraclavicular tumor at age 4. This was resected, along with two cords of the brachial plexus. She has survived 10 years after multiple-drug chemotherapy. The fourth patient had no tumor recurrence in her neck but developed a malignant schwannoma in her leg 12 years later. This required three operations to obtain tumor-free margins, and she is free of tumor and now off chemotherapy 2 years after the operation.

Since 1954, there have been 16 patients diagnosed as having schwannoma or neurofibrosarcoma at our hospital. Half also had von Recklinghausen's disease. Five children who had small, localized, completely resected lesions are either alive or lost to follow-up. Six who had extensive cervicomediastinal lesions have died, most before the advent of chemotherapy. Five more who had extensive, even partially resected disease are alive and free of disease for at least 10 years. Chemotherapy clearly has been beneficial to these patients. The drug regimens were not standard but included vincristine, cyclophosphamide, and doxorubicin.

REFERENCES

1. Hochberg FH, DaSilva AB, Goldabini, et al: Gastrointestinal involvement in Von Recklinghausen's neurofibromatosis. Neurology 24:1144, 1974
2. Terberg JC, Winters K: Plexiform neurofibromatosis of the colon as a cause of congenital mega colon. Am J Surg 109:663, 1965
3. Takehaski M, Ketsumoto K, Yokoyoma J, et al: Plexiform neurofibromatosis of the ileum in an infant. J Pediatr Surg 12:1571, 1977
4. Adkins JC, Ravitch M: The operative management of Von Recklinghausen's neurofibromatosis in children with special reference to lesions of the head and neck. Surgery 82:342, 1977
5. Ducatman B, Scheithauer B, Piepgras D, Reiman H: Malignant peripheral nerve sheath tumors: A clinicopathologic review of 120 cases. Cancer 57:2006, 1986
6. Sordillo P, Helson L, Hajdu S, et al: Malignant schwannoma—clinical characteristics and response to therapy. Cancer 47:2503, 1981
7. Raffensperger JG, Cohen R: Plexiform neurofibroma in childhood. J Pediatr Surg 7:144, 1972

54
Tumors of the Thyroid

The pathology and clinical findings of thyroid tumors in children are comparable to those found in thyroid tumors of young adults. Girls are affected more often than boys, but the sexual differences are not so marked in patients with a history of exposure to radiation. Carcioma may appear in thyroglossal duct cysts and in an undescended thyroid, but the most important etiologic factor in the development of both benign and malignant tumors of the thyroid gland is prior exposure to irradiation. Many reports over the past 35 years have clearly demonstrated this correlation.[1-4] In these reports the radiation most often was administered to the thymus gland but was also directed to the tonsils, adenoids, and acne. The time interval between exposure to the radiation and development of a thyroid tumor varies from 5 to 35 years. The current multimodal treatment of pediatric cancer increases the risk for the future development of thyroid neoplasms.[5] Among our own patients, one 14-year-old boy with cyanotic cardiac disease developed thyroid cancer after extensive exposure to diagnostic x-ray procedures. Another developed carcinoma of the thyroid 7 years after treatment for Hodgkin's disease of the neck, and a third boy developed an adenoma following radiation treatment for a neuroblastoma. The U.S. Department of Health, Education and Welfare has issued a booklet with suggestions for finding patients who may be at risk for radiation-induced tumors. The booklet also covers the indicated investigations and treatment.[6]

PATHOLOGY

Table 54–1 lists the pathology found in 58 children, aged 2 weeks to 17 years, who were operated on for tumors of the thyroid gland at the Children's Memorial Hospital between 1953 and 1987. From this review of our own material, we can surmise that a solitary mass in the thyroid gland has about a 50/50 chance of being malignant. During the newborn period, a diffusely enlarged thyroid can occur secondary to maternal ingestion of antithyroid drugs. In infancy, a teratoma is probably the most likely cause for a discrete thyroid mass.[7]

The benign adenomas are well encapsulated and present a uniform appearance on cut section (Fig. 54–1). A careful search must be made for capsular and blood vessel invasion. If these characteristics are absent in examining sections, the pathologist may confidently diagnose a nodule as benign.

Papillary adenocarcinoma, often with elements of follicular carcinoma in the same lesion, accounts for 75 to 80 percent of malignant thyroid tumors in childhood.[8] Grossly, this tumor is poorly encapsulated and infiltrates the thyroid lobe.[9] The opposite lobe is involved in 85 percent of cases.[10] Metastases occur first to the tracheoesophageal and jugular and later to other groups of nodes, including those on the contralateral side. Metastases to the lung are more common with follicular tumors. Microscopically, the papillary adenocarcinoma is well differentiated, with frondlike papillae supported on fibroconnective tissue stalks. There is often an intermixture of a follicular pattern, but the clinical behavior of a mixed tumor is that of a papillary tumor. Medullary carcinoma accounts for only 1 percent or less of thyroid tumors in children, but this lesion is interesting because of its familial incidence and its association with other endocrine tumors, such as pheochromocytomas and parathyroid adenomas. This tumor arises from the C cells diffusely spread throughout the thyroid gland and so is multicentric in origin. Further, the diagnosis can be made in patients with no clinically detectable tumor by radioimmunoassay of serum and urine calcitonin.[11]

TABLE 54–1. THYROID TUMORS AT CHILDREN'S MEMORIAL HOSPITAL, 1953–1987

Malignant		Benign	
Type	*Number*	*Type*	*Number*
Papillary adenocarcinoma	22	Adenoma	11
Follicular carcinoma	7	Fetal adenoma	1
		Hyperparathyroid adenoma	5
		Microfollicular adenoma	1
Total	29	Follicular adenoma	3
		Thyroiditis	2
		Cyst	4
		Teratoma	2
		Total	29

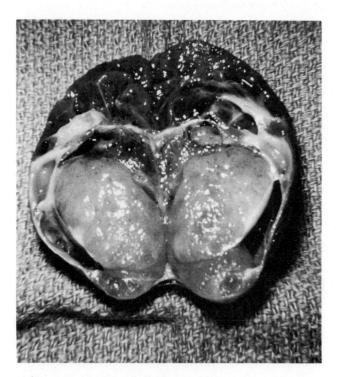

Figure 54–1. A benign thyroid adenoma. Grossly, the tumor is well encapsulated and uniform in appearance.

CLINICAL FINDINGS

A child with thyroid cancer may have a nodule within the gland, or the first sign may be an enlarged lymph node secondary to metastases. Diffuse enlargement of the gland is most likely due to chronic lymphocytic thyroiditis or the simple goiter common in teenage girls. Thyroid function studies and a determination of antithyroid antibodies are helpful in differentiating malignant from benign lesions, and percutaneous needle biopsy has been shown to be safe in children.[12]

Any solitary mass in the thyroid must be removed for histologic study. A chest x-ray and a radioactive scan are performed preoperatively, primarily to evaluate the lobe opposite the clinically involved lobe. Cancer, benign adenoma, and simple cysts will all show up as cold spots on the scan. Ultrasonography will demonstrate cystic lesions, but we have found both adenomas and carcinomas in the walls of cysts.

TREATMENT

The proper surgical management of thyroid carcinoma must be based on the known high incidence of involvement of the opposite lobe and the pattern of lymph node metastases. An analysis of 346 cases in 6 series of carcinoma of the thyroid in children revealed a 75 percent incidence of cervical lymph node metastases.[13–18] Thus, the ideal therapy for a papillary, follicular, or mixed type carcinoma is excision of the lobe containing the mass, subtotal or total removal of the opposite lobe, and excision of the juxtaesophageal and paratracheal lymph nodes. Paloyan et al. recommended total thyroidectomy for radiation-induced tumors.[19] They found carcinoma in both lobes in 45 percent of patients, and in 4 patients carcinomas were found in the lobe contralateral to the one containing the palpable nodule.[19] Unfortunately, the unpleasant sequelae of total thyroidectomy—namely, the increased risk of injury to the recurrent laryngeal nerves and the parathyroid glands—may outweigh the risk of leaving some tumor. The decision to perform a subtotal or total resection of the contralateral lobe must rest on a definitive diagnosis of carcinoma. Abnormalities in the contralateral lobe on the preoperative scan would be an indication for its subtotal removal.

If excised lymph nodes definitely contain thyroid tissue, the diagnosis is obviously cancer.

In the usual situation, we remove the entire lobe on the involved side, taking great care to identify and to avoid injury to the parathyroid glands. The lobe is then hemisected in the operating room and examined grossly and microscopically by the pathologist. If it is possible to make a definitive diagnosis of carcinoma by frozen section, a subtotal resection is performed, leaving a small posterior rim of tissue on the opposite side. All enlarged lymph nodes that can be reached through the standard collar incision are removed. If these nodes are positive for tumor on frozen section, the incision may be extended in order to remove all possible nodes from both sides of the neck. This is not a radical node dissection. The sternocleidomastoid muscle and jugular veins are left. If the pathologist cannot make a definitive diagnosis of carcinoma on the basis of the frozen section, the isthmus and the medial portion of the opposite gland are removed for biopsy. If the lesion does turn out to be a carcinoma, the opposite lobe is examined clinically and with scans at frequent intervals. It is unlikely that a small residual tumor will harm the patient, provided it is excised as soon as it becomes clinically apparent.

The recurrent laryngeal nerves should not be sacrificed if they are invaded by tumor because postoperative treatment with thyroid extract is effective in suppressing further tumor growth.

Since medullary carcinoma is definitely multicentric in origin, total thyroidectomy is indicated.[20] Children with multiple endocrine neoplasia are known to develop medullary carcinoma of the thyroid. Therefore, thyroidectomy should be performed, based on an increase in the plasma immunoreactive calcitonin.[21] All 14 patients who had occult medullary carcinomas resected before the onset of clinical disease were free from disease at follow-up, whereas 3 patients with clinical disease had persistent metastatic lesions.

The specific surgical anatomy and the techniques of thyroid surgery are well described in the usual texts on adult surgery and are particularly well covered in the monograph by Sedgwick.[22] Even experienced surgeons are well advised to review the many variations in the surgical anatomy of the recurrent laryngeal nerves, as well as the location of the parathyroid glands, before undertaking a major operation on the thyroid gland.

All children who have been operated on for thyroid cancer are given doses of thyroid extract to suppress the thyroid-stimulating hormone secretion by the pituitary. Radioactive iodine therapy will clear lung metastases that are resistant to thyroid extract if the tumor will take up a tracer test dose. Lymph nodes that enlarge after the initial operation should be excised in further "berry-picking" operations.

The prognosis for the usual cancer of the thyroid in children is excellent. In the series of 346 cases previously mentioned, there were only 6 deaths due to the original malignancy.

REFERENCES

1. Clark DE: Association of irradiation with cancer of the thyroid in children and adolescents. JAMA 159:1007, 1955
2. Rooney DR, Powell RW: Carcinoma of the thyroid in children after x-ray therapy in early childhood. JAMA 169:1, 1959
3. Fisher JN: Cancer in the irradiated thyroid. N Engl J Med 292:975, 1975
4. Refetoff S, Harrison J, Karaufliki BT, et al: Continuing occurrence of thyroid carcinoma after irradiation of the neck in infancy and childhood. N Engl J Med 292:171, 1975
5. Jane D, King D, Boles T: Secondary thyroid neoplasms in pediatric cancer patients: Increased risk with improved survival. J Pediatr Surg 19:855, 1984
6. HEW: Irradiation-related Thyroid Cancer. Washington, D.C., U.S. Dept. of Health, Education and Welfare, Public Health Service Publication NIH 77, 1976, p 1120
7. Numanoglu I, Aksu Y, Mutaf O: Teratoma of the thyroid gland in newborn infants. J Pediatr Surg 5:381, 1970
8. Rosvoll RV, Winship T: Cancer in the thyroid in children. Thyroid Cancer. In Hedinger CE (ed): Proceedings of a Conference Organized by the International Union Against Cancer. Switzerland, Springer-Verlag, 1968. UICC Monograph Series 12:75, 1969
9. Dehner LP: Pediatric Surgical Pathology. St. Louis, Mosby, 1975, p 410
10. Clark RL, White EC, Russell WO: Total thyroidectomy for cancer of the thyroid: Significance of intraglandular dissemination. Am Surg 149:858, 1959
11. Melvin KEW, Miller HH, Tashjian AH: Early diagnosis of medullary cancer of the thyroid gland by means of calcitonin assay. N Engl J Med 285:1115, 1971
12. Weitzman JJ, Ling SM, Kaplan SA, et al: Percutaneous needle biopsy of goiter in childhood. J Pediatr Surg 5:251, 1970
13. Exelby PE, Frazell EL: Carcinoma of the thyroid in children. Surg Clin North Am 49:249, 1969
14. Buckwalter JA, Thomas CG, Freeman JB: Is childhood thyroid cancer a lethal disease? Ann Surg 181:632, 1975
15. Harness JK, Thompson NW, Nishiyama RH: Childhood thyroid carcinoma. Arch Surg 102:278, 1971
16. Liechty RD, Safaie-Shirazi S, Soper RT: Carcinoma of the thyroid in children. Surg Gynecol Obstet 134:595, 1972
17. Tawes RL, DeLorimier AA: Thyroid carcinoma during youth. J Pediatr Surg 3:210, 1968
18. Hayles AB, Johnson ML, Beahrs OH, et al: Carcinoma of the thyroid in children. Am J Surg 106:735, 1963
19. Paloyan E, Lawrence AM, Brooks MH, et al: Total thy-

roidectomy and parathyroid autotransplantation for radia-tion-associated thyroid cancer. Surgery 80:70, 1976

20. Leape LL, Miller HH, Graze K, et al: Total thyroidectomy for occult familial medullary carcinoma of the thyroid in children. J Pediatr Surg 11:883, 1976

21. Telander R, Zimmerman D, Van Heerden J, Sizemore G: Results of early thyroidectomy for medullary thyroid carcinoma in children with multiple endocrine neoplasia type 2. J Pediatr Surg 21:1190, 1986

22. Sedgwick CE: Surgery of the Thyroid Gland. Philadelphia, Saunders, 1974, vol 15

55
Tumors of the Salivary Glands

True neoplasms of the salivary glands are extremely rare in the pediatric age group. Vascular malformation and inflammatory lesions are more common and must be differentiated from tumors to avoid unnecessary surgery. An analysis of 430 salivary gland lesions in children from the Armed Forces Institute of Pathology revealed that 262 were nonneoplastic, cystic, or inflammatory lesions.[1] In this review, there were 114 benign tumors, including vascular malformations, and 54 malignant tumors. Intraoral mucoceles (retention cysts involving the minor salivary glands) were the most common, especially on the lower lip. In our experience, the simple retention cysts have required only drainage or excision. The parotid gland is far more often involved with hemangiomas, inflammatory lesions, and true tumors than are the submaxillary or sublingual glands. It is likely that inflammatory lesions, especially recurrent parotitis, are more frequent than the review would lead one to suspect, since few of these require an operation. A computed tomography (CT) scan, particularly when combined with a sialogram, will reliably differentiate tumors from inflammatory conditions of the parotid gland.

HEMANGIOMA

A parotid hemangioma behaves in a fashion similar to that of hemangiomas in other superficial areas. It occurs as a bulky, rapidly enlarging swelling of the parotid gland. There is usually involvement of the overlying skin, so that the diagnosis is obvious (Fig. 55–1). Hemangiomas in this area are a serious cosmetic problem, but attempts at surgical removal, irradiation, or chemotherapy are contraindicated. Spontaneous regression occurred in 8 of 10 cases reported by Williams.[2] In our experience, these lesions commence to involute and disappear by the time the patient is 2 to 5 years of age. Hemangioen-

dotheliomas are firm, rubbery masses within the gland. Discoloration of the overlying skin or signs of an increased blood supply are not as obvious as with the cavernous hemangioma. Pressure on the mass may squeeze out the blood. A biopsy is indicated if the lesion cannot be differentiated from a tumor. Most hemangioendotheliomas spontaneously resolve. If they have not disappeared by 4 years of age, we recommend surgical excision.

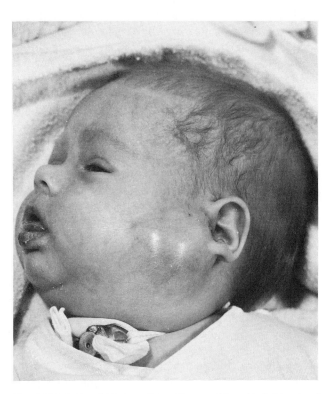

Figure 55–1. Parotid hemangioma. The overlying skin is tense and shining and has numerous blood vessels.

CYSTIC HYGROMAS

Congenital lymphangiomas contain multiple cystic spaces of varying size that intertwine between the lobes of the parotid gland and the branches of the facial nerve. The diagnosis is based entirely on palpation of a soft, fluctuant, transilluminating mass. Surgical excision is required for cure. However, excision of these lesions, which in other locations are easily removed, involves a technically extremely difficult dissection of the parotid gland and facial nerve. These structures must be approached with the same precautions in identifying and protecting the nerve as in any other operation on the parotid gland.

INFLAMMATORY LESIONS

The first episode of tenderness and swelling in the parotid gland is usually termed epidemic parotitis, or mumps. Usually the same gland is involved and is firm to nodular on palpation. There are few systemic signs of infection and minimal discomfort in the gland itself. The swelling diminishes within 2 or 3 days but may recur after intervals of weeks or even months. Physical examination during an acute episode reveals minimal redness about Stenson's duct and enlarged lymph nodes. Katzen, in his review of 45 patients with idiopathic recurrent parotitis, found that virtually 100 percent of his patients were spontaneously cured by the age of 15 years.[3] Antibiotics and other conservative measures have no influence on the acute attack and are of no value in preventing future episodes. The etiology of this recurrent parotitis of childhood is unknown and has been variously termed Mikulicz's disease and benign lymphosialdoenopathy.[4] An operation is rarely, if ever, indicated. If the gland remains enlarged and firm after several recurrent episodes in a teenage child, we advise superficial parotidectomy only to remove the undesirable facial swelling. At operation, the gland is fibrotic and densely adherent to the facial nerve. On histologic examination, there are microabscesses, epithelial hyperplasia, and lymphocytic infiltration, and the acini are atrophic or disrupted.

EPITHELIAL TUMORS OF THE SALIVARY GLANDS

The pleomorphic adenoma, or mixed tumor, is the most common tumor of the salivary glands. The largest series was 30 patients collected over 25 years at the University of Michigan.[5] Although the mixed tumor may occur in infants, the usual age range is 10 to 13 years. The incidence is equal in males and females. The lesion occurs as a painless, discrete mass that usually is movable. The lack of tenderness, induration, or inflammation of Stenson's duct should differentiate a tumor from recurrent parotitis. At operation, the pleomorphic adenoma is unencapsulated and may be isolated, and it will have both cystic and solid areas. This is a pleomorphic tumor containing both columnar and squamous epithelial cells. Special stains are required to demonstrate the mucus-containing cells, which confirm the diagnosis. As in the adult, an incomplete excision will lead inevitably to local recurrence. Other adult forms of parotid gland carcinomas also occur in older children. One in particular, the acinic cell carcinoma, appears to have some predilection for younger girls.[6] Parotid gland tumors are radioresistant. Consequently, complete surgical removal is indicated. Wide local excision, including at least the superficial lobe of the gland, is sufficient for mixed tumors. There may be irregular projections of the tumor outside its smooth exterior that also must be excised. The rare, more highly malignant parotid gland tumors may require sacrifice of all or portions of the facial nerve. Later, the nerve may be grafted, or reconstructive cosmetic surgery may be performed.

PAROTID OPERATIONS

Lesions about the angle of the mandible, in the lateral portion of the face, or within the parotid gland are likely

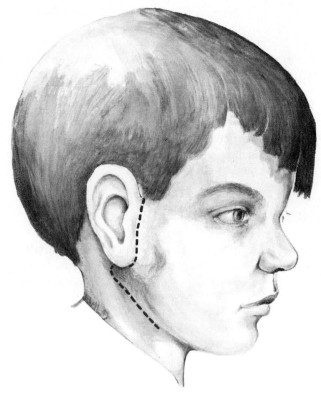

Figure 55–2. Incision for parotidectomy.

to involve branches of the facial nerve. Lymphangiomas and hemangiomas in particular infiltrate tissues from the subcutaneous layers through to bone, distorting normal anatomy. Consequently, wide exposure and careful identification and dissection of the facial nerve are the primary consideration. The patient is positioned on the operating table with the shoulders slightly elevated and the head turned away from the lesion. The endotracheal tube must exit away from the sterile field, which includes the entire lateral face and especially corners of the eye and mouth. Magnification with binocular loupes or the operating microscope is helpful, and a nerve stimulator is invaluable in identifying tiny branches of the facial nerve.

An S-shaped incision carried anterior to the ear and curved posteriorly behind the tragus provides adequate exposure, with excellent healing and a minimally exposed scar (Fig. 55–2). The anterior flap of skin is retracted with double-pronged skin hooks at right angles to the skin. With this technique, small vessels are identified and coagulated with a bipolar electrosurgical unit. In operations for tumors of the parotid gland itself, expo-

sure of the main trunk is feasible and safe. The facial nerve is found deep and cephalad to the anterior lower border of the mastoid process as it emerges from the stylomastoid foramen. In gaining access to the nerve trunk, the ear lobe is elevated after the anterior flap is raised. The external jugular vein and the greater auricular nerve course vertically directly over the access route to the facial vein and must be divided (Fig. 55–3). The inferior-posterior margin of the gland is then grasped, retracted forward, and separated from the sternocleidomastoid muscle, which originates from the mastoid process. The cartilage of the external auditory meatus is followed by spreading the blades of the scissors between the gland and the ear in the direction of the nerve trunk. The scissors should not penetrate more deeply than the plane of the lateral surface of the mastoid process. The gland must be separated from the mastoid process and the auditory canal over a broad, shallow area in order to avoid working into a deep hole. In a small infant, the facial nerve may be no more than 1 to 1.5 mm in diameter. Consequently, progress must be painstaking, and every suspicious strand of tissue is stimulated, check-

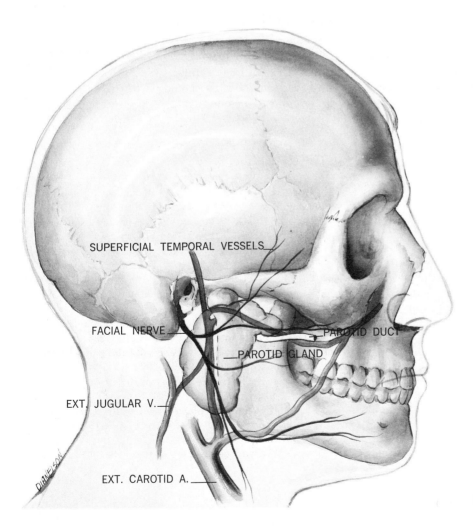

SUPERFICIAL TEMPORAL VESSELS

FACIAL NERVE

PAROTID DUCT

PAROTID GLAND

EXT. JUGULAR V.

EXT. CAROTID A.

Figure 55–3. Anatomy of the facial nerve.

ing carefully for twitching of the eye or mouth. Once the main nerve trunk has been identified, the superficial lobe of the parotid is removed by following the nerve and its branches peripherally with continuous upward traction on the gland and division of all strands of tissue that will not separate bluntly.

Lymphangiomas in particular may involve only one trunk of the facial nerve, or they may be so diffuse as to severely distort the anatomy, making identification of the main trunk hazardous. Frequently, the nerve is inextricably surrounded by daughter cysts of a lymphangioma, in which case the safest course is to merely open and drain the cysts and leave them attached to the nerve. Even so, the nerve must be identified and often is found in a peripheral location. Fortunately, there are several sites where it may be reliably identified, especially with the aid of a nerve stimulator. Shortly after leaving the skull, it enters the parotid substance and divides into the temporofacial and cervicofacial divisions. These give rise to the tertiary branches within the parotid. It is necessary to have this pattern of division well in mind before commencing the operation. When the anatomy has been worked out in a cadaver, dissection in this region can be performed with more confidence. Peripherally, there are three sites in which the facial nerve branches are sufficiently constant to provide for safe exposure. The best method of exposing the entire nerve in a retrograde manner is to pick up the mandibular ramus or even the entire cervicofacial division at the lower pole of the parotid gland just anterior to the posterior facial vein, which makes its exit from the gland in this area. The posterior facial vein is large and easily identified and has a constant relationship to the lower division of the facial nerve. It is deep to the nerve and runs in the same direction, just parallel to the ramus of the mandible. Consequently, the nerve must be found superficial to both this vein and the facial artery, which occurs more distally along the mandible. Once the lower division of the nerve has been identified, it may be followed back to the main trunk or distally along the mandible. At this point, the nerve has a variable location within 1 cm above or below the mandible itself (Fig. 55–4). Furthermore, the nerve may lie within or under a thick platysma muscle or may be immediately subcutaneous to a poorly developed platysma. These important facts must be kept in mind when commencing the dissection about a cystic hygroma whose upper extent is the mandibular ramus. A branch of the facial nerve also runs along the upper border of Stenson's duct at the anterior border of the parotid. This duct, which can be palpated in its subcutaneous position before elevation of the flaps, can be used to locate the small nerve that accompanies

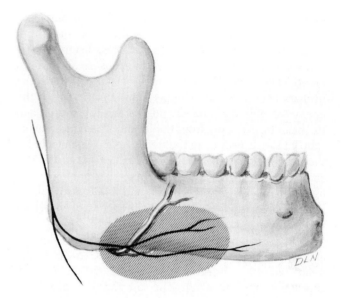

Figure 55–4. Relationships of the mandibular branch of the facial nerve.

it. Both of these structures lie within a fascial sheath that surrounds the facial muscles. They are usually not elevated with the skin flaps if care is taken in the initial dissection. The monograph by Anderson and Byars and the articles on the technique by Beahrs and Chong and by Woods and Beahrs should be consulted for further details on the technique of parotid gland operations.[7–9]

REFERENCES

1. Krolls SO, Trodahl JN, Boyers RC: Salivary gland lesions in children: A survey of 430 cases. Cancer 30:459, 1972
2. Williams HG: Hemangiomas of the parotid gland in children. Plast Reconstr Surg 56:29, 1975
3. Katzen M: Recurrent parotitis in children. S Afr J Surg 7:37, 1969
4. Nash L, Morrison LF: Asymptomatic chronic enlargement of the parotid gland. Ann Otol Rhinol Laryngol 58:646, 1949
5. Malone B, Baker S: Benign pleomorphic adenomas in children. Ann Otol Rhinol Laryngol 93:210, 1984
6. Ali J, Riese K: Acinic cell cancers of the parotid gland in children. Clin Pediatr 14:1111, 1975
7. Anderson R, Byars LT: Surgery of the Parotid Gland. St. Louis, Mosby, 1965
8. Beahrs H, Chong C: Management of the facial nerve in parotid gland surgery. Am J Surg 124:473, 1972
9. Woods L, Beahrs OH: A technique for the rapid performance of parotidectomy. Surg Gynecol Obstet 142:87, 1976

SECTION VI

Gastrointestinal Hemorrhage

The spectrum of diseases that cause gastrointestinal bleeding in children not only is unlike that seen in adults but also varies within different pediatric age groups. Cancer of the gastrointestinal tract is rare, but medical diseases and coagulation disorders are sufficiently common that the surgeon must be wary of operating on a child for bleeding without complete preoperative studies.

One must make every effort to determine the volume and character of the bleeding. The extent to which one studies a child, as well as making the correct diagnosis, hinges on whether there were only a few drops of blood on the surface of the stool or a large quantity of dark blood mixed with the feces. It is also necessary to be sure there is actual bleeding. Children who ingest large amounts of red Kool-Aid will have loose, red stools not unlike those seen with an intussusception. Beets, tomatoes, and chocolate also color the stool. Before embarking on extensive studies, the "blood" must be tested chemically, and a dietary history must be obtained. A history of drug ingestion, particularly of aspirin, is important.

Direct inspection of the blood will provide a clue to its source and will aid in deciding whether the blood is from the upper or lower gastrointestinal tract. Hematemesis always indicates a bleeding point proximal to the ligament of Treitz. Bright red blood originates from the anorectal area. On the other hand, massive upper gastrointestinal hemorrhage stimulates peristalsis so that unaltered blood does not appear in the stool. Brick-red blood is characteristic of a Meckel's diverticulum, and bloody mucus or a currant jelly stool is a classic sign of an intussusception. Acute bloody diarrhea results from shigellosis or other enteric infection, whereas chronic diarrhea with recurrent rectal bleeding suggests ulcerative colitis. In general, the darker the blood, the higher its origin in the gastrointestinal tract.

The volume of blood lost is estimated by direct observation of stool or vomitus as well as of the child's vital signs. Pallor, tachycardia, a depressed urinary output, and a dropping hematocrit are signs of considerable blood loss. Bleeding of this magnitude is associated with a Meckel's diverticulum, intestinal duplication, a stress peptic ulcer, and esophageal varices. One can quickly eliminate lesions proximal to the ligament of Treitz by the insertion of a nasogastric tube during the acute bleeding episode. If there is a return of clear, bile-stained fluid, the hemorrhage is in the small bowel or colon. On the other hand, if blood or coffee-ground material returns through the tube, one should leave the tube in place to quantitate the hemorrhage and to provide a means of alkaline irrigation. Physical signs that aid in the diagnosis include the melanin spots of the Peutz-Jeghers syndrome and superficial hemangiomas, bruises, and petechiae, which suggest a coagulation disorder. A palpable spleen in the presence of upper gastrointestinal hemorrhage is practically diagnostic of portal hypertension and esophageal varices. Visual inspection of the anus may reveal an anal fissure, cryptitis, or even a severe diaper rash that oozes blood. A rectal examination will detect 60 to 75 percent of juvenile polyps.

There is often a tendency to rush into diagnostic studies in a child with gastrointestinal bleeding, when a thoughtful evaluation of the history and physical examination is indicated. This push to do something results in hasty or poorly performed studies. For example, barium in the gastrointestinal tract will obscure the radioisotope material used to diagnose ectopic gastric mucosa. Thus, a hastily ordered upper gastrointestinal study will postpone the diagnosis of Meckel's diverticulum. Conservative treatment with rest, sedation, transfusions, and antacids rather than an immediate operation is indicated in children with upper gastrointestinal bleeding. Thus, there is no need to perform emergency upper endoscopy. Clots often obscure the visual field, making a diagnosis difficult or impossible. When the bleeding has been controlled by conservative means and endoscopy is indicated, it can be carried out under optimum conditions. Colonoscopy is not the first procedure when polyps are suspected in the colon. An air contrast barium enema may demonstrate a single juvenile polyp within easy reach of the simple, inexpensive rigid proctoscope. Celiac and mesenteric arteriograms are last resort studies when all others are normal and the bleeding seems to originate from the small intestine or liver.

It is rarely necessary to operate on a child for gastrointestinal bleeding without first localizing the exact source of hemorrhage. As a general rule, if the child has required transfusions equal to his or her own blood volume to maintain stable vital signs and is continuing to bleed, an operation is in order unless there are medical contraindications, such as a coagulation disorder. When there has been chronic or repetitive blood loss with no changes in the vital signs or blood count, an operation is never indicated without a specific diagnosis.

56
Rectal Bleeding in Infancy

Hematemesis or black stool in a newborn infant is often caused by swallowed maternal blood. The infant has no change in vital signs and appears perfectly healthy except for the bleeding. The Apt and Downey test distinguishes adult from fetal hemoglobin and makes the diagnosis.[1] It is performed by mixing 1 part bloody stool or vomitus with 5 parts of water. This mixture is centrifuged for 1 or 2 minutes at 2000 rpm. The supernatant is mixed with 1 ml of 0.1 percent normal sodium hydroxide. Fetal hemoglobin remains pink, whereas adult hemoglobin changes to a dirty brown color. In our experience and according to that of others, gastrointestinal hemorrhage in the neonate is most often due to a coagulation disorder and is usually controlled with conservative treatment without a specific diagnosis.[2,3] Hemorrhage has occurred in infants born to mothers who ingested salicylates just before delivery.[4] Initial treatment consists of giving 1 mg vitamin K daily and correction of other coagulation abnormalities. Fresh whole blood and fresh frozen plasma are administered to maintain vital signs and urinary output. The blood is warmed before administration, especially if large amounts are given rapidly. A nasogastric tube is inserted and irrigated with 1 percent sodium bicarbonate if blood is present. Continuous irrigation of the tube provides an index to the rapidity of bleeding.

Massive, unrelenting hemorrhage is unusual. We have found duodenal ulcers in some infants after cessation of bleeding and observed a hemangioma in another baby who first bled during the neonatal period. In one rare situation in which bleeding was not controllable by the usual means, transumbilical arteriography demonstrated a bleeding gastric ulcer, which was sutured.[5] We also have observed massive hemorrhage before complete rupture of the greater curvature of the stomach. Pneumoperitoneum finally prompted the laparotomy. If more than 50 ml of blood per hour is required to maintain an infant's vital signs or if the infant's total blood volume has been replaced, an operation is indicated. The stomach and duodenum may be explored through a vertical right paramedian or midline incision. If there is no obvious external lesion, one should open the stomach and duodenum and search for a discrete ulcer. In the neonatal period, simple suture-ligation of the ulcer and its vessel is all that is indicated.

We have observed one newborn infant with rapid, massive gastric hemorrhage. After the second blood volume replacement, attempted endoscopy demonstrated a massive clot just below the esophagogastric junction. At laparotomy, the clot filled the entire stomach, and no specific bleeding site was found. Bleeding did not recur after removal of the clot and irrigation of the stomach with saline.

ANORECTAL FISSURES

Minor degrees of bright red rectal bleeding in babies from the newborn period to 1 year are almost certainly caused by anal fissure. First, the baby passes a hard stool, which tears the sensitive squamous-lined anal canal. There is anal spasm and pain with each bowel movement. The baby learns to hold back stool and becomes more constipated. A vicious cycle of hard stools, bleeding, and pain takes place. An anal fissure is never seen in breast-fed infants, since they have soft stools. The diagnosis is made by placing the infant prone on the table under a good light. The buttocks are gently spread apart until the anal canal is clearly visible. Most babies help by straining down a bit at this point. Fissures occur posteriorly and vary from chronic, indurated raw lesions to acute ulcers with inflammation (Fig. 56–1). One should demonstrate the fissure to the mother to reassure her that no further studies are indicated to determine the

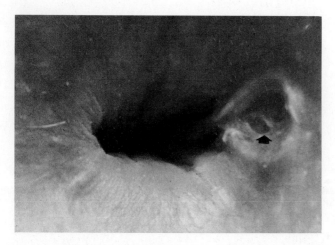

Figure 56–1. Anal ulcer demonstrated by spreading the buttocks.

source of bleeding. Treatment consists of keeping the stools soft by feeding the baby a teaspoonful of mineral oil and prune juice daily until the fissure has healed. Local applications of zinc oxide or other soothing ointments also is helpful. Perhaps 1 in 100 anal fissures

becomes chronic and recalcitrant to conservative therapy. It then becomes necessary to dilate the rectum under general anesthesia and excise the chronic scar tissue down to the superficial sphincter muscle. In older children, anal fissues are associated with leukemia. These are recalcitrant, burrowing lesions that cause sepsis and often fail to heal even after a diverting colostomy.

REFERENCES

1. Apt L, Downey WS: Melena neonatorum: The swallowed blood syndrome. J Pediatr 47:6, 1955
2. Stanley-Brown E, Stevenson SS: Massive gastrointestinal hemorrhage in the newborn infant. Pediatrics 35:482, 1965
3. Sherman NJ, Clathworthy HW Jr: Gastrointestinal bleeding in neonates: A study of 94 cases. Surgery 62:614, 1967
4. Haslam RR, Ekert H, Gillam G: Hemorrhage in a neonate due to maternal ingestion of salicylate. J Pediatr 84:556, 1974
5. Fliegel CP, Herzog B, Signer E, Nars P: Bleeding gastric ulcer in a newborn infant diagnosed by transumbilical aortography. J Pediatr Surg 12:589, 1977

57
Polyps of the Gastrointestinal Tract

The most common intestinal polyp in childhood is the juvenile or inflammatory polyp. Unlike colonic polyps in adults, juvenile polyps have no malignant potential. They are composed of connective tissue with large numbers of lymphocytes, plasma cells, polymorphonuclear leukocytes, and some eosinophils. Granulation tissue, and not epithelium, covers the polyp's surface. Obstruction of the orifices of the intestinal glands by inflammatory tissue results in the formation of cystic spaces (Fig. 57–1). From 70 to 85 percent of juvenile polyps are found within 20 cm of the anus, or within reach of the proctoscope. Some 75 percent are solitary, and it is extremely rare to find more than three polyps scattered throughout the colon. They range in size from 1 to 5 cm and grossly resemble a raspberry on a pedicle.

SIGNS AND SYMPTOMS

Between the ages of 2 and 6 years, the most common cause of rectal bleeding is the juvenile polyp. Characteristically, there are a few drops of bright to dark red blood on the surface of the stool, which lightly stains the toilet water. When the polyp outgrows its blood supply, it spontaneously sloughs off its stalk, causing a single brisk bleeding episode. Prolapse is the next most common symptom of juvenile polyps (Fig. 57–2). The parents state that a mass of tissue appears at the anus during straining at stool. Polyps in the descending or transverse colon may cause cramping pain due to peristaltic activity and traction on the polyp, but in the usual case, there is only painless bleeding. On physical examination, the child is healthy, and the polyp usually can be felt on rectal examination. Such children are rarely anemic, which fact gains significance in differential diagnosis from other, more serious lesions. An air contrast barium enema will demonstrate polyps above the rectum with great accuracy (Fig. 57–3).

TREATMENT

Juvenile polyps are removed through the proctoscope. If polyps remain higher in the colon, they may be safely observed, since in children less than 10 years of age

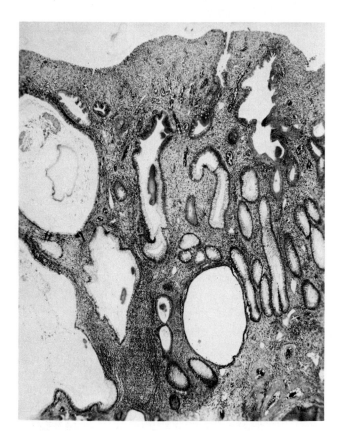

Figure 57–1. Photomicrograph of a juvenile polyp with granulation tissue and cystic spaces.

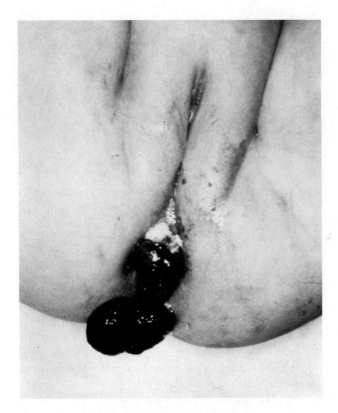

Figure 57–2. Prolapsed juvenile polyp.

the other polyps can be assumed to have a similar histology. They will eventually outgrow their blood supply and spontaneously autoamputate. Alternatively, juvenile colonic polyps may be removed with a flexible fiberoptic colonoscope.[1–3] This procedure may be performed at

the same time as the proctoscopic examination if no polyps are found in the rectum or if the barium enema demonstrates other colonic polyps. There is increased risk of colonic perforation when polyps are removed above the peritoneal reflection. If removal is not possible by snare and cautery, the pedicle is transected with the biopsy forceps close to the polyp and then coagulated.

Following proctoscopy, children are sent home immediately on awakening from the anesthetic. If colonoscopy has been performed, the patient is given only clear liquids by mouth and observed overnight in the hospital.

PROCTOSCOPIC EXAMINATION

Proctoscopy is a basic examination for any child with rectal bleeding, since almost all mucosal and polypoid lesions of the colon may be diagnosed by visual observation, biopsy, and culture of stool and mucus for ova and parasites. If a polyp is found, it is removed with a snare and cautery.

Although an adequate proctosigmoidoscopy may be performed on a conscious child as an outpatient procedure, we much prefer to perform the first diagnostic examination with the child under a general anesthetic. This is particularly important if one is to remove a polyp. At best, the procedure is uncomfortable, and unless the child is perfectly cooperative, it is easy to miss a polyp. Further, after removal of a polyp, there is sometimes bleeding, which requires further coagulation, pressure, and observation. In the operating room, one is more likely to have suction, electrocoagulation, and functioning biopsy forceps than in the outpatient department.

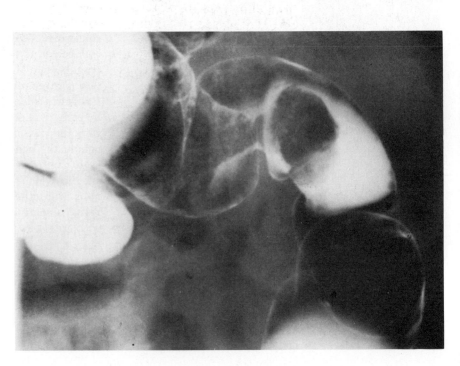

Figure 57–3. Barium enema illustrating a large pedunculated juvenile polyp in the sigmoid colon. The polyp was later removed by colonoscopy.

The child is given a phosphosoda enema the evening before and another the morning of the examination. The jackknife, head-down position is ideal. Frequently, a rectal polyp can be seen and removed by inserting two retractors into the anal canal. The polyp is then grasped with a forcep and pulled down, its pedicle is ligated, and it is amputated. Otherwise, the standard adult-sized proctoscope is inserted and advanced 20 to 25 cm. Higher polyps are grasped with a forceps and drawn into a wire snare, which electrocoagulates the pedicle as it amputates the polyp. The snare must catch the pedicle immediately beneath the polyp. It is easy to put too much traction on the polyp, tent up the bowel wall, and perforate the colon with the snare. If a polyp is not seen at first, a second and third insertion of the instrument may be performed, since the child is asleep.

JUVENILE POLYPOSIS

Although the usual juvenile or inflammatory polyp is solitary, or at most accompanied by a few scattered lesions in the colon, occasionally the entire bowel may be studded with juvenile polyps. This is an extremely rare condition that causes chronic bleeding, anemia, diarrhea, and protein loss. Infants have died from this benign disease as a result of severe anemia and malnutrition.[4,5] Furthermore, juvenile and adenomatous polyps may exist simultaneously in the same patient and may occur in families.[6]

On proctoscopic examination, the lumen of the

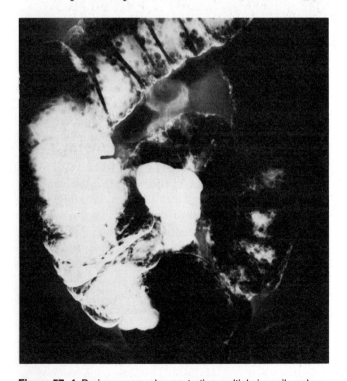

Figure 57–4. Barium enema demonstrating multiple juvenile polyposis.

bowel is filled with hundreds of pedunculated polyps. A barium enema reveals involvement of the entire colon (Fig. 57–4). Microscopically, these polyps are indistinguishable from the common juvenile or inflammatory polyp. The severe symptoms are due to their number. These children require support with transfusions and total intravenous nutrients, followed by a total colectomy with an endorectal ileal pull-through, just as for familial polyposis.

ADENOMATOUS POLYPS

Adenomatous polyps are rare in children. Kottmeier and Clathworthy found only 3 patients with this lesion in a group of 50 children with colonic polyps.[7] One of their patients developed carcinoma in a polyp at the age of 12 years. In another study, adenomas were found in 5 children less than 10 years of age during a period when 187 children were found with juvenile polyps. In this same study, adenomas became more prevalent in patients between 10 and 20 years of age.[8] Adenomatous polyps are true neoplasms and are more likely to be sessile than pedunculated. Microscopically, there is regular proliferation of glands supported on a thin, vascular, connective tissue stroma. The surface is covered with columnar epithelium rather than the granulation tissue seen in juvenile polyps. The small but definite possibility of an adenomatous polyp in a child requires tissue study of any lesion above the reach of a proctoscope. This is an indication for colonoscopy and biopsy. If an adenoma is biopsied, it should be removed by operation and resection.

FAMILIAL MULTIPLE POLYPOSIS

Familial adenomatous polyposis of the colon is inherited as a simple autosomal dominant trait. Each child of an affected parent has a 50 percent chance of inheriting the disease. Cases do occur sporadically without a family history.[9] The polyps in this disease are limited to the colon and rectum. They are too numerous to count, since the entire mucosa is studded with sessile polyps. In adults these polyps are usually no more than 0.5 cm in diameter, and some are no more than a tiny excrescence 1 mm or so above the mucosa (Fig. 57–5). There are no extracolonic manifestations of this disease. Although symptoms of familial polyposis may not appear until the third decade of life, we have observed diarrhea, bleeding, and abdominal pain in children as young as 10 years of age. Other children are asymptomatic but are subjected to proctoscopic examination because a parent was known to have the disease. Eventually, every untreated patient with familial polyposis of the colon

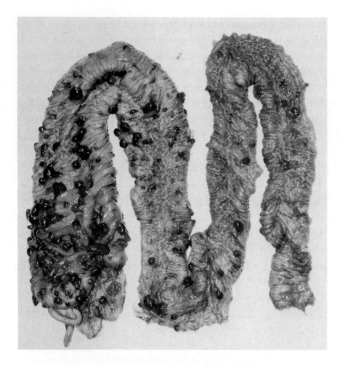

Figure 57–5. Resected colon demonstrating familial polyposis.

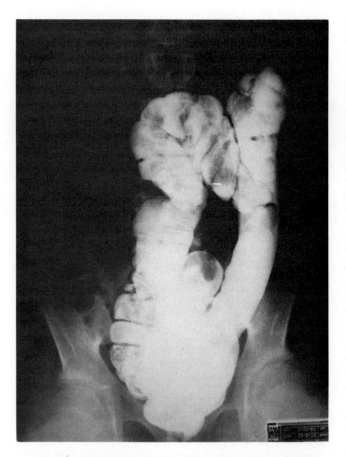

Figure 57–6. Barium enema illustrating familial polyposis.

will develop an adenocarcinoma of the colon. Bussey's study points out that adenocarcinoma occurs an average of 20 years earlier in these patients than in persons without polyposis,[9] and cancer has occured in teenage children with this disease.[10]

The diagnosis is made by the proctoscopic observation of myriads of sessile polyps covering the wall of the colon. On barium enema examination, the entire colon is seen to be studded with polyps (Fig. 57–6). A biopsy demonstrates the typical features of an adenomatous polyp. Grossly, only hyperplastic lymphoid follicles will resemble multiple polyposis. Children with this disease have symptoms of diarrhea and bleeding at a younger age than those with familial polyposis, and on proctoscopic examination, the polyps are smooth and pale or white.[11,12] The diagnosis is made by observing an umbilicated appearance of the polyps on barium enema examination and by a biopsy that demonstrates only aggregates of hyperplastic lymphoid follicles.[13] Lymphoid hyperplasia may occur in the ileum of a patient with colonic polyposis. Consequently, ileal lesions must not be resected on their gross appearance because lymphoid hyperplasia is benign and regresses spontaneously.[14]

Treatment

The presence of symptoms and the known risk of carcinoma of the colon in children with familial polyposis are indications for removal of the colon when the diagno-

sis is made. Although some surgeons recommend total colectomy with a permanent ileostomy, we do not consider this operation necessary. The choice of operation is between subtotal resection of the colon, with anastomosis of the ileum to the remaining 10 cm of rectum, and resection of the colon, with an endorectal pull-through of the ileum to the dentate line. This sphincter-saving operation suggested by Ravitch and Sabiston was applied to children by Shirazi and Soper.[15,16]

From a technical standpoint, the low anterior resection is an easier operation, with fewer potential complications than the endorectal pull-through. Although there have been scattered observations that rectal polyps will regress following a low anterior resection, this has not been our observation.[17,18] A child whose rectum has been left in place must return for examination and fulguration of remaining polyps at intervals of 6 months to 1 year. In a study at the Mayo Clinic, 31 patients who had polyps remaining in the rectum developed cancer. In this study, none of the patients who did not initially have rectal polyps, but who had lesions higher in the colon, developed a malignancy in the rectum.[19] Total colectomy with an endorectal pull-through is now the generally accepted operation for children with familial polyposis.[20]

Preparation for Surgery. The child is admitted to the hospital several days in advance of the operation and given an elemental diet, together with a mechanical bowel preparation. All feedings are stopped 48 hours before operation, and intravenous fluids are given. On the day before surgery, four doses of neomycin are given by mouth to provide a total of 100 mg/kg body weight. Blood transfusions are given as indicated to correct anemia.

Technique. The child is placed in the lithotomy position for easy access to the abdomen and perineum. The rectum is then irrigated with a solution of povidone-iodine and saline and swabbed with povidone-iodine-soaked sponges. A left paramedian incision is made because this provides easy access to the pelvis and leaves the left lower quadrant free for a temporary ileostomy if there are anastomotic complications.

The small bowel is minimally handled and covered with warm, moist pads while the colon is mobilized, commencing with the cecum. As soon as the right colon has been mobilized, the mesenteric vessels at the ileocecal junction are isolated, ligated, and divided. The ileum is divided between a double row of staples and the proximal end is further closed with interrupted sutures, which are cut long. The colon is progressively mobilized, with isolation and ligation of its mesenteric vessels. The inferior hemorrhoidal artery is spared in order to provide a blood supply to the muscular cuff of rectum that is left behind after stripping out the mucosa. Commencing 10 cm proximal to the peritoneal reflection, the bowel is dissected close to its muscular wall to avoid damage to pelvic nerves. With the bowel held up on traction, the muscular wall is clamped with two allis forceps, which are then held up to apply traction to the intervening bowel (Fig. 57-7). The muscle layers of the colon are then divided down to the submucosa in a longitudinal direction. Pressure, traction, and suction are necessary to keep this incision free of blood so that the submucosal layer may be recognized. The edges of the muscle are held up with the allis forceps, and the mucosa is separated by scissors dissection. All of the blood vessels that traverse the submucosa are electrocoagulated. Once the dissection is underway, the scissors are exchanged for moistened Kuttner dissectors. An assistant must be careful to coagulate each strand of tissue that does not separate easily with blunt dissection because these are small vessels. It occasionally is necessary to clamp and ligate a larger vessel. Continued traction is maintained on the mucosal tube, but the cuff of muscle is allowed to retract away from the mucosa as the dissection proceeds deeper

into the pelvis. It is possible to continue the dissection all the way to the dentate line, but we prefer to precisely dissect the intact mucosa away from the squamous epithelium and perform the last portion of the operation by dissecting the mucosa up from below. When the last of the mucosa has been dissected free from the muscular cuff, all bleeding must be controlled with coagulation or, if the vessel has retracted into the muscle, by suture-ligation. The muscular cuff must be absolutely dry before the ileum is pulled through. Six to eight sutures are then placed about the circumference of the muscle cuff 2 cm above the dentate line. These are left long with their needles attached and held aside with hemostats (Fig. 57-7E-G). While one operator is placing these sutures, another mobilizes the terminal ileum until there is enough length to reach the anus. The ileum is then brought down, and the sutures previously placed through the muscle of the rectal cuff are inserted into the seromuscular layer of the small intestine. These sutures stabilize the bowel and take tension off the one layer of sutures, which are then placed through the full thickness of the ileum into the internal sphincter and through the dentate line. Polyglycolic acid sutures remain for at least 2 weeks, allowing sufficient time for healing. At the end of the operation, a central hyperalimentation line is placed percutaneously into either the subclavian or jugular vein.

Postoperative Care. The nasogastric tube is left in place for at least 5 or 6 days to ensure prolonged decompression of the small bowel. The child is given nothing by mouth for another 5 days before clear liquids are offered. During this time, nutrition is maintained with intravenous alimentation. Most children will commence to pass liquid stools by the fifth day. Before the oral feedings, the child is given oral diphenoxylate hydrochloride with atropine (Lomotil, Searle). This medication controls diarrhea and allows the child to have 6 to 10 soft stools a day after being on complete oral nutrition. The number of stools rapidly lowers, unlike patients with ulcerative colitis. Most of our patients have no more than 3 or 4 stools a day 6 months after the operation. There does not seem to be any indication for the more complex S or J pouches.

PEUTZ-JEGHERS SYNDROME

Intestinal polyposis associated with mucocutaneous pigmentation was first noted by Peutz in 1921 and later established as a specific entity by Jeghers et al. in 1949.[21,22] This is an autosomal dominant disorder, but sporadic nongenetically caused cases are found, especially in children.[23] The polyps in Peutz-Jeghers syndrome are hamartomas, which occur principally in the

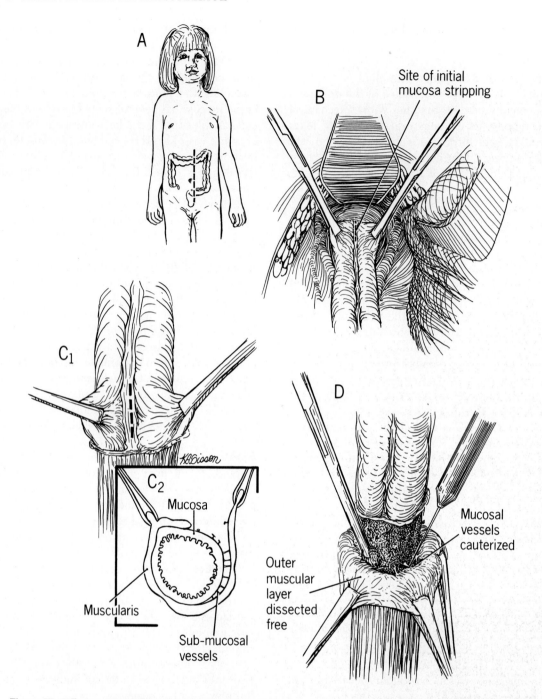

Figure 57–7. Endorectal pull-through for familial polyposis. The same technique for removing the mucosa is applicable to children with familial polyposis, imperforate anus, and perhaps ulcerative colitis. This illustration depicts the endorectal and ileal pull-through portion of the operation for a child with familial polyposis. The entire colon has been mobilized up to step **B.** A vertical incision is made through the muscle down to the mucosa (**C₁, C₂**). The dissection is then carried around the mucosal sleeve. The submucosal vessels are coagulated and divided. The dissection is continued toward the anus until the entire mucosal cuff has been removed to the pectinate line **D.** (Continued)

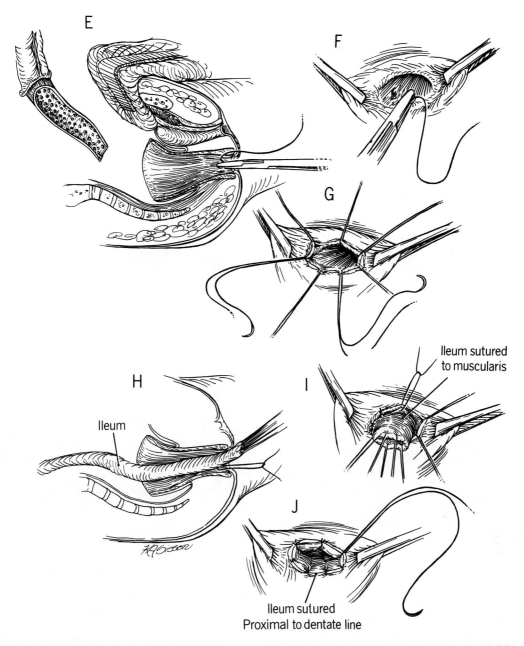

E

F

G

Ileum sutured
to muscularis

H

Ileum

I

J

Ileum sutured
Proximal to dentate line

Figure 57–7 (Cont.). E, F, and **G.** Placement of sutures through the remaining muscular wall. These are left long and then passed through the seromuscular layers of the ileum. The operation is completed by suturing the full thickness of the ileum 1 cm proximal to the dentate line **(H, I, J).**

small intestine but are found also in the colon, stomach, and duodenum. Grossly, the typical polyp is the color of intestinal mucosa, lobulated, and on a pedicle (Fig. 57–8). Closer observation of the mucosa will, however, demonstrate other small sessile growths. Microscopically, the polyp is composed of normal-appearing glands with epithelial cells common to that portion of the gastrointestinal tract. Bands of smooth muscle representing the muscularis mucosa course though the polyp. In children, polyps grow rapidly, especially in the small intestine. In adults, there is evidence that the size of polyps

remains stationary or will even regress. Among 222 recorded cases, malignancy was found in 28, or 12.5 percent.[24] Three of these patients were teenage children with stomach carcinoma. Nongastrointestinal tract cancers developed in 10 of 31 patients in another series.[25] Thus, the overall incidence of cancer in patients with Peutz-Jeghers syndrome is 18 times greater than in the general population.

Children with Peutz-Jeghers syndrome have iron deficiency anemia from chronic slow blood loss, which produces occult blood in the stool but rarely produces

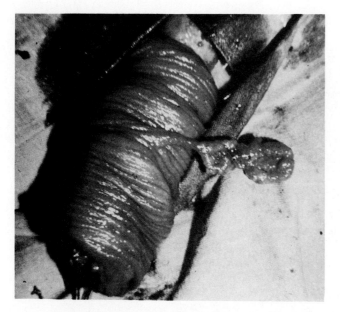

Figure 57–8. Polyp of the Peutz-Jeghers syndrome.

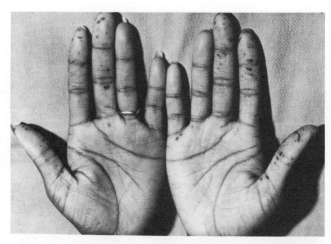

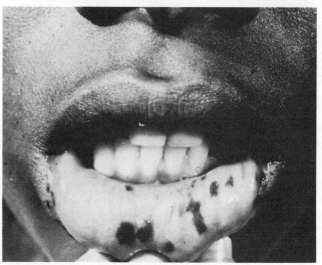

Figure 57–9. Pigmentation of Peutz-Jeghers syndrome on the palms (**top**) and buccal mucosa (**bottom**).

gross bleeding. Recurrent abdominal pain from intussusception, which leads to complete obstruction and often a gangrenous intestine, is the second major clinical problem. The melanin spots appear on the lip of the affected child by the time he or she is 1 to 2 years old. As the child grows older, pigmentation appears on the buccal mucosa and on the palmar surfaces of the fingers (Fig. 57–9). Diagnostic studies include roentgenograms of the stomach, small bowel, and colon, with endoscopic examination of the colon and stomach. These studies are indicated to determine the extent of the disease and to follow up on the afflicted children, who are at risk to develop cancer of the gastrointestinal tract.

Treatment

In the past, surgical therapy has been advised only for intussusception and refractory anemia.[26] This policy may lead to recurrent irreducible intussusceptions causing repeated intestinal obstruction and the short gut syndrome. We have taken a more aggressive approach to this disease by attempting to remove as many polyps as possible, even at repeated operations, in order to avoid anemia and recurrent intussusception. The entire intestinal mucosa may be observed and all polyps removed by intussuscepting the bowel by means of three or four enterotomies placed at intervals from the ligament of Treitz to the ileocecal valve (Fig. 57–10). The pedicles of larger polyps are suture-ligated, and those of smaller polyps are electrocoagulated. After the diagnosis is made, these patients must be followed for life with stool studies for occult blood, hemoglobin determinations, and when indicated, roentgen and endoscopic studies.

OTHER INHERITED POLYPOSIS SYNDROMES

Watne has reviewed the various syndromes associated with intestinal polyps, with particular reference to the extraintestinal manifestations of these diseases that lead to diagnosis.[20] Most of these syndromes occur in adults, but they should be kept in mind when dealing with children who have intestinal polyposis. Gardner's syndrome consists of adenomatous polyps involving primarily the colon, with osteomas and cortical thickening of the bone and such soft tissue lesions as epidermoid cysts, endocrine neoplasms, lipomas, fibromas, and, after an operation, wound fibromatosis and desmoid tumors. Gardner's syndrome is inherited as a simple autosomal dominant trait. Turcot's syndrome consists of intestinal polyposis and brain tumors, and the Cronkhite-Canada syndrome features polyposis alopecia and cutaneous hyperpigmentation.

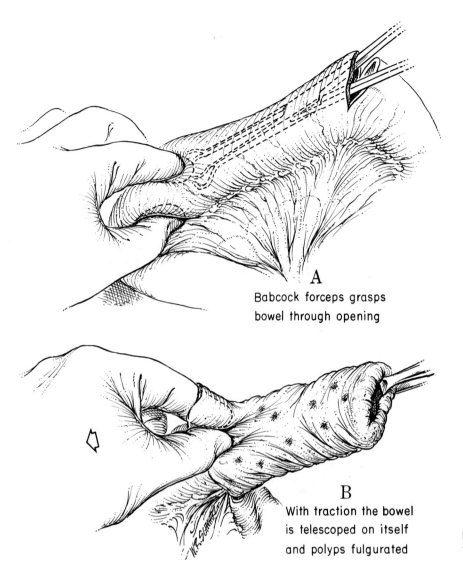

A

Babcock forceps grasps
bowel through opening

B

With traction the bowel
is telescoped on itself
and polyps fulgurated

Figure 57–10. Technique for intussuscepting
the small bowel for the removal of polyps.

REFERENCES

1. Holgersen LO, Mossberg SM, Miller RE: Colonoscopy for rectal bleeding in childhood. J Pediatr Surg 13:83, 1978
2. Nelson EW Jr, Rodgers BM, Zawatzky L: Endoscopic appearance of auto-amputated polyps in juvenile polyposis coli. J Pediatr Surg 12:773, 1977
3. Gleason WA Jr, Goldstein PD, Shatz BA, Tedesco F: Colonscopic removal of juvenile colonic polyps. J Pediatr Surg 10:519, 1975
4. Soper RT, Kent TH: Fatal juvenile polyposis in infancy. Surgery 69:692, 1971
5. Sachatello CR, Griffen WO Jr: Hereditary diseases of the gastrointestinal tract. Am J Surg 125:198, 1975
6. Velcek FT, Coopersmith IS, Chen CK, et al: Familial juvenile adenomatous polyposis. J Pediatr Surg 11:781, 1976
7. Kottmeier PK, Clathworthy HW Jr: Intestinal polyps and associated carcinoma in childhood. Am J Surg 110:709, 1965
8. Mazier W, MacKeigan J, Billingham R, Dignan R: Juvenile polyps of the colon and rectum. Surg Gynecol Obstet. 154:829, 1983
9. Bussey HRJ: Familial Polyposis Coli: Family Studies in Histopathology, Differential Diagnosis, and Results of Treatment. Baltimore, Johns Hopkins University Press, 1975
10. Peck DA, Watanabe KS, Trueblood HW: Familial polyposis in children. Dis Colon Rectum 15:23, 1972
11. Collins JO, Falk M, Gribone R: Benign lymphoid polyposis of the colon. Pediatrics 38:877, 1966
12. Louw JH: Polypoid lesions of the large bowel in children with references to benign lymphoid polyposis. J Pediatr Surg 3:195, 1968
13. Capitanio MA, Kirkpatrick JA: Lymphoid hyperplasia of the colon in children. Radiology 94:323, 1970
14. Dorazio RA, Whelan TJ Jr: Lymphoid hyperplasia of the

terminal ileum associated with familial polyposis coli. Ann Surg 171:300, 1970

15. Ravitch MM, Sabiston DC: Anal ileostomy with preservation of the sphincter. Surg Gynecol Obstet 84:1095, 1947

16. Shirazi SS, Soper RT: Endorectal pull-through procedure in the surgical treatment of familial polyposis. J Pediatr Surg 8:5, 1973

17. Localio SA: Spontaneous disappearance of rectal polyps following subtotal colectomy and ileo proctoscopy for polyposis of the colon. Am J Surg 103:81, 1962

18. Shepherd JA: Familial polyposis of the colon with special reference to regression of rectal polyposis after subtotal colectomy. Br J Surg 58:85, 1971

19. Moertel CG, Hill JR, Adson MA: Management of multiple polyposis of the large bowel. Cancer 28:160, 1971

20. Watne A: The syndromes of intestinal polyposis. Curr Probl Surg 24:320, 1987

21. Peutz J: Very remarkable case of familial polyposis of mucous membrane of intestinal tract and nasopharynx accompanied by peculiar pigmentations of skin and mucous membrane. Ned Voor Maandshr Geneesik 10:134, 1921

22. Jeghers H, McKusick VA, Katz KH: Generalized intestinal polyposis and melanin spots of the oral mucosa, lips and digits: A syndrome of diagnostic significance. N Engl J Med 241:933, 1031, 1949

23. Yusowitz P, Hobson R, Ruymann F: Sporadic Peutz-Jeghers syndrome in early childhood. Am J Dis Child 128:709, 1974

24. Utsunomiya J, Gocho H, Miyanaga T, et al: Peutz-Jeghers syndrome: Its natural course and management. Johns Hopkins Med J 136:71, 709, 1975

25. Giardiello F, Welsh S, Hamilton S, et al: Increased risk of cancer in the Peutz-Jeghers syndrome. N Engl J Med 316:1511, 1987

26. Beck A, Jewett TC: Surgical implications of the Peutz-Jeghers syndrome. Ann Surg 165:299, 1967

58
Stress Bleeding and Peptic Ulcer

Hematemesis and melena, either singly or combined, are obvious signs of bleeding from above the ligament of Treitz. Bright red blood may appear in the stool also when there is a brisk hemorrhage. A nasogastric tube inserted during the bleeding episode will localize bleeding to the esophagus, stomach, or duodenum. A history of liver disease or a palpable spleen suggests portal hypertension. In older children, chronic pain or bleeding points to a chronic peptic ulcer. The recent ingestion of aspirin or alcohol points to gastritis, and a past history of vomiting may lead to the diagnosis of gastroesophageal reflux and esophagitis. Do not forget to look in the nose or throat.

STRESS BLEEDING

Critically ill children, particularly those with hypoxia, head injuries, sepsis, posterior fossa brain tumors, and burns, are liable to develop upper gastrointestinal hemorrhage during the course of their illness. Multiple factors are involved, but as yet, the etiology of stress bleeding is unknown. Mucosal hypoxia, secondary to shock and decreased visceral blood flow, as well as gastric hypersecretion and alterations in mucus production all have been implicated. The term "stress ulcer" often is used, but these patients are just as likely to have diffuse erosions of the stomach as a discrete ulcer. Ulcers are more likely to occur in association with neurologic problems. These lesions, or Cushing's ulcer, seem to be associated with increased acid production.[1] They may bleed or perforate and are more likely to be in the duodenum than the stomach.[2] Ulcers occurring with burns and Cushing's ulcer also are more likely to be single.[3-5] Ulcers associated with burns and neurologic damage may perforate

as well as bleed, another indication that they are discrete, deep lesions.

Infants and children under 1 year of age seem more likely to develop a solitary ulcer secondary to stress, and otherwise healthy newborns may bleed from or perforate an ulcer[6-9] (Fig. 58–1). Perhaps the stress of birth initiates the ulcer; however, during the first few days of life, acidity in the stomach is at adult levels. In our own review of 80 children with complications of peptic ulcers, there were 21 infants under 14 days of age.[10] Thirteen had perforated gastric ulcers, and there were 4 perforated and 4 bleeding duodenal ulcers. There were 18 perforated and 16 bleeding duodenal ulcers in babies between 2 weeks and 1 year of age. Most of these were premature infants who had suffered repeated stress.

Bleeding in older children with a severe medical illness is as likely to originate from diffuse gastric erosions as from a specific lesion. We must make every effort to prevent stress bleeding in critically ill children. A continuous milk drip with antacid medication has dramatically reduced stress bleeding in children with burns. Whether or not increased gastric acid is responsible for bleeding in these patients, it is the only factor we can control. The gastric pH should be kept above 6 with antacids or IV H_2-receptor blocking agents. At our hospital, these measures are used routinely in all children with posterior fossa brain tumors, head injuries, complicated medical problems, especially those requiring steroid therapy. Aluminum antacids cause constipation, and we have had one patient develop a small bowel obstruction because of an antacid impaction.[11] For this reason, one should alternate an aluminum gel with a magnesium-containing antacid; in children with an ileus, 10 to 15 ml is injected into the tube, then aspirated after 10 mintues. Histamine-$_2$ antagonists inhibit secretion of acid from the pari-

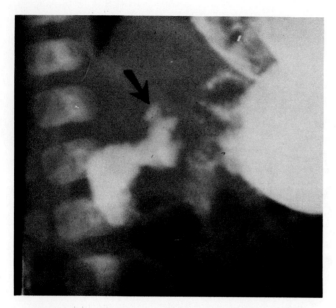

Figure 58–1. Bleeding duodenal ulcer in a 5-day-old baby.

etal cells. These drugs are effective, but they do not take the place of antacid medication. Ranitidine should be given rather than cimetidine because the latter drug can cause thrombocytopenia and diminish hepatic microsomal activity, and it interacts with other drugs.[12]

Treatment

The appearance of hematemesis, melena, or a bloody return from a gastric tube in an already ill child requires vigorous treatment. It is essential to prevent the accumulation of clots in the stomach by irrigation of the gastric tube with an alkaline solution, such as 1 percent sodium bicarbonate or lactated Ringer's solution. One to two milligrams of ranitidine is given every 8 hours to maintain an alkaline stomach pH. Two large intravenous lines are required for the transfusion of blood and blood products, and an arterial line often is necessary to monitor the blood gases and arterial pressure.

These patients frequently require ventilator support and multiple drugs for their primary disease. All drugs must be reviewed to obviate adverse interactions. The administration of fresh frozen plasma and platelets is often necessary to correct coagulation defects. When there is massive hemorrhage, a physician must stay at the bedside to continually monitor bleeding and the volume of transfusion necessary to maintain the pulse, blood pressure, capillary refill, and urinary output.

If the bleeding stops spontaneously and the child remains stable, endoscopy is indicated to determine the bleeding site to better treat the child in case of rebleeding. The esophagus, stomach, and duodenum must all be searched for a specific bleeding site. Most often, however, all one sees is small superficial erosions or inflammation of the stomach mucosa. As long as the

bleeding stops, conservative treatment is continued regardless of the endoscopic findings. When there is continued hemorrhage, blood and clots obscure the site of bleeding so that endoscopy and radiologic studies are almost useless.

Emergency angiography has been helpful in localizing the site of bleeding in adults.[13] Angiography and balloon embolization of the gastroduodenal artery have been successful in a 1-year-old child.[14] However, Gelfoam embolization and selective vasopressin infusion failed in 4 of 10 patients with stress bleeding,[15] and 1 of the patients suffered a thrombosed femoral artery secondary to the procedure. We have had no experience with angiography in patients with stress bleeding because the volume rather than the site of bleeding determines the necessity for operation.

The decision to operate on these children is difficult. When bleeding continues after the transfusion of one blood volume, it is time to operate. Distention of the stomach with a blood clot occurs with rapid bleeding and is another indication for surgery.[16] If the volume of blood lost is slowing or is intermittent, we tend to continue with conservative therapy. When the decision to operate has been made, endoscopy is carried out in the operating room. This will rule out bleeding from the esophagus and may give some idea of the source of the bleeding. If endoscopy demonstrates diffuse gastric oozing, we prefer to continue with nonoperative therapy.

An upper midline incision provides easy access to the stomach and duodenum. The stomach is opened, and all blood is irrigated and aspirated. The duodenum is then packed with sponges, and the interior of the stomach is inspected. If nothing is found, the pylorus and duodenum are irrigated, aspirated, and inspected. If an ulcer is found, it is sutured. One may stop at this point, but a vagotomy and a pyloroplasty are indicated if the child's underlying stressful disease is likely to persist. It is difficult to know what to do with diffuse gastric oozing from multiple small erosions. Gastric devascularization by dividing the gastroepiploic and left gastric artery has been successful in a neonate.[17] Morden et al. carried out extensive gastric resections in 6 of their 8 children with multiple ulcers.[15] Two of these children died as a result of their original disease. One of the survivors had a mild dumping syndrome.

In our series, one gastric resection was performed in a 16-year-old girl who had varicella after a renal transplant. She had diffuse gastric bleeding and died after the operation. In our hospital, we currently prefer vagotomy and pyloroplasty.

CHRONIC PEPTIC ULCER

Approximately one third of children who develop peptic ulcers have a family history of ulcer.[18,19] This may be important in diagnosis, since younger children do not give a typical history of ulcer pain. In the preschool child, the pain is periumbilical and is worsened by meals. The typical ulcer pain that is relieved by food or milk does not become prominent before 10 or 12 years of age. One of our patients consumed several quarts of milk a day and would regularly get up at night to drink milk because he felt hungry. Both his father and grandfather had been operated on for duodenal ulcers. The diagnosis can be made with considerable accuracy with the aid of roentgenograms alone; endoscopy is indicated only if there is a major episode of bleeding with negative x-rays (Fig. 58–2). Medical therapy consists of antacids in the form of magnesium–aluminum gel (2 ml/5 kg) given 1 and 4 hours after meals, with another dose at bedtime. Either cimetidine or ranitidine is safe and effective in these children.

Episodes of bleeding in this group of patients will respond to medical therapy, but bleeding from an ulcer in a child is a poor prognostic sign. Children who have a definite ulcer with pain severe enough to interfere with normal childhood activities, two or more episodes of hemorrhage, and any evidence of obstruction are candidates for an operation. Before surgery, the family is urged to reduce emotional stress in the child's environment and to intensify medical therapy. The same boy whose father and grandfather had ulcers was the pitcher for his Little League baseball team, a boy scout, and on the swimming team, took tennis lessons, and made straight As in school. He developed refractory duodenal obstruction at 12 years of age.

There is clearly a greater need for surgical therapy in children who are eventually referred to a medical center than in the general pediatric population. There was a 50 percent recurrence rate in 109 children seen at the Mayo Clinic when the disease first appeared in childhood. Of 35 patients seen at the Toronto Children's Hospital, 43 percent required an operation. Ravitch has recommended more aggressive surgical therapy in children with duodenal ulcers who show a poor response to medical therapy.[20,21] Approximately 15 percent of children who develop duodenal ulcers eventually will require an operation.[22]

Vagotomy and pyloroplasty constitute the procedure of choice for chronic duodenal ulcers. If there is a gastric ulcer or if there is severe scarring of the duodenum or pylorus, an antral resection with a vagotomy is satisfactory. Neither procedure interferes with future growth and development. Children under 1 year of age have tolerated the operation without difficulty. We have been unable to identify symptoms recognizable as the dumping syndrome in following these children for up to 15 years.

ZOLLINGER-ELLISON SYNDROME

The Zollinger-Ellison syndrome consists of intractable peptic ulceration, gastric hypersecretion, and a gastrin-secreting pancreatic islet cell tumor. There were 28 case histories of children in the Zollinger-Ellison Tumor Registry in 1982.[23]

Pathology

The primary lesion is a functioning gastrin-producing tumor that metastasizes to the liver and the celiac lymph nodes. The tumor itself, although malignant, is rarely the cause of death and may regress after a total gastrectomy. The ulcer is found most often in the duodenum but may be gastric or jejunal. There is thickening and hypertrophy of the gastric mucosa, but there are no other anatomic changes in the gastrointestinal tract. The associated endocrine tumors found in adults have not been observed in children.

Symptoms

Children with the Zollinger-Ellison syndrome have a history of unremitting abdominal pain that is poorly controlled by medical therapy. This symptom may go on for as long as 2 years before the ulcer perforates or bleeds. Diarrhea is less frequent in children than in adults.

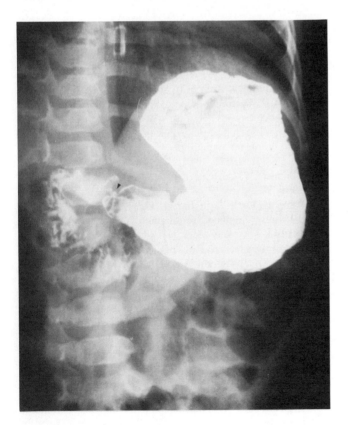

Figure 58–2. Chronic channel ulcer in a 10-year-old boy who had several episodes of hemorrhage.

TABLE 58–1. GASTRIC ACIDITY IN NORMAL CHILDREN

Age	Mean Basal pH	Basal Acid Output (mEq/10 kg per hour)	Maximal Acid Output After Histamine (mEq/10 kg per hour)
3–12 months	3.01	0.34	2.39
1–3 years	2.54	0.38	2.44
3–6 years	2.60	0.37	2.58
6–12 years	2.07	0.45	2.62

Data from *Kopel and Barbero*.[24]

Diagnosis

Roentgenographic studies demonstrate hypertrophied gastric rugal folds with increased secretions, duodenal hypomotility, and jejunal hypermotility. Usually, a deep ulcer crater is seen. A gastric analysis should always be performed in a child with a recalcitrant peptic ulcer. Certainly this test is indicated before surgical therapy. The gastric analysis is of no help in distinguishing normal children from those with ulcers, but it leads the way to a diagnosis of Zollinger-Ellison syndrome. Children with this disease have a gastric output of 1 to 2 liters of fluid per day, with total acid values ranging from 23 to 164 mEq.

Gastric acidity is measured by passing a radiopaque catheter into the most dependent portion of the stomach under fluoroscopic control. The stomach is irrigated with water and emptied. The tube is then connected to a source of low, continuous suction. Aliquots may be taken at hourly intervals, or a 12-hour aspirate may be examined. Kopel and Barbero determined values for gastric acidity in normal children (Table 58–1).[24]

In the Zollinger-Ellison syndrome, the basal acid output is elevated, but since there is already maximal stimulation, there is no response to histamine. The serum gastrin levels also are elevated; in borderline or doubtful cases, the serum gastrin may be stimulated with a calcium infusion.[25]

Treatment

In the past, total gastrectomy with removal of the primary tumor and all possible metastases was the treatment of choice. Cimetidine has now been shown to be effective in controlling the gastric hypersecretion. Adult patients who respond to H_2-receptor antagonists are operated on to remove the primary tumor and all possible metastases.[26] A total gastrectomy is performed only if there is an inadequate response to drug therapy. However, according to the results found in the Zollinger-Ellison Tumor Registry, total gastrectomy may be more advantageous and safer than a lifetime of drug therapy.

GASTRITIS

When an episode of gastrointestinal hemorrhage subsides on administration of medical therapy, we obtain roentgenograms the next day. In the past, when this study failed to demonstrate an ulcer or varices, we were at a loss for a diagnosis. Endoscopy currently is the most reliable single diagnostic technique in establishing a diagnosis of gastritis or diffuse gastric ulceration.[27,28] Two of our patients who bled massively had a history of aspirin ingestion. Both had small punctate hemorrhages on the gastric mucosa, with no evidence of an ulcer. Our diagnosis was "aspirin gastritis." No further therapy was required, and so far both patients have been asymptomatic.

REFERENCES

1. Norton L, Greer J, Eisemon B: Gastric secretory response to head injury. Arch Surg 101:200, 1970
2. Lewis E: Gastroduodenal ulcerations and hemorrhages of neurogenic origin. Br J Surg 60:279, 1973
3. Krasna J, Schneider K, Becker J: Surgical management of stress ulcers in childhood: report of five cases. J Pediatr Surg 6:301, 1977
4. Abramson P: Cushing ulcer in childhood. Surgery 55:321, 1964
5. Curci M, Little K, Sieber W, Kiesewetter W: Peptic ulcer disease in childhood reexamined. J Pediatr Surg 11:329, 1976
6. Lyday JE, Markarian M, Rhoads JE: Perforated duodenal ulcer in a 2100 gram female infant, with survival. Am J Surg 97:346, 1959
7. Thompson NW, Tuburgen DG, Yull AB: Duodenal ulcer in the newborn infant. Arch Surg 90:233, 1965
8. Groom RD, Thomas CG Jr: Hemorrhage from duodenal ulceration in the newborn: Case report. South Med J 65:185, 1972
9. Bell M: Keating J, Ternberg J et al: Perforated stress Ulcers in infants. J Pediatr Surg 16:998, 1981
10. Raffensperger JG, Condon JB, Greengard J: Complications of gastric and duodenal ulcers in infancy and childhood. Surg Gynecol Obstet 123:1269, 1966

11. Hurley JK: Bowel obstruction occurring in a child during treatment with aluminum hydroxide gel. J Pediatr 92:592, 1978
12. Gilman A, Goodman L, Rall T, et al. (eds): Goodman and Gilman's The Pharmacological Basis of Therapy, 7th ed. New York, Macmillan, 1985, pp 624–627
13. Keller FS, Rosch J: Value of angiography in diagnosis and therapy of acute upper gastrointestinal hemorrhage. Dig Dis Sci 26:785, 1981
14. Janik J, Culhom J, Filler R, et al: Balloon embolization of a bleeding gastroduodenal artery in a one year old child. Pediatrics 67:671, 1981
15. Morden R, Schullinger J, Mollitt D, Sontulli T: Operative management of stress ulcers in children. Ann Surg 196:18, 1982
16. Glasow P, Murphy D, Bloss R, et al: Massive upper gastrointestinal hemorrhage in an infant following cardiac surgery. J Pediatr Surg 22:1005, 1987
17. Udassin R, Nissan S, Lernau O, et al: Gastric devascularization—an emergency treatment for hemorrhagic gastritis in the neonate. J Pediatr Surg 18:579, 1983
18. Nuss D, Lynn HB: Peptic ulcerations in childhood. Surg Clin North Am 51:945, 1971
19. Roy CC, Silverman A, Cozzetto FJ: Pediatric Clinical Gastroenterology. St. Louis, Mosby, 1975, p 155
20. Seagram CF, Stephens CA, Cunning WA: Peptic ulceration at the Hospital for Sick Children, Toronto, during a 20-year period, 1949–69. J Pediatr Surg 8:407, 1973
21. Ravitch MM, Duremides G: Operative treatment of chronic duodenal ulcer in childhood. Ann Surg 171:641, 1970
22. White A, Carachi R, Young D: Duodenal ulceration presenting in childhood: long-term follow-up. J Pediatr Surg 19:6, 1984
23. Wilson S: The role of surgery in children with the Zollinger-Ellison syndrome. Surgery 92:682, 1982
24. Kopel FB, Barbero G: Gastric acid secretion in infancy and childhood. Gastroenterology 52:1101, 1967
25. Schwartz DL, White JJ, Saulsbury F, Haller JA Jr: Gastrin response to calcium infusion: an aid to the improved diagnosis of Zollinger-Ellison syndrome in children. Pediatrics 54:599, 1974
26. Bumpils S, Landon J, Mignon M, Hervoir P: Results of surgical management in 92 consecutive patients with Zollinger-Ellison syndrome. Ann Surg 194:692, 1981
27. Gleason WA Jr, Tedesco FJ, Keating JP, Goldstein PD: Fiberoptic gastrointestinal endoscopy in infants and children. J Pediatr 85:810, 1974
28. Cox K, Ament M: Upper gastrointestinal bleeding in children and adolescents. Pediatrics 63:408, 1979

59
Portal Hypertension

The spectrum of diseases causing portal hypertension is considerably different in children than in adults. In our own patients during the past 20 years, there were 20 with extrahepatic portal vein obstruction and 30 with liver disease. The incidence of portal vein thrombosis in infancy seems to be declining, possibly as a result of more cautious use of the umbilical vein in neonates. At the same time, as more children survive with biliary atresia and cystic fibrosis of the pancreas, more tend to develop intrahepatic portal vein obstruction. Regardless of etiology, portal hypertension results in massive upper gastrointestinal hemorrhage from esophageal varices.

EXTRAHEPATIC PORTAL VEIN OBSTRUCTION

Portal vein obstruction has been attributed most often to omphalitis, exchange transfusion, or neonatal sepsis.[1-3] Presumably, thrombosis of the vein is followed by recanalization, with the development of cavernous transformation of the vein into a number of small channels. Only 5 of our own 20 patients with extrahepatic obstruction had a history of umbilical vein catheterization, and none had sepsis. Only 32 percent of 47 cases reported from the Pittsburgh Children's Hospital showed a history of omphalitis or neonatal sepsis; there was no definite etiology in the rest.[4] There is some evidence that portal vein obstruction has a congenital basis. Three of our patients had other vascular anomalies, and in one surgical case, as well as in two patients on whom autopsies were performed, there was either stenosis or atresia of the portal vein without evidence of inflammation. The portal vein develops from the right and left vitelline veins, which form an anastomotic plexus around developing liver cells. Cross anastomoses develop be-

tween these two channels during rotation of the gut.

The right vitelline vein persists and receives blood through its dorsal anastomosis with the left vitelline vein. Congenital obstruction may develop at any of these normal embryologic junction points.[5,6] Some splenoportograms show structures resembling the original double vitelline vein system (Fig. 59–1). Caucasian children appear to have a definite predilection for developing extrahepatic portal vein obstruction. Perhaps this is another factor supporting the theory of a congenital basis for this disease.

Signs and Symptoms

Although there may be a history of jaundice or ascites in infancy, the first symptom is usually a sudden massive hemorrhage when the child is between 2 and 6 years of age. The first and subsequent bleeding episodes often are precipitated by a febrile illness, such as an upper respiratory infection or gastroenteritis. There may be a history of aspirin ingestion. Between episodes of hemorrhage, children with extrahepatic portal vein obstruction are well. Their growth and development are normal. On physical examination, there is invariably an enlarged, firm spleen. There are often hematologic signs of hypersplenism, with platelet counts as low as 75,000 and white blood counts of 2000 to 3000. Fortunately, this degree of hypersplenism rarely if ever causes symptoms and must not be considered as an indication for splenectomy. The liver is normal on palpation, and liver function tests are normal.

In our patients, the diagnosis of esophageal varices has been made with the aid of a barium swallow in every case. Roentgenograms demonstrate clusters of enlarged veins in the distal esophagus and often in the fundus of the stomach (Fig. 59–2). In doubtful cases, the diagnosis may also be made with esophagoscopy and confirmed with splenoportography. Although splenopor-

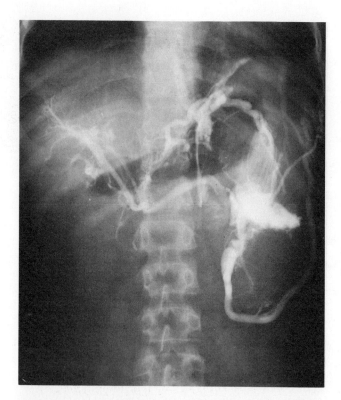

Figure 59–1. Double portal veins, resembling the vitelline system. Note the huge splenic collaterals. The patient had a central splenorenal shunt at 13 years of age, with one incident of minor postoperative bleeding.

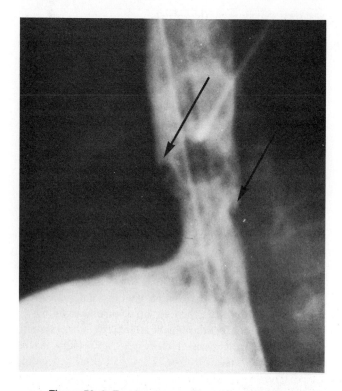

Figure 59–2. Esophagogram with esophageal varices.

tography is not necessary to make the diagnosis of portal hypertension, it is required to map the portal bed in order to determine the exact site of obstruction when planning an operation. Even if an operation is not immediately indicated, a splenoportogram will provide information that may prove valuable in the management of future episodes of hemorrhage.

The natural history of extrahepatic portal vein obstruction in children has been reviewed in considerable detail by Fonkalsrud et al. and Cohen and Mansour.[7,8] Only 2 of the 69 patients reviewed by Fonkalsrud et al. died as a result of bleeding; both lived in remote communities and were not able to receive medical care. Sixteen of the patients in this study survived without any operation. Cohen and Mansour confirmed these observations and noted that bleeding episodes became less frequent during the teen years. Thus, there is good evidence for the natural development of retroperitoneal shunts that direct blood away from the esophageal varices.

INTRAHEPATIC PORTAL HYPERTENSION

Any chronic liver disease that results in fibrosis or cirrhosis eventually will cause portal hypertension. Patients with such disease are clearly distinguished from those with extrahepatic portal obstruction by the history of liver disease, usually with jaundice and occasionally with ascites. On physical examination, the liver is firm and enlarged, and the child may show other signs of chronic illness, such as muscle wasting and poor development. Liver function tests usually are abnormal, but in congenital fibrosis or cystic disease, they are surprisingly normal.

Cystic disease of the liver usually is associated with polycystic kidneys. Even though the liver is enlarged and firm, its function is well maintained. This ailment is apparently a familial variant of congenital hepatic fibrosis.[9,10] The increased portal pressure in the afflicted patients is caused by severe distortion of the fine architecture of the liver. A liver biopsy demonstrating bands of fibrous tissue and cystic spaces confirms the diagnosis. A splenoportogram demonstrates distortion of the finer vein radials within the liver, but the main portal vein is normal. A portosystemic shunt offers safe and effective decompression in these patients, since liver function is well preserved.[11–13] On the other hand, a shunt should not be performed if there is declining liver function and a transplant might be indicated.

CYSTIC FIBROSIS OF THE PANCREAS

With improved nutritional and pulmonary care, children with cystic fibrosis of the pancreas are living longer, and approximately 2 percent develop portal hypertension.[14] The liver disease consists of focal biliary cirrhosis, with plugging of the bile ducts by inspissated secretions. Schuster et al. defined the indications for surgery in this group of patients. When there are esophageal varices, a shunt should be performed before pulmonary decompensation. Ascites, jaundice, and advanced pulmonary sepsis are contraindications to a shunt.

Preoperative care has consisted of tracheotomy a week before surgery, vigorous postural drainage, pulmonary toilet, and antibiotics. With this regimen, Schuster et al. reported that 16 children of 35 operated on were alive at the time of the report (for 1 month to 15 years after operation). Both portacaval and splenorenal shunts were used in these patients. Now, sclerotherapy is the treatment of choice.

BILIARY ATRESIA

Portal hypertension has become the principal threat to children who have had an otherwise successful operation for biliary atresia. Even those children who have excellent bile drainage and are free from jaundice or cholangitis have developed some degree of portal hypertension, as manifested by a firm, enlarged spleen and esophageal varices. The fibrosis invariably associated with biliary atresia results in progressive narrowing of the intrahepatic portal veins. This process is usually progressive, although improvement in portal hypertension has been reported, possibly as a result of improved liver histology or the development of spontaneous shunts.[15] One of our patients died 15 years after successful bile drainage with variceal hemorrhage and liver failure, and another developed variceal bleeding with liver failure and died. Two others with biliary atresia underwent liver transplantation after they developed bleeding from varices, one at 20 years of age and another 3 years after she had required transthoracic ligation of varices. Altman recommended an interpositional mesocaval shunt with a segment of jugular vein in these patients.[16]

Portosystemic shunting is no longer appropriate for children with biliary atresia. Many eventually will become candidates for liver transplantation, and the complications of portal hypertension can be controlled by variceal sclerotherapy and splenic artery embolization.[17]

SPLENOPORTOGRAPHY

Percutaneous splenoportography is a safe and accurate technique for demonstrating the portal system.[18] Coagulation studies should be performed, and blood should be available for possible transfusion. The platelet count should be at least 100,000 and the prothrombin time within normal limits. Although it is possible to perform the study under sedation, we prefer to use general anesthesia to prevent motion and to stop all respiratory movements during the injection. The left flank and abdomen are sterilized and draped. An 18-gauge spinal needle is attached to a length of plastic tubing and then to a syringe containing saline. The spleen is palpated and stabilized with one hand while the needle is inserted through the 8th or 9th intercostal space to a depth of 2 to 3 cm into the spleen. There must be a free drip of blood from the needle before the injection. A common mistake is to insert the needle too low and traverse the splenic substance. The resultant injection will be intraperitoneal rather than into the spleen. If desired, the splenic pulp pressure may be measured with a manometer; the normal range is 8 to 14 cm of saline. After the injection of 20 to 30 ml of 50 percent sodium diatrizoate solution, sequential films are obtained at intervals of 1 to 2 seconds. We have observed no complications as a result of splenoportography.

If splenoportography is not feasible, the portal system may be visualized by celiac and mesenteric artery injection. In addition, we inject a peripheral mesenteric vein at the time of operation to visualize the mesenteric vein as well as the mesenteric–splenic–coronary vein junction.

TREATMENT

The treatment of variceal hemorrhage in children is a difficult, frustrating experience. Those with underlying liver disease are chronically ill with poor nutrition and coagulation problems, and sometimes other organ systems are involved as well. Portal hypertension with esophageal varices and hypersplenism are major complications. Children with extrahepatic portal vein obstruction often are the picture of health between episodes of bleeding. They want to lead normal lives, yet there is always the threat of a terrifying hemorrhage.

Stress, intercurrent infections, coughing, and aspirin ingestion may precipitate a bout of hemorrhage.[19] We must repeatedly warn against giving these children aspirin. It is wise to keep them on a bland diet and antacids. Respiratory infections are treated with bedrest, humidity, cough suppressants, antibiotics, and increased doses of antacids.

Individual episodes of bleeding may commence with melena or hematemesis. The child's blood is promptly typed and crossmatched, coagulation studies are performed, and transfusions of whole blood or packed cells with fresh frozen plasma are given. Mild bleeding may be handled with bedrest and antacid therapy in additon to transfusion. It is my own distinct impression that hemorrhage is aggravated by coughing, agitation, straining, and crying. Consequently, these children require heavy sedation, particularly before the passage of a nasogastric tube, drawing of blood, or other painful procedures. If there is hematemesis, a soft plastic nasogastric tube is passed and irrigated with 1 percent sodium bicarbonate. These measures will control hemorrhage in most cases. If bleeding continues, the next step is the intravenous administration of vasopressin to reduce splanchnic blood flow.[20] The initial dose is 0.2 units/ml per minute, but this concentration may be increased. Careful monitoring is required because the side effects of vasopressin include fluid overload and hyponatremia.

Continued bleeding requires the passage of a well-lubricated child-sized Sengstaken-Blakemore tube. The gastric balloon is inflated and drawn up against the esophagogastric junction under x-ray control. The esophageal balloon is then inflated. The position of the tube is maintained by having the child wear a football helmet, with the tube tied to the faceguard. The tube is irrigated to remove blood and clots from the stomach, the child is kept sedated, and saliva is aspirated from the esophagus with another tube. Obviously, pulmonary aspiration and pneumonia are major complications. The balloon is deflated 12 to 24 hours after bleeding has stopped. It is left in place another 24 hours, then carefully removed after the child has taken a few sips of mineral oil to prevent pulling a clot away from a varix.

If bleeding recurs or is not controlled by these measures, the child is taken to the operating room, and flexible endoscopy is carried out under general anesthesia. Endoscopy will confirm the presence of varices, and a search is made for another source of bleeding, such as gastric varices or an ulcer. This is difficult and frustrating when there is continued bleeding because blood and clots obscure vision. Eight patients in our series have required emergency transthoracic ligation of varices. The left chest is opened, and the lower third of the esophagus is opened longitudinally. If necessary, the esophagus is mobilized through the hiatus to allow suture-ligation of all varices. This operation has controlled the acute hemorrhage in all patients, and all patients survived. It has the additional advantage of leaving the abdomen free for a future liver transplantation or a shunt operation if necessary.

Once the first episode of bleeding has been controlled, the child must be assessed to determine the best therapy to prevent future bleeding episodes. Bleeding seems to be more frequent and severe when it commences in younger children. It is also more severe in children who have had previous failed shunts, particularly if a splenectomy was performed. Current studies indicate that injection of the varices with a sclerosing agent through an endoscope should be carried out immediately after the first bleeding episode.

Sclerotherapy

Several series of both adult and pediatric patients have demonstrated the safety and effectiveness of treating esophageal varices by the injection of sclerosing solutions through an esophagoscope.[21–24] Sclerotherapy has successfully controlled acute bleeding episodes and, in a follow-up of 16 patients from 5 to 30 years, was more successful than portosystemic shunts in patients with both intrahepatic and extrahepatic portal block in all age groups.[25] Lilly uses a slotted rigid esophagoscope and 5 percent sodium morrhuate for injection.[23] Under a general anesthetic, the instrument is passed under direct vision to the esophagogastric junction, then withdrawn until a varix is trapped in the slot. The injection is performed with a long, 25-gauge needle. Blanching and ballooning of the varix indicate a successful injection. The esophagoscope is then advanced and rotated approximately 120 degrees to compress the infected varix. It is again withdrawn until another varix protrudes into the slot; then it too is injected. Three to four varices are injected at each session with 1 to 5 ml of sodium morrhuate. Lilly reinjects children who are actively bleeding at 2 to 3 day intervals until hemorrhage ceases. Others are injected at intervals of 6 weeks to 3 months. One of Lilly's 25 patients died as a complication of therapy and three died of the disease. The rest have survived without bleeding.

Howard et al. obtained equally good results using a flexible endoscope in 57 consecutive children.[26] The mean number of injections to obliterate varices was 4.7 in the children with extrahepatic obstructions and 5.7 in those with intrahepatic disease. In this series, 12 children, or 23 percent of the total, developed esophageal ulcers, and 5 had strictures after healing of their ulcers. Vane and Boles commenced their program of variceal injection using a rigid esophagoscope and then changed to a flexible instrument.[27] They reported seeing one esophageal ulcer before they switched to a more dilute sclerosing agent (1.5 percent sodium tetradecylsulfate). They inject only 1.25 ml of solution into each varix at a time. Eleven of their 13 children survived and are free from further episodes of bleeding.

The flexible instruments have several advantages over a rigid esophagoscope. It is much easier to see and accurately inject the varices because of the superior optical system. Our technique is to position the flexible esophagoscope just proximal to a varix in the lower third of the esophagus. The sheathed needle is passed through the instrument until it is visible in the field. The needle is then unsheathed, and while the operator guides the needle with the tip of the esophagoscope, an assistant, observing through the teaching head, jabs the needle into the varix and injects. Bleeding from the needle hole is irrigated and aspirated, and when the field is clear, another injection is made. All reports of sclerotherapy have stressed the need for repeated, frequent injections to obliterate varices. Failure to understand this has led to failure in our own hands.

The complications of sclerotherapy include transient chest pain, perforation, pleural effusion, pericardial effusion, esophageal ulcers, strictures, esophagitis, and profuse bleeding occurring during the procedure.[28–31] There is one report of transverse myelitis and permanent paraplegia in a 4-year-old girl.[32] These complications can be reduced by using no more than 1.5 ml of solution for each injection and doing no more than four injections at one time. Antibiotics should be given for 24 hours and no food or fluid allowed by mouth until the day after the injection.

Even if sclerotherapy offers only temporary control of variceal hemorrhage, children with extrahepatic portal hypertension can be more easily carried over until they are old enough to undergo a successful portosystemic shunt. The benefits may be even greater in patients with liver disease because a shunt operation makes an eventual liver transplant more difficult. Sclerotherapy combined with splenic embolization to control hypersplenism may eliminate completely the need for surgery in these children.[33]

Surgical Management

Many procedures have been described to control esophageal varices by paraesophageal ligation of veins, esophageal transection, and gastric devascularization. These operations are performed through the abdomen and often require the use of stapling instruments.[34,35] Two of these operations have been performed in our hospital, and bleeding recurred in both. Transthoracic ligation is just as effective in emergency control of bleeding and has the advantage of avoiding a laparotomy in case a future liver transplant or a shunt operation is necessary. Further, sclerotherapy appears to be just as effective in controlling varices, and a major operation can be avoided.

Portosystemic shunts. Operations designed to divert blood from the portal to the systemic venous system were the mainstay of surgical therapy for portal hypertension in children for more than 25 years. The problem is more difficult in children with extrahepatic portal vein obstruction because the portal vein is not available for the usual portacaval shunt. Further, in small children, the splenic and mesenteric veins are small. In a combined series of 148 patients, Fonkalsrud found rebleeding in 45 percent of children with various types of shunts.[36] The longer patients are followed, the higher is the incidence of bleeding. One of my patients rebled 12 year after a splenorenal shunt; he was listed a "success" in previous reports. Not only are the long-term results

in control of hemorrhage open to question, but also portosystemic shunts may be followed by encephalopathy.[37]

Even the distal splenorenal shunt eventually steals blood flow to the liver by collaterals.[38] The possibility of a future liver transplant is another contraindication to a portosystemic shunt. Despite these problems, shunts are still indicated in selected patients. These patients include those with recurrence of bleeding after a trial of sclerotherapy, particularly children with an extrahepatic block or with intrahepatic block but with otherwise good liver function, who may be expected to live a number of years without a transplant. There is less risk of encephalopathy in children with portal vein thrombosis. We have not observed this complication in our children, several of whom are successful in high school or college.

Most surgeons in this country prefer to postpone shunt surgery until the mesenteric or splenic vein is at least 1 cm in diameter or the child is approaching 10 years of age. Bismuth et al. of France, however, have performed shunts in 90 children, and only 5 have thrombosed their shunts.[39] In their hands, shunts are possible when the vein is only 4 mm in diameter. Shunt patency occurred in 70 of 76 patients reported by Alvarez et al.[40] The operations in this series were carried out in young children, often after only one episode of bleeding. The operations performed were almost equally divided between central splenorenal and mesocaval shunts. There was no variceal hemorrhage or encephalopathy seen after surgery in this series. The excellent results in these two series from France are unique and have not been duplicated in the United States.

The choice of a shunt in any individual patient should be governed by the largest of available veins as seen on radiologic studies. Obviously, no operation is perfect. If the splenoportogram reveals a segment of portal vein, portacaval shunt may be feasible (Fig. 59–3). Martin has successfully anastomosed a short stub of portal vein just beyond the junction of the splenic and superior mesenteric veins to either the inferior vena cava or the left renal vein.[41] Since the portal vein is already obstructed and the liver function is normal, there is minimal ammonia toxicity after complete portal diversion. Figure 59–4 illustrates an end-to-side shunt using the junction of the superior mesenteric and splenic veins. In most cases, the splenoportogram will not demonstrate a usable portal vein. Some form of splenorenal or mesocaval shunt, then, offers the best hope of preventing future hemorrhage. The criteria for a successful operation include leaving the spleen in place and making an anastomosis with a portal vessel that is at least 1 cm in diameter. The anastomosis must lie in an anatomic situation where it will not be kinked or obstructed by other viscera.

The end-to-side central splenorenal shunt originally described by Clatworthy and Delorimer requires a sple-

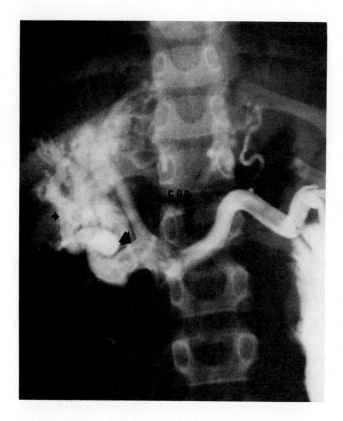

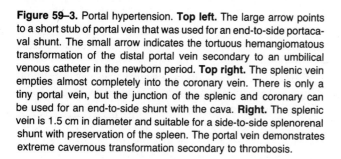

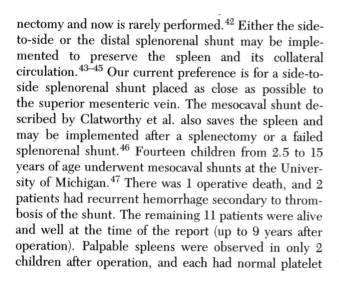

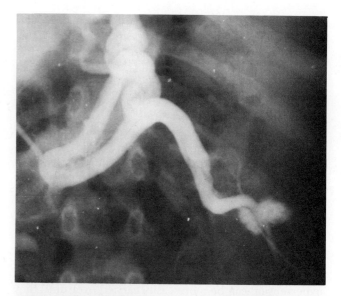

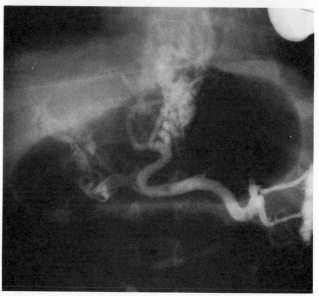

Figure 59–3. Portal hypertension. **Top left.** The large arrow points to a short stub of portal vein that was used for an end-to-side portacaval shunt. The small arrow indicates the tortuous hemangiomatous transformation of the distal portal vein secondary to an umbilical venous catheter in the newborn period. **Top right.** The splenic vein empties almost completely into the coronary vein. There is only a tiny portal vein, but the junction of the splenic and coronary can be used for an end-to-side shunt with the cava. **Right.** The splenic vein is 1.5 cm in diameter and suitable for a side-to-side splenorenal shunt with preservation of the spleen. The portal vein demonstrates extreme cavernous transformation secondary to thrombosis.

nectomy and now is rarely performed.[42] Either the side-to-side or the distal splenorenal shunt may be implemented to preserve the spleen and its collateral circulation.[43–45] Our current preference is for a side-to-side splenorenal shunt placed as close as possible to the superior mesenteric vein. The mesocaval shunt described by Clatworthy et al. also saves the spleen and may be implemented after a splenectomy or a failed splenorenal shunt.[46] Fourteen children from 2.5 to 15 years of age underwent mesocaval shunts at the University of Michigan.[47] There was 1 operative death, and 2 patients had recurrent hemorrhage secondary to thrombosis of the shunt. The remaining 11 patients were alive and well at the time of the report (up to 9 years after operation). Palpable spleens were observed in only 2 children after operation, and each had normal platelet

counts. Auvert and Weisgerber compared 46 mesocaval shunts with 75 splenorenal shunts and concluded that comparable results could be obtained with either shunt when the vein diameter was at least 1 cm, but that the mesocaval shunt had a better chance of remaining patent in cases where it was necessary to use a smaller vessel.[48]

Technique. A long midline incision has the advantage of providing access for any of the possible shunts. There is also less bleeding, and the same incision may be used again if the first shunt fails. All these operations require meticulous suture ligation of mesenteric and retroperitoneal tissues because the electrocautery will not control thin-walled collateral vessels. The side-to-side splenorenal shunt requires less dissection and is technically easier than any of the other procedures. We choose this proce-

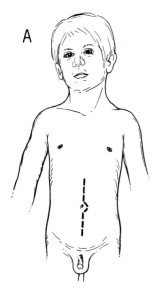

A

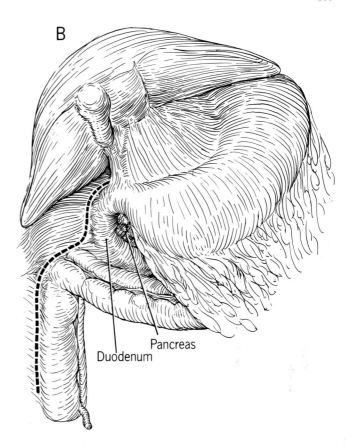

B

Pancreas

Duodenum

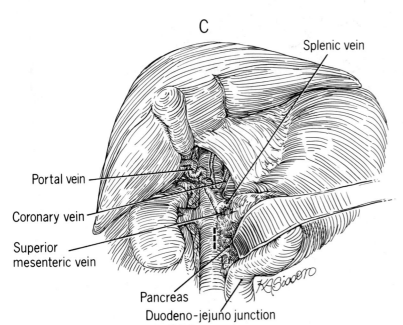

C

Splenic vein

Portal vein

Coronary vein

Superior
mesenteric vein

Pancreas

Duodeno-jejuno junction

Figure 59–4. The usual portacaval shunt is impossible in the child with a thrombosis of the vein, but Martin has shown that there is often a stub of vein at the junction of the splenic, superior mesenteric, and coronary veins that can be anastomosed end-to-side to either the vena cava or the left renal vein. **A.** We prefer an extended midline incision for all shunting procedures. **B.** The duodenum and colon are reflected to the left to expose the inferior vena cava. Further dissection behind the pancreas reveals the junction of the splenic and superior mesenteric veins. There are many fine blood vessels that must be coagulated or ligated in the periotoneum, but once the areolar tissue layers are entered, there is minimal bleeding. **C.** The renal veins, vena cava, and portal vein are all exposed. (Continued)

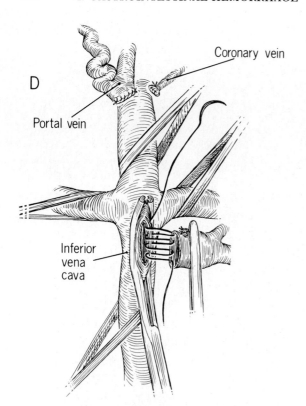

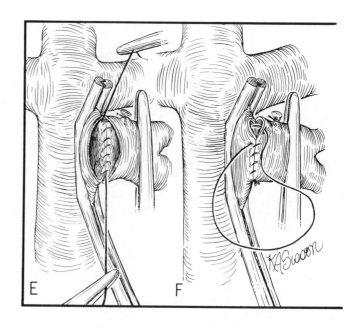

Figure 59–4 (cont). D. All vessels in the field are encircled with loops, and the inferior vena cava is clamped with a curved Potts or Satinsky vascular clamp. The posterior row of sutures is placed to evert the intima of the veins. **E.** When the posterior continuous suture is pulled down, the veins are approximated. The ends are then tied. **F.** The anastomosis is completed with another continuous suture.

dure when the splenic vein is at least 1 cm in diameter. The transverse colon is held up, and the ligament of Treitz and the inferior mesentric vein are identified (Fig. 59–5). The duodenojejunal junction is reflected to the right, and the mesocolon is incised. The inferior mesenteric vein is then traced up beneath the pancreas to its junction with the splenic vein. The pancreas is reflected upward; even in the presence of portal hypertension, this is a relatively avascular plane. The splenic vein is then isolated with narrow slips of Penrose drain and dissected toward its junction with the superior mesenteric vein. Small branches are suture-ligated. When the splenic vein has been isolated and dissected between the inferior and superior mesenteric veins, the left renal vein is isolated and dissected from the inferior vena cava to its bifurcation at the renal hilum. The renal artery is then looped so that it may be occluded with a bulldog clamp during the anastomosis. The splenic artery may be ligated and divided to help decompress the enlarged spleen, since the spleen will receive sufficient arterial supply through the short gastric vessels. When a sufficient length of each vein has been obtained for an anastomosis 2.5 to 3 cm long, the vessels are either circled with loops or held together with vascular clamps. This may require ligation and division of the inferior mesen-

teric vein. The anastomosis is then performed with 6–0 polypropylene sutures. The distal splenorenal shunt may be performed through the same retropancreatic approach (Fig. 59–6).

The mesocaval shunt is performed by anastomosing the end of the inferior vena cava or left iliac vein to the side of the superior mesenteric vein. If the mesenteric vein was not well visualized by splenoportography or if the spleen has been removed previously, it is necessary to cannulate a distal mesenteric vein and inject contrast material in order to visualize the superior mesenteric vein at the time of operation. The right colon is reflected to the left, and the posterior peritoneum is opened until the vena cava can be dissected from the junction of the common iliac vessels to the renal veins. After elevation of the cava with a Penrose drain, all lumbar veins are suture-ligated and divided. The right iliac vein is divided between vascular clamps and closed with a continuous vascular suture. A 2 to 3 cm stump of left iliac vein is left attached to the cava to provide the additional length required for a tension-free anastomosis. The superior mesenteric vein is isolated just beneath the pancreas. The end of the cava or left iliac vein is then brought through a defect in the mesocolon and around the duodenum until it reaches the mesenteric vein. If possible,

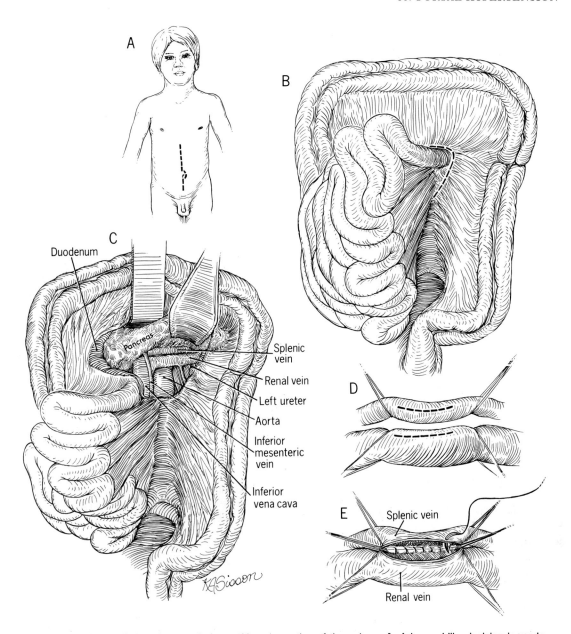

Figure 59–5. Side-to-side splenorenal shunt with preservation of the spleen. **A.** A long midline incision is made. **B.** The colon is elevated to expose the ligament of Treitz and the inferior mesenteric vein, which will lead to the splenic vein. The duodenum is mobilized and moved to the right. **C.** The dissection continues beneath the pancreas, which is elevated with a retractor to demonstrate the splenic vein. The renal vessels are immediately adjacent to the splenic vein. **D.** After the veins are isolated, they are encircled with loops and anastomosed. The left renal artery must be occluded with a bulldog clamp during the anastomosis. **E.** The anastomosis is performed with 6–0 polypropylene sutures.

the mesenteric vein is only partially occluded with a curve-toothed vascular clamp. The anastomosis is then made with continuous polypropylene sutures.

The results in any shunt operation are improved by meticulous microvascular techniques. A continuous suture is satisfactory for the posterior layer, but interrupted sutures anteriorly allow a larger anastomosis that can grow with the child. The absence of recurrent variceal bleeding is the best sign of a successful shunt. Diminution of spleen size, increase in the thrombocyte count, and the absence of varices as seen by endoscopy or x-ray also are indications of shunt patency. Ultrasonography is helpful in evaluating flow through the shunt and vessel size.[49]

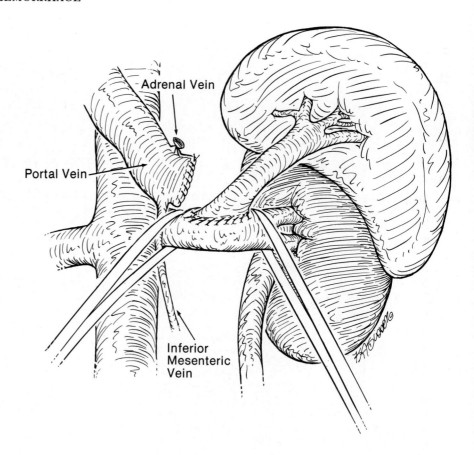

Figure 59–6. The distal sphlenorenal shunt may be performed if a side-to-side anastomosis causes kinking or torsion.

REFERENCES

1. Clatworthy HW Jr, Boles ET: Extrahepatic portal bed block in children: Pathogenesis and treatment. Ann Surg 150:371, 1959

2. Thompson EN, Sherlock S: The etiology of portal vein thrombosis with particular reference to the role of infection and exchange transfusion. J Med 33:465, 1964

3. Oski FA, Allen DM, Diamond LK: Portal hypertension: A complication of umbilical vein catheterization. Pediatrics 31:297, 1963

4. Ehrlich F, Pipatanagul S, Sieber WK, Kiesewetter WB: Portal hypertension: Surgical management in infants and children. J Pediatr Surg 9:283, 1974

5. Marks C: Developmental basis of the portal venous system. Am J Surg 117:671, 1969

6. Kingsley FJ, Brown A: A clinical syndrome associated with a rare anomaly of the vena portal system. Surg Gynecol Obstet 18:520, 1944

7. Fonkalsrud EW, Myers NA, Robinson MJ: Management of extrahepatic portal hypertension in children. Ann Surg 180:487, 1974

8. Cohen D, Mansour A: Extrahepatic portal hypertension: Long-term results. Prog Pediatr Surg 10:129, 1977

9. Bradford WD, Bradford JW, Porter FS, et al: Cystic disease of the liver and kidney with portal hypertension. Clin Pediatr 7:299, 1968

10. Kerr DNS, Harrison CV, Sherlock S, et al: Congenital hepatic fibrosis. J Med 30:91, 1961

11. Herman RE, Hawk WA: Congenital hepatic fibrosis as a cause of portal hypertension: Report of two cases. Surgery 62:1095, 1967

12. Kupper F, Laissue J, Hoffman E, et al: Congenital fibrosis of the liver. Helv Paediatr Acta 24:38, 1969

13. Boley SJ, Arlen M, Mogilner LJ: Congenital hepatic fibrosis causing portal hypertension in children. Surgery 54:356, 1963

14. Schuster SR, Shwachman H, Toyama WM, et al: The management of portal hypertension in cystic fibrosis. J Pediatr Surg 12:201, 1977

15. Odievre M: Long-term results of surgical treatment of biliary atresia. World J Surg 2:589, 1978

16. Altman RP: Portal decompression by interposition mesocaval shunt in patients with biliary atresia. J Pediatr Surg 11:809, 1976

17. Lilly J, Stellin G: Variceal hemorrhage in biliary atresia. J Pediatr Surg 19:476, 1984

18. Kreel L: Radiology of the portal system. Gut 11:620, 1970

19. Grosfeld JL, Phelps TO, Jesseph JM: Effect of stress and aspirin on extrahepatic portal hypertension in rats. J Pediatr Surg 10:609, 1975

20. Chojkier M, Groszmann RJ, Atterbury CE, et al: A controlled comparison of continuous intraarterial and intravenous infusion of vasopressin in hemorrhage from esophageal varices. Gastroenterology 77:570, 1979

21. Terblanche J, Northorer, Burnma P, et al: A prospective controlled trial of sclerotherapy in the long-term manage-

ment of patients after esophageal variceal bleeding. Surg Gynecol Obstet 148:323, 1979

22. Lewis J, Chung R, Allison J: Sclerotherapy of esophageal varices. Arch Surg 115:476, 1980

23. Lilly J: Endoscopic sclerosis of esophageal varices in children. Surg Gynecol Obstet 152:513, 1981

24. Reilly J, Schade R, Ruh M, Vanthiel D: Esophageal variceal sclerosis. Surg Gynecol Obstet 155:497, 1982

25. Spence R, Johnston G, Odling-Smee G, Rodgers H: Bleeding esophageal varices with long-term follow-up. Arch Dis Child 59:336, 1984

26. Howard E. Stamatokis J, Mowat A: Management of esophageal varices in children by injection sclerotherapy. J Pediatr Surg 19:2, 1984

27. Vane D, Boles E, Clatworthy H: Esophageal sclerotherapy: an effective modality in children. J Pediatr Surg 20:703, 1985

28. Atkinson J, Wooley M: Treatment of esophageal varices by sclerotherapy in children. Am J Surg 146:103, 1983

29. Tabibian N, Schwartz J, Smith J, Graham O: Cardiac tamponade as a result of endoscopic sclerotherapy: Report of a case. Surgery 102:546, 1987

30. Evans C, Jones D, Cleary B: Oesophageal varices treated by sclerotherapy: A histopathological study. Gut 23:615, 1982

31. Barsoum M, Moore H, Boulous F: The complications of injection sclerotherapy of bleeding oesophageal varices. Br J Surg 69:79, 1982

32. Seidman E, Weber A, Morin E: Spinal cord paralysis following sclerotherapy for esophageal varices. Hepatology 4:950, 1984

33. Kumpe D, Rumack E, Pretorius D: Partial splenic embolization in children with hypersplenism. Radiology 155:357, 1985

34. Sugiura M, Futagawa S: Further evaluation of the Sugiura procedure in the treatment of esophageal varices. Arch Surg 112:1317, 1977

35. Bessa S, Helmy I, Haman S: Esophageal transection by the EEA stapler for bleeding esophageal varices in schisto-somal hepatic fibrosis. Surg Gynecol Obstet 166:19, 1988

36. Fonkalsrud E: Surgical management of portal hypertension in children. Arch Surg 115:1042, 1980

37. Voorhees AB, Chaitman E, Schneider S: Portal-systemic encephalopathy in the noncirrhotic patient: Effects of portal-systemic shunting. Arch Surg 107:659, 1973

38. Belghiti J, Gremier P, Norel O: Long-term loss of Warren's shunt selectivity. Angiographic demonstration. Arch Surg 116:1121, 1981

39. Bismuth H, Franco D, Alagile D: Portal diversion for portal hypertension in children, the first ninety patients. Ann Surg 192:18, 1980

40. Alvarez F, Bernoud O, Brunell F: Portal obstruction in children: results of surgical portosystemic shunts. J Pediatr 103:703, 1983

41. Martin LW: Changing concepts of management of portal hypertension in children. J Pediatr Surg 7:559, 1972

42. Clatworthy HW Jr, Delorimer HA: Portal decompression procedures in children. Am J Surg 107:447, 1964

43. Krasna I, Kark A: Side-to-side splenorenal shunt for portal hypertension in a child. J Pediatr Surg 7:369, 1972

44. Mitra SK, Kumar V, Datta DV, et al: Extrahepatic portal hypertension: a review of 70 cases. J Pediatr Surg 12:51, 1978

45. Maksoud J, Mies S: Distal splenorenal shunt (DSS) in children. Analysis of the first 21 consecutive cases. Ann Surg 195:401, 1982

46. Clatworthy HW Jr, Wall T, Watman RN: A new type of porto-to-systemic venous shunt for portal hypertension. Arch Surg 11:588, 1955

47. Lambert MJ, Tank ES, Turcotte JG: Late sequelae of mesocaval shunts in children. Am J Surg 127:19, 1974

48. Auvert J, Weisgerber G: Immediate and long-term results of superior mesenteric vein-inferior vena cava shunt for portal hypertension in children. J Pediatr Surg 10:901, 1975

49. Rodgers B, Kouda J: Real-time ultrasound in determination of portasystemic shunt patency in children. J Pediatr Surg 16:968, 1981

60
Meckel's Diverticulum

The diverticulum named after Johann Meckel, a German anatomist, is the most common congenital anomaly of the intestine. It is present in approximately 2 percent of the population, is within 2 feet of the ileocecal valve, and is usually no more than 2 inches in length. Although a Meckel's diverticulum may produce an intestinal obstruction or perforate, simulating an appendicitis, hemorrhage is its most important clinical presentation.

PATHOLOGY

Meckel's diverticulum is caused by an incomplete obliteration of the vitelline or omphalomesenteric duct. If this remnant of the primitive yolk stalk remains intact, there will be a patent connection between the ileum and the umbilicus, draining stool. A fibrous remnant connecting the bowel with the umbilicus is often the site of a volvulus. The true Meckel's diverticulum arises from the antimesenteric border of the lower ileum. It is usually obvious on inspection, but the diverticulum may be folded to one side of the bowel and lie within the mesentery. The blood supply of the diverticulum is derived from the vitelline arteries, paired vessels that run on either side of the mesentery, surround the vitelline duct, and ramify on the yolk sac. Normally, the left vitelline artery atrophies while the right forms the superior mesenteric artery. Any omphalomesenteric duct remnant will be supplied by the right vitelline artery, which arises as an end-artery from the superior mesenteric artery. Occasionally, this vessel is separate from the main portion of the mesentery as a mesodiverticular band, which can trap a loop of bowel and produce an obstruction (Fig. 60–1). Rutherford and Akers studied 147 surgical specimens and found heterotopic tissue in 57 percent. In autopsy specimens of patients in whom the diverticulum had been asymptomatic, there was only a 6 percent incidence of heterotopic tissue.[1] The types of ectopic tissue found were as follows:

Gastric mucosa	51
Pancreatic tissue	10
Colon mucosa	2
Jejunal mucosa	1
Duodenal mucosa	1

The ectopic gastric acid-secreting mucosa at the tip of a Meckel's diverticulum may result in a peptic ulcer, either adjacent to the ectopic mucosa or in the ileum. These ulcers are deep and can erode into a major mesenteric artery. The resultant bleeding is similar to that found in a peptic ulcer in that it usually becomes self-limiting as the vessel contracts and the ulcer fills in with clot. Rebleeding, however, is the rule.

SIGNS AND SYMPTOMS

The pattern of bleeding is similar to that found in any other peptic ulcer. It is episodic rather than chronic and may be massive. Classically, the mother finds a large, brick-red, bloody stool in the diaper. The infant becomes pale and has tachycardia, and the bleeding stops spontaneously. It is unusual to see bright red blood with clots, and tarry stools are even less common. Bleeding is more likely to be severe in children under 2 years of age, and boys are affected more often than girls by a ratio of 3:1. In our experience, Caucasians are affected much more frequently than blacks. The magnitude of the bleeding episode is gauged by the child's vital signs, the drop in hematocrit and hemoglobin, and the volume of blood required for transfusion. The bleeding stops spontaneously, often by the time the child is admitted to the hospital. We have operated on only one child

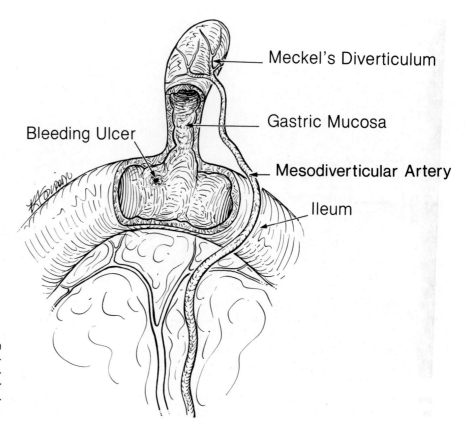

Figure 60–1. Although the most common symptom of Meckel's diverticulum is bleeding, it may also cause an intestinal obstruction, either secondary to a mesodiverticular band or as a leading point in an intussusception.

for uncontrolled bleeding during the first episode. The usual diagnostic studies—proctoscopy, barium enema, and an upper gastrointestinal series–sometimes performed to rule out other causes of hemorrhage are normal. In 1967, Harden et al. demonstrated that technetium-99m was concentrated in the gastric mucosa.[2] In 1970, Jewett et al. identified uptake by Meckel's diverticulae on abdominal scans after the injection of sodium pertechnetate Tc-99m.[3] Later, there were reports of both false positive and false negative scans, possibly because of technical difficulties and overlap of the bladder over the area of the diverticulum.[4,5] Further reports have indicated that the radionuclide may be taken up by intussusceptions, hemangiomas, and duplications of the small bowel and that laxatives or recent barium studies distort the findings.[6] Refinements in imaging technique have improved the accuracy of imaging to nearly 100 percent.[7] Since this is a safe, noninvasive technique, it should be used in children with unexplained gastrointestinal bleeding.

MANAGEMENT

When the diagnosis of a Meckel's diverticulum is suspected on the basis of episodic, brick-red rectal bleeding, the child is admitted to the hospital. Upper gastrointestinal hemorrhage is ruled out by the passage of a nasogastric tube. Plasma or blood transfusions are given to maintain the child's vital signs and hematocrit. An operation is undertaken during the first bleeding episode only if transfusions equivalent to 50 percent of the child's blood volume are required to maintain vital signs—this is practically never the case. Usually, the bleeding ceases and the hemoglobin stabilizes. At that point, diagnostic studies are carried out. If the technetium scan is positive, the child is submitted to surgery as an elective procedure after the hemoglobin level has returned to normal. If the scan is negative, the parents are warned about the possibility of a Meckel's diverticulum. If there is a second acute bleeding episode, we advise an operation.

Operative Technique

When preoperative studies have ruled out the possibility of hemorrhage from the esophagus and stomach, as well as from the colon, the small intestine may be explored through a small subumbilical transverse incision. The small bowel is explored by tracing the ileum proximal from the ileocecal junction. A bleeding diverticulum will be slightly inflamed and edematous (Fig. 60–2). A bluish color within the bowel distal to the diverticulum testifies to the presence of intraluminal blood. A bleeding diverticulum should be widely excised with adjacent ileum because the ulcer may be adjacent to, rather than within, the diverticulum. A wide V excision leaving the mesenteric border of the ileum is satisfactory if one is sure

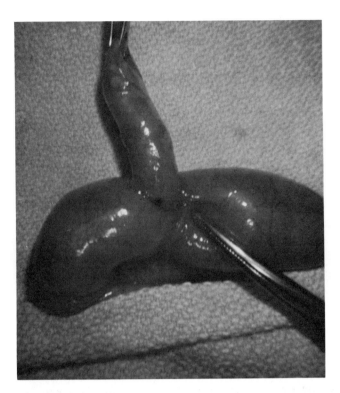

Figure 60–2. Meckel's diverticulum. At operation there was an ulcer in the ileum (tip of hemostat).

that the ulcer is within the resection. Otherwise, a formal small intestinal resection is indicated. The open technique has the advantage of allowing one to see the ulcer, thus ensuring its resection. The appendix also is removed. An asymptomatic Meckel's diverticulum found incidentally at another operation may be safely resected with the closed technique.

RESULT

When the indicated criteria for operation have been strictly observed, either a Meckel's diverticulum or some other specific bleeding point (such as an intestinal duplication or a hemangioma) will be found. When an operation is carried out for hemorrhage, there is little postoperative morbidity and no mortality. Deaths reported as resulting from Meckel's diverticulum have not been related to hemorrhage but rather to neglected intestinal obstruction with intestinal infarction.

REFERENCES

1. Rutherford RB, Akers DR: Meckel's diverticulum: A review of 148 pediatric patients with special reference to the pattern of bleeding and to mesodiverticular bands. Surgery 59:618, 1966
2. Harden RM, Alexander WD, Kennedy I: Isotope uptake and scanning of stomach in man with ^{99m}Tc-pertechnetate. Lancet 1:1302, 1967
3. Jewett TC Jr, Duszynski DO, Allen JE: The visualization of Meckel's diverticulum with ^{99m}Tc-pertechnetate. Surgery 68:567, 1970
4. Rosenthal L, Henry JN, Murphy DA, Freeman LM: Radiopertechnetate imaging of the Meckel's diverticulum. Radiology 105:371, 1972
5. Chandhuri TK, Christie JH: False positive Meckel's diverticulum scan. Surgery 71:313, 1972
6. Duszynski DO: Radionuclide imaging of gastrointestinal disorders. Semin Nucl Med 11:383, 1972
7. Ho JE, Konieczny KM: The sodium pertechnetate Tc-99m scan: An aid in the evaluation of gastrointestinal bleeding. Pediatrics 56:34, 1975

61

Unusual or Unexplained Gastrointestinal Bleeding

Roentgenograms and endoscopy will reveal the site of bleeding in the upper and lower gastrointestinal tracts with a great deal of accuracy. The diagnosis of a Meckel's diverticulum can be made on the basis of significant episodic bleeding and the technetium scan. Diagnostic problems arise when the clinical picture is atypical for Meckel's diverticulum, and the routine roentgenographic and endoscopic studies are negative. Shandling demonstrated that a diagnostic laparotomy in this situation will reveal a source of hemorrhage in only half the children operated on.[1] A diligent clinical examination, coagulation studies, and, on occasion, mesenteric and celiac arteriography will reveal the cause of hemorrhage in the vast majority of children. A laparotomy should be undertaken only in the event of life-threatening, unexplained bleeding.

ESOPHAGUS AND STOMACH

Specific lesions of the esophagus that may cause hemorrhage include ectopic gastric mucosa and esophagitis from reflux. Each of these lesions can be diagnosed by x-ray and endoscopic studies. Specific diseases of the stomach and duodenum that cause bleeding are quite rare in the pediatric age group. Fortunately, they too are easily diagnosed by clinical and roentgenographic studies and, particularly, with endoscopy. These include duplications, hamartomas with ulceration, teratomas, diverticuli, and lymphomas of the stomach (Fig. 61–1).

These lesions may all be treated with a local or segmental gastric resection. Menetrier's disease consists of hyperplastic gastric rugae that cause upper abdominal pain, hematemesis, and edema with ascites because of hypoalbuminemia.[2] The hypertrophic rugae are seen easily on roentgenograms, and the diagnosis is confirmed by endoscopy and biopsy, which is particularly important

in ruling out lymphoma and eosinophilic gastritis. One of our patients required a partial gastrectomy because of persistent bleeding. A second child recovered with transfusions and hyperalimentation, and a repeat gastrointestinal x-ray 11 months later was normal. Hereditary hemorrhagic telangiectasia may occur with nosebleeds or intermittent hematemesis. Some children have visible cutaneous telangiectasia, but, in others, endoscopy with biopsy is essential to make the diagnosis.[3] (Fig. 61–2).

SMALL INTESTINE

When a site of bleeding from the stomach or duodenum has been excluded and there is nothing to suggest a colon lesion, we can assume that the bleeding originates from the small intestine. If there are no systemic signs of disease, such as cutaneous hemangiomas, neurofibromatosis or the melanin spots of the Peutz-Jeghers syndrome, one should first do a nuclear scan to look for a Meckel's diverticulum. This also would reveal ectopic gastric mucosa in a duplication or ectopic gastric mucosa elsewhere in the small bowel. If this study is negative, sometimes a Tc-99m sulfur colloid flow study will reveal a blush at the bleeding site.[4] Ordinarily, however, this study will be of no benefit in children unless there is a 500 ml loss of blood in 24 hours. Small bowel barium studies also are unlikely to be helpful but might reveal a lymphoma or other tumor. Persistent bleeding even with a negative or an equivocal workup is an indication for surgical exploration. This may be the only way to diagnose small bowel ulcerations.[5]

Intestinal hemangiomas are an important source of both recurrent and chronic bleeding. Abrahamson and Shandling reviewed 65 cases of intestinal hemangiomatosis and described a triad of symptoms.[6] All of their pa-

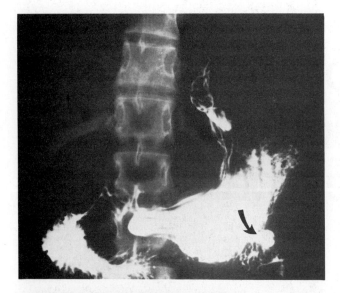

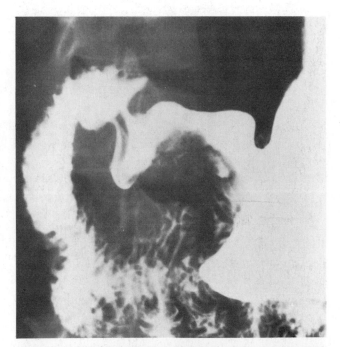

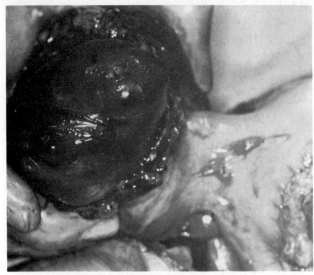

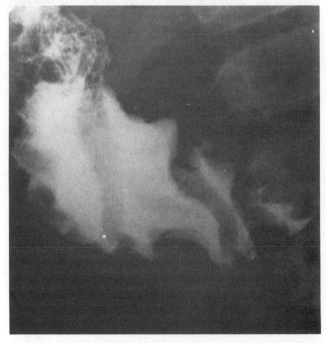

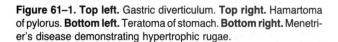

Figure 61–1. Top left. Gastric diverticulum. **Top right.** Hamartoma of pylorus. **Bottom left.** Teratoma of stomach. **Bottom right.** Menetrier's disease demonstrating hypertrophic rugae.

tients had had gastrointestinal bleeding, 49 percent had cutaneous hemangiomas, and phleboliths were seen frequently on plain roentogengrams of the abdomen (Fig. 61–3). Mellish removed 200 hemangiomas from one child and another required five operations to control bleeding.[7] The possibility of an arteriovenous malformation or hemangioma is one of the prime indications for mesenteric and celiac angiography in children, although most of these lesions are found in adults.[8] In our experience, two of four children with proven intestinal hemangiomas had cutaneous lesions, and a third had chronic blood

loss and anemia, but the hemangioma finally became the lead point for an intussusception. A mesenteric arteriogram made the diagnosis in the fourth child after she had undergone a negative laparotomy elsewhere. Intestinal telangiectasia also may occur in children with Turner's syndrome and gonadal aplasia. A buccal smear for sex chromatin will in most cases confirm the diagnosis.[9] At operation, hemangiomas may be obvious because of enlarged mesenteric feeding vessels (Fig. 61–4). Others may require diligent search with transillumination of the bowel to find small lesions. A preoperative

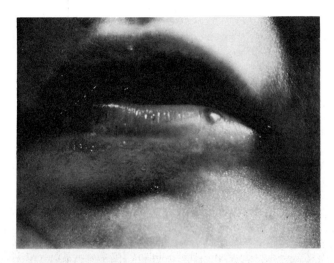

Figure 61–2. Hemangioma on the lip of a 4-month-old baby who had persistent occult rectal bleeding. Exploration revealed a hemangioma of the ileum.

mesenteric arteriogram is helpful in localizing the lesions. The management of a child with multiple hemangiomas is further complicated by excessive consumption of platelets and other coagulation components. One must be prepared to transfuse fresh whole blood, and administra-

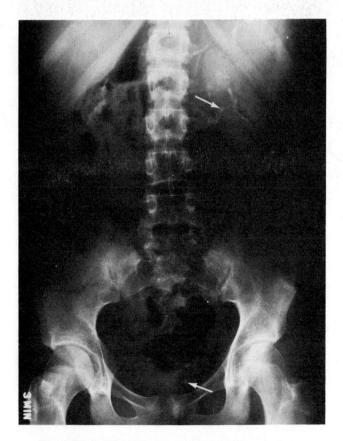

Figure 61–3. Phleboliths in gastrointestinal hemangiomas.

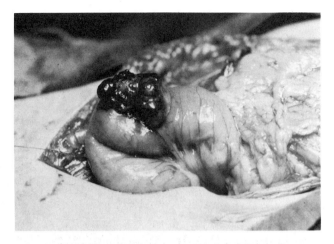

Figure 61–4. Jejunal hemangioma at operation.

tion of platelets and heparinization may be indicated during the postoperative period.[10]

SYSTEMIC DISEASES

In addition to the specific lesions that may bleed, there are a large number of systemic diseases that may be accompanied by gastrointestinal bleeding. One of the more common causes of chronic blood loss and anemia is intolerance of the protein in cow's milk.[11–13] There may be either occult or gross rectal bleeding with mucus in the stools and diarrhea. The onset of symptoms usually occurs within the first 6 weeks of life. The afflicted infants may have recurrent respiratory infections, otitis media, wheezing, and atopic dermatitis. Sigmoidoscopy reveals an edematous colon with petechial hemorrhages. Stool smears reveal increased eosinophils. High milk antibody titers may be found, but the diagnosis rests on the subsidence of symptoms after the elimination of milk from the diet.

The Wiskott-Aldrich syndrome is a sex-linked recessive disorder of boys, characterized by dermatitis and bloody diarrhea. Afflicted patients are thrombocytopenic because of increased platelet destruction.[14,15]

The hemolytic uremic syndrome is characterized by fever, purpura, hemolytic anemia, and neurologic problems. Occlusion of small vessels in multiple organs, including the gastrointestinal tract, results from disseminated intravascular coagulation.[16–18] Early in the disease, there may be massive lower intestinal hemorrhage that simulates ulcerative colitis. Infarction of a segment of intestine may occur, but the syndrome must be recognized and the coagulation disorder treated before any surgical intervention.

Gastrointestinal hemorrhage may accompany both the Ehlers–Danlos syndrome and pseudoxanthoma

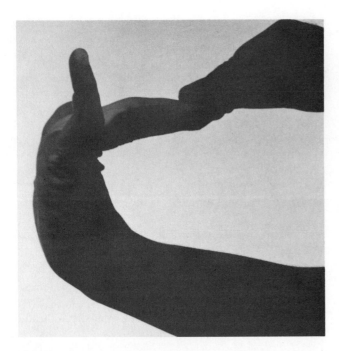

Figure 61–5. Hypermobile joints associated with the Ehlers–Danlos syndrome.

elasticum.[19-21] One of our patients was operated on (after he had lost 100 ml of blood) with the mistaken diagnosis of a Meckel's diverticulum before his abnormal joint mobility was observed (Fig. 61–5).

Parasitic and infectious diseases must be considered, particularly in children who have recently immigrated from or traveled in tropical countries. Hollander et al. described a Puerto Rican infant who had massive intestinal hemorrhage secondary to hookworm infestation.[22] Obviously, it behooves the physician to obtain fresh stool specimens for ova and parasites when studying a child with unexplained rectal bleeding. This can most conveniently be done at the time of proctoscopy.

We have mentioned aspirin, that ubiquitous medication, in reference to gastritis and esophageal varices. The ingestion of therapeutic doses of aspirin in normal children is possibly one of the most common causes of unexplained gastrointestinal bleeding.[23] It is apparent that aspirin both causes local gastric irritation and interferes with the coagulation mechanism.

CONCLUSION

Gastrointestinal bleeding can be an exasperating problem in children. It is alarming to the parents, and often the pediatrician and then the surgeon are drawn into extensive studies that turn up nothing. A careful history and physical examination, with coagulation studies, roentgenograms, and, occasionally, endoscopic study, with "tincture of time" will solve most of these problems, obviating the need for an exploratory laparotomy, which is often fruitless and may be harmful.

REFERENCES

1. Shandling B: Laparotomy for rectal bleeding. Pediatrics 35:787, 1965
2. Kraut J, Powell R, Hruby M, Lloyd-Still J: Menetrier's disease in childhood: Report of two cases and a review of the literature. J Pediatr Surg 16:707, 1987
3. Mestre J, Andres J: Hereditary hemorrhagic telangiectasia causing hematemesis in an infant. J Pediatr 101:577, 1982
4. Alavi A: Scintigraphic demonstration of acute gastrointestinal bleeding. Gastrointest Radiol 5:208, 1980
5. Sunaryo F, Boyle J, Ziegler M, Heyman S: Primary nonspecific ileal ulceration as a cause of massive rectal bleeding. Pediatrics 68:247, 1981
6. Abrahamson J, Shandling B: Intestinal hemangiomata in childhood, a syndrome for diagnosis: A collective review. J Pediatr Surg 8:4, 1973
7. Mellish RW: Multiple hemangiomas of the gastrointestinal tract in children. Am J Surg 121:412, 1971
8. Cavett CM, Selby JH Jr, Hamilton JL, Williamson JW: Arteriovenous malformation in chronic gastrointestinal bleeding. Ann Surg 185:116, 1977
9. Redondo D, Swenson O: Gastrointestinal bleeding associated with gonadal aplasia. Surgery 61:285, 1967
10. Jona JZ, Kwan HC, Bjelan M, Raffensperger JG: Disseminated intravascular coagulation after excision of giant hemangioma. Am J Surg 127:588, 1974
11. Freier S, Kletter B: Milk allergy in infants and young children. Clin Pediatr 9:449, 1970
12. Gryboski JC: Gastrointestinal milk allergy in infants. Pediatrics 40:354, 1967
13. Eastham EJ, Walker WA: Effect of cow's milk on the gastrointestinal tract: A persistent dilemma for the pediatrician. Pediatrics 60:477, 1977
14. Krivit W, Good RA: Aldrich's syndrome (thrombocytopenia, eczema, and infection in infants). J Dis Child 97:137, 1959
15. Baldini MG: Nature of the platelet defect in the Wiskott–Aldrich syndrome. Ann NY Acad Sci 201:434, 1972
16. Ekberg M, Nilsson IM, Dennebert T: Coagulation studies in hemolytic uremic syndrome and thrombotic thrombocytopenic purpura. Acta Med Scand 196:373, 1974
17. Olgaard K, Madsen S, Jacobsen SV: Recurrent attacks of hemolytic anemia, thrombocytopenia and uremia—hemolytic uremic syndrome? Acta Med Scand 196:541, 1974
18. Berman W Jr: The hemolytic-uremic syndrome: Initial clinical presentation mimicking ulcerative colitis. J Pediatr 81:275, 1972
19. Beighton PH, Murdoch JL, Votteler T: Gastrointestinal complications of the Ehlers-Danlos syndrome. Gut 10:1004, 1969

20. Eddy DD, Farber EM: Pseudoxanthoma elasticum. Arch Dermatol 86:729, 1962

21. McEntyre RL, Raffensperger JG: Surgical complications of Ehlers–Danlos syndrome in children. J Pediatr Surg 12:531, 1977

22. Hollander M, Tabingo R, Stankewick WR: Successful treatment of massive intestinal hemorrhage due to hookworm infection in a neonate. J Pediatr 82:332, 1973

23. Bergman GE, Philippidis P, Naiman JL: Severe gastrointestinal hemorrhage and anemia after therapeutic doses of aspirin in normal children. J Pediatr 88:501, 1976

SECTION VII

Anomalies of the Gastrointestinal Tract

This section deals with the anomalies of the gastrointestinal tract, most of which are obstructive lesions occurring anywhere from the stomach to the anus. This important group of diseases accounts for a major portion of the operations performed in newborn infants.

When there is an atresia or other form of complete obstruction, the symptoms commence soon after birth. Surprisingly, a partial obstruction may be tolerated well for months or even years. Thus, a child with a duodenal stenosis or Hirschsprung's disease may present a diagnostic problem at an age well beyond the newborn period. Anomalies of intestinal rotation and fixation are notorious in this regard because the child's symptoms may be relatively mild and intermittent until there is an abdominal catastrophe, such as a midgut volvulus or a complete intestinal obstruction. Intestinal duplications, although congenital, often produce symptoms in older infants or children. These fascinating lesions must be considered in a child with an unexplained intestinal obstruction, mass, or bleeding.

We have included a chapter on the management of infants with short gut syndrome (Chapter 69) because some infants with intestinal atresia are left with barely enough intestine to sustain life. The principles of management of the baby with a short gut apply to every newborn who has had an intestinal resection. The same principles of care, involving refinements in both enteral and parenteral nutrition, that have allowed us to maintain infants with extensive intestinal resections have brought to light a new and poorly understood group of diseases, which at this time, for lack of a better term, are called "functional intestinal obstructions." The afflicted patients are infants who clinically and radiologically appear to have mechanical intestinal obstructions. Yet at exploration the bowel is grossly in continuity. Thus far, studies of intestinal innervation have failed to shed much light on these problems. Formerly, these infants died from malnutrition soon after an exploratory operation. They now survive for indefinite periods of time with parenteral nutrition. We have included these diseases in the chapter on uncommon forms of neonatal intestinal obstruction (Chapter 68) because these infants are almost always operated on at some point in the course of their disease, and it behooves surgeons to recognize the problem as one for which we have no surgical cure.

Hirschsprung's disease is a classic, major problem in pediatric surgery. This many-faceted problem may occur as an intestinal obstruction in a newborn baby and should be considered in the differential diagnosis of constipation in older children. The pediatric surgical literature is replete with articles and textbooks that delve with great detail into the pathology, diagnosis, and treatment of this disease. This disease continues to be a highly controversial subject. We have merely summarized the salient features of Hirschsprung's disease in the light of our extensive personal experience with large numbers of patients, many of whom have been followed for over 40 years.

At the Children's Memorial Hospital, we have benefited from the contributions of Doctors Willis Potts, Orvar Swenson, and Douglas Stephens to our knowledge of anomalies of the anus and rectum. This is another controversial area in pediatric surgery. Consequently, we have merely attempted to distill the experience at our own hospital.

Embryology is the basic science of this section, in that it will provide the reader with knowledge in understanding the pathogenesis of these congenital intestinal lesions. It is especially important to understand rotation and fixation of the intestine in relation to volvulus, atresia, and intestinal hernias. Some of this information is also discussed in Chapter 23, since the umbilicus is the central point of intrauterine intestinal development.

62
Intestinal Obstruction in the Neonate

Vomiting, abdominal distention, and failure to pass normal meconium stools are, in varying degrees, symptoms common to the various forms of intestinal obstruction seen in newborn infants. The vomitus is usually but not always bile-stained. The loss of gastric, biliary, pancreatic, and intestinal secretions rapidly leads to hypovolemia, dehydration, and acid-base imbalance. Further, the aspiration of vomitus causes airway obstruction, followed by a chemical and bacterial pneumonia. Abdominal distention is directly proportional to the level of the obstruction. When it is severe, the diaphragms are elevated and respiration is impaired. The gastrointestinal tract is sterile at birth, but as the baby is born, he or she will aspirate bacteria. These swallowed organisms reach the obstruction, proliferate, and cause sepsis as they enter the circulation through a frank perforation or through damaged intestinal mucosa. This sequence of events can be forestalled by prompt diagnosis, preoperative resuscitation, and an operation that relieves the obstruction. Early diagnosis rests on a high index of suspicion among nurses and physicians who care for newborn infants. Resuscitation commences with the passage of a gastric tube and the administration of intravenous fluids and antibiotics. Relief of the obstruction and restoration of continuity of the gastrointestinal tract poses a major challenge for the surgeon.

Table 62–1 presents a record of 346 cases of neonatal intestinal obstruction requiring surgery at the Children's Memorial Hospital in Chicago from July 1970 through 1987. During this period, there were few changes in surgical technique from previous years, but our ability to provide long-term nutritional and respiratory support has improved.

ETIOLOGY

The orderly development of the gastrointestinal tract is sufficiently well understood that plausible though often controversial explanations may be offered for the errors in development that result in congenital obstructions.[1] The most critical period commences with the fifth week of embryologic life, when the elongation of the midgut, which comprises the intestine from the duodenum to the midtransverse colon, begins to grow at a more rapid rate than the embryo. The growing intestine pushes out into the coelom of the yolk stalk, where its apex is still connected by the omphalomesenteric duct. With continued elongation of the intestine, all the bowel supplied by the superior mesenteric artery lies outside the embryonic cavity. During the tenth week, the intestine normally returns to the abdominal cavity. During this phase of development, intestinal rotation results in the eventual normal placement of the prearterial loop, which includes the duodenojejunal junction, to the left of the superior mesenteric artery and the postarterial loops (or the ileocecal portion) to the right. This normal process of intestinal rotation is accompanied by fixation of the bowel to the posterior abdominal wall. The abnormalities, which are described in more detail in this and later chapters, take place during the critical tenth week, when the bowel is returning to the abdominal cavity.

There has been some controversy about a possible phase of epithelial occlusion of the gastrointestinal tract. Tandler observed epithelial occlusion of the duodenum in embryos during the sixth to the seventh weeks and concluded that membranous atresias may result from a failure of recanalization.[2] These observations were confirmed by Lynn and Espinas, who studied 68 human embryos.[3] There was evidence of epithelial plugging of the lumen of the duodenum in 20 specimens. In 6 other specimens, epithelial occlusion was observed at various levels of the jejunum, ileum, and colon.

Atresias of the small intestine also may be explained as the result of an intrauterine vascular accident.[4,5] Louw and Barnard performed the classic experiments, which consisted of ligating the mesenteric vessels of fetal pups

TABLE 62–1. NEONATAL INTESTINAL OBSTRUCTIONS, 1970–1987

Level of Obstruction	Patients Alive	Patients Dead, and Cause of Death
Pyloric web	3	1 Epidermolysis bullosa
Malrotation, duodenal obstruction	60	1 Trisomy 13
Gangrenous volvulus, with malrotation	11	5 Total intestinal gangrene
Duodenal atresia, stenosis, annular pancreas	109	4 Not operated, Down's syndrome 2 Heart disease, Down's syndrome 1 SIDS[a] (home) 1 TEF 2 Multiple anomalies
Jejunal atresia, stenosis	50	1 Pierre-Robin syndrome with aspiration 1 Delayed diagnosis, perforation with sepsis 1 Short gut, sepsis, bleeding at 1 year
Ileal atresia and stenosis	25	1 Multiple atresia 1 Gastroschisis 1 Short gut, died with liver disease at 8 months
Colon atresia	14	1 Leakage at colostomy closure
Simple meconium ileus	17	1 Premature infant, sepsis
Meconium ileus with perforation, gangrene	7	2 Sepsis, shock
Small left colon syndrome, operated by error	2	
Intussusception	2	
Unusual	5	4 Intestinal hypoperistalsis and malrotation
Hirschsprung's disease	40	1 Overwhelming enterocolitis, not operated 1 Total aganglionosis, delayed diagnosis, sepsis
Total	345	33 deaths—90% survival

[a] SIDS, sudden infant death syndrome; TEF, tracheoesophageal fistula.

to demonstrate the pathogenesis of intestinal atresia.[6] Initially, after mesenteric vessel ligation, the devitalized intestine disintegrates. Since the intestine is sterile, there is only meconium peritonitis, which clears, leaving a few adhesions and the sealed ends of the bowel. The pathology is identical to that seen in most infants with jejunal–ileal atresia. The clinical evidence that supports the theory of an intrauterine vascular accident is the finding of squamous epithelium and lanugo hair distal to the atresia. This indicates that at one time the intestine was patent to swallowed amniotic fluid.[7] Further evidence found at operation consists of an anomaly of rotation, varying degrees of peritonitis, and loss of mesenteric vessels. Intrauterine volvulus, incarceration of the intestine in the umbilical ring, and intussusception have all been implicated in atresia.[8–10]

Intestinal obstruction also may be associated with cystic fibrosis of the pancreas, a systemic genetic disease. Finally, congenital absence of ganglion cells in the myenteric plexus, or Hirschsprung's disease, is an important cause of intestinal obstruction in the neonate. Even though the diagnosis may not be made until much later, a careful history will reveal that the infant failed to pass meconium during the first 24 hours of his life.

MATERNAL FACTORS

Hydramnios during pregnancy is a sign of an abnormal fetus. In one series of 74 mothers with polyhydramnios during pregnancy, 27 percent of the infants had severe congenital abnormalities—8 percent had gastrointestinal tract obstructions. Fetal ultrasonography is particularly indicated in mothers with polyhydramnios. In many centers, this test is becoming a part of routine prenatal care. The diagnosis of intestinal atresia can be made with great accuracy before the baby is born, ensuring speedy care at birth.[12,13] Maternal viral infections, diabetes, and eclampsia during the first trimester are also associated with a higher incidence of abnormal infants.

The maternal ingestion of drugs may cause symptoms in the infant that simulate an intestinal obstruction. The administration of magnesium sulfate to eclamptic women is associated with hypermagnesemia, which depresses smooth muscle activity in the baby.[14] The symptoms of lethargy, respiratory depression, and failure to pass meconium must be differentiated from those due to a mechanical obstruction. Maternal narcotic addiction has long been known to cause abdominal distention and vomiting in the newborn.[15,16] The family history is important as well because if a sibling has had a birth defect, especially cystic fibrosis of the pancreas or Hirschsprung's disease, the chances that another baby will be affected are increased.

SIGNS AND SYMPTOMS

Any newborn infant who vomits, spits up, or regurgitates must be carefully examined. The first question is, "What color is the vomitus?" Green or bile-stained vomitus must be considered the result of a mechanical obstruction or some other serious illness. A baby with a high obstruction, such as duodenal atresia, will vomit earlier than a baby with a low obstruction. Abdominal distention is another sign. Abdominal distention present at the time of birth is more likely due to ascites or an abdominal mass than to an obstruction, but with a low obstruction, distention develops during the first 24 to 48 hours of life. Babies with an upper intestinal obstruction may have only minimal signs of abdominal distention and may actually have a scaphoid abdomen after vomiting or gastric decompression. The normal infant will pass 50 to 250 g of dark green, tenacious meconium stool within the first 24 hours. Preterm infants, weighing 1500 g at birth, commonly have a delayed passage of the first stool. Twenty percent will have no stool during their first 48 hours. This is particularly true of those who have the respiratory distress syndrome, which delays intestinal motility.[17] A baby with an atresia may still pass a few plugs of gray, puttylike material, which may even be bile-stained. Thus, one must make careful inquiries into the character and volume of the stool before deciding that it is normal meconium.

PHYSICAL EXAMINATION

Simple observation of the neonate is very rewarding. Lethargy and hypotonia may be the earliest signs of sepsis secondary to intestinal perforation and peritonitis. A respiratory rate over 40 breaths/minute or retractions suggests pneumonia or a pool of vomitus in the pharynx. One should observe specifically for stigmata of Down's syndrome and other genetic abnormalities, as well as for obvious congenital defects, such as an imperforate anus. When one defect is found, others must be suspected. Jaundice frequently is associated with high intestinal obstruction. Examination of the abdomen commences with observation for distention, asymmetry, cyanosis, enlarged veins, and peristaltic waves. Visible peristalsis is normal in small, premature infants who have thin abdominal walls. Light palpation is necesasry to feel dilated loops of intestine, areas of increased density, or discrete masses, such as meconium ileus, a mass of necrotic bowel, or a duplication of the intestine. Tenderness, the all-important sign of perforation or intestinal gangrene, is difficult to evaluate in a small infant. The baby who cries, grimaces, or pulls up the legs during abdominal palpation is saying, "My tummy is tender." Infants never exhibit abdominal rigidity, but distention with a gray, ecchymotic appearance of the abdominal wall is practically diagnostic for intestinal necrosis. Auscultation of the abdomen is not as helpful in the evaluation of a newborn as in an older child. However, the total absence of intestinal sounds may help when the diagnostic possibilities are paralytic ileus caused by sepsis, central nervous system damage, and mechanical obstruction. Ascitic fluid transmits the cardiac sounds to the abdomen. A distended scrotum is another sign of intraperitoneal fluid secondary to an intestinal perforation. A rectal examination with the fifth finger is always performed. This will rule out an imperforate anus hidden in a deep anal cleft. The passage of copious amounts of green meconium after the examination rules out an atresia but not Hirschsprung's disease. The presence of a bit of gray material suggests an obstruction, whereas the passage of a firm, white plug, followed by normal meconium, is compatible with either the meconium plug syndrome or Hirschsprung's disease. An obstruction at any level will result in a small, unused rectum that feels tight on the examining finger. The rectosigmoid angle is so low in a newborn that there is often the sensation of a stenosis or even complete rectal obstruction at the tip of the finger.

The physical examination is not complete without the passage of a nasogastric tube. This simple maneuver will rule out choanal and esophageal atresia, and the aspiration of copious amounts of thick green material practically clinches the diagnosis of an intestinal obstruction. After choanal atresia is excluded, the tube is removed and reinserted through the infant's mouth, so that the nasal passage remains unobstructed for respiration. If there are signs of sepsis, the gastric aspirate is stained for bacteria and then cultured.

RADIOLOGIC EVALUATION

Upright and supine roentgenograms of the abdomen are most valuable in the diagnosis of neonatal intestinal obstruction. No other radiologic study is required in the majority of cases. A normal infant swallows air with his first breath.[18] Air reaches the proximal bowel within 30 minutes and the colon 3 to 4 hours later. It should be possible to identify air in the rectum by 6 and certainly by 12 to 18 hours of age. There are no air–fluid levels in the upright view of a normal infant. A clear distinction between the small and large bowel is extremely difficult during the neonatal period, since the haustrations of the colon, the mucosal folds of the small bowel, and other distinguishing features are not readily apparent. Gas normally is present throughout the small intestine until the child is 1.5 to 2 years of age. Infants with respiratory distress or an H-type tracheoesophageal fistula may swallow a large amount of air, which causes intestinal distention. On the other hand, newborn infants with central nervous system damage and those born to heavily sedated mothers experience delayed passage of gas through the intestine. The initial roentgenogram should also include the chest to rule out other lesions and to check on the proper placement of the gastric tube and any vascular catheter that may have been inserted.

Dilated loops of intestine with air–fluid levels are characteristic of intestinal obstructions. An upper gastrointestinal series with contrast material adds nothing to plain films with swallowed air for contrast. Furthermore, anything given to the infant can be vomited and aspirated. The only indication for an upper gastrointestinal examination is a partial obstruction that cannot be definitely diagnosed on the plain films. In this situation, the baby's vomitus is at first clear and then bile-stained. The plain roentgenograms demonstrate gas throughout the abdomen, possibly with only a suggestion of duodenal dilatation. This clinical situation is most common with partial duodenal obstruction due to a malrotation. As we will see later, a contrast enema is indicated for the baby who has signs of a low intestinal obstruction, in order to differentiate among ileal atresia, meconium ileus, and Hirschsprung's disease. The barium enema will also definitely make the diagnosis of colon atresia, and a Gastrograffin enema is therapeutic for meconium ileus.

In addition to clinical and roentgenographic evaluation, the following studies are performed on every infant with an intestinal obstruction requiring an operation. Tests for blood glucose, bilirubin, blood urea nitrogen, and hematocrit and blood typing and crossmatching are performed on the baby's admission to the surgical nursery. Serum electrolyte evaluations are most helpful in the treatment of an infant who has been vomiting for several days, but these are not routinely performed before an operation unless there is dehydration, convulsions, twitching, or other signs of metabolic disturbance. Platelet counts and blood cultures are obtained if there is evidence of sepsis or intestinal perforation.

RESUSCITATION

Fluid resuscitation is most important and must be carried out before operation. When the vomitus and gastric aspirate are bile-stained, lactated Ringer's solution in 10 percent glucose with additional potassium is the usual replacement fluid. The volume and rate of administration are based on the clinical signs of hypovolemia and weight loss from birth. Weight loss is most reliable in infants with an upper intestinal obstruction. With lower obstructions, fluid is sequestered in loops of bowel and is lost to the circulation even though weight loss is minimal. When it is anticipated that an intestinal anastomosis will be made, the infant is given therapeutic doses of an aminoglycoside and penicillin or ampicillin before operation. With the exception of infants who have signs of peritonitis or gangrenous intestine, several hours or days may be profitably spent in preoperative preparation. The correction of hyperbilirubinemia, hypoglycemia, respiratory distress, and electrolyte disturbances have decreased anesthetic complications and improved survival. One milligram of vitamin K is given before operation.

REFERENCES

1. Gray SW, Skandalakis JE: Embryology for Surgeons. Philadelphia, Saunders, 1972, pp 129–36
2. Tandler J: Zur Entwicklungsgeschichte des menschlichen duodenum in Fruben embryonelsadien. Morph Johrb 29:186, 1900
3. Lynn HB, Epinas EE: Intestinal atresia: An attempt to relate location to embryologic processes. Arch Surg 79:357, 1959
4. Louw JH: Congenital intestinal atresia and stenosis in the newborn: Observation on its pathogenesis and treatment. Ann R Coll Surg Engl 25:209, 1959
5. Louw JH: Jejuno-ileal atresia and stenosis. J Pediatr Surg 1:8, 1966
6. Louw JH, Barnard CN: Congenital intestinal atresia: An attempt to relate location to embryologic processes. Observations on its origins. Lancet 2:1065, 1955
7. Santulli TV, Blanc WA: Congenital atresia of the intestine: Pathogenesis and treatment. Ann Surg 154:939, 1961
8. Grosfield JL, Clatworthy HW Jr: The nature of ileal atresia due to intrauterine intussusception. Arch Surg 100:714, 1970
9. Todani T, Tabuchi K, Tanaka S: Intestinal atresia due to intrauterine intussusception: Analysis of 24 cases in Japan. J Pediatr Surg 10:445, 1975
10. Shafie M, Waag KL, Spitz L: Ileal atresia secondary to antenatal strangulation by a ruptured omphalocele. J Pediatr Surg 7:64, 1972
11. Moya F, Apgar V, Janes HS, Berrien L: Hydramnios and congenital anomalies: Study of a series of patients. JAMA 173:1552, 1960

12. Samuel N, Dicker D, Feldberg D, Goldman J: Ultrasound diagnosis and management of fetal intestinal obstruction and volvulus in utero. J Perinat Med 12:333, 1984
13. Kurjak A, Gugolja D, Kuglar A, Latin V: Ultrasound diagnosis and perinatal management of surgically correctable fetal malformations. Ultrasound Med Biol 10:443, 1984
14. Sokal MM, Koenigsberger MR, Rose JS, et al: Neonatal hypermagnesemia and the meconium plug syndrome. N Engl J Med 286:823, 1972
15. Reddy AM, Harper RG, Stern G: Observation on heroin and methadone withdrawal in the newborn. Pediatrics 48:353, 1971
16. Zelson C, Rubio E, Wasserman E: Neonatal narcotic addiction: 10-year observation. Pediatrics 48:178, 1971
17. Jhaveri M, Meenakshik W, Savitri P, Kumar M: Passage of the first stool in very low birthweight infants. Pediatrics 79:1005, 1987
18. Boraedis AC, Gershon-Cohen J: Aeration of respiratory and gastrointestinal tracts during the first minutes of neonatal life. Radiology 67:407, 1956

63
Pyloric and Duodenal Obstruction

PYLORIC ATRESIA

Congenital pyloric atresia accounts for less than 1 percent of all gastrointestinal tract anomalies. The diagnosis is often delayed because the vomitus is not bile-stained. Thus, the physician is misled into thinking that the vomiting is on a functional rather than a mechanical basis. There is a solid mucosal diaphragm that may be the result of a vascular or mechanical injury to the fetus (Fig. 63–1).[1–5] There is a familial occurrence, and an autosomal recessive transmission is suspected. This lesion must be differentiated from a perforated antral membrane, which causes a partial obstruction in older children and which may be confused with pyloric stenosis. One of our patients with pyloric atresia also had epidermolysis bullosa, an association that has been observed by others.[6,7] The lesion may be familial. Malheur et al. described atresia of the pylorus and the first part of the duodenum in seven children from three families.[8] The plain roentgenogram will demonstrate a dilated stomach with no distal air.

Treatment

At operation, the exact location of the web is found by advancing a firm, 14 French catheter, which has been passed through the mouth by the anesthesiologist, to the obstruction. A vertical incision is then made from the stomach to the duodenum, crossing the web, which is then excised. Bleeding is controlled, and the mucosa is approximated with a continuous 5-0 catgut suture. The vertical incision is then closed horizontally to further enlarge the pyloroduodenal junction. A gastroduodenostomy is indicated only when the stomach and duodenum are completely separated. A gastrojejunostomy should never be performed because of the risk of a marginal ulcer and the blind loop syndrome.

DUODENAL ATRESIA AND STENOSIS AND ANNULAR PANCREAS

Symptoms, roentgenographic findings, and treatment are the same for all of the intrinsic duodenal obstructions. The obstruction occurs below, at, or above the ampulla of Vater, but in most cases early biliary vomiting, the hallmark of duodenal obstruction, indicates an obstruction below the bile duct.

Pathology

Intrinsic duodenal obstructions vary from a narrowing of the lumen, which will admit swallowed gas and small amounts of secretions but not formula, to complete discontinuity of the duodenum and jejunum. Most commonly, the duodenum and jejunum are in continuity, and the intrinsic obstruction is a membranous web.

Annular pancreas is a ring or collar of pancreatic tissue that encircles the second portion of the duodenum. The ring may be incomplete, consisting of two arms of the pancreas that fail to meet anteriorly. A pancreatic duct, most probably the accessory duct of Santorini, lies within the anterior portion of a complete ring. There is no satisfactory explanation for an annular pancreas. In order for an annular pancreas to produce an obstruction, there must be an associated stenosis or atresia. Furthermore, in our own series of 24 infants and children afflicted with annular pancreas, 18 had severe associated congenital anomalies, such as Down's syndrome, tracheoesophageal fistula, and cyanotic heart disease. It has been associated with congenital absence of the gallbladder and obstruction of the bile duct.[9,10] The duodenum above the obstruction becomes tremendously enlarged and is often half the size of a normal newborn infant's stomach. The wall of the duodenum is thickened because of obstructed peristaltic activity. The continued

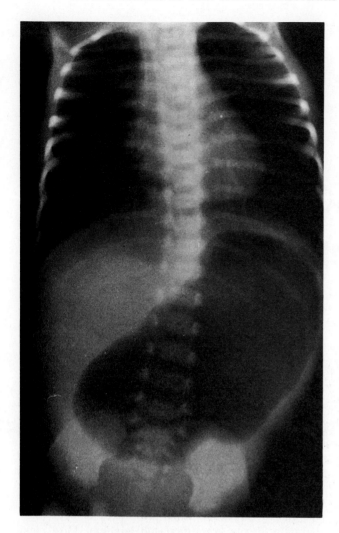

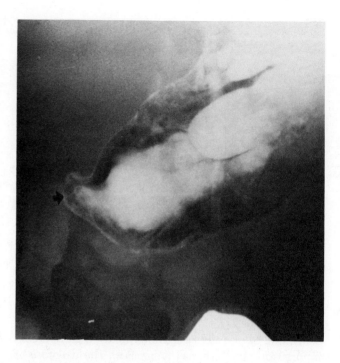

Figure 63–1. Pyloric atresia in an infant with epidermolysis bullosa. Air distention is limited to the stomach, with no distal gas. **Left.** Supine film. **Above.** Barium study. The arrow indicates the pyloric web.

peristaltic activity also may produce an important variation of the simple membranous obstruction, termed the "windsock" duodenum by Bill and Pope in 1954 (Fig. 63–2).[11] As can be seen in the illustration, the duodenum is dilated below the point of obstruction due to the prolapsing membrane. Because of this, anastomoses have been performed in the duodenum below the membrane.[12,13]

Associated Anomalies

Congenital anomalies in other organ systems are found in approximately half the babies with duodenal stenosis and atresia.[14,15] Table 63–1 lists the anomalies found in a series of 503 cases of duodenal stenosis and atresia, collected from the Surgical Section of the American Academy of Pediatrics.[16] Reports from Australia and England confirm this experience. The incidence of Down's syndrome in our series of cases is 40 percent, which is

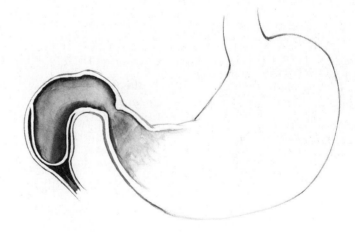

Figure 63–2. The windsock duodenal web. In a case such as this, the duodenum is dilated, and if the duodenum is opened below the web, it is possible to mistakenly perform an anastomosis below the obstruction.

>>><>n<>An<> An<> An infant who vomits bile and also has the stigmata of Down's syndrome almost certainly has a duodenal obstruction. The diagnosis is made by finding the classic double bubble sign on an upright roentgenogram. Supine films are more difficult to interpret because there is no air–fluid level (Fig. 63–4). A partial duodenal obstruction, whether due to an intrinsic stenosis, annular pancreas, or a malrotation, will cause some gastric and perhaps duodenal dilatation to appear on the plain x-ray, with gas below the level of obstruction. In this situation, a cautiously performed barium swallow will demonstrate the partial obstruction (Fig. 63–5).

A partial duodenal obstruction may not cause symptoms for many years. The first will be an episode of vomiting, with green-tinged vomitus. Close questioning and examination will usually reveal evidence of chronic poor nutrition, but unless there is a secondary peptic ulcer there is, suprisingly, no pain. Figure 63–6 illustrates a hugely dilated duodenum in a 12-year-old girl who had suffered from recurrent episodes of vomiting for over a year. At operation, there was an intraluminal web with a 3 mm opening.

Treatment

Intrinsic duodenal obstruction definitely is not a surgical emergency. Since there is no concern over peritonitis or gangrenous intestine, all possible metabolic and respiratory complications may be corrected before operation. We treated a premature infant with the respiratory distress syndrome with assisted ventilation and total intravenous alimentation for 3 weeks before operation for a

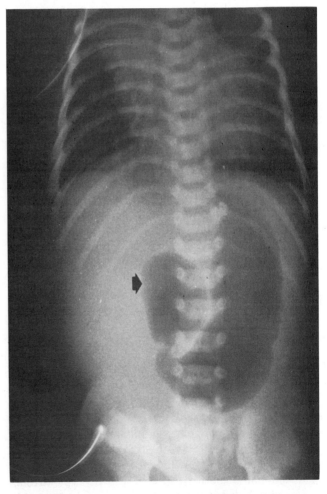

Figure 63–3. This is an obstruction of the first portion of the duodenum above the bile ducts, one of the rare instances in which an infant with an obstruction does not vomit bile. The arrow marks the duodenal bulb.

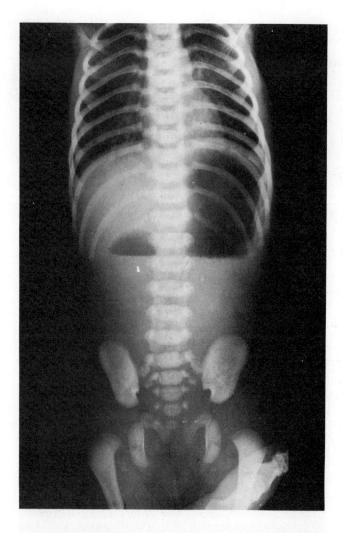

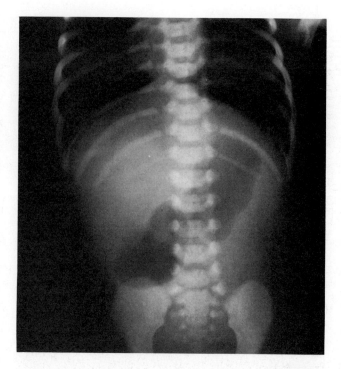

Figure 63–4. Left. This is the classic double bubble sign of duodenal atresia, seen on an upright x-ray. **Above.** A supine film demonstrates the dilated stomach and duodenum; it does not show air–fluid levels.

duodenal atresia. At least half of our infants with duodenal obstruction are jaundiced, and anesthesia and blood transfusion would further increase their bilirubin levels. In these cases, the infant is properly hydrated and treated with phototherapy until the indirect bilirubin is below 10 mg/100 ml. There are two options in the surgical treatment of intrinsic duodenal obstruction.

1. Direct excision of an obstructing web with plastic repair of the duodenum (Fig. 63–7)
2. Bypass of the obstruction with a duodenoduodenostomy (Fig. 63–8)

Operation. A transverse, supraumbilical incision provides excellent exposure of the duodenum and the rest of the small intestine. Initially, the small bowel is eviscerated onto warm moist packs so it can be explored for other sites of obstruction. If there is a malrotation, the cecum and ascending colon are freed from the right side of the abdomen and moved to the left. By also freeing the rudimentary ligament of Treitz, the entire duodenum may be seen. Often, there is a high, or mobile,

cecum that also facilitates exposure of the duodenum. The gallbladder is observed, and one must be certain that there is no preduodenal portal vein. The anesthesiologist is asked to pass a firm, size 14, red rubber catheter into the stomach. This is then grasped and directed into the duodenum. If the duodenum is in continuity and there is no annular pancreas, the catheter will stop at the site of an intraduodenal web (Fig. 63–7). The web often will protrude down the bowel lumen beyond what appears to be a ring of tissue at its base. The duodenum is held up with stay sutures, and a vertical incision is made directly over the web, which will be covered with mucosa on either side. It is now extremely important to identify the ampulla of Vater, which may be at any location, on either side of the web. If there is a small fenestration in the web, the ampulla most often is on the medial posterior edge of the opening. Magnifying loupes are helpful, and the gallbladder may be squeezed to observe drops of bile from the ampulla. To be certain, it is cannulated with a size 3.5 plastic feeding tube. With this accomplished, a V-shaped portion of the web is excised, and its edges are sutured to control hemor-

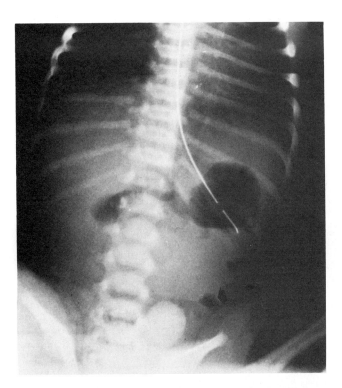
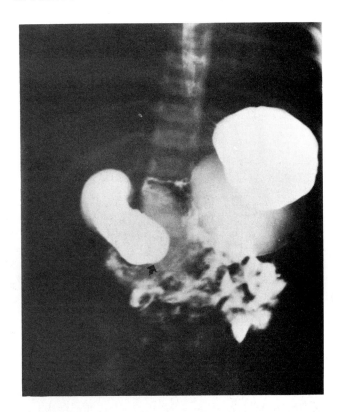

Figure 63–5. With a partial duodenal obstruction, the roentgenograms demonstrate a variable degree of gastric and duodenal obstruction, with some air below the duodenum. A barium study is necessary to confirm the diagnosis. **Left.** Plain film showing minimal duodenal distention and a few bubbles of air in the small intestine. **Right.** A barium swallow outlines the dilated duodenum, which ends in a rounded, sacklike configuration. Air and barium are also seen in the distal small bowel. This infant had a windsock web with a small central opening.

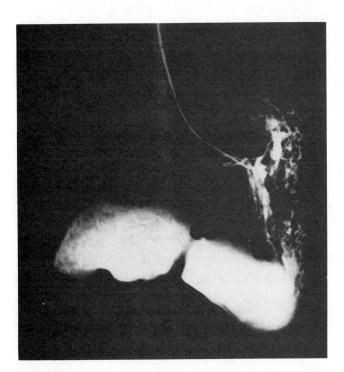

Figure 63–6. Upper gastrointestinal examination of a 12-year-old girl who suffered from episodic vomiting. She had an intraluminal duodenal web.

rhage. The vertical incision is now closed transversely with one layer of interrupted 5-0 or 6-0 nonabsorbable sutures.

A duodenoduodenostomy is chosen when there is either an annular pancreas or a visible separation of the two ends of the duodenum or if one cannot be sure that a web is present (Fig. 63–8). The entire duodenum is exposed by reflecting the hepatic flexure of the colon downward. The obstruction is again identified by the passage of a firm catheter. Stay sutures are inserted to mark the ends of a transverse incision at the most dependent portion of the dilated duodenum. The distal, collapsed duodenum is then mobilized and brought up to lie, without kinking, next to the dilated proximal bowel. Sutures are inserted and tied at either end of the proposed suture line; then parallel incisions are made in the proximal and distal bowel. The anastomosis must be made as large as possible—twice the width of the distal bowel is a good rule of thumb. The posterior sutures are placed and tied. Before closure of the anterior layer, a catheter must be passed distally and saline injected while the operator is searching for another obstruction. In addition, a catheter must be passed into the stomach to avoid the terrible embarrassment of making an incision below a web. An anterior row of interrupted sutures

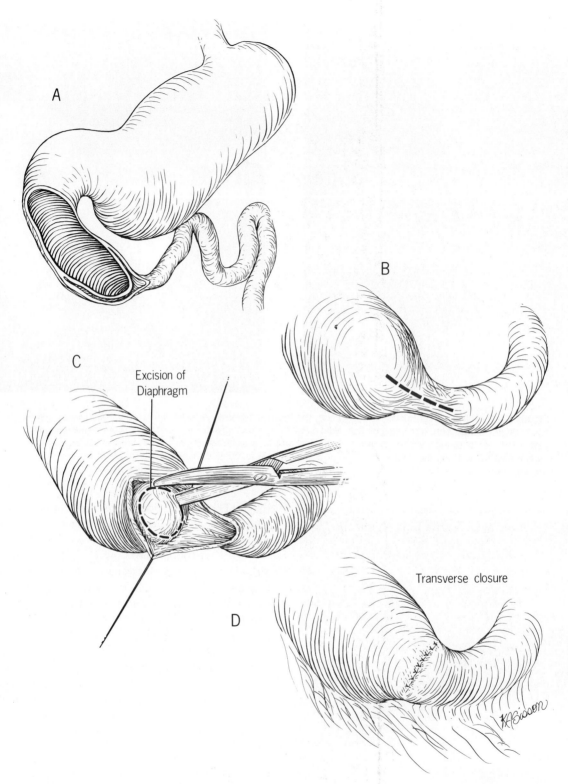

Figure 63–7. A. Duodenotomy with excision of a windsock web. **B.** The incision must be placed directly over the web, which is localized by passing a catheter from the stomach. **C.** Great care must be taken to identify the ampulla of Vater before excision of a duodenal web. **D.** The duodenum is then closed transversely.

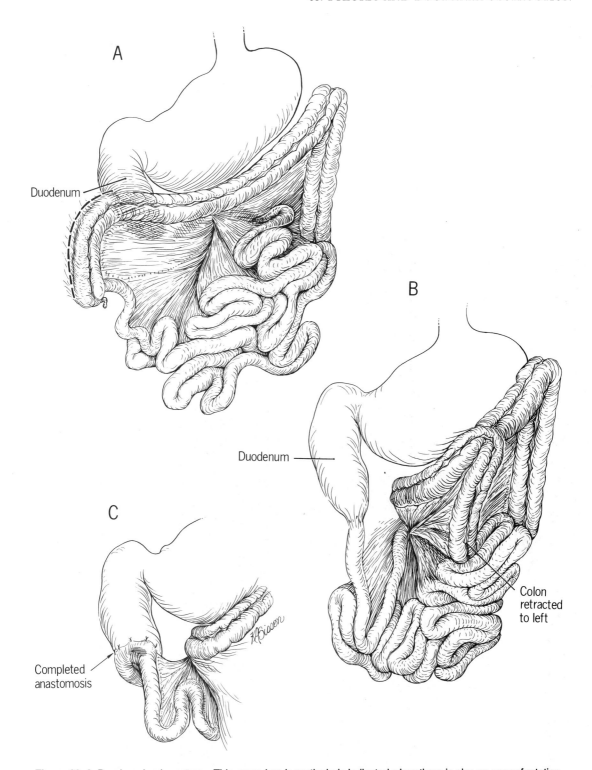

Figure 63–8. Duodenoduodenostomy. This procedure is particularly indicated when there is also an error of rotation because the colon is already away from the duodenum, which pursues a straight course down the right gutter.

will invert the seromuscular layer. The loops of intestine are carefully replaced into the abdomen, with one last look at the area of anastomosis to see if there is kinking that would obstruct. Postoperative recovery of function can be slow if the duodenum was hugely dilated before

the operation. Bile-stained material will return from the tube for prolonged periods of time, but if the abdomen is scaphoid and if stool is passed in response to a rectal examination, the orogastric tube may be removed. If there is no vomiting, small feedings are started the next day. Most often, these infants will tolerate full oral feedings within 5 to 7 days after the operation. If there is recurrent vomiting, gastric retention, and roentgenographic evidence of a dilated, atonic, poorly functioning duodenum, its size can be reduced and function restored by a tapering duodenoplasty.[17-19] This is performed by exposing the length of duodenum from the pylorus to the anastomosis and opening the duodenum anteriorly. If the anastomosis is widely patent, it is left alone, a longitudinal wedge of duodenum is removed, and the incision is closed.

In our series of 109 infants with duodenal atresias, stenosis, and annular pancreas, 4 were not operated on because of Down's syndrome. These infants died. At this time, Down's syndrome is no longer even considered a reason not to operate. There were 5 other deaths due to associated anomalies, and 1 infant died at home, presumably of sudden infant death syndrome. There was a 94 percent survival rate in the 105 infants operated on.

Long-term results in children with duodenal atresia depend on the presence or absence of coexisting congenital anomalies, particularly Down's syndrome.[20] Children with no other defects have normal gastrointestinal function with normal growth and development. However, cholelithiasis has been observed in 2 patients, 9 and 16 years after their operation for duodenal atresia.[21] Each had a stenotic distal common bile duct. In 1977, the first survivor of an operation for duodenal atresia was 60 years old, alive and well.[22]

REFERENCES

1. Ducharme JC, Bensoussan AL: Pyloric atresia. J Pediatr Surg 10:149, 1975
2. Tan K-L, Murugasu JJ: Congenital pyloric atresia in siblings. Arch Surg 105:100, 1973
3. Bronsther B, Nadeau MR, Abrams MW: Congenital pyloric atresia: A report of three cases and a review of the literature. Surgery 69:130, 1971
4. Becker JM, Schneider KM, Fischer AF: Pyloric atresia. Arch Surg 87:413, 1963
5. Wurtenberger H: Gastric atresia. Arch Dis Child 36:161, 1961
6. Korber JS, Glasson MJ: Pyloric atresia associated with epidermolysis bullosa. J Pediatr 90:600, 1977
7. Rosenbloom M, Ratner M: Congenital pyloric atresia in epidermolysis bullosa hepatitis in premature siblings. J Pediatr Surg 22:374, 1987
8. Malheur RE, Salem G, Mishalany H, et al: Pyloroduodenal atresia: A report of three families with several similarly affected children. Pediatr Radiol 3:1, 1975
9. Merrill JR, Raffensperger JG: Pediatric annular pancreas: Twenty years' experience. J Pediatr Surg 11:921, 1976
10. Heij H, Niessen G: Annular pancreas associated with congenital absence of the gallbladder. J Pediatr Surg 22:1033, 1987
11. Bill AH Jr, Pope WM: Congenital duodenal diaphragm. Surgery 35:482, 1954
12. Haller JA Jr, Cahill JL: Combined congenital gastric and duodenal obstruction: Pitfalls in diagnosis and treatment. Surgery 63:503, 1968
13. Swartz RM, Hunter MT, Hartz CR: Reoperation for congenital duodenal diaphragm. Ann Surg 177:441, 1973
14. Young DG, Wilkinson AW: Abnormalities associated with neonatal duodenal obstruction. Surgery 63:832, 1968
15. Reid IS: The pattern of intrinsic duodenal obstructions. Aust NZ J Surg 42:349, 1973
16. Fonkalsrud EW, et al: Congenital atresia and stenosis of the duodenum. Pediatrics 43:79, 1969
17. Sherman JO, Schulten M: Operative correction of duodenomegaly. J Pediatr Surg 9:461, 1974
18. Adzick N, Harrison M, Delorimer A: Tapering duodenoplasty for megaduodenum associated with duodenal atresia. J Pediatr Surg 21:311, 1986
19. Ein S, Shandling B: The late nonfunctioning duodenal atresia repair. J Pediatr Surg 21:798, 1986
20. Stauffer UG, Irving I: Duodenal atresia and stenosis: Long-term results. Prog Pediatr Surg 10:49, 1977
21. Tan H, Jones P, Auldist A: Gallstones and duodenal atresia. Ann Acad Med Singapore 14:604, 1985
22. Madsen CM: Duodenal atresia: 60 years of follow-up. Prog Pediatr Surg 10:61, 1977

64 Malrotation

The term "malrotation" should be reserved for the classic form of duodenal obstruction described by Dr. William Ladd, in which folds of peritoneum running from the cecum to the posterior abdominal wall cross the duodenum.[1] The dudoenum is obstructed by the peritoneal folds and is kinked secondary to its partial rotation to the left. A nongangrenous midgut volvulus accompanies most typical malrotations.

There are many variations of abnormal intestinal rotation, one of which is nonrotation, in which the entire colon and terminal ileum are on the left side of the abdomen, with the duodenum–jejunum on the right. Nonrotation is seen in infants with gastroschisis, omphaloceles, and Bochdalek hernias as well as in asymptomatic older children. The cecum may be in the right upper quadrant, with a normally rotated duodenum. This condition is usually asymptomatic and is frequently seen in infants with biliary atresia. Abnormalities of intestinal fixation, which is the final phase of rotation, account for paraduodenal and paracecal internal hernias as well as the mobile cecum. Nonrotation often is seen in association with intestinal atresia, and a mobile cecum is necessary for an intussusception.[2] We have seen two neonates treated for malrotation who later proved to have Hirschsprung's disease.

EMBRYOLOGY

Intestinal rotation involves the midgut, which becomes the duodenum, small intestine, and colon up to its mid-transverse portion. The superior mesenteric artery, which supplies this portion of the bowel, is the pivotal point about which rotation occurs. The midgut has become differentiated from the foregut and hindgut in the 5 mm embryo, or at about the fourth week of embryonic life. At this time, the gut commences to elongate from a straight-line structure and herniates into the yolk stalk or umbilical cord. The developing liver and left umbilical vein push the duodenojejunal loop down and to the right. Thus, the duodenum initially lies to the right of the superior mesenteric artery. In the 25 to 30 mm embryo, the duodenojejunal loop rotates counterclockwise beneath the artery, where it becomes attached at the ligament of Treitz.[3,4] At this time, loops of small intestine and the cecal segment are still within the umbilical cord. Continued elongation of the intestine takes place while it is outside the abdominal cavity. During the tenth intrauterine week, the coelomic cavity has enlarged sufficiently to permit the return of the intestine. Snyder and Chaffin dissected a 37 mm embryo that demonstrated partial return of the bowel.[5] In their specimen, the duodenojejunal junction was already fixed into its normal position, and jejunal loops had returned to the abdomen, leaving the distal ileum and cecum still in the umbilical stalk. As the ileum and colon (postarterial segment) return to the abdominal cavity, they lengthen to form the splenic flexure and rotate counterclockwise over the superior mesenteric artery until the cecum and terminal ileum lie to the right and the transverse colon is in front of the artery. As it initially returns to the abdomen, the cecum is at the level of the iliac crest. Further growth of the ascending colon increases the distance between the cecum and the liver. Fixation of the intestine commences during the 11th week of life and continues until the postnatal period. In this process, the intestine develops a broad attachment to the posterior abdominal wall, from the ligament of Treitz to the cecum. Abnormalities in fixation result in volvulus or internal hernias.[6]

PATHOLOGY

In complete nonrotation, there is a common mesentery that is not fixed to the posterior abdominal wall. The ileum, at the point of a Meckel's diverticulum, represents the apex of the bowel. The cecum is either in the midabdomen or to the left of the superior mesenteric artery. The duodenum pursues a straight course down the right gutter of the abdomen. This pathology is most typically seen in babies with gastroschisis or omphaloceles.

The pathologic findings in malrotation are variable, but in essence the cecum is found in the right upper quadrant or midabdomen. Bands from the cecum or ascending colon cross the duodenum to the posterolateral abdominal wall. The duodenum lies beneath these bands.[7] As it is traced distally from the pylorus, it is seen to be dilated and curving toward the left. At a point corresponding to the duodenojejunal junction, it narrows and is kinked. The terminal ileum is bound to the proximal jejunum by adhesions, or abnormal peritoneal bands. This creates a narrow pedicle, which with the complete lack of intestinal fixation causes a volvulus in a complete 360 degree clockwise twist. There may even be more than one twist. The duodenal obstruction appears to be more related to the volvulus and to its kinking than to the transduodenal, or Ladd's, bands. The volvulus results in dilated veins and lymphatics in the mesentery and, occasionally, chyle in the peritoneal cavity. Congenital bands obstructing the duodenum may occur in the absence of malrotation.[8]

DIAGNOSIS

Most infants with malrotation vomit bile during their first month of life. There may be a complete obstruction during the first day or two after birth, but this is unusual and should alert the surgeon to an accompanying intraduodenal web even when a malrotation is found. The typical baby takes feedings well and then commences to spit up, until finally he or she vomits green material, and the diagnosis is made. On physical examination, the abdomen rarely is distended because the obstruction is high and the stomach is decompressed by vomiting. Plain films of the abdomen that demonstrate a dilated duodenum or double bubble are diagnostic of a duodenal obstruction, and no further studies are indicated. There is more often a relatively normal intestinal gas pattern with only a suggestion of a dilated duodenum. In this situation, an upper gastrointestinal examination is indicated, rather than a barium enema.

The upper gastrointestinal study affords direct evidence of a partial duodenal obstruction, whereas a barium enema is more difficult to interpret. The ascending colon may be shifted medially, but if barium refluxes into the terminal ileum it will be difficult to localize the cecum.[9] On the other hand, in Simpson et al.'s series, the correct diagnosis of malrotation was made in 22 of 23 patients by use of the upper gastrointestinal examination.[10] Char-

acteristically, the proximal duodenum is dilated. Distally it resembles a corkscrew, and as barium trickles through, the small intestine is seen to occupy the right side of the abdomen (Fig. 64–1).

In older children, there may be recurrent bouts

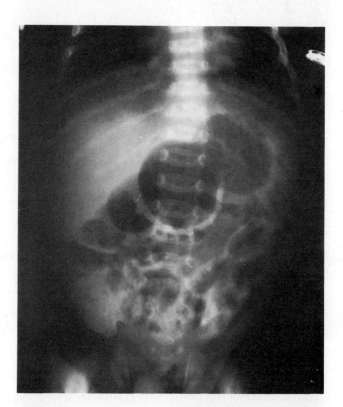

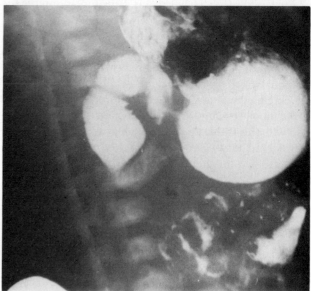

Figure 64–1. This 8-day-old boy first began to spit up his formula and by the sixth day was vomiting bilious material. **Top.** The plain film demonstrates dilatation of the stomach and duodenum, but there is distal gas. **Bottom.** Barium fills the stomach and proximal duodenum but only trickles through a tapered narrowing in the descending duodenum. This is characteristic of malrotation.

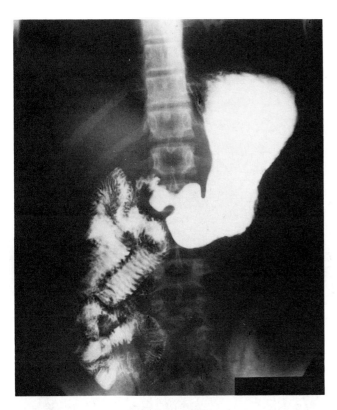

Figure 64–2. Upper gastrointestinal series of a 16-year-old boy with mild, recurrent abdominal pain. There was no nausea or vomiting. On barium enema, his colon was nonrotated. His upper gastrointestinal series demonstrates no obstruction, but the entire small bowel is on the right side of the abdomen.

of colicky abdominal pain, and some have histories of episodic bilious vomiting. Episodes of diarrhea and evidence of malabsorption also have been reported as a result of malrotation. Roentgenograms that demonstrate a partial duodenal obstruction are clearly compatible with these symptoms, but it is more difficult to correlate the child's complaints with the x-ray when there is no duodenal obstruction and only evidence of a nonrotated colon (Fig. 64–2).

TREATMENT

An infant with a symptomatic malrotation is operated on as soon as fluid and electrolyte deficits are corrected. A size 14 rubber tube is inserted through the mouth to decompress the stomach and is later used to ensure patency of the duodenum. A transverse supraumbilical incision will provide adequate exposure. On opening the abdomen, one sees only small bowel, which lies over the cecum and ascending colon. The entire mass of viscera is lifted from the abdomen and placed on warm, moist pads. At the narrowed base of the mesen-

tery, there are usually one or more loops of bowel that appear to lie transversely. This is a volvulus, which must be reduced by a counterclockwise derotation of the bowel (Fig. 64–3A). The cecum is then held up and to the left by an assistant. This demonstrates the Ladd's bands, peritoneal folds that cross the duodenum to the posterior lateral abdominal wall (Fig. 64–3B). These are elevated from the duodenum with tissue forceps and divided with scissors. When all of these folds and strands of connective tissue have been divided, the duodenum may be traced from the pylorus to the jejunum. Frequently, the terminal ileum is attached by peritoneal bands to the proximal jejunum. These must be cautiously divided, with care not to injure the mesenteric vessels. This is an important step, because the juxtaposition of the ileum and the jejunum form a pivotal point for a future volvulus. At the end of this dissection, the intestine with its mesentery should be spread out like an apron over the anterior abdominal wall (Fig. 64–3C). With this completed, the duodenum is again inspected. Further dissection of its lateral wall to divide small strands of fibrous tissue is necessary to completely straighten out kinks that could cause continued obstruction. The duodenum will still tend to curve to the left because it is held attached to the head of the pancreas by its blood supply. When the duodenum is as straight as possible, the previously placed firm catheter is advanced through the pylorus, down the duodenum, and on into the jejunum. This step rules out intrinsic webs. When patency has been proven, the rubber catheter is withdrawn and replaced with a small, plastic gastric tube. If the infant is in good condition, an appendectomy is performed. Return of the intestine commences, first placing the duodenum and jejunum in the right gutter of the abdomen. This loop is followed by others in an orderly fashion until the terminal ileum and cecum are placed in the left upper or midabdomen. Postoperatively, the gastric tube is left on gravity drainage until the infant has passed a stool and drainage has diminished.

RESULTS

All of the 21 infants operated on at our hospital for simple malrotation since 1970 have survived. Malrotation with gangrenous volvulus or other anomalies results in some fatalities. Most associated anomalies involve the gastrointestinal tract.[11]

Postoperatively, adhesive intestinal obstruction is the most common complication after operative repair of a malrotation. Approximately half of the children we have seen with an adhesive intestinal obstruction had a malrotation. This complication may be reduced by using the utmost gentleness in handling the bowel and by replacing it carefully into the abdominal cavity.

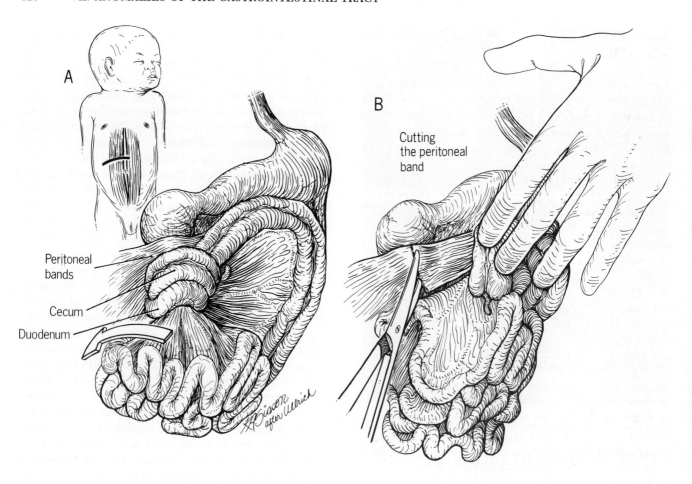

A

Peritoneal
bands

Cecum

Duodenum

B

Cutting
the peritoneal
band

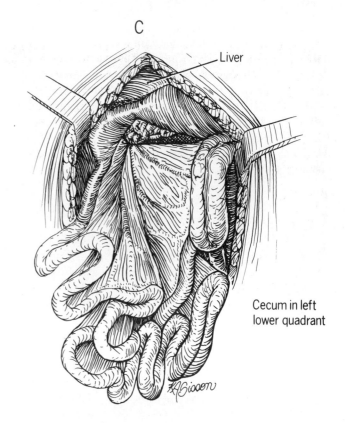

C

Liver

Cecum in left
lower quadrant

Figure 64–3. A. The entire small bowel is elevated from the abdomen, the volvulus is identified, and the entire pedicle of the bowel is rotated to the right. **B.** An assistant then picks up the cecum to place the Ladd's bands on a stretch so they may be identified and divided. **C.** When the operation is completed, the duodenum is straight and the small bowel hangs over the abdominal wall like an apron. The base of the mesentery has been widened to prevent a future volvulus.

MALROTATION WITH GANGRENOUS VOLVULUS

Small segments of localized gangrene are unusual in infants with malrotation. When there is at least 75 cm of uninvolved intestine, the gangrenous segment is resected and a primary end-to-end anastomosis is performed. Unfortunately, the most common situation is a newborn infant who is distended at birth. The combination of abdominal distention, green vomiting, and bloody stools makes the diagnosis of intestinal gangrene. In addition, the abdomen has a bluish gray appearance and is rigid. These infants are in shock and require large volumes of blood and colloid and electrolyte solutions for resuscitation. At operation, the entire small bowel is usually gangrenous (Fig. 64–4). We have been able to save up to 20 cm of jejunum by untwisting the volvulus, injecting a local anaesthetic into the base of the mesentery, and then closing only the abdominal skin. The infant is supported with antibiotics and more fluids, including low molecular weight dextran, and the abdomen is reopened in 18 to 24 hours. If any bowel appears viable at this point, it is saved. The obviously gangrenous bowel is resected, and the two ends are exteriorized. The infant is then kept on intravenous hyperalimentation until the two ends of the bowel can be anastomosed. In our hands, this technique has saved only those infants who have 25 or more cm of viable intestine with an intact ileocecal valve. All of the complications of abnormal intestinal rotation seen in infants may occur in older

children and even in adults.[12] The usual history is one of recurrent abdominal pain with asymptomatic intervals. If the pain is associated with vomiting and roentgenographic findings of a partial duodenal obstruction, the diagnosis and treatment are essentially the same as described for an infant. Unfortunately, the first indication may be the sudden onset of abdominal pain with shock. We have observed four children, aged 4, 12, 13, and 16 years, with abdominal distention, vomiting, and roentgenographic signs of a small intestinal obstruction. Each had a gangrenous midgut volvulus. Three died, and one is still alive on home hyperalimentation.

The diagnosis in other children may be more difficult. Some who are ultimately found to be suffering from malrotation have been diagnosed as having psychosomatic vomiting or abdominal pain. Others may have chronic diarrhea and malabsorption due to a partial volvulus. Properly performed roentgenographic studies of the gastrointestinal tract should lead to the correct diagnosis. A child with vague abdominal pain, which on history seems to be of clear psychogenic origin, is occasionally found to have a nonrotated colon. It is very difficult to correlate symptoms with x-ray findings. If we are to explain the pain on the basis of a volvulus, that pain should be severe and episodic, not daily, mild, and vague. The diagnosis is strengthened if the pain is associated with vomiting. Duodenal obstruction is obviously a clear indication for operation, but if the only positive finding is nonrotation of the colon, the indications for an operation are not so clear. In each of two children, a volvulus of the terminal ileum and cecum was noted on fluoroscopy in the course of a barium enema examination. At operation, the ileum and cecum were bound together, producing a narrow pedicle of bowel that twisted easily. The bowel was separated, and the cecum was sutured to the left lateral abdominal wall. We are currently following three other children with nonrotation of the colon whose symptoms were quite vague. All these improved with family counseling for emotional problems involving the children and their families. The parents as well as the child were warned, however, of the possibility and the signs of a volvulus.

Although internal hernias are congenital lesions resulting from a failure of fusion with the mesocolon and the posterior abdominal wall, they are rarely seen in childhood.[13,14] Failure of fusion of the descending mesocolon results in a hernia sac that extends from the ligament of Treitz to behind the descending mesocolon. This is termed a "left paraduodenal hernia." Its opening is bounded on the left by the inferior mesenteric vein and the ascending branch of the left colic artery. A right paraduodenal hernia extends behind the transverse and ascending mesocolon. Its opening is bounded by the superior mesenteric artery and vein. The boundaries of these hernias are of surgical significance because of

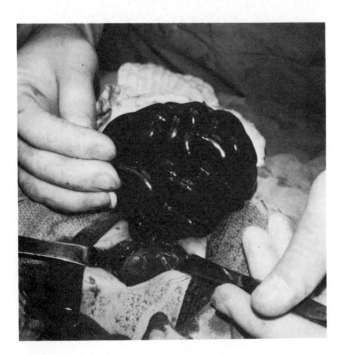

Figure 64–4. Loops of gangrenous small intestine secondary to a midgut volvulus.

the risk of injury to one of these major vessels. The diagnosis of an internal hernia is usually made at laparotomy for an intestinal obstruction. In retrospect, there may be a history of postprandial pain before the acute episode. On physical examination, there may be a suggestion of a mass. Roentgenograms demonstrate an intestinal obstruction and, possibly, displacement of either the colon or the stomach. Treatment consists of reduction of the trapped bowel and obliteration of the hernia sac.

REFERENCES

1. Ladd WE: Congenital obstructions of the duodenum in children. N Engl J Med 206:277, 1932
2. Filston H, Kirks D: Malrotation—the ubiquitous anomaly. J Pediatr Surg 16:614, 1981
3. Frazer JE, Robbins JH: On factors concerned in causing rotation of the intestine in man. J Anat Physiol 50:75, 1915
4. Snyder WH, Chaffin L: Embryology and pathology of the intestinal tract: Presentation of 40 cases of malrotation. Ann Surg 140:368, 1954
5. Snyder WH, Chaffin L: An intermediate stage in the return of the intestines from the umbilical cord: Embryo 37 mm. Anat Rev 113:451, 1952
6. Estrada RL: Anomalies of Intestinal Rotation and Fixation. Springfield, Thomas, 1958
7. Ladd WE, Gross R: Abdominal Surgery of Infancy and Childhood. Philadelphia, Saunders, 1941, p 55
8. Wayne ER, Burrington JD: Extrinsic duodenal obstruction in children. Surg Gynecol Obstet 136:87, 1973
9. Berdon WE, Baker DH, Bull S, Santulli T: Midgut malrotation and volvulus (which films are most helpful?). Radiology 96:375, 1970
10. Simpson AJ, Leonidas JC, Krasna I, et al: Roentgen diagnosis of midgut malrotation: Value of upper gastrointestinal radiographic study. J Pediatr Surg 7:243, 1972
11. Stewart DR, Colodny AL, Daggett WC: Malrotation of the bowel in infants and children: A 15-year review. Surgery 79:716, 1976
12. Gohl ML, DeMeester TR: Midgut nonrotation in adults: An aggressive approach. Am J Surg 129:319, 1975
13. Rubin SZ, Ayalon A, Berlatzky Y: The simultaneous occurrence of paraduodenal and paracecal herniae, presenting with volvulus of the intervening bowel. J Pediatr Surg 11:205, 1976
14. Lough JO, Estrada RL, Wigglesworth W: Internal hernia into Treves' field pouch: Report of two cases and review of the literature. J Pediatr Surg 4:198, 1969

65
Jejunoileal Atresia and Stenosis

The various forms of small intestinal obstruction illustrated in Figure 65–1 represent gradations in severity, from a web to atresia with loss of the increasing length of bowel. The V-shaped gap in the mesentery is evidence of an intrauterine vascular accident. The vascular accidents are usually attributed to an intrauterine volvulus. However, maternal factors, such as the ingestion of cafergot, and anaphylactic shock also have caused fetal vascular insufficiency and atresia.[1,2] Associated anomalies of rotation vary from simple lack of fixation of the cecum to nonrotation of the bowel with an obviously gangrenous volvulus. The most dramatic form of intrauterine vascular accident is that illustrated in Figure 65–2, in which there is a proximal jejunal atresia with complete loss of continuity in the mesentery. The entire intestine supplied by the superior mesenteric artery distal to the ileocolic vessel is missing. The distal ileum has no mesentery but is coiled about its single vessel as a helix. This abnormality has been described with such picturesque terms as "Christmas tree deformity" and "apple peel small bowel," as well as simply jejunal atresia with absent mesentery and a helical ileum.[3,4] Christmas tree deformity is an excellent descriptive term because of the resemblance of the abnormality to coils of tinsel wrapped about a fir tree, the trunk of which represents the single blood vessel. This condition has occurred in families and may be transmitted by an autosomal recessive gene.[5]

Jejunoileal atresias differ from duodenal obstructions in their high incidence of multiple obstructions. The incidence of multiple atresias varies from 6 percent in the series of 587 cases collected from the Surgical Section of the American Academy of Pediatrics to 22 percent of 105 cases studied at the Liverpool Neonatal Center.[6,7] The actual incidence of multiple atresias in the United States is closer to 10 or 12 percent.[8] Multiple atresias may consist of only the intraluminal web below an obvious atresia or a localized series of short segments of intestine pinched off to resemble a string of pearls. The most unusual form of multiple atresia was reported by Guttman et al. in 1973.[9] The entire length of the bowel was occluded by multiple webs only a few centimeters apart. This lesion is hereditary and reportedly occurs most frequently in a group of related French Canadian families.[9–11] A gross section of the bowel, through the cordlike segments, reveals multiple tiny holes or cleftlike spaces lined with ulcerated mucosa. There is severe inflammation of the mucosa with inflammatory cells and a chalklike, calcified debris in the bowel wall. These lesions appear to be postinflammatory, with no vascular component. This form of atresia appears to be hereditary, and thus far all reported infants with it have died.[12]

The intestine proximal to an atresia is hugely distended. The tip is bulbous, thickened, and edematous (Fig. 65–3). Perforation may occur secondary to vascular insufficiency and overdistention. In addition to overdistention of the proximal gut, Touloukian and Hastings found evidence in 19 newborn infants with jejunoileal atresia of villous hypertrophy in both the proximal and distal atretic segments.[13] They speculated that an increase in villous length might represent an attempt to compensate for intestinal loss after a vascular accident. Not only is the proximal bowel distended, but experiments with animals have demonstrated both hypertrophy and hyperplasia of muscle cells in the proximal obstructed bowel segment.[14] Even with muscular hyperplasia and increased strength of peristalsis, the muscular contractions are never sufficient to achieve effective propulsion. In the experimental model, this hyperplasia is reversible, suggesting that we might be able to save more of the grossly dilated bowel in babies whose intestinal length is severely compromised.

ASSOCIATED ANOMALIES

Unlike duodenal atresia, infants with jejunoileal atresia have few defects in other organ systems, and none of

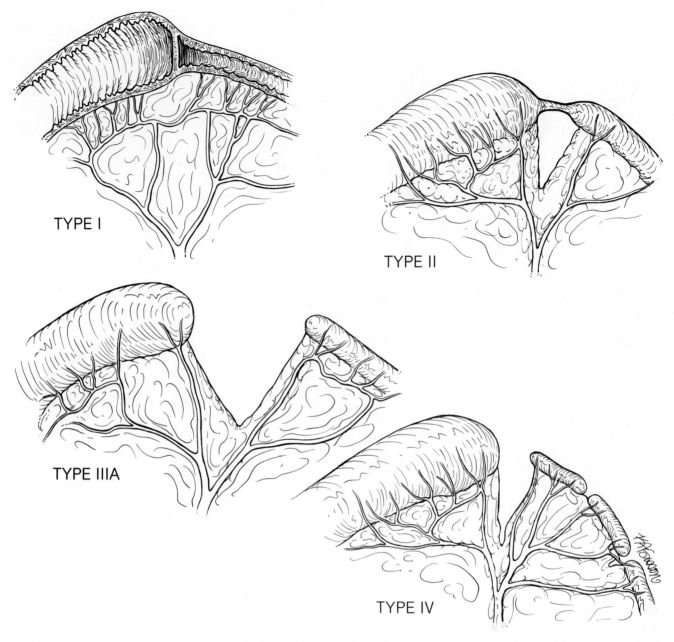

Figure 65–1. Types of small intestinal atresia.

our patients with this disease have had Down's syndrome. Unfortunately, cystic fibrosis of the pancreas is associated with localized volvulus and atresia with sufficient frequency to warrant a sweat chloride test for every baby with an atresia. When examination of the distal collapsed bowel reveals firm plugs of puttylike meconium, requiring vigorous irrigation, the presumptive diagnosis of meconium ileus and cystic fibrosis can be made at the operating table, even though the primary pathology is an atresia. Ileal atresia also has been associated with long-segment Hirschsprung's disease.[15] All resected tissue,

particularly bowel distal to the atresia, should be studied for ganglion cells.

DIAGNOSIS

All babies with small bowel atresia vomit bile and have varying degress of abdominal distention. Roentgenograms demonstrate dilated loops of intestine with air–fluid levels on upright films (Fig. 65–4). When there is considerable distention and multiple loops of dilated

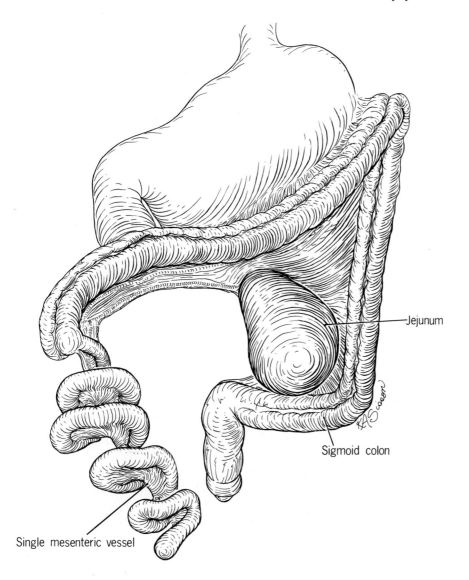

Jejunum

Sigmoid colon

Single mesenteric vessel

Figure 65–2. Christmas tree deformity. There is jejunal atresia with loss of the midgut down to the terminal ileum.

bowel, the differential diagnosis must include Hirschsprung's disease and meconium ileus. A contrast enema is helpful in differentiating these lesions (Fig. 65–5). An upper gastrointestinal study should never be performed on an infant with the clinical and roentgenographic signs of small bowel obstruction. This study is indicated only in the older child suspected of having an anomaly of rotation or an intestinal stenosis. Rickham and Johnston observed a complete obstruction from inspissated masses of barium in the ileum and colon of an otherwise normal premature infant.[16]

TREATMENT

Since problems with other organ systems are unusual and there is an increased danger of perforation and peritonitis in small intestinal atresias, preoperative studies

and treatment should be carried out so that the infant may be operated on within a few hours of diagnosis. If there are signs of perforation, we give large boluses of plasma and electrolyte solutions as needed until the vital signs, arterial blood pressure, and acid-base balance are stable, and then operate as soon as possible.

The transverse upper abdominal incision described for duodenal atresia is also satisfactory for atresias of the small bowel and colon. Adhesions resulting from an intrauterine perforation are divided so the entire intestine may be eviscerated onto warm, moist pads. The bowel is then inspected from the duodenum to the sigmoid colon for the atresia, secondary obstructions, anomalies of rotation, and mesenteric defects. The intestinal length is measured along the antimesenteric border with suture material, which is in turn measured against a centimeter rule. The newborn infant normally has about 250 cm of small bowel. In many patients with atresias,

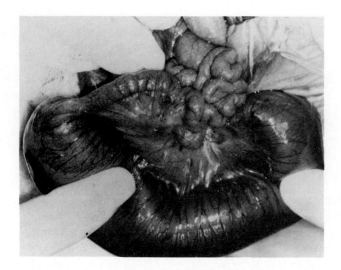

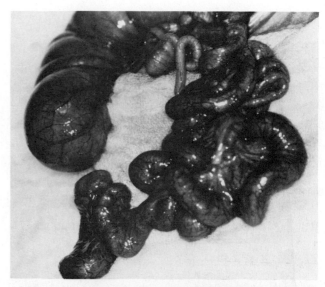

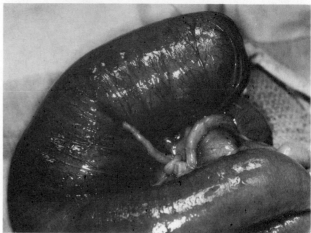

Figure 65–3. Top left. An intestinal atresia due to an intraluminal web. The bowel is in continuity, but the proximal intestine is hugely dilated. **Top right.** A Christmas tree defect. There is no intestinal continuity, and the proximal jejunum is five times the size of the ileum. **Bottom left.** Ileal atresia, demonstrating the huge disparity between the proximal and the distal bowel.

the intestinal length is shorter than normal. The first step is to decompress the proximal intestine by advancing the orogastric tube into the duodenum and applying suction. In addition, a large-bore needle is inserted into the bulbous end of the atresia to aspirate air and secretions. The second important step is the insertion of a needle into the distal blind loop to inject air and saline with a syringe (Fig. 65–6). This distends the distal bowel, loosens plugs of meconium, and demonstrates secondary atresias. The most difficult problem in the management of ileal or jejunal atresia is deciding what to do with the bulbous proximal bowel. If it is left and a direct anastomosis is made, the dilated bowel will never develop effective peristalsis, and there will be a prolonged period of functional obstruction. This problem may be solved by resecting the proximal dilated bowel back to nearly normal size intestine, and then an end-to-end anastomosis is carried out (Fig. 65–6). This procedure continues to be our choice for the vast majority of intestinal atresias. It is particularly successful in ileal atresia or any situation in which the original vascular accident did not destroy

excessive lengths of intestine. If, after the proposed resection, there is 70 cm of intestine left with the ileocecal valve, one can expect prompt return of function and normal absorption. We have attempted to exteriorize the proximal blind loop with various forms of double-barreled jejunostomies or with one of the chimney operations.[17] In our hands, these procedures have allowed survival, but the total length of hospital stay was longer than when a direct anastomosis was performed. We no longer recommend any exteriorization procedure unless there has been preoperative perforation or gangrene of the bowel with a compromised blood supply.

Tapering the bowel by resecting a segment along the antimesenteric border had been recommended as a way to maintain bowel length and to improve peristalsis in the proximal segment.[18] In our hands, the resection has caused considerable blood loss, and one infant developed a postoperative leak at the junction of the two suture lines. Simple plication of the bowel without resection is the best solution when one wants to salvage intestinal length and to create a functional end-to-end

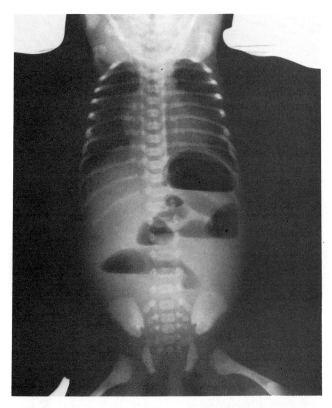

Figure 65–4. This upright roentgenogram shows multiple air–fluid levels. This is pathognomonic for a jejunal atresia. There is no reason to perform barium studies.

anastomosis.[19] This procedure is most useful in high jejunal atresias, when the dilatation goes all the way back into the duodenum, making it impossible to resect back to intestine of a suitable caliber. By reflecting the colon to the left, the distal duodenum and the entire proximal jejunum may be plicated. Nonabsorbable sutures should be used (Fig. 65–7).

After either resection or a tapering procedure, a primary, open anastomosis is performed. The intestine is never clamped and should be handled with the fingers. Forceps are used only to stabilize tissue and to pick up the needle. Tissue reaction and edema at the anastomosis are further minimized by the use of a single layer of interrupted 5-0 or 6-0 Teflon-coated dacron suture material. Care must be taken to make sure that seromuscular approximation is achieved without bits of mucosa peaking through the suture line. The end sutures used for traction in lining up the two lumina are reinforced because traction may cause these end sutures to cut through and leak. If possible, the mesentery is approximated with the same interrupted sutures used in the anastomosis. There is no mesentery to approximate in the Christmas tree defect.

Multiple atresias, if confined to localized areas, are resected, and an anastomosis is performed. Several anastomoses are preferable to an extensive resection that would leave the infant with a severely shortened bowel and malabsorption.

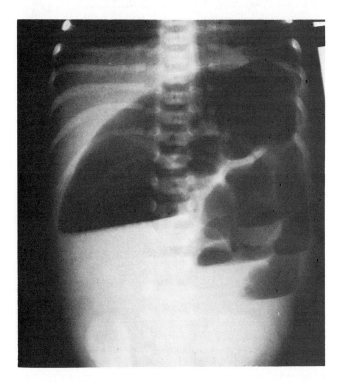

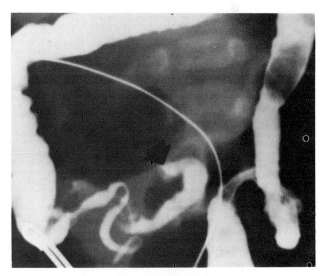

Figure 65–5. Left. This plain roentgenogram demonstrates a dilated small intestine, which could represent an atresia, meconium ileus, or even Hirschsprung's disease, since it is difficult to differentiate a dilated loop of small bowel from the colon. **Right.** The barium enema demonstrates a collapsed colon with reflux of barium into narrow loops of ileum. This confirms the diagnosis of a low atresia.

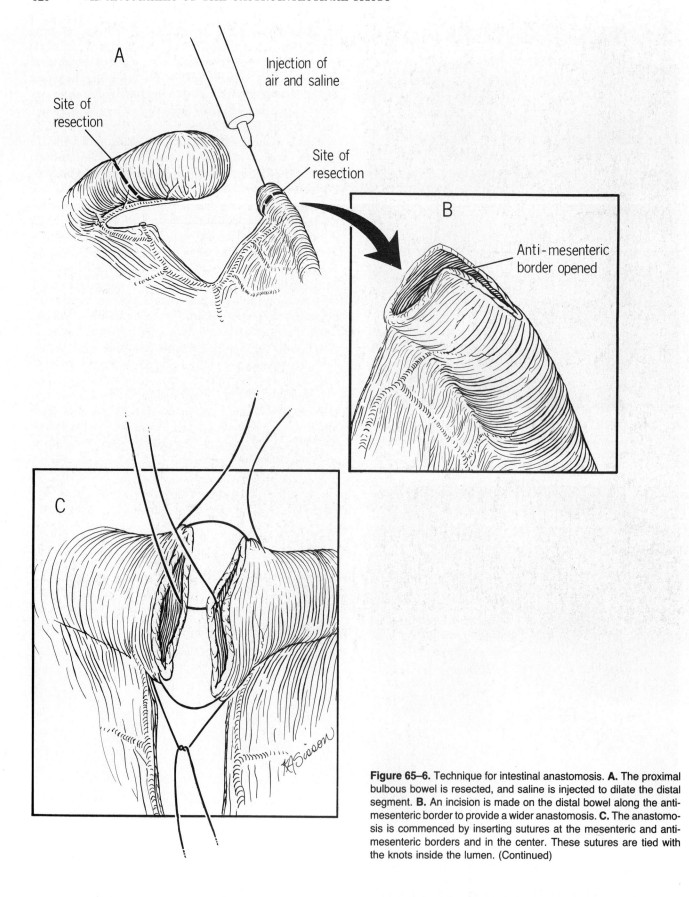

Figure 65–6. Technique for intestinal anastomosis. **A.** The proximal bulbous bowel is resected, and saline is injected to dilate the distal segment. **B.** An incision is made on the distal bowel along the anti-mesenteric border to provide a wider anastomosis. **C.** The anastomosis is commenced by inserting sutures at the mesenteric and anti-mesenteric borders and in the center. These sutures are tied with the knots inside the lumen. (Continued)

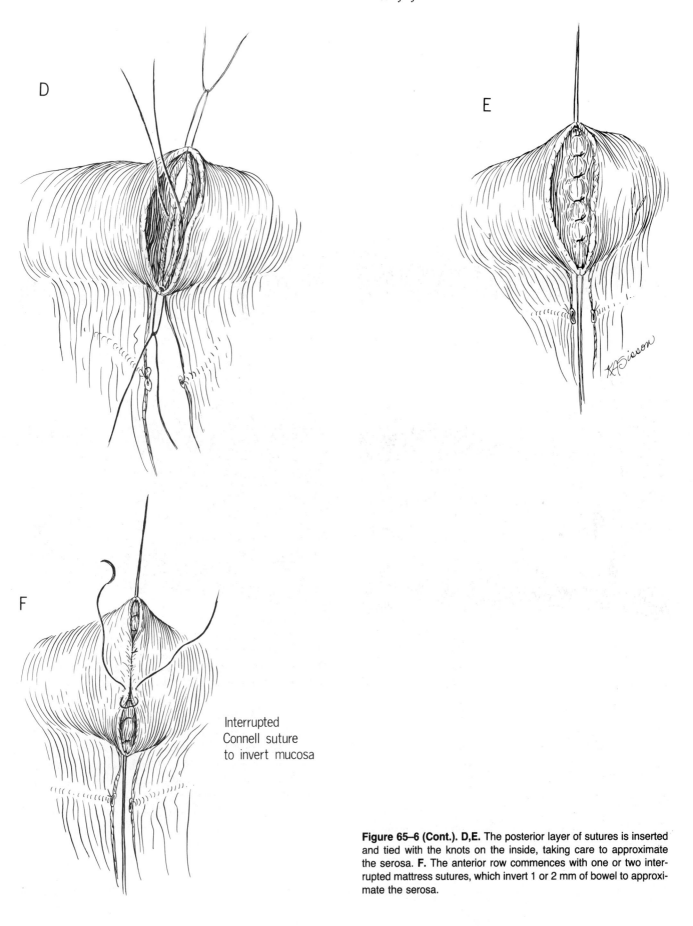

Interrupted
Connell suture
to invert mucosa

Figure 65–6 (Cont.). D,E. The posterior layer of sutures is inserted and tied with the knots on the inside, taking care to approximate the serosa. **F.** The anterior row commences with one or two interrupted mattress sutures, which invert 1 or 2 mm of bowel to approximate the serosa.

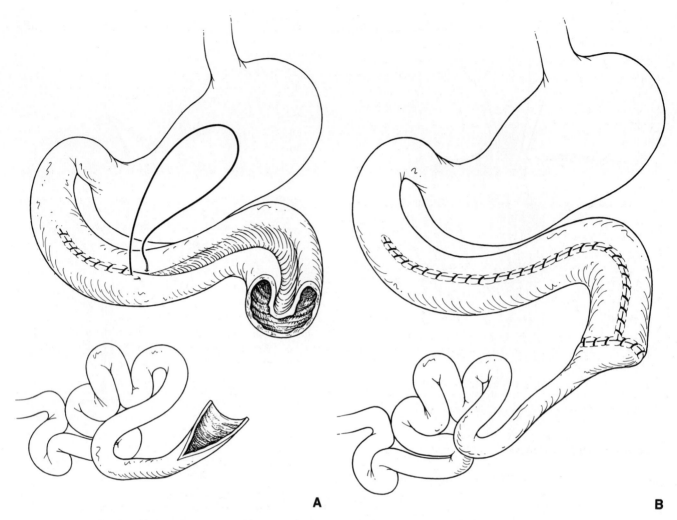

A   **B**

Figure 65–7. A. The proximal dilated bowel is opened at the tip and tapered with a continuous suture back to near normal-size intestine. **B.** After tapering the proximal bowel and spatulating the distal intestine, an end-to-end anastomosis can be carried out. The junction of the two suture lines should be reinforced with an additional suture.

POSTOPERATIVE CARE

Gastric drainage, antibiotics, and peripheral intravenous alimentation are continued in the postoperative period. Rectal irrigations with 15 to 20 ml normal saline are begun on the third day in order to dislodge plugs of meconium from the colon and to stimulate peristalsis. The baby's abdomen is carefully measured at the umbilicus each time the nursing shift changes. If there is any change in the baby's condition, lethargy, unstable temperature, increase in abdominal girth, increase in the gastric drainage, or signs of hypovolemia, the diagnostic possibilities include an anastomotic leak or necrotizing enterocolitis. If studies, such as the chest roentgenogram, blood culture, spinal tap, and serum electrolyte test, fail to demonstrate any other cause for the infant's deterioration, reexploration is indicated. Roentgenograms rarely demonstrate free air because, when an anastomosis does leak, it is usually small and partially sealed off. When found early, the anastomosis usually can be reinforced and saved. Otherwise, exteriorization is indicated. When drainage from the orogastric tube diminishes and the infant has stooled, oral feedings are offered. This is a critical time in the postoperative period. There is the risk of fluid overload if intravenous fluids are continued at the maintenance rate and the infant takes in considerable oral feedings. If the feedings are not tolerated, there is also the risk of vomiting and aspiration. Every effort should be made to have the mother pump her breasts, since human milk is tolerated much better than any formula. If breast milk is unavailable, a lactose-free formula containing medium-chain triglycerides and a protein hydrolysate is offered. If there is malabsorption, hyperalimentation must be continued, and elemental formulas may be tried. We have had to reoperate on four of our infants with jejunal atresia, twice to plicate the proximal dilated bowel, once for postoperative necrotizing enterocolitis, and once to bypass an obstruction of the common bile duct that must have been caught in the suture line after a high resection of a dilated duodenum. Our current survival rate for 75 infants with jejunal–ileal atresias is 92 percent.

The prognosis for infants with jejunoileal atresia depends on the length of intestine remaining after the operation. One of our survivors, a boy who is now 12 years old and perfectly normal, was left with 31 cm of small intestine, including his distal ileum and the ileocecal valve. There are also reports of children surviving with only 26 cm of bowel.[20] These babies must be followed for a number of years because some nutritional deficiencies, as of vitamin B_{12}, may not become evident until the fetal stores have been used.

REFERENCES

1. Graham J, Marin-Padilla M, Huefnagel D: Jejunal atresia associated with cafergot ingestion during pregnancy. Clin Pediatr 22:226, 1983
2. Olsen H, Flom S, Kierney S: Identical twins with malrotation and type IV jejunal atresia. J Pediatr Surg 11:1015, 1987
3. Weitzman JJ, Vanderhoof RS: Jejunal atresia with agenesis of the dorsal mesentery with "Christmas tree" deformity of the small intestine. Am J Surg 111:443, 1966
4. Zerella JT, Martin LW: Jejunal atresia with absent mesentery and a helical ileum. Surgery 80:550, 1976
5. Seashore J, Collins F, Markwitz R, Seashore M: Familial apple peel jejunal atresia: Surgical, genetic and radiologic aspects. Pediatrics 80:540, 1987
6. DeLorimier AA, Fonkalsrud EW, Hays DM: Congenital atresia and stenosis of the jejunum and ileum. Surgery 65:819, 1969
7. Shafie ME, Rickham PP: Multiple intestinal atresias. J Pediatr Surg 5:655, 1970
8. Martin LW, Zerella JT: Jejunoileal atresia: A proposed classification. J Pediatr Surg 11:399, 1976
9. Guttman FM, Braun P, Garance PH: Multiple atresias and a new syndrome of hereditary multiple atresias involving the gastrointestinal tract from stomach to rectum. J Pediatr Surg 8:633, 1973
10. Wald ER, Levine MM: Multiple gastrointestinal atresias, with intraluminal calcifications and cystic dilatation of bile ducts: A newly recognized entity resembling "a string of pearls." Pediatrics 57:268, 1976
11. Rittenhouse EA, Beckwith JB, Chappel JS, Bill AH: Multiple septa of the small bowel: Description of an unusual case, with review of the literature and consideration of etiology. Surgery 71:371, 1972
12. Teja K, Schnatterly P, Shaw A: Multiple intestinal atresias: Pathology and pathogenesis. J Pediatr Surg 16:194, 1981
13. Touloukian RJ, Hastings KW: Intrauterine villus hypertrophy with jejunoileal atresia. J Pediatr Surg 8:799, 1973
14. Cloutier R: Intestinal smooth muscle response to chronic obstruction: Possible applications in jejunoileal atresia. J Pediatr Surg 10:3, 1975
15. Garderer M, Rothstein F, Izant R: Ileal atresia with long-segment Hirschsprung's disease in a neonate. J Pediatr Surg 19:15, 1984
16. Rickham PP, Johnston JH: Neonatal Surgery. New York, Appleton-Century-Crofts, 1969, p 323
17. Ahlgren L: Apple peel jejunal atresia. J Pediatr Surg 22:451, 1987
18. Weber T, Vane D, Grosfeld J: Tapering enteroplasty in infants with bowel atresia and short gut. Arch Surg 117:684, 1982
19. DeLorimier A, Harrison M: Intestinal plication in the treatment of atresia. J Pediatr Surg 18:734, 1983
20. Rickham PB, Irving I, Shmerling DH: Long-term results following extensive small intestinal resection in the neonatal period. Prog Pediatr Surg 10:65, 1977

66

Meconium Ileus, Meconium Peritonitis, and the Meconium Plug Syndrome

Normal meconium consists of bile pigments and salts together with desquamated epithelial cells and sebaceous material that the fetus swallows with amniotic fluid. Usually from 50 to 250 g of meconium are passed during the first 24 hours of life. The meconium diseases discussed in this chapter cannot be separated into neat classifications. We thought for a long time that the meconium plug syndrome was never associated with cystic fibrosis of the pancreas. However, 6 of our 25 babies initially given this diagnosis eventually had a positive sweat test for cystic fibrosis. We have also seen 3 babies who were initially thought to have meconium ileus because of their thick tenacious meconium who did not have cystic fibrosis. These were small, premature infants who simply had poor peristalsis with inspissated meconium. One was even operated on because of a mistaken diagnosis. Fewer than half of the babies operated on in our hospital for meconium peritonitis have cystic fibrosis. Most commonly, they have a perforated intestinal atresia or have had an idiopathic intestinal perforation early in intrauterine life. Cystic fibrosis, however, is the common thread through all these diseases and must always be considered.

MECONIUM ILEUS

Abnormally thick, viscid, inspissated meconium is packed in the distal ileum in 15 percent of children born with cystic fibrosis of the pancreas. In cystic fibrosis (mucoviscidosis), all mucus-secreting glands are abnormal. The inspissated meconium has an increased protein content and abnormal mucoproteins.[1,2] In addition, the lack of pancreatic enzymes contributes to the abnormality of the meconium. Meconium ileus has also been reported in infants who had normal sweat electrolytes and who demonstrated no subsequent signs of cystic fibrosis.[3,4]

The situation is sufficiently rare, however, that several sweat chloride tests must be performed and a long-term follow-up carried out before the diagnosis of cystic fibrosis can be safely dismissed in a baby who has had meconium ileus.

Pathology

The ileum in meconium ileus is dilated, thick-walled, and packed with viscid stool. (Fig. 66-1). The bowel narrows distally so that the terminal 15 to 20 cm of the ileum is the thickness of a pencil. This portion of the bowel is packed with dense meconium, which clings tenaciously to the intestinal mucosa. Perforation of a localized gangrenous volvulus is a complication in approximately 50 percent of infants with meconium ileus.[5] Grossly, a similar picture is seen in babies who have aganglionosis of the entire colon and terminal ileum. The differential diagnosis can be made with certainty only by a microscopic examination of the intestine for ganglion cells.

Diagnosis

A family history is important because cystic fibrosis is an autosomal recessive genetic abnormality. Even if there are no signs of an intestinal obstruction, a sweat chloride test must be performed on all siblings of a child with known cystic fibrosis. One mother who had a baby with meconium ileus made the diagnosis in her second child by noting the salty taste of his skin when she first held him in the nursery.

Abdominal distention and bilious vomiting appear during the first few hours after birth. Firm loops of bowel that indent on palpation are found on abdominal examination. Abdominal radiographs are characteristic because swallowed air mixes with meconium in the proximal bowel to impart a soap bubble or ground glass appearance to the plain roentgenograms. In addition, the thick

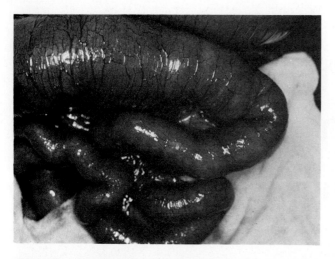

Figure 66–1. The intestine in meconium ileus gradually tapers to the thickness of a pencil at the terminal ileum. At this point, the meconium has the consistency of putty.

meconium fails to layer out into clear air–fluid levels when the infant is held upright. Thus, the supine and upright films demonstrate dilated loops of intestine, but not the air–fluid levels typically seen with atresias. (Fig. 66–2). It is important to suspect meconium ileus on clini-

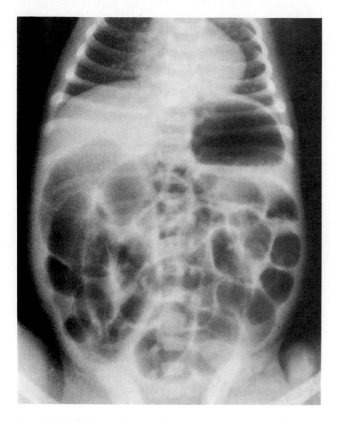

Figure 66–2. This upright roentgenogram demonstrates an air–fluid level in the stomach, but there are none in the remainder of the bowel because the meconium is too thick to layer out with the air.

cal and preliminary radiologic investigation because an immediate operation is no longer required for simple meconium ileus. A contrast study of the colon is definitely indicated, not only to confirm the diagnosis but for treatment as well.

Treatment

Uncomplicated meconium ileus may be relieved with Gastrografin enemas.[6–8] Gastrografin is an aqueous solution of methylglucamine diatrizoate that contains a wetting agent, Tween 80. It is radiopaque and has an osmolarity of 1800. For use as a therapeutic enema, it is diluted to half strength with water. As it comes in contact with the bowel, mucosal fluid is drawn out of the extravascular space into the intestinal lumen. This extravasation of fluid, along with the wetting agent, loosens and liquefies the inspissated meconium. Since fluid is lost to the circulation, the vital signs are carefully monitored and Ringer's lactate solution or plasma is given intravenously. Only those infants who show no signs of abdominal tenderness or free intraperitoneal air or fluid are candidates for this treatment. They are prepared with an orogastric tube and intravenous fluids before the enema. We prefer to use a straight catheter rather than a Foley balloon because an inflated 5 ml bag can split the rectum if it is advanced too far. We have seen two rectal perforations with a balloon catheter. Ein et al. reported bowel perforations in 5 of 22 patients in whom a balloon catheter was used.[9] A size 12 or 14 soft, straight rubber catheter is inserted into the rectum and taped in place. The buttocks are then taped together, although even with these precautions, some Gastrografin leaks out the anus. Perhaps this is a good way to prevent high pressure build-up within the bowel lumen. Half-strength Gastrografin is then injected with a 50 ml syringe under fluoroscopic control. The narrow, unused colon is first outlined (Fig. 66–3). Considerable resistance is encountered, but with persistence Gastrografin will reach the terminal ileum, where large plugs of meconium are outlined. Success is nearly assured if the material can be refluxed into the dilated ileum. After the first enema, the baby is allowed to evacuate the Gastrografin and is kept warm in a portable incubator for a half-hour or so. Then the procedure is repeated. Meconium loosened with the first enema is often evacuated at this time. The infant is returned to the nursery, where rectal irrigations with 1 percent acetylcysteine in normal saline are implemented, again with a rubber catheter and syringe. Often administration of another Gastrografin enema 6 to 8 hours later completes the evacuation of all the thickened meconium and the distention is relieved. Daily enema treatments are continued until the infant spontaneously passes meconium, and the abdominal distention is relieved. If there are no signs of intestinal perforation or gangrene, we have persisted for as long as a week. These infants

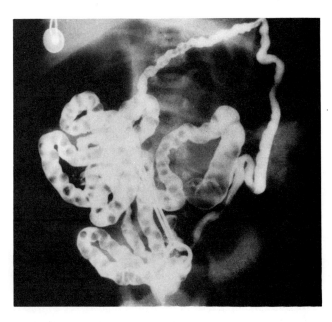

Figure 66–3. Gastrografin enema outlining a microcolon and pellets of hard meconium in the ileum.

must be evaluated at frequent intervals and should show gradual improvement. Intravenous hyperalimentation is continued until the baby can take full oral feedings.

Surgical Therapy

Since adopting the Gastrografin–acetylcysteine enema technique, we have operated only on infants with perforations or volvulus or those for whom we made an incorrect initial diagnosis of atresia.

When conservative management fails or when a

baby with a simply meconium ileus is operated on in error, the dilated distal ileum, which is packed with thick meconium, is lifted out of the abdomen onto warm, moist pads with great care. Rough handling will split the serosa. The dilated intestine is opened on its antimesenteric border, and a catheter is advanced proximally and then held in place with an assistant's fingers. One percent acetylcysteine is then injected into the bowel lumen through the catheter. Acetylcysteine (Mucomyst) is a proteolytic enzyme that rapidly liquefies the inspissated meconium. In animal studies, a 4 percent solution caused no intestinal mucosal damage and was clinically effective.[10-12] In our experience, the 1 percent solution has been equally effective.

The injection of Mucomyst quickly liquefies the thickened meconium in the dilated bowel. The pellets of meconium in the distal ileum are the consistency of concrete and take longer to loosen. After two or three injections of the solution, through the catheter which is passed to the ileocecal valve, one can pass a 5 or 6 Fogarty catheter, inflate the balloon, and pull back the semiliquefied pellets. This procedure is less traumatic than milking the bowel (Fig. 66–4). When the meconium has been removed, the enterotomy is closed. Formerly, we and most surgeons thought that it was necessary to resect the dilated bowel. Bishop and Koop described an end-to-side chimney type of anastomosis that allowed further irrigation of the distal bowel[13] (Fig. 66–5). The tendency to conservative therapy and the avoidance of stomas was furthered by Harberg et al.'s report that a simple T-tube enterostomy and irrigations was sufficient.[14] We have had only 1 infant of 17 treated who died with simple meconium ileus. This was a 950 g

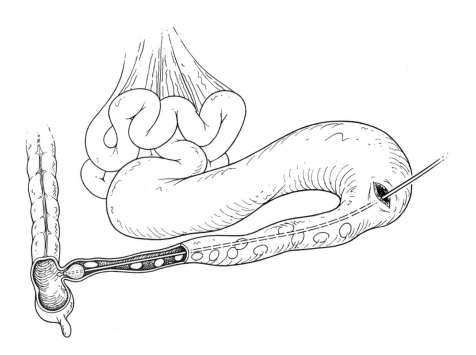

Figure 66–4. Meconium pellets may be removed from the ileum by irrigation and by withdrawing an inflated Fogarty catheter.

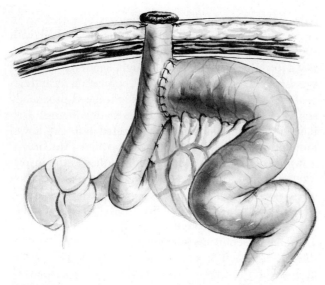

Figure 66–5. Bishop–Koop end-to-side enteroenterostomy with distal venting.

infant who died 3 weeks after the operation with sepsis. Similar results were obtained in an almost identical group of patients at the Montreal Children's Hospital.[15]

Complicated Meconium Ileus
The weight of the dilated bowel filled with meconium predisposes to volvulus formation and intrauterine perforation. The findings at operation include frankly gangrenous intestine or, if the volvulus occurred early, an atresia. There are often vascular adhesions in the abdomen, and the distal bowel is packed with hard pellets of meconium. In this situation, resection of nonviable bowel with the creation of a double-barreled stoma is the safest course to follow. The distal bowel is then irrigated with acetylcysteine until it is patent. The infant is supported with fluid replacement and hyperalimentation. Often the stoma can be closed within 3 to 4 weeks.

Postoperative Care. In addition to the usual hyperalimentation and gastric drainage, infants with meconium ileus are subjected to vigorous therapy to prevent the pulmonary complications of cystic fibrosis. These infants are kept in maximum humidity, turned from side to side every hour, and stimulated to cry. Gentle pulmonary physiotherapy and postural drainage to loosen secretions are commenced as soon as the postoperative condition permits, usually on the second or third postoperative day. During the first week of life, a sweat test for chloride levels may be inaccurate. The pilocarpine iontophoresis technique, however, can be used.[16] A sweat chloride level of up to 35 mEq/liter is normal, but most children with cystic fibrosis will have values as high as 60 mEq/liter. This test should be repeated at least twice to be certain of the diagnosis. When admin-

istration of a normal cow's milk formula is commenced in a baby with cystic fibrosis, it is necessary to provide extra pancreatic enzymes, as with a quarter of a teaspoonful of Viokase twice daily. There is some disadvantage to starting pancreatic enzymes during the neonatal period because some children become allergic to them. For that reason, a protein hydrolysate formula (such as Pregestimil) is given, since it will not require additional pancreatic enzymes for digestion and absorption. Human breast milk appears to be well tolerated without the addition of pancreatic enzymes.

Before discharge, the mother is taught how to administer physiotherapy and postdural drainage. Immediate referral to a cystic fibrosis clinic is helpful for the parents as well as the child. The current immediate survival rate with either nonoperative or surgical methods is approaching 100 percent. The long-range prognosis for children with cystic fibrosis is also improving. Schwachman reported on 10 adults who were operated on for muconium ileus. All survived to at least 28 years old and lived relatively normal lives.[17] The child with cystic fibrosis will encounter further surgical problems, including atelectasis, bronchiectasis, hemoptysis, pneumothorax, and portal hypertension. The equivalent of meconium ileus is seen in older children who for one reason or another have failed to take sufficient pancreatic extract.[18] The normal liquid contents of the terminal ileum become thick and puttylike, just as in neonatal meconium ileus. The result is an intestinal obstruction. This syndrome should respond to Gastrografin and acetylcysteine enemas. If it does not, an operation is indicated to clear out the dense, obstructing masses of stool.

MECONIUM PERITONITIS

Meconium peritonitis is the term applied to any antenatal intestinal perforation. The perforation may occur secondary to a meconium ileus or to an intestinal atresia. In some cases, there is no obvious explanation other than a possible localized vascular accident. When the perforation occurs early in embryonic life, the meconium causes an inflammatory reaction and calcification within the peritoneal cavity.[19] Since the processus vaginalis is open until the seventh month, meconium may escape into the scrotum and cause a calcified mass that may simulate a testicular tumor.[20] The typical infant with calcified meconium peritonitis vomits bile and has abdominal distention and all the other signs of an intestinal obstruction. Abdominal roentgenograms demonstrate air–fluid levels diagnostic of an obstruction with calcification (Fig. 66–6). At operation, there are adhesions and frequently a localized mass of intestine encased in a dense inflammatory reaction and calcium. On rare occasion, one sees scattered calcification on a roentgenogram and no signs

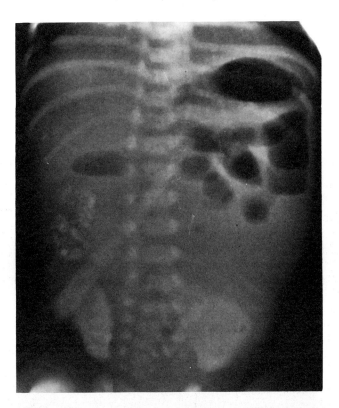

Figure 66–6. This x-ray demonstrates calcification, which is diagnostic of an early intrauterine perforation of the bowel. There are also air–fluid levels diagnostic of an obstruction.

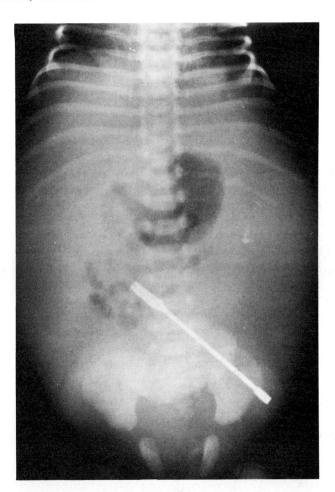

Figure 66–7. A late antenatal intestinal perforation. The abdomen is filled with fluid, and the bowel floats in the center of the abdomen.

of an obstruction. We operated on two older children, 6 months and 2 years of age, who had adhesive obstructions with intraperitoneal calcification. One can only guess that these two children started with a mild meconium peritonitis that ultimately resulted in an intestinal obstruction. In yet another variation of meconium peritonitis, there is both calcification and free fluid within the peritoneal cavity. The intestine is matted together against the posterior abdominal wall, and the fluid is encapsulated in a dense shell of adhesions.[21] Infants with this affliction are born with abdominal distention due to the intraperitoneal fluid. When an operation is delayed, they soon show free air layered out into the intraperitoneal fluid. At operation, after a painstaking dissection through the adhesions to find the bowel, one finds a rosette of open mucosa, usually in the terminal ileum. It is necessary to dissect out the entire length of small bowel, irrigate away plugs of meconium from the lumen, and exteriorize the perforation.

When the antenatal perforation occurs late in intrauterine life, there is no calcification, although the infant is born with a hugely distended abdomen that interferes with respiration (Fig. 66–7). The abdomen is dull to percussion, and there is bulging of the flanks. Roentgenograms demonstrate an almost totally opaque abdomen with little intestinal gas. Prompt abdominal paracentesis is essential for decompression of the abdomen and relief of the respiratory distress. There is usually a thick green fluid within the peritoneal cavity. In our experience, children with this form of late meconium peritonitis have all had an associated meconium ileus. The intestinal perforation may be at any location. With distal perforations, we resect the area and perform an ileostomy. With more proximal perforation, we have successfully resected back to relatively normal intestine and performed a direct end-to-end anastomosis.

MECONIUM PLUG SYNDROME

The meconium plug syndrome is a rare, benign form of colon obstruction in the neonate that bears no relationship to meconium ileus. We have studied 25 infants with the meconium plug syndrome. Associated problems that may contribute to the syndrome include a 36 percent incidence of prematurity and a 50 percent incidence of maternal complications. Six of these infants, or 25 percent, later were diagnosed as having cystic fibrosis.[22] The only abnormality in these infants is a firm, white plug of mucus that is sufficiently tenacious to block the colon. These babies have abdominal distention, but vomiting is unusual because the problem is so easily relieved. Plain roentgenograms demonstrate distended loops of intestine, but a barium enema is diagnostic when the barium outlines a long radiolucency within the descending colon.[23] The plug is almost always passed after the barium enema or a simple saline rectal irrigation. Immediately after the plug is expelled, the infant passes normal meconium and is well thereafter. In retrospect, some children who were originally thought to have a simple meconium plug syndrome actually had Hirschsprung's disease.[24] For this reason, we now routinely perform a rectal suction biopsy to search for ganglion cells in Meissner's plexus before these infants leave the nursery. In addition, because of the possibility of cystic fibrosis, we also obtain a sweat chloride test. It is dangerous to make a diagnosis of meconium plug syndrome without being absolutely certain the infant does not have either Hirschsprung's disease or cystic fibrosis.

REFERENCES

1. Buchanan DJ, Rapoport S: Chemical comparison of normal meconium and meconium from a patient with meconium ileus. Pediatrics 9:304, 1952
2. Knauff RE, Adams JA: Meconium protein and mucoproteins in meconium ileus. Proc Soc Exp Biol Med 127:801, 1968
3. Rickham PP, Boeckman CR: Neonatal meconium obstruction in the absence of mucoviscidosis. Am J Surg 109:173, 1965
4. Dolan TF Jr, Touloukian RJ: Familial meconium ileus not asociated with cystic fibrosis. J Pediatr Surg 9:821, 1974
5. O'Neill JA Jr, Grosfeld JL, Boles ET Jr, Clatworthy HW Jr: Surgical treatment of meconium ileus. Am J Surg 119:99, 1970
6. Noblett HR: Treatment of uncomplicated meconium ileus by Gastrografin enema: A preliminary report. J Pediatr Surg 4:190, 1969
7. Frech RS, McAlister WH, Ternberg J, Strominger D: Meconium ileus relieved by 40 percent water-soluble contrast enemas. Radiology 94:341, 1970
8. Wagget J, Bishop HC, Koop CE: Experience with Gastrografin enema in the treatment of meconium ileus. J Pediatr Surg 5:649, 1970
9. Ein S, Shandling B, Reilly B, Stephens C: Bowel perforation with nonoperative treatment of meconium ileus. J Pediatr Surg 22:146, 1987
10. Schiller M, Grosfeld JL, Morse TS: Nonoperative treatment of meconium ileus: An experimental study in rats. Am J Surg 122:22, 1971
11. Shaw A: Safety of N-acetylcysteine in treatment of meconium obstruction in the newborn. J Pediatr Surg 4:119, 1969
12. Meeker IA Jr, Kincannon WN: Acetylcysteine used to liquefy inspissated meconium causing intestinal obstruction in the newborn. Surgery 56:419, 1964
13. Bishop HC, Koop CE: Management of meconium ileus: Resection, Roux-en-y anastomosis and ileostomy irrigation with pancreatic enzymes. Ann Surg 145:410, 1957
14. Harberg F, Senekjian E, Pokorny J: Treatment of uncomplicated meconium ileus via a T-tube ileostomy. J Pediatr Surg 16:61, 1981
15. Nguyen L, Youssef S, Guttman F, et al: Meconium ileus: Is a stoma necessary? J Pediatr Surg 21:766, 1986
16. Gibson LE, Cooke RE: Test for concentration of electrolytes in sweat in cystic fibrosis of pancreas utilizing pilocarpine by iontophoresis. Pediatrics 23:545, 1959
17. Shwachman H: Meconium ileus: Ten patients over 28 years of age. J Pediatr Surg 18:570, 1983
18. Cordonnier JD, Izant RJ Jr: Meconium ileus equivalent. Surgery 54:667, 1963
19. Steinfield JB, Harrison RB: Extensive intramural calcification in a newborn with intestinal atresia. Radiology 107:405, 1973
20. Thompson RB, Rosen DI, Gross DM: Healed meconium peritonitis presenting as an inguinal mass. J Urol 110:364, 1973
21. Kolawole TM, Bankole MA, Olurin EO, et al: Meconium peritonitis presenting as giant cysts in neonates. Br J Radiol 46:964, 1973
22. Olson M, Luck S, Lloyd-Still J, Raffensperger J: The spectrum of meconium disease in infancy. J Pediatr Surg 17:479, 1982
23. McKity VG, Hoogman JE, Paciulli J: Meconium blockage syndrome. Radiology 88:740, 1967
24. Ellis DG, Clatworthy HW: The meconium plug syndrome revisited. J Pediatr Surg 1:54, 1966

67
Colon Atresia

_____ *Randall W. Powell*

Atresia of the colon is the least common form of congenital intestinal atresia, accounting for 5 to 15 percent of reported cases.[1] A review of our patients with colon atresias operated at Children's Memorial Hospital from 1947 (when Dr. Potts performed the first successful anastomosis in an infant with an atresia of the transverse colon[2]) through 1978 yielded 19 patients. Ten patients in that series were seen in the 1970s. Since that review, 4 new patients have been treated, for a total of 23 with colon atresia.

PATHOLOGY

Of these 23 atresias, 14 occurred in the ascending colon, 1 in the transverse colon, and 8 in the descending colon. In 12 cases, the blind, dilated proximal bowel was separated from the distal colon by a V-shaped defect in the mesentery. This pathology was most commonly seen in the ascending colon, which was hugely dilated because of the blind loop effect between the atresia and the competent ileocecal valve. In these cases, the colon was absent up to the splenic flexure or descending colon, suggesting that the thrombosis of the middle colic artery accounted for the atresia and mesenteric defect. In 6 cases, there was only a web obstructing the lumen, and in 2, the blind ends were connected with a fibrous cord. Tremendous distention of the blind loop between the ileocecal valve and the atresia results in a thin-walled atonic structure that may become ischemic and perforated.[3] There is probably a greater disparity in size between the proximal and distal segments of colon than in any other form of intestinal atresia, yet the ileum proximal to the ileocecal valve often is of normal size. (Fig. 67-1).

ASSOCIATED DEFECTS

Of our 23 patients, 8 had associated lesions. Two had congenital ophthalmic defects, 1 a bladder exstrophy, and 1 had a duodenal and 1 a jejunal atresia. One baby had a gastroschisis with both a colon atresia and a jejunal atresia, and 2 babies with gastroschisis had left colon atresias. Two infants have been reported as having associated Hirschsprung's disease.[4,5]

DIAGNOSIS

An infant with colon atresia develops severe abdominal distention, often with palpable intestinal loops, during the first 24 hours of life. The baby passes no meconium. Vomiting may be delayed because the remarkable intestinal distention results in the prompt passage of a gastric tube, which returns bile-stained material but fails to relieve the distention. Plain roentgenograms reveal dilated loops of intestine with air–fluid levels. A single, long air–fluid level in a hugely dilated segment of bowel is almost diagnostic for atresia of the transverse colon.[6] A barium enema will accurately locate the obstruction and will differentiate colon atresia from Hirschsprung's disease, meconium ileus, and atresias of he small bowel (Fig. 67–2). When the column of barium pushes against a membranous obstruction, one may see a windsock sign.[7,8]

TREATMENT

An operation is urgent, since the closed loop obstruction results in severe distention with danger of intestinal perforation.[9,10] A transverse upper abdominal incision

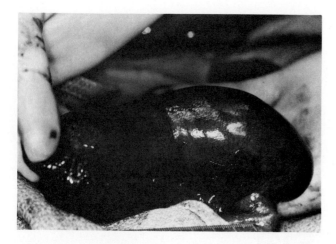

Figure 67–1. The cecum and ascending colon are hugely dilated. This creates great disparity in size, and if a colostomy is performed, there is a tendency toward prolapse.

allows excellent exposure unless the atretic distal segment is very short. If it appears that the distal segment is in the descending or sigmoid colon, a left paramedian incision is necessary if an anastomosis is planned.

The proximal dilated colon may be managed either with an end colostomy with later anastomosis or by resec-

tion and primary anastomosis. Although a colostomy would appear to be a safe procedure, two of our patients treated with colostomy performed on a severely dilated colon developed severe prolapse of the bowel. Further, in both patients, the severe dilatation failed to resolve within 12 months. One child had a prolonged anastomotic dysfunction that required frequent rectal irrigations, and another died following closure of the colostomy and anastomosis of the bowel. Primary resection of the proximal dilated colon to the ileum with a primary ileotransverse colostomy is the treatment of choice when the atretic segment is in the ascending or transverse colon.[11-16] When the atresia is in the descending or sigmoid colon, we perform a colostomy and at 1 year of age resect the colostomy and distal collapsed bowel down to the rectal ampulla. In cases where the distal segment is short, it is helpful to have the mother irrigate the rectum with saline for several weeks before the operation in order to dilate and stretch the short distal segment.

RESULTS

Only 2 of our 23 patients since 1947 have died. One had multiple anomalies, and the other's death was secondary to an anastomotic leak after colostomy closure.

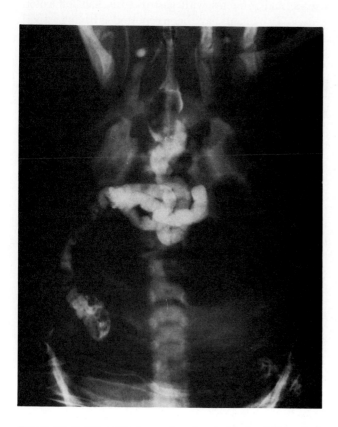

Figure 67–2. The colon is small and ends blindly at the splenic flexure. The dilated, air-filled cecum is to the right.

REFERENCES

1. Powell RW, Raffensperger JG: Congenital colonic atresia. J Pediatr Surg 17:166, 1982
2. Potts WJ: Congenital atresia of intestine and colon. Surg Gynecol Obstet 85:14, 1947
3. Moore TC: Atresia of the colon at the splenic flexure with absence of the distal colon and ischemic destruction of the proximal colon. J Pediatr Surg 13:89, 1978
4. Hyde GA Jr, Delorimier AA: Colon atresia and Hirschsprung's disease. Surgery 69:976, 1968
5. Haffner JF, Schistad G: Atresia of the colon combines with Hirschsprung's disease: A case report. J Pediatr Surg 4:560, 1964
6. Boles ET Jr, Vassey LE, Ralston M: Atresia of the colon. J Pediatr Surg 11:69, 1976
7. Blank E, Afshani E, Girdany BR, Pappas A: "Windsock sign" of congenital membranous atresia of the colon. Am J Roentgenol Radium Ther Nucl Med 120:330, 1974
8. Coryllos E, Simpson J: Congenital atresia of the colon: Review of the literature and report of two cases. Dis Colon Rectum 5:37, 1962
9. Lanigan MW: Congenital atresia of the colon: A review and a case report. Aust NZ J Surg 45:170, 1975
10. Lee SS, Kim KY, Hong PW: Congenital atresia of the colon. JAMA 202:1148, 1967
11. Hardin CA, Friesen SR: Congenital atresia of the colon: Report of two cases. Arch Surg 80:616, 1960

12. Sturim HS, Ternberg JL: Congenital atresia of the colon. Surgery 59:458, 1966

13. Benson CD, Lotfi MW, Brough AJ: Congenital atresia and stenosis of the colon. J Pediatr Surg 3:253, 1968

14. Coran AG, Eraklis AJ: Atresia of the colon. Surgery 65:828, 1969

15. Freeman NV: Congenital atresia and stenosis of the colon. Br J Surg 53:595, 1966

16. Defore WW Jr, Garcia-Rinaldi R, Mattox KL, Harberg FJ: Surgical management of colon atresia. Surg Gynocol Obstet 143:767, 1976

68

Uncommon Forms of Neonatal Bowel Obstruction

Vomiting and abdominal distention in the neonate are usually caused by one of the diseases discussed previously. However, other types of obstruction should be mentioned. They may simulate other diseases, and a discussion of rare cases may be of help to a puzzled surgeon. In addition to unusual mechanical obstructions, which are relieved by an operation, there are cases of disordered peristalsis in which the intestinal dysfunction remains completely unexplained. Some of these cases present recognizable syndromes, and the afflicted infants can be kept alive for prolonged periods with intravenous hyperalimentation.

TUMORS

The most common tumors of the small bowel in children are hemangiomas. These cause bleeding but rarely obstruction. We observed one 2-month-old baby whose history of recurrent abdominal pain went back to her first week of life. She had an angiomatous malformation of the ileum that caused recurrent intussusceptions. Tunell reported a hemangioendothelioma of the pancreas that first obstructed the common bile duct and then the duodenum.[1] The mass was bypassed with a gastrojejunostomy and a cholecystojejunostomy. It was then treated with radiation and steroids. Roth and Farinacci reported on jejunal leiomyosarcoma in a newborn infant who had an intestinal obstruction at birth.[2]

INTUSSUSCEPTION

Although intussusception is the most common cause of intestinal obstruction in infants between 6 and 12 months of age and is an accepted etiology of intestinal atresia, it practically never occurs in the newborn period. Only

one was seen at the Cook County Hospital over a period of 15 years, with an average of 14,000 deliveries a year, and two were seen at the Children's Memorial Hospital during the past 17 years. In a review of 26 cases reported before 1962, vomiting and bloody stools were the only symptoms of neonatal intussusception. The incidence of polyps and intestinal duplications was higher in neonates than in older children, and intestinal resection was required in 12 babies.[3] Yoo and Touloukian reported a single case and again reviewed the literature in 1974.[4] Even though there are clear signs of an intestinal obstruction, there are few specific indications of intussusception.[4] Hydrostatic reduction is contraindicated because of the increased risk of perforation in the neonate and the higher incidence of small bowel rather than ileocolic lesions. Irreducible and gangrenous intussusceptions are more frequent in neonates than in older children, which is perhaps due to delay in diagnosis.

SEGMENTAL DILATATION

The absence of musculature in any portion of the intestinal tract leads to localized dilatation of the affected segment with obstruction because of lack of peristalsis. This lesion has been described in the duodenum, jejunum, ileum, and colon.[5-9] Irving and Lister summarized the features of 15 cases.[10] Clinically, these babies have distended, tympanitic abdomens and vomiting. Plain radiographs demonstrate a few dilated loops of bowel with one hugely distended segment containing an air–fluid level. In reported cases, there was no question about the clinical diagnosis of intestinal obstruction, although Hirschsprung's disease was considered in infants with segmental dilatation of the colon. At operation, the proximal intestine is normal, with an abrupt transition to an enormously distended, thinned-out segment. Distally, there is another abrupt transition to bowel of normal caliber. If the lesion occurs in the duodenum or small bowel, the muscular coats are either absent or atrophic. If it occurs in the colon, the muscle is hypertrophic. Other unusual microscopic features found by Irving and Lister include heterotopic tissue resembling the esophagus and lung. In the 15 cases summarized there were a variety of associated defects, including omphalocoele, malrotation, exstrophy of the bladder, and meningocoele.

Treatment consists of excision of the dilated segment and end-to-end anastomosis. It would be wise to obtain a rectal biopsy that demonstrates ganglion cells before making this diagnosis in the colon.

NEONATAL SMALL LEFT COLON SYNDROME

The small left colon syndrome is a functional obstruction of the colon that is only slightly different from the meconium plug syndrome and Hirschsprung's disease (Fig. 68–1). Before Davis et al. coined the term in 1974, we had operated on three infants with the clinical and radiographic signs of an aganglionic segment of colon up to the splenic flexure.[11] Two had severely distended abdomens and had resisted saline irrigations. The third had perforated cecum and at operation had what appeared to be a classic zone of transition to a narrowed aganglionic descending colon. Transverse colostomies were performed on the first two and a cecostomy on the third. When rectal biopsies were obtained before a proposed pull-through operation, all three patients were found to have normal ganglion cells, and all had normal function following closure of their colostomies.

Infants with this problem have the clinical and radiographic signs of a low intestinal obstruction. A contrast enema demonstrates a colon that is narrow to the splenic flexure with a zone of transition to a transverse colon that is two to three times the diameter of the sigmoid. The radiographic picture is indistinguishable from that of a long-segment aganglionosis. A similar radiographic picture is seen in the meconium plug syndrome, except that the contrast material outlines radiolucent plugs.

Almost all infants with small left colons are born to diabetic mothers. In fact, as many as 40 percent of infants born to diabetic mothers have this syndrome in varying degrees.[12] An effort has been made to correlate the fall in blood glucose experienced by infants of diabetic mothers with a corresponding increase in glucagon secretion, which in turn inhibits colon peristalsis.[13] This theory will be difficult to prove, since some infants who appear to have this syndrome do not have diabetic mothers. Regardless of the etiology, the small left colon syn-

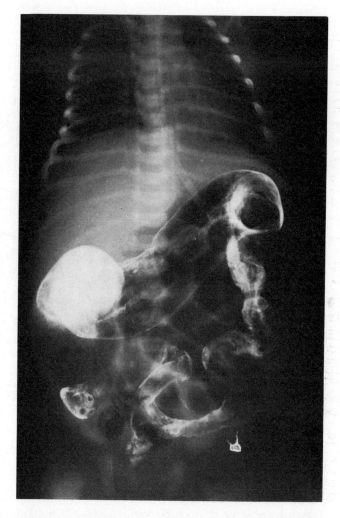

Figure 68–1. The small left colon syndrome. This infant's grandmother had diabetes, but his clinical and roentgenographic findings were indistinguishable from those in Hirschsprung's disease. The descending colon was narrow in comparison with the transverse colon. The ganglion cells in the rectal biopsy ruled out Hirschsprung's disease.

drome is potentially very serious. Three of four patients in one series had cecal or ileal perforations, and two died.[14]

Except in cases with a history of a diabetic mother, it is not possible at first to definitely distinguish between a long-segment Hirschsprung's disease, small left colon syndrome, and the meconium plug syndrome. The first treatment in all three diseases is a continuation of the diagnostic contrast enema with a second enema of Gastrografin under fluoroscopic control. This procedure along with saline irrigations in the nursery should relieve the obstruction in all three conditions. With the known complication of cecal perforation in mind, there should be no hesitation in performing a prompt colostomy if the obstruction is not relieved by these means. One should obtain a rectal suction biopsy first.

MILK BOLUS OBSTRUCTION

Intestinal obstruction caused by impacted milk curds in the terminal ileum would not occur if every infant was fed human breast milk. In an effort to speed weight gain in premature infants, formulas have been developed that contain 24 to 28 cal/ounce and correspondingly high levels of milk protein solids. The clinical picture involves a premature infant started on high calorie feedings during the first day or so of life, often before the passage of normal meconium stools. Within 5 to 14 days, the infant develops abdominal distention and vomits. Plain roentgenograms demonstrate a ground glass appearance due to the inspissated milk.[15] Contrast enemas demonstrate intraluminal filling defects in the terminal ileum and colon not unlike those seen in meconium ileus. However, the inspissated milk is not adherent to the mucosa.[16]

Milk curd obstruction results from a combination of the premature infant's poor peristalsis and inability to digest the increased concentration of protein.[17,18] If treatment with gastric drainage, intravenous fluids, and a Gastrografin enema fails to relieve the obstruction, an operation is necessary, manually removing the firm bolus through an enterotomy.

FUNCTIONAL INTESTINAL OBSTRUCTION

Sepsis, hypothyroidism, adrenal insufficiency, hypokalemia, and maternal drug ingestion may simulate a neonatal mechanical obstruction.[19–21] A needless laparotomy in an infant with any of these medical conditions could be disastrous. Although infants with these diseases have abdominal distention and vomiting, as well as roentgenograms that demonstrate dilated loops of intestine, they will usually pass some stool. In addition, the septic baby will be lethargic and hypotensive and will show thermal instability. Any of these signs is an indication for culture of the blood and spinal fluid. Unless there is some evidence of perforation or nonviable intestine, an operation should be delayed pending the results of these tests and a trial of antibiotic therapy. Babies with adrenal insufficiency may have a flank mass in addition to abdominal distention. Low levels of serum sodium and chloride, despite adequate replacement, provide the real clue to diagnosis. Hypothyroidism closely mimics Hirschsprung's disease, with delayed passage of stool, but the baby may also be sluggish and hypotonic, with a large fontanelle and prolonged jaundice.[22] Although an inspired guess often is necessary to make the diagnosis, several states now require routine screening of all newborns for hypothyroidism.

INTESTINAL PSEUDO-OBSTRUCTION

There is a small group of patients who clinically have an intestinal obstruction but who have no mechanical, metabolic, or drug problem. The very worst of these syndromes develop during the neonatal period, but there are milder degrees of the disease that have onset later in childhood and cause symptoms for many years. The first of these patients were reported on by the Pittsburgh Children's Hospital.[23] All were male, 5 were premature, and 1 had a diabetic mother. The findings at operation varied, but some had dilated, thin-walled intestine as far as the terminal ileum, where the bowel tapered into a narrow, collapsed area. This gross finding suggested total colon aganglionosis. However, a proximal ileostomy was of no benefit to these babies, and at autopsy, all had ganglion cells throughout their colons. There would appear to be a spectrum of severity, since Byrne et al. found 3 babies who became symptomatic during the neonatal period and 4 more whose symptoms did not develop until 7 years of age.[24] Of the 3 symptomatic during the neonatal period, all had abdominal distention and vomiting and clinical courses marked by periods of slight improvement, followed by recurrent episodes that increased in severity and frequency until no diet or formula was tolerated. There is no evidence of malabsorption in such cases, but studies demonstrate poor esophageal motility, delayed gastric emptying, and to-and-fro peristalsis in dilated loops of small intestine. No muscular or neuronal abnormalities were found in light or electron microscope studies of the duodenum or small bowel. Kapila et al. carried out extensive pharmacologic studies in one neonate with similar findings.[25] Carbachol, neostigmine, metaclopramide, pheloxybenzamine (alpha blocker), propranolol (beta blocker), and Senokot failed to stimulate effective peristalsis. The bowel musculature demonstrated in vitro insensitivity to acetylcholine. Intramuscular injections of cerulein (0.5 μg/kg), an extract from the skin of an Australian frog, resulted in peristalsis and ileostomy drainage in one baby. While taking this medication, the child was able to tolerate oral feedings and gain weight until she died with a gangrenous adhesive intestinal obstruction at 1 year of age.

Ten neonates with this syndrome were studied at the Toronto Children's Hospital.[26] Patients were studied with rectal manometry, rectal biopsy, and barium studies. In 5, there were changes in the smooth muscle of the bowel wall, suggesting a primary intestinal myopathy. Specific therapy was of no particular value in these patients, but some improved spontaneously after long-term support with hyperalimentation. Six of the patients survived.

NEURONAL INTESTINAL DYSPLASIA

Some infants with pseudo-obstruction have defects in their ganglion cells. They do not have typical Hirschsprung's disease because ganglion cells are present. Neuronal intestinal dysplasia is characterized pathologically by hyperplasia of the myenteric plexus, with an increase of acetylcholinesterase activity and the formation of giant ganglia.[27] When the neuronal abnormality is localized to the rectum and sigmoid, the symptoms consist of diarrhea, bloody stools, and abdominal distention. There is ulceration of the rectal mucous membrane resembling ulcerative colitis. When the condition is localized, rectal irrigations or a colostomy is curative. Unfortunately, the abnormality may extend to the entire small bowel and is fatal.

We have detailed studies of 3 patients, all girls, who had abnormal ganglion cells throughout their bowel. The first was a newborn girl with distended loops of small intestine whose barium enema demonstrated a microcolon. At operation, the ileum tapered from distended, thin-walled bowel to an airless, collapsed termi-

nal ileum and colon. Multiple biopsies demonstrated normal ganglion cells in the colon, but in the ileum, there were only scattered clusters of abnormal ganglion cells. In other areas of the small intestine, the ganglion cells were more numerous than usual, but the normal nerve fibers were absent in these areas. An ileostomy performed at 1 week of age never functioned. She was unable to tolerate any feeding, including human breast milk and died at 4 months, when her family elected to discontinue hyperalimentation. The second patient was also a healthy, full-term girl. She vomited all her early feedings and developed abdominal distention. Her x-rays demonstrated dilated loops of intestine, and the working diagnosis was total colonic aganglionosis (Fig. 68–2). The rectal biopsy demonstrated ganglion cells, which on close study appeared to be immature. At operation, the terminal ileum and colon were collapsed, but abnormal ganglion cells were present throughout the bowel (Fig. 68–3). There were weak peristaltic contractions in response to direct electrostimulation in the terminal ileum, and an ileostomy was performed. The patient improved and eventually was weaned off hyperalimentation to breast milk feedings. At 2 years of age, she was still on breast milk and thriving. Repeat biopsies were thought to show improvement in the rectal ganglion cells, but there was no change in the rest of the colon. The ileum was then anastomosed to the distal rectum.

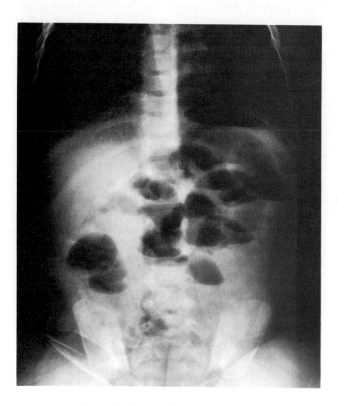 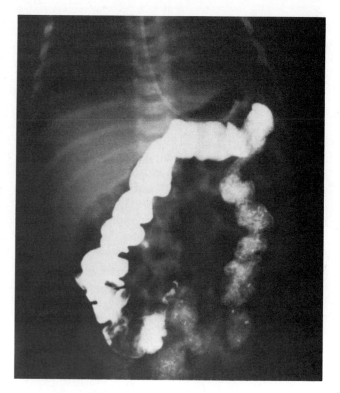

Figure 68–2. Left. Dilated small bowel with air–fluid levels. Right. Barium is still in the colon after 48 hours. Child was thought to have total colon Hirschsprung's disease, but ganglion cells were present.

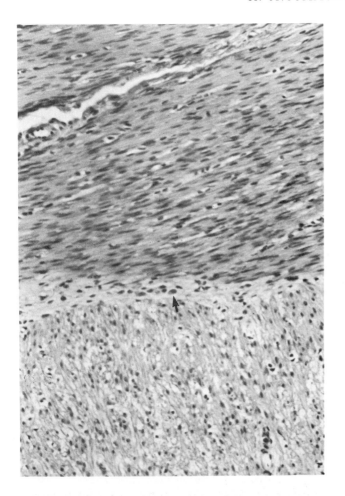

Figure 68–3. The arrow points to a rare small, abnormal ganglion cell in Auerbach's plexus. There were also degenerating nerves. The immature ganglion cells were positively identified by electron microscopy but were displaced into the muscle.

At 5 years of age, the ileostomy was reestablished because of progressively more severe bouts of distention and vomiting. The child continues to do well with the ileostomy at 7 years of age. Another girl had a history of encephalitis following a live measles vaccination at 5 years of age. She had normal intestinal function until she gradually became constipated at 8 years of age, after she had recovered from the encephalitis. The constipation increased in severity. At 9 years of age, a barium enema demonstrated what appeared to be a typical transition zone from a dilated transverse colon to a narrow descending and sigmoid colon. Biopsy of this child's colon demonstrated total degeneration of the ganglion cells in Auerbach's plexus from the sigmoid colon to the rectum, although the ganglion cells in Meissner's plexus were normal. Multiple other biopsies demonstrated small, pyknotic ganglion cells in the remaining colon and ileum. Biopsies of the upper small intestine demonstrated less severe changes. This child also developed achalasia of the esophagus, further demonstrating a dif-

fuse abnormality of motility. She was treated with an ileostomy and, during 8 years of observation, has had repeated bouts of distention with watery diarrhea. X-rays have demonstrated to-and-fro peristalsis in the small intestine. She has survived to age 25 with the aid of frequent hospitalization for hyperalimentation. This child's clinical course resembles Chagas' disease, but several antibody titers have been found to be normal. Perhaps the live measles vaccination was responsible for central vagal degeneration.

The Megacystis-Microcolon-Intestinal Hypoperistalsis Syndrome

The most recently described syndrome of intestinal hypoperistalsis involves a large, distended bladder, microcolon, and nonrotation of the midgut. The small intestine is about one third the normal length, and there is no mesenteric fixation. The 5 patients described by Berdon et al. and Amoury et al. were all girls; 2 were siblings.[28,29] We have encountered one newborn girl with the megacystis-microcolon-intestinal hypoperistalsis syndrome and one boy with identical intestinal findings but a normal bladder. This patient had two siblings, both boys, who had died with the same syndrome. Clinically, such infants have abdominal distention and bilious vomiting. Roentgenograms demonstrate a hugely distended bladder that displaces the bowel. At operation, the bladder is large and thick-walled and the intestine is nonrotated. Our patients, as well as those reported in the literature, have died despite the creation of stomas and pharmacologic attempts to stimulate bowel peristalsis. Electron microscopic examinations of the ileum and urinary bladder have demonstrated vacuolar degeneration in the smooth muscle cells and increased connective tissue between the cells. The ganglion cells are normal, and acetylcholinesterase activity is normal. Intestinal motility studies demonstrate only a few contractions of low amplitude. Puri et al. have coined the term "neonatal hollow visceral myopathy" to decribe this syndrome.[30] These pathologic findings are similar to but far more severe than those found in older children and adults with the syndrome of chronic intestinal pseudo-obstruction.[31,32] Visceral myopathy also may be familial, perhaps transmitted as an autosomal dominant trait.[33]

SUMMARY

All of these syndromes are poorly understood and few are helped by an operation. The surgeon, however, has an extremely important role in the diagnosis and management of these patients. In the newborn infant, when the diagnosis of a mechanical obstruction is unclear but an operation seems indicated, the surgeon must think of these lesions. First, it is essential to obtain biopsies and frozen section examinations to rule out Hirschsprung's disease. Next, sufficient biopsy material should be taken from all segments of the intestine so that electron microscopic and biochemical studies can be made. If a portion of the intestine has peristalsis, a stoma may be made at that point. In general, however, these babies are best served with long-term hyperalimentation, and possibly a venting gastrostomy, in the hope that they will improve spontaneously.[34] There is now 1 reported case of an 11-year-old boy with chronic pseudointestinal obstruction who improved after an IV bolus of 0.15 mg/kg of cisapride. The improvement was maintained by rectal administration of the same drug. Cisapride is a benzamide derivative that stimulates motor activity of the entire gut and is 100 times more potent than metoclopramide. It acts by enhancing acetylcholine release at the myenteric plexus.[35]

REFERENCES

1. Tunell WP: Hemangioendothelioma of the pancreas obstructing the common bile duct and duodenum. J Pediatr Surg 11:827, 1976
2. Roth D, Farinacci CJ: Jejunal leiomyosarcoma in a newborn. Cancer 3:1039, 1950
3. Talwalker VC: Intussusception in the newborn. Arch Dis Child 37:203, 1962
4. Yoo RP, Touloukian RJ: Intussusception in the newborn: A unique clinical entity. J Pediatr Surg 9:495, 98, 1974
5. Ravitch MM: An unusual cause of neonatal intestinal obstruction: Congenital absence of the duodenal musculature. Surgery 58:1022, 1965
6. Komi N, Kohyama Y: Congenital segmental dilatation of the jejunum. J Pediatr Surg 9:409, 1974
7. Carroll RL Jr: Absence of musculature of the distal ileum: A cause of neonatal intestinal obstruction. J Pediatr Surg 8:29, 1973
8. Swenson O, Rathauser F: Segmental dilatation of the colon: A new entity. Am J Surg 97:734, 1959
9. Brawner J, Shafer AD: Segmental dilatation of the colon. J Pediatr Surg 8:957, 1973
10. Irving IM, Lister J: Segmental dilatation of the ileum. J Pediatr Surg 12:103, 1977.
11. Davis WS, Allen RP, Favara BE, Slovis TC: Neonatal small left colon syndrome. Am J Roentgenol Radium Ther Nucl Med 120:322, 1974
12. David WS, Campbell JB: Neonatal small left colon syndrome. Am J Dis Child 129:1024, 1975
13. Philippart AI, Reed JO, Georgeson KE: Neonatal small left colon syndrome. J Pediatr Surg 10:733, 40, 1975
14. Stewart DR, Nixon GW, Johnson DG, Condon VR: Neonatal small left colon syndrome. Ann Surg 186:741, 1977
15. Cook RC, Rickham PP: Neonatal intestinal obstruction due to milk curds. J Pediatr Surg 4:599, 1969
16. Cremin BJ, Smythe PM, Cywes S: The radiological appearance of the "inspissated milk syndrome": A cause of intestinal obstruction in infants. Br J Radiol 43:856, 1970
17. Graivier L, Harper NG, Currarino G: Milk-curd bowel obstruction in the newborn infant. JAMA 238:1050, 1977
18. Lewis CT, Dickson JA, Swain VA: Milk bolus obstruction in the neonate. Arch Dis Child 52:68, 1977
19. Raffensperger J, Johnson FR, Greengard J: Nonmechanical conditions simulating obstructive lesions of the intestinal tract in the newborn infant. Surgery 49:696, 1961
20. Ueda T, Okamoto E, Seki Y: Nonmechanical intestinal obstruction simulating surgical emergency in the newborn infant. J Pediatr Surg 3:676, 1968
21. Solomon JR: Functional intestinal obstruction in the newborn. Progressive Pediatric Surgical Congress, Melbourne 1:38, 1970
22. Boruchow IB, Miller CD, Fitts WT: Paralytic ileus in myxedema. Arch Surg 92:960, 1966
23. Sieber WK, Girdany BR: Functional intestinal obstruction in newborn infants with morphologically normal gastrointestinal tracts. Surgery 53:357, 1963
24. Byrne WJ, Cipel L, Euler AR, et al: Chronic idiopathic intestinal pseudo-obstruction syndrome in children—clinical characteristics and prognosis. J Pediatr 90:585, 1977
25. Kapila L, Haberkorn S, Nixon HH: Chronic adynamic bowel simulating Hirschsprung's disease. J Pediatr Surg 10:885, 1975
26. Bagwell C, Filler R, Cutz E, et al: Neonatal intestinal pseudo-obstruction. J Pediatr Surg 19:732, 1984
27. Scharli A, Meier-Ruge W: Localized and disseminated forms of neuronal intestinal dysplasia mimicking Hirschsprung's disease. Pediatr Surg 16:164, 1981
28. Berdon WE, Baker DH, Blanc WA, et al: Megacystis-microcolon-intestinal hypoperistalsis syndrome: A new cause of intestinal obstruction in the newborn: report of radiologic findings in five newborn girls. Am J Roentgenol Radium Ther Nucl Med 126:957, 1976
29. Amoury RA, Fellows RA, Goodwin CD, et al: Megacystis-microcolon-intestinal hypoperistalsis syndrome: A cause of intestinal obstruction in the newborn period. J Pediatr Surg 12:1063, 1977
30. Puri P, Lake B, Gorman F, et al: Megacystis-microcolon-intestinal hypoperistalsis syndrome: A visual myopathy. Pediatr Surg 18:64, 1983
31. Schoffler M, Lowe M, Bill A: Studies of idiopathic intestinal pseudo-obstruction: I. Hereditary hollow visceral myopathy: clinical and pathological studies: Family studies. Gastroenterology 73:327, 1977
32. Anvras S, Mitros F, Soper R, Pringle K: Chronic intestinal pseudo-obstruction in young children. Gastroenterology 91:62, 1986
33. Mayer EA, Schoffler M, Rotter J, et al: Familial visceral neuropathy with autosomal dominant transmission. Gastroenterology 91:15, 1986
34. Pitt H, Mann L, Berquist W, et al: Chronic intestinal pseudo-obstruction management with TPN and a venting gastrostomy. Arch Surg 120:614, 1985
35. Cohen N, Booth I, Parashar K, Corkery J: Successful management of idiopathic intestinal pseudo-obstruction with cisapride. J Pediatr Surg 23:229, 1988

69
Short Gut Syndrome

"Short gut syndrome" is an imprecise term used to describe rapid intestinal transit, inadequate digestion, and malabsorption in patients who have had a massive intestinal resection. In neonates, this is usually the result of a gangrenous midgut volvulus, extensive intestinal atresia, necrotizing enterocolitis, or Hirschsprung's disease involving the entire colon and terminal ileum.

The loss of up to 50 percent of the small intestine, which in the newborn infant leaves approximately 125 cm of bowel, requires no special postoperative management, particularly when the ileocecal valve is retained. Such a patient will require only the usual postoperative fluid and electrolyte management and should tolerate normal feedings. If there is diarrhea or malabsorption, a search must be made for some other problem, such as a blind loop syndrome, anastomotic stricture, or a specific absorption problem (such as lactose deficiency). There are reports of adults who have maintained marginal survival on oral intake following anastomosis of the distal duodenum to the transverse colon.[1] Long-term follow-up studies also indicate that adolescents and adults can live after the anastomosis of 45 cm of jejunum to the transverse colon or with the retention of 30 cm of small bowel with an intact ileocecal valve.[2,3] Wilmore, by reviewing reports on 50 infants up to 2 months of age who had massive intestinal resections, correlated the factors that led to survival.[4] Some 21 infants had 38 to 75 cm of residual bowel with intact ileocecal valves. There was only 1 death, and this was due to a second obstruction. Of 14 babies with 15 to 38 cm of residual bowel, 7 survived. There were no survivors among those who had less than 40 cm of small intestine and no ileocecal valve or less than 15 cm of small bowel with an intact valve. The mean birth weight of survivors with 15 to 38 cm of bowel was 3.1 kg, whereas the nonsurvivors had a mean weight of 2.3 kg. One infant with 11 cm of jejunum and an intact ileocecal valve has survived but is mentally and physically retarded.[5] The prognosis depends not only on the length of remaining bowel but also on its quality. Intestine damaged by ischemia, particularly by necrotizing enterocolitis (NEC), requires a longer recovery period. Some infants with an apparent adequate length of bowel never develop the ability to absorb even the simplest of nutrients.

The anatomic and functional differences between the jejunum and ileum require that the surgeon not only measure and record the total length of residual bowel but that the length of the jejunal and ileal segments be recorded separately, along with the presence or absence of the ileocecal valve. The proximal 40 percent of the small bowel is jejunum and the rest is ileum, but the jejunum has twice the diameter of the ileum, and its circular folds are more numerous. Normally, such water-soluble substances as simple sugars, vitamins, and electrolytes are absorbed in the duodenum and proximal jejunum. Fats, proteins, and fat-soluble vitamins are digested first and then absorbed in the ileum. The reabsorption of bile salts by the ileum and their recirculation to the liver and thence back into the intestine play an important role in the digestion and absorption of fats. The ileum has a greater functional reserve than the jejunum and can compensate for loss of the proximal bowel. Thus, absence of proximal intestine is better tolerated than loss of the ileum.

PATHOLOGY

The diarrhea and malabsorption seen after the loss of critical lengths of small intestine are due to a decrease in absorptive surface area and decreased transit time from the stomach to the anus. Gastric hypersecretion has been demonstrated following intestinal resection.[6–8] This has been associated with hypersecretion of gastrin, but Scully et al. found no correlation with either gastrin levels or hypersecretion in neonates who had experienced massive resections.[9] However, their patients were receiving hyperalimentation, which depresses gastric secretion. The outpouring of gastric acid into the small intestine has three deleterious effects. First, the intestinal mucosa suffers injury so that the adaptive process of mucosal hypertrophy is damaged. Acid inactivates lipase and trypsin, which interferes with fat and protein digestion. Finally, the high solute load of the secretions may result in an osmolar diarrhea, whereby the intestinal tract secretes rather than absorbs water and electrolytes. Soon after intestinal resection, particularly after loss of the ileocecal valve, bacterial contamination of the upper intestine further damages the mucosa. Buildup of bile acids because of the loss of the ileum's active transport process for their absorption causes irritation of the colon and a potent cathartic effect. In addition, the pool of bile salts available for liver secretion into the upper intestine is decreased. This results in failure of solubilization of long-chain fatty acids and monoglycerides.[10] Disturbances in the enterohepatic circulation of bile salts after ileal resection also are associated with cholelithiasis.[11] Sugar intolerance is relatively common following any gastrointestinal surgery in the neonate. After intestinal obstruction, there is a 30 percent incidence of intolerance to either lactose or sucrose.[12,13] In the short gut syndrome, damage to the brush border of the mucosa by bacterial contamination and hyperacidity particularly impairs digestion of disaccharides because the enzymes necessary to this digestion normally are concentrated in the upper bowel.

ADAPTIVE MECHANISMS

Although intravenous nutrition and supportive therapy can prolong life in infants with massive intestinal resection, the ultimate growth, development, and quality of life of these infants depend on the capacity of the remaining intestine to compensate for loss of its absorptive surface. Experiments with animals, along with radiographic studies and repeat operations, have clearly demonstrated the increase in length and caliber of the bowel.[14,15] The dilated loops of intestine that are seen several years after resection may simulate an intestinal obstruction. Absorption also is enhanced by growth of villi, which can result in a fourfold increase of the absorptive surface.[16] The longer villi are the result of an actual increase in the number of cells, which is probably due to a more rapid rate of cell migration from the crypts.[17–19] The ileum has a greater capacity for compensation than has the jejunum.[20] The ileum can increase its absorption of substances that require no special transport mechanisms, and it retains the ability to absorb bile acids and

vitamin B_{12}, which require special transport systems.[21,22] Other than the functional demand that regulates such related phenomena as liver regeneration following resection and hypertrophy of a contralateral kidney after nephrectomy, there is no satisfactory explanation for the changes seen in the bowel following resection.

DIAGNOSIS

There is no doubt about the diagnosis when the surgeon who performed the original resection has carefully measured the residual bowel and continues to care for the infant. Frequently, however, patients are transferred from one institution to another, and it is easy for a diagnosis of short gut syndrome to be applied inappropriately. The measurement of transit time with a nonabsorbable marker (such as charcoal or carmine red) will rule out partial obstructions or a blind loop. An upper gastrointestinal study with a small bowel follow-through should further document the length of the residual bowel and demonstrate any obstruction or internal fistula. This study is also helpful in planning therapy to study specific problems of digestion and absorption. The stools are tested for sugar at frequent intervals, especially when oral feedings are being increased. Intolerance to sugar can be studied further with a lactose absorption test. Normally, the ingestion of 2 g lactose per kg body weight will increase the blood sugar by at least 25 mg/100 ml. Fecal fat and bile acid measurements are useful in documenting choleretic enteropathy. The measurement of gastric acid secretion by removing a 12-hour sample through a gastric tube on low suction is of value in documenting gastric hypersecretion. Blood counts and serum electrolyte studies are carried out along with other indicated metabolic studies at weekly intervals or more often as indicated.

TREATMENT

More than anything else, successful treatment of an infant with a major intestinal resection requires the patience and devotion of physicians and nurses. The potential advantages of each change in diet or medication must be weighed against a possible deleterious effect on the normal adaptive mechanisms. This is particularly true when another surgical procedure is being considered. Only one change in therapy should be made at a time, and these changes at suitable intervals. At least 2 or 3 days should elapse before something new is commenced or the previous change is discontinued. Although total intravenous alimentation is necessary for survival of infants with the short gut syndrome, infants with only 15 to 30 cm of intestine were known to survive before the introduction of this mode of therapy, at a time when only routine fluids and blood and plasma transfusions were available.[23,24] By trial and error, clinicians found that by starting and gradually increasing oral feedings soon after the operation, diarrhea slowly subsided. Most used a formula low in fat but high in carbohydrates and protein. Frequently, patients would be given two to three times the usual volume of formula, despite diarrhea.

Currently, intravenous nutrition or hyperalimentation is the cornerstone of therapy for infants with the short gut syndrome. During the first 3 or 4 postoperative days, fluid therapy is maintained to provide for maintenance water and electrolyte requirements and to cover losses through gastric drainage. Hyperalimentation is then commenced and increased so that the infant gains weight at a normal rate. A Broviac catheter inserted into the external jugular vein and tunneled to the midchest provides the best long-term access in these children. Initially, the solution is run continuously, but cycling is commenced so that by the time the child is ready for home care, the total parenteral nutrition (TPN) solution is given intermittently, often only at night. It is paradoxical that although hyperalimentation has been hailed as life-saving in patients with the short gut syndrome, intravenous alimentation may slow the migration of epithelial cells and leads to a significant reduction in mucosal thickness in laboratory animals.[25,26] Oral feeding is more effective than total intravenous nutrition in maintaining mucosal protein, DNA, and disaccharidase activity in the bowel mucosa of these animals.[27] These observations may not be applicable to humans, but they do indicate the importance of starting some oral feeding as soon as possible.

Dietary Therapy

In planning dietary therapy, one must consider not only caloric intake and fluid volume but also the fat content, the type of sugar contained, and the osmolarity of the formula. Most standard infant formulas contain lactose and approximately 3.5 percent fat and cow's milk protein. Artificial formulas containing lactose and cow's milk protein are almost never tolerated by these infants, yet human breast milk, which does contain lactose, is almost universally beneficial. Every mother should be encouraged to breast-feed her baby, but this is particularly important in infants with intestinal resections. If breast milk is unavailable, our preference is to commence feeding with Pregestimil (Mead-Johnson). This formula contains hydrolyzed casein as a source of protein, sucrose, and fat in the form of medium chain triglyceride (MCT) oil. The feedings are commenced with 5 ml of a half-strength formula that provides 10 cal/ounce, every 3 hours. If this is tolerated, the feedings are advanced in increments of 5 to 10 ml/feeding/day until the infant's

fluid volume requirements are set. The concentration is then increased to 15 cal/ounce and finally to 20 cal/ounce. If diarrhea commences or if the baby develops abdominal distention, the volume and concentration are decreased for a few days and then once again increased. Those infants who cannot tolerate Pregestimil may be able to absorb an elemental diet consisting of amino acids, glucose, minerals, and vitamins.[28,29] Unfortunately, the osmolar load of an elemental diet requires that the formula be diluted to 7 to 10 cal/ounce when it is first started. Initially, the elemental diet is better tolerated when given by a slow, continuous intragastric drip at a rate of 1 ml/kg per hour. If there is no diarrhea, the volume and the concentration are consecutively increased. Eventually, as the intestine adapts over a period of weeks or months, the concentration is increased to 20 cal/ounce. As adaptation progresses, oral feedings are given every 3 hours in addition to the continuous tube feedings, they are gradually substituted until the baby can take all his feedings orally. Often, progress with feedings is so slow that only 1 ml/hour can be added over the course of several days. When persistent diarrhea does occur, it is necessary to cut back on the feedings and to increase the volume of intravenous fluids. The change from an elemental diet to an infant formula also must be made slowly. We begin by adding oral Pregestimil at one or two feedings a day while the continuous tube feedings are still in progress. Often this process continues after the infant has been discharged to home care. Banana flakes and rice cereal are the first foods other than formula that are introduced. Later, the usual baby foods are begun, one at a time and in teaspoon amounts until they have been tolerated for several days without diarrhea. Eventually, children who survive are able to take a diet that is normal except that it excludes such roughage as corn and beans.

Drug Therapy

Drug therapy includes agents to decrease motility, antacids to reduce the consequences of gastric hypersecretion, antibiotics when bacterial overgrowth in the intestine is suspected, and cholestyramine to bind bile acids. It is difficult to evaluate the efficacy of any therapy in the short gut syndrome because of variations in the natural compensatory mechanisms. Often a drug is considered to have no effect when in fact it was not given in the proper dosage or over a sufficiently long period of time. Loperimide in doses of 0.5 mg/kg per day is the most effective drug to control intestinal motility. This dose may be increased if a rapid transit time interferes with its absorption. Cholestyramine is a chloride salt of a basic anion exchange resin containing quaternary ammonium groups that bind bile acids and prevent their cathartic effect on the colon.[30] In addition, this drug binds endotoxin produced by bacteria in the bowel.[31] It is useful in many diarrheal conditions, particularly after ileal resection.[32–34] We have found, as have others, that the combination of oral cholestyramine and paregoric is particularly useful.[35] In order to be most effective, cholestyramine must be given before a meal. Otherwise, bile acids will reach the colon before they can be bound. There is no recommended dosage for infants and children, but we start with 100 mg/kg per day in divided doses and increase to three times this much. In tube-fed infants, the cholestyramine is dissolved in water and given every 3 hours. Questran, the Mead-Johnson product, contains 3 g of sucrose for each gram of active cholestyramine. This, of course, alters the dosage, and the sucrose itself may not be well tolerated. Cimetidine or ranitidine is indicated to protect the upper intestinal mucosa from gastric acid.[36]

The care of these infants is frustrating and tedious. It is not surprising, therefore, that many operations have been devised to slow the transit time or to increase the mucosal surface area.[37–40] Many operations that show promise in the dog laboratory are useless or even dangerous in patients! The reversal of a short segment of intestine to slow peristalsis has been attempted.[41] In our hands, it has been of no benefit. If the ileocecal valve is missing, the creation of an antirefluxing nipple valve to prevent the reflux of colonic bacteria into the small bowel may be of some use.[42,43] Even when these procedures have been reported to be of benefit in humans, however, it is difficult to know if the success of the operation was not the result of continued medical therapy and bowel maturation.

Many of the problems seen in this group of patients are caused by prolonged hospitalization, exposure to infections, and the prolonged use of tube feeding. Plans should be made for home care of these infants as soon as possible. This includes training the parents in the care of the central venous line and the management of gradually increased enteral feedings. Prolonged tube feeding should be avoided, because eventually, when the infant can tolerate oral feedings, he or she simply will not suck, chew, or swallow. Postuma et al. outlined the details of care in one infant with 13 cm of small bowel who survived with normal motor, intellectual, and emotional development.[44] This infant was given frequent oral feedings of human breast milk as soon as intestinal function commenced. He was discharged from the hospital on home parenteral nutrition and was given small amounts of rice, banana, and pureed meats at 6 months of age.

Complications and setbacks in the group of patients are frequent. A touch of epidemic diarrhea or an upper respiratory infection can cause explosive diarrhea, requiring the resumption of TPN. Intestinal losses of electrolytes cause episodic acidosis, and problems with the central venous line require catheter changes. The prognosis for these infants is improving. Their adaptation to total enteral feedings often takes place at about the time when the caloric requirements per unit of body mass normally are decreasing.[45] After the child is able to tolerate a complete enteral diet, one must be alert to the development of specific nutritional deficiencies, particularly vitamin D, calcium, phosphorus, and vitamin B$_{12}$. Supplements, particularly of MCT oil, to supply fats may be required indefinitely. Rickham et al. followed 9 patients for 10 to 18 years and found that they were essentially normal.[46] Our patients, however, all are in the lower percentiles for height and weight. Those infants who have succumbed have not died of malnutrition but of liver disease associated with a prolonged lack of oral intake and TPN.

REFERENCES

1. Kinney JM, Goldwyn RM, Barr JS Jr, Moore FD: Loss of the entire jejunum and ileum, and the ascending colon: Management of a patient. JAMA 170:529, 1962
2. Meyer HW: Extensive resection of small and large intestine: A further 22-year follow-up report. Ann Surg 168:287, 1968
3. Anderson CM: Long-term survival with 6 inches of small intestine. Br Med J 1:419, 1965
4. Wilmore DW: Factors correlating with a successful outcome following extensive intestinal resection in newborn infants. J Pediatr 80:88, 1977
5. Kurz R, Saver H: Treatment and metabolic findings in extreme short bowel syndrome with 11 cm jejunal remnant. J Pediatr Surg 18:257, 1983
6. Aber GM, Ashton F, Carmalt MH, Whitehead TP: Gastric hypersecretion following massive small-bowel resection in man. Am J Dig Dis 12:785, 1967
7. Avery GB, Randolph JG, Weaver T: Gastric response to specific disease in infants. Pediatrics 38:874, 1966
8. Straus E, Gerson CD, Valow RS: Hypersecretion of gastrin associated with short bowel syndrome. Gastroenterology 66:175, 1974
9. Scully JM, Lynch FJ, Passaro E, Dudgeon DL: Serum gastrin concentration in infants with short gut syndrome. J Pediatr Surg 11:315, 1976
10. Hofmann AF, Grundy SM: Abnormal bile salt metabolism in a patient with extensive lower intestinal resection. Clin Res 13:254, 1965
11. Pellerin D, Bertin P, Nihoul-Fekete CL, Ricour CL: Cholelithiasis and ileal pathology in childhood. J Pediatr Surg 10:35, 1975
12. Burke V, Anderson CM: Sugar intolerance as a cause of protracted diarrhea following surgery of the gastrointestinal tract in neonates. Aust Paediatr J 2:219, 1966
13. Howat JM, Aaronson I: Sugar intolerance in neonatal surgery. J Pediatr Surg 6:719, 1971
14. Bell MJ, Martin LW, Schubert WK, et al: Massive small-bowel resection in an infant: Long-term management and intestinal adaptation. J Pediatr Surg 8:197, 1973
15. Benson CD, Lloyd JR, Krabbenhoft KL: The surgical and

metabolic aspects of massive small bowel resection in the newborn. J Pediatr Surg 2:227, 1967

16. Flint JM: The effect of extensive resections of the small intestine. Bull Johns Hopkins Hospital 23:127, 1962

17. Weser E, Hernandez HM: Studies of small bowel adaptation after intestinal resection in the rat. Gastroenterology 60:69, 1971

18. Porus RL: Epithelial, hyperplasia following massive small bowel resection in man. Gastroenterology 48:753, 1965

19. Weinstein LD, Shoemaker CP, Hersh T, et al: Enhanced intestinal absorption after small bowel resection in man. Arch Surg 99:560, 1969

20. Dowling RH, Booth CC: Functional compensation after small-bowel resection in man. Lancet 2:146, 1966

21. Perry PM, White J, Dowling RH: Bile salt absorption following small bowel resection in the rat. Gut 13:845, 1972

22. MacKinnon AM: Intestinal adaptation of vitamin B_{12} absorption. Clin Sci 42:29, 1972

23. Lawler WH, Bernard HR: Survival of an infant following massive resection of the small intestine. Ann Surg 155:204, 1962

24. Pilling GP, Cresson SL: Massive resection of the small intestine in the neonatal period: Report of two successful cases and review of the literature. Pediatrics 19:940, 1957

25. Feldman EJ, Dowling RH, McNaughton J, et al: Effects of oral versus intravenous nutrition on intestinal adaptation after small bowel resection in the dog. Gastroenterology 70:712, 1976

26. Eastwood GL: Small bowel morphology and epithelial proliferation in intravenously alimented rabbits. Surgery 82:613, 1977

27. Levine GM, Derren JJ, Steiger E, et al: Role of oral intake in maintenance of gut mass and disaccharidase activity. Gastroenterology 67:975, 1974

28. Weinberger M, Rowe MJ: Experience with an elemental diet in neonatal surgery. J Pediatr Surg 8:175, 1973

29. Thompson WR, Stephens RV, Randall HT, Bowen JR: Use of the "space diet" in the management of a patient with extreme short bowel syndrome. Am J Surg 117:449, 1969

30. Thompson WG: Cholestyramine. Can Med Assoc J 104:305, 1971

31. Nolan JP, Ali M: Effect of cholestyramine on endotoxin toxicity and absorption. Am J Dig Dis 17:161, 1972

32. Hofmann AF, Poley JR: Role of bile acid malabsorption in pathogenesis of diarrhea and steatorrhea in patients with ileal resection. Gastroenterology 62:918, 1972

33. Tamer MA, Santora TR, Sandberg DH: Cholestyramine for intractable diarrhea. Pediatrics 53:217, 1974

34. Hofmann AF, Poley JR: Cholestyramine treatment of diarrhea associated with ileal resection. N Engl J Med 281:397, 1969

35. Nagaraj HS, Cook L, Canty TG, Haight G: Oral cholestyramine and paregoric therapy for intractable diarrhea following surgical correction for catastrophic disease of the GI tract in neonates. J Pediatr Surg 11:795, 1976

36. Cortot A, Fleming R, Malagelada J: Improved nutrient absorption after cimetidine in short bowel syndrome with gastric hypersecretion. N Engl J Med 300:79, 1979

37. Hutcher NE, Mendez-Picon G, Salzberg AM: Prejejunal transposition of colon to prevent the development of short bowel syndrome in puppies with 90% small intestine resection. J Pediatr Surg 8:771, 1973

38. Binnington HB, Tumbleson ME, Ternberg JL: Use of jejunal venomucosa in the treatment of the short gut syndrome in pigs. J Pediatr Surg 10:617, 1975

39. Cywes S: The surgical management of massive bowel resection. J Pediatr Surg 3:740, 1968

40. Glick P, deLorimer A, Adzick N, Harrison M: Colon interposition: an adjuvant operation for short gut syndrome. J Pediatr Surg 19:719, 1984

41. Warden JM, Wesley J: Small bowel reversal procedure for the "short gut" baby. J Pediatr Surg 13:321, 1978

42. Sadri D: Construction of an ileocecal valve and its role in massive resection of the small intestine. Surg Gynecol Obstet 152:310, 1984

43. Grieco G, Reyes H, Ostrovsky E: The role of a modified intussusception jejunocolic valve in short bowel syndrome. J Pediatr Surg 18:354, 1983

44. Postuma R, Moroz S, Friesen F: Extreme short bowel syndrome in an infant. J Pediatr Surg 18:264, 1983

45. Cooper A, Floyd T, Ross A, et al: Morbidity and mortality of short bowel syndrome acquired in infancy: an update. J Pediatr Surg 19:711, 1984

46. Rickham PP, Irving I, Shmerling DH: Long-term results following extensive small intestinal resection in the neonatal period. Prog Pediatr Surg 10:65, 1977

70
Hirschsprung's Disease

_____ *Orvar Swenson and John G. Raffensperger*

Congenital megacolon, or Hirschsprung's disease, is one of the classic problems in pediatric surgical practice. It enters into the differential diagnosis of newborn infants with intestinal obstruction as well as the perplexing problem of an older child with recalcitrant constipation. Furthermore, our understanding of this fascinating entity, from the original, clinical, gross autopsy descriptions to the current histochemical and functional studies, mirrors the progress of all medical practice.

Although there were references to patients with megacolon before 1886, it was Harald Hirschsprung, a Danish pediatrician, who first described it as a distinct clinical entity.[1] His two patients died at 8 and 11 months, respectively, with unrelenting constipation, malnutrition, and enterocolitis. During the early 1900s, there were a number of theories for the etiology of the disease, but the concept that gained most support was that of neural imbalance, producing malfunction in the entire large intestine. This concept resulted in attempts to treat Hirschsprung's disease with drugs and sympathectomy.[2,3] The long-term results of patients treated in this manner were unsatisfactory.[4] Consequently, treatment evolved to resection of the massively dilated portion of the bowel, with anastomosis of apparently normal proximal bowel to the remaining sigmoid.[5,6] The initial improvement in these patients was transient—they again developed constipation with massive bowel dilatation and hypertrophy.

Reports of an absence of ganglion cells in the distal colon were not fully appreciated, and the absence even was attributed to stasis and fecal impaction.[7-9] This was the prevailing situation when Swenson began his studies of Hirschsprung's disease in 1945. He saw a 4-year-old child with progressive, life-threatening abdominal dis-

tention make a surprisingly prompt, complete recovery after a sigmoid colostomy. Since the child had regained good health, the family requested that the colostomy be closed, and this was done. However, despite vigorous treatment with drugs, a lumbar sympathetic block, and spinal anesthesia, the child became progressively worse, and 16 months later a transverse colostomy was made. There was again a prompt recovery. Two additional patients with congenital megacolon responded in a similar manner when their colostomies were closed. The explanation for this recovery following colostomy appeared to be a functional defect in the distal colon. This prompted a critical review of barium enemas in patients with congenital megacolon. All of the patients showed narrow, irregular distal colonic segments, which varied in length. Colonic peristaltic tracings demonstrated propulsive waves descending through the left colon in normal subjects. A study of five patients with Hirschsprung's disease showed normal contractions in the left colon that did not continue into the rectosigmoid. Resected specimens of distal colon that were defective in peristalsis demonstrated an absence of ganglion cells. This established the fact that the aganglionic bowel was defective in function and could be cited as the cause of Hirschsprung's disease.[10-12] Swenson's work was confirmed by others who reported the absence of ganglion cells in the distal bowel in children with Hirschsprung's disease.[13-15]

PATHOPHYSIOLOGY

The intrinsic autonomic nervous system of the bowel consists of three distinct plexuses of ganglion cells with their neural connections. Auerbach's plexus lies between the circular and longitudinal muscles, Henle's, or the deep submucosal, plexus is along the inner margin of the circular muscularis propria, and Meissner's plexus lies immediately beneath the muscularis mucosa (Fig. 70–1).[16] Sympathetic fibers originating from cells in the prevertebral parasympathetic ganglia enter the bowel wall and end in a fibrillar network about the intrinsic ganglion cells. Cholinergic fibers from the vagal and pelvic outflow also terminate in the intrinsic plexus, primarily in the distal rectum and internal sphincter.[17,18] The ganglion cells constitute the intrinsic neuroregulatory apparatus of the bowel.[19] Longitudinal sections through the distal rectum have demonstrated the absence of ganglion cells in Auerbach's plexus to 1.4 cm above the pectinate line in normal patients. The submucosal plexus terminates an average of 2 mm proximal to Auerbach's plexus, and there is an additional 0.5 cm of distal rectum with a diminished number of ganglion cells.[20,21] This normal absence or paucity of ganglion cells for 2 cm above the pectinate line indicates the necessity of taking a diagnostic rectal biopsy above this point.

In classic Hirschsprung's disease, the ganglion cells are asbsent from all three plexuses. The space normally occupied by ganglion cells is taken up by large, longitudinally oriented nerve fibers. There is a transition zone between the normal and aganglionic bowel, which contains reduced numbers of cells. Grossly, this zone is a tapered section from the dilated to the contracted bowel.

Histochemical studies have shown an increase in the number and size of cholinergic and adrenergic fibers in the aganglionic segment. The concentration of acetylcholine in the aganglionic bowel is 2 to 9 times higher than in the normal colon.[22] Thus, the aganglionic bowel does not have normal cholinergic receptors. The abnormal bowel also has a higher concentration of catecholamine-containing nerve fibers. Touloukian et al. found the tissue concentration of norepinephrine in aganglionic segments to be nearly 3 times that of normal bowel, evidence for adrenergic hyperactivity.[23] In vitro studies and electrical field stimulation confirm the excess release of acetylcholine and that the nonadrenergic inhibitory system is absent.[24-26] The adrenergic system is unable

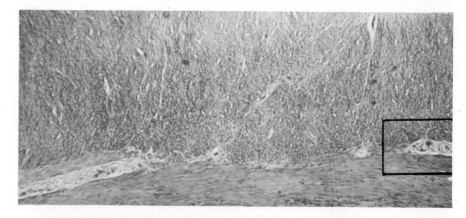

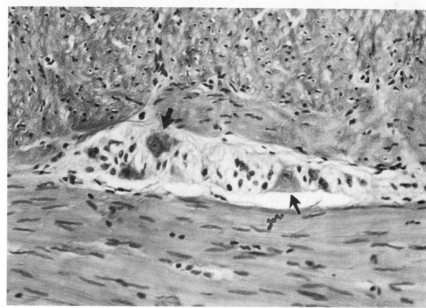

Figure 70–1. Auerbach's plexus, containing ganglion cells. **Top:** The longitudinal and transverse muscle layers are visible; the ganglion cells are in between. **Bottom:** Higher power magnification of the ganglion cells.

to effect muscle relaxation by direct action on the muscle in spite of the elevated norepinephrine concentrations. The absent cholinergic ganglion cells prevent coordinated peristalsis, and cholinergic nerves from the sacral parasympathetic plexus directly stimulate muscle cells, producing unchecked contraction.[27] The intramural nonadrenergic inhibiting neurons of Auerbach's plexus are absent, so any stimulus to relaxation of the circular muscle fibers also is lost. The result of this autonomic imbalance is a constant state of contraction in the aganglionic bowel and internal sphincter. Peristaltic waves from normal bowel stop at the aganglionic segment, and the internal sphincter remains spastic despite pressure stimulation in the rectum.

Extent of Aganglionosis

We have analyzed data in 880 cases collected from seven centers throughout the world. In 75 percent of the patients, the aganglionic segment extended into the sigmoid colon, whereas in only 2 percent was the total colon or portions of the terminal ileum aganglionic. Total intestinal aganglionosis also has been reported.[28,29] We have not personally observed ultrashort Hirschsprung's disease but believe that if one does a very low biopsy, the normally aganglionic internal sphincter could be misinterpreted. We have now observed one histologically proven skip area, in which the transverse colon contained ganglion cells, whereas both the distal and proximal colon were aganglionic. Other reports of skip areas have indicated that the transverse colon contained ganglion cells and could be used in the pullthrough operation.[30,31]

There are two embryologic explanations for the presence of ganglion cells in the bowel. The most commonly accepted theory suggests that the ganglion cells are derived from the vagal neural crest and that the neuroblasts are distributed to the bowel by a craniocaudal migration during the 5th to the 12th weeks of gestation.[32] The neuroblasts initially appear in the myenteric plexus just outside the circular muscle layer and later migrate across muscle to submucosa. The earlier this caudal migration of neuroblasts is arrested, the longer is the aganglionic segment. Smith confirmed these studies and observed the postnatal development of ganglion cells, especially in premature babies.[33] This theory of craniocaudal migration explains the absence of ganglion cells at the distal end of the alimentary tract but leaves the nagging question of how skip areas can occur. It is possible that the distal bowel is innervated from the caudal portion of the neural crest.[34]

EPIDEMIOLOGY

The incidence of Hirschsprung's disease is not known precisely but is about 1 in 5000 live births. In our review of 880 cases, 81.1 percent occurred in males, and 88.3 percent of the cases were in Caucasians. There is a familial tendency. Richardson and Brown found 57 cases in 24 families.[35] One mother had six sons by three different fathers, all afflicted with the disease. In our series, the disease was found in 1.3 percent of the children's parents, and 0.5 to 1.0 percent occurred in siblings. Bodian and Carter reviewed the basis for genetic and familial transmission and found it unaffected by maternal age or birth order.[36] The disease appears to be an autosomal recessive and sex-linked trait. If the first child is a girl with a long segment disease, the chances are increased that her siblings will be affected. In our series, one mother with a sigmoid lesion had twin girls, both with total colon aganglionosis. Another had four children, three of whom had Hirschsprung's disease.

ASSOCIATED DEFECTS

Down's syndrome occurred in 4.2 percent of our patients, and associated cardiac and urologic defects were rare. Hirschsprung's disease is even more rarely linked with other intestinal anomalies, such as atresia or malrotation.[37,38] Always examine the distal resected bowel in atresias for ganglion cells! Wardenburg's syndrome, consisting of a characteristic facial deformity, congenital deafness, and extensive areas of white hair, also has been associated with Hirschsprung's disease.[39] This is not surprising, since this disease also arises from an abnormal development of the neural crest. The association of megacolon and piebald hair also occurs in a strain of mice.[40]

DIAGNOSIS

The signs and symptoms of Hirschsprung's disease are highly variable. On the one hand, it may appear in the newborn period with acute signs of abdominal distention, vomiting, and failure to pass meconium. On the other hand, the disease may persist untreated into adult life. However, all of the 26 patients (aged 17 to 62 years) reported by Todd had symptoms since birth.[41] Not only do the symptoms date from birth, but when birth histories are available, 94 percent of infants with Hirschsprung's disease are seen to have had delayed passage of meconium. This is the cardinal symptom that, if appreciated, allows diagnosis in the neonatal period. Frequently, the initial passage of meconium is stimulated by a rectal examination or an enema. If the diagnosis is not made at that time, there may be a period in which the baby has constipation but moves the bowels in response to formula changes or suppositories. Either this constipation will progress to severe obstruction, or the infant will develop enterocolitis. The enterocolitis associated with Hirschsprung's disease is poorly understood but is associated with fever, vomiting, progressive abdominal distention, and, paradoxically, explosive diarrhea. As the disease progresses, peristalsis diminishes and then stops. At this point of intestinal decompensation, there is massive abdominal distention. In previous years, when it usually went unrecognized, this condition carried an 80 percent mortality. Intestinal perforation and peritonitis may occur secondary to Hirschsprung's disease. In our series of 880 patients, there were 25 intestinal perforations, and we have seen 2 cases of appendicitis in neonates with Hirschsprung's disease.

In the usual case, abdominal distention and constipation wax and wane in response to formula changes, enemas, and laxatives. If the mother breast-feeds, the symptoms will be ameliorated, only to commence again when formula is substituted for breast milk. The mother may hear loud borborygmi, and the infant may have episodic vomiting when the feces is severely impacted. In the older child, there is typically severe abdominal distention with dilated loops of intestine outlined on the thin abdominal wall. Fecal soiling is generally absent in older children but may occur in 4 percent of patients, especially with short segment disease. On physical examination, a visible and palpable transverse colon with an explosive passage of stool in response to a rectal examination suggest Hirschsprung's disease. In older children, the abdominal distention is associated with an increased anteroposterior diameter of the chest, and there are palpable fecal impactions in the abdomen. Occasionally, these impactions are so huge they are thought to be tumors, but an impaction will indent on finger pressure. Classically, the rectum will be empty. Small amounts of stool were found in 40 percent of the author's patients, and 15 percent had rectal impactions. The first diagnostic test in most children should be a plain supine and upright film of the abdomen (Fig. 70–2). In the newborn, it is difficult to distinguish small intestinal distention from colonic distention, but in older infants, one often can identify a dilated segment of transverse colon crossing the upper abdomen.

The barium enema is a diagnostic tool, but its limitations must be appreciated. Errors in interpretation of the barium enema rest on two factors: the age of the patient and the length of the aganglionic segment. In infants less than 1 month old, the proximal bowel has not yet dilated in contrast to the aganglionic zone. The x-ray diagnosis in the neonate is improved by obtaining a film 24 hours later that shows retained barium. Furthermore, the small left colon syndrome, hypothyroidism, and the meconium plug syndrome may all be confused with Hirschsprung's disease.

A baby with a total colon aganglionosis may be diagnosed as normal or as having a proximal small bowel obstruction because the entire colon is small but is not a true microcolon. In older children, there is difficulty with the diagnosis of short segment disease because the

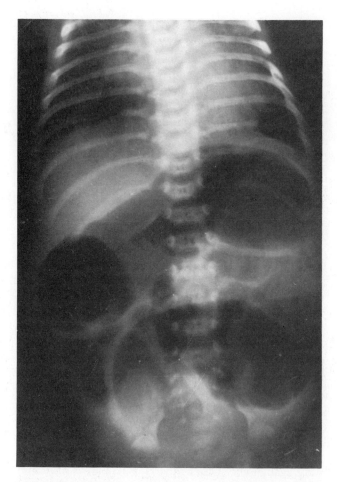

Figure 70–2. Supine film of the abdomen with hugely dilated loops of intestine. It is difficult to distinguish dilated small bowel from dilated large bowel. Here the upper loop is the transverse colon.

column of barium may obscure a narrow rectal segment. This fact accounts for the 6 percent rate of inaccurate diagnosis by barium enema in children over 1 year of age. With the barium enema, one typically observes dilated bowel proximal to a narrow segment. This is best appreciated on a lateral film of the barium-filled rectum (Fig. 70–3). Failure to evacuate the barium is another consistent finding in cases of congenital megacolon. Irregular, spiculated mucosa is caused by intercurrent enterocolitis (Fig. 70–4). A typical history, together with barium enema demonstration of an unequivocal narrow distal segment, precludes a need for further diagnostic tests.

More specific tests are indicated in newborn infants in whom the radiologic findings are atypical, as well as in the occasional older child who is thought to have psychogenic constipation but whose history or barium enema examination is atypical. The most reliable diagnostic test is the full-thickness rectal wall biopsy, and the microscopic study for ganglion cells (Fig. 70–5).[42] This test requires hospitalization for 2 to 3 days and adminis-

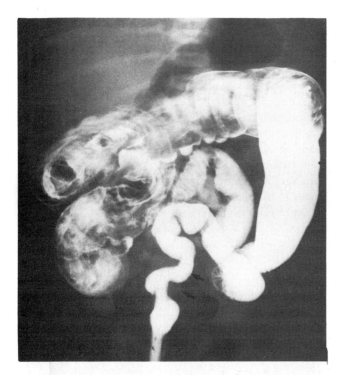
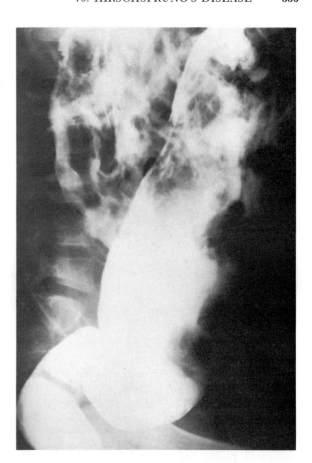

Figure 70–3. Classic barium enemas demonstrating the proximal dilated and the distal contracted segments diagnostic of Hirschsprung's disease in older children.

tration of a general anesthetic. The child is prepared with rectal irrigations and oral cathartics until the colon is emptied. The biopsy is performed with the child in an exaggerated lithotomy position. A headlight is extremely helpful. The rectum is vigorously dilated and further cleansed with saline and povidone-iodine irrigations. Small retractors are inserted into the rectum to expose the posterior rectal wall. Two traction sutures are placed 2 to 3 cm above the mucocutaneous line, and traction prolapses the full thickness of the rectal wall into the operative field. A third suture is placed through the rectal wall between and above the traction sutures. The biopsy is then taken with scissors. The first cut is aimed to penetrate through the rectal wall, after which the scissors are spread outside the muscular layers. Bleeding vessels are controlled with electrocoagulation so that the two layers of muscle wall can be clearly identified. A 0.5 by 1 cm segment of tissue is then removed with the suture, after which the rectal muscle and mucosa are closed separately. A frozen section is performed immediately to ensure that the specimen is adequate. If there are no ganglion cells on the frozen section, we may proceed with a colostomy under the

same anesthetic, if indicated. An experienced pathologist can make a definitive diagnosis, providing the biopsy is taken proximal to the area where ganglion cells are normally sparse or absent. The only disadvantage to a full-thickness biopsy is scarring, which may hinder the definitive resection.

Biopsy of the mucosa and the submucosa is easier to perform and, with experience, will yield results that are nearly as satisfactory as those obtained with a full-thickness biopsy. A mucosal biopsy may be obtained in a neonate or small infant by having a nurse hold the child by the legs in the lithotomy position. The anus is then spread with an anal speculum, and a specimen of mucosa is obtained with a laryngeal or any short biopsy forceps.[43] The technique of rectal biopsy has been further simplified by the use of an intestinal suction biopsy capsule.[44,45] We currently use a 4.7 mm capsule with the following technique. Rectal irrigations are given until the rectum is clean to digital palpation. When the test is performed on outpatients, these irrigations may be given by the mother at home. The capsule is inserted into the anal canal for a distance of 5 to 6 cm, with the knife of the capsule closed. The capsule is opened when

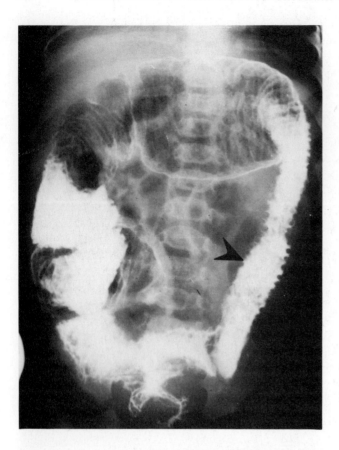

Figure 70–4. The narrow aganglionic segment extends to the splenic flexure. In addition, the descending colon is spiculated. This is typically observed in babies with the enterocolitis associated with Hirschsprung's disease.

it is in the proper position, and negative pressure of at least 20 mm of mercury is applied for several seconds. This allows time for the mucosa and submucosa to be pulled into the capsule. The knife is pulled shut, and the capsule is removed from the rectum. The biopsy is then teased out of the capsule with a needle and placed on a plastic film. It is helpful to examine the biopsy with a magnifying lens to make sure that a bit of submucosa is included in the specimen. The specimen is oriented with the mucosa down. It must be kept as flat as possible and immediately fixed in Bouin's solution. It is helpful to obtain at least two biopsies in case the first one is not satisfactory. In normal pastients, ganglion cells are readily found in a properly obtained submucosal biopsy. As many as 20 to 50 sections may be required to confirm the presence of ganglion cells, which are smaller and more difficult to identify than in the Auerbach's plexus. No errors of interpretation were found in a series of 42 patients when two adequate specimens from each patient were examined.[46] In Hirschsprung's disease, no ganglion cells are found, but in the typical patient, nerve trunks are identified. The rectal suction biopsy has proved to be most valuable in the exclusion

of Hirschsprung's disease, especially in the newborn infant who has had a delayed passage of meconium. We now perform this test on all infants for whom the diagnosis of meconium plug syndrome has been suggested. The rectal suction biopsy is not so helpful in excluding Hirschsprung's disease in older children, who may have a short segment lesion. In such cases, the mucosa is thickened, and it is more difficult to obtain a sufficiently thick specimen. In these patients, we continue to prefer the full-thickness biopsy, which can be extended to an anorectal myotomy if there are no ganglion cells on the frozen section. We are not willing at this time to make a definitive diagnosis of Hirschsprung's disease in any patient solely on the basis of an absence of ganglion cells in a suction biopsy. Histochemical techniques add to the accuracy of light microscopy.[47,48] Normal patients show barely detectable acetylcholinesterase activity in the intestinal submucosa. When ganglion cells are absent, there is an overabundance of acetylcholine and, consequently, of the corresponding enzyme, acetylcholinesterase. When acetylcholinesterase stains are used, it is necessary to look at only one section to make a definitive diagnosis. There is an additional factor: stains for acetylcholinesterase are positive findings, whereas the absence of ganglion cells may mean only that one has not looked at enough material.

Measurements of anorectal pressure also have been used to diagnose Hirschsprung's disease. In normal patients, distention of the rectum produces an involuntary relaxation of the internal sphincter with synchronous contraction of the external sphincter. This reflex relaxation of the internal sphincter appears to be mediated through the intramural ganglia. In Hirschsprung's disease, the internal sphincter fails to relax in response to balloon distention of the rectum.[49,50] Using a simplified triple balloon system and a water manometer, distention of the rectal balloon with 10 to 15 mm of water results in a gradual fall of internal sphincteric pressure (2 to 4 cm of water in normal children).[51] In our experience, it has been difficult to place accurately the recording balloons or an open system within the internal sphincter. Furthermore, crying and abdominal straining may produce false results. In the newborn period, when one would like to make the diagnosis of Hirschsprung's disease without resort to a biopsy, the anorectal reflex is poorly developed. Holschneider et al. have demonstrated that the normal rectoanal reflex does not develop until 12 days of age.[52] In a highly sophisticated study conducted in a special manometric laboratory, there were 10 false positive and 8 false negative results in 229 examinations. There was a 26 percent error rate in infants under 1 month of age.[53] Although the accuracy of manometry increases with patient age, it is never sufficiently accurate to make a definitive diagnosis of Hirschsprung's disease without confirmatory biopsy evidence. The his-

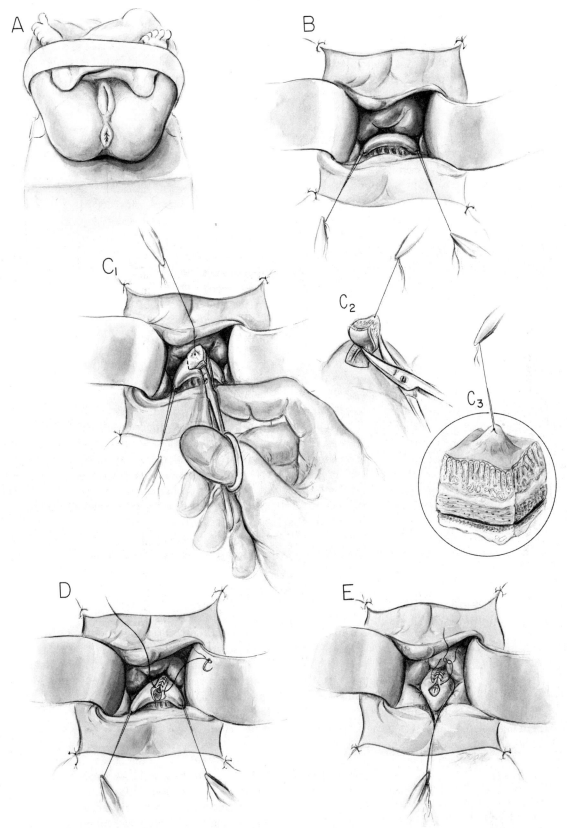

Figure 70–5. Technique for a full-thickness rectal biopsy. The full-thickness rectal wall 2 to 3 cm above the pectinate line is prolapsed into the field with traction sutures. The biopsy must include both the circular and longitudinal muscle layers to encompass the Auerbach's plexus. All sutures must be mounted on the smallest half-Fergusson needle to allow turning within the narrow confines of the rectum. The muscle is closed with 5-0 polyglyconate sutures.

tory, physical examination, and barium enema are just as accurate in determining the need for biopsy in the older child. Consequently, manometry is at best only a rough screening test. The rectal suction biopsy is simple and fast and provides a greater degree of accuracy in the diagnosis of Hirschsprung's disease than do other preliminary tests.

TREATMENT

A variety of operations have been developed for the cure of Hirschsprung's disease. They are all designed to bring bowel containing normal ganglion cells down to the distal rectum. This can be accomplished as a primary procedure in a child over 1 year of age and in good nutritional condition whose colon is not excessively dilated. When the diagnosis is made in small infants or when the bowel is tremendously dilated, temporization is indicated to allow the child to grow normally and to reduce the size of the colon. The choice of treatment depends on the child's age and general condition. However, either prolonged rectal irrigations or a colostomy will be indicated before the definitive operation. Rectal irrigations are indicated to decompress the neonate while awaiting a definitive diagnosis, to treat enterocolitis, and to remove fecal impactions in older children.

When the diagnosis is made in a child whose only symptom is constipation and who has never had enterocolitis, it is possible to avoid a colostomy if the mother is willing to give rectal irrigations until her baby is a year old.

An irrigation is not an enema! Saline is instilled into the rectum through a rubber catheter with a syringe. In a newborn, a size 16 catheter is inserted for several centimeters. Saline (15 to 20 ml) is instilled into the rectum with a syringe and then allowed to run out through the catheter by gravity. The procedure continues as long as stool is returned and is repeated several times a day until the infant's bowel has decompressed. In older children, a well-lubricated, size 20–28 French catheter is used, and 50 to 100 ml of saline is injected each time. It frequently is necessary to provide half-hour irrigation sessions several times a day to rid a child of a large impaction. During this time, oral mineral oil and mineral oil retention enemas are given to soften the impaction. Once the impaction has been broken up, once-daily irrigations are sufficient to keep the bowel empty. A child who is 4 to 6 months old is admitted to the hospital and irrigated until completely deflated. During this time, the mother is taught how to give the irrigations. Many children are then sent home, with the provision that if the mother cannot keep the bowel deflated, a colostomy will be performed. However, if the infant has enterocoli-

tis, the irrigations are used along with total IV alimentation to improve the baby's general condition and to deflate the overdistended bowel until a colostomy can be performed. Hyperalimentation is continued after the colostomy is performed because some infants continue to have diarrhea and vomiting whenever oral feedings are commenced.

A colostomy is indicated in any child who has had enterocolitis, in younger children when irrigations fail, and in older children who are malnourished and have hugely distended colons. The colostomy should be placed just proximal to the transition zone in the most distal portion of the bowel with normal ganglion cells. The location of the incision is determined by observing the location of the transition from dilated to narrow bowel via barium enema. In the usual case, a left lower quadrant, muscle-splitting incision will expose this area. A biopsy must be taken of the bowel wall to accurately determine the proper colostomy site. The biopsy site is chosen by observing the apparent transition zone; an extramuscular biopsy will avoid contamination with intestinal contents. This is accomplished by placing two traction sutures so as to stabilize the colon wall. Two incisions are then made one-quarter of an inch apart down to the mucosa, and with scissors dissection, a strip of muscle is excised, leaving the mucosa intact. The muscular defect is then closed with silk sutures. When no ganglion cells are found on a frozen section, another more proximal biopsy is taken. A colostomy is made at the point where the pathologist finds ganglion cells.

A blindly placed transverse colostomy should be avoided because in 10 percent of patients the aganglionosis extends across the ascending colon. Furthermore, a transverse colostomy attaches the colon to the anterior abdominal wall, and there may be insufficient length of bowel to extend to the perineum during the reconstruction. Even if the bowel distal to the stoma is long enough, it is small in diameter, and when anastomosed to the rectal stump, it is more likely to stricture. Finally, if the colostomy is left in place, a third operation will be necessary for its closure.

Evisceration of small intestine through the colostomy site is a constant hazard in neonates. Consequently, the bowel is sutured to the peritoneum and fascia. A loop colostomy with the bowel over a rod is preferable because of the ease with which it can be taken down. If the bowel is greatly dilated, it may be opened after it has been sutured to the fascia. Otherwise it is opened after 8 to 12 hours to allow time for a seal to develop about the bowel. When the rod is removed a week later, the colon is completely divided and a bridge of fibrous tissue has developed that will prevent prolapse. The resection is delayed until the child weighs 15 to 20 pounds (Fig. 70–6).

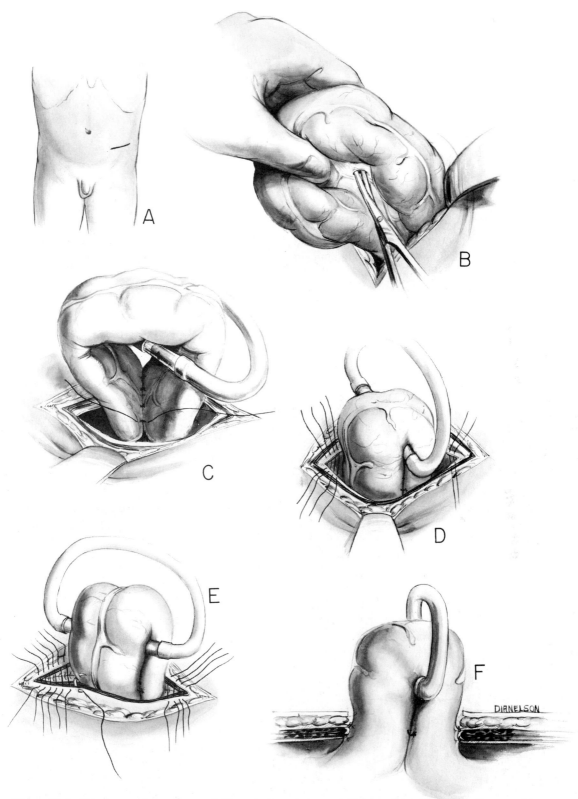

Figure 70–6. Colostomy using a glass rod. The colostomy is opened 12 hours later. This allows the wound to seal before it is exposed to stool.

The Swenson Pullthrough

Children who must undergo colon resection are given only clear liquids and an elemental diet by mouth for 3 days before surgery. Rectal irrigations are carried out until the colon is completely emptied. If there is a colostomy, both the proximal limb and distal limb are irrigated until the bowel is clean. Parenteral antibiotics are given the morning of surgery.

Technique The abdomen and perineum are prepared with povidone-iodine, and the rectum is again irrigated after the child is under anesthesia. The rectum may be further cleansed with povidone-iodine swabs. A small, Silastic Foley catheter is inserted into the bladder for decompression during the operation and for the first 3 to 4 postoperative days. The patient is positioned on the operating table to provide simultaneous exposure of the perineum and abdomen (Fig. 70–7). During the initial portion of the operation, the perineum is covered with sterile drapes that can be removed. If the child has a colostomy, the opening is detached from the skin and closed. The drapes, gown, and gloves are changed, and the colostomy opening may then be dissected from the peritoneum and fascia within the abdomen without contamination.

A left rectus, retracting incision is advantageous because the splenic flexure can be more easily mobilized. A transverse incision limits the proximal dissection. Once the abdomen is opened, the sigmoid colon is delivered into the wound (Fig. 70–8). If there has been a previous colostomy and there are biopsy-proven ganglion cells, this opening is used for the pullthrough. Otherwise, it is necessary to use the most distal bowel to contain ganglion cells as demonstrated by biopsy. The proximal line of resection above this point is selected and the bowel is divided between Kocher clamps or staples. One or more sigmoidal arteries are then divided to provide a length of bowel sufficient to reach the perineum. At this point, it may be necessary to mobilize the splenic flexure to provide adequate length. The marginal vessels must be preserved to maintain vigorous blood supply at the anastomotic site. When the lesion is in the transverse colon, it is necessary to ligate and divide the middle colic artery so that the right colon may be turned down to the perineum.

The pelvic dissection is commenced by dividing the peritoneum along the rectosigmoid and the rectum. These incisions, which commence laterally, are united in the cul-de-sac anterior to the rectum. The vas deferens and ureters are identified and observed in the course of the peritoneal incision and the pelvic dissection. At this point, if there is a large bulky segment of bowel, it may be divided at the rectosigmoid junction and removed (Fig. 70–9). This segment of bowel may be examined by frozen section for the presence of ganglion cells if no previous biopsies were obtained. The superior hem-

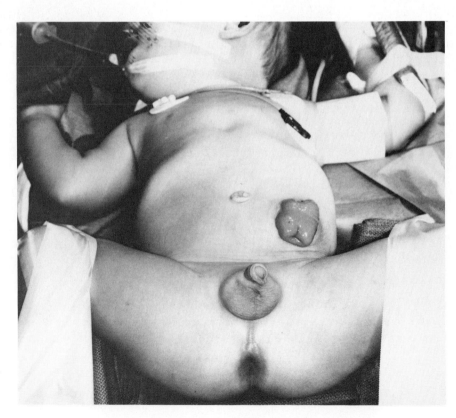

Figure 70–7. The child is positioned to allow access to the perineum and abdomen. Soft, padded saddle-type holders support the legs.

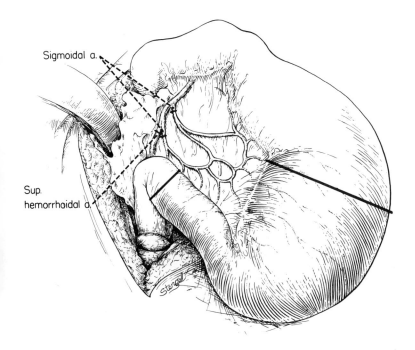

Figure 70–8. The dilated sigmoid colon has been drawn into the wound. The dark lines indicate the portion of the bowel to be removed first in order to provide more room for the pelvic dissection. The superior hemorrhoidal artery is ligated to diminish bleeding during the pelvic dissection.

orrhoidal artery, but not the vein, is ligated at this point to reduce bleeding during the subsequent pelvic dissection, which is brought right to the bowel wall at a point well superior to these vessels. The entire subsequent dissection is kept immediately on the muscular wall of the bowel. It is necessary to make a definite effort to dissect through the surrounding fatty tissue until the muscle fibers of the bowel are identified. If this is not done, and if the dissection is performed outside this plane, one may damage the urinary bladder innervation (Fig. 70–10). It is also helpful to free the peritoneum on each side in the pelvis so that it can be sutured to the anterior peritoneum adjacent to the abdominal inci-

sion. This will effectively wall off the small intestine from the field. The dissection through the pelvis is kept immediately on the bowel wall by separating tissue with the scissors to identify the blood vessels entering the bowel wall. As each vessel is identified, it is clamped with a long, curved hemostat and divided. These vessels may be coagulated on the bowel side and ligated on the pelvic side. Alternatively, vessels are coagulated with bipolar forceps flush with the bowel wall and then divided. This portion of the operation is tedious, and an assistant should hold the tissue up on traction, while the bowel is held the opposite direction, so as to allow identification and control of all vessels.

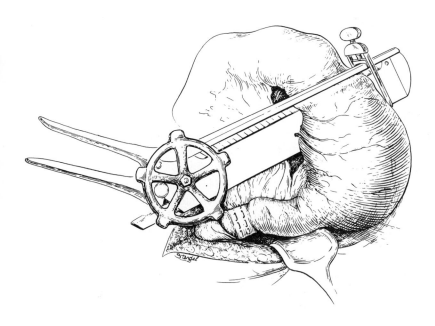

Figure 70–9. The dilated segment of bowel is removed after stapling with the von Petz or other device to diminish spilling of colonic contents.

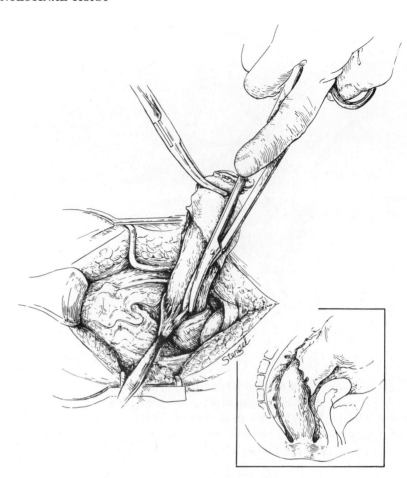

Figure 70–10. After dissection of the pelvic peritoneum, the rectum is held upward with vigorous traction. An assistant holds the perirectal tissue on a stretch with long-tissue forceps. This figure demonstrates small blood vessels that must be either clamped and then tied on the pelvic side or coagulated flush with the colon. This meticulous dissection continues flush with the bowel wall to the perineum.

Frequently, the dissection is kept so close to the bowel wall that a small divot of muscle is taken along with the vessel on the bowel side. When the dissection has reached the perineum, the surgeon leaves the abdominal field, and the perineum is exposed. The extent of dissection may be estimated by having an assistant palpate the depths of the wound while the surgeon examines the rectum. However, it is impossible to accurately judge the extent of the dissection until the rectum has been prolapsed through the anal canal.

The patient is now placed in the Trendelenburg position for better exposure of the perineum. After a vigorous dilatation, a long, curved clamp is inserted through the anal canal, and an assistant places the closed rectal stump within the jaws of the clamp (Fig. 70–11). The rectal stump is then everted. If it has been dissected sufficiently, traction on the rectum and countertraction on the perianal skin will expose the mucocutaneous line. This is important only posteriorly and laterally (Fig. 70–12). If the bowel has not been freed sufficiently, the rectal stump is returned to the abdominal cavity for further dissection. The distal dissection must be precise because if insufficient bowel is resected, there will be a recurrence of symptoms.

When the prolapsed rectum has been sufficiently

freed, the perineal field is again prepared and draped so that a small area of perineal skin is exposed around the anus. A cut is made anteriorly through the rectal wall about 2 to 3 cm from the dentate line, extending halfway through the rectal circumference. A clamp is inserted through this opening to grasp multiple sutures placed through the cut end of the proximal colon (Fig. 70–13). Before the proximal colon is pulled down, the assistant cleans 1 to 2 cm of the mesentery to facilitate the anastomosis. When the proximal colon is pulled through, the mesenteric border must extend 2 to 3 cm beyond the rectal incision, without tension and with an adequate blood supply. Unless these conditions are met, there is danger of poor anastomotic healing and leakage. If necessary, the proximal colon is returned to the abdomen for more dissection to provide sufficient length.

When the proximal colon is of proper length and the pathologist has definitely identified ganglion cells in the proximal end of the resected specimen, the anastomosis is started (Fig. 70–14). It is often helpful to place a fine traction suture anteriorly through the mucosa of the rectum to clearly expose the muscular coat (Fig. 70–14A). Interrupted sutures are placed through the cut muscular edge of the rectum and the muscular coat

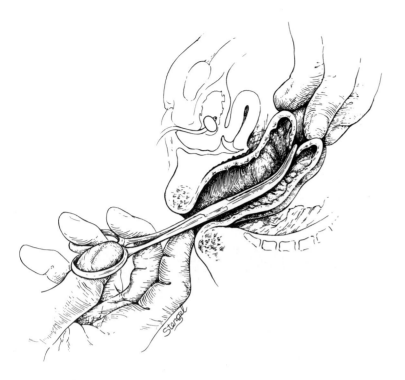

Figure 70–11. The surgeon passes a long, curved clamp up the rectum, and an assistant inverts bowel into the clamp for eversion of the rectal stump.

of the prolapsed colon. These sutures are not cut but are placed in a clamp so that retraction of the rectal stump does not occur and exposure is improved (Fig. 70–14B). The amputation of the rectum is completed after sutures have been completed on the anterior half (Fig. 70–14C, D). The cut is placed posteriorly within 0.5 cm of the mucocutaneous margin. We use absorbable 5-0 or 4-0 polydioxone sutures for both the muscle and

mucosal layers. Care must be taken not to fold in a portion of the proximal colon and thereby leave excessive space between sutures. If the circumference of the proximal colon is larger than that of the distal everted rectal stump, the sutures must be placed slightly further apart in the proximal colon to compensate for the discrepancy. When all the sutures have been placed, the proximal bowel is opened along half its circumference. Some su-

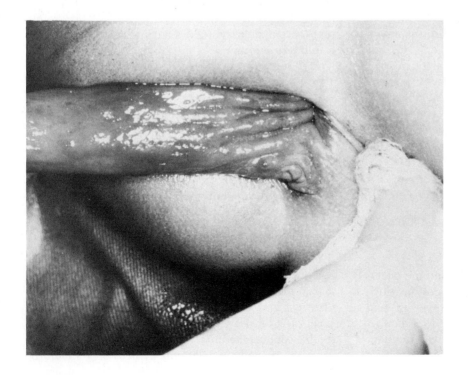

Figure 70–12. The prolapsed rectum must be everted sufficiently to clearly demonstrate the posterior dentate line. If this is not possible, the bowel is returned to the abdomen for further dissection.

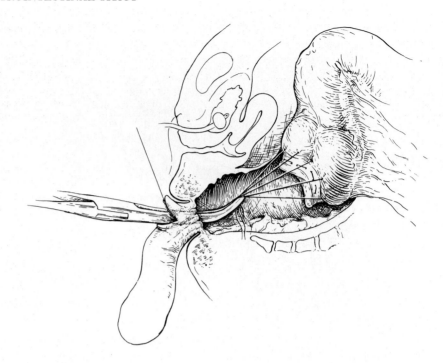

Figure 70–13. An incision has been made through the anterior half of the prolapsed rectum. At this point, a clamp is passed through the incision into the pelvis. An assistant then places sutures from the cut edge of the colon into the clamp, and the proximal bowel is pulled through to the perineum.

tures are cut, but enough are left to provide traction to allow accurate approximation of the mucosa. These sutures also are held to prevent the anastomosis from retracting into the pelvis. As more mucosal sutures are placed, the muscular sutures are cut. It is helpful to place sutures at each quadrant; while these are held outward on traction, the intervening tissue can be easily seen and accurately sutured. When all of the mucosal sutures have been placed, they are cut, allowing the anastomosis to retract back into the pelvis. While one team makes the anastomosis, an assistant closes the pelvic peritoneum and the abdominal incision. The anastomosis itself is aseptic until the proximal colon is opened, and at this point the pelvis is protected from contamination by the first row of interrupted sutures. In order to prevent cross-contamination, two separate instrument tables may be used for the abdominal and perineal portions of the operation, respectively. In recent years, one of us (JGR) has removed the appendix and left a No. 16 catheter with multiple holes in the ascending colon for postoperative decompression.

POSTOPERATIVE CARE

When the bowel has been well prepared and the operation has been performed properly, the postoperative course is benign. The Foley catheter is removed, and liquids may be offered by mouth within 2 to 3 days. A cecostomy tube is left on gravity drainage, with frequent saline irrigations, to drain liquid stool, preventing colonic distention and pressure on the suture line. The child

is given a liquid diet and advanced to full feedings as tolerated. Broad-spectrum antibiotics, which are started immediately preoperatively, are continued for 5 days after surgery. By that time, if the child is afebrile and tolerating feedings, he or she is discharged home. Two weeks later, a rectal examination is performed during an outpatient visit. If healing is satisfactory, the child is seen for follow-up visits at intervals. All patients are evaluated continuously for difficulties in bowel habits. Diarrhea may be secondary to a lactose or other sugar intolerance, and acute diarrhea with distention sometimes accompanies episodic infectious diarrheas or upper respiratory infections.

COMPLICATIONS AND RESULTS

We have now evaluated the immediate and long-term results of 880 patients operated on in seven pediatric surgical centers from 1947 to 1986. The most dangerous immediate postoperative complication is leakage at the suture line, which occurred in 5.6 percent of the 880 patients and led to a pelvic abscess in 3.3 percent. If there is any unexplained rise in temperature, lower abdominal tenderness, or distention, a leak should be suspected. A rectal examination may reveal a boggy, tender mass, or there may be generalized peritonitis. An immediate contrast enema should be performed through a small, well-lubricated catheter. After injection of a water-soluble contrast medium, one can see the leak on fluoroscopy. An immediate colostomy or ileostomy should be performed to prevent chronic pelvic infection, stricture,

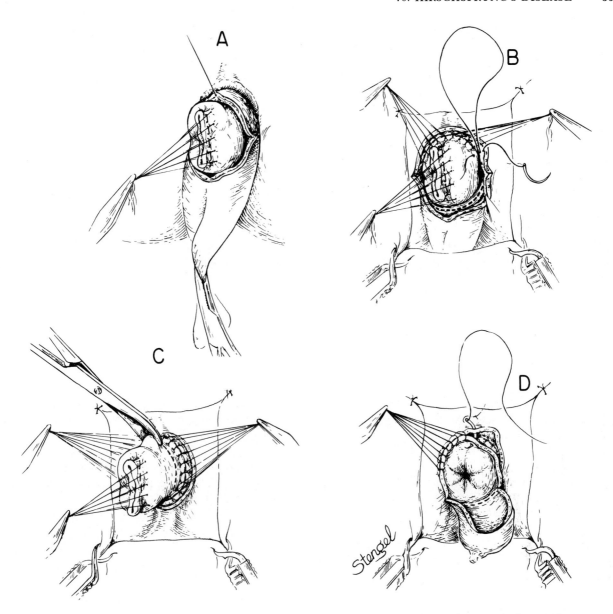

Figure 70–14. The anastomosis is performed in two layers, with 5-0 silk sutures used to the muscular layer and 4-0 chromic catgut or polyglycolic acid sutures used on the mucosa. **A.** Exposure of the muscularis is improved with a stay suture placed through the mucosa anteriorly. **B.** The first sutures placed through the muscularis are held on traction to improve exposure. **C.** After all of the necessary sutures have been placed in the muscularis, the proximal bowel is cut back to the suture line. **D.** The mucosal sutures are held on outward traction to prevent the anastomosis from slipping back into the pelvis until completion of the suture line.

and damage to the perineal muscles. We have observed one patient with a generalized peritonitis, but no leak was seen on x-ray, and she recovered after abdominal drainage, antibiotics, and a colostomy. In our earlier series, it appeared that anastomotic leaks were more common in children with Down's syndrome and in those who had not undergone a preoperative colostomy. In this entire group of patients, dating back to 1947, including a group of operations carried out in the newborn period, there were 21 deaths, a mortality rate of 2.4 percent. The mortality rate has decreased to 1.2 percent during the past two decades.

Enterocolitis occurred at some point in the course of the disease in 12 percent of the study group and accounted for 8 deaths. Six percent of patients have had dilatations for strictures, and 1.5 percent have required surgical excision of a severe stricture. In the long-term study of 880 patients treated since 1947, 87 percent report having normal bowel movements. Eight percent have some degree of constipation requiring the occasional use of either laxatives or enemas. Soiling was associated with some degree of constipation in 8 percent of the group. One hundred forty-two patients are now married, and 183 children have resulted from these marriages.

There has been no long-term urinary complication, and no defects in ejaculation have been reported. Other surgeons have reported equally good results.[54,55]

Enterocolitis

An infant with Hirschsprung's disease may have massive abdominal distention, paradoxical diarrhea, and sepsis. There are tremendous losses of fluids and electrolytes, and in the past, these infants had a high mortality rate. We have had one 3-day-old infant who was dead on arrival at our hospital. The colon proximal to the aganglionic zone was massively distended and ulcerated at autopsy. Milder cases are not so dramatic but are likely to occur during bouts of upper respiratory infections or concomitant with community epidemics of diarrhea. The clinical picture simulates that of a mechnical intestinal obstruction, but a rectal examination releases huge amounts of fluid and gas. Often, after the passage of a rectal tube, the abdomen deflates like a punctured automobile tire. This, of course, suggests that the spastic internal sphincter is at fault. The syndrome may occur even after the infant has a colostomy and is seen in the postoperative period after a pullthrough procedure.

Infants who are fed human breast milk almost never suffer from enterocolitis. In fact, human breast milk feeding relieves the distention and constipation of some cases of Hirschsprung's disease as well, obviating the need for a colostomy.

After a pullthrough operation, some children suffer with bouts of bloating, borborygmi, and diarrhea. This, perhaps is not enterocolitis; at least it is not an infectious enterocolitis but is caused by a spastic obstructing internal sphincter. None of the recommended pullthrough procedures ablate the internal sphincter for fear of creating incontinence. Therefore, a short length of aganglionic rectum always remains. DeLorimer correctly stated, "I suggest that we need to change the term enterocolitis to simply SOS, or the syndrome of the obstructing sphincter."[56] There may, however, be an infectious component to some cases because stasis anywhere in the gastrointestinal tract leads to bacterial overgrowth. Investigators at the Great Ormond Street Hospital have isolated *Clostridium difficile* from 10 of 13 children with enterocolitis.[57] The age distribution suggested that this organism may play an etiologic role, particularly in children under 3 years of age.

When a child has symptoms suggestive of enterocolitis or distention, the first treatment should be a rectal examination and the passage of a rectal tube. A nasogastric tube is placed for further decompression, and the infant is given replacement and maintenance IV fluids. Often, a bolus of plasma or albumin is necessary to treat hypovolemia. The stools are cultured and tested for reducing substances to rule out bacterial diarrhea and lactose intolerance. If *C. difficile* is cultured, vancomycin

should be given at first, and later, cholestyramine may be effective in binding the toxins. One or more vigorous rectal dilations under anesthesia will often relieve the symptoms.

Total Colon Aganglionosis

Hirschsprung's disease that involves the entire colon and varying portions of the small intestine presents quite different problems from the classic case. The diagnosis is much more difficult, and early studies included many patients in whom the diagnosis was not made until autopsy. The incidence is now estimated to be between 5 to 7 percent of all cases of Hirschsprung's disease.[58,59] These infants vomit bile-stained material shortly after birth but do not have severe abdominal distention. Some will pass stool, particularly after enemas. Plain films of the abdomen demonstrate nonspecific, dilated small bowel. Often the radiologic diagnosis is ileus or partial small bowel obstruction. A barium enema is nondiagnostic because the colon is of normal size. The suspicion of Hirschsprung's disease is heightened if the flexures are shortened and if barium refluxes into dilated ileum. The clinical and radiologic picture may be confused with meconium ileus. X-rays taken 24 hours after the barium enema will demonstrate residual barium in a contracted colon (Fig. 70–15). A rectal suction biopsy should be carried out promptly in any infant with unusual signs or symptoms of intestinal obstruction. Strangely enough, cases of total colon aganglionosis have been reported in older children.[60]

The findings at laparotomy are confusing to the surgeon who expects to find atresia or stenosis. There is no obvious mechanical obstruction. The colon is collapsed, and there may be a transition zone to distended bowel in the ileum. A preoperative rectal biopsy will spare considerable confusion at the operating table. Biopsies for frozen sections must be taken from the wall of the sigmoid, transverse colon, and cecum to establish the diagnosis and to rule out a skip area. Another biopsy is taken from the transition zone or dilated bowel to determine the length of the ganglionic bowel.

In prior years, an ileostomy was performed and, later, some type of pullthrough procedure. As many as 50 percent of infants would die from sepsis, malnutrition, and electrolyte loss while they had the ileostomy. The mortality rate was higher the longer the length of aganglionic bowel.[61] An ileoanal anastomosis after a Swenson pullthrough resulted in normal growth and development of several patients, but more were troubled with episodic diarrhea and poor growth. In an effort to increase the absorptive surface of the bowel, Martin advocated a Duhamel type pullthrough with a long lateral anastomosis between the aganglionic and ganglionic bowel.[62]

Martin's procedure improved absorption and survival rate but has been followed in some instances by

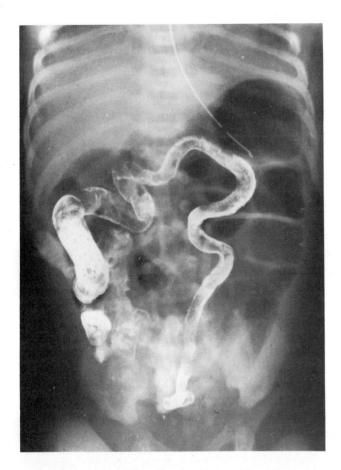

Figure 70–15. Total aganglionosis of the colon. The bowel is narrowed, and the flexures are shortened. The small bowel is dilated with air. Biopsy of the cecum is necessary to confirm the diagnosis, since this picture is similar to that of any small bowel obstruction in the neonate. The shortened flexures are suspicious, however.

enterocolitis.[63] The terminal ileum and the right side of the colon are more important from the standpoint of absorption than the rest of the colon. The attachment of a patch graft of either ileum or cecum improves absorption, and the composite of aganglionic and ganglionic bowel does not interfere with motility.[64,65] Kimura et

al. have now reported 7 patients who had colonic aganglionosis with from 5 to 40 cm of involved ileum who were operated on using their technique. Several months after the patch graft, a Swenson type of pullthrough is performed, using a segment of bowel containing ganglion cells distal to the patch graft. The Soave type of pullthrough procedure also has been used following a patch graft of ileum and right colon.[66,67]

Our own preference is to use the Kimura operation with a Swenson pullthrough. We have now applied the right colon patch and have completed the pullthrough in four children. In all patients, there was a reduction in stool output, and the consistency changed from watery to pasty after the second stage. Clearly, in these patients, absorption was improved. In one child, the patch consisted of terminal ileum, cecum, and up to the right transverse colon. He had two bouts of distention after the pullthrough, which responded to rectal dilatations. In retrospect, the patch may have been too long.

At this time, we recommend the following procedures. An ileostomy is created at the level determined to have ganglion cells by frozen section (Fig. 70–16). No aganglionic bowel is resected. The infant is treated from the onset with TPN and, when tolerated, an elemental diet. The permanent sections are reviewed to confirm the frozen section diagnosis. If the infant will tolerate oral feedings and can be weaned from TPN, nothing further is done in the neonatal period. Unfortunately, if more than the distal few centimeters of ileum are involved, there will be a profuse watery output of stool from the stoma requiring continuation of TPN. If this occurs, the infant should be promptly reoperated on, and a patch of aganglionic terminal ileum, cecum, and ascending colon should be sutured onto the ileum (Fig. 70–17). In our hands, this has promptly decreased the stool output, so the infant can tolerate oral feedings. The Swenson pullthrough may then be deferred to 1 year of age. Kimura has now followed four patients from 5 to 8 years. None has experienced enterocolitis, and

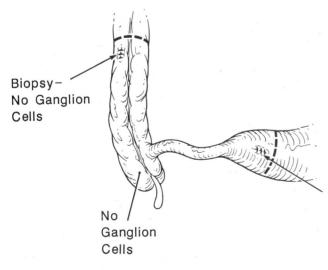

Biopsy– No Ganglion Cells

No Ganglion Cells

Biopsy With Ganglion Cells, Site Of Ileostomy

Figure 70–16. Biopsies are taken from the ileum just proximal to the transition zone. If ganglion cells are present, an ileostomy is performed.

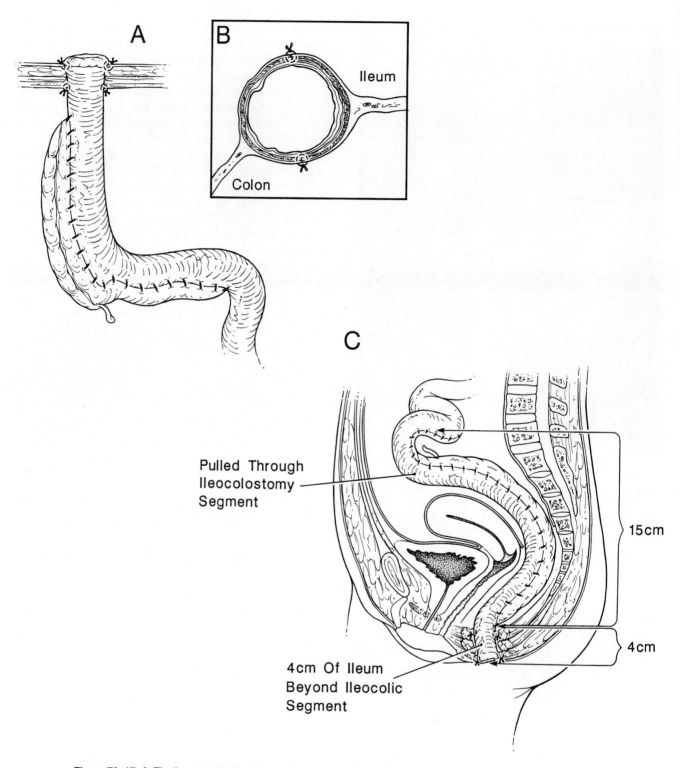

Figure 70–17. A. The ileostomy is taken down, and a side-to-side anastomosis between the terminal ileum containing ganglion cells is made to the aganglionic cecum and ascending colon. Six centimeters of ileum projects beyond the patch up ascending colon. This is brought out as another ileostomy. **B.** Cross section demonstrating the combined aganglionic cecum with the ileum. **C.** At 1 year of age, a Swenson pullthrough is performed, pulling through the terminal ileum with the cecal patch.

they average one to four bowel movements a day. On fluoroscopic examination, bowel motility in the patched segment was normal.

Total intestinal aganglionosis has been considered incompatible with long-term survival without TPN. Zeigler has carried out a myotomy by removing a 1 cm wide segment of muscle from the antimesenteric side of aganglionic jejunum. The infant then had 60 cm of small bowel distal to the ligament of Treitz, which ended with a stoma. By 18 months, the infant was able to tolerate 75 percent of her total caloric intake enterally, and she was at the 97th percentile for height and weight.[68] At the time of this writing, the infant is 2½ years old and has had a pullthrough operation. She has had some enterocolitis but is able to tolerate most of her caloric intake in the form of an elemental diet, plus table food (M. Zeigler, personal communication).

Older Children

There are special problems in the diagnosis and management of Hirschsprung's disease in older children. The diagnosis may become confused with other forms of megacolon, particularly psychogenic constipation. A detailed history and physical examination must be carried out to determine the time of onset of the child's bowel difficulties. When the onset of constipation is at birth or shortly afterward, Hirschsprung's disease must be a strong consideration. A history of constipation commencing after the switch from breast milk feedings to formula also is suggestive. On the other hand, when constipation commences at 2 or 3 years of age, coincident with toilet training, this diagnosis is unlikely. Children with Hirschsprung's disease are more likely to have a distended abdomen, with spindly legs and arms, than are children with common constipation. The rectal examination is most important. Inspect first for signs of an anteriorly displaced anus, anal stenosis, or spinal cord lesion. If there is a smear of feces around the anus, the diagnosis is more likely encopresis than an organic lesion. With Hirschsprung's disease, there is classically an empty rectum, with a fecal impaction palpated at a high level. Unfortunately, a very small percentage of children with a very short aganglionic segment will have fecal soiling and stool palpable in the ampulla of the rectum. A barium enema is the most important examination, since this will demonstrate the narrow aganglionic rectum. With short segment disease, the barium study may demonstrate only a megacolon with no transition segment. If there is a suspicion of Hirschsprung's disease, we proceed to a full-thickness biopsy to determine the presence of ganglion cells. A suction biopsy may not cut a deep enough specimen to see the submucosa. Rectal pressure studies are no more accurate than the history and barium enema. One must perform a test that is absolutely accurate to decide on the proper treatment.

If the barium enema suggests a short aganglionic segment and if a frozen section reveals absent ganglion cells, one may proceed with an anorectomyomectomy.[69,70] In this procedure, the child is placed in the lithotomy position, the rectum is irrigated, and a vigorous rectal dilatation is performed. Retractors placed supriorly and laterally will expose the posterior rectal walls. A transverse incision is made through the mucosa 2 cm above the dentate line. The mucosa is then undermined to expose the underlying circular muscle fibers. A 1 cm segment of muscle is taken for biopsy. If this demonstrates no ganglion cells, a 1 cm wide strip of muscle is excised from the posterior rectal wall for as far as one can dissect, usually about 6 cm. The muscle is then left open, but the mucosa is loosely sutured in place, and a small drain is left under the mucosa for 24 hours. In our hands, this operation has helped relieve postoperative obstructive symptoms but has failed in two patients with what was thought to be short segment disease. In one child, the operation was performed when he was 4 years of age. He returned at age 8 and required an abdominoperineal pullthrough. The other was 14 years old when his disease was first diagnosed. He was asymptomatic after the myectomy until age 25. At age 28, a Swenson pullthrough operation was performed. Starling et al. also reported a 6-year improvement, then recurrence of symptoms after myectomy in a 9-year-old boy.[71] An anorectal myectomy will provide temporary relief of symptoms, but for permanent cure, a pullthrough operation appears to be indicated.

In Sherman et al.'s series of 880 patients, 332 were over 2 years of age at the time of their pullthrough operation, 78 were 6 to 10 years old, and 80 were over 11. Only 55 of these 332 patients required a colostomy before the pullthrough operation. The decision to perform a colostomy before the pullthrough operation depends on the patient's nutritional status and the size of the dilated bowel. In some older children, the bowel is so packed with stool that disimpaction and enemas under general anesthesia are required. If the parents are willing to give effective rectal irrigations for several months, it frequently is possible to carry out a primary pullthrough. However, when the sigmoid is massively distended, we have preferred to determine the upper extent of the aganglionic segment at laparotomy, then resect the massively dilated, hypertrophied sigmoid colon and bring out a proximal end colostomy that is of nearly normal size. It is foolhardy to attempt a colostomy in the massively distended bowel because once the colon shrinks down in size, the bowel will likely prolapse. Also, even with a colostomy, the massively distended intestine functions poorly. Resection back to normal size bowel at the first operation, leaving the distal aganglionic segment closed, makes the pullthrough operation much easier.

Psychogenic Constipation

Constipation is a frequent problem among children of all ages. The parents often are upset out of all proportion to the degree of the child's illness. They often are referred for surgical consultation because the family pediatrician is at his wits' end and needs help. Frequently, these children arrive with a stack of x-rays purporting to demonstrate megacolon. Usually, a careful history will rule out Hirschsprung's disease without resorting to further tests. An excessive intake of cow's milk with too little variety of other foods will produce simple constipation. Other causes include hypothyroidism, spinal cord defects, anal fissures, and anal stenosis.

When the onset is in later childhood, with a past history of normal bowel movements, it is rare to find an organic lesion. These children may have a history of fecal soiling as the primary complaint, and it is only after performing a rectal examination that the bowel is found to be impacted with stool.

A careful history often will reveal that the mother forced early toilet training at about the same time a new baby made his appearance or when there was a major family upheaval, such as a move to a new home or a divorce.[72] The age of onset of encopresis ranges from 4 to 13 years but is usually during the early, preschool years.[73] The family thinks the child is having great pain and suffering when moving the bowels when actually the patient struggles to hold back bowel movements by tightening the buttocks. He or she turns red in the face, stiffens, and, in general, frightens the parents. Detailed studies of these children have not revealed consistent data concerning intestinal transit time or evidence for motor abnormalities of the anorectal musculature.[74] In a detailed study of 38 encopretic children, however, 63 percent were unable to relax the external anal sphincter during attempts at defecation. More importantly, in this study, a high percentage of these children were depressed, socially withdrawn, or delinquent or had overt major psychiatric problems.[75] To make matters worse, their parents view these children with disgust and often hostility. Treatment starts with an explanation that the child could not help himself or herself at the onset of the problem and that now the rectum is so distended it will not respond to the normal urge to defecate. The object of medical treatment is to empty the rectum and colon so the bowel can be restored to a more normal size. Hopefully, this will restore the normal defecatory reflex. A high-fiber diet is the basis of treatment. Excessive amounts of milk and cheese are eliminated from the diet, and whole grain cereals, such as bran, are emphasized. Corn, beans, salads, all vegetables with the skins left in place, raw celery, raw carrots, and other perfectly logical dietary items are suggested. Popcorn is well accepted and is an excellent source of fiber. It is necessary to remove the fecal impaction with frequent soapsuds enemas. Once the impaction has been removed, soiling stops, and the child commences to have a better self-image. In addition to the diet and enemas, either mineral oil or milk of magnesia is prescribed. Sometimes, initially, as much as 4 to 6 ounces of mineral oil a day is necessary; the dosage is then tapered over a period of months.

Treatment failures are frequent. In one study, there was an almost 25 percent failure rate in keeping clinic appointments.[76] A telephone follow-up and enthusiasm on the part of the physician are essential to success. During the entire treatment process, one must work to dispel the hostility between the parents and the child. It helps to have the child assume responsibility for as much of his or her own treatment as possible. Psychotherapy may become necessary because some children are severely disturbed, and the vigorous treatment plan directed at the symptom may only aggravate the psychologic problem.

ALTERNATIVE OPERATIONS FOR HIRSCHSPRUNG'S DISEASE

There have been a number of modifications of the Swenson technique to minimize the pelvic dissection. The Duhamel procedure consists of resection of the bowel down to the peritoneal reflection, where the distal rectum is closed.[77] A tunnel is then made behind the rectum. The proximal bowel with ganglion cells is brought through this tunnel to the distal rectum. An end-to-side anastomosis is made to the back wall of the rectum. Initially, a long stump of rectum was left above the anastomosis, which accumulated stool. A number of modifications have been devised, including the use of modified crushing clamps and stapling devices to obliterate the septum between the normal and the aganglionic bowel.[78–80]

The endorectal pullthrough was adopted for Hirschsprung's disease by Soave in a further effort to minimize or eliminate the pelvic dissection.[81] In the initial description of this operation, the pulled-through bowel was left hanging out the anus until it adhered to the rectal cuff. Boley modified this by making a primary anastomosis of the pulled-through bowel to the anus.[82] Regardless of how the operation is performed, an aganglionic cuff of rectum is left around the pulled-through bowel, and the internal sphincter is left completely in place. In 1984, Soave reviewed his 20-year experience with the endorectal pullthrough.[83] He provided a very precise illustrated guide to his operation and a follow-up of his 271 patients. Most of his early complications, cuff abscesses, retraction, and residual aganglionic segments, were eliminated in later patients. Postoperative enterocolitis was cured with rectal dilatations. Seventy-three of his patients were followed for 15 years or longer and are essentially normal.

Holschneider has exhaustively reviewed the various operations and has found comparable results.[84] An experienced surgeon who brings bowel with normal ganglion cells down to the anus and who does some procedure to overcome the internal sphincter spasm without destroying its function can expect at least 85 percent of his or her patients to have essentially normal bowel movements over the long term.

REFERENCES

1. Hirschsprung H: Stuhltragheit Neugeborener in Folge von Dilatation and Hypertrophie des colon. Jahrb 8: Kinderh 27:1, 1887.

2. Law JL: Treatment of megacolon with acetylbeta methylcholine bromide. Am J Dis Child 60:262, 1940

3. Wade RB, Rogale ND: Operative treatment of Hirschsprung's disease: a new method with explanation of technique and results of operation. Med J Aust 1:137, 1927

4. Ross JP: The results of sympathectomy. Br J Surg 23:438, 1935

5. Whitehouse F, Bargan JA, Dixon CF: Congenital megacolon: favorable end results of treatment by resection. Gastroenterology 1:922, 1943

6. Grimson KS, Vandergrift HN, Dratz HM: Surgery in obstinate megacolon: one-stage resection and ileosigmoidostomy. Surg Gynecol Obstet 80:164, 1945

7. Tiffin ME, Chandler LR, Faber HK: Localized absence of ganglion cells of the myenteric plexus in congenital megacolon. Am J Dis Child 59:1071, 1940

8. Ehrenpreis T: Megacolon in the newborn. Acta Chir Scand [Suppl] 94 (112), 1946

9. Adamson WAD, Aird I: Megacolon evidence in favor of neurogenic origin. Br J Surg 20:200, 1933

10. Swenson O, Bill AH: Resection of rectum and rectosigmoid with preservation of the sphincter for benign spastic lesions producing megacolon. Surgery 24:212, 1948

11. Swenson O, Rheinlander HF, Diamond I: Hirschsprung's disease: a new concept in etiology—operative results in 34 patients. N Engl J Med 241:551, 1949

12. Swenson O, Neuhauser EBD, Picket LK: New concepts in the etiology, diagnosis, and treatment of congenital megacolon. Pediatrics 4:201, 1949

13. Zulzer WW, Wilson JL: Functional intestinal obstruction on a congenital neurogenic basis in infancy. Am J Dis Child 75:40, 1948

14. Whitehouse FW, Kernahan JW: Myenteric plexus in congenital megacolon. Arch Intern Med 82:75, 1948

15. Bodian M, Stephens JD, Ward BCH: Hirschsprung's disease and idiopathic megacolon. Lancet 1:6, 1949

16. Gunn H: Histological and histochemical observations on the myenteric and submucosal plexuses of mammals. J Anat 102:223, 1968

17. Jacobowitz D: Histochemical studies of the autonomic innervation of the gut. J Pharmacol Exp Ther 149:358, 1965

18. Garrett JR, Howard ER, Lausdale JM: Myenteric plexus in the hind gut of the cat. J Physiol (London) 226:103, 1972

19. Baumgarten HG, Holstein AF, Stelzner F: Nervous elements in the human colon of Hirschsprung's disease. Virchow's Arch Pathol 358:113, 1973

20. Aldridge R, Campbell P: Ganglion cell distribution in the normal rectum and anal canal: a basis for the diagnosis of Hirschsprung's disease by anorectal biopsy. J Pediatr Surg 3:475, 1968

21. Weinberg AG: The anorectal myenteric plexus: its relation to hypoganglionosis of the colon. Am J Clin Pathol 54:637, 1970

22. Ikawa H, Yokoyama J, Morikama Y, et al: A qualitative study of acetylcholine in Hirschsprung's disease. J Pediatr Surg 15:48, 1980

23. Touloukian RJ, Aghajanian G, Roth RH: Adrenergic hyperactivity of the aganglionic colon. J Pediatr Surg 8:191, 1973

24. Larsson L, Malmfors G, Wahlestedt C, et al: Hirschsprung's disease: a comparison of the nervous control of ganglionic and aganglionic smooth muscle in vitro. J Pediatr Surg 22:431, 1987

25. Nirasawa Y, Yokoyama J, Ikawa H, et al: Hirschsprung's disease: catecholamine content, alpha-adrenoreceptors and the effect of electrical stimulation in aganglionic colon. J Pediatr Surg 21:136, 1986

26. Hanani M, Lerner O, Zamir O, Nissan S: Nerve-mediated responses to drugs and electrical stimulation in aganglionic muscle segments in Hirschsprung's disease. J Pediatr Surg 21:848, 1986

27. Holschneider A: Hirschsprung's disease. Stuttgart, Hippocrates Verlag; New York, Thieme-Stratton, 1982, p 37

28. Camiano D, Ormsbee H, Polito W: Total intestinal aganglionosis. J Pediatr Surg 20:456, 1985

29. Ziegler M, Ross A, Bishop H: Total intestinal aganglionosis: a new technique for prolonged survival. J. Pediatr Surg 22:82, 1987

30. Martin L, Buchino I, LeCoultre C, et al.: Hirschsprung's disease with skip area (segmental aganglionosis). J Pediatr Surg 14:686, 1979

31. Chadarevian J, Slim M, Akel S: Double zonal aganglionosis in long segmental Hirschsprung's disease with a "skip area" in the transverse colon. J Pediatr Surg 17:195, 1982

32. Okamoto E, Veda T: Embryogenesis of intramural ganglia of the gut and its relation to Hirschsprung's disease. J Pediatr Surg 2:437, 1967

33. Smith B: Pre- and postnatal development of the ganglion cells of the rectum and its surgical implications. J Pediatr Surg 3:386, 1968

34. Okamoto E, Satani M, Kuwata K: Histologic and embryologic studies on the innervation of the pelvic viscera in patients with Hirschsprung's disease. Surg Gynecol Obstet 155:823, 1982

35. Richardson W, Brown I: Hirschsprung's disease in infants and children. Ann Surg 28:142, 1962

36. Bodian M, Carter CO: A family study of Hirschsprung's disease. Am Hum Genet 26:261, 1963

37. Gauderer M, Rothstein F, Izant R: Ileal atresia with long-segment Hirschsprung's disease in a neonate. J Pediatr Surg 19:15, 1984

38. Kilcoyne R, Taybi H: Conditions associated with congenital megacolon. Am J Roentgenol Radiother Nucl Med 108:615, 1970

39. Currie A, Haddad M, Honeyman M, Buddy S: Associated developmental abnormalities of the anterior end of the neural crest: Hirschsprung's disease–Wardenburg's syndrome. J Pediatr Surg 21:248, 1986

40. Bielschowsky M, Schofield G: Studies on megacolon in piebald mice. Aust J Exp Biol Med Sci 40:395, 1962

41. Todd I: Adult Hirschsprung's disease. Br J Surg 64:311, 1977

42. Swenson O, Fisher J, MacMahon J: Rectal biopsy as an aid in the diagnosis of Hirschsprung's disease. N Engl J Med 253:632, 1955

43. Shandling B, Auldist A: Pinch biopsy for the diagnosis of Hirschsprung's disease. J Pediatr Surg 7:546, 1972

44. Dobbins WO, Bill AH: Diagnosis of Hirschsprung's disease excluded by rectal suction biopsy. N Engl J Med 272:990, 1965

45. Aldridge RT, Campbell PE: Ganglion cell distribution in the normal rectum and anal canal: a basis for the diagnosis of Hirschsprung's disease by anorectal biopsy. J Pediatr Surg 3:475, 1968

46. Campbell P, Noblet H: Experience with the rectal suction biopsy in the diagnosis of Hirschsprung's disease. J Pediatr Surg 4:510, 1969

47. Meier-Ruge W, Lutterbeck P, Harsog B, et al: Acetylcholinesterase activity in suction biopsies of the rectum in the diagnosis of Hirschsprung's disease. J Pediatr Surg 7:11, 1972

48. Elema J, Vries J, Vos L: Intensity and proximal extension of acetylcholinesterase activity in the mucosa of the rectosigmoid in Hirschsprung's disease. J Pediatr Surg 8:361, 1973

49. Lawson J, Nixon HH: Anal canal pressures in the diagnosis of Hirschsprung's disease. J Pediatr Surg 2:544, 1967

50. Schnaufer I, Talbert J, Haller JA: Differential sphincteric studies in the diagnosis of anorectal disorders of childhood. J Pediatr Surg 2:538, 1967

51. El-Shafie, Suzuki H, Schanufer I, et al: A simplified method of anorectal manometry for wider clinical application. J Pediatr Surg 7:230, 1972

52. Holschnieder A, Kellner E, Streibl P, et al: The development of anorectal continence and its significance in the diagnosis of Hirschsprung's disease. J Pediatr Surg 11:151, 1976

53. Mernier P, Marechel J, Mollard P. Accuracy of the manometric diagnosis of Hirschsprung's disease. J Pediatr Surg 13:411, 1978

54. Puri P, Nixon HH: Long-term results of Swenson's operation for Hirschsprung's disease. Prog Pediatr Surg 10:87, 1977

55. Neilson O, Madson L: Twenty-five-year follow-up after Swenson's operation for Hirschsprung's disease. Prog Pediatr Surg 10:97, 1977

56. DeLorimer A: Discussion of Hirschsprung's disease. Am J Surg 152:55, 1986

57. Thomas D, Ferino D, Bayston R, et al: Enterocolitis in Hirschsprung's disease: a controlled study of the etiologic role of Clostridium difficile. J Pediatr Surg 21:22, 1986

58. Kleinhous S, Boley S, Sheron M: Hirschsprung's disease: a survey of the members of the surgical section of the American Academy of Pediatrics. J Pediatr Surg 14:588, 1980

59. Ikeda K, Goto S: Diagnosis and treatment of Hirschsprung's disease in Japan. An analysis of 1628 patients. Ann Surg 199:400, 1984

60. Fekete N, Ricour C, Martelli H, et al: Total colonic aganglionosis (with or without ileal involvement): a review of 27 cases. J Pediatr Surg 21:251, 1986

61. Ikeda K, Goto S: Total colonic aganglionosis with or without small bowel involvement: an analysis of 137 patients. J Pediatr Surg 21:319, 1986

62. Martin LW: Total colonic aganglionosis preservation and utilization of the entire colon. J Pediatr Surg 17:635, 1982

63. Davies M, Cywes S: Inadequate pouch emptying following Martin's pull-through procedure for intestinal aganglionosis. J Pediatr Surg 18:14, 1983

64. Kottmeier P, Jonglo B, Valeck F, et al: Absorptive function of the aganglionic ileum. J Pediatr Surg 16:275, 1981

65. Kimura K, Nishijima E, Muraji T, et al: Extensive aganglionosis: further experience with the colonic patch graft procedure and long-term results. J Pediatr Surg 23:52, 1988

66. Boley S: A new operative approach to total aganglionosis of the colon. Surg Gynecol Obstet 159:481, 1984

67. Stringel G: Extensive intestinal aganglionosis including ileum: a new surgical technique. J Pediatr Surg 667, 1986

68. Zeigler M, Ross A, Bishop H: Total intestinal aganglionosis: a new technique for prolonged survival. J Pediatr Surg 22:82, 1987

69. Nisson S, Bar-Maur JA: Changing trends in presentation and management of Hirschsprung's disease. J Pediatr Surg 6:10, 1971

70. Lynn HB, van Hiedren JA: Rectal myectomy in Hirschsprung's disease: a decade of experience. Arch Surg 110:991, 1975

71. Starling J, Croum R, Thomas C: Hirschsprung's disease in young adults. Am J Surg 151:104, 1986

72. Bellman M: Studies on encopresis. Acta Pediatr Scand [Suppl] 70:170, 1960

73. Levine M: Children with encopresis: a descriptive analysis. Pediatrics 56:412, 1975

74. Corazzari E, Cucchiara S, Staiano A, et al: Gastrointestinal transit time, frequency of defecation and anorectal manometry in healthy and constipated children. J Pediatr 106:379, 1985

75. Loening-Bouck V, Cruikshank B, Savage C: Defecation dynamics and behavior profiles in encopretic children. Pediatrics 80:672, 1987

76. Katz C, Drongowski R, Coran A: Long-term management of chronic constipation in children. J Pediatr Surg 22:976, 1987

77. Duhamel B: A new operation for the treatment of Hirschsprung's disease. Arch Dis Child 35:38, 1960

78. Wilcox M, Bill A: Experimentation with the Duhamel operation for the treatment of congenital megacolon. J Pediatr Surg 7:168, 1972

79. Soper RT, Miller F: Modification of the Duhamel proce-

dure: elimination of rectal pouch and colorectal septum. J Pediatr Surg 3:372, 1968

80. Steichen F, Talbert JL, Ravitch MM: Primary side-to-side colon rectal anastomosis in the Duhamel operation for Hirschsprung's disease. Surgery 64:475, 1968

81. Soave F: Die Nahtose Colon-Anastomosis nach Extramucoser Mobilierung und Herbzielung des Rectosigmoids zur chirugischen Behouslung des M. Hirschsprung. Zentralbl Chir 88:31, 1963

82. Boley SJ: New modification of surgical treatment of Hirschsprung's disease. Surgery 56:1015, 1964

83. Soave F: Endorectal pullthrough: 20 year experience. Address of the guest speaker, APSA, 1984. J Pediatr Surg 20:568, 1984

84. Holschneider A: Hirschsprung's diseases. Stuttgart, Hippokrates Verlag; New York, Thieme-Stratton, 1982, pp 155–201

71
Duplication of the Alimentary Tract

The term "duplication of the alimentary tract" is applied to cystic and tubular structures that are in intimate contact with portions of the gut, from the mouth to the anus.[1-4] The variety and anatomic location of duplications are illustrated in Figure 71–1. The most common type consists of a cystic, endothelium-lined structure enclosed in a common muscular wall with its adjacent segment of gut. Other types include tubular structures lying on the mesenteric side of the bowel, which may be blind at either end or may communicate with the bowel. The endothelial lining is usually from the adjacent gut, but it may contain heterotopic tissue. Gastric mucosa, which is most commonly found in foregut anomalies and tubular duplications of the small intestine, results in peptic ulceration and hemorrhage (Fig. 71–2). Tubular duplications that arise at right angles to the bowel may be better termed "giant diverticulae" but are by common usage considered to be duplications. This type is most likely to extend from the abdomen through the diaphragm and into the mediastinum. There is also a rare form of duplication that occurs within the mesentery but is separate from the intestinal wall (Fig. 71–3). These lesions have a muscular wall and an endothelial lining and must be differentiated from simple mesenteric cysts, which are soft, thin-walled structures containing clear fluid or chyle. These lesions also can be classified as lymphangiomas and may become so large as to simulate ascites. They remain asymptomatic, although extensive lymphangiomas involving the mesentery and bowel may cause a protein-losing enteropathy.

There is no unified embryologic explanation for all duplications, but Gray and Skandalakis have summarized the most likely theories as follows.[5]

1. Small intramural duplications arise from a persistent embryonic diverticulum or from incomplete recanalization.
2. Tubular duplications lying close to the gut and sharing a common muscular wall may result from the formation of a septum that divides the bowel into two parallel tubes.
3. Cystic and tubular duplications with independent muscular coats, as well as the giant diverticulae, are dorsal enteric remnants of early adhesions between the gut and the more dorsal structures.
4. Antimesenteric cystic duplications of the midgut are vitelline duct remnants.
5. Presacral enteric cysts are remnants of the embryonic tailgut.

Males are more frequently affected with duplications. Hemivertebrae and intestinal and anal malformations are commonly associated anomalies. Occasionally two duplications are found in the same patient, and there has been one report of a "triple duplication."[6] In adults, squamous cell carcinomas have arisen in duplications of the colon and small bowel.[7,8]

Duplications produce a bizarre range of symptoms and findings, depending on their location and whether they are cystic or tubular. There may be unexplained abdominal pain, intestinal obstruction, gastrointestinal bleeding, or constipation. Lesions originating in the gastrointestinal tract may extend through the diaphragm to cause respiratory symptoms. They rarely cause problems during the neonatal period, but in our hospital, their progressive symptoms result in a diagnosis during the first months of life.

Abdominal ultrasonography is the most useful imaging study to detect duplications. It will differentiate cystic from solid lesions and will demonstrate the intimate association between the duplication and the bowel wall. It is the only study required to make a diagnosis in many cases. Plain films of the abdomen demonstrate intestinal obstructions caused by intestinal duplications, but the traditional barium studies are rarely indicated. Techne-

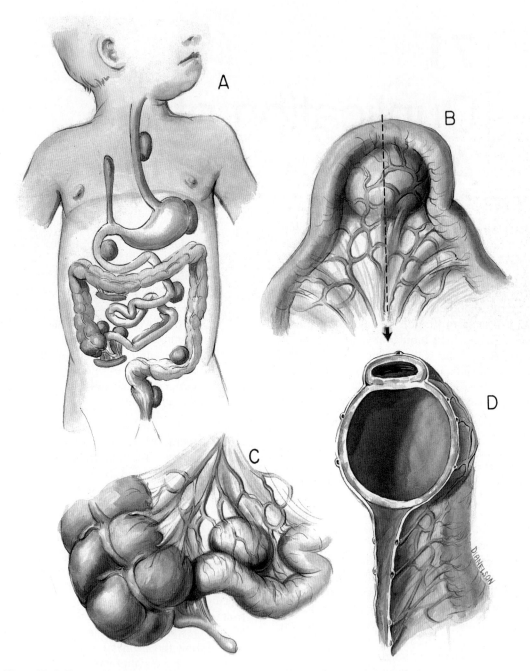

Figure 71–1. Types of intestinal duplications. **A.** These are the many varieties of duplications and giant diverticulae that may be found. **B,C,** and **D.** Common cystic duplication, which may produce a mere abdominal mass or an intestinal obstruction, either by pressure or as a leading point in an intussusception.

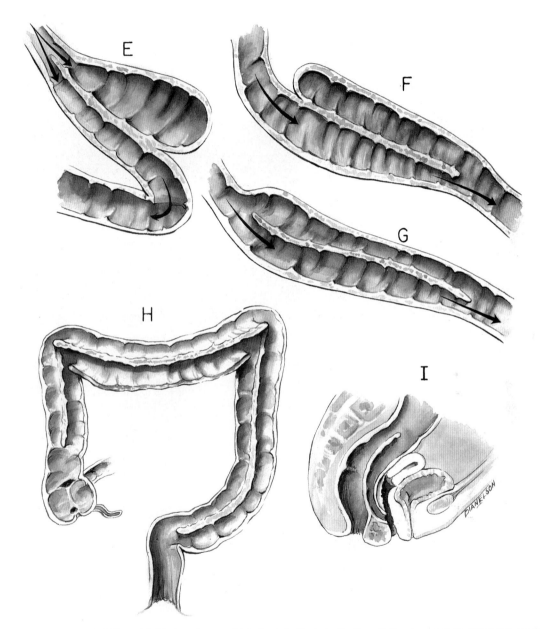

Figure 71–1. E,F,G,H, and **I.** Various types of tubular intestinal duplications that may occur in either the small intestine or the colon.

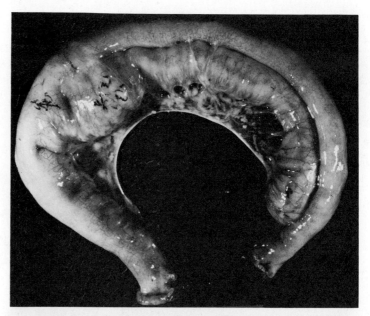

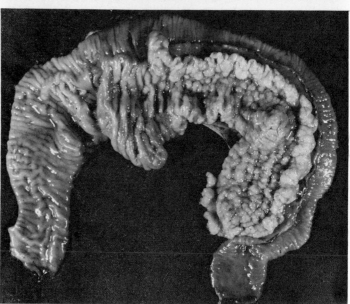

Figure 71–2. Top. Tubular duplication of the ileum. **Bottom.** This duplication contains gastric mucosa, which has caused intestinal bleeding.

tium scans will demonstrate gastric mucosa in bleeding lesions. Computed tomography (CT) scans of the abdomen may be required to solve puzzling cases that are not delineated completely by ultrasonography. The differential diagnosis before operation usually includes mesenteric cysts in cases of mass lesions and a Meckel's diverticulum when there is bleeding. Each requires an operation, and the final diagnosis should be made based on findings in the operating room. Frozen sections are helpful, particularly in establishing the type of mucosa lining the cyst duplication.

DUPLICATIONS OF THE STOMACH

Duplications of the stomach vary from those that are larger than the child's stomach to small, submucosal cysts. A small duplication of the pylorus will cause obstruction and vomiting during the first weeks of life, simulating a pyloric stenosis. The mass feels like the typical olive, and the roentgenogram may resemble that with a pyloric stenosis.[9–13] The small cysts near the pylorus may be completely excised, after which the defect in the stomach may be closed. Most duplications occur

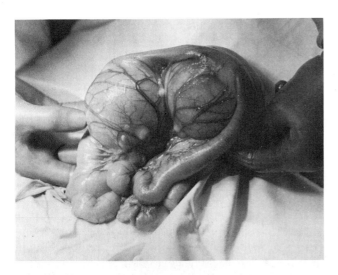

Figure 71–3. A large cystic duplication of the ileum that was partly within the mesentery. Such cysts are thick-walled, which differentiates them from the thin, translucent mesenteric cysts.

on the greater curvature and produce vomiting or pain. They are palpable as smooth, movable masses in the abdomen. Small lesions may be totally excised, but the excision of large duplications may require extensive gastric resection. It is preferable to remove all the duplication except that adjacent to the stomach wall. At that point, the mucosa is stripped away from the underlying muscle.[14] This technique leaves the entire stomach intact. Duplications of the stomach are lined with gastric mucosa and consequently may ulcerate and erode into the abdominal wall, pancreas, or through the diaphragm into the lung.[15–17] Afflicted children may have gastrointestinal bleeding and a noticeable mass, requiring resection of the duplication with repair or resection of adjacent organs.

DUPLICATIONS OF THE DUODENUM

Duodenal duplications most commonly occur on the posterior wall of the descending duodenum.[18,19] Small duplications of the duodenum can remain asymptomatic for years but most often produce a partial duodenal obstruction with a palpable mass.[20] Fifteen percent of duodenal duplications contain gastric mucosa and can result in peptic ulceration with perforation or hemorrhage.[21]

The usual duodenal duplication that projects into the lumen is in intimate contact with the pancreas and the common bile duct. Duplications in this area actually may arise from the pancreas, even though they are lined with gastric mucosa.[22,23] They cause recurrent abdominal pain, and there may be transient elevations of the serum amylase. Ultrasonography and CT demonstrate a cystic

lesion in intimate contact with the stomach, duodenum, and head of the pancreas. Intraoperative cholangiography is essential to determine the relationship of the cyst to the common bile and pancreatic ducts. Some of these lesions can be completely excised, but it may be better to do a partial excision, then excise only the lining mucosa that is adherent to the duodenum or pancreas.

DUPLICATIONS OF THE SMALL INTESTINE

Cystic duplications most often occur in the terminal ileum. They may impinge on the bowel and cause intestinal obstruction during the neonatal period, or they may remain asymptomatic until they become leading points of intussusceptions. These lesions, as well as short tubular duplications, are resected with the adjacent intestine. Tubular duplications occur on the mesenteric side, where they share their blood supply with the intestine. They may communicate with the normal bowel, either caudally or distally. When there is no communication, they fill with secreted mucus and cause pain and a mass. They are serious and life-threatening when they contain gastric mucosa and involve large portions of normal bowel. When these gastric-lined duplications communicate with the normal bowel, they cause ulceration and hemorrhage. The same thing happens if a communication is formed surgically between the duplication and the adjacent bowel. In one case, it was possible to resect the gastric mucosa, which was localized to the distal end of the duplication, and to anastomose the remainder to normal bowel.[24] Wrenn described an ingenious solution to the problem of gastric mucosa in long tubular duplications.[25] He stripped the gastric mucosa from the duplication, which extended almost the entire length of the small bowel, through multiple incisions into the seromuscular layer. The muscular wall containing the blood supply to the normal bowel was left intact. The child has remained symptom-free.

In some cases, the tubular duplication has a partially separate mesentery, or a cleavage plane can be established between the duplication and the small bowel mesentery to allow a complete resection.[26] This is an area that requires individualized surgical management and ingenuity in the operating room.

DUPLICATIONS OF THE COLON

Duplications of the colon contain only colonic epithelium. Symptoms are the result of obstruction, not ulceration. Cystic duplications of the sigmoid or rectum compress the bowel within the pelvis and produce obstruction and progressive constipation.

A longitudinal septum may separate the normal colon from a long tubular duplication. The proximal ends of both the duplication and the normal bowel communicate with duplicated segments of the ileum. If the distal end of the duplication is blind, stool accumulates in the pouch and produces a huge, impressionable mass.[27] Constipation is produced because the distended duplication obstructs the normal lumen. A rectal examination may disclose the bulging mass. Treatment consists of making an anastomosis between the distal end of the duplication and the normal bowel. Tubular duplications of the colon also may be associated with duplications of the genitourinary system, with the duplication and normal bowel opening side-by-side on the perineum.[28,29] The normal bowel may end at a normally placed anus, whereas the duplication terminates in a rectovaginal or rectourethral fistula.[30] One of our patients with an imperforate anus had a longitudinal duplication of the rectum. The septum was divided to make a single lumen at the time of colostomy closure.

A presacral cystic duplication of the rectum will cause constipation and urinary obstruction by virtue of being wedged into the pelvic inlet (Fig. 71–4). It can be palpated just within the rectum as a smooth, firm mass that bulges into the lumen. It is difficult to differentiate this mass from a presacral teratoma. We performed an abdominoperineal resection with a Swenson pull-through anastomosis on one child with a duplication. This left her with poor fecal control because the cyst was intimately involved with the levator ani and the internal sphincter muscle. A better approach would be transrectal aspiration with a syringe and needle to prove the cystic nature of the lesion, followed by either excision of the wall between the rectum and the duplication, with suture of the mucosal layers, or presacral resection of the cyst mucosa, leaving the muscle intact.

One can see from this discussion that duplications of the gut represent a diverse group of lesions. Small lesions in readily accessible areas (such as the terminal ileum) may be excised along with adjacent intestine. In other locations, resection of the duplication would endanger adjacent structures. In such situations, if there is no gastric mucosa, the duplication may be safely anastomosed to adjacent bowel. If the presenting symptom is bleeding, one can assume the presence of gastric mucosa. If resection is contraindicated, the mucosa may be stripped away, leaving the muscular wall intact.

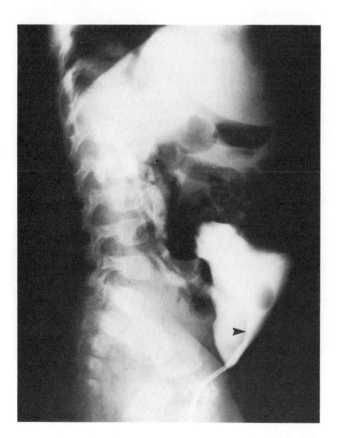

Figure 71–4. Forward displacement of the bladder by a cystic duplication of the rectum. The presenting complaint in this case was urinary retention.

REFERENCES

1. Gross RE, Holcomb GW Jr, Farber S: Duplications of the alimentary tract. Pediatrics 9:449, 1952
2. Mellish RWP, Koop CE: Clinical manifestations of duplication of the bowel. Pediatrics 27:397, 1961
3. Sieber WK: Alimentary tract duplications. Arch Surg 73:383, 1956
4. Grosfeld JD, O'Neill AA, Clatworthy HW Jr: Enteric duplications in infancy and childhood: an 18-year review. Ann Surg 172:83, 1970
5. Gray SW, Skandalakis JE: Embryology for Surgeons. Philadelphia, Saunders, 1972, p 174
6. Sherman NJ, Morrow D, Asch MA: Triple duplication of the alimentary tract. J Pediatr Surg 13:187, 1978
7. Adair H, Trowell J: Squamous cell carcinoma arising in a duplication of the small bowel. J Pathol 133:25, 1981
8. Hickey W, Corson J: Squamous cell carcinoma arising in a duplication of the colon: case report and literature review of squamous cell carcinoma of the colon and of malignancy complicating colonic duplication. Cancer 47:602, 1981
9. Anas P, Miller RC: Pyloric duplication masquerading as hypertrophic pyloric stenosis: case reports. J Pediatr Surg 6:664, 1971
10. Grosfeld JL, Boles E, Reiner C: Duplication of the pylorus in the newborn: a rare case of gastric outlet obstruction. J Pediatr Surg 5:365, 1970
11. Thorbjarnarson B, Haynes LL: Duplication of the stomach: a report of two cases in infants. Surgery 44:585, 1958
12. Kammerer GT: Duplication of the stomach resembling hypertrophic pyloric stenosis. JAMA 207:2101, 1969

13. Bommen M, Singh M: Pyloric duplication in a preterm infant. J Pediatr Surg 19:158, 1984
14. White JJ, Morgan WW: Improved operative technique for gastric duplication. Surgery 67:522, 1970
15. Cloutier R: Pseudocyst of the pancreas secondary to gastric duplication: case reports. J Pediatr Surg 8:67, 1973
16. Parker BC, Guthrie J, France NE, Atwell JD: Gastric duplications in infancy. J Pediatr Surg 7:294, 1972
17. Shochat SJ, Strand RD, Fellows KE, Folkman J: Perforated gastric duplication with pulmonary communications: a case report. Surgery 70:370, 1971
18. Inovye WY, Farrell C, Fitts WT Jr, et al: Duodenal duplication: case report and literature review. Ann Surg 162:910, 1965
19. Leenders EL, Osman MZ, Sukarochana K: Treatment of duodenal duplications with international review. Am Surg 36:368, 1970
20. Ackerman NB: Duodenal duplication cysts: diagnosis and operative management. Surgery 76:330, 1974
21. Dickinson WE, Weinberg SM, Vellios F: Perforating ulcer in a duodenal duplication. Am J Surg 122:418, 1971
22. Black P, Welch K, Eroklis A: Juxtapancreatic intestinal duplications with pancreatic ductal communication: a cause of pancreatitis and recurrent abdominal pain in childhood. J Pediatr Surg 21:257, 1986
23. Hoffman M, Sugerman J, Herman D, Turner M: Gastric duplication cyst communicating with aberrant pancreatic duct: a rare cause of recurrent acute pancreatitis. Surgery 101:369, 1987
24. Niesche JW: Duplication of the small bowel with peptic ulcer perforation. Aust NZ Surg 42:356, 1973
25. Wrenn E: Tubular duplication of the small intestine. Surgery 52:494, 1962
26. Norris R, Brereton R, Wright V, Cudmore R: A new surgical approach to duplications of the intestine. J Pediatr Surg 21:167, 1986
27. Soper RT: Tubular duplication of the colon and distal ileum: case report and discussion. Surgery 63:998, 1968
28. Beach PD, Wright RH Jr, Deffer PA: Duplication of the primitive hindgut of the human being: An 8-year follow-up of a previous case report. Surgery 66:405, 1969
29. Ravitch MD, Scott WW: Duplication of the entire colon, bladder and urethra. Surgery 34:843, 1953
30. McPherson AG, Trapnell JE, Airth GR: Duplication of the colon. Br J Surg 56:138, 1969

72
Anorectal Anomalies

The intestine of humans has evolved to such a high state of efficiency that the waste products of digestion can be retained and then evacuated, privately and in the proper place, whether behind a bush or on a gold-plated commode. Considerable emotion is aroused by toilet training, which is one of the first adaptions a child is expected to make in the process of becoming "civilized." Successful training is a source of pride for both the infant and his parents. Conversely, a child who is incontinent because of an anatomic defect causes intense embarrassment, is ridiculed by his peers, and is sent home from school because he smells bad. The surgeon who cares for a baby with an imperforate anus has a tremendous responsibility. Success or failure is not measured simply by survival but by long-term functional results.

Historically, malformations of the anogenital region have always aroused feelings of horror. This is well expressed on a stone slab from the library of King Assurbanipal of Nineveh:

> When a women bears a child whose anus is closed,
> then the whole land will suffer the want of food.

Scharli has traced the treatment of anorectal anomalies through antiquity, commencing with the above quotation.[1] Throughout recorded history, physicians, midwives, and laymen have successfully treated low lesions by rupturing the anal membrane with the finger or an instrument. High lesions usually were treated by the blind insertion of a trocar into the perineum, although Amusset successfully freed the bowel and sutured it to the skin in 1835.[2] A colostomy was suggested by Littre in 1710, but wasn't successfully performed in an infant until 1793.[3,4]

The first textbook of pediatric surgery in the English language, *The Surgical Diseases of Children*, was written by John Cooper Forster in 1860. He clearly recognized low lesions that could be reached through a perineal incision. Quite wisely, he recommended the Littre operation, or colostomy, for high pouches associated with urinary tract fistulas.

Rudolph Matas, the versatile New Orleans surgeon best known for his work with aneurysms, recommended a sacroperineal approach and extensively reviewed the literature on anorectal anomalies in 1896.[5] The report by Ladd and Gross was a milestone.[6] They proposed a classification that is still used by some surgeons and outlined a reasonable plan of treatment. The mortality rate at that time for all anorectal anomalies was 26 percent. The simultaneous abdominal and perineal approach advocated by Rhoads et al. for males with high lesions was the next advance.[7] This operation remained the standard from the time of its introduction in 1948 until the early 1960s. At about that time, surgeons in the United States became aware of the work of Douglas Stephens in Australia, who clearly demonstrated the importance of the puborectalis muscle in the development of fecal continence. Currently, all surgeons are striving to achieve a better understanding of the anatomy and physiology of the anorectal mechanism in order to improve functional results.

There is a wide variety of anorectal anomalies, which are difficult to understand, let alone treat successfully. In this chapter we first present the normal physiology of continence, then discuss the classification and pathologic anatomy of these lesions, and finally discuss treatment. The reader is advised to refer to the illustrations continually in order to understand the terms used as well as the skeletal anatomic reference points.

NORMAL CONTINENCE

The anal canal is surrounded by intertwining involuntary and voluntary sphincters that provide a fine degree of control of the passage of flatus and stool. The internal sphincter is an extension and thickening of the inner circular layer of the bowel wall. It extends just beneath the mucosa of the bowel distal to the pectinate line. This muscle is the most important factor in anorectal resistance to defecation, since it is normally tonally contracted to occlude the anal canal. This has been demonstrated by measuring the continuous electrical potential of this muscle and the bowel wall. The internal sphincter relaxes in response to rectal distention to initiate the act of defecation.[8] Although the internal sphincter is a continuation of the rectal wall, it contains few ganglion cells, responding instead to cholinergic and adrenergic fibers.

The pelvic diaphragm, which consists of an interlocked group of muscular, fascial and fibrous components attached to the bony pelvis, supports the abdominal viscera and provides the voluntary musculature essential for full continence. The levator ani muscles arise from the pelvis and converge in a funnel-shaped ring about the anal canal and rectum. The levator muscles, particularly the puborectoanalis, interlace with the deepest fibers of the internal sphincter, especially posteriorly.[9] The levator ani is subject to normal variations, but in most cases the uppermost fibers consist of the pubococcygeus and iliococcygeus muscles. These anchor the perineal body in front of the rectum, pass laterally around the upper rectum to insert on the coccyx, and reach as far cranially as the obturator foramen. The puborectoanalis fibers form the most important component of the anorectal sling and compose the most significant muscle in anorectal anomalies. The puborectalis arises from the pubis anteriorly and passes about the urethra in males and the vagina in females, joining posterior to the rectum. This muscle forms a sling about the rectum, almost at right angles to the anorectal junction. It is intimately attached to the rectum and is inferiorly intertwined with the annular deep fibers of the external sphincter. The puborectalis can squeeze the rectum posteriorly against the immobile pubis as well as exerting a strong lateral force. The fibers of the puborectalis arise more laterally in the female. Radiologically, the upper border of the levator sling corresponds to a line drawn from the midpoint of the pubis anteriorly to just beneath the fifth sacral vertebra. This is known as the P-C line. The inferior limits of the puborectalis extend just beyond the lowermost point of the ischium.

Waldeyer's fascia is a peripherally sited extraperitoneal septum that blends superiorly with the levator muscles. Inferiorly, it becomes continuous with the rectovesical septum and the white line of the pelvic fascia. This fascia, or septum, carries the pelvic nerve plexus deriving from the hypogastric nerves, the sacral sympathetic chain, and the nervi erigentes. All the vessels and nerves serving the broad ligament in the female and the bladder, ureters, prostate, and seminal vesicles travel through Waldeyer's layer.

Continence is dependent on the existence of an intact nervous arc between the sensory receptors within the anal canal and the pelvic musculature, as well as on the central nervous system and the nerve endings in the muscles that control continence. These mechanisms have been studied by dissection, anorectal balloon pressure studies, electromanometry, histochemistry, and clinical examination.[10-19]

There is a profusion of nerve endings in the anal canal, as well as such organized nerve structures as Meissner's corpuscles and the end-organs of Krause in the subepithelial tissues. Thus, the skin-lined anal canal plays an important part in the more discriminating and sensitive aspects of continence. The pelvic musculature, particularly the puborectalis sling, is able to perceive pressure. Normally, distention of the rectum causes relaxation of the internal sphincter but contraction of the external sphincter. This is supported by the observation that when the rectum is resected for purposes other than imperforate anus, the patient retains the sensation of fullness in the pelvis, as well as continence. The second, third, and fourth sacral segments of the spinal cord are responsible for perineal cutaneous sensation as well as sensation from the rectum, anus, bladder, and urethra. The sympathetic nerves arise from the second, third, and fourth lumbar segments and the preaortic plexus in front of the fifth lumbar vertebra. These plus the parasympathetic nerves from the third and fourth sacral plexuses are responsible for creating normal, organized peristalsis through the myenteric plexus within the bowel wall. Branches from the anterior roots of the third and fourth sacral nerves are the main pathways for innervation of the levator ani muscles. They course laterally in Waldeyer's fascia. The pudendal nerve also courses laterally to innervate the puborectalis muscles. Fortunately, the levator muscles will continue to function even if only the third (or even the second) sacral vertebra is intact.

The pelvic and sacral nerve plexuses are closely applied to the wall of the bowel and the posterior and lateral walls of the bladder. When the bowel has failed to descend through the levator muscles, these nerves, especially the nervi erigentes, pursue a more midline course than normal and are vulnerable to injury during surgical procedures.

Every surgeon who has studied these problems in detail has concluded that the puborectalis muscle and infolded perineal skin provide sensation and that the puborectalis is the chief muscle of continence following operation on a child with a high rectal pouch. Although the external anal sphincter may be poorly developed in infants afflicted with imperforate anus, it should be preserved.[20]

EMBRYOLOGY

Differences of opinion arise among students of embryology concerning normal embryologic development because deductions must be made concerning a dynamic ongoing process from static observations of individual specimens. It is even more difficult to relate normal embryologic events to individual anomalies. The surgeon who has some knowledge of embryology, however imperfect or controversial, will be better prepared to understand the relationship of the anus and rectum to surrounding structures and to the fistulas that so frequently connect the rectum to the genitourinary system.

The major events in the development of the anus and rectum take place between the fourth fetal week and the sixth fetal month, times corresponding to a crown–rump length of 4 to 200 mm. The upper rectum and sigmoid colon are derived from the hindgut, which in the 4 mm embryo joins the allantois and the mesonephric ducts to form the cloaca. The division of the cloaca forms the portion of the rectum extending from the upper part of the anal canal to the peritoneal reflection. Failure of division of the cloaca into the urogenital tract and rectum results in the high and intermediate anorectal anomalies. In the 5 mm embryo, the cloaca extends caudally into the tail stalk of the embryo (Fig. 72–1 A,B). On the ventral surface of the body wall, the cloacal membrane represents a thin area where entoderm and ectoderm are fused without intervening mesoderm (Fig. 72–1 C,D). As the embryo develops, this cloacal membrane moves posteriorly and inferiorly. The urorectal fold or septum divides the cloaca into rectum and urogenital tract by two processes.[21] First, there is downgrowth of mesoblastic tissue in the cranial to caudal direction. This is Torneaux's septum, which stops its downgrowth at the level of the verumontanum or the müllerian tubercle (Fig. 72–1E). This point is of great significance because it is here where most rectourethral fistulas occur in the male. Below this point, the urorectal septum consists of an ingrowth of mesenchyme from a lateral direction that fuses in the midline. This is called Rathke's fold. There appears to be unanimity on this twofold process of descent and ingrowth of the urorectal septum.[22,23] However, authors differ in their explanations of the development of the perineum and the ultimate separation of the anus from the urogenital tract. Stephens refers to an external cloaca, whereas DeVries thinks that an external cloaca occurs only in birds.

Not only is there a difference in terminology among various authors, but the problem is compounded because of the obvious perineal differentiation between the sexes. Anal tubercles, two protruding bumps of tissue, develop just beneath the fetal tail at approximately the 10th week. The cloacal membrane, which commences on the ventral body wall, migrates posteriorly until it becomes deeply set in the perineum in a buildup of mesoderm. The final process of partitioning of the anus from the urogenital tract is a combination of growth of the urorectal and uroanal septum and ingrowth of the genital folds. The genital tubercle that becomes the phallus is anterior. The inner and outer genital folds form between these structures (Fig. 72–1F$_{4,5}$). In the male, the inner genital folds fuse, covering the posterior portion of the urogenital sinus and forming the bulbous and penile portions of the urethra. In the female, these folds form the labia minora. The outer genital folds fuse caudally in the male to form the scrotum and the median perineal raphé, whereas in females the outer genital folds become the labia majora. The junction of the inner genital folds in the female forms the fourchette. The elongation of the genital folds and the fusion of the anal tubercles about the anus complete the separation of the anus and rectum from the genitourinary tract. The cloaca and the depressed anal pit, which is lined with ectoderm, are finally joined by the atrophy and breakdown of the anal membrane. This junction marks the pectinate line. The low and intermediate anomalies represent a failure of posterior migration of the anus away from the urogenital sinus.[24] This explains the relatively rare rectobulbar fistula in the male and the common low anovestibular and anoperineal fistulas in the female. In either sex, simple failure of degeneration of the anal membrane results in anal agenesis without a fistula. Defects of septation of the cloaca leading to high female anomalies are extremely rare in comparison with the frequency of high rectovesical or rectourethral fistulae in the male. There are many varieties of cloacal defects in which the rectum joins with the vagina and urethra to form a common channel. An important observation is the frequent association of failure of fusion of the müllerian ducts leading to bicornuate uteri and septate or separate vaginas with the female cloacal lesion. Stephens offers the following explanation for this obvious sexual difference in incidence of the high anomalies. The descent of the müllerian ducts in the female occurs long after the partitioning of the cloaca by the urogenital septum. If the partitioning fails to occur in the female, the müllerian ducts relentlessly descend on the undivided cloaca and carry through to the perineum. Thus, the rectum is carried along with the descent of the müllerian ducts to arrive at or very near the perineum. It is almost as if nature made sure that the genital tract would reach the perineum to propagate the race regardless of the social consequence of an abnormally placed anus. Stephens has correlated a number of birth defects, such as torticollis, flattening of the skull, dislocated hip, and clubfoot, with anorectal and other perineal anomalies. These could be deformations as a result of intrauterine pressure rather than

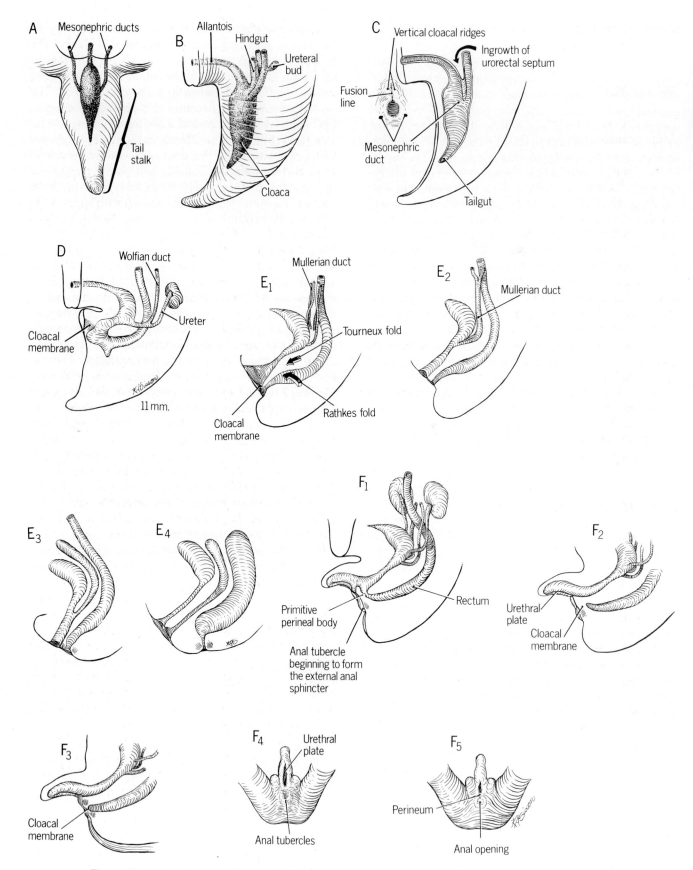

Figure 72–1. Normal anorectal embryology, illustrating the separation of the cloaca into the urogenital system and the rectum. The anus forms on the perineum from the anal tubercles.

defects of embryologic development (F.D. Stephens, personal communication).

PATHOLOGY

The variety of classifications and differences in terminology has caused considerable confusion in describing the pathology of anorectal anomalies. The terms "imperforate anus," "rectourethral fistula," and "rectovaginal fistula" are not sufficiently precise to define a lesion in any individual child. That a lesion is low usually implies that the defect may be repaired from a perineal approach, whereas a high lesion requires a more extensive operation. This simple approach to classification creates problems because it does not take into consideration the relation of the rectum or anus to the levator ani musculature. It has led to surgical disasters when a perineal operation has been used for a lesion that we would now consider intermediate between a truly low or perineal lesion and one that requires an abdominal operation. In 1984, an international group of surgeons developed a simplified classification for the most common anorectal anomalies. The lesions included in this classification are illustrated in Figure 72–2 (see color insert).

In this discussion of pathology, the reader should continually refer to the classification and the diagrams of individual lesions.

LESIONS IN THE MALE

In low lesions, the rectum has penetrated the levator sling, often leaving the internal sphincter perfectly intact. In mild degrees of anal stenosis, there is a ring of fibrous tissue at the pectinate line that can cause constipation. A completely covered anus consists of a heaped-up mass of tissue covering the anus in the form of a bucket handle. With diligent probing, one may find a small opening just lateral to the midline. In the male, an anterior perineal, or covered, anus may occur anterior to the normal anus; often a tiny opening is found on the scrotum. These fistulas may not be evident on casual examination, especially immediately after birth.

Intermediate Lesions

In these rare anomalies, the rectum has descended through the puborectalis muscle to within a centimeter or so from the perineal skin. There is often a deep anal dimple and an excellent external sphincter muscle that is in continuity with the levator complex. In most cases, a small fistula runs forward from the rectal pouch to the bulbar portion of the urethra. These lesions often are associated with a hypospadias or split scrotum. We have observed only five cases of rectobulbar fistula during

the past 10 years. Anal agenesis without fistula in males is even more unusual but is seen in children with Down's syndrome.

It is difficult to differentiate intermediate from high lesions in boys. Ultrasonography has proven accurate in determining the distance from the pouch to the skin surface but will not demonstrate the fistula. This requires a carefully performed urethrogram with lateral films. If there is doubt about the presence of a fistula or the level of the pouch, it is safer, in the newborn period, to perform a colostomy. This will allow time for careful studies to accurately determine the pouch level and the presence of a fistula.

High Lesions

The most difficult anorectal anomaly in males is anorectal agenesis with a fistula to the prostatic urethra. Rarely, there is a fistula to the bladder. The blind rectal pouch lies above the levator sling. The correct term is "anorectal agenesis" if the blind rectum has no communication with the urinary tract. Usually, however, there is a fistula to the posterior urethra adjacent to the ejaculatory ducts. The fistula varies in size, and the lack of meconium in the urine or the inability to find a fistula radiographically does not rule out the presence of a small tract. The fistula usually is very short, with the bowel in intimate relationship to the urethra. Occasionally, because of the upward angulation of the urethra at the point of entrance of the fistula, a catheter or sound will preferentially enter the rectum rather than the bladder. Fistulas higher in the urethra and connected to the bladder are rare. The puborectalis sling encircles the urethra just distal to the rectourethral fistula. On radiologic studies, the bowel is above the pubococcygeal line and is, therefore, completely supralevator. There is no internal sphincter, and the external sphincter is variable.

LESIONS IN THE FEMALE

Low Lesions

All low lesions in the female have a fistula or connection to the perineum. Anal stenosis is simply a narrowing of the anus at its normal location, all sphincters are intact, and a minor anoplasty or dilatation is all that is necessary. The term "anocutaneous fistula" includes conditions formerly diagnosed as "anterior ectopic anus" or "anoperineal fistula." The opening may be normal in size but is more often stenotic. It is skin lined, or there may be a slight mucosal ectropion. Sphincter function is normal. There is a spectrum of lesions up to the anovestibular fistula, all of which have squamous epithelium between the anal opening and the vestibule. Thus, when the fistula is opened posteriorly with a cutback operation, there is a perineal body and a good distance from the anal opening to the vagina. I have observed a 20-year-old woman with an anterior anocutaneous fistula who was asymptomatic.

Stephens and Smith considered the anovestibular fistula to be the most common anal deformity in the female child.[25] The rectal orifice is not visible on inspection of the perineum. It is necessary to separate the labia and examine the back wall of the vestibule and vagina with a small nasal speculum. The orifice is surrounded by moist epithelium, and its upper end is immediately adjacent to vaginal epithelium. A probe or catheter inserted into the opening tends to aim toward the anal dimple. When there is a normal-appearing hymen, the rectal opening is either on the perineum or in the posterior part of the vestibule.[26] All patients without hymens had cloacal deformities. The puborectalis surrounds the rectum in an anovestibular fistula, and the external sphincter mechanism is well developed.

Intermediate Lesions
The differentiation between an anovestibular and a rectovestibular fistula is extremely difficult. The opening is at the same location as an anovestibular fistula, but there is a long, thin track extending upward to the pouch along the back wall of the vagina. The fistula, but not the rectum itself, has penetrated through the levator and puborectalis muscles. The external sphincter is variable. A catheter or probe introduced into the fistula goes upward and cannot be palpated at the anal dimple. If a small Foley catheter is inserted into the fistula and on into the rectum, the balloon is blown up and traction is placed on the catheter. The distance from the opening to the balloon represents the length of the tract. It may also be delineated by the injection of contrast material and roentgenograms.

The opening of a low rectovaginal fistula may be seen with a good light and a nasal speculum, higher on the posterior vaginal wall. Anal agenesis without a fistula in girls is extremely rare, but we have seen six, all in girls with Down's syndrome.

High Lesions
When there is anorectal agenesis with a high vaginal fistula, the opening is usually just distal to the uterine cervix. In addition, there is a high incidence of associated upper urinary tract defects as well as a spectrum of genital lesions, often including a vaginal septum and double uteri. The bowel ends above the levator complex, and all the spincter muscles are poorly developed. The puborectalis hugs the back wall of the vagina below the fistula. Rectal atresia without a fistula is associated with a deep anal dimple surrounded by well-developed muscles. This anomaly, rare in the United States, is seen with some frequency in India.

Cloaca
The intestinal, genital, and urinary tracts join to form a common channel, the cloaca, that empties through a single perineal orifice. The variations are infinite and complex. The channel may be short enough to discern the urethral, vaginal, and rectal openings with a speculum, or the canal may extend well up into the abdomen. The most serious lesions are those associated with vaginal obstruction, which produce a hydrometrocolpos. Externally, there are malformed labioscrotal folds lying lateral to a normal or enlarged phallic structure. When both meconium and urine issue from the single perineal orifice, the diagnosis is made in the neonatal period. Figure 72–3 illustrates the most common types of cloaca. The levator sling encircles the distal single channel and the external sphincter muscle is poorly developed. Figure 72–4 illustrates the cross-sectioned pelvis of a 4-month fetus, showing a cloacal defect in relation to the pelvic skeleton. Rectovesical fistula may occur in the female only in the presence of an absent or divided vagina and uterus.

Miscellaneous
Imperforate anus associated with cloacal exstrophy is discussed in Chapter 91. Other variations include the H-type rectovaginal fistula in girls, which consists of a 2 to 3 mm connection between the rectum and the vestibule but with a normal anal opening. Our one patient with this lesion had an associated esophageal atresia and fistula. Urethroanal fistulas in boys usually connect the membranous urethra with the anus just proximal to the pectinate line.[27] The urethra distal to the fistula may be stenotic or absent, so urine is passed through the wide open fistula into the rectum. Rectovesical fistulas without imperforate anus also have been observed.[28]

INCIDENCE OF TYPES

A survey of the Surgical Section of the American Academy of Pediatrics for the years 1965 through 1969 reviewed 1142 children.[29] Of 661 males, 328 (50 percent) had supralevator lesions, in contrast to 90 (19 percent) of 481 females. Fistulas of various forms were found in 72 percent of the males and 90 percent of the females. Classification of patients seen at our hospital is shown in Table 72–1.

A familial history of anorectal anomalies is unusual. The risk of a family having a subsequent infant with the same anomaly is about 1 percent.[30,31] As many as four children with anorectal anomalies have been born to the same family, and several families have been reported with children having multiple anomalies involving the anus, hands, and feet.[32–35] Anorectal anomalies would

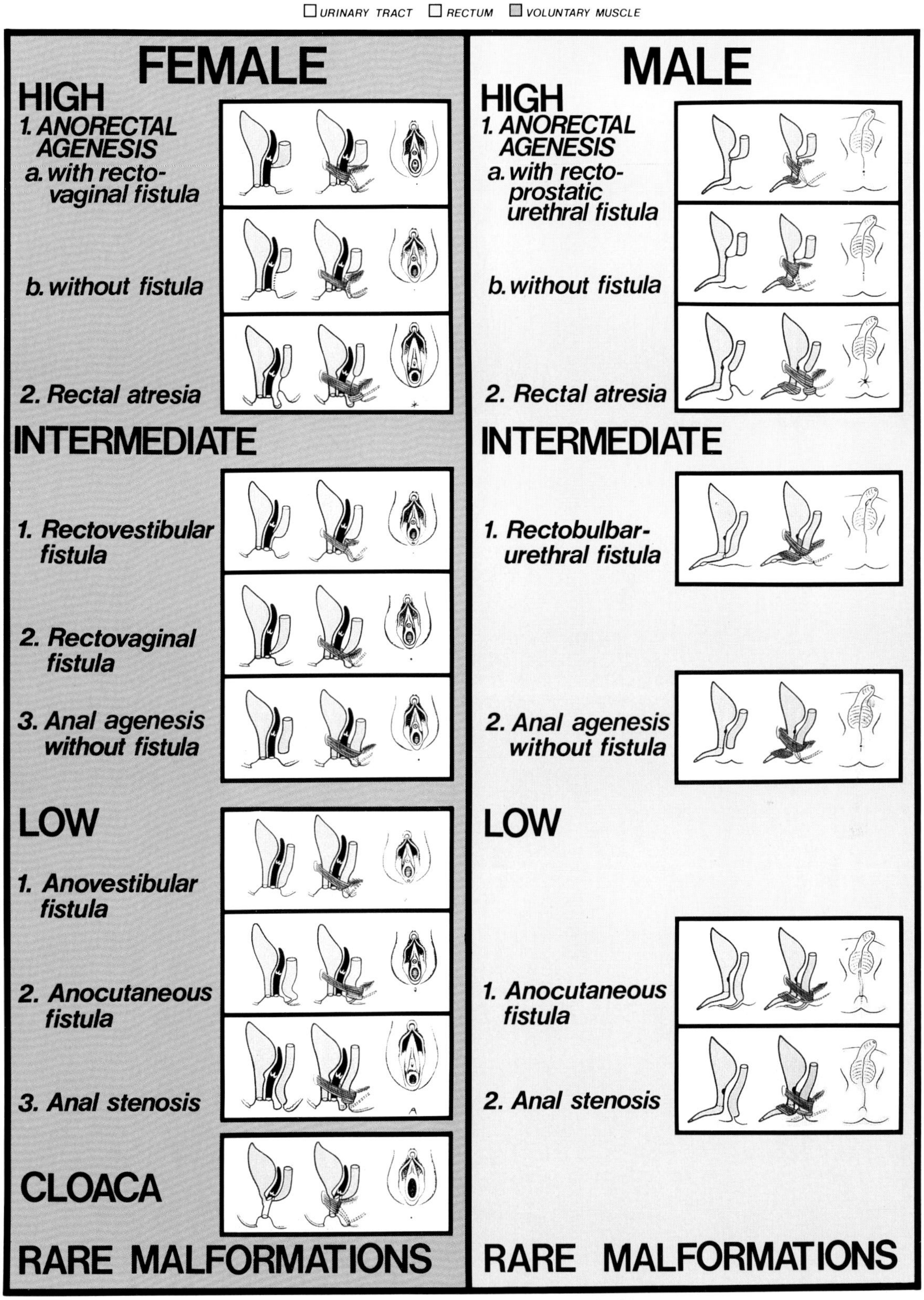

Prepared by Kascot Media Inc. for the Department of Surgery, Children's Memorial Hospital, Chicago, Illinois, U.S.A.

Figure 72–2. Classification of anorectal malformations—1984.

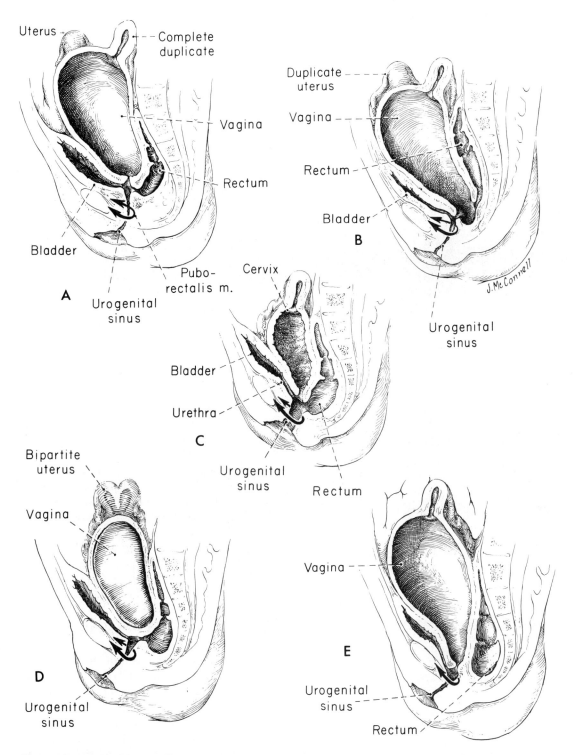

Figure 72–3. A through E. Five cloacal anomalies that vary in the height of the insertion of the rectum into the vagina (also called urogenital sinus). In each of these defects, the puborectalis surrounds the urogenital sinus. The vagina is invariably septate with either bipartite or duplicate uterus.

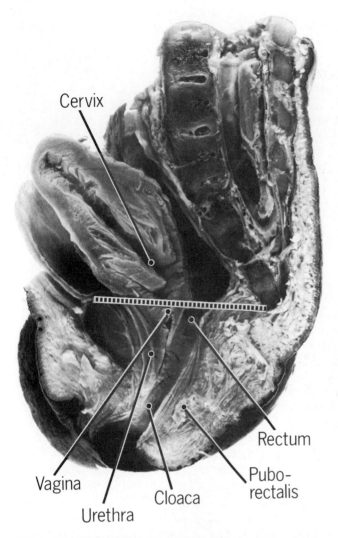

Figure 72–4. Cross-section of a 4-month fetus with a cloacal deformity. The puborectalis is seen adjacent to the urogenital sinus. The rectum ends above the pubococcygeal line. (*Specimen prepared by Rowena Spencer, M.D.*)

TABLE 72–1. ANORECTAL ANOMALIES: CHILDREN'S MEMORIAL HOSPITAL, 1970–1986

Males		Females	
Low	53	Low	49
Intermediate	6	Intermediate	14
High	73	high	7
Total	132	Cloaca	14
		Total	84

appear to be autosomal recessive when genetically linked.

ASSOCIATED MALFORMATIONS

Hasse found a 41.6 percent incidence of associated anomalies in other organ systems in a study of 1420 patients

TABLE 72–2. INCIDENCE OF ASSOCIATED ANOMALIES IN 1420 PATIENTS WITH ANORECTAL MALFORMATIONS

Type or Location of Defect	Number of Patients	%
Urogenital	278	19.7
Extremities and spine	188	13.1
Cardiovascular	113	7.9
Gastrointestinal	89	6.0
Esophageal atresia and esophagotracheal fistula	65	5.6
Abdominal wall	28	1.9
Hare lip and cleft palate	23	1.5
Mongolism	22	1.5
Meningomyelocele	7	0.4
Others	114	8.2

Data from Hasse.[36]

(Table 72–2).[36] In three reported series, unilateral agenesis of the kidney was the most common single defect, occurring in 8 to 10 percent of the infants surveyed.[37,38] Other urinary defects included renal dysplasia, hydronephrosis secondary to ureteropelvic obstruction, and horseshoe kidneys. In a series at the Children's Memorial Hospital (Table 72–3), the incidence of urinary anomalies was 54 percent for supralevator defects and 16 percent for the low lesions.[39] Essentially all of the females we have seen with cloacal abnormalities have had ectopic ureters or agenesis of a renal unit. Cardiovascular malformations were found in 12 percent of 222 infants with imperforate anus studied at the Boston Children's Hospital, an incidence 20 times that expected in normal children. The most common lesions were tetralogy of Fallot and ventricular septal defect.[40]

Fifteen of our 216 infants with anorectal anomalies, or 7 percent, had associated esophageal atresia. This frequent association of rectal and esophageal anomalies is not surprising, since the embryonic division of the foregut into trachea and esophagus occurs at about the same time and is similar to the division of the cloaca.[41] Atresias and intestinal malrotation occur sporadically and are often first identified on an invertogram, which seems extremely confusing until an upright film of the abdomen is obtained. Malformations of the colon are of specific interest because atresia or aganglionosis interferes with successful rectal repair. Singh et al. reported 10 cases of colon atresia, all from one localized area in India with a large Punjabi population.[42] Fifty-six cases of congenital short colon have been reported from India as well.[43] In these children, the entire colon was a huge pouch measuring 8 to 15 cm, which attached to the urinary tract in boys or to a cloaca in girls. This syndrome accounted for 8.3 percent of all anorectal anomalies seen. At our hospital, there has been only one such case during the past 10 years, indicating great regional variations

TABLE 72–3. ANOMALIES ASSOCIATED WITH ANORECTAL MALFORMATIONS AT CHILDREN'S MEMORIAL HOSPITAL, 1970–1977

Type and Number of Malformations	Associated Anomalies and Number of Patients
Male	
Low lesions (13)	Inguinal hernia (2)
	Hypospadius (2)
	Bilateral ureteral reflex (1)
Intermediate (4)	Prune belly, megaurethra, open urachus (1)
	Severe gastroesophageal reflux, ureteral reflux (1)
High (29)	Ureteral reflux (3)
	Bilateral renal dysplasia (1)
	Dysplasia with pelvic kidney (1)
	Absent kidney (1)
	Absent kidney, VSD, bilateral clubfeet (1)
	Ureteral reflux, TEF, VSD, clubhand (1)
	TEF (1)
	Dislocated hips (1)
H type (1)	Urethral stricture (1)
Female	
Low (13)	Duplication of genitalia, absent kidney (1)
	Duplication of genitalia, epispadius (1)
	TEF (1)
	Aganglionosis, distal bowel (1)
	VSD, subaortic stenosis (1)
	Hemisacrum, neurogenic bladder (1)
Intermediate (8)	Ureteral reflux (unilateral) (1)
	Hydronephrosis, neurogenic bladder, esotropia (1)
	PDA (1)
High (rectovaginal) (3)	Bicornuate uterus (1)
	Absent kidney (1)
	Absent kidney, hemisacrum (1)
Cloacal (7)	Pseudotruncus absent radius (1)
	Absent kidney (1)
	Ureterouterine fistula (1)
	Bilateral ureteral reflux (1)
	Unilateral ureteral reflux (1)

PDA, patent ductus arteriosus; TEF, tracheo-esophageal fistula; VSD, ventricular septal defect.

in types. Hirschsprung's disease with aganglionosis of the rectum above the fistula does occur.[44–46] However, the fistula itself—particularly the long, slender, rectovestibular fistula—does not normally contain ganglion cells. Biopsies of this area may be confusing. Hirschsprung's disease should be suspected when there is severe constipation in the postoperative period, particularly if roentgenograms demonstrate a narrow rectal zone rather than the typical dilated rectum seen in many children with constipation following anorectal procedures.

Skeletal Defects

Stephens and Smith found that sacral anomalies fell into two groups, with agenesis of either the entire sacrum or of its segments, respectively.[47] Development processes of the sacrum, levator musculature, and sacral nerves are closely related. In the report of Stephens and Smith on 246 patients, 51 patients had sacral anomalies, and in 12 the defect seriously impaired function. Deficiencies of the fourth and fifth sacral segments allow normal innervation, but progressive absence of the third and fourth segments leads to defective bladder innervation and incontinence of urine and stool. Other vertebral defects, consisting of hemivertebrae or missing vertebrae, are important because they may cause scoliosis, particularly as the child approaches puberty. One should obtain roentgenograms of the entire spine after the newborn infant has been stabilized and the intestinal obstruction has been relieved in order to document these additional problems. Dislocated hips and extremity defects usually are obvious on clinical examination and can be confirmed with appropriate roentgenographic studies (Fig. 72–5).

Neurologic defects have a tremendous effect on the ability of a child to become continent. One should suspect spinal cord abnormalities in children who have obvious lumps, hemangiomas, or sinus tracts in the midline of the back. Other physical signs of neurologic deficit include clubfeet and motor weakness or sensory loss in the lower extremities. X-ray evidence of vertebral changes or sacral dysplasia indicate the need for neurologic studies. Carson et al. found a 30 percent incidence of abnormal sacra in 97 patients treated for anorectal abnormalities. The incidence was 48 percent in children with high anomalies.[48] Eight of nine patients who had a myelogram had spinal cord lesions, consisting of a tethered cord or lipomyelomeningocele. The tethered spinal cord is the result of an abnormal fixation that prevents the cord's rostral migration. This results in a short cauda equina and stretching of the spinal cord, with gradual loss of function. In our hospital, 16 patients with anorectal abnormalities have been identified with spinal cord abnormalities. Six had a cloacal exstrophy, four had a high lesion, and six had a low imperforate anus. Five had progressive lower extremity motor and sensory changes, and two who had previously developed continence for stool became incontinent of both stool and urine. Spinal cord anomalies are so important in this group of patients that every newborn with an anorectal anomaly should have an ultrasonographic examination of the spinal canal. In older children, magnetic resonance provides the best imaging of the spinal cord.

Local perineal lesions include masses of lipomalike tissue, hemangiomas, and duplications of the genitalia (Fig. 72–6). These lesions should be excised before rectal repair to allow healing of suture lines without fecal con-

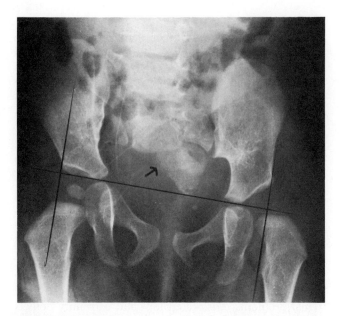

Figure 72–5. Hemisacrum with a left, flat acetabulum in a girl with a rectovestibular fistula.

tamination. In fact, when there is a complex duplication involving the genitalia and anus, a colostomy should be performed before perineal reconstruction even if the child has been moving her bowels through an adequate perineal fistula.

Black and Sherman at our hospital made a serendipi-

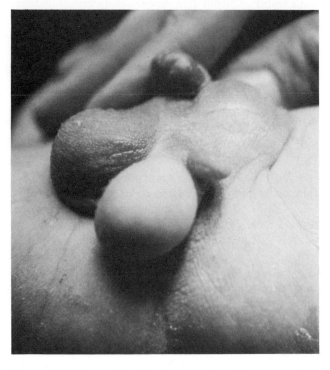

Figure 72–6. Mass of fibrofatty tissue on the perineum associated with an imperforate anus.

tous observation on the association of Down's syndrome with a specific lesion (personal communication). Eight boys and six girls with Down's syndrome had an anal atresia without genitourinary fistula. This observation came about through ultrasonographic examination of the perineum in the neonatal period. Some had undergone a needless colostomy when all that was required was a perineal anoplasty. Perhaps not every child with Down's syndrome will have this specific lesion, but it is sufficiently common that it must be considered in all cases.

DIAGNOSIS

An absent or anomalous anus usually is so obvious that it is discovered in the delivery room. A deep anal pit may hide a complete membrane, however, and a rectal atresia consisting of a web several centimeters above the anus may also be overlooked until it is noted that the infant is distended and has not passed meconium.

The diagnosis of low, or translevator, lesions can often be made by physical examination of the perineum. The baby must be held in the lithotomy position in a good light. Lacrimal duct probes, a number 5 French feeding tube, a curved hemostat, and a nasal speculum are the only instruments required. In the male, one searches from the anal dimple forward along the median raphe to the tip of the penis for a fistulous tract. The pits on either side of a bucket handle defect in the male are carefully examined and probed, searching for a small tract that leads to the rectum. Similarly, in the female one searches for an ectopic opening on the perineum and within the vestibule (Fig. 72–7). It often is necessary to spread the labia with a small nasal speculum or a curved hemostat to demonstrate the ectopic anus. When an opening has been found, it may be explored with a lacrimal probe, or the catheter may be inserted and irrigated until meconium is obtained.

The diagnosis of a perineal fistula may be extremely difficult in the male during the first 24 hours of life. The examination should be repeated several times, because at first the fistula may be occluded by debris, and later, mucus will distend the fistula, producing epithelial pearls, and often one will find a speck of meconium that was not present initially (Fig. 72–8).

In females, one can differentiate between a cloaca and a high rectovaginal fistula by observing the urethra (Fig. 72–9). With a cloaca, there is only one opening on the perineum, and catheterization reveals both meconium and urine. There is usually an enlarged clitoris just above the single perineal orifice. If there is an identifiable urethra in the normal location and a vagina that contains meconium, the infant has a rectovaginal fistula and not a cloaca. An abdominal mass with a cloaca is a hydrometrocolpos.

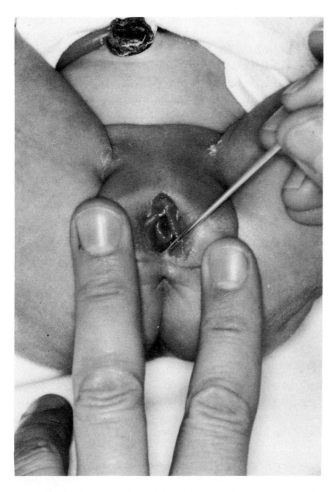

Figure 72–7. Anovestibular fistula. Note the probe in the anal orifice and the deep anal dimple.

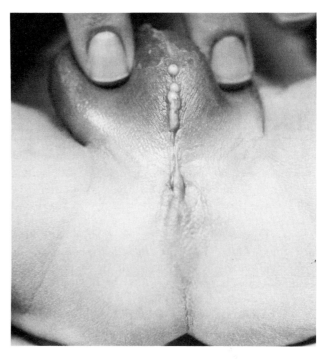

Figure 72–8. Male infant with a perineal fistula extending to the scrotum. The epithelial pearls did not become evident until the boy was 24 hours old.

Examination of the perineum also will provide information concerning sacral innervation and muscular development. A deep anal dimple exhibiting a strong muscle reaction to a pin prick suggests normal innervation. Contraction of the levator ani will pull the anal dimple forward, but a circumferential puckering at the site of the dimple is an indication of superficial external sphincter fibers. A flat perineum with no anal dimple and poor muscular response to a pin prick is a sign of defective perineal innervation. A slow dribble of urine or a distended bladder provides further proof of poor innervation. A soft mass located in the posterior perineum and extending onto the sacrum may very well represent a lipomeningocele with severe sacral deformities. Protruding knobs of tissue in the vicinity of the anal dimple that demonstrate muscular activity can be classified as retained anal tubercles with remnants of external sphincter muscle. Poor development of the labia, signs of ambiguous genitalia, and, in the male, undescended testicles are further evidence of a severe defect.

A complete physical examination must be carried out, including the passage of a nasogastric tube to rule out an esophageal atresia. The abdomen is specifically examined for distention and palpable enlargement of the kidneys or bladder. The urine is examined for squamous epithelial cells and meconium.

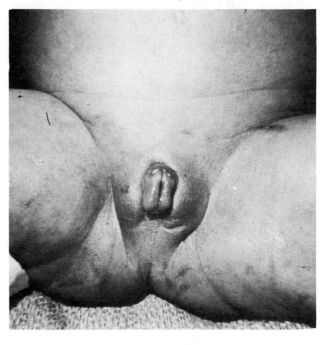

Figure 72–9. Cloaca. Note the malformed labia. There is only one perineal opening.

The upside-down x-ray originally described by Wangensteen and Rice has been the classic method for determining the distance from the blind rectal pouch to a marker placed on or within the anal dimple.[49] With this technique, the baby is placed upside down, and a marker is taped to the anal dimple. Roentgenograms then allow one to measure the distance between the marker and the blind pouch (Fig. 72-10). With the rare, high rectal atresia without fistula, a radiopaque catheter is inserted into the anus against the rectal membrane. Since 18 to 20 hours are required for gas to reach the distal rectum, no decision should be made about the level of the rectal pouch for at least 24 hours. During this interval, the infant should be allowed to become mildly distended before a gastric tube is inserted to remove swallowed air, and the infant is maintained in a prone position with a pad under the hips to elevate the buttocks. This position places a rectal pouch at the highest level of the gastrointestinal tract. A number 5 French radiopaque feeding tube is placed in the male urethra for a simultaneous urethrogram. A physician (preferably the responsible surgeon) must accompany the infant to the x-ray department to personally supervise the study. We prefer to securely tape a small bit of lead deep within the anal dimple, taking at least one x-ray while pressure is applied to the dimple with the tip of a curved hemostat. The baby is then carefully held upside down by a lead-shielded technician or nurse for at least 3 minutes while the x-ray plates are being arranged. The baby's hips are kept slightly extended and not flexed, and the x-ray beam is centered over the greater trochanter of the femur. The baby must be held exactly at a right angle to the x-ray plate to prevent distortion of the pelvic anatomy. Stephens prefers to smear barium paste over the dimple to outline the natal cleft. Several roentgenograms are obtained because contraction of the levator muscles occludes the rectum, forcing the gas higher into the pelvis and giving an impression of a high pouch. The additional time required for more x-rays allows more gas to percolate up through the sticky meconium to outline the very distal portion of the pouch.

A prone, cross-table lateral film is an excellent alternate to the standard invertogram.[50] It is the study of choice if the infant has a tracheoesophageal fistula because the inverted position allows the free flow of gastric juice into the lungs. For a cross-table lateral, the infant is positioned prone on the x-ray table, with padding under the lower abdomen to raise the hips. This is really just an extension of the knee–chest position previously described. Pelvic and perineal real-time ultrasonography also provides excellent information about the location of the rectal pouch. Currently, we carry out both ultrasonography and the prone, cross-table roentgenogram for comparison and to obtain as much preoperative information as possible. We have been able to perform a perineal anoplasty in all infants in whom ultrasonography demonstrated a pouch within 1 cm of the skin. Some authors have recommended the injection of a water-soluble contrast material through the perineum into the distal pouch for definitive diagnosis.[51,52] With this technique, a needle sheathed with a plastic cannula is advanced into the perineum under fluoroscopic control until the blind pouch is punctured and meconium is aspirated. The needle is then withdrawn, leaving the plastic cannula. From 3 to 5 ml of 20 percent Hypaque is then injected.

None of these techniques is completely accurate. The information from several studies, especially the ultrasound and invertogram studies, must be correlated with clinical findings. If there is any doubt about the level of the lesion, a colostomy should be performed.

After the inverted x-rays are completed, a voiding cystogram is obtained to demonstrate a fistula. Voiding x-rays demonstrate urinary tract abnormalities such as ureteral reflux, urethral stricture, and a connection between the ureter and the vas deferens. Once it is filled with either air or contrast material, the blind rectal pouch

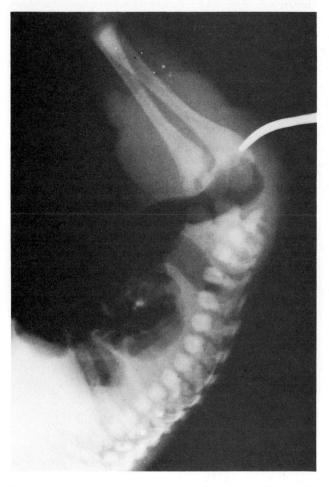

Figure 72–10. A simple anal membrane indented by the tip of a hemostat.

is located in relation to the pubococcygeal line or to the I-point of the ischium. If the sacrum is poorly developed, the pubococcygeal (P-C) line may be determined by commencing from the midpoint of the pubis anteriorly and transecting the junction of the upper and lower three quarters of the ischium. It is essential to have a straight lateral view of the pelvis with the hips extended in order to properly evaluate these pelvic skeletal landmarks. Supralevator lesions are identified when the blind rectal pouch ends above the P-C line. The bowel in intermediate lesions extends to a line drawn through the most inferior portion of the ischium, parallel to the P-C line.

Other Studies

During the neonatal period, either at the same time as the other x-ray studies or before the infant's discharge from the hospital, the following studies are obtained: echocardiography, ultrasonography of the genitourinary system and the spine.

TREATMENT

Low Lesions

Male. A perineal anoplasty is performed in boys when there is definite evidence of a fistulous tract, either at the anal dimple or forward on the perineum, or if there is a bulging anal membrane. The infant may be operated on under either local or general anesthesia in the lithotomy position. The fistula is located and dilated with lacrimal duct probes. Anterior perineal fistulas are then opened over the probe by cutting down with the sharp pointed tips of fine dissecting scissors. As the fistula reaches the anal canal, it widens, and large amounts of thick, sticky meconium must be aspirated and irrigated. The anal canal is opened, and the mucosa and skin are loosely approximated with 4-0 absorbable sutures. The epithelium remaining on the perineum is left alone. Severe anal stenosis at the anal dimple is opened with a V-Y plasty, but a complete anal membrane is opened with cruciate incisions with flaps of skin sutured up into the anal canal. Postoperatively, these patients require dilatation until the anal canal will accept the index finger with ease.

Female. Minimal degrees of anterior displacement of the anus in girls require no treatment if the fifth finger can be inserted into the anal canal. Otherwise dilatation may be required. More anterior displacement of the anus or anal stenosis can be treated with the V-Y operation, a modification of the simple anal cutback favored by most British pediatric surgeons. In the cutback operation, scissors are inserted into the fistula, and the opening is enlarged toward the normal anal site with a single cut. Dilatation is required afterward. We favor the V-Y modification because by first reflecting the posteriorly based, V-shaped wedge of skin, one can see the fibers of the external sphincter muscle. These fibers may be pushed backward and saved, so that only the fistulous tract itself is involved in an incision straight back to normal rectal mucosa. The V-shaped flap of skin is then sutured into the mucosal incision. This provides a skin-lined anal canal, and obviates the need for prolonged rectal dilatation (Fig. 72–11).

The anovestibular fistula is too far forward and too close to the vagina for a cutback operation. It is absolutely essential to differentiate between an anovestibular and an anorectal lesion because an anorectal fistula requires a colostomy and later repair. If the baby is full term and without any other birth defects, an anoperineal repair may be carried out during the neonatal period. If the infant moves her bowels without constipation or difficulty, the operation is delayed to at least 3 months of age.

Anoplasty

The identification of the external sphincter is the first step in any rectal pullthrough operation (Fig. 72–12). Always warn the anesthesiologist against giving muscle relaxants until all elements of the muscle complex have been identified by nerve stimulation. Two responses will be seen on initial electrical stimulation of the perineal skin. There is a forward contraction of the perineum and a circular contraction of the external sphincter muscle around the anal dimple. This point is marked and checked several times. The initial midline skin incision is carefully thought out and marked with a pen (Fig. 72–12A). It is centered over the contracting fibers of the external sphincter and must be as long as half the circumference of the bowel. At either end of this incision, triangular shaped wedges of skin are removed (Fig. 72–12B). The two lateral flaps of skin are then elevated from the muscle fibers. These flaps must be long enough to line the anal canal to the depth of the external sphincter muscle to prevent mucosal prolapse after the final repair. The nerve stimulator is again used to guide the dissection through the exact center of the contracting muscle fibers. This delicate stage of the operation is done with the aid of magnifying loupes and a head light. The tunnel is gradually deepened to 1.5 or 2 cm and enlarged by opening and closing the tips of fine dissecting scissors. This canal through the external sphincter is gradually stretched until, at the end of the operation, it will accommodate the pulled-through rectum. The skin flaps then are sutured up to the bowel wall. Closure of the triangular skin defect forces the flaps up the anal canal (Fig. 72–12C–F). This perineal procedure is the first step in all the operations described here.

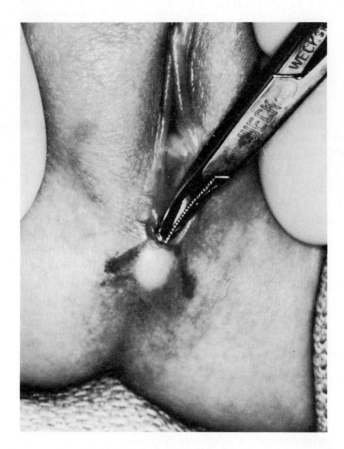 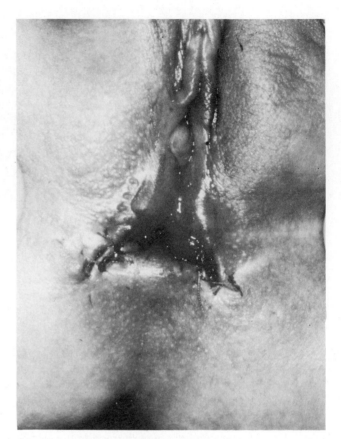

Figure 72–11. Left. V-Y plastic repair of an anovestibular fistula. The skin flap is outlined with ink. **Right.** The flap is sutured into the anal canal.

Technique of Perineal Anoplasty for Anovestibular Fistula.

The baby is placed in an exaggerated lithotomy position, the external sphincter is found with the nerve stimulator, and the midline incision is made as described in Figure 72–12. An incision is then made around the ectopic anus, and its edge is transfixed with a number of 6-0 sutures (Fig. 72–13). The anterior and posterior sutures are held on traction with separate hemostats so that it is possible to open the fistula from time to time to determine how close one's dissection is to the bowel wall (Fig. 72–13B). The incision about the fistula is extended laterally for no more than a quarter of an inch. It is best to dissect on the wall of the bowel anteriorly to gradually separate the bowel from the vagina. Apply downward traction on the bowel while an assistant elevates the vaginal wall with small skin hooks (Fig. 72–13D). The dissection is then carried laterally and posteriorly to separate the bowel from the levator muscle. This is extremely difficult because muscle slips from the puborectalis intermingle with the outer muscle layer of the bowel wall. It is easy at this point to inadvertently dissect outside the levator sling. When the bowel is free for 3 or 4 cm and with traction on the sutures, the bowel is brought down to the anal dimple (Fig. 72–13E). The lowermost fibers of the puborectalis are stretched backward to accommodate the angulated position of the bowel as it diverges from the posterior wall of the vagina. The rectum is thus acutely angulated by the puborectalis sling. In order to bring the skin flaps up to form a deep anal cleft, a series of sutures are taken through the subcutaneous tissue of the skin flaps, after which a bite is taken through the levator sling and then the seromuscular wall of the bowel. When these sutures are tied, the skin is secured to the levator sling as well as to the bowel. This allows the formation of a skin-lined anal canal. Finally, excess mucosa is trimmed away, and the skin flaps are sutured to the bowel mucosa with 4-0 sutures. These must be tied loosely over the tips of a hemostat so they will not cut through during the period of postoperative edema.

In our hands, this operation has often turned out to be more difficult than here described. If the lesion is the slightest bit higher than anticipated, it will be necessary to dissect the bowel up almost to the peritoneal reflection. If one dissects too closely to the bowel, there is the risk of perforation and reformation of the fistula.

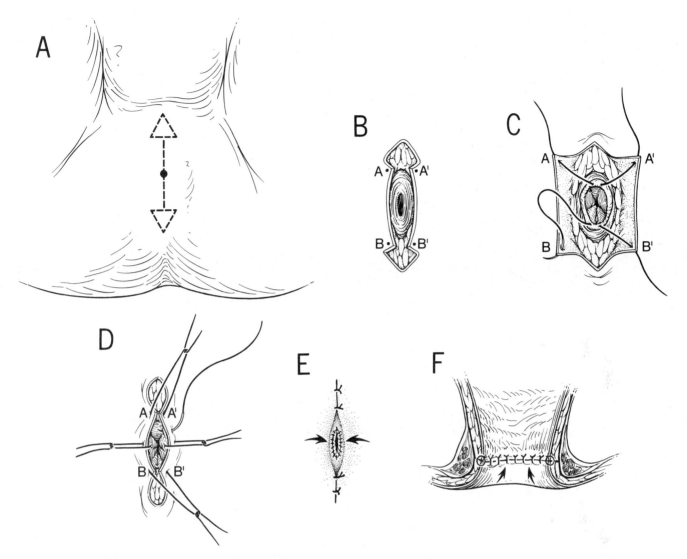

Figure 72–12. The Nixon technique to obtain a skin-lined anus. Removal of two triangles of skin from either end of the incision forces skin up through the external sphincter muscle to meet the bowel. This procedure is followed as the first and last step in all the operations described here.

On the other hand, if one leaves more tissue on the bowel side, the levator muscles are injured. For these reasons, one must select patients for this operation with extreme care. The most feared immediate complication is complete separation and retraction of the bowel. If this occurs, the infant must be immediately reoperated on, more bowel freed, and a new anastomosis made. Minor degrees of separation between the skin and mucosa will heal without difficulty.

At 10 days to 2 weeks, the infant is returned to the operating room for inspection and the first dilatation. If healing is complete, gentle, progressive dilatations are continued with flexible rubber esophageal dilators until the anus will easily take first the fifth and then the index finger. These children must be followed very closely, and constipation must be prevented with diet and mineral oil.

Anal Agenesis Without Fistula. Even though this is classified as an intermediate lesion, it can be cured with a perineal anoplasty during the neonatal period. One must be absolutely certain that there is no fistula to the urethra. The operation is carried out with the infant in the lithotomy position. A urethral catheter is inserted in boys. The external sphincter muscle is identified with the nerve stimulator and marked. The skin incision illustrated in Figure 72–12 is made, and the fibers of the external sphincter are gradually separated. The incision is deepened in the midline until the bulging pouch is encountered. If the pouch is not

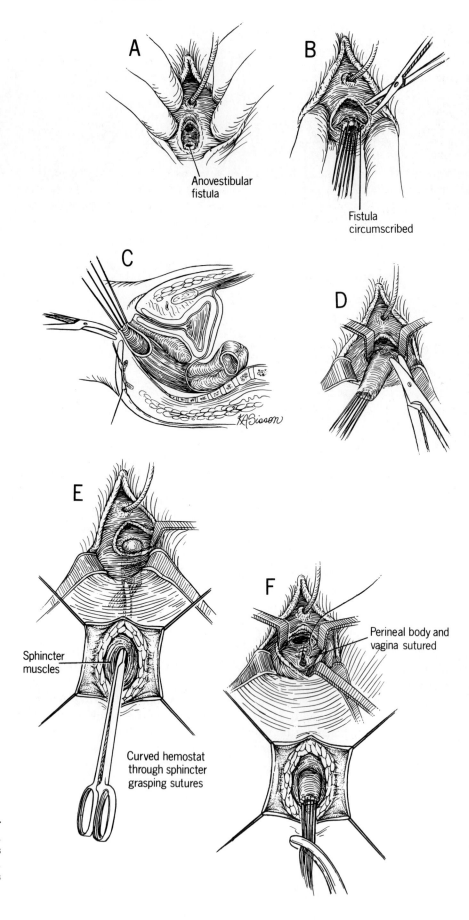

Figure 72–13. Perineal anoplasty or transplantation of an anovestibular fistula. The incision described in Figure 72–12 is made over the external sphincter muscle, and after the bowel is transplanted, skin flaps are sutured up to the new rectum.

found within 1.5 cm, either the diagnosis or the plane of dissection is wrong. Sufficient length of the pouch is freed until the skin flaps can be sutured to the wall of the bowel without tension.

Colostomy

Infants with intermediate or supralevator lesions require a colostomy in the neonatal period and repair at 12 to 15 months of age. A satisfactory colostomy must completely divert the fecal stream. Furthermore, since the dilated bowel will become considerably smaller after it is decompressed, the peritoneum and fascia must be sutured to the seromuscular layer of the bowel to prevent

herniation of small intestine around the stoma. Finally, there must be sufficient length of bowel distal to the colostomy for the repair.

There are several advantages to the technique illustrated in Figure 72–14. There is sufficient bowel distal to the left transverse colon so that the splenic flexure may be mobilized in order to obtain more length at the time of rectal pullthrough. The two limbs are completely separated by a bridge of abdominal wall, and the mucosa is immediately everted and sutured to the skin. This prevents serositis and decreases the incidence of colostomy strictures. In addition, the incision is well away from that used in the final repair.

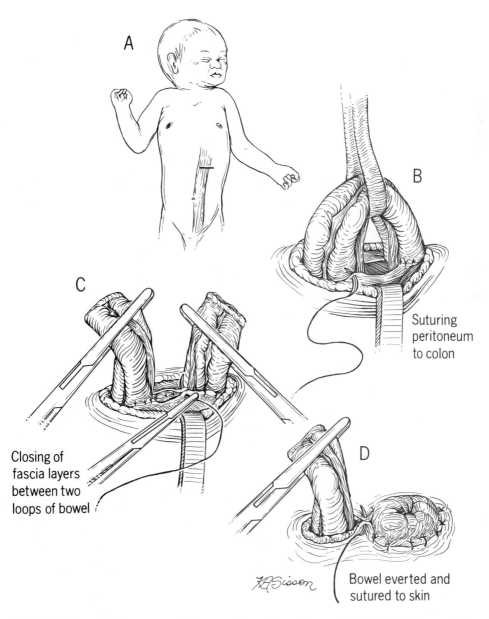

Figure 72–14. This is a left transverse colostomy performed through a small incision that is remote from the eventual pullthrough. Immediate maturation of the colostomy prevents serositis and allows earlier discharge of the patient.

The left transverse colostomy can be performed under either local or general anesthesia. A 3 cm transverse skin incision is made about half way between the umbilicus and the costal margin. Frequently, the dilated transverse colon is palpable. It is important to make the incision directly over the colon to minimize handling of the small bowel. The colon is drawn into the wound, and one or two mesenteric vessels adjacent to the bowel wall are ligated and divided to create a small mesenteric defect. A catheter is placed through this defect for traction. Care must be taken not to injure the marginal vessels. The peritoneum and fascia are then sutured in layers to the seromuscular layer of the bowel wall. If these sutures penetrate the lumen, one can expect a fistula and possibly a deep wound infection. Two clamps are placed across the bowel wall, which is divided. Peritoneum, fascia, and skin are then closed between the two loops. The bowel is everted and loosely sutured to the skin. The completed colostomy should protrude from the abdominal wall for at least 1 cm, and the proximal loop should be just large enough to accept a size 18 French catheter. Meconium is irrigated from each limb of the colostomy. A moistened sponge held in place with Montgomery straps will control oozing from the bowel edges during the next several days, and the distal limb of the colon is irrigated with 1 percent neomycin in saline to minimize the risk of urinary tract infection from retained stool. Colostomy care consists of careful cleansing and drying of the skin, which is protected with zinc oxide paste. A second diaper wrapped around the infant's abdomen collects stool. Unfortunately, a few liquid stools on unprotected skin will result in weeping dermatitis. If *Candida* is cultured, nystatin ointment is indicated. Steroid ointments are helpful to clear up a persistent rash. Some mothers prefer to use a colostomy bag with a karaya ring.

Infants with rectourinary tract fistulas are at risk to develop infections, especially if there are other urinary anomalies, such as vesicoureteral reflux. These babies are maintained on suppressive antibiotics, and periodic urine cultures guide more specific therapy. Infants with severe reflux associated with persistent infection may require an antireflux operation. Hyperchloremic acidosis secondary to the absorption of urine from the rectum is an indication for complete repair at an earlier age.

Intermediate Lesions

Male. A boy with anal agenesis and a rectobulbar fistula should have a colostomy performed in the newborn period and the definitive operation delayed until he is about 1 year old. It is perfectly feasible, and perhaps preferable, to operate on a boy with this lesion with an anterior perineal operation. With the fistula, however, the bowel is densely adherent to the urethra and is difficult to separate. Most surgeons prefer a sacroperineal pullthrough.

Technique of the Sacral Approach. The sterile skin preparation must include the abdomen, the perineum, the back, and the legs at least to the knees (Fig. 72–15). A size 10 or 12 metal sound is inserted into the urethra. It should be possible to palpate the sound in the bladder, which is held in place with multiple turns of Steristrips. The child is then turned onto his abdomen and supported in the knee–chest position. He is draped so that the urethral sound is in the sterile field.

The anal dimple is localized with the nerve stimulator, and a skin incision is made at the point of maximum contraction. A second incision is made from over the coccyx to within 3 cm of the first incision. The coccyx is held up with forceps, and the dissection is deepened in the midline through fatty tissue interlaced with loose muscle fibers. In order to avoid damage to the lower portion of the levator sling, the dissection can be directed superiorly toward the rectal pouch. The rectum is mobilized by dissecting immediately on its wall, circumferentially and superiorly away from the fistula. One continually palpates in the depth of the wound for the metal sound in the urethra. When the rectum is separated from the urethra, it is encircled with a slip of Penrose drain, and traction is applied upward and away from the fistula. A right-angled clamp is opened and closed to separate the rectum from the urethra anteriorly and from the puborectalis posteriorly. The dissection posterior to the rectum continues until the tip of the clamp is palpated at the exact center of the external sphincter as demonstrated by the nerve stimulator. The center of the external sphincter is opened until a tunnel is made through this muscle and into the space anterior to the puborectalis. The fibers of these muscles are in continuity and must be carefully identified with the nerve stimulator. A Penrose drain is then draw through the tunnel. All further dilatations of the puborectalis tunnel are carried out through the Penrose drain. These dilatations must be performed slowly and gently and preferably from above to avoid tearing the lowermost fibers of the muscle. Traction on the Penrose drain through the tunnel elevates the sling so that the bowel may be dissected distally to its fistula with the urethra. The bowel also may be opened to identify the fistula from within. By frequently palpating the sound, the urethra can be identified and the fistula divided, leaving enough tissue for a two-layer closure. When the fistula has been divided and closed, the sound is replaced with a Foley catheter. More proximal dissection may then be required to mobilize sufficient bowel to reach the perineum. The skin is then sutured to the levator muscle and the bowel wall to create a skin-lined anal canal, as previously de-

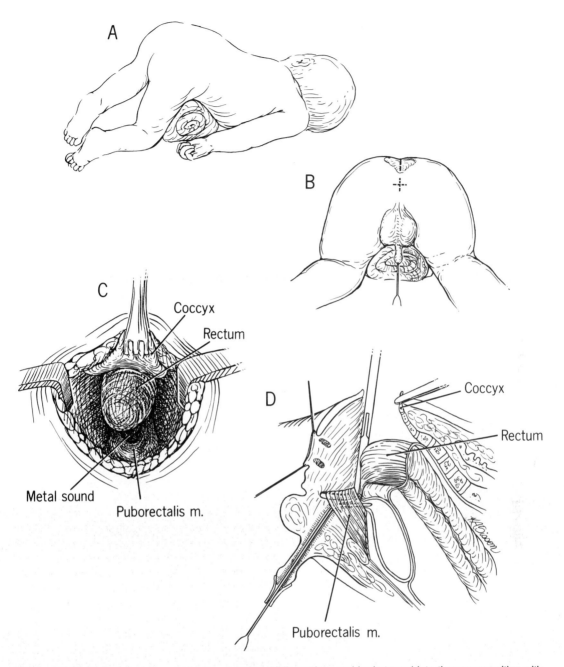

Figure 72–15. A, B. A metal sound is placed in the child's urethra, and he is turned into the prone position with his buttocks elevated on sterile sheets. The external sphincter is located with a nerve stimulator and the previously described cruciate incision is made. **C.** An incision is then made over the coccyx, which can either be removed or elevated with an Allis forceps. **D.** The dissection is deepened until the posterior rectal wall is seen. By palpating the urethral sound, the dissection is continued directly on the urethra within the puborectalis muscle. When the tip of the forceps can be palpated through the anal incision, the tunnel is completed. A Penrose drain is drawn through the tunnel, and further stretching of the puborectalis is carried out within the drain. The fistula is then dissected and detached from the rectum, and the bowel is pulled through the tunnel and sutured to the skin flaps.

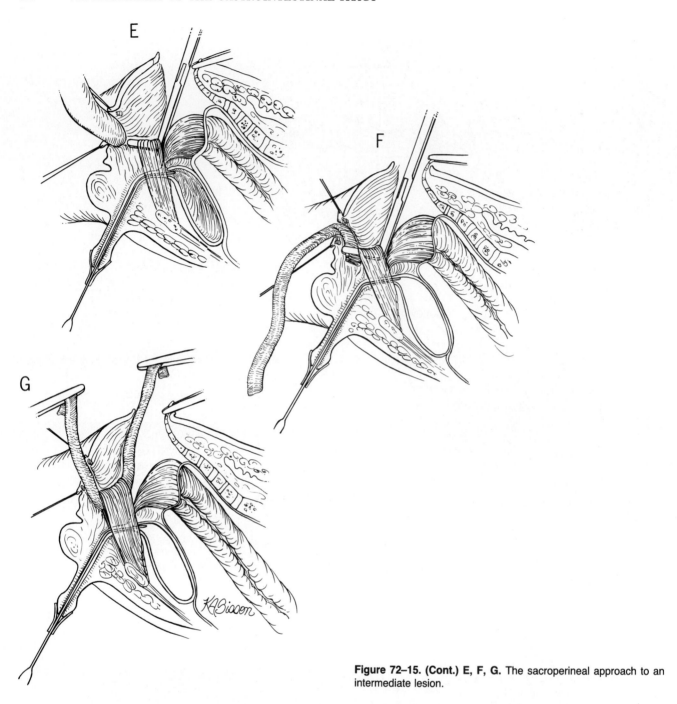

Figure 72–15. (Cont.) E, F, G. The sacroperineal approach to an intermediate lesion.

scribed. Rectal dilatations are commenced within 10 days to 2 weeks, and the colostomy is closed after 2 to 3 months.

Female. The endorectal pullthrough described by both Rehbein and Roumualdi completely obviates injury to the levator sling and pelvic nerves.[53,54] This operation is particularly well suited to the female with an intermediate lesion.

Technique of the Endorectal Pullthrough. The child is placed in a lithotomy position by taping the legs onto sandbags. This provides simultaneous access to the perineum and abdomen. After electrostimulation, skin flaps are made, and the external sphincter muscle is carefully identified and dissected as in Figure 72–12. This dissection must be completed before the child is given muscle relaxants for the abdominal portion of the operation.

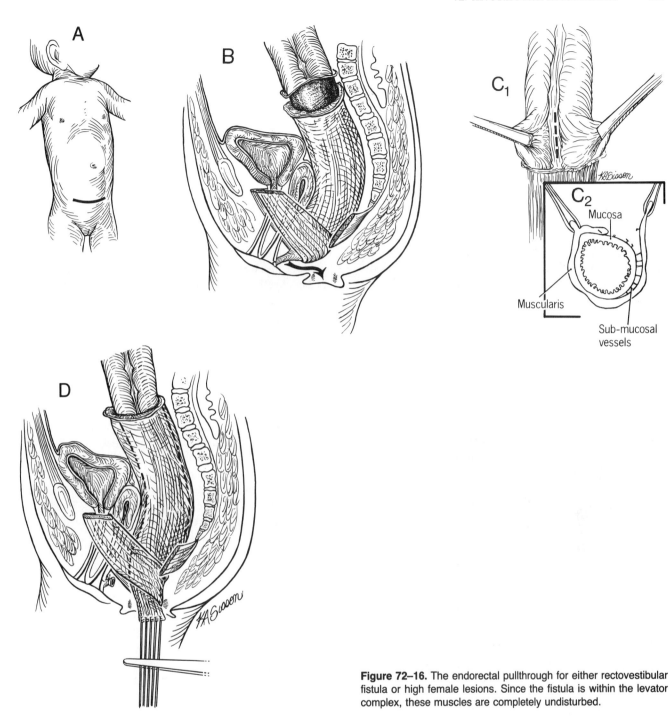

Figure 72–16. The endorectal pullthrough for either rectovestibular fistula or high female lesions. Since the fistula is within the levator complex, these muscles are completely undisturbed.

After opening of the abdomen, the small bowel is packed into the upper abdomen, and the ureters are identified. The uterus and vagina are held forward with traction sutures to expose the rectum and sigmoid, which are mobilized to the peritoneal reflection. At this point, the seromuscular layer of the rectum is incised down to the mucosa. This must be done carefully to avoid penetrating the mucosa. Bleeding must be meticulously controlled with the bipolar electrocautery (Fig. 72–16). When the proper submucosal plane is located, the mu-

cosa is stripped away from the muscle with a Küttner dissector.

With careful dissection, the submucosal vessels are easily visible and are coagulated by an assistant before they are divided. When a circumferential core of mucosa has been stripped away from the muscle, it is clamped and divided. Then, with upward traction on the mucosa, the dissection is carried down to the junction of the bowel and the vagina. If necessary, the last centimeter or so can be dissected from below. There is then left a muscular tunnel with an intact Aurbach's plexus that traverses the levator sling. The incision into the anal dimple is deepened through the fibers of the external sphincter. A curved hemostat is directed anteriorly to the muscular tunnel. This dissection is relatively superficial so as to avoid damage to the distal fibers of the puborectalis. The rectosigmoid is then freed sufficiently to draw it through the muscular tunnel to the perineum. The previously described skin–mucosal anastomosis is then made.

Supralevator Lesions

Male. A high anorectal agenesis with a rectoprostatic urethral fistula is difficult to treat. No two surgeons agree on the best operation, and arguments over the merits of the various procedures have spawned bitter feuds among otherwise pleasant people. DeVries has reviewed the evolution of surgery for imperforate anus through the centuries.[55] The pendulum has swung from purely perineal approaches to the abdominoperineal pull-through and now back to a perineal operation. Each new operation, as it is enthusiastically introduced by its inventor, is hailed as a great step forward. Within 10 years, when the results are in, the operation is criticized, and the surgical community embraces a new operation. There are many problems in evaluating the operations available for these unfortunate infants. Some authors artfully mix their results in low and intermediate with high lesions. Others, in fine print, eliminate patients with neurologic problems, mental retardation, or multiple anomalies. Finally, there is a tremendous variation in the available sphincteric musculature. In some, the perineum shows an active response to stimulation with a pin prick or the nerve stimulator. These patients will have well-developed muscles and a better outcome than the poor child with little or no musculature. CT scan evaluation of the pelvis and a greater awareness of associated spinal cord lesions will aid in sorting out these problems.

We have arrived at the operation described here because it allows for an accurate identification of the plane immediately behind the urethra, which is within the levator sling–puborectalis muscle complex. The external sphincter muscle is identified and is in plain view for accurate dissection. The abdominal incision allows for resection of the bulbous, poorly functioning terminal rectum, while leaving a cuff of smooth muscle containing Auerbach's plexus. Also, if a portion of the rectum has descended, the upper levators are completely undisturbed. Since there is no dissection along the base of the bladder or upper urethra, damage to the nerves in this area is avoided. Finally, an intact tube of bowel is placed next to the urethral fistula. This operation differs from the abdominoperineal pullthrough described previ-

ously only by the anteriorly placed perineal incision. This is the anterioperineal abdominal pullthrough described by Mollard et al. and later by Martin-Laberge et al.[56,57]

Procedure. The operation is performed when the child is about 1 year old (Fig. 72–17). Both the proximal and distal colostomy must be liberally irrigated with saline for several days. While the child is on the operating table, the stomas are again irrigated with dilute povidone-iodine. The anesthesiologists are warned not to paralyze the child until after all nerve stimulation and muscle identification are complete. The child is placed in an exaggerated lithotomy position, and the entire abdomen and perineum are prepared and draped into a single field. A metal sound or a firm, plastic catheter is placed in the urethra. This step is essential. Sometimes the catheter goes through the fistula into the bowel, in which case a cystotomy is performed, and the catheter is passed from the bladder out the urethra.

Mollard et al. originally described a transverse skin incision immediately posterior to the scrotum and then a second incision over the external sphincter. It is more convenient to use a single vertical incision that exposes both the external sphincter and the anterior gateway to the urethra. Kite-shaped excisions of skin from either extremity of the incision allow the creation of two skin flaps that, when sutured up to the bowel, provide a skin-lined anal canal (Figure 72–17A–J).

The surgeon is comfortably seated, and both the surgeon and assistant wear magnifying loupes. The lowermost fibers of the puborectalis muscle are identified with the nerve stimulator and are pushed back from the urethra. Maintain the dissection directly on the urethra, which must be in sight at all times. The bulbocavernous muscle is left undisturbed (Fig. 72–17D). This dissection must be painstaking and unhurried. The jaws of a small dissection scissors are opened and closed to open a straight path behind the urethra. Lateral deviations will injure the muscle sling. The nerve stimulator is used constantly to identify the muscles. On stimulation, the muscle sling contracts forward toward the pubis. As the dissection proceeds, the incision is held open with narrow retractors inserted on either side. It continues until the pouch is reached or until the surgeon can no longer proceed under direct vision. Bleeding is controlled with pressure or with the cautious application of an accurately directed bipolar electrocoagulation unit.

If there is a deep anal dimple, stimulation usually will demonstrate the center of contraction of the superficial sphincter fibers. This is difficult when the external sphincter is poorly developed and represented only by stray muscle fibers coursing from back to front in fat. The center of the external sphincter is deepened with blunt dissection. This is straight in as long as one can

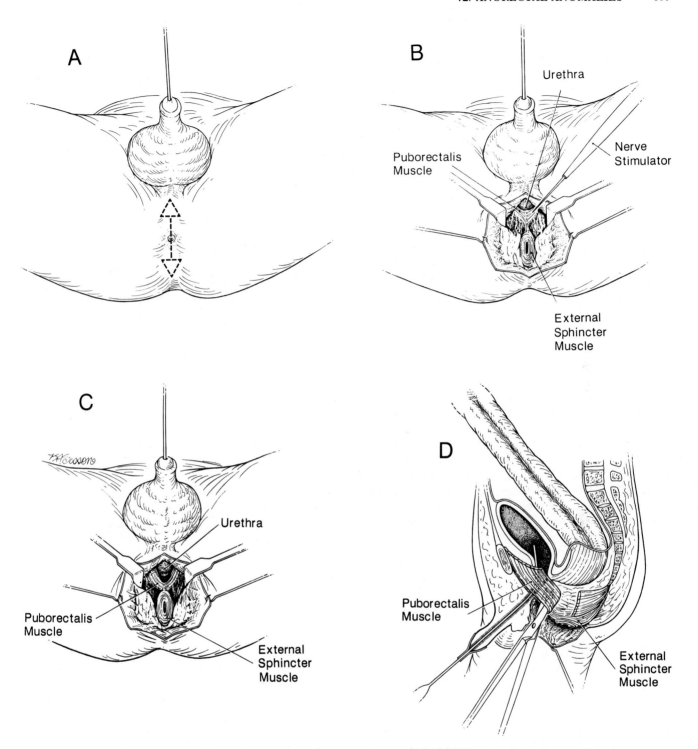

Figure 72–17. Technique for the anterior abdominoperineal pullthrough. After opening the perineum with Nixon's incision, all muscles are identified with the nerve stimulator. The dissection within the puborectalis is immediately on the urethra, which must be under direct vision. The abdominal portion of the operation consists of either freezing the distal bowel or, as illustrated here, using an endorectal dissection. The pulled-through bowel rather sharply angles backward in its course from the puborectalis through the external sphincter.

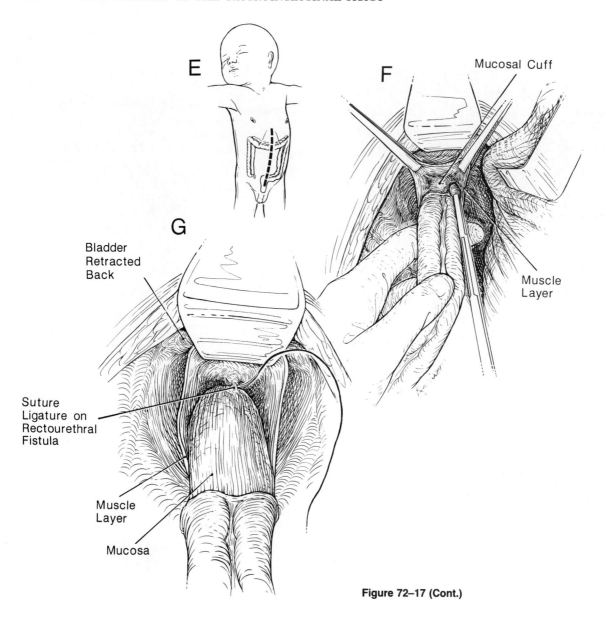

Figure 72–17 (Cont.)

identify circular fibers; then it is angled anteriorly to meet the previous dissection. A Penrose drain is placed through this tunnel, and the abdomen is opened. After a brief abdominal exploration, pack the small bowel into the upper abdomen, exposing the rectum and sigmoid. The left transverse colostomy is well out of the way, leaving plenty of bowel between it and the pelvis. Suture the bladder forward to improve exposure and identify both ureters. The sigmoid and upper rectum are mobilized to the pelvic peritoneal reflection. At that point, the small collapsed intestine balloons out into the dilated terminal rectum.

The previously described endorectal dissection is carried out by freeing the mucosa from the muscular cuff (Fig. 72–17F,G). Vessels are identified and controlled with the bipolar coagulation unit. If the fistula

is so high that it enters the bladder, there is no point to the endorectal dissection, but in the usual case, the fistula will be found to the urethra, which is again identified by palpating the sound. The fistula is suture-ligated and divided. At this point, the muscular cuff of the rectum is intact. The surgeon then shifts back to the perineum and, under direct vision, passes a long, curved hemostat upward along the posterior wall of the urethra, within the levator sling, until the tip of the instrument indents the bowel wall (Fig. 72–17H). The pouch is opened on the hemostat, and a Penrose drain is passed through the tunnel, connecting the abdomen with the anterior peroneal incision (Fig. 72–17I) The peroneal end of the drain is then placed through the tunnel made in the external sphincter. The tunnel is gently enlarged by passing flexible, lubricated Tucker esophageal dilators

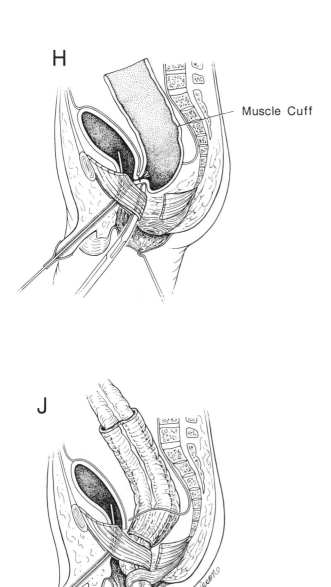

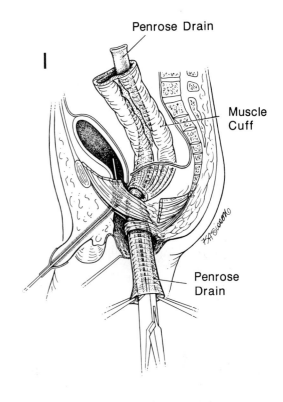

Figure 72–17 (Cont.)

through the Penrose drain. The size of the eventual tunnel is that of a 9 or 10 Hegar dilator. Since the dilated megarectum has been removed by the endorectal dissection, the bowel may now be drawn through the tunnel with long sutures passed through the Penrose drain (Fig. 72–17J). If the tunnel is so narrow that the bowel becomes ischemic, it is again gently dilated. The bowel pursues a course through the levator sling, then angles backward through the external sphincter. Closure of the kite-shaped incisions forces skin flaps up the anal canal to meet the bowel, where they are sutured by taking bites through skin, sphincter muscle, and the bowel wall.[58]

Ten to 14 days after the operation, the new anus is examined and gently dilated under anesthesia. Flexible dilators must be used because the bowel is angulated rather sharply. The colostomy may be closed any time after the new rectum has been dilated to accept the surgeon's finger.

Females. Girls with anorectal agenesis are handled in a similar fashion, except that the dissection proceeds along the back wall of the vagina to maintain a tunnel within the puborectalis–levator sling.

Cloaca. There are several ways in which the rectum, vagina, and urethra may join into a common tract. In the most common type, the three join at the same level, at the apex of the cloaca. The cloaca may be so short that, with a nasal speculum, one can identify the three orifices. The vagina may be absent or hypoplastic, a variant of the Mayer-Rokitansky syndrome. Even when the vagina is absent, there often are rudimentary fallopian tubes and a uterus. In this situation, the rectum may join with the bladder or urethra to form a rectourinary sinus. In this case, the posterior wall of the cloaca is lined with colon mucosa and the anterior wall with urinary tract epithelium. In one of our patients, the cloaca consisted of the rectum, displaced forward to the location of the vagina, and the urethra was only a little posterior. In her final repair, the cloaca was left to function as a vagina, and the bowel was divided above the cloaca and pulled through the levator sling to its normal location. The most serious types of cloacal malformations include varying degrees of hydrocolpos because of either vaginal obstruction or the preferential drainage of urine into the dilated vagina. Associated malformations of the urinary tract were found in 13 of 15 of the original patients we studied.[59] The incidence of associated defects rises in direct proportion to the complexity of the lesion.

These infants should be evaluated in the neonatal period to determine the extent of the defect. A wide-open single orifice on the perineum often will drain urine and meconium sufficiently well to allow complete radiologic, CT, and endoscopic studies. On the other hand, in two of our infants, the hydrocolpos was so large that the diaphragms were elevated and the lungs were compressed. They required endotracheal intubation, ventilation, and immediate abdominal vaginostomy. In both of these infants, the tiny perineal orifice barely admitted a probe.

All infants with a cloaca should have a completely divided transverse colostomy during the neonatal period. While the baby is in the operating room, the perineal opening should be further studied by probing and endoscopy. If the perianal opening is anterior and probing demonstrates a thin membrane covering the vestibule, as with an adherent labia, this may be cut back to uncover a urogenital sinus and perhaps low-lying orifices of the vagina and rectum. This allows the child to urinate or at least to have intermittent catheterization. Unfortunately, a dilated, undrained vagina is a continuing source of urinary tract infection, which results in deteriorating renal function. Originally, we recommended a combined vaginal and rectal pullthrough in the newborn period in order to ensure complete separation of the three tracts. We now believe that a hydrocolpos should be opened and explored through a low abdominal incision. A transvaginal septum is excised with the cautery, and the vagina is drained by suturing it to the skin of the abdominal wall. This ensures tubeless free drainage of the vagina and bladder. The repair of the cloacal defect

is delayed until the girl is over 1 year old. At that time, all the genital, rectal, and urinary defects should be repaired in one operation. The repair of the most common anomaly is illustrated in Figure 72–18. The most difficult part of the operation is closing the vaginal fistula to the urinary tract. The bladder must be opened, and a catheter is guided down the common channel and secured in place. The vagina is opened widely, and the anterior wall is retracted up and out of the wound. The vaginal opening is then circumscribed, and the vaginal wall is separated from the cloaca. The mucosa of the fistula is closed with interrupted 3-0 polyglycolic acid sutures. Adjacent fibrous tissue or the muscular wall of the vagina is sutured, and, finally, the vaginal mucosa is firmly closed. A tunnel is made directly along the back wall of the cloaca in order to stay within the levator muscle. The rectum and the posterior wall of the vagina are brought through this tunnel and sutured to skin flaps on the perineum.

The entire original cloaca is left as the urethra. There are many variations of this operation. The perineal portion of the dissection should remain anterior, immediately on the cloaca. In two patients, we have been able to separate the vagina from the cloaca with this anterior perineal approach, but a combined abdominal incision allows much more accurate delineation of the anatomy and is necessary for mobilization of the rectum. Pena and deVries and Nakayama et al. have successfully corrected cloacal anomalies through a posterior sagittal approach.[60,61] Three of the seven patients treated by Nakayama et al. developed urethrovaginal fistulas despite the excellent exposure afforded by this approach.

Hendren has described his extensive experience with cloaca malformations.[62–64] He stresses the necessity of repairing all malformations of the rectum, vagina, and urinary tract in one operation. When necessary, he has used an isolated segment of colon to replace an absent or hypoplastic vagina. He has been able to achieve an anatomic correction in essentially all of his 64 patients.

Posterior Sagittal Anorectoplasty

DeVries and Pena have reintroduced the repair of almost all anorectal anomalies through an extended perineal operation.[65,66] This operation is carried out after a sigmoid colostomy, with the patient in a prone jackknife position. The authors stress the use of electrostimulation to accurately identify all available muscles. The midsagittal incision is made from the midsacrum to the perineum, anterior to the anal dimple. This incision divides the coccyx and is carried through the layers of connective tissue, the levator ani muscle, and the center of the external sphincter, which these authors found to be fused with the lowermost fibers of the puborectalis muscle. Each muscle layer is identified, divided, and retracted laterally until the bowel is exposed. The dissection tra-

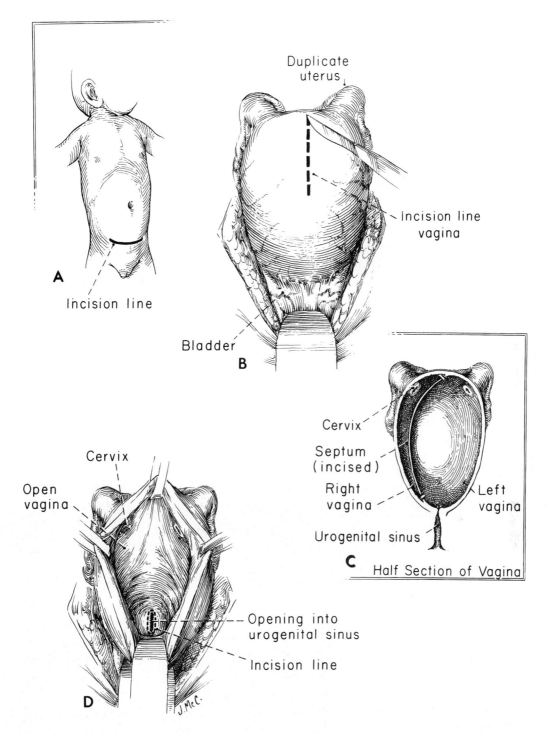

Figure 72–18. Correction of a cloaca. The abdomen is opened through a transverse lower abdominal incision, and the much distended vagina is brought into the operative field. If there is a vaginal septum, it is excised. A catheter is passed through the urogenital sinus, and the fistula between the vagina and the sinus is circumscribed and closed with three layers of polyglycolic sutures. The rectum is separated from the back wall of the vagina, and the vagina and rectum are pulled through the puborectalis tunnel to the perineum.

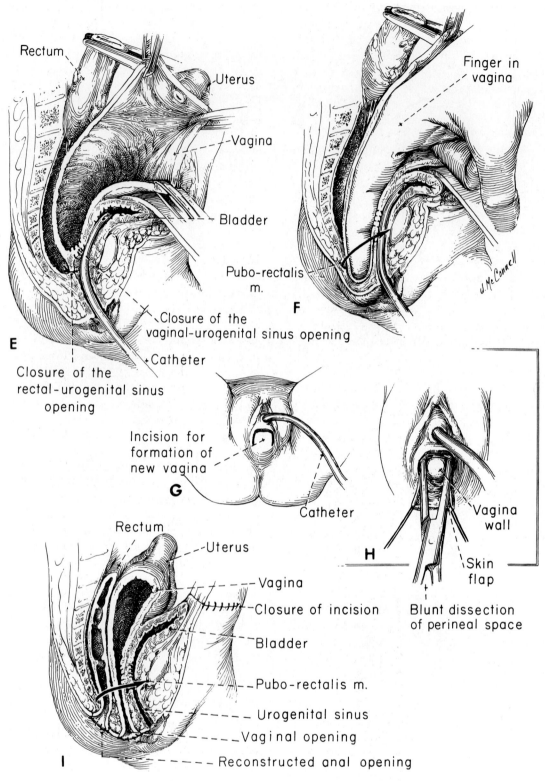

Rectum

Uterus

Vagina

Bladder

Closure of the
vaginal-urogenital sinus opening

Catheter

E

Closure of the
rectal-urogenital sinus
opening

Finger in
vagina

Pubo-rectalis
m.

F

J. McConnell

Incision for
formation of
new vagina

G

Catheter

Vagina
wall

H

Skin
flap

Blunt dissection
of perineal space

Rectum

Uterus

Vagina

Closure of incision

Bladder

Pubo-rectalis m.

Urogenital sinus

Vaginal opening

Reconstructed anal opening

I

Figure 72–18. (Cont.).

verses the pelvic nerve plexus that surrounds the terminal rectum. These nerves are cut, as is all the extrinsic blood supply to the rectum. Any genitourinary fistula is dissected and divided from within the rectum, and some intestinal muscle is left attached to the urethra in the area of the fistula in males. Pena removes a wedge from the anterior bowel and narrows it to the size of a 9 to 10 Hegar dilator, whereas deVries takes a wedge from the posterior surface to avoid suture line apposition to the urethral fistula. The bowel is then placed within the muscle layers, which are closed and attached to the rectal wall. This operation is well described, and Pena has made several films illustrating its essential details. Many surgeons are now using this operation because it is possible to accurately identify all muscles, and there is a minimum of prolapse. It is too early to evaluate the operation properly, but my objection at this time rests on possible damage to the nerve plexus during dissection around the bowel and the possibility of disruption of suture lines in muscles that are devoid of fascia. There is also the risk of intestinal ischemia and refistulization because of apposed suture lines. Nakayama et al. reviewed the complications in 23 patients with the posterior sagittal anorectoplasty.[67] There was an 18 percent complication rate in primary operations and a 33 percent rate in secondary procedures. These complications included refistulization to the urethra and multiple rectoperineal fistulas. Pena and deVries have forced everyone to restudy the perineal musculature and to focus more attention on the external sphincter muscle.

POSTOPERATIVE CARE

During the first 4 or 5 days after any anoplasty, it is convenient to suspend the infant's legs in a simplified form of Bryant's traction. The buttocks may be left on the bed, but the anus is exposed and kept clean with saline-soaked cotton balls. The infant receives routine postoperative care. At about the tenth postoperative day, the rectum is gently dilated with a flexible mercury esophageal bougie, with the child under general anesthesia. Further dilatations are carried out at intervals by the surgeon until the mother can dilate the new anus with her fifth and then her index finger. The surgeon must continue to observe the child as an outpatient at frequent intervals until the anus will accept the index finger and is soft and pliable. The colostomy is closed 2 to 3 months after the rectal repair.

After colostomy closure, a few children have loose stools and excoriated skin. Dietary manipulation, which includes avoidance of fruits and the addition of yogurt or skim milk, is sometimes helpful. Perineal excoriations require frequent experiments with different regimens and ointments. Zinc oxide paste works as well as any-

thing, and the mother should be encouraged to expose the perineum to the air without a diaper during nap time.

Parents of children with low lesions treated by an anoplasty are encouraged to commence toilet training at the usual age. With high lesions, if the child has a palpable contracting puborectalis muscle, toilet training may be attempted within 1 year after colostomy closure. The child is placed on the toilet once or twice a day and is encouraged to push and is rewarded if he or she passes a stool. If these efforts meet with resistance, training is postponed for another 3 to 6 months. A well-knit, stable family with an intelligent mother will have much more success than a family experiencing emotional problems.

The goal should be to achieve continence before the child starts school. As soon as the child can understand, he or she is taught to squeeze on the examiner's finger. This consists of a voluntary contraction of the puborectalis and gluteal muscles, which tightens the anal canal. Once the child understands what is expected, he or she performs the exercises several times a day, especially when feeling an abdominal cramp or pressure sensation in the rectum. The exercises are combined with efforts to firm the stools. Most children learn to avoid corn, beans, and other foods that produce a loose stool. Loperamide has produced continence in children who have been unable to control a loose stool. We have continued patients on this drug for several years, after which it is used only for diarrhea. If the child is still soiling, the next step is to empty the bowel with either a suppository or enema in the hope that the child will stay clean the rest of the day. The mother is given a syringe and a catheter and told to administer a small castile soap enema while the child lies on the side. During the enema, the child is told to squeeze to hold in the fluid. It is helpful to demonstrate this to the parents in the outpatient department. These efforts are continued until the child is socially continent and stops soiling underwear. Continued, frequent supervision by the surgeon is essential until the child is fully continent. This continued support is as important as the operation.

COMPLICATIONS

Twelve of 216 patients treated at our hospital from 1970 to 1986 have died, a mortality rate of 5 percent. Ten of these deaths occurred during the neonatal period secondary to associated congenital malformations. One infant died of unknown cause at home 1 month after his colostomy. One 2 year old died with sepsis after his second pullthrough, performed because at the first operation, the distal rectum had become ischemic and fibrosed to a solid cord.

Intraoperative urethral tears are treated with a suprapubic cystotomy to drain the bladder. A soft Silastic stent is placed in the urethra and firmly sutured to the suprapubic tube so it cannot be removed accidentally. The stent is left in place for a minimum of 2 weeks, and then a cystogram is performed through the cystotomy tube. In three of our patients, the urethra has healed without incident, and all three children are continent of urine.

In four of our patients operated on between 1970 and 1977, the blood supply of the pulled-through bowel appeared to be marginal at the time of operation. During the next several days, the bowel became obviously necrotic. In two, a prompt reexploration, closure of the colostomy, and pullthrough of well-vascularized colon salvaged the situation. In two others, the bowel became a fibrotic strand, and a second, very difficult pullthrough was performed a year later. This complication is best handled with an immediate reoperation when the tunnel is still easily found.

Fistulas have recurred in two patients. In one, the child had a congenitally short colon and a J pouch, created when a stapled suture line was pulled through. He required redivision of the fistula with protection by an ileostomy. The second occurred in a girl who had her distal bowel tapered with staples. The staples may not have been at fault in these two patients, but they are no longer allowed in our operating rooms!

Two children, both with associated sacral and urinary tract anomalies, developed neurogenic bladder after a pullthrough. Both now require intermittent catheterization.

SECONDARY OPERATIONS

In most anoplasties, the bowel mucosa is sutured directly to the skin after the creation of various types of local flaps. This often results in the prolapse of rectal mucosa.

Nixon's anoplasty has prevented this in recent years. The problems remain, however, in older patients. Simple excision of the mucosa with the advancement of small local flaps invariably results in a recurrence. Millard and Rowe solved the problem by using two long skin flaps to line the anal canal.[68] These flaps will not only cure the ectopic mucosa but will also relieve strictures at the mucosa–skin junction. The first flap is based posteriorly, and the second is 1.5 cm wide and 5 cm long from skin medial to the scrotum or labia. After excision of the prolapsed mucosa and incision of the skin–mucosa junction, the posterior flap is sutured inside the canal to break up strictures, whereas the second, long flap spirals inside the canal. Both this operation and that described by Caovette-Laberge et al. take skin remote from the anus to break up the lines of tension, thus preventing recurrence of the prolapse.[69]

Unless there are associated problems or a lack of motivation, children with low or intermediate lesions should attain fecal continence by 3 years of age. Children whose fecal incontinence continues beyond 5 years of age require special attention. The surgeon should personally assess the family situation, emotional problems, and diet. When dietary manipulation, drugs to firm the stools, and enemas fail to achieve complete continence, the child should be studied with rectal pressure manometry and a CT scan of the perineum to evaluate the strength of the sphincters and the position of the bowel relative to the levator sling and external sphincter (Figs. 72–19, 72–20, 72–21, 72–22, 72–23). If the bowel is misplaced relative to the sphincter mechanism, it may be repositioned by one of several operations, or the levator muscle may be plicated and tightened.[70,71] Pena identified several errors in the original operation, when he reoperated via a posterior sagittal approach.[72] These included anterior or lateral displacement of the rectum relative to the muscle complex and megarectum. Five of his eight patients had excellent results after reoperation, and three were improved. The operation involved com-

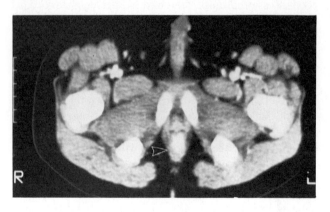
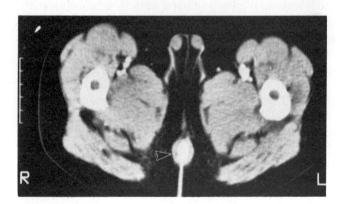

Figure 72–19. CT scans showing normal anatomy. **Left.** Normal puburectulis muscle. **Right.** Normal external sphincter.

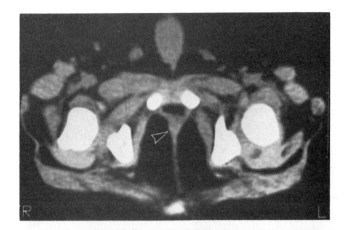
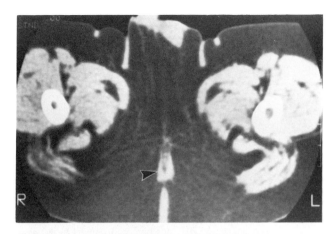

Figure 72–20. Preoperative CT scans of pelvis. **Left.** The arrow points to a thin, almost atrophic levator ani muscle. **Right.** The external sphincter muscle is also thin. This is the picture seen in children who clinically have a flat bottom or sacral abnormalities.

plete mobilization of the rectum, tapering a megarectum and resuturing the levator sling and external sphincter to surround the bowel. The anterior perineal approach to reoperation, when the puborectalis has been missed, offers the same advantages as it does in primary operations.[73] The bowel can be mobilized for a considerable distance without further damage to the sphincter complex, then redirected through a tunnel immediately behind the vagina or urethra.

In our own studies of persistent incontinence, factors such as spinal cord anomalies, mental retardation, and emotional problems are common. Furthermore, when

CT scans demonstrate that the sphincter muscles are absent or hypoplastic, a local reoperation is of no benefit. In these patients, the gracilis muscle sling, described by Pickrell et al., is helpful.[74] Scharli performed 27 gracilis muscle transplant operations. Some patients also had release of their levator muscles as well and all were improved.[75] The gracilis transplant was termed "vital." In our hands, the gracilis transplant has helped 5 of 10 children achieve continence. In 1, infection ruined the operation, and the rest were helped but not cured.

The operation should be performed only in children who are old enough to be completely cooperative and

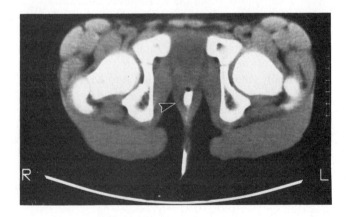
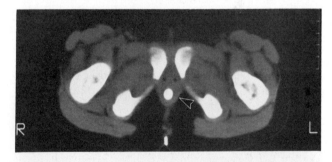
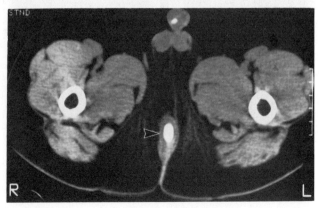

Figure 72–21. Postoperative CT scans demonstrating anatomically intact levator muscles. **Top left.** A 6-year-old boy with good muscle contraction with the palpating finger; correlates with the CT scan. **Top right.** A 4-year-old girl with rectum accurately within the levator muscles, who is toilet trained. **Right.** CT scan demonstrating accurate placement of rectum within a good external sphincter muscle.

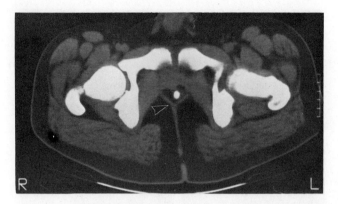 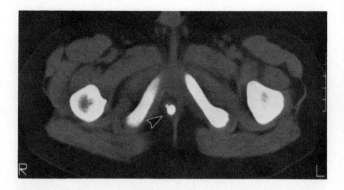

Figure 72–22. Postoperative CT scans of pelvis. **Left.** Thin levator muscle in a 10-year-old boy who became continent with diet, enemas, and Lomotil by 5 years of age. **Right.** The levator muscle is absent on one side. There was also a unilateral sacral anomaly.

who have failed to benefit from a careful medical regimen. Children who have an associated neurogenic problem with no discernible levator action are the best candidates, providing they have normally innervated legs. Postoperative infection is disastrous. Consequently, these children must have either a preliminary colostomy or prolonged mechanical bowel preparation. At operation, the bowel is irrigated with povidone-iodine to further ensure a clean operative field. As originally described by Pickrell et al., the gracilis muscle is freed from its insertion and attachments, and the patient is put in the lithotomy position (Fig. 72–24). It is possible to perform the entire operation with the child in the lithotomy position if the lower leg is suspended from a support in such a way that the knee is in the operative field. The muscle is found through an incision over its distal third in the thigh. Then, with traction, its insertion on the pes anserinus is found. As much tendon length as possible is preserved. The muscle is freed up to the insertion of its blood and nerve supply in its upper third. The muscle and tendon are then drawn through a perineal incision

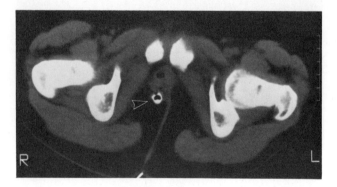

Figure 72–23. CT scan of pelvis. This 12-year-old girl had a cloacal defect. Both on CT scan and at perineal reexploration, half of the levator appears to be absent. She is completely continent with enemas.

and tunneled about the anus. The muscle and tendon are drawn tightly about the anus and firmly sutured to the ischial tuberosity with heavy sutures. The muscle should be tight enough to occlude the anus but relaxed when the leg is abducted. Secondary tightening of the sling was necessary in one patient.

Immediately after the operation, loperamide or codeine is given, along with a high-residue diet. When the child feels intraabdominal pressure, he or she is placed on the toilet and urged to push. Persistent constipation may be secondary to a stricture, overlooked Hirschsprung's disease, or a massively overdistended rectosigmoid (Fig. 72–25). The huge fecal impactions in these children also lead to urinary tract obstruction and infections. This condition has been called the "terminal fecal reservoir syndrome" and has been attributed to rectal inertia.[76] The distal bowel is dilated and atonic from the very beginning and, thus, should be either resected or tapered at the original operation.

Initially, the constipation is treated with diet, mineral oil, and enemas in the hope of reducing the distended bowel. If the size of the bowel does not decrease after prolonged therapy, it may be resected and a new pullthrough performed.[77] The endorectal pullthrough has the advantage of causing no additional damage to the sphincter mechanism or to the pelvic nerve plexus.

EVALUATION AND RESULTS

Children with low and intermediate lesions achieve continence rapidly. By the time they reach school age, they are essentially normal. There has been great controversy about how children with high lesions should be evaluated. In comparing the results obtained by different surgeons or different operations, it is necessary to consider the original classification of the lesion, associated defects, and age of the patient. Manometric and radiologic studies

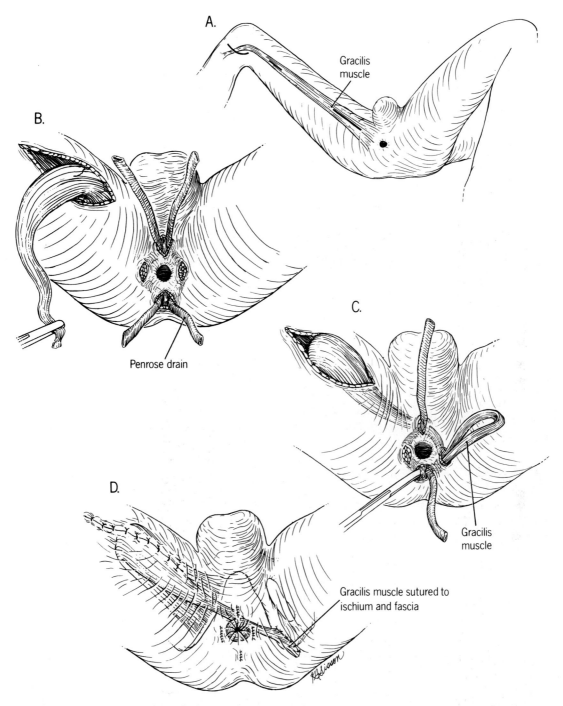

Figure 72–24. The gracilis sling. The child is placed in lithotomy position with exposure of the knee. The gracilis muscle is isolated through three incisions. Its tendon is divided flush with the tibia. The muscle is mobilized up to its nerve and blood supply. The tendon is then passed around the rectum through tunnels made with blunt dissection. Penrose drains are passed through these tunnels as a guide for the muscle. The tendon of the gracilis is sutured to the ischial tuberosity through an incision made directly over the bone. The muscle sling must be pulled as tightly as possible.

merely test the ability of the puborectalis and levator muscles to occlude the rectum against a column of barium or to exert pressure on an inflated catheter. Since the child must cooperate to carry out these tests, they are of little value during the critical preschool years. The clinical evaluation is most accurate. The history and examination will determine the degree of continence. At each postoperative visit, the family is questioned about the child's ability to move the bowels and how long the child can go without diapers or with clean underwear.

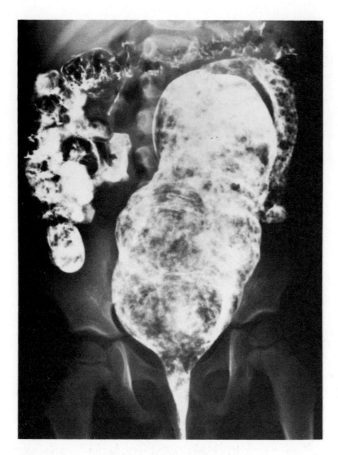

Figure 72–25. Massively distended recto sigmoid in a 12-year-old girl who had a rectovestibular fistula repaired without resection of the terminal bulbous rectum.

There are degrees from clean to total fecal incontinence. The proposals from an international meeting on anorectal anomalies stress the clinical evaluation and provide a guide for a continence score.[78]

Continence Score

	With/without Drugs	With/without Constipation
Normal		
Mucus staining		
Fecal soiling		
Incontinence		

Scoring: 0—never, 1—rarely, 2—frequently, 3—continuously

Four stages are classified. It is essential to note if constipation is coexisting or if drugs are necessary to achieve a certain degree of continence.

The rectal examination will provide further evidence of the child's degree of continence. Observe for fecal smearing about the anus, the condition of the underwear,

and any degree of mucosal prolapse or stricture. The digital examination should note the resting tone of the sphincter muscles as well as the child's ability to contract voluntarily on command. With a cotton swab, examine for sensation of the skin of the perineum as a measure of sacral innervation and, then, after inserting the swab into the rectum, apply pressure to measure propioceptive sensation.

We have now studied 28 children, ages 4 to 16 years, with CT scans. They were a minimum of 3 years postsurgical repair of high lesions. Twenty-two also have had manometry, so we could correlate the results of these tests with the clinical evaluation. The CT was performed with a rectal catheter in place using 10 mm collimation and gantry angulation parallel to the pubococcygeal line. The anorectal muscles were evaluated with an overall score of 1 through 5 with particular attention to the position of the pullthrough. Figure 72–21 A, B and C illustrates a child with a score of 5. There is an intact, thick puborectalis–levator with a good external sphincter muscle. Figure 72–22 A and B demonstrates the poorest appearance of the muscles, with a score of 1. The pullthrough has missed the levator sling complex and the external sphincter muscle. The CT appearance of the anorectal muscles correlated closely with manometric pressures in 17 children. Those with good muscle anatomy had the best resting pressures and could produce the best voluntary squeeze. Those with missed or deficient muscles had weak or absent pressures. The poorest correlation between the clinical assessment and CT was in five children under 6 years of age. They had adequate muscles on CT but were poorly continent. On the other hand, in two children ages 10 and 14, the CT demonstrated poor muscles, yet both had learned bowel control. These studies confirm the lack of correlation between a child's ability to voluntarily squeeze on the examiner's finger with the child's continence. The available sphincters are striated, voluntary muscles that the child must learn to use.

Nine children in this group continue to be incontinent. Two regressed from continence, one because of recalcitrant constipation and the other following repair of a tethered spinal cord. One girl originally operated on for a complex cloacal defect is incontinent at age 15 and essentially ignores her condition. All of these nine patients have other major congenital defects.

The results of clinical examinations in any individual will vary over the course of years. Some children regress at times of emotional distress, but there is usually gradual improvement in all parameters, particularly at puberty.[79,80] In a long-term follow-up of 61 children with high lesions, Templeton and Diteshien found a 58 percent continence rate between 10 and 16 years and a 64 percent rate at 17 to 24 years.[81] These results are impressive, since they were obtained in patients operated on before our understanding of the role of the puborectalis. Unfortunately, the quality of life as measured by ability to interact in society decreased in the older patients.[82] In girls, this decrease in the quality of life may be a reflection of associated anomalies of the genital tract that become important during adolescence. There is a persistent vaginal anomaly in as many as 25 percent of girls with anorectal anomalies.[83] Two of our own patients with cloacal anomalies have had tuboovarian abscesses after they commenced having menses.

FISTULA IN ANO

Perianal fistulas that appear during the first months of life undoubtedly are congenital lesions. The only finding may be a small, uninfected dimple lateral to the anus.

However, the first symptom may be a firm, tender, red swelling, indicating secondary infection (Fig. 72–26). Bilateral fistulas are not uncommon. The diagnosis is made by inspection. Treatment consists of warm, moist dressings with local cleanliness and incision and drainage if there is a definite abscess. Most of these fistulas will close spontaneously, but if there is a repeated bout of infection, an operation is indicated. With the patient under general anesthesia, the internal opening of the fistula is found at the dentate line. A probe is passed from the inside out, and the tract is laid open. The entire tract is superficial to the external sphincter and is, in fact, in the subcutaneous tissue. Postoperatively, the mother is instructed to separate the incision and to apply a topical antibiotic ointment until healing takes place. If the skin closes over before healing from the bottom, the fistula will recur.

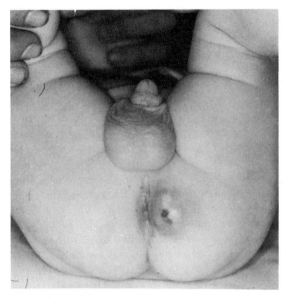

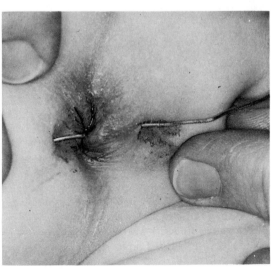

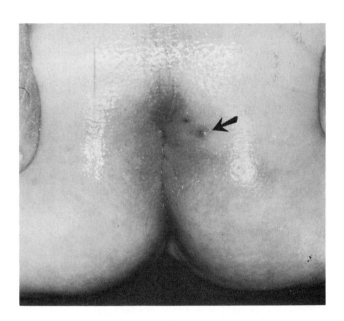

Figure 72–26. Top left. A perianal abscess, which is frequently the presenting sign of a fistula in ano. **Top right.** An uninfected fistula in ano. **Bottom left.** A probe demonstrating the fistulous tract to the mucocutaneous junction.

REFERENCES

1. Scharli AF: Malformations of the anus and rectum and their treatment in medical history. Prog Pediatr Surg 11:141, 1978
2. Amusset JZ: Histoire d'une operation d'anus artificiel pratiqué avec success par un neuveau procede, dans un cas d'absence congenital d'anus. Gazette Medical de Paris, 28, November 1835
3. Littre M: Histoire de l'Academie des Sciences. 1710, p 36
4. Duret C: Racevil Periodique de la Societé de Medicin de Paris 4:45, 1978
5. Matas R: The treatment of congenital ano-rectal malformations. Trans Am Surg Assoc 15:453, 1896
6. Ladd WE, Gross RE: Congenital malformations of anus and rectum: Report of 162 cases. Am J Surg 23:167, 1934
7. Rhoads JE, Pipes RL, Randall JP: A simultaneous abdominal and perineal approach in operations for imperforate anus with atresia of the rectum and rectosigmoid. Ann Surg 127:552, 1948
8. Holschneider AM: The problem of ano-rectal continence. Prog Pediatr Surg 9:85, 1976
9. Wilson PM: Anchoring mechanisms of the anorectal region. S Afr Med J 41:1127, 1138, 1967
10. Duthie HL, Gairus FW: Sensory nerve endings and sensations in the anal canal in man. Br J Surg 47:585, 1960
11. Scott JES: The anatomy of the pelvic anatomic nervous system in cases of high imperforate anus. Surgery 45:1013, 1959
12. Stelzner F: The problem of continence in ano-rectal surgery. Chirurgia 28:155, 1957
13. Nixon HH, Callaghan RP: Defects in operations for imperforate anus. Dis Colon Rectum 7:459, 1964
14. Bennett RC: Sensory receptors in the ano-rectum. Aust NZ J Surg 42:42, 1972
15. Stephens FD: Nervous pathways in anorectal control. Aust NZ Surg 42:45, 1972
16. Shepherd JJ: The nerve supply of the internal anal sphincter. Aust NZ J Surg 42:50, 1972
17. Varma KK: The role of the voluntary anal sphincter in the maintenance of fecal control in normal and abnormal states. Aust NZ J Surg 42:52, 1972
18. Kiesewetter WB, Nixon HH: Imperforate anus: its surgical anatomy. J Pediatr Surg 2:60, 1967
19. Schnaufer L, Talbert J, Haller JA, et al: Differential sphincter studies in the diagnosis of ano-rectal disorders of childhood. J Pediatr Surg 2:538, 1961
20. Smith IE, Gross RE: The external anal sphincter in cases of imperforate anus: A pathologic study. Surgery 49:807, 1961
21. Arey LB: Developmental Anatomy. Philadelphia, Saunders, 1952
22. Stephens FD, Smith ED: Ano-rectal Malformations in Children. Chicago, Year Book, 1971, p 122
23. de Vries PA, Friedland GW: The staged sequential development of the anus and rectum in human embryos and fetuses. J Pediatr Surg 9:755, 1974
24. Bill AH, Johnson RJ: Failure of migration of the rectal opening as the cause for most cases of imperforate anus. Surg Gynecol Obstet 106:643, 1958
25. Stephens FD, Smith ED: Ano-rectal Malformations in Children. Chicago, Year Book, 1971, p 109
26. Bill AH, Hall DG, Johnson RJ: Position of rectal fistula in relation to the hymen in 46 girls with imperforate anus. J Pediatr Surg 10:361, 1975
27. Stephens FD, Donnellan WL: "H-type" urethroanal fistula. J Pediatr Surg 12:95, 1977
28. Burger J, Barnes J: Congenital rectovesical fistula in the absence of imperforate anus. J Pediatr Surg 22:349, 1987
29. Santulli TV, Schullinger JN, Kiesewetter WB, Bill A: Imperforate anus: A survey from the members of the Surgical Section of the American Academy of Pediatrics. J Pediatr Surg 6:484, 1971
30. Anderson RC, Reed SC: The likelihood of recurrence of congenital malformations. Lancet 74:175, 1954
31. Murken JD, Albert A: Genetic counseling in cases of anal and rectal atresia. Prog Pediatr Surg 9:115, 1976
32. VanGelder DW, Kloepfer HW: Familial anorectal anomalies. Pediatrics 27:334, 1961
33. Winkler JM, Weinstein ED: Imperforate anus and heredity. J Pediatr Surg 5:555, 1970
34. Naveh Y, Freidman A: Familial imperforate anus. Am J Dis Child 130:441, 1976
35. Townes PLT, Brocks ER: Hereditary syndrome of imperforate anus with hand, foot, and ear anomalies. J Pediatr 81:321, 1972
36. Hasse W: Associated malformations with anal and rectal atresia. Prog Pediatr Surg 9:100, 1976
37. Singh MP, Haddadin A, Zachary RB, Pilling DW: Renal tract disease in imperforate anus. J Pediatr Surg 9:197, 1974
38. Wiener ES, Kiesewetter WB: Urologic abnormalities associated with imperforate anus. J Pediatr Surg 8:151, 1973
39. Belman AB, King LR: Urinary tract abnormalities associated with imperforate anus. J Urol 108:823, 1972
40. Greenwood RD, Rosenthal A, Nadas AS: Cardiovascular malformations associated with imperforate anus. J Pediatr 86:576, 1975
41. Pierkarsky DH, Stephens FD: The association and embryogenesis of tracheoesophageal and anorectal anomalies. Prog Pediatr Surg 9:63, 1976
42. Singh A, Singh R, Singh A: Short colon malformation with imperforate anus. Acta Paediatr Scand 66:589, 1977
43. Narasimharroa K, Yadav K, Mitra S, Pathak J: Congenital short colon with imperforate anus (pouch colon syndrome). Ann Pediatr Surg 159, 1984
44. Shafie ME: Congenital short intestine with cystic dilation of the colon associated with ectopic anus. J Pediatr Surg 6:67, 1971
45. Kiesewetter WB, Sukarochana K, Sieber WK: The frequency of aganglionosis associated with imperforate anus. Surgery 58:877, 1965
46. Vanhoutte JJ: Primary aganglionosis associated with imperforate anus. Review of the literature pertinent to one observation. J Pediatr Surg 4:468, 1969
47. Stephens FD, Smith ED: Ano-rectal Malformations in Children. Chicago, Year Book, 1971, p. 281

48. Carson J, Barnes P, Tunnell W, et al: Imperforate anus: The neurologic implication of sacral abnormalities. J Pediatr Surg 19:838, 1984

49. Wangensteen OH, Rice CO: Imperforate anus: A method of determining the surgical approach. Ann Surg 92:77, 1930

50. Narasimharao K, Prasad G, Kataringa S, et al: Prone cross-table lateral view: An alternative to the invertogram in imperforate anus. Am J Radiol 140:227, 1983

51. Murugasu JJ: A new method of roentgenological demonstration of anorectal anomalies. Pediatr Surg 68:706, 1970

52. Wagner ML, Harbert FJ, Kumar APM, Singleton EB: The evaluation of imperforate anus utilizing percutaneous injection of water-soluble iodide contrast material. Pediatr Radiol 1:34, 1973

53. Rehbein F: Imperforate anus: Experiences with abdomino-perineal and abdomino-sacro-perineal pullthrough procedures. J Pediatr Surg 2:99, 1967

54. Roumualdi P: Eine Neve Operations—Technik fur die Behandlung einiger rectommissbild ungen. Langenbecks Arch Chir 296:371, 1960

55. deVries P: The surgery of anorectal anomalies: Its evolution with evaluation of procedures. Curr Probl Surg 21: May 1984

56. Mollard P, Marechal J, deBeaujeu M: Surgical treatment of high imperforate anus with definition of the puborectalis sling by an anterior perineal approach. J Pediatr Surg 13:499, 1978

57. Martin-Laberge J, Bose O, Yazbeck S, et al: The anterior perineal approach for pullthrough operations in high imperforate anus. J Pediatr Surg 18:774, 1983

58. Daries M, Cywes S: The use of a lateral skin flap perineoplasty in congenital anorectal malformations. J Pediatr Surg 19:577, 1984

59. Raffensperger JG, Ramenofsky M: The management of a cloaca. J Pediatr Surg 8:647, 1973

60. Pena A, deVries P: Posterior sagittal anorectoplasty: Important technical considerations and new applications. J Pediatr Surg 17:796, 1982

61. Nakayama D, Snyder H, Schnaufer L, et al: Posterior sagittal exposure for reconstructive surgery for cloacal anomalies. J Pediatr Surg 22:588, 1987

62. Hendren WA: Urogenital sinus on anorectal malformations: Experience with 22 cases. J Pediatr Surg 15:628, 1980

63. Hendren WH: Further experience in reconstructive surgery for cloacal anomalies. J Pediatr Surg 17:695, 1982

64. Hendren WH: Repair of cloacal anomalies: Current techniques. J Pediatr Surg 21:1159, 1986

65. deVries P: The surgery of anorectal anomalies. Curr Prob Surg 21:44, 1984

66. deVries P, Pena A: Posterior sagittal anoplasty. J Pediatr Surg 17:638, 1982

67. Nakayama D, Templeton J, Ziegler M, et al: Complications of posterior sagittal anorectoplasty. J Pediatr Surg 21:488, 1986

68. Mollard D, Rowe M: Plastic surgical principles in high imperforate anus. Plast Reconst Surg 69:399, 1982

69. Caovette-Laberge L, Yazbeck S, Laberge J, Duchamel J: Multiple-flap anoplasty in the treatment of rectal prolapse after pullthrough operations for imperforate anus. J Pediatr Surg 22:65, 1987

70. Kottmeier PK: A physiological approach to the problem of anal incontinence through use of the levator ani as a sling. Surgery 60:1262, 1966

71. Puri P, Nixon HH: Levatorplasty: A secondary operation for fecal incontinence following primary operation for anorectal agenesis. J Pediatr Surg 11:77, 1976

72. Pena A: Posterior sagittal anorectoplasty as a secondary operation for the treatment of fecal incontinence. J Pediatr Surg 18:762, 1983

73. Bass J, Yazbeck S: Reoperation by anterior perineal approach for missed puborectalis. J Pediatr Surg 22:761, 1982

74. Pickrell KL, Bradbent TR, Masters W, et al: Construction of a rectal sphincter and restoration of anal continence by transplanting the gracilis muscle. Ann Surg 135:853, 1952

75. Scharli A: Anorectal incontinence: Diagnosis and treatment. J Pediatr Surg 22:693, 1987

76. Brent L, Stephens FD: Primary rectal ectasia: A quantitative study of smooth muscle cells in normal and hypertrophied human bowel. Prog Pediatr Surg 9:41, 1976

77. Powell R, Sherman J, Raffensperger J: Megarectum: A rare complication of imperforate anus repair and its surgical correction by endorectal pullthrough. J Pediatr Surg 17:786, 1982

78. Stephens FD, Smith DE: Classification, identification and assessment of surgical treatment of anorectal anomalies. Pediatr Surg Int 1:200, 1986

79. Kiesewetter WB, Chung JHT: Imperforate anus: A 5- to 30-year follow-up perspective. Prog Pediatr Surg 10:111, 1977

80. Nixon HH, Puri P: The results of anorectal anomalies: A 13- to 20-year follow-up. J Pediatr Surg 12:27, 1977

81. Templeton J, Diteshien J: High imperforate anus—quantitative results of long-term fecal continence. J Pediatr Surg 20:645, 1985

82. Ditesheim J, Templeton J: Short-term vs. long-term quality of life in children following repair of high imperforate anus. J Pediatr Surg 22:581, 1987

83. Fleming S, Hall R, Gysler M, McLorie G: Imperforate anus in females: Frequency of genital involvement, incidence of associated anomalies and functional outcome. J Pediatr Surg 21:146, 1986

SECTION VIII

Peritonitis in Infancy

The clinical diagnosis of peritonitis is considerably more difficult to make in infants than in older children. A small infant with far-advanced peritoneal inflammation may only wince or draw up the legs in response to abdominal palpation, whereas an older child will respond more decisively to the resultant pain. The entities discussed in this section represent a variety of peritoneal diseases peculiar to the newborn or very young infant. Necrotizing enterocolitis commences with mucosal inflammation and ulceration. At this stage, it often can be treated successfully with gastric drainage, antibiotics, and parenteral nutrition. When the disease progresses through the wall of the bowel with either perforation or gangrene, it becomes a surgical problem. Thus, the decision for surgical intervention depends on one's ability to elicit abdominal tenderness. When a perforation occurs after the infant has swallowed air, a roentgenogram will demonstrate free air in the peritoneal cavity. This is the second cardinal sign of peritonitis in infancy, which is why we must stress the importance of obtaining either an upright x-ray or a cross-table lateral film for any patient with abdominal symptoms.

With peritonitis, there is an outpouring of intestinal contents from the perforation into the peritoneal cavity. This rapid fluid shift depletes the intravascular volume and causes abdominal distention with respiratory distress because of elevation of the diaphragms. These physiologic changes require rapid fluid therapy and, occasionally, a paracentesis to relieve the distention and a laparotomy to either close or exteriorize the perforation.

A perforation that occurs in early fetal life, due to intestinal infarction or volvulus, behaves in an entirely different fashion. The meconium, which is present in the intestine at 4 months of intrauterine life, enters the peritoneal cavity, causing an intense but sterile reaction with dense adhesions and calcification. The perforation itself is sealed, and the infant develops symptoms and signs of an intestinal obstruction at birth. When the perforation occurs later in fetal life, the peritoneal cavity fills with meconium and a peritoneal exudate. On examination, the baby will have a hugely distended abdomen. This form of meconium peritonitis has more of the characteristics of ascites than the usual picture with acute peritonitis. A simple paracentesis will determine the specific diagnosis, and the removal of peritoneal fluid will relieve diaphragmatic pressure.

When bile or urine leaks into the peritoneal cavity, there is minimal reaction, with distention, bulging, flanks, and a fluid wave on examination. Roentgenograms demonstrate air-filled loops of intestine floating in the central portion of the distended abdomen. A paracentesis will lead to a definitive diagnosis.

73

Necrotizing Enterocolitis

———— *Richard Ricketts*

Necrotizing enterocolitis (NEC) has never been reported in stillborn infants, and, therefore, it is an acquired rather than a congenital disease. Its clinical spectrum varies from one with mild abdominal distention, ileus, occult blood in the stools, and pneumatosis coli to one with fulminant sepsis and shock from widespread intestinal necrosis.[1] NEC has become the single most common surgical emergency in newborns, and it is the major cause of death among neonates who undergo surgical procedures.[2]

Genersich, in 1891, reported what was probably NEC in a 2-day-old infant dying with inflammation and perforation of the ileum.[3] Rossier et al. first used the term "necrotizing enterocolitis" in 1959, and Berdon et al. and Mizrahi et al., in 1964 and 1965, reported the first series of cases of NEC in the United States.[4–6] Despite a considerable experience with NEC since then, the pathogenesis of the disease has not been fully established.

PATHOGENESIS

Three main factors—ischemic damage to the intestine, bacterial colonization, and a substrate—acting alone or in combination create the setting in which NEC occurs.[7–9] Nearly all experimental models for NEC use ischemia as a primary initiating factor for development of the disease.[10] Clinically, intestinal ischemia can occur as a result of vasospasm (diving reflex or selective mesenteric ischemia, umbilical artery catheterization, hypothermia), thrombosis (exchange transfusions, polycythemia), or low flow states (hypotension, patent ductus arteriosus, asphyxia, respiratory distress syndrome).[1,2,7]

These circumstances that can lead to intestinal ischemia are found in a majority of infants with NEC, but they also occur with equal frequency in matched controls, thus minimizing their role as primary etiologic factors.[11–13]

Although no specific etiologic organism has been identified with NEC, there is substantial evidence to support the role of bacteria in the pathogenesis of the disease: (1) epidemics of NEC are aborted by standard infection control measures, (2) NEC outbreaks are sometimes associated with specific bacterial pathogens, (3) identical organisms are recovered from the blood, peritoneal cavity, and resected intestine from NEC patients, (4) increased amounts of bacterial toxins are recovered from patients with NEC as compared to controls, and (5) NEC epidemics are suppressed with specific oral antibiotics.[14–18] Furthermore, the presence of hydrogen gas within the lumen and cysts of pneumatosis intestinalis supports the role of bacteria, since the only source of hydrogen gas in humans is bacterial fermentation.[1,19] Musemeche et al., in an experimental model evaluating the relative contributions of ischemia, bacteria, and substrate to the pathogenesis of NEC, found that the presence of bacteria was the most crucial to the development of bowel necrosis.[20]

Ninety to ninety-five percent of infants in whom NEC develops have been fed a commercial formula.[1,9] The formula serves as a substrate for bacterial proliferation. In addition, direct intestinal mucosal injury may be caused by the high osmolarity of formulas or by a feeding schedule that is advanced too rapidly.[1,21] However, attempts to prevent NEC by delaying oral feedings or by advancing feedings slowly in premature infants have yielded conflicting results in lowering the incidence of the disease.[22–24] Barlow et al. showed that fresh breast milk was protective against the development of NEC experimentally.[25] Breast milk supplies the infant with secretory IgA, which the newborn lacks, as well as with breast milk macrophages.[2] Perhaps for these reasons, NEC rarely develops in infants fed exclusively fresh breast milk. Banked, frozen, or heated breast milk has no protective effects.[1,7] The disease does occur, however, in a small number of patients who have never been fed or who have been fed breast milk alone.[1,26]

It is difficult to develop a unifying theory for the pathogenesis of NEC that explains the development of the disease in the enterally fed, high-risk neonate as well as in the healthy term infant or in the unfed infant. In most cases, the disease occurs when the bowel is immature, before an age equivalent of 35 to 36 weeks gestation. This age is associated with rapid maturation of the gastrointestinal tract and with a markedly declining incidence of NEC.[27] Thus, the immature bowel may have a limited response to injury from various causes, one of which is the syndrome of NEC.[1,9] The mature bowel, on the other hand, or the bowel that has not been exposed to enteral feeding, can also develop NEC after exposure to quantitative extremes of the three main etiologic factors—severe ischemia, highly pathogenic flora, or marked excess of a substrate. For example, NEC caused by *Clostridium*, a highly pathogenic organism, occurs more commonly in term infants than among preterm infants.[7,28] Similarly, NEC in unfed infants occurs primarily, if not exclusively, from ischemic insult.[26] Thus, according to Kosloske, NEC in all settings can be explained by the simultaneous occurrence of at least two of the three main etiologic factors[7] (Fig. 73–1).

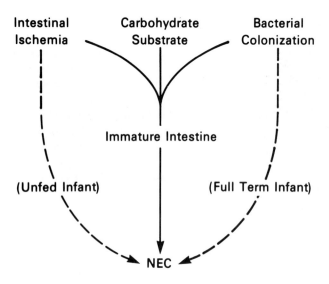

Figure 73–1. Pathogenesis of necrotizing enterocolitis.

PATHOLOGY

Initially there are distended loops of intestine with serosal edema, hemorrhage, and peritoneal fluid. The serosa is dull and covered with fibrinous exudate. Mucosal ulceration and transmural necrosis then occur (Fig. 73–2). As the disease progresses, relatively normal segments of the bowel may alternate with irregular gray or reddish black blotches, which represent transmural necrosis and hemorrhage. The process is usually segmental and circumferential but may be confined to the antimesenteric border. Bubbles of air are seen under the serosa and in the mesentery. Some areas balloon out, with the bowel held together only by the serosa. The ileum is involved in 86 percent, the colon in 74 percent, and the jejunum in 28 percent of patients.[29] Twelve to thirty-eight percent of patients will have necrosis of the entire small bowel.[30,31] The stomach and duodenum rarely are involved.

Histologic examination confirms necrosis of the entire bowel wall.[32] There are inflammatory cells and bacteria in all layers of the intestine, which present a ghostlike appearance on the microscopic slide (Fig. 73–3). Some areas, especially in the infants who die rapidly, may show surprisingly little inflammatory reaction, in which case some pathologists may diagnose autolysis rather than NEC. Air bubbles often are seen. Later in the course of the disease there will be a fibroplastic proliferation with submucosal granulation tissue and proliferating epithelium. These affected areas may progress to stricture formation.[33]

DIAGNOSIS

NEC occurs primarily in premature infants with a mean gestational age of 31 weeks and mean birth weight of 1460 g.[34] Only 7 to 10 percent of cases occur in full-term infants,[27,34] in whom there is usually a history of significant respiratory distress, congenital heart disease, polycythemia, or hypoglycemia.[35,36] An identical clinical picture and pathology have been observed in older infants with severe diarrhea, hypovolemia, and low cardiac output. The incidence of NEC varies from 0.8 to 8 percent of all admissions to newborn intensive care units,[22,37–40] averaging 2 to 4 percent. The incidence in low birth weight infants (<1500 g) is 3 to 8 percent.[11–13,41]

The mean age of diagnosis is 7 days. Wilson et al. found that as birth weight increases, the age of onset of NEC decreases so that only 6 percent of infants with a birth weight greater than 1500 g have onset of disease after 10 days of age compared to over 50 percent of

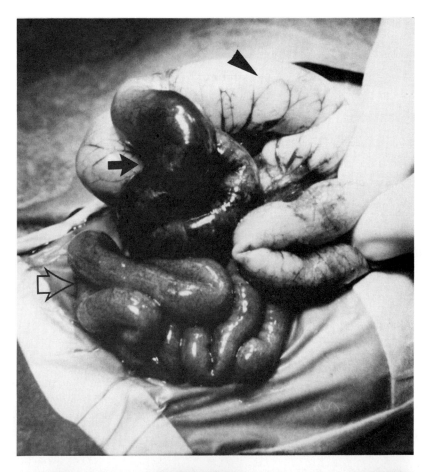

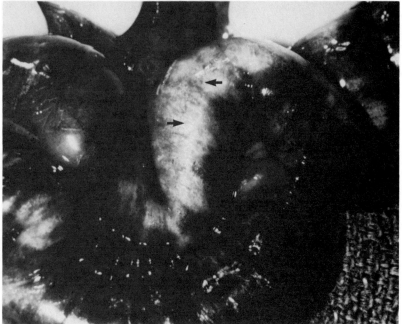

Figure 73–2. Top. Long segment of distended loop of ileum. The arrows point to a darkened, congested loop and to one that is pale and ischemic. **Bottom.** Pale ischemic bowel held together only with serosa.

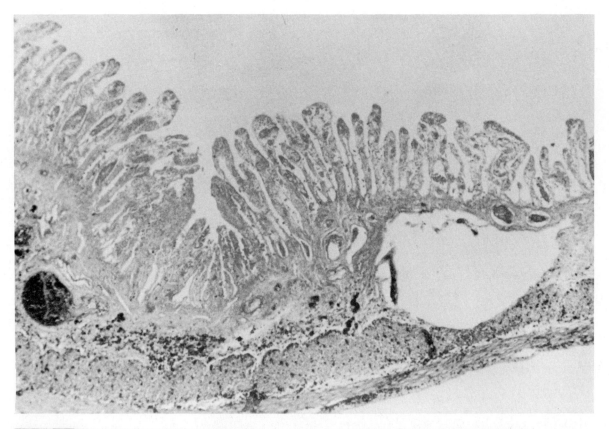

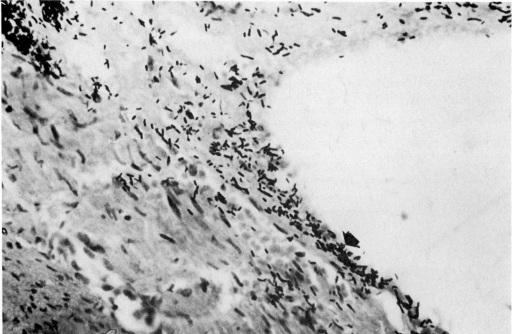

Figure 73–3. Microscopic appearance of intestine resected in a premature infant with NEC. **Top.** The serosa is ghostlike. There are air bubbles between the mucosa and the serosa, indicating the necrosis of the muscularis. **Bottom.** A large pocket of pneumatosis surrounded by *Clostridium* organisms (arrow).

infants weighing less than 1500 g at birth.[27] NEC occurring in the first day of life is rare and is usually found in larger, full-term infants who have respiratory distress or who have received exchange transfusions for polycythemia.[42]

The initial findings are abdominal distention with increased gastric aspirate that may be clear, bloody, or bilious. Meconium has been passed in nearly all infants (unlike Hirschsprung's disease, where 90 percent have delayed evacuation).[43] Bloody or nonbloody diarrhea, although an integral part of infectious forms of enterocolitis (i.e., staphylococcal), is seen in less than 25 percent of infants with NEC. Gross or occult gastrointestinal bleeding is more common. Localized abdominal erythema and induration, with mild to marked abdominal tenderness, are signs of associated peritonitis. With advanced disease, there is marked abdominal distention, bilious emesis, rapid deterioration, and shock. The differential diagnosis includes a midgut volvulus (which is characterized clinically by bloody diarrhea and radiographically by a gasless abdomen), sepsis with a paralytic ileus, and Hirschsprung's disease. Abdominal roentgenograms at intervals of 4 to 6 hours are essential, not only for the initial diagnosis but also to evaluate the results of therapy (Fig. 73–4). Pneumatosis intestinalis or bubbles of subserosal air identified on plain abdominal roentgenograms are essential for the diagnosis.[44,45] Gas also may embolize through the mesenteric vein to the liver to outline the portal system; this is an ominous radiologic sign.[39,46] Portal vein ultrasonography is more sensitive than radiographs in detecting the presence of portal vein gas. Abdominal ultrasonography, therefore, has the potential to lead to earlier diagnosis and treatment.[47,48] Infants on high pressure ventilators may develop pneumatosis and pneumoperitoneum secondary to air being forced down from the mediastinum.[49,50] Cultures are obtained of the blood, urine, cerebrospinal fluid, and, in some cases, peritoneal fluid. Blood gas determinations, white blood cell counts with differentials, hematocrits, platelet counts, electrolytes, and coagulation studies (PT, PTT) are determined initially and then serially to follow the results of medical therapy.[51]

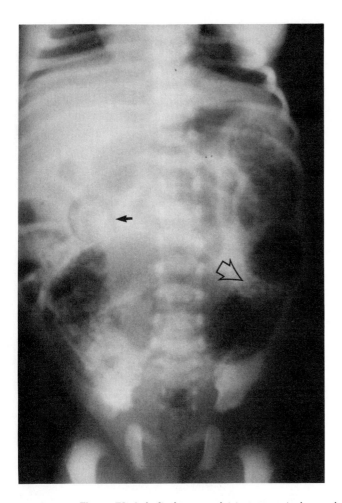
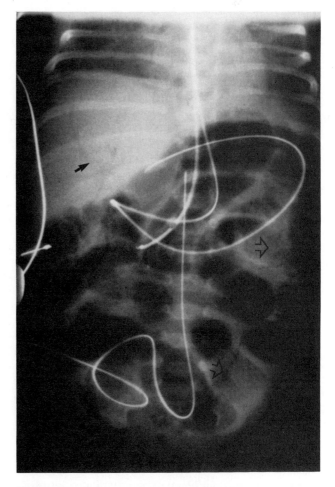

Figure 73–4. Left. Arrows point to pneumatosis, or air within the wall of the bowel. **Right.** Air is visible in the portal vein, as are pneumatosis and dilated loops of bowel.

MEDICAL TREATMENT

As soon as the diagnosis of NEC is suspected, all oral feedings are discontinued, and an orogastric tube is passed to decompress the gastrointestinal tract. IV fluid, colloid, and blood are given to maintain a urine output of 1.5 to 2.0 ml/kg/hour.[2] Intubation and assisted ventilation often are required because of lethargy, sepsis, and massive abdominal distention. Systemic antibiotics to cover for both gram-positive and gram-negative organisms are provided for 10 to 14 days for infants with "definite" NEC, as defined by Bell et al.[52] A shorter course is appropriate for those with "suspected" NEC who improve within 24 to 48 hours.[9] Stone et al., in a study on perforated NEC, never cultured anaerobic organisms if the perforation occurred before the eighth day of life.[15] Hence, anaerobic coverage is not indicated unless an anaerobe is cultured from the blood or peritoneal fluid or unless the onset of the disease is beyond the age of 10 days, in which case the infant may be colonized by anaerobic flora.[7] Enteral antibiotics are not indicated, since they do not alter the course of the disease and since they may actually injure the mucosa because of their hyperosmolarity.[1,9] Parenteral nutrition is provided to supply the infant with 110 to 150 kcal/kg/day. Since epidemics of NEC are well documented, infection control measures, such as strict handwashing and cohorting of patients and personnel, are instituted.[9] Frequent examination and serial monitoring of the acid-base status, coagulation profile, electrolyte status, and abdominal radiographs are an integral part of the medical therapy to determine the infant's response to treatment and the need for surgery.[51]

Bowel rest and antibiotics are continued for 10 to 14 days after the resolution of pneumatosis.[1] Feedings are then commenced with a dilute, lactose-free formula of low osmolarity. The feedings are slowly increased in concentration and volume as the enteral nutrition is reduced.

Although intestinal strictures can develop in infants treated successfully medically,[1,9,53] we do not perform routine gastrointestinal contrast studies unless symptoms, such as abdominal distention, vomiting, obstipation, or occult bleeding, occur.

SURGICAL TREATMENT

Surgery will be required in 31 to 57 percent of infants with NEC.[31,37,40,41,54,55] Kosloske et al. evaluated 10 clinical radiologic and laboratory criteria for surgery and found that (1) pneumoperitoneum, (2) a positive paracentesis, (3) erythema of the abdominal wall, (4) a fixed abdominal mass, and (5) a persistently dilated intestinal loop on serial radiographs were valid indications for sur-

gery. Clinical deterioration, abdominal tenderness, lower gastrointestinal bleeding, ascites, and severe thrombocytopenia were not reliable indicators of intestinal gangrene and, thus, the need for surgery.[56] Our approach has been to consider pneumoperitoneum as the only absolute indication for surgery. If the infant deteriorates under maximal medical support or develops one of the many relative indications for surgery (abdominal wall erythema, fixed intestinal loop, fixed tender mass, portal vein gas,[39] or refractory acidosis,[57] a paracentesis is performed to confirm the suspicion of intestinal gangrene. A positive tap (more than 0.5 ml of yellow-brown fluid or the presence of bacteria on gram stain) reliably indicates intestinal necrosis and the need for surgery.[58,59] A negative tap justifies continued medical treatment and reevaluation. Most of these infants will recover, although some will require surgery anyway for persistent clinical deterioration or massive abdominal distention[59] (Fig. 73–5).

The abdomen is entered through a supraumbilical transverse incision. Aerobic and anaerobic cultures are obtained from the peritoneal fluid. The entire gastrointestinal tract from the stomach to the rectum is inspected. The standard surgical treatment of NEC is resection of all necrotic intestine, exteriorization of the viable ends, and preservation of as much potentially viable bowel as possible to prevent development of the short gut syndrome.[2,30,40,60] Approximately 12 to 38 percent (average 19 percent) of infants will have such extensive intestinal necrosis that future survival on enteral nutrition alone would be impossible.[30,31,39,40,51,60] The bowel is returned to the abdominal cavity, the parents are counseled, and the infant is allowed to expire humanely. In some infants, extensive ischemic bowel, which has the potential for

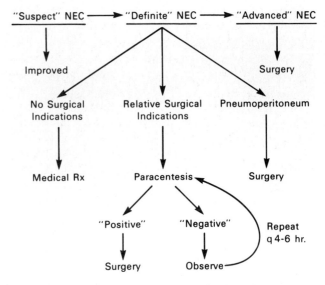

Figure 73–5. An algorithm to guide treatment of an infant with NEC.

recovery after intestinal decompression and continued vigorous medical support, is found. A proximal jejunostomy will protect the distal bowel, and a planned second-look laparotomy may be performed 24 to 48 hours later. Approximately 70 percent of these infants will be salvaged.[30,60,61]

In infants with localized NEC, perforated and gangrenous bowel is resected using multiple segmental resections as necessary to preserve intestinal length. Small foci of necrotic bowel can be imbricated with transversely oriented seromuscular sutures in order to avoid unnecessary resection. The ends of the bowel are then exteriorized as separate stomas or as a Mikulicz enterostomy either through the lateral margin of the laparotomy incision or through a separate incision.[30,40,60,62] Harberg et al. recommended resection with primary anastomosis in all infants operated on for NEC.[63] Pokorny et al., in a large series of infants operated on for NEC, found this approach to be acceptable in approximately 50 percent of infants.[41] Before closure, the abdominal cavity is copiously lavaged with warm saline and antibiotic solution. The fascia is closed in two layers with continuous absorbable sutures, and the skin is loosely approximated with interrupted fine nylon sutures.

Other procedures for acute NEC include proximal diversion via a jejunostomy for infants with extensive ischemia without necrosis[64] and peritoneal drainage under local anesthesia for markedly unstable neonates weighing less than 1000 g.[65,66] The latter technique has been found to be a valuable adjunct in the preoperative resuscitation of infants with advanced NEC.[54] In addition, 16 to 40 percent of infants treated with peritoneal drainage may recover completely without the need for further surgery.[54,60]

Postoperatively, patients are maintained on ventilatory support, parenteral nutrition, and antibiotics. Antibiotics are adjusted as necessary when culture results are available. Oral feedings are resumed when normal gastrointestinal function returns but not sooner than 7 days after surgery. Parenteral nutrition is continued until the infant demonstrates sustained weight gain on enteral nutrition alone. Infants with ileostomies lose the ability to absorb salt and water in the colon. This results in a chronic salt-and-water-losing state that cannot be normalized until intestinal continuity is reestablished.[67] These infants demonstrate growth retardation, which is reversed once the stoma is closed. These observations have led to the recommendation for early elective closure of enterostomies in these infants (no sooner than 4 weeks after the initial operation).[62,68]

Postoperative stricture formation occurs in 12 to 42 percent (average 28 percent) of patients.[30,37,40,54,62] These are generally in the defunctionalized colon and must be identified by contrast enema before stoma clo-

sure. There is a lower incidence of stricture formation after primary anastomosis or early enterostomy closure, perhaps as a result of self-dilatation of inflammatory strictures by the passage of enteric contents.[62,63]

Recent series of surgical experience with NEC report survival rates of from 50 percent to 73 percent.[30,31,39,41,54,59,60] Those infants who have localized disease and who are, therefore, candidates for a definitive surgical procedure have a 70 to 82 percent survival rate.[30,31] Long-term follow-up on neonates weighing less than 1000 g or having a gestational age less than 31 weeks indicates a high (24 percent) late mortality rate. These infants may also have late morbidity resulting from complications of sepsis, total parenteral nutrition (TPN)-related cholestasis, short gut syndrome, and chronic pulmonary disease.[69] However, the incidence of these complications is no higher than for those resulting from prematurity, respiratory distress syndrome, or other problems present before the onset of NEC[9,51,70-73] and, thus, should not discourage one from treating these infants aggressively.

In the 7½ years from July 1980 through December 1987, the author has operated on 91 infants with NEC according to the algorithm depicted in Figure 73–5. This represents approximately one half of the infants with NEC seen during that time period. The remaining patients were treated successfully medically. The patients' weights, the indication for surgery, and the survival rate are shown in Table 73–1. Two thirds of the infants weighed less than 1500 g, and one quarter weighed less than 1000 g. Overall, one half of the infants were operated on because of a positive paracentesis. This was particularly evident in the ≤1000 g infants where a positive paracentesis was the indication for surgery in 63 percent of the patients. The 1001 to 1500 g infants had the highest

TABLE 73–1. RESULTS OF SURGICAL TREATMENT FOR NEC USING THE STANDARD ALGORITHM (FIG. 73–5). JULY 1980–DECEMBER 1987

Weight (g)	Number (%)	Indication for Surgery (%)		Survival Number (%)
≤ 1000	24 (26)	Perf[a]	6 (25%)	14 (58)
		Para	15 (63%)	
		Other	3 (12%)	
1001–1500	36 (40)	Perf	22 (61%)	27 (75)
		Para	14 (39%)	
		Other	0	
> 1500	31 (34)	Perf	10 (32%)	25 (81)
		Para	17 (55%)	
		Other	4 (13%)	
Total	91 (100)	Perf	38 (42%)	66 (72.5)
		Para	46 (50%)	
		Other	7 (8%)	

[a] Perf, perforation; Para, positive paracentesis.

perforation rate (61 percent). Overall survival for these 91 infants was 72.5 percent, being lowest for the ≤1000 g infants (58 percent) and highest for the >1500 g infants (81 percent). There were 25 deaths; of these, 13 (14 percent of the entire group) had total bowel involvement with NEC and, therefore, had exploratory laparotomy only, since a definitive procedure was not possible. If these 13 infants are excluded, the overall survival for the 78 infants having a definitive surgical procedure was 85 percent. The other deaths were caused by complications of NEC (6), respiratory failure (4), congenital heart disease (1), and TPN sepsis (1).

PREVENTION

Even with modern intensive support, NEC has a significant morbidity and mortality. Substantial improvement in survival is dependent on improved preventive measures. The best preventive approach is to minimize the prematurity rate and the severity of perinatal asphyxia. In a multicenter study evaluating the effect of antenatal corticosteroids on lung development, a strikingly decreased incidence of NEC was noted in those receiving steroids when compared to controls not receiving steroids.[74] Whether antenatal treatment of high-risk neonates with steroids is warranted or efficacious remains to be seen. Once a premature infant has been delivered, however, the possibilities for prevention include (1) the use of fresh breast milk, (2) prophylactic oral antibiotics, and (3) delayed introduction of feedings.

Fresh breast milk has many excellent cellular and humoral immunologic properties that may protect the intestinal mucosa against NEC.[75-77] Unfortunately, it may not be feasible for the mother to provide a sufficient volume of unprocessed (fresh) breast milk on a daily basis. If the mother's breast milk is frozen or heat-sterilized, the protective benefits against NEC are destroyed. Although fresh donor breast milk can sometimes be obtained, there is a theoretical risk of graft versus host reaction. The use of fresh breast milk feedings continues to be an experimentally documented but clinically impractical preventive measure.

Prophylactic administration or oral antibiotics has been tried in an effort to decrease the incidence of NEC. The results have been inconsistent, with some studies showing prevention of NEC[78,79] and others showing no difference.[18,80] Furthermore, sepsis and meningitis from an unusual organism, such as *Staphylococcus epidermidis*, have been reported following the prophylactic use of oral antibiotics.[81]

Delayed introduction of oral feedings also has been evaluated in the prevention of NEC. Slower introduction of full calories orally decreased the incidence of NEC in one study,[82] whereas in another it made no difference.[24] Withholding enteral feedings entirely for 2 weeks in hopes of reducing the incidence and severity of NEC also has had conflicting results, showing benefit in one study[22] and no benefit in another.[23]

In summary, the best preventive approach for NEC is better perinatal care, resulting in deliveries associated with less perinatal asphyxia and a greater degree of maturity. In the meantime, a high degree of suspicion, early diagnosis, and appropriate medical and surgical management are necessary to maximize the outcome of a disease that has been a significant cause of morbidity and mortality in the neonatal intensive care unit patient.

REFERENCES

1. Kliegman RM, Fanaroff AA: Necrotizing enterocolitis. N Engl J Med 310:1093, 1984
2. Kosloske AM: Necrotizing enterocolitis in the neonate. Surg Gynecol Obstet 148:259, 1979
3. Genersich A: Bauchfellentzundung beim Neugebornen in Folge von Perforation Des ileums. Virchows Arch Pathol Anat 126:485, 1891
4. Rossier A, Sarrut S, Delplanque J: L'enterocolite ulceronecrotique du premature. Ann Pediatr 6:1428, 1977
5. Mizrahi A, Barlow O, Berdon W, et al: Necrotizing enterocolitis in premature infants. J Pediatr 66:697, 1965
6. Berdon WE, Grossman H, Baker DH, et al: Necrotizing enterocolitis in the premature infant. Radiology 83:879, 1964
7. Kosloske AM: Pathogenesis and prevention of necrotizing enterocolitis: a hypothesis based on personal observation and a review of the literature. Pediatrics 74:1086, 1984
8. Milner ME, de la Monte SM, Moore GW, Hutchins GM: Risk factors for developing and dying from necrotizing enterocolitis. J Pediatr Gastroenterol Nutr 5:359, 1986
9. Walsh MC, Kliegman RM: Necrotizing enterocolitis: treatment based on staging criteria. Pediatr Clin North Am 33:179, 1986
10. Topalian SL, Ziegler MM: Necrotizing entercolitis: a review of animal models. J Surg Res 37:320, 1984
11. Stoll BJ, Kanto QP Jr, Glass RI, et al: Epidemiology of necrotizing enterocolitis: a case control study. J Pediatr 96:447, 1980
12. Kanto WP Jr, Wilson R, Breart GL, et al: Perinatal events and necrotizing enterocolitis in premature infants. Am J Dis Child 141:167, 1987
13. Kliegman RM, Hack M, Jones P, Fanaroff AA: Epidemiologic study of necrotizing enterocolitis among low-birth-weight infants. J Pediatr 100:440, 1982
14. Han VKM, Sayed H, Chance GW, et al: An outbreak of *Clostridium difficile* necrotizing entercolitis: a case for oral vancomycin therapy? Pediatrics 71:935, 1983
15. Stone HH, Kolb LD, Geheber CE: Bacteriologic considerations in perforated necrotizing enterocolitis. South Med J 72:1540, 1979
16. Cashore WJ, Peter G, Lauermann M, et al: Clostridia colonization and clostridial toxin in neonatal necrotizing enterocolitis. J Pediatr 98:308, 1981

17. Grylack L, Scanlon JW: Prevention of necrotising enterocolitis with gentamicin. Lancet 2:506, 1977

18. Hansen TN, Ritter DA, Speer ME, et al: A randomized, controlled study of oral gentamicin in the treatment of neonatal necrotizing enterocolitis. J Pediatr 97:836, 1980

19. Engel RR, Virnig NL, Hunt CE, Levitt MD: Origin of mural gas in necrotizing enterocolitis. Pediatr Res 7:292, 1973

20. Musemeche CA, Kosloske AM, Bartow SA, Umland ET: Comparative effects of ischemia, bacteria, and substrate on the pathogenesis of intestinal necrosis. J Pediatr Surg 21:536, 1986

21. Goldman HI: Feeding and necrotizing enterocolitis. Am J Dis Child 134:553, 1980

22. Gregory JR, Campbell JR, Harrison MW, Campbell TJ: Neonatal necrotizing enterocolitis. A 10-year experience. Am J Surg 141:562, 1981

23. LaGamma EF, Ostertag SG, Birenbaum H: Failure of delayed oral feedings to prevent necrotizing enterocolitis. Am J Dis Child 139:385, 1985

24. Ostertag SG, LaGamma EF, Reisen CE, Ferrentino FL: Early enteral feeding does not affect the incidence of necrotizing enterocolitis. Pediatrics 77:275, 1986

25. Barlow B, Santulli TV, Heird WC, et al: An experimental study of acute neonatal necrotizing enterocolitis: the importance of breast milk. J Pediatr Surg 9:587, 1974

26. Marchildon MB, Buck BE, Abdenour G: Necrotizing enterocolitis in the unfed infant. J Pediatr Surg 17:620, 1982

27. Wilson R, Kanto WP Jr, McCarthy BJ, et al: Short communication. Age at onset of necrotizing enterocolitis: an epidemiologic analysis. Pediatr Res 16:82, 1982

28. Kosloske AM, Ball WS Jr, Umland E, Skipper B: Clostridial necrotizing enterocolitis. J Pediatr Surg 20:155, 1985

29. Santulli TV, Schullinger JN, Heird WC, et al: Acute necrotizing enterocolitis in infancy: a review of 64 cases. Pediatrics 55:376, 1975

30. Ricketts RR: Surgical therapy for necrotizing enterocolitis. Ann Surg 200:653, 1984

31. Cikrit D, Mastandrea J, West KW, et al: Necrotizing enterocolitis: factors affecting mortality in 101 surgical cases. Surgery 96:648, 1984

32. Larroche J-C: Developmental Pathology of the Neonate. Amsterdam, Excerpta Media, North-Holland Biomedical Press, 1977, p 141

33. Joshi VV, Winston YE, Kay S: Neonatal necrotizing enterocolitis: histologic evidence of healing. Am J Dis Child 126:113, 1973

34. Kliegman RM, Fanaroff AA: Neonatal necrotizing enterocolitis: a nine-year experience. Am J Dis Child 135:603, 1981

35. Polin RA, Pollack PF, Barlow B, et al: Necrotizing enterocolitis in term infants. J Pediatr 89:460, 1976

36. Wilson R, del Portillo M, Schmidt E, et al: Risk factors for necrotizing enterocolitis in infants weighing more than 2000 grams at birth: a case-control study. Pediatrics 71:19, 1983

37. Dudgeon DL, Schneider PA, Colombani P, et al: Neonatal necrotizing enterocolitis: an update. South Med J 77:1389, 1984

38. Teasdale F, Le Guennec J-C, Bard H, et al: Neonatal

necrotizing enterocolitis: the relation of age at the time of onset to prognosis. J Can Med Assoc 123:387, 1980

39. Kennedy J, Holt CL, Ricketts RR: The significance of portal vein gas in necrotizing enterocolitis. Am Surg 53:231, 1987

40. Beasley SW, Auldist AW, Ramanujan TM, Campbell NT: The surgical management of neonatal necrotizing enterocolitis, 1975–1984. Pediatr Surg Int 1:210, 1986

41. Pokorny WJ, Garcia-Prats JA, Barry YN: Necrotizing enterocolitis: incidence, operative care, and outcome. J Pediatr Surg 21:1149, 1986

42. Thilo EH, Lazarte RA, Hernandez JA: Necrotizing enterocolitis in the first 24 hours of life. Pediatrics 73:476, 1984

43. Touloukian RJ: Neonatal necrotizing enterocolitis: an update on etiology, diagnosis, and treatment. Surg Clin North Am 56:281, 1976

44. Yu VYH, Tudehope DI, Gill GJ: Neonatal necrotizing enterocolitis: radiological manifestations. Aust Paediatr J 13:200, 1977

45. Reyna R, Soper RT, Condon RE: Pneumatosis intestinalis: report of twelve cases. Am J Surg 125:667, 1973

46. Cikrit D, Mastandrea J, Grosfeld JL, et al: Significance of portal vein air in necrotizing enterocolitis: analysis of 53 cases. J Pediatr Surg 20:425, 1985

47. Lindley S, Mollitt DL, Seigbert JJ, Golladay ES: Portal vein ultrasonography in the early diagnosis of necrotizing enterocolitis. J Pediatr Surg 21:530, 1986

48. Merritt CRB, Goldsmith JP, Sharp MJ: Sonographic detection of portal venous gas in infants with necrotizing enterocolitis. AJR 143:1059, 1984

49. Lee SB, Kuhn JP: Pneumatosis intestinalis following pneumomediastinum in a newborn infant. J Pediatr 79:813, 1971

50. Steves M, Ricketts RR: Pneumoperitoneum in the newborn infant. Am Surg 53:226, 1987

51. O'Neill JA Jr, Holcomb GW: Surgical experience with neonatal necrotizing enterocolitis (NNE). Ann Surg 189:612, 1979

52. Bell MJ, Ternberg JL, Feigin RD, et al: Neonatal necrotizing enterocolitis. Therapeutic decisions based upon clinical staging. Ann Surg 187:1, 1978

53. Born M, Holgersen LO, Shahrivar F, et al: Routine contrast enemas for diagnosing and managing strictures following nonoperative treatment of necrotizing enterocolitis. J Pediatr Surg 20:461, 1985

54. Cheu HW, Sukarochana K, Lloyd DA: Peritoneal drainage for necrotizing enterocolitis. J Pediatr Surg 23:557, 1988 (in press)

55. Kliegman RM, Fanaroff AA: Neonatal necrotizing enterocolitis: a nine-year experience. Am J Dis Child 135:608, 1981

56. Kosloske AM, Papile L-A, Burstein J: Indications for operation in acute necrotizing enterocolitis of the neonate. Surgery 87:502, 1980

57. Buras R, Guzzetta P, Avery G, Naulty C: Acidosis and hepatic portal venous gas: indications for surgery in necrotizing enterocolitis. Pediatrics 78:273, 1986

58. Kosloske AM, Lilly JR: Paracentesis and lavage for diagnosis of intestinal gangrene in neonatal necrotizing enterocolitis. J Pediatr Surg 13:315, 1978

59. Ricketts RR: The role of paracentesis in the management of infants with necrotizing enterocolitis. Am Surg 52:61, 1986

60. Kosloske AM: Surgery of necrotizing enterocolitis. World J Surg 9:277, 1985

61. Weber TR, Lewis JE: The role of second-look laparotomy in necrotizing enterocolitis. J Pediatr Surg 21:323, 1986

62. Musemeche CA, Kosloske AM, Ricketts RR: Enterostomy in necrotizing enterocolitis: an analysis of techniques and timing of closure. J Pediatr Surg 22:479, 1987

63. Harberg FJ, McGill CW, Saleem MM, et al: Resection with primary anastomosis for necrotizing enterocolitis. J Pediatr Surg 18:743, 1983

64. Martin LW, Neblett WW: Early operation with intestinal diversion for necrotizing enterocolitis. J Pediatr Surg 16:252, 1981

65. Ein SH, Marshall DG, Girran D: Peritoneal drainage under local anesthesia for perforations for necrotizing enterocolitis. J Pediatr Surg 12:963, 1977

66. Janik JS, Ein SH: Peritoneal drainage under local anesthesia for necrotizing enterocolitis (NEC) perforation: a second look. J Pediatr Surg 15:565, 1980

67. Rothstein FC, Halpin TC Jr, Kliegman RJ, Izant RJ Jr: Importance of early ileostomy closure to prevent chronic salt and water losses after necrotizing enterocolitis. Pediatrics 70:249, 1982

68. Gertler JP, Seashore JH, Touloukian RJ: Early ileostomy closure in necrotizing enterocolitis. J Pediatr Surg 22:140, 1987

69. Cikrit D, West KW, Schreiner R, Grosfeld JL: Long-term follow-up after surgical management of necrotizing enterocolitis: sixty-three cases. J Pediatr Surg 21:533, 1986

70. Abbasi S, Pereira GR, Johnson L, et al: Long-term assessment of growth, nutritional status, and gastrointestinal function in survivors of necrotizing enterocolitis. J Pediatr 104:550, 1984

71. Hack M, Gordon D, Jones P, Fanaroff A: Necrotizing enterocolitis (NEC) in the VLBW: an encouraging follow-up report [Abstract]. Pediatr Res 15:534, 1981

72. Schullinger JN, Mollitt DL, Vinocur CD, et al: Neonatal necrotizing enterocolitis. Survival, management, and complications: a 25-year study. Am J Dis Child 135:612, 1981

73. Stevenson DK, Kerner JA, Malachowski N, Sunshine P: Late morbidity among survivors of necrotizing enterocolitis. Pediatrics 66:925, 1980

74. Bauer CR, Morrison JC, Poole WK, et al: A decreased incidence of necrotizing enterocolitis after prenatal glucocorticoid therapy. Pediatrics 73:682, 1984

75. Pitt J, Barlow B, Heird WC: Protection against experimental necrotizing enterocolitis by maternal milk. I: Role of milk leukocytes. Pediatr Res 11:906, 1977

76. Liebhaber M, Lewiston NJ, Asquith MT, et al: Alterations of lymphocytes and antibody content of human milk after processing. J Pediatr 91:897, 1977

77. Goldman AS: Human milk, leukocytes, and immunity. J Pediatr 90:167, 1977

78. Egan EA, Mantilla G, Nelson RM, Eitzman DV: A prospective controlled trial of oral kanamycin in the prevention of neonatal necrotizing enterocolitis. J Pediatr 89:467, 1976

79. Grylack LJ, Scanlon VW: Oral gentamicin therapy in the prevention of neonatal necrotizing enterocolitis: a controlled double-blind trial. Am J Dis Child 132:1192, 1978

80. Rowley MP, Dahlenberg GW: Gentamicin in prophylaxis of neonatal necrotizing enterocolitis. Lancet 2:532, 1978

81. Conroy MM, Anderson RS, Cates KL: Complications after use of prophylactic oral kanamycin in preterm infants. Presented at Midwest Society for Pediatric Research, St. Louis, Missouri, 1977.

82. Book LS, Herbst JJ, Jung AL: Comparison of fast and slow feeding rate schedules to the development of necrotizing enterocolitis. J Pediatr 89:463, 1976

74
Gastrointestinal Perforation

Perforations of the gastrointestinal tract may occur in the neonate anywhere from the stomach to the rectum. Aside from necrotizing enterocolitis, perforations may occur secondary to intestinal obstruction, ischemia, overdistention, a gangrenous volvulus, or in association with drug therapy.[1-4]

Although pneumoperitoneum is universally seen in gastrointestinal perforations regardless of etiology, we discuss the pathology of those lesions according to the organ involved. Our experience with perforations of the gastrointestinal tract, exclusive of necrotizing enterocolitis over a period of years, from the Cook County and Children's Memorial Hospital are listed according to site of perforation.

Site of Perforation	Number of Cases
Stomach	15
Duodenum	10
Small bowel	14
Cecum	9
Colon	5
Rectosigmoid	8

PERFORATION OF THE STOMACH

The most common perforation of the stomach is a laceration of the greater curvature, which commences near the gastroesophageal junction and extends halfway to the pylorus. These linear tears are ragged, the edges of the mucosa are hemorrhagic, and the muscle has usually retracted back a bit from the edge of the mucosa. Difficult deliveries are common in this group of infants. Furthermore, in our own and two other series, there was a predominance of black infants.[5,6] It is possible that if a baby has swallowed meconium and is then "squeezed" during delivery the stomach would rupture. Further evidence for the rupture theory, or overdistention, is that other babies required vigorous resuscitation with a mask and ventilation, which could have distended their stomachs. Experimental work in seven neonatal stomachs recovered at autopsies demonstrated that the stomach ruptured at pressures approximating 120 to 180 mm Hg. The ruptures were identical to those we see at operation. This was confirmed by another study, in which the stomachs ruptured with the application of 3.4 to 7 pounds/square inch.[7]

We have seen exactly the same lesion in a 2-month-old infant who was struck in the abdomen after he had taken a full bottle of milk. Two of our patients had massive upper gastrointestinal hemorrhage for several hours before developing free air in the abdomen. Perforation of the stomach secondary to passage of stiff nasogastric tubes was a problem at one time, but we have not observed this type of perforation since the introduction of soft plastic drainage and feeding tubes. Such drugs as tolazoline may cause gastric perforations in infants being treated for pulmonary hypertension.

PERFORATION OF THE DUODENUM

Four full-term newborns in our series who were otherwise healthy had typical anterior duodenal ulcers with perforation. The holes were simply closed with patches of omentum. None of the children had any further gastrointestinal problems. Perforated duodenal ulcers were formerly seen as a semiterminal event in hypoxic premature infants. However, the advent of mechanical ventilation seems to have eliminated this complication. The perforation in one of our patients was proximal to a stenosis of the second portion of the duodenum.

PERFORATION OF THE SMALL INTESTINE

Small bowel perforations usually are secondary to mechanical obstructions, such as atresia with gangrene or meconium ileus. Several infants, however, have had punched-out holes in the terminal ileum. This condition is not associated with necrotizing enterocolitis, Meckel's diverticulum, or distal obstruction. The etiology of these perforations remains a mystery, although there is some evidence that a *Pseudomonas* intestinal infection can produce this lesion. The perforations caused by meconium ileus result in severe meconium peritonitis.

PERFORATION OF THE CECUM

Perforation of the cecum or appendix in a neonate must be attributed to distal Hirschsprung's disease until proven otherwise.[8,9] Several of our patients had a history of constipation before their sudden deterioration, and at operation, the typical narrowed sigmoids were found. The small left colon syndrome also may cause cecal perforation.

PERFORATION OF THE RECTOSIGMOID

Unfortunately, most perforations in the rectosigmoid area are iatrogenic.[10-12] Four of our cases were caused by diagnostic barium enemas. If the balloon of a Foley catheter is inflated in a small rectum, a longitudinal tear will result. Under fluoroscopy, one sees barium extravasating into the peritoneal cavity. This complication occurred once in our experience during an attempt to treat meconium ileus with Gastrografin irrigations. Other causes of perforations in this area are mishaps with rectal thermometers and enema tubes.

DIAGNOSIS

An infant who is born with a distended abdomen that is dull to percussion has either a large intraabdominal tumor or meconium peritonitis. Distention of the scrotum with fluid suggests free meconium in the peritoneal cavity. An immediate paracentesis will make the diagnosis and at the same time improve the baby's respirations. An infant who is doing well and suddenly develops abdominal distention that is tympanitic to percussion most likely has an intestinal perforation. In other infants, the signs of perforation either are masked by or are secondary to the primary intestinal obstruction. A perforation with an enema tip or a thermometer will cause irritability,

increasing abdominal distention, and often sepsis. A baby with a perforation will become hypovolemic, pale, and tachycardic and will have rapid respirations. Any infant with abdominal signs or symptoms, particularly an increase in abdominal distention, must have abdominal roentgenograms made. Large amounts of free air in the peritoneal cavity may be observed on flat films of the abdomen because the falciform ligament is outlined. This air gives the abdomen a football shape (Fig. 74–1). An upright roentgenogram of the abdomen will detect as little as 3 ml of free air in the peritoneal cavity. However, if the infant is too ill to be held upright, free air may be detected just as well on a cross-table lateral film. This may be obtained at the infant's bedside with a portable machine. A large amount of free air in the peritoneal cavity with a paucity of intestinal gas suggests a gastric rather than an intestinal perforation. With distal perforation, there will be an air–fluid level in the stomach.[13]

The pressure of pneumoperitoneum does not necessarily mean that there is an intestinal perforation. Premature infants with the respiratory distress syndrome may develop interstitial pulmonary air, which dissects through the mediastinum into the retroperitoneal space.[14] The air then breaks through into the peritoneal cavity. In this situation, the abdomen remains soft, and there is no general deterioration in the infant's condition. Since the air collects under the anterior abdominal wall while the infant is in a supine position, it is perfectly safe to aspirate the air with a small needle, and if one desires, the abdomen may be lavaged with sterile saline through a plastic cannula. If there is only air and no bile or purulent fluid, one may confidently rule out a perforated viscus and merely continue to observe the infant. In our experience, the air reabsorbs as the pulmonary condition improves.

TREATMENT

These infants must be prepared for operation as rapidly as possible. Increments of colloids (20 ml/kg) and electrolyte solutions are given to replace fluid sequestered in the peritoneal cavity. In addition, broad-spectrum antibiotics are administered before operation. A gastric tube is inserted, aspirated with a syringe, and placed on gravity drainage. Respiratory distress caused by severe abdominal distention may be relieved by aspirating the abdominal air with a syringe and needle.

Since it is often difficult to predict the location of the perforation, the abdomen should be explored through a vertical paramedian incision, which can be extended to the xiphoid to repair a high perforation of the stomach or to the lower abdomen to exteriorize a segment of intestine. Perforations of the stomach and duodenum are closed. Gastric tears require debridement of devital-

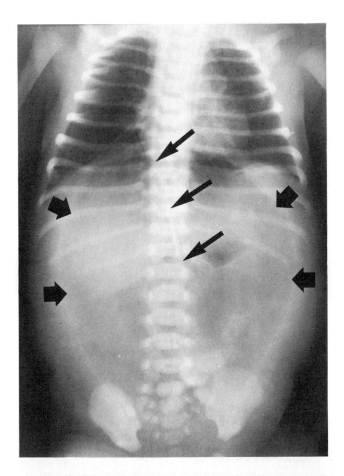

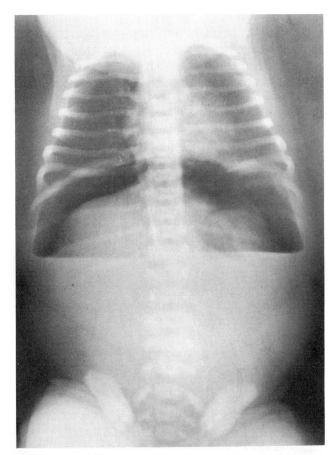

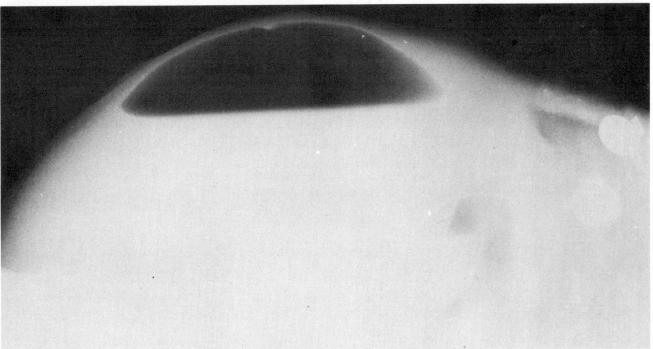

Figure 74–1. Pneumoperitoneum in a neonate, secondary to a gastric perforation. Note the paucity of gastric and intestinal air in the films. **Top left.** A supine film with air outlining the falciform ligament and the football sign. **Top right.** An upright roentgenogram that clearly demonstrates an intraperitoneal air–fluid level. **Bottom.** A cross-table lateral view will also demonstrate the air and an air–fluid level.

ized tissue and closure of the stomach with two layers of nonabsorbable suture material, which invert several millimeters of viable gastric tissue. Duodenal perforations are usually small and are either sutured transversely or covered with a tag of omentum. Proximal small intestine perforations usually are secondary to an atresia or volvulus. Treatment of the primary lesion involves resection and an end-to-end anastomosis. We strongly believe that perforations of the terminal ileum, cecum, and colon must be exteriorized because of the great likelihood of a distal obstruction. The bowel with the perforation is brought outside the abdomen through a separate incision and sutured to the peritoneum and fascia. Perforations of the rectum are treated with a drain down to the peritoneal reflection and a proximal, completely diverting colostomy. A rectal biopsy of ganglion cells must be performed before closure of any exteriorized distal perforation or colostomy.

In addition to closure or exteriorization of the perforation, we lavage the peritoneal cavity with a warm antibiotic solution. Postoperative antibiotic therapy is continued and altered when results of cultures taken at the operation become available.

REFERENCES

1. Grund K, Dzieniszewski G: Gastrointestinal perforations in the newborn. Z Kinderchir 32:56, 1981
2. Bell MJ: Perforation of the gastrointestinal tract and peritonitis in the neonate. Surg Gynecol Obstet 160:20, 1985
3. Lloyd JR: Etiology of gastrointestinal perforations in the newborn. J Pediatr Surg 4:77, 1969
4. Nagaraj H, Sandhu A, Cook L, et al: Gastrointestinal perforation following endomethacin therapy in very low birth weight infants. J Pediatr Surg 16:1003, 1981
5. Holgerson L: The etiology of spontaneous gastric perforation of the newborn: a re-evaluation. J Pediatr Surg 16:608, 1981
6. Rosser S, Clark C, Elechi E: Spontaneous neonatal gastric perforation. J Pediatr Surg 17:390, 1982
7. Houck W, Griffin J: Spontaneous linear tears of the stomach and newborn. Ann Surg 193:763, 1981
8. Martin LW, Perrin EV: Neonatal perforation of the appendix in association with Hirschsprung's disease. Ann Surg 166:799, 1967
9. Soper RT, Opitz JM: Neonatal pneumoperitoneal and Hirschsprung's disease. Surgery 51:527, 1963
10. Becker MH, Genieser NB, Clerk A: Perforation of the colon during barium enema. NY State J Med 67:278, 1967
11. Fonkalsrud EW, Clatworthy HW Jr: Accidental perforation of the colon and rectum in newborn infants. N Engl J Med 272:1097, 1965
12. Wolfson JJ: Rectal perforation in infants by thermometer. Am J Dis Child 111:197, 1966
13. Pochaczevsky R, Bryk D: New roentgenographic signs of neonatal gastric perforation. Radiology 102:145, 1972
14. Hall RT, Holder TM, Amory RA: Pneumoperitoneum with chronic respiratory disease in neonate. Pediatrics 511:933, 1973

75
Neonatal Ascites

Ascites in older children is usually caused by a medical illness, such as nephrosis, heart failure, or cirrhosis of the liver. Peritoneal fluid in a newborn or young infant is almost always from a perforation in the genitourinary, biliary, or gastrointestinal tract. Hemolytic disease of the newborn, syphilis, peritonitis secondary to a ruptured ovarian cyst, and chyle leakage are other rare causes of ascites.

Neonatal ascites may cause dystocia, and the abnormal abdominal distention can be recognized on roentgenograms or sonography of the fetus in the last trimester of pregnancy.[1,2]

PHYSICAL SIGNS

Abdominal distention, bulging flanks, and shifting dullness are the usual signs of free intraperitoneal fluid. When the abdomen is tensely distended, the signs of ascites are difficult to elicit, but there will be generalized dullness to percussion, and the breath sounds and heart tones will be readily audible over the abdomen. Fluid in a hernia sac and edema of the scrotum may tip off the diagnosis (Fig. 75–1). On clinical grounds alone, we have mistaken ascites for low intestinal obstruction because fluid-filled loops of intestine present similar physical signs. Because of the possible serious underlying disease and respiratory distress caused by the elevated diaphragms, it is urgent to proceed rapidly with diagnostic tests and surgical treatment.

ROENTGENOGRAPHIC SIGNS

Free fluid in the peritoneal cavity separates the air-filled loops of bowel and produces a generalized haze on plain roentgenograms (Fig. 75–2). There also will be bulging of the flanks, and loops of intestine will tend to conglomerate together and float in the midabdomen.[3] Scattered calcification is diagnostic of meconium peritonitis. Finally, in comparison of the clinical findings with the roentgenograms, the abdominal distention is seen to be out of proportion to the amount of gas and fluid within the bowel. This observation helps rule out an intestinal obstruction. An ultrasound examination of the abdomen will reveal small amounts of fluid with great accuracy. The ultrasound study will reveal hydronephrosis or a distended bladder and dilatation of the bile ducts and will differentiate localized fluid in an ovarian or mesenteric cyst from ascites. When the roentgenographic studies and physical examination clearly indicate ascites, a paracentesis should be performed. Enough fluid should be removed to relieve the baby's respiratory distress. Clear or light yellow fluid is probably urine, green fluid can come only from an intestinal perforation, and a golden yellow color indicates bile. The character of the fluid will determine the need for an immediate operation or further studies.

In 1894, Fordyce reviewed 64 infants with fetal and neonatal ascites.[4] Of these, 17 had associated urinary tract anomalies. Since then, others have reported the association of fetal ascites with posterior urethral valves in boys.[5–7] Linde reported on an infant girl with ascites secondary to unilateral ureteral stenosis.[8] We have observed one infant with urinary ascites from a bladder that perforated secondary to obstruction from a sacrococcygeal teratoma. North et al. could find no definite connection between the urinary tract and the peritoneal cavity; they thought that the fluid was a transudate.[9] However, our radiologic studies, as well as those of others, indicate a definite perforation of the kidney and the overlying peritoneum.

Since urine formation commences during the third trimester of intrauterine life, obstruction leads to in-

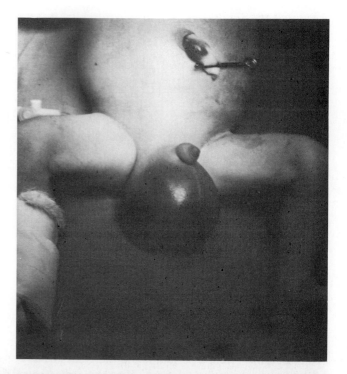

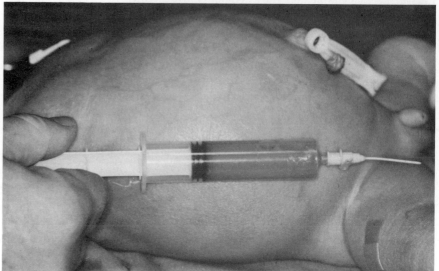

Figure 75–1. Top. Newborn infant with massive ascites due to meconium peritonitis. Note the distended scrotum. **Bottom.** Aspiration with a plastic-sheathed cannula will provide the diagnosis. The substance shown is green meconium.

creased hydrostatic pressure, which may cause perforation before birth. Birth trauma may provide the final sudden increased pressure needed to rupture the kidney. The perforation occurs in the most damaged kidney, particularly on the side with more severe ureteral reflux.

DIAGNOSTIC APPROACH

When the paracentesis shows clear yellow fluid, an immediate renal ultrasound examination is indicated. This may demonstrate bilateral nonvisualization of the kidneys

or hydronephrosis. An IV pyelogram may demonstrate contrast material in the peritoneal cavity or the halo sign of extravasated dye about the kidney.[10] The gravity cystogram is most important. Under meticulously sterile conditions, one should insert a number 5 feeding tube into the urethra and allow the contrast material to drip from a height of 24 inches. Several anterioposterior and oblique films should be exposed while the bladder is being filled. These films should demonstrate the trabeculated bladder, ureteral reflux, and hydronephrosis with extravasation (Fig. 75–3). If the infant voids after withdrawal of the catheter, it should be possible to see the

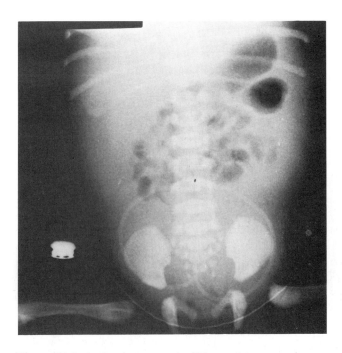

Figure 75–2. Ascites in a neonate. This roentgenogram demonstrates loops of small intestine floating in the middle portion of the abdomen.

posterior urethral valves on further roentgenograms. While the radiologic workup is in progress, one should obtain serum electrolytes and the blood urea nitrogen (BUN). It is also helpful to know the blood pH and base deficit, since many of these infants are severely acidotic and rapidly become uremic. Electrolyte studies on the ascitic fluid and urine may help determine a plan of fluid therapy.

TREATMENT

The initial paracentesis will improve the baby's condition by revealing respiratory distress, and an indwelling catheter will temporarily overcome the urinary obstruction. Reaccumulation of peritoneal fluid after a paracentesis may result in hypovolemia, whereas rapid relief of the urinary obstruction results in a prompt diuresis of dilute urine. These factors make control of the baby's fluid and electrolytes difficult. It is necessary to monitor the hematocrit, body weight, and serum electrolytes. Observation of the central venous pressure also is helpful. Plasma is best for correction of hypovolemia, and sodium bicarbonate should be given to correct acidosis.

The obstruction may be relieved temporarily with catheter drainage; later the urethral valves may be removed endoscopically. The extravasated fluid may resorb or will require aspiration. Cywes et al. reported two survivors after bilateral loop ureterostomies and liberal drainage of the peritoneum and perirenal spaces.[11]

Frequent urine cultures and vigorous antibiotic therapy are essential. The ultimate prognosis of these babies will depend on how well the ureter can regain peristalsis as well as on the degree of initial kidney destruction.

BILE ASCITES

Bile ascites, or peritonitis, is secondary to perforation of the bile ducts. This is such a rare lesion that it is seldom considered in the differential diagnosis of an infant with abdominal distention. In 1983, there were only 67 cases reported in the English literature, and an earlier report from Japan recorded 132 cases worldwide.[12,13]

Pathology
Borde and Cotoni reviewed 4 cases of their own and 41 from the literature.[14] Of these patients, 36 had perforations of the bile duct, 6 had anomalies of the ductal system, and 11 had cholelithiasis. Peterson suggested that the perforation in such cases occurs at a congenitally weak point proximal to an obstruction in the common bile duct.[15]

Moore and Cameron carefully reviewed, by correspondence with authors, the pathology and the outcome in 77 patients.[16] In 39 percent, the onset of symptoms was in the first 2 weeks, and by 1 month of age, 61 percent were symptomatic. The site of operation was at the junction of the cystic and hepatic ducts in the majority and on the anterior surface of the duct in 75 percent. In my 1 patient, mucosa at the site of perforation had everted as a tiny red bud. Not only is there ascitic fluid in the peritoneal cavity, but there are also adhesions and an edematous mass about the portal triad. It is possible that small perforations become encapsulated and eventually become variants of choledochal duct cysts.

Diagnosis
During the first few weeks of life, there may be fluctuating jaundice and pale stools. Gradually, the abdomen becomes distended, and by 6 weeks of age, free fluid is detectable. Respiratory distress becomes a problem as the abdominal distention progresses. Most infants are apathetic, refuse to eat, and lose weight. Jaundice should draw attention to the biliary tract, but occasionally ascites may be the only finding. When the physical examination and findings on plain films of the abdomen suggest ascites, a paracentesis should be performed. The fluid is golden yellow—the presence of bile should differentiate this disease from the ascites associated with cirrhosis.

When ultrasonography demonstrates ascites and a peritoneal tap demonstrates bile, the next study should be a cholescintography. There are now several radiophar-

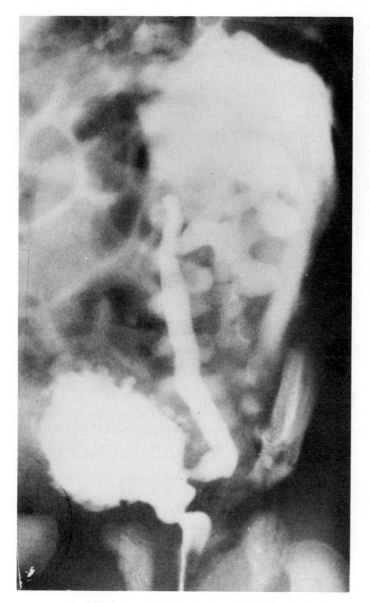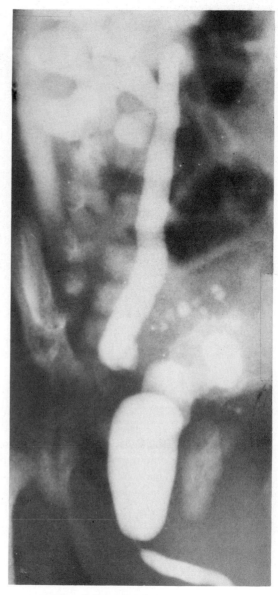

Figure 75–3. Left. Cystourethrogram in a newborn infant with ascites, demonstrating a trabeculated bladder and ureteral reflux. Contrast material has escaped from the kidney into the retroperitoneal tissue. **Right.** The oblique view demonstrates a posterior urethral valve.

maceuticals that, when given IV, are excreted by the liver.[17,18] These studies demonstrate extravasation of contrast out of the bile ducts into the peritoneal cavity. It also may be possible to identify an obstruction of the bile duct.

Treatment

Dissection in the porta hepatis in these infants is difficult because of edema and inflammation in response to the bile leak. Once the perforation is found, a small plastic catheter may be inserted proximal and distal, searching for an obstruction. Contrast material injected distally may reveal an obstruction. In addition, an operative

cholangiogram through the gallbladder will demonstrate the bile ducts and distal obstruction. Most authors have inserted a cholecystectomy tube and either closed or drained the perforation. Moore and Cameron are concerned about the possibility of an ongoing inflammatory destructive cholangitis in the bile duct, which may lead to obliteration or a choledochal duct cyst.[16] However, only 5 of 56 patients who had suture, drainage, and a cholecystostomy required a second operation. This operation, then, should be the primary emergency procedure. The child must be followed closely, with repeat cholangiograms to detect further obstruction that would require a bypass operation.

REFERENCES

1. Hadlouk R, Deter J, Garcia-Pratt P: Fetal ascites not associated with Rh incompatibility: recognition and management with sonography. AJR 134:1225, 1980

2. Radnab HM: Dystocia due to fetal abdominal enlargement. Obstet Gynecol 19:481, 1962

3. Baghdassarian OM, Koehler PR, Schultze G: Massive neonatal ascites. Radiology 76:586, 1962

4. Fordyce W: Intrauterine ascites: its obstetrical significance and pathology. Teratologia 1:61, 1894

5. Moncada R, Wang JJ, Love L, Bush I: Neonatal ascites associated with urinary outlet obstruction (urine ascites). Radiology 90:1165, 1968

6. France NE, Back EH: Neonatal ascites associated with urethral obstruction. Arch Dis Child 29:565, 1954

7. Swain VA, Tucker S, Stimmler L, France NE: Perinatal ascites due to extravasation of urine from ruptured kidneys. Clin Pediatr (Phila) 4:199, 1965

8. Linde NC: Neonatal ascites and urinary tract obstruction. Acta Paediatr Scand 55:345, 1966

9. North A, Frederick W, Eldridge DM, Talpey WB: Abdominal distention at birth due to ascites associated with obstructive uropathy. Am J Dis Child 111:613, 1966

10. Dockray KT: Perirenal contrast medium. A new roentgenographic sign of neonatal urinary ascites. JAMA 193:1121, 1965

11. Cywes S, Wynne JM, Louw JH: Urinary ascites in the newborn, with a report of two cases. J Pediatr Surg 3:350, 1968

12. Stringel G, Mercer S: Idiopathic perforation of the biliary tract in infancy. J Pediatr Surg 18:546, 1983

13. Ohkawa H, Takahashi H, Maie M: A malrotation of the pancreatic–biliary system as a cause of perforation of the biliary tract in childhood. J Pediatr Surg 12:541, 1977

14. Borde J, Cotoni A: Peritoneal biliary effusion and perforation of the biliary ducts in infants. Ann Chir Infant 7:287, 1966

15. Peterson G: Spontaneous perforation of the common bile duct in infants. Acta Clin Scand 110:192, 1955

16. Moore T, Cameron R: Spontaneous perforation of the extrahepatic biliary tract in infancy and childhood. Pediatr Surg Int 1:206, 1986

17. Stringel G, Mercer S: Idiopathic perforation of the biliary tract in infancy. J Pediatr Surg 18:546, 1983

18. Kolbe A, Bearer B, Rosenbaum R, Hill J: Diagnosis of spontaneous perforation of the biliary tract in the newborn. J Pediatr Surg 21:1139, 1986

SECTION IX

Jaundice in Infancy

Nearly every newborn infant has some degree of physiologic jaundice. In addition to this, many medical diseases involve the liver and cause jaundice. Infants with biliary atresia are otherwise well during their first few weeks of life. Thus, the diagnosis is almost always delayed. This is unfortunate because the liver becomes progressively damaged.

Unfortunately, few infants with biliary atresia have a dilated common bile duct suitable for anastomosis to the gastrointestinal tract with any hope of complete success. In the past, we and most other pediatric surgeons performed a liver biopsy and an operative cholangiogram to confirm the diagnosis and then meticulously dissected the structures in the porta hepatis. If there was no dilated bile duct, the abdomen was closed, and the baby was sentenced to a slow death. We were dubious about the benefits of portoenterostomy but were spurred on by the results of other surgeons, such as Dr. R. Peter Alt-man. We have performed portoenterostomies on all infants with "inoperable" biliary atresia for the past 10 years. We were further persuaded that this was the correct course to follow when we found dilated ducts in the portal areas of the livers of four infants who died after negative explorations. It is possible to obtain bile drainage from the liver with reduction of the serum bilirubin in many children. We have demonstrated connections between bile ducts within the liver and the bowel by transhepatic cholangiography performed after the operation. Unfortunately, some children develop ascites, portal hypertension, and episodes of sepsis in a manner similar to that of patients who are merely explored. However, we firmly believe that the operation should be offered because it relieves the terrible pruritis that plagues children with atresias who are not operated on. Furthermore, there are a few children who appear to be cured by this operation.

SECTION IX

Jaundice in Infancy

76
Biliary Atresia

_____ *Frederick M. Karrer and John G. Raffensperger*

Biliary atresia is an enigma. We are not absolutely certain about its etiology and despite advances in surgical management, there is still no cure for these unfortunate infants. Previously, such terms as "operable" or "correctable" were used to describe infants with a patent bile duct outside of the liver that could be used for anastomosis to a segment of the bowel. These terms are no longer applicable, since some infants with only microscopic remnants of bile ducts at the hilus of the liver are "operable" in the sense that a proper operation may secure bile flow. The incidence of biliary atresia is approximately 1 in 25,000 live births, and it does not appear to have a racial predilection.[1,2]

PATHOLOGY

The pathology of biliary atresia depends somewhat on the age of the infant at the time of diagnosis. From about 2 weeks to about 3 months, a period of time when the diagnosis is usually made, one finds a grossly enlarged, firm liver with a distinctly greenish hue. There is some variation in the extrahepatic bile ducts. Most commonly, the gallbladder is small but contains a lumen, and the entire extrahepatic biliary system consists of only fibrous cords. These may be so small that they barely can be found with magnification. The gallbladder and cystic and distal common ducts may be patent, but nothing is found from the hilum of the liver to the cystic duct. In perhaps 5 percent of patients, a patent duct, variable in size, is found at the hilum of the liver, which may or may not connect with the intrahepatic distal system. There is some overlap with choledochal duct cysts when the extrahepatic duct is dilated. If a dilated duct is completely obstructed, the term "biliary atresia" is applicable.

There is no generally accepted classification for the many variations in extrahepatic ductal anatomy seen in biliary atresia, but the most common types are diagrammed in Figure 76–1. Most important in the pathology of extrahepatic biliary atresia is the presence of microscopic bile ducts, embedded in a mass of fibrous tissue at the hilus of the liver. Often, the obstructed ducts may be traced to this fibrous mass. Serial sections taken through this tissue have demonstrated minute connections to the intrahepatic bile ducts.[3,4] This observation is the basis for the operations currently in use for biliary atresia.

The size of these microscopic ducts varies from definite structures measuring 150 microns in diameter and having an epithelial lining to unlined slitlike spaces in the fibrous tissue (Fig. 76–2). The ducts are smaller and unlined in infants older than 3 months of age. Better bile flow is seen postoperatively, when definite ducts are lined with epithelium.[5] Microscopic study of the liver reveals cholestasis in the form of yellow or brown pigment within bile canaliculi and in the interlobular bile ducts. Giant cell transformation of the bile ducts often is seen, but the most striking finding is distortion of portal areas by fibrous tissue. Fibrosis is found in all livers of children with biliary atresia, regardless of age, although it is milder in younger infants. Serial liver biopsies have demonstrated persistent fibrosis, even when bile flow adequate to completely clear the child's jaundice is obtained at operation. In some children, the fibrosis progresses to cirrhosis regardless of treatment.

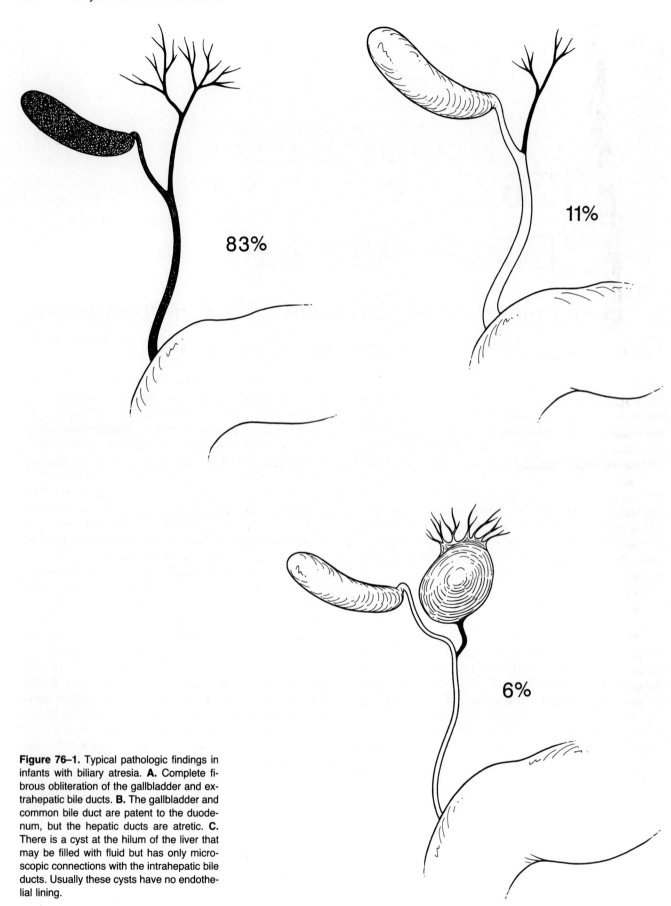

Figure 76–1. Typical pathologic findings in infants with biliary atresia. **A.** Complete fibrous obliteration of the gallbladder and extrahepatic bile ducts. **B.** The gallbladder and common bile duct are patent to the duodenum, but the hepatic ducts are atretic. **C.** There is a cyst at the hilum of the liver that may be filled with fluid but has only microscopic connections with the intrahepatic bile ducts. Usually these cysts have no endothelial lining.

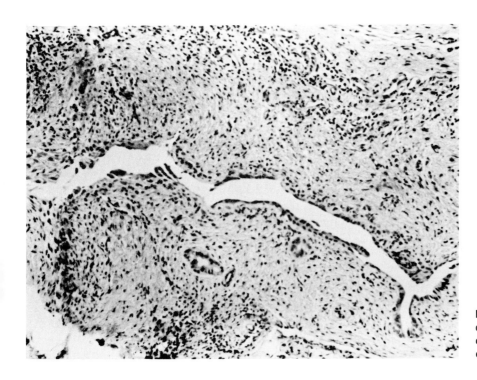

Figure 76–2. Section through porta hepatis demonstrating fibrous tissue and small bile ducts. The slitlike space is partially lined with endothelium.

ETIOLOGY

Examination of tissues resected at the time of operation reveals inflammation and progressive fibrosis. This information, together with the fact that there are children who had definite bile-stained stools at birth, and then progressed to biliary obstruction, has led to the theory that biliary atresia is not a single embryologic event but rather an ongoing inflammatory or infectious process that has its onset in the prenatal period or shortly after birth. There may be a causal relationship between the reovirus type 3 and biliary atresia, since, in one series, 68 percent of infants with biliary atresia had antibodies to this virus and it produces biliary atresia in weanling mice.[6,7]

The appearance of biliary atresia in only one of a set of identical twins is further evidence for an acquired rather than a genetic basis for the disease.[8] A cluster of babies born with biliary atresia in rural Texas also suggests an infectious or environmental etiologic agent.[9]

Associated defects with biliary atresia are uncommon but include anomalies of intestinal rotation and preduodenal portal vein.[10] In our series, we have observed associated imperforate anus, esophageal atresia, and cyanotic heart disease.

DIAGNOSIS

Neonates are often mildly jaundiced because of immature hepatic function, and infants may have prolonged jaundice from sepsis, metabolic errors, or hemolysis or, in later infancy, secondary to a lack of oral intake and total parenteral nutrition (TPN). The baby with biliary atresia will be mildly jaundiced at birth. The icterus deepens but may not be observed immediately, particularly in darker-skinned babies. It is sometimes difficult to determine if the stools are acholic because various formulas will color the stools yellow, and oral iron darkens the stool. Unlike infants with hepatitis, babies with biliary atresia are perfectly well except for the jaundice. They eat normally, gain weight, develop, and in general appear to be healthy. This is a useful differential point because other diseases that cause jaundice usually impair growth and development. Every persistently jaundiced infant must be studied with a battery of tests to rule out unusual infections, such as toxoplasmosis, rubella, cytomegalovirus infection, herpes, and syphilis. These are lumped together as the TORCH titers. In addition, each baby is screened for alpha $_1$-antitrypsin deficiency.[11] Most often, by the time the child is seen by a surgeon, the more common, medical causes for jaundice have been ruled out and the diagnosis lies between biliary atresia and neonatal hepatitis. In the past, there was no good way to differentiate these two problems without an open liver biopsy and an operative cholangiogram.

The two most important tests are ultrasound and radionuclide hepatobiliary imaging and excretion studies using ^{99m}Tc PIPIDA or DISIDA.[12,13] Ultrasonography will accurately identify dilated obstructed bile ducts (Fig. 76–3). The ultrasound examination will often demonstrate the gallbladder, which may contract after feeding if the distal duct is intact, even when there is proximal atresia. The ^{99m}Tc-IDA derivatives are rapidly extracted

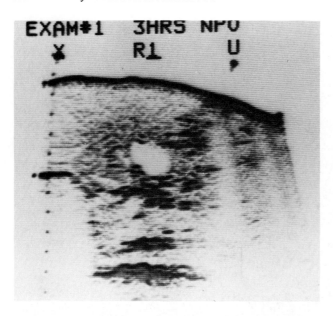

Figure 76–3. Ultrasound study demonstrating a cyst at the hilum of the liver.

from the blood by the hepatocytes and excreted into the bowel through the biliary ducts. Most of the IV administered tracer is seen in the liver within 30 minutes. When there is hepatocellular disease, there is delay in liver uptake, but with biliary obstruction, the material accumulates in the liver, but none appears in the bowel. It is then excreted through the kidneys. The value of this test is enhanced by giving the infant 5 mg/kg of phenobarbital per day for 5 days before the nuclear excretion study. Phenobarbital increases bilirubin conjugation and excretion and has a choleretic effect, independent of its function as an inducer of hepatic enzymes.[14] Phenobarbital thus enhances and accelerates the liver's uptake of ^{99m}Tc-IDA analogs but has no effect on their excretion in babies with biliary atresia.

The complete evaluation of a jaundiced infant should be completed within the length of time it takes to do the phenobarbital loading and hepatobiliary scan. If there is excretion on the scan, a percutaneous needle biopsy of the liver is indicated for definitive diagnosis. Failure of excretion most often indicates a diagnosis of extrahepatic biliary atresia and is an indication for an operation. Unfortunately, even the hepatobiliary scan will not diagnose intrahepatic atresia of the bile ducts, a condition that is not benefited by an operation. This condition is also known as Alagille's syndrome or arteriohepatic dysplasia.[15,16] Thus, before operation, each infant must be critically evaluated for this diagnosis. They have heart disease, most often pulmonary artery stenosis, and a characteristic facial appearance consisting of a high prominent forehead, a pointed chin, and deep-set eyes. A percutaneous liver biopsy should be performed rather than an open operation. Eventually, a liver transplanta-

tion may be indicated in these children because of advancing liver disease and the development of hepatocarcinoma.[17] The biopsy in these infants reveals a paucity of intrahepatic ducts and an absence of ductular proliferation, characteristic of extrahepatic atresia.

TREATMENT

Before operation, each infant must have coagulation defects corrected with vitamin K and transfusions of fresh frozen plasma. A gastric tube is placed before the induction of anesthesia, and it is helpful to deflate the colon with a rectal tube and enemas. Broad-spectrum antibiotics are started when the child reaches the operating room.

Technique

A transverse, right subcostal incision extended to the left of the midline, which transects the round ligament, allows mobilization of the liver and retraction of the stomach and intestine for optimal visualization of the porta hepatis. A wedge biopsy of the liver is obtained and examined by frozen section to affirm the diagnosis. This biopsy is particularly important to rule out intrahepatic atresia, which is a contraindication to the Kasai type of operation. The gallbladder may be almost normal in size and distended with white mucus when the distal bile duct is patent. More often, the gallbladder is small and hidden in a fissure. After the liver biopsy has been obtained, secure a size 5 French plastic feeding tube in the gallbladder with double ties. Contrast material, such as Omnipaque, is injected into the gallbladder, and the cholangiogram is obtained (Fig. 76–4). If ducts are seen in the liver in continuity with the gallbladder and duodenum, nothing further is done. Often, the gallbladder is completely fibrous, with no lumen. If this is the case, a cholangiogram is unnecessary, and the operation is continued. Each structure in the porta hepatis is meticulously examined and identified. The hepatic artery, its branches, and the portal vein are encircled with tapes. Magnifying loupes and perfect lighting are essential for the identification and dissection of the fibrous remnants of the bile ducts (Fig. 76–5). It is helpful to keep the gallbladder in continuity with the ductal structures for traction as the dissection approaches the hilus of the liver. Often, the fibrous cords will bifurcate and with magnification can be seen to enter the liver to the right and left. This phase of the operation is critical! Steady retraction on the liver, perfect light, and magnification are essential to accurate dissection. The mass of fibrous tissue and ductal remnants are elevated so the posterior dissection reaches back between the bifurcation of the portal vein. Laterally, it extends out to the secondary branches of the hepatic arteries (Fig. 76–6). Thus,

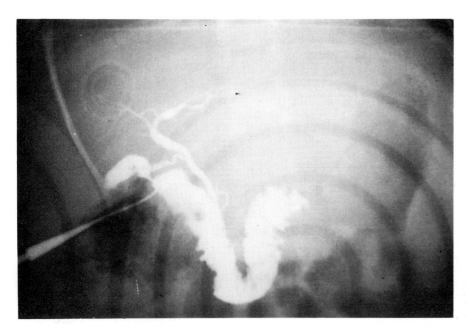

Figure 76–4. Operative cholangiogram demonstrating a normal gallbladder and bile ducts.

one hopes to find all patent ducts that reach the hilum. It is necessary to divide small branches from the portal vein during this dissection. Ligatures should never be used to control bleeding for fear of including a bile duct. Pressure with a sponge and judicious use of the bipolar electrocoagulation unit are usually sufficient to obtain hemostasis.

Suruga et al. use 10 power magnification to visualize the bile ducts so they can limit the dissection.[18] They believe that this reduces scarring at the anastomosis. Kimura et al. studied the level of resection and found their best results were obtained when the fibrous mass was resected either flush with the liver substance or

including a fragment of liver.[19] When 2 to 3 cm of liver was removed, there was more bleeding, but no bile flow was obtained. Frozen section studies may determine the level of microscopic bile ducts and the optimum depth of dissection.[20] In our hospital, the fibrous tissue with a thin rim of liver is included with the specimen. Stay sutures placed along the posterior and lateral rim are helpful when making the anastomosis. Occasionally a bile cyst is encountered at the liver hilum. In the past, an anastomosis was made directly to the cyst, and long-term bile flow was obtained. Results are improved by resecting these cysts and carrying out a standard portoenterostomy, since Lilly et al. have demonstrated

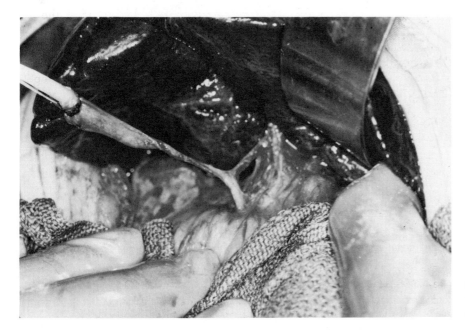

Figure 76–5. The gallbladder is held up on traction and the fibrous duct may be seen entering the porta hepatis.

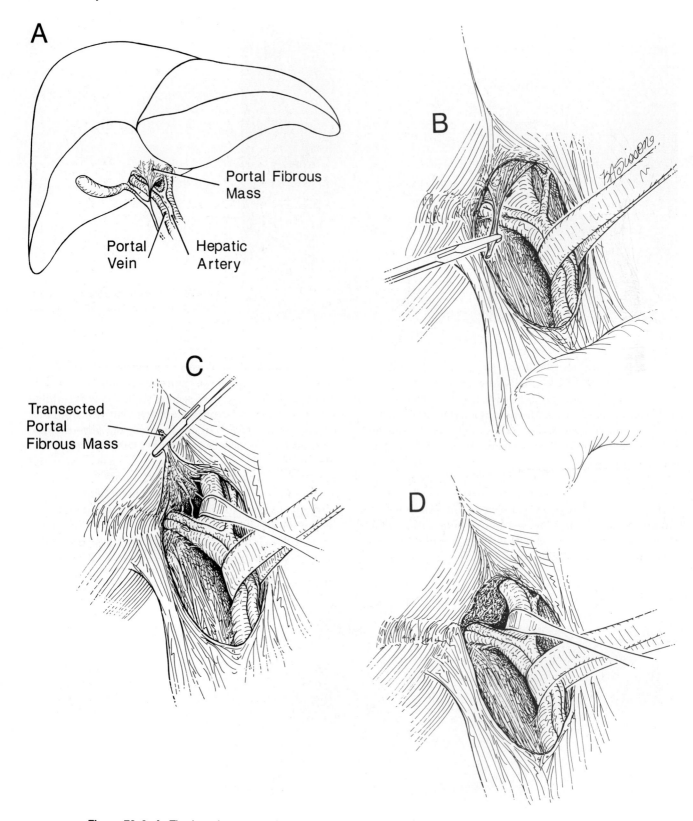

Figure 76–6. A. The hepatic artery and portal vein are identified and encircled with a tape. Then the fibrous mass of hepatic duct is dissected into the hilum of the liver by traction on the gallbladder. **B.** The hepatic duct fibrous mass has been transected so it can be dissected laterally to the first branches of the hepatic arteries. **C.** The fibrous mass is elevated, and the portal vein is retracted inferiorly to allow complete posterior dissection of the fibrous tissue. Note the small branches of the portal vein, which must be coagulated. **D.** Retraction of the portal vein demonstrates the raw area of liver left by resection of the fibrous mass containing minute bile ducts.

E

F.

1.5cm

Valve

Liver

Jejunal
Interposition

G

Duodenum

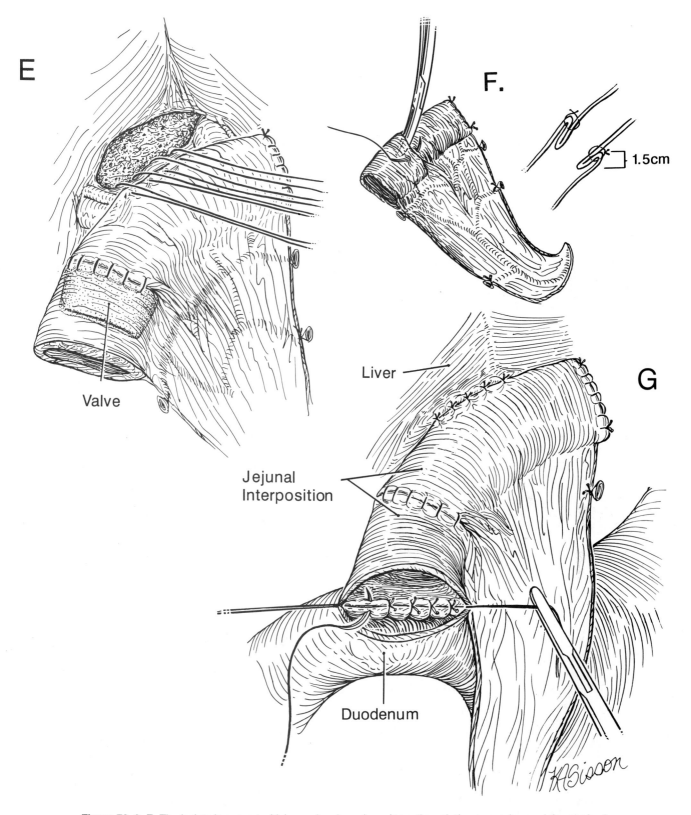

Figure 76–6. E. The isolated segment of jejunum has been brought up through the mesocolon, and the proximal end has been closed with a continuous suture. Interrupted 6-0 polydioxone sutures are placed through an incision in the jejunum and the posterior rim of liver between the bifurcation of the portal vein. The anastomosis is completed after opening the jejunum and suturing the anterior layer of jejunum to the liver capsule. **F.** A 1 to 1.5 cm intussusception is created in the conduit to prevent reflux. **G.** The liver anastomosis is complete, and the anastomosis to the second portion of the duodenum is in progress.

that the cyst has no epithelial lining.[21] When the portal dissection is completed, a warm, moist sponge is applied to control bleeding and a loop of jejunum is identified for the bile conduit.

Originally, Kassai et al. drained bile into the bowel with a traditional Roux-en-Y loop. They later modified this by exteriorizing one limb of the loop so bile could drain to the exterior through a stoma.[22,23] There are now innumerable modifications of the Roux-en-Y loop to drain bile to the outside in an attempt to reduce the incidence of cholangitis. Lilly and Altman use a double-barrelled stoma so bile can be reinserted through a tube.[24] Sawaguchi et al. use a short isolated loop of jejunum to drain bile from the porta hepatis to a skin stoma. Later, when bile flow has been established, the jejunal loop is reanastomosed to the jejunum just beyond the ligament of Treitz.[25]

Our preference is to use an isolated 10 cm segment of jejunum interposed between the liver and duodenum with a 1 cm intussuscepted valve to prevent reflux (Fig. 76–6 E,F,G). The proximal end of the loop is closed with an inverting, continuous suture because an end-to-side anastomosis lies better at the porta hepatis. The antimesenteric side of the bowel is opened and placed adjacent to the liver. The posterior sutures first pick up the jenunum; then the needle is passed through the cut edge of liver well back between the branches of the portal vein. The previously placed stay sutures are useful to pull up and identify this rim. Laterally, the suture line extends to the secondary branches of the hepatic arteries to ensure inclusion of the right and left ducts. Anteriorly, the suture line continues around the open jejunum, taking bites through the cut anterior margin of the liver. We prefer absorbable 6-0 monofilament sutures to avoid leaving a foreign body in a potentially contaminated area. This is not true of mucosa-to-mucosa anastomosis. The jejunum is sutured to the porta hepatis in the hope that bile ducts will drain. After healing by secondary intention, the junction between bile ducts and jejunum will become covered by endothelium.

The second portion of the duodenum is then mobilized so an anastomosis can be made between it and the segment of jejunum. The valve is made by intussuscepting 1 cm of bowel into itself with forceps and a row of nonabsorbable sutures. The abdomen may be closed without drainage after this procedure.

When the cholangiogram demonstrates a patent duct between the gallbladder and duodenum, the gallbladder itself may be turned down and used for the portoenterostomy. Lilly and Stellin advise leaving a plastic tube in the gallbladder for drainage because the distal duct is too small to carry the flow of bile.[26] This operation has a lower incidence of postoperative cholangitis than has the Roux-en-Y loop and its many modifications. Unfortunately, it is difficult to maintain the blood supply

of the gallbladder, and turning it down to the portal area tends to kink the cystic duct. The size of the gallbladder is not always large enough to cover the dissected porta hepatis. Since the interposed jejunal loop with a valve has essentially eliminated cholangitis, there is little indication for the gallbladder conduit.

POSTOPERATIVE CARE

The stomach is decompressed with a nasogastric tube until there are peristaltic sounds and a stool is passed. There is great rejoicing when lovely green bile appears in the tube! We continue broad-spectrum antibiotics for a week after the operation, then administer trimethoprim-sulfamethoxazole (TMP-SMZ) 5 mg/25 kg/day for a year after the operation. There is, however, no evidence that prophylactic antibiotics prevent cholangitis. As soon as oral feedings are tolerated, prednisone 2 mg/kg/day is started and continued for a month, then is slowly tapered. Steroids have a choleretic effect on bile flow, and there is some hope that they decrease scar formation at the anastomosis. Children who have good bile flow and become anicteric have no special nutritional requirements. However, if there is a deficiency of bile acid secretion, the digestion and absorption of fats and fat-soluble vitamins is impaired. A formula, such as Pregestamil, contains medium-chain triglycerides that are easier to absorb than fats. It is necessary to supplement the diet with water-soluble vitamins. When nutritional deficits are severe, it may be necessary to give these vitamins parenterally. Although the value of administering phenobarbital to these children is doubtful, we continue to give it during the first year because of its choleretic effect.

COMPLICATIONS

Cholangitis has been reported to follow operations for biliary atresia in as high as 50 to 100 percent of patients.[27–29] It is the most important factor in determining the prognosis of infants who have cleared their jaundice and have good bile flow following a Kasai type of operation. Cholangitis may occur anytime after the operation, but the first bout is usually within a month. After a year, if there is good bile flow, episodes may decrease. Cholangitis is recognized when there is an episode of fever with recurrence of jaundice, elevation of liver enzymes, leukocytosis, and acholic stools. Blood and liver biopsy cultures are positive for enteric organisms, evidence that this is ascending cholangitis from the gut.[30,31] It is difficult to differentiate other febrile illnesses from cholangitis because we have observed transient jaundice in children with a viral illness who had negative blood and liver cultures and who became well without antibiotics. Localized edema may temporarily obstruct ducts in the hilum of the liver.

Cholangitis is treated with IV antibiotics, including at least one that has significant biliary excretion, such as ampicillin, cephalosporin, TMP-SMZ, or an aminoglycoside. A short course of high-dose prednisone has been beneficial, perhaps by reducing edema in the porta hepatis.[32] Reoperation to eliminate cholangitis is indicated if ultrasound examination or a transhepatic cholangiogram reveals poorly drained bile lakes within the liver. These may be drained by anastomosis to the original loop of bowel. Excision of granulation tissue and microabscesses at the portoenteric anastomosis occasionally has been helpful in eliminating a focus of infection.[33] Absorbable sutures at this site would logically reduce the incidence of prolonged local infection.

Experimentally and in several small series of cases, the addition of either an intussuscepted antireflux valve or a spur between the Roux-en-Y loop and the jejunum has reduced the incidence of cholangitis.[34-37] Exteriorization of the draining limb of bowel does not decrease the incidence of cholangitis and has many other complications, including electrolyte loss and variceal hemorrhage from the stoma site.

In adults, exclusion of bile from the duodenum by the use of a Roux-en-Y loop results in a 5 percent incidence of duodenal ulcer and fat malabsorption.[38] The interposed jejunal loop prevents these complications, and, in addition, the duodenum has a lower concentration of bacteria, another possible factor in preventing cholangitis. Simply stated, the operation described here more nearly duplicates normal anatomy than any other. We have carried out this operation in 27 children; 12 are now 1½ to 8 years old and continue to be jaundice free. Two of these patients had one episode each of cholangitis proven by blood or liver culture. One had a febrile episode treated with steroids and antibiotics but with negative cultures. These children are jaundice free and have had no more episodes of jaundice or fever. Before use of the intussuscepted valve, 1 of our patients had recurrent bouts of cholangitis and multiple liver abscesses and died at 3 years of age.

REOPERATION

Since the portoenterostomy is not a direct mucosa-to-mucosa anastomosis, healing is by secondary intention, with the possibility that scar tissue will form to obstruct the small bile ducts before endothelialization has taken place. Thus, when the operation results in a good flow of bile, which then ceases, with recurrence of jaundice, several surgeons have reported successful bile drainage after a second operation. There are few indications for reoperation, particularly since another operation will result in more adhesion that will make a future liver transplant more difficult. Only 6 of 32 patients reoperated on by Kasai et al. became free of jaundice after a second operation.[39] Resection of scar tissue at the anastomotic site resulted in bile flow in only 4 of 11 patients reported by Hata et al., and no child in either group was benefited by a second operation when there was poor bile flow the first time.[40] Specific indications for a second operation include demonstration of obstructed, dilated intrahepatic bile ducts by ultrasonography or cholangiogram, cholelithiasis, and a sudden cessation of bile flow.[41,42] We reoperated upon 2 of our 27 patients. A bile lake was found and successfully drained in one, while the other had no bile drainage after the second operation. One other patient was found to have a thin layer of scar tissue obstructing the bile ducts. This scar could have been removed at a second operation.

RESULTS

The Kasai operation is one of the great advances in pediatric surgery. Formerly, only 5 percent or less of infants with biliary atresia had a duct in the porta hepatis that could be used for an anastomosis, and only a few of those patients survived for long periods of time. All children who had no bile ducts at operation had the incision closed without any attempt at cure. They died with liver failure, sepsis, ascites, or portal hypertension. Initially, in this country, many surgeons questioned the value of the Kasai operation. During the past 10 years, the results have improved to the point where approximately 40 to 50 percent of infants who have this operation are alive with bile flow more than 1 year after operation.[43-46]

In 1983, Kasai had 41 jaundice-free survivors, or 27 percent of his patients, who were 5 to 28 years old.[47] Unfortunately, children who survive more than 5 years may still develop portal hypertension secondary to continuing hepatic fibrosis.[48] In this country, Altman and Levy obtained extended bile drainage in 81 of 100 patients, and 30 were jaundice free from 1 to 9 years after operation.[49] All reports stress the importance of early diagnosis and operation, since children operated on after 10 weeks of age have a significantly poorer prognosis. Canty was able to establish bile drainage in 17 of 18 infants operated on before 10 weeks of age and in only 2 of 7 operated on after that time.[50]

Our own results in a small series mirror the overall experience. From 1979 to 1986, we used the valved conduit in 27 children, operated on between 1½ and 4 months of age. Twelve are alive, well, and jaundice free from 1½ to 8 years of age. They are not completely normal, since they have firm, palpable livers, and in about half, the spleen is enlarged. Liver biopsies have shown continued fibrosis with mild cholestasis. In only 4 children was there no perceptible postoperative bile flow. All of these patients died from 4 months to 3 years after their operation. Eleven children had some bile flow; 2 died with congenital heart disease, and 1 died with a gangrenous midgut volvulus. Two are alive after liver transplantation, and 1 died after a transplant. The rest died by 1½ years of age from liver failure. These results from our own patients suggest that if a child has good bile flow and is anicteric at 1 year of age, he or she has an excellent opportunity for prolonged life, although the child is always at risk from chronic liver disease. We should be able to determine the child's prognosis and ultimate need for a liver transplant within a few weeks after the operation.

Long-term survivors after the Kasai operation may have delayed mental and motor development. This may be related to delay in diagnosis and treatment or to nutritional deficiencies, especially of vitamin E.[51,52]

HEPATIC TRANSPLANTATION

Despite the advances in therapy for biliary atresia, many children succumb to their disease unless the diseased organ can be replaced by hepatic transplantation. The dramatic improvement in survival after liver transplantation using cyclosporine A immunosuppression supports the feasibility of the procedure for biliary atresia.[53] We believe that liver transplantation is not an alternative to hepatic portoenterostomy but rather a complementary operation. Limitations in the number of infant donors preclude transplantation of all infants with biliary atresia as a primary procedure. Many infants who do not undergo a Kasai operation will die before transplantation can be accomplished. For those children with progressive liver failure post-Kasai, we should strive to optimize their condition before transplantation.[54] Deficiencies of fat-soluble vitamins (A, D, E, K) occur commonly, owing to reduced bile excretion, and require supplementation. Nutritional deficiencies of fat calories can be corrected by replacing long-chain triglycerides with formula containing medium-chain triglycerides, e.g., Portagen or Pregestamil. Adequate protein–calorie intake may necessitate nocturnal nasogastric feeding as the liver disease progresses. Salt restriction may be mandated by the presence of ascites and protein restriction by encephalopathy. Complications of portal hypertension, such as bleeding esophageal varices, should preferrentially be managed without shunting. Endoscopic sclerotherapy may avoid the need to shunt these patients, thereby sparing the portal vein for the liver replacement procedure and avoiding scarring from repeated laparotomies. Similarly, hypersplenism can be treated by embolization rather than splenectomy. Repeated operations on the porta hepatis should be avoided except in the case of a child with a good result (anicteric with good bile drainage) who suddenly has an obstruction, usually in association with cholangitis.

The preoperative evaluation of children for liver transplantation should begin early. In this way, their course can be followed closely and optimized to achieve maximal growth and survival. The modalities used in this assessment are shown in Table 76–1. The most important factors predicting early death are serum cholesterol less than 100 mg/dl, history of ascites, indirect bilirubin greater than 3 mg/dl, and PTT greater than 20 seconds.[55] The only absolute contraindications to transplantation are unresectable or metastatic malignancy, progressive incurable nonhepatic disease, or lack of informed consent. Other relative contraindications include portal vein thrombosis, active intraabdominal sepsis, multiple abdominal operations, HIV or HBsAg positivity, and severe mental retardation.[56]

The technical aspects of hepatic transplantation in children differ little from those in adults. In the donor operation, the celiac axis and superior mesenteric artery are removed in continuity with the entire abdominal and thoracic aorta. This segment of aorta is sometimes used as a conduit.[57] The transplant operation has become well standardized since the original reports.[58,59] The actuarial survival rates are approximately 75 percent in the cyclosporine era.[60] Even infants (under 1 year of age) can be transplanted with similar success.[61] Liver transplantation is a viable therapeutic option for those children with biliary atresia and progressive liver failure. For those children in whom biliary drainage is not achieved or those with significant parenchymal damage,

TABLE 76–1. PRETRANSPLANT EVALUATION

Measures to confirm diagnosis
    Hepatitis screen, alpha-₁-antitrypsin level and phenotype, ceruloplasmin, antimitochondrial antibody, ANA, ASMA, LE preparation, iron, iron binding capacity, ferritin
Measures to assess liver function
    Liver enzymes, coagulation profile, bilirubin, fasting ammonia, cholesterol triglycerides, galactose elimination, aminopurene demethylation, indocyanine green clearance
Measures of suitability for transplant
    Antiviral antibody titers: CMV, EBV, VZV, HSV, HIV
    Routine cultures: blood, urine, sputum, ascites, stool
    Ultrasound of liver and portal vein, possible angiography
    Neuropsychologic evaluation
Nutritional assessment
    Triceps skinfold thickness, total protein, albumin, transferrin, total lymphocyte count, serum vitamin levels, bone survey
Immunologic evaluation
    ABO blood typing, HLA and DR typing, quick PRA (cytotoxic antibody screen), T cell, B cell, and T cell subset quantitation, quantitative immunoglobulins

liver transplantation should be considered as part of ongoing care.

REFERENCES

1. Shim W, Kasai M, Spence M: Racial influence on the incidence of biliary atresia. Prog Pediatr Surg 6:53, 1974
2. Suzuki H: Incidence of biliary atresia in Sendai in proceedings of the International Symposium on Cholestasis. Univ of Tokyo Press, 1978
3. Kasai M, Ohi R, Chiba T: Intrahepatic bile ducts in biliary atresia. In Proceedings of the International Symposium on Cholestasis. Tokyo, University of Tokyo Press, 1979
4. Chandra R, Altman R: Ductal remnants in extrahepatic biliary atresia: a histopathologic study with clinical correlations. J Pediatr 93:196, 1978
5. Ohi R, Shikes R, Stellin G, Lilly J: In biliary atresia duct histology correlates with bile flow. J Pediatr Surg 19:467, 1984
6. Glaser J, Balistravi W, Morecki R: Role of reovirus type 3 in persistent infantile cholestasis. J Pediatr 105:912, 1984
7. Bangaru B, Morecki R, Glaser J, et al: Comparative studies of biliary atresia in the human newborn and reovirus-induced cholangitis in weanling mice. Lab Invest 43:456, 1980
8. Moore T, Hyman P: Extrahepatic biliary atresia in one human leukocyte to antigen identical twin. Pediatrics 76:604, 1985
9. Strickland A, Shannon K: Studies in the etiology of extrahepatic biliary atresia: time space clustering. J Pediatr 100:749, 1982
10. Lilly J: Surgical hazards of co-existing anomalies in biliary atresia. Surg Gynecol Obstet 139:49, 1974
11. Nobbia G, Hadchovel M, Odievre M, Alagille D: Early assessment of evolution of liver disease associated with alpha1-antitrypsin deficiency in childhood. J Pediatr 102:661, 1983
12. Majd M, Reba R, Altman P: Hepatobiliary scintography with 99mTC-DIPIDA in the evaluation of neonatal jaundice. Pediatrics 67:140, 1981
13. Spivak W, Sarkor S, Winter D, et al: Diagnostic utility of hepatobiliary scintagraphy with 99mTC-DISIDA in neonatal cholestasis. J Pediatr 110:855, 1987
14. Capron J, Erlinger S: Barbiturates and biliary function. Digestion 23:43, 1975
15. Alagille D, Odievre M, Gautier M, et al: Hepatic ductular hypoplasia associated with characteristic facies. Vertebral malformations, retarded physical, mental and sexual development and cardiac murmur. J Pediatr 86:63, 1975
16. Markowitz J, Daum F, Kahn E, et al: Arteriohepatic dysplasia. Pitfalls in diagnosis and management of hepatology 3:74, 1983
17. Kaufman S, Wood P, Shaw B, et al: Hepatocellular carcinoma in a child with the Alagille syndrome. Am J Dis Child 141:698, 1981
18. Suruga K, Kono S, Miyano T, et al: Treatment of biliary atresia: microsurgery for hepatic portoenterostomy. Surgery 80:558, 1976
19. Kimura K, Tsuqawa C, Kubo M, et al: Technical aspects of hepatic portal dissection in biliary atresia. J Pediatr Surg 14:27, 1979
20. Altman R, Lilly J: Technical details in the surgical correction of extrahepatic biliary atresia. Surg Gynecol Obstet 140:953, 1975
21. Lilly J, Hall R, Vasquez-Estevez J, et al: The surgery of "correctable" biliary atresia. J Pediatr Surg 22:522, 1987
22. Kasai M, Kimura K, Asakura Y, et al: Surgical treatment of biliary atresia. J Pediatr Surg 3:665, 1968
23. Kasai M, Suzuki H, Ohashi E, et al: Technique and results of operative management of biliary atresia. World J Surg 2:571, 1978
24. Lilly J, Altman R: Hepatic portoenterostomy (the Kasai operation) for biliary atresia. Surgery 78:76, 1975
25. Sawaquichi S, Nakajo T, Hori T: Surgical treatment of biliary atresia by making a temporary external biliary fistula. J Jpn Surg Soc 1317, 1968
26. Lilly J, Stellin G: Catheter decompression of hepatic portocholecystostomy. J Pediatr Surg 17:904, 1982
27. Kobayashi A, Utsunomiya T, Ohbe T Shimuza K: Ascending cholangitis following hepatic portoenterostomy for biliary atresia. J Pediatr 99:656, 1981
28. Barkin R, Lilly J: Biliary atresia and the Kasai operation: continuing care. J Pediatr 96:1015, 1980
29. Ecoffey C, Rothman E, Bernard O, et al: Bacterial cholangitis after surgery for biliary atresia. J Pediatr 3:824, 1981
30. Hitch D, Lilly J: Identification, quantification and significance of bacterial growth within the biliary tree after Kasai's operation. J Pediatr Surg 13:563, 1978
31. Brook J, Altman P: The significance of anaerobic bacteria in biliary tract infection after hepatic portoenterostomy for biliary atresia. Surgery 95:281, 1984
32. Karrer F, Lilly J: Corticosteroid therapy in biliary atresia. J Pediatr Surg 20:693, 1985
33. Graeve A, Volpicelli N, Kosloske A: Endoscopic reconalization of a portoenterostomy. J Pediatr Surg 17:901, 1982
34. Chin-Che-Chang: An antireflux spur valve in Roux-Y anastomosis. J Jpn Soc Pediatr Surg 18:73, 1982
35. Donanoe P, Hendren W: Roux-en-Y on-line intussusception to avoid ascending cholangitis in biliary atresia. Arch Surg 118:1091, 1983
36. Tanaka K, Satomura K, Ohnishi S: A new operation for biliary atresia. J Jpn Soc Pediatr Surg 16:227, 1980
37. Shim W, Jin-Zhe Z: Antirefluxing Roux-en-Y. Biliary drainage valve for hepatic portoenterostomy: animal experiments and clinical experiments. J Pediatr Surg 20:689, 1985
38. Pappolordo G, Correnti S, Moborham S, et al: Long-term results of Roux-en-Y hepaticojejunostomy and hepaticojejunoduodenostomy. Ann Surg 196:149, 1982
39. Ohi R, Henamatsu M, Mochizuki I, et al: Reoperation in patients with biliary atresia. J Pediatr Surg 20:256, 1985
40. Hata Y, Uchino J, Kasai Y: Revision of portoenterostomy in congenital biliary atresia. J Pediatr Surg 20:217, 1985
41. Frietas L, Gauthier F, Valayer J: Second operation for biliary atresia. J Pediatr Surg 22:857, 1987
42. Warlin S, Sty J, Starshak R, et al: Intrahepatic biliary tract abnormalities in children with corrected extrahepatic biliary atresia. J Pediatr Gastroenterol Nutr 4:537, 1985

43. Smith E, Carson J, Tunell W, et al: Improved results with hepatic portoenterostomy. Ann Surg 195:746, 1982

44. Suruga K, Miyano T, Arai T, Deguchi E: A study on hepatic porto-enterostomy for the treatment of biliary atresia. Surg Gynecol Obstet 159:53, 1984

45. McClement J, Howard E, Mowat A: Results of surgical treatment for extrahepatic biliary atresia in the United Kingdom 1980–82. Br Med J 290:345, 1985

46. Andrews H, Zwiren G, Caplan D, Ricketts R: Biliary atresia: an evolving perspective. South Med J 79:581, 1986

47. Kasai M: Advances in treatment of biliary atresia. Jpn J Surg 13:265, 1983

48. Kobayashi A, Itabashi F, Ohbe Y: Long-term prognosis in biliary atresia after hepatic portoenterostomy: analysis of 35 patients who survived beyond 5 years. J Pediatr 105:243, 1984

49. Altman R, Levy J: Biliary atresia. Pediatr Ann 14:481, 1985

50. Canty T: Encouraging results with a modified Sawaguchi hepatoportoenterostomy for biliary atresia. Am J Surg 154:19, 1987

51. Burgess D, Martin H, Lilly J: The development status of children undergoing the Kasai operation for biliary atresia. Pediatrics 70:624, 1982

52. Stewart S, Vang R, Waller D, et al: Mental and motor development correlates in patients with end-stage biliary atresia awaiting liver transplantation. Pediatrics 79:882, 1987

53. Starzl TE, Iwatsuki S, Van Thiel DH: Evolution of liver transplantation. Hepatology 2:614, 1982

54. Lilly JR, Karrer FM: Contemporary surgery of biliary atresia. Pediatr Clin North Am 32:1233, 1985

55. Malatack JJ, Schaid JD, Urbach AM, et al: Choosing a pediatric recipient for orthotopic liver transplantation. J Pediatr 111:429, 1987

56. Esquivel CO, Iwatsuki S, Gordon RD, et al: Indications for pediatric liver transplantation. J Pediatr 6:1039, 1987

57. Starzl TE, Hakala TR, Shaw BW, et al: A flexible procedure for multiple cadaveric organ procurement. Surg Gynecol Obstet 158:223, 1984

58. Starzl TE, with assistance of Putnam CW: Experience in Hepatic Transplantation. Philadelphia, Saunders, 1969

59. Starzl TE, Iwatsuki S, Esquivel CO, et al: Refinements in the surgical technique of liver transplantation. Semin Liver Dis 5:349, 1985

60. Andrews WS, Wanek EA: Pediatric liver transplantation: a three-year experience. J Pediatr Surg (in press) J Pediatr 24:77, 1989

61. Esquivel CO, Koneru B, Karrer F, et al: Liver transplantation before 1 year of age. J Pediatr 110:545, 1987

77
Congenital Dilatation of the Bile Ducts

PATHOLOGY

The classic choledochal duct cyst consists of a rounded cystic dilatation of the common bile duct with distal narrowing. The hepatic ducts often are normal. In addition, Alonso-Lej et al. and later Klotz et al. included various types of biliary atresia, diverticulae, and dilatations of the intrahepatic bile ducts in their classification of choledochal cysts.[1,2] There is a form of cystic dilatation of the bile duct that occurs in early infancy with jaundice. This has been referred to as an "infantile" type of choledochal cyst. However, in some reported cases, there has been complete obstruction, and the course of these babies is similar to that of babies with biliary atresia. This should be classified as an extrahepatic biliary atresia. Other forms of bile duct dilatation have been referred to as "fusiform," "cylindrical dilatation," or "forme frust" choledochal cyst.[3-5] These classifications could be abandoned and all simply termed "congenital dilatation of the bile duct." There would be less confusion, since the pathology, etiology, and treatment of all these lesions are similar, and they are part of a spectrum of the same disease. The common bile duct dilatation varies from a maximum of 2 or 3 cm to a giant cyst containing a liter or more of bile. Distally, the duct narrows abruptly, but in the usual case, there is no anatomic obstruction. The cystic duct and gallbladder are distended, and the hepatic ducts vary in their involvement. Caroli described localized dilatations of the hepatic ducts that resemble a chain of lakes.[6] Caroli's disease may coexist with dilatation of the common bile duct or may exist independently. There is a predisposition to cholangitis, abscess, and stone formation even after adequate drainage of the hepatic ducts in Caroli's disease. Perhaps this condition is a link between congenital cystic dilatation of the common bile duct and liver cysts.[7]

Regardless of the gross appearance, microscopic examination of the duct wall in all these lesions is the main justification for grouping them together. Even in very young infants, the wall of the cyst is fibrous, and there are changes in the epithelium. In older patients, the epithelium is ulcerated, desquamated, and infiltrated with inflammatory cells. Often, there is no visible epithelium, only a thick fibrous wall. Epithelial metaplasia and cancer in situ also have been seen in adults.[8,9]

Abnormalities of the choledochopancreatic duct junction are almost universally seen in all forms of congenital cystic dilatation of the bile duct.[10-13] A variety of anomalies has been identified in this area, the most common being a right angle junction between the common bile duct and the pancreatic duct (Figs. 77–1, 77–2). A high entry of the pancreatic duct into the bile channel has also been noted (Fig. 77–3). The pressure in the pancreatic duct is higher, and, therefore, pancreatic juice drains into the biliary system. An elevated amylase level often is found in the duct at the time of operation. Attacks of pain with an elevated serum amylase level are attributed to pancreatitis in these children when in fact, they may have a normal pancreas. The elevated serum amylase is possibly due to its absorption from the damaged bile duct.[14] Anastomosis of the pancreatic duct to the gallbladder or bile duct in experimental animals produces a lesion identical to cystic dilatation of the bile duct in humans.[8,15] Even though the abnormal choledochal–pancreatic junction with reflux of pancreatic juice is the most likely etiology of these lesions, this may not be the entire story. Simple ligation of the bile duct in newborn animals produces a similar picture.[16] Also, by

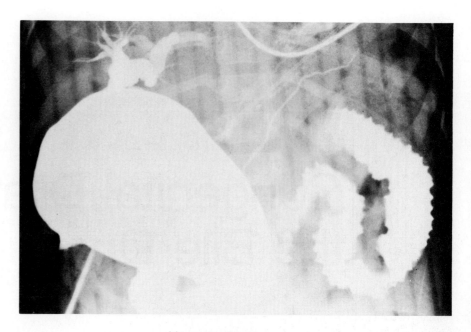

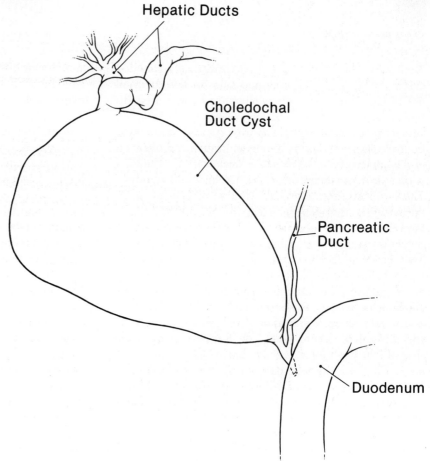

Hepatic Ducts

Choledochal
Duct Cyst

Pancreatic
Duct

Duodenum

Figure 77–1. Top. Operative cholangiogram of a classic choledochal duct cyst, demonstrating the giant dilatation of the common bile duct, with lesser dilation of the hepatic ducts. There is drainage of contrast medium into the duodenum, and the pancreatic duct is visualized. **Bottom.** Diagram of **top.**

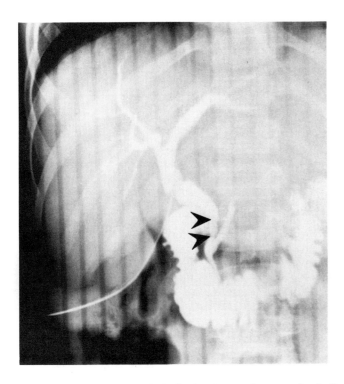 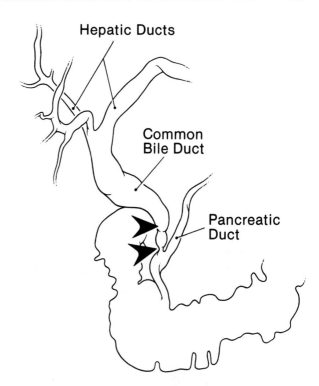

Figure 77–2. Left. Cholangiogram demonstrating fusiform dilatation or a forme fruste choledochal duct cyst. The arrows point to the insertion of the pancreatic duct into the common bile duct. **Right.** Diagram of **left.**

fetal ultrasonography, choledochal duct cysts have been diagnosed as early as the third trimester of pregnancy in the human fetus. Amylase does not appear in pancreatic secretions until after 1 month of age in full-term babies, although there are other proteolytic pancreatic enzymes present in the newborn.[17] The complications of congenital cystic dilatation of the bile duct include perforation during infancy, progressive biliary cirrhosis with portal hypertension, and biliary stone formation.[18–20] The most significant delayed complication is cancer of the bile duct. There is a 17.5 percent incidence of cancer developing in choledochal duct cysts reported in the Japanese literature.[21] The risk of malignant disease in young patients is much higher than in normal individuals. Sarcoma botryoides has developed in the cyst wall of a 4-year-old child, and the mean age of cancer detection is 35 years.[22] Almost all of the reported cases of carcinoma developed after a previous drainage procedure had been performed without resection of the cyst.

DIAGNOSIS

The classic triad of an abdominal mass, pain, and jaundice is rarely seen during childhood. Congenital cystic dilatation of the bile ducts may remain asymptomatic for many years. On the other hand, prolonged jaundice in the neonatal period may lead to the diagnosis. Episodic ab-

dominal pain, which may be vague and diffuse, is the most common presenting symptom. In older children, there may be a history of jaundice. The numbers of children diagnosed as having congenital cystic dilatation of the bile duct has risen dramatically with the widespread use of abdominal ultrasonography. This test should be carried out in any child with unexplained abdominal symptoms. It is worthwhile to perform serum amylase studies during acute episodes of pain and complete liver function tests once the diagnosis is suspected. The ultrasound study will reliably reveal minimal dilatation of the bile ducts and will accurately define the extent of the disease (Fig. 77–4). If there is doubt, for example, it may be difficult to distinguish a duplication of the duodenum from a cyst, a technetium excretion scan (HIDA or DISIDA) will outline the biliary tract. These two studies provide sufficient information about the bile ducts to proceed with an operation. Further definition of the anatomy is obtained with an operative cholangiogram, obviating the need for retrograde endoscopic cholangiography.

TREATMENT

Resection of the cyst with some form of internal drainage of the hepatic ducts into the intestine is the preferred treatment for all forms of cystic dilatation.[23–25] In the

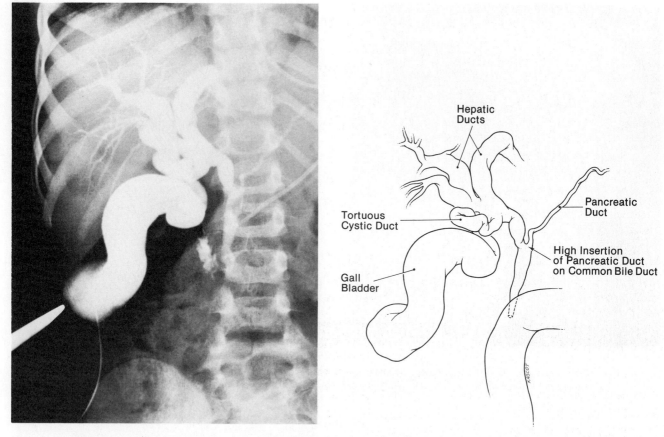

Figure 77–3. Left. Cholangiogram demonstrating a mildly dilated common bile duct with a high insertion of the pancreatic duct. The gallbladder is hugely distended, and the cystic duct is elongated and tortuous. **Right.** Diagram of **left.**

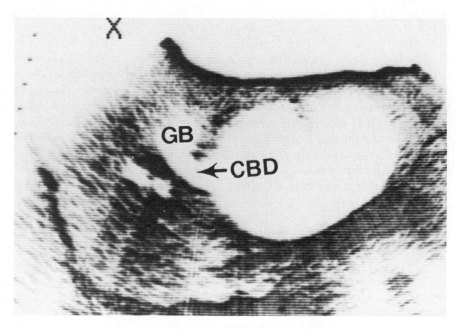

Figure 77–4. Ultrasound examination demonstrating a typical dilatation of the common bile duct, or choledochal duct cyst.

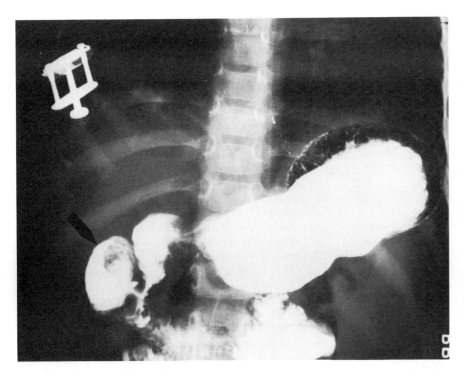

Figure 77–5. Postoperative upper gastrointestinal series demonstrating the antireflux valve in the isolated segment of jejunum that prevents reflux into the biliary tract. Barium fills the duodenum and the conduit up to the valve (arrow).

past, internal drainage without resection of the cyst led to long-term complications, including malignancy, stone formation, stricture, and cirrhosis. In our hands, simple choledochoduodenostomy for a minimally dilated common duct led to recurrent pain because of sludge and debris in the retained duct distal to the anastomosis in one girl 12 years after the operation.

Most surgeons now recommend resection of the cyst with anastomosis of the proximal hepatic duct to a Roux-en-Y loop. Our preference is for drainage into an isolated jejunal segment interposed between the hepatic duct and the duodenum with a 1 cm intussuscepted valve to prevent reflux (Fig. 77–5).

Technique

The child is positioned on an x-ray plate, and a preliminary film is taken after induction of anesthesia. A right subcostal or transverse incision as described for biliary atresia is made. Immediately after inspection of the pathology, a tube is sutured into the gallbladder and bile is aspirated. A sample may be sent for amylase determination, and then a cholangiogram is performed after the injection of contrast medium into the biliary system. We must visualize the entire ductal system in order to evaluate the intrahepatic bile ducts as well as the pancreaticobiliary junction. It is necessary to be absolutely certain about the location of the pancreatic duct before excision of the cyst. In all of our patients, we have first identified and isolated the hepatic artery and the portal vein, then removed the cyst completely. The distal end of the duct is closed just proximal to the pancreatic junction. Proximally, the lesion is resected to the hepatic ducts, removing the gallbladder and cystic duct as well. A frozen section should be made at the proximal end to determine if there is normal mucosa at the site of anastomosis. The hepatic ducts may be opened longitudinally or sutured together to make a common opening for the bowel anastomosis. This point is essential to avoid anastomotic stricture. An alternative technique to resect the cyst is to remove as much as possible, then take out only mucosa, leaving the fibrotic wall attached to the portal vessels. After resection of the bile duct, the isolated segment of jejunum is brought up through the mesocolon. The proximal bile duct is anastomosed end-to-side to the bowel, which is then sutured to the second portion of the duodenum. Absorbable 5-0 plastic sutures are used for each anastomosis. It has not been necessary to drain the wound or the bowel loop.

RESULTS

In our series of 14 patients using the isolated jejunal segment, there has been 1 anastomotic stricture that required reoperation. All other patients are clinically well on follow-up from 1 to 10 years. Repeat ultrasonography has not demonstrated dilatation of intrahepatic ducts, and there have been no episodes of cholangitis. The long-term prognosis will depend on the condition of the hepatic ducts. If there is associated Caroli's disease, the risk of cholangitis and abscess is higher. Time will tell if cancer will develop in the residual hepatic ducts. Ricketts has observed similar excellent results using the identical operation (R. Ricketts, personal communication). In the United States, follow-up after cyst excision has not been long enough to completely evaluate the procedure, but the long-term results in Japan appear to be excellent.

REFERENCES

1. Alonso-Lej F, Rever W, Pressagno DJ: Congenital choledochal cyst, with a report of 2 and an analysis of 94 cases. Int Abstr Surg 108:1, 1959
2. Klotz D, Cohn B, Kottmeir P: Choledochal cysts: diagnostic and therapeutic problems. J Pediatr Surg 8:271, 1973
3. Todani T, Watanabe Y, Fujii T, et al: Cylindrical dilatation of the choledochus: a special type of congenital bile duct dilatation. Surgery 98:964, 1985
4. Raffensperger J, Given G, Warrner R: Fusiform dilation of the common bile duct with pancreatitis. J Pediatr Surg 8:907, 1973
5. Lilly J, Stellin G, Karrer F: Forme fruste choledochal cyst. J Pediatr Surg 20:449, 1985
6. Caroli J: Diseases of the intrahepatic bile ducts. Isr J Med Sci 4:21, 1968
7. Barnes J, Polo J, Sanabia J, et al: Congenital cystic dilation of the intrahepatic bile ducts (Caroli's disease): report of a case and review of the literature. Surgery 85:589, 1979
8. Oguchi Y, Okada A, Nakamura T, et al: Histopathologic studies of congenital dilation of the bile duct as related to an anomalous junction of the pancreaticobiliary ductal system: clinical and experimental studies. Surgery 103:168, 1988
9. Komi N, Tamura T, Tsuge S, et al: Relation of patient age to premalignant alterations in choledochal cyst epithelium: histochemical and immunohistochemical studies. J Pediatr Surg 21:430, 1986
10. Babbit D, Starshak R, Sty J: Choledochal cyst pathogenesis, diagnosis and surgical implications. Appl Radiol Nov–Dec:125, 1981
11. Todani T, Watanabe Y, Fujii T, et al: Anomalous arrangement of the pancreaticobiliary ductal system in patients with a choledochal cyst. Am J Surg 147:672, 1984
12. Iwai N, Tokiwa K: Sphincter function of the bile duct in patients with congenital choledochal dilatation. J Jpn Soc Pediatr Surg 22:688, 1986
13. Ono J, Sakoda K, Akita H: Surgical aspect of cystic dilation of the bile duct: an anomalous junction of the pancreaticobiliary tree in adults. Ann Surg 195:203, 1982
14. Ohkawa H, Sawaguchi S, Khali B, et al: Cholangio-venous reflux as a cause of recurrent hyperamylasemia in choledochal dilatation with anomalous pancreaticobiliary ductal union: an experimental study. J Pediatr Surg 20:53, 1985
15. Miyano T, Suruga K, Shimomura H, et al: Choledochopancreatic elongated common channel disorders. J Pediatr Surg 19:165, 1984
16. Spitz L: Experimental production of cystic dilatation of the common bile duct in neonatal lambs. J Pediatr Surg 12:39, 1977
17. Howell C, Templeton J, Weiner S, et al: Antenatal diagnosis and early surgery for choledochal cyst. J Pediatr Surg 18:387, 1983
18. Donahoe P, Hendren W: Bile duct perforation in a newborn with stenosis of the ampulla of vater. J Pediatr Surg 11:823, 1976
19. Martin L, Rowe G: Portal hypertension secondary to choledochal cyst. Ann Surg 190:638, 1979
20. Harris V, Ramilo J, Radhakrishnan J: Choledochal cyst with cholelithiasis: 15 year follow-up. J Pediatr Surg 14:191, 1979
21. Todani T, Watanabe Y, Toki A, Urushihara N: Carcinoma related to choledochal cysts with internal drainage operations. Surg Gynecol Obstet 164:61, 1987
22. Tsuchiya R, Harada N, Ito T, et al: Malignant tumors in choledochal cysts. Ann Surg 186:22, 1977
23. Ishida M, Tsuchida Y, Saito S, Hori T: Primary excision of choledochal duct cysts. Surgery 68:884, 1970
24. Lilly J: The surgical treatment of choledochal cyst. Surg Gynecol Obstet 149:36, 1979
25. Saing H, Tam P, Lee J, Pe-Nyun P: Surgical management of choledochal cysts: a review of 60 cases. J Pediatr Surg 20:443, 1985

SECTION X

Respiratory Distress

From the first gasp and cry, the normal newborn infant quickly adapts to extrauterine existence. The infant's respiratory tract undergoes considerable change to make these adaptations. The normal neonate breathes 40 to 60 times per minute with a tidal volume of approximately 15 ml. The infant is an obligatory nose breather whose tongue is large in comparison to the oral pharynx. He or she breathes primarily with the diaphragm, since the ribs are nearly horizontal and the intercostal muscles are poorly developed. The trachea lacks firm cartilaginous support for several months and is only 4 to 6 mm in diameter.

Respiratory distress in the newborn infant is most often due to the idiopathic respiratory distress syndrome, or hyaline membrane disease. There are, however, a number of mechanical problems that the surgeon can relieve. These include airway obstructions anywhere from the nose to the bronchi, compression of lung tissue by air, fluid, or blood in the pleural cavities, anatomic defects in the diaphragm, and intrinsic pulmonary lesions that compress normal lung tissue or alter pulmonary blood flow.

In this section, we consider primarily those conditions that affect the newborn, but almost every lesion presented here can and does affect older children as well. Thus, not only are the principles of airway care similar for older children, but many of the lesions are as well.

The symptoms of respiratory distress are completely nonspecific. Babies as well as older children respond to respiratory insufficiency with tachypnea, retractions, and finally cyanosis. Since breathing and eating are so closely related, some infants with major airway problems show only tachypnea and poor feeding. It would appear that beyond a certain respiratory rate (approximately 70 to 80), babies cannot breathe and swallow at the same time. Cyanosis without respiratory distress suggests a congenital cardiac defect with a right-to-left shunt. At the same time, tachypnea and air hunger may also be secondary to heart failure.

The clinical examination of a newborn with respiratory distress commences with observation of the baby's head and neck. Several lesions are obvious. A receding jaw with a retrodisplaced tongue is diagnostic for the Pierre Robin syndrome, and a large tongue obstructing the airway may be secondary to hemangioma, hygroma, or the muscular hypertrophy seen in Beckwith's syndrome. Drooling of saliva should automatically make one think of esophageal atresia. Tumors in the neck, such as hygromas, congenital goiter, or a second branchial cleft cyst, may compress the trachea. All of these cervical lesions are treated with prompt surgical excision, but it must be realized that a large hygroma in the neck is often associated with similar tissue in the pharynx and larynx. Palpation of the oral cavity at the base of the tongue will reveal an obstructing thyroglossal duct cyst at the foramen cecum. This can be differentiated from an ectopic thyroid, which represents failure of the gland's descent, by pulling the tongue forward and aspirating the cyst with a syringe and needle. The next step is the passage of a size 8 French plastic feeding tube through each nostril and down the esophagus into the stomach. Confirmation of the passage of this tube with a roentgenogram rules out choanal and esophageal atresia. If the tube stops in the nose, the baby may have choanal atresia and will need an oral airway while the diagnosis is confirmed with the injection of contrast material into the nasal cavity.

Palpation and ausculation of the chest are performed, specifically to find gross shifts of the mediastinum by noting the position of the apex beat. It is difficult for any but an experienced examiner to deduce such information from auscultation of the lungs. Breath sounds are readily transmitted even when there is a complete lung collapse. This rapid clinical examination is completed by observation of the abdomen. A scaphoid abdomen with an enlarged chest is a classic indication of a foramen of Bochdalek diaphragmatic hernia. On the other hand, abdominal distention and elevation of the diaphragms will hinder respiration just as much as an intrinsic pulmonary problem.

The next step consists of radiologic evaluation of the chest and upper airway. This is a most important x-ray, which must be obtained with perfect technique and then correctly interpreted because nothing delays a diagnosis quite so much as a "negative" or incorrect x-ray report. Portable films are generally not satisfactory. Consequently, arrangements must be made to properly support the infant while he or she is in the x-ray department. A posteroanterior, lateral, upright chest film is obtained. The lateral film should be taken with the baby's head and neck extended and the shoulders held down. This provides an anterolateral view of the trachea and is an excellent technique for finding lesions in the neck

or mediastinum that compress the airway. If the radiopaque catheter is clearly in the stomach, ruling out an esophageal atresia, a barium swallow may reveal either a vascular ring that compresses both the trachea and esophagus or an H-type tracheoesophageal fistula. During these initial diagnostic maneuvers, the baby should be nursed in a heated, humidified incubator with oxygen concentrations determined by blood gas analysis. Mucus is suctioned from the oropharynx, and if the patient is not making satisfactory respiratory efforts at that point, endotracheal intubation and respiratory support are indicated. An airway obstruction that is not demonstrated by these studies will require endoscopy. A poor cry or stridor is an indication of a vocal cord lesion or laryngeal stenosis. Wheezing occurs with obstructive lesions in the trachea or bronchi. Laryngoscopy and bronchoscopy should be carried out in the operating room, with preparations made for immediate endotracheal intubation or tracheotomy if a serious obstructive lesion is found. The lesions discussed in the following chapters are in themselves rare and unusual. The examiner is unlikely to overlook these problems if he or she follows the aforementioned sequence of clinical, radiologic, and endoscopic routes to a correct diagnosis.

78

Upper Airway Obstruction in the Newborn

_____ *Lauren D. Holinger*

Obstruction of the upper respiratory system in the newborn is an acute emergency, requiring immediate and accurate diagnosis and treatment. Cyanosis due to obstruction of the repiratory tract must be differentiated from lesions of the cardiovascular, gastrointestinal, and central nervous systems (Table 78–1). Lesions of the cardiovascular and central nervous systems can be ruled out if the cyanotic infant is making a vigorous effort to breathe. Lesions such as subdural hematoma (in association with a birth injury) or cerebral agenesis may result in decreased respiratory drive and apnea because of an abnormality of the respiratory center. In such cases the infant is flaccid and unresponsive and reflexes are severely impaired or absent. Cardiovascular anomalies cause cyanosis because of shunts or cardiac decompensation. As with central lesions, the infant breathes quietly. Auscultation may reveal a cardiac murmur, irregular rate or rhythm, and enlargement or displacement of the heart. Only with respiratory tract obstruction will the cyanotic infant be making strenuous and active respiratory effort. In this case, respirations are labored. Dyspnea is associated with suprasternal and epigastric retractions, agitation, wheezing, and stridor. The infant is tachypneic. A respiratory rate over 60 is distinctly abnormal.[1]

Consideration must be given to determine whether the airway obstruction involves the pleural cavities (as in spontaneous pneumothorax or Bochdalek diaphragmatic hernia), the lungs (as in hyaline membrane disease, idiopathic lobar emphysema, or agenesis of a lung), or the airway itself. This chapter is concerned primarily with those lesions that compromise the airway itself (Table 78–2).

If the newborn infant is severely obstructed, he or she must be immediately suctioned and the tongue pulled forward. This assures a patent airway above the larynx. If the obstruction persists, a laryngoscope with a straight blade is used to lift the base of tongue and epiglottis to visualize the larynx. If the larynx is patent, a small (2.0) endotracheal tube is placed carefully between the vocal cords and into the midtrachea. If the infant remains in severe distress after suctioning, it is concluded that the problem is related to the lungs or pleural cavities, and a chest x-ray is obtained immediately. Appropriate treatment is determined by the roentgenogram.

When the obstruction is less severe and time permits a more orderly approach, the infant is observed carefully. Cyanosis is seen most readily in the perioral region and the nails of the fingers and toes. Pulse and respiratory rates are noted. Gross deformities—such as micrognathia and Pierre Robin syndrome, cleft lip and palate, or a

TABLE 78–1. DIFFERENTIAL DIAGNOSIS OF CYANOSIS IN THE NEWBORN

Central nervous system: Apnea
    Maternal anesthesia
    Congenital anomaly
    Birth trauma
Cardiovascular system
    Congenital heart disease
Gastrointestinal system
    Gastroesophageal reflux
    Tracheoesophageal fistula
Respiratory system
    Airway obstruction

TABLE 78–2. AIRWAY OBSTRUCTION IN THE NEWBORN

Nose
  Congenital nasal deformities (agenesis, vestibular atresia, deviated septum)
  Traumatic nasal deformities (displaced nasal septum, septal hematoma, nasal fracture)
  Stuffy nose syndrome (turbinate hypertrophy)
  Bilateral choanal atresia
Pharynx
  Nasopharyngeal mass (encephalocele, teratoma, glioma, adenoids)
  Facial retrusion (craniofacial anomalies: Crouzon's syndrome, Apert's syndrome)
  Pierre Robin syndrome (glossoptosis, micrognathia)
  Base of tongue mass (lingual thyroid, thyroglossal duct cyst, lingual tonsil hypertrophy)
  Neurologic lesions (IX, X)
  Hypertrophy of tonsils and adenoids
  Peritonsillar abscess, lateral pharyngeal space abscess
  Retropharyngeal mass (abscess, tumor)
Larynx
  Laryngomalacia
  Neurologic lesions (vocal cord paralysis)
  Subglottic stenosis
  Cartilagenous stenosis
    Cricoid cartilage deformity
    Trapped first tracheal ring
  Soft tissue stenosis
  Webs, atresia
  Neoplasms
    Hemangioma (subglottic)
    Lymphangioma (cystic hygroma)
    Recurrent respiratory papillomatosis
  Cleft larynx and other anomalies
Tracheobronchial tree
  Tracheomalacia, bronchomalacia
  Vascular anomalies (aberrant innominate artery, double aortic arch, pulmonary artery sling)
  Tracheoesophageal fistula and esophageal atresia
  Tracheal webs and stenoses
  Accessory bronchi and lobes
  Foregut cysts (bronchogenic cysts, esophageal duplication)
  Pulmonary sequestration

mass in the neck that may compress the airway—are readily observed. The index finger may be used to palpate for a mass in the base of the tongue or nasopharynx. If placing the infant in a supine position or pulling the tongue forward relieves the obstruction, small catheters may be placed through each nostril to check the patency of the posterior choanae. A lateral soft tissue x-ray of the head, neck, and chest and a standard posteroranterior chest film are obtained. These studies quickly define gross abnormalities of the chest, abdomen and nasopharynx. They are most important in supplementing auscultation of the chest, which is extremely difficut in a struggling newborn (Fig. 78–1). The lateral film of the chest, head, and neck is most productive when taken with the head and neck extended and the shoulders down and back. Lesions in the nasopharynx, base of tongue,

and larynx often can be identified and compression of the trachea can be observed. Passage of a small radiopaque feeding tube through the mouth to the stomach will rule out esophageal atresia. If the tube does not pass or if there is continued aspiration of secretions, a small swallow of barium may delineate an esophageal stenosis, tracheoesophageal fistula, vascular rings, that compress the trachea and esophagus, or neurologic lesions that affect cranial nerves IX and X, producing aspiration and dysphagia. The radiologist must also look for gastroesophageal reflux, which may produce symptoms of coughing, choking, aspiration pneumonia, and respiratory arrest in infants.[2]

Prenatal ultrasonography can detect fetal anomalies, including cervical tumors that cause neonatal airway obstruction. When a potential airway obstruction is detected by prenatal diagnosis, an elective cesarean section allows preparation for establishing an airway in the delivery room. We have observed an infant with a cervical teratoma that was diagnosed by prenatal ultrasonography. In this case, we were prepared with laryngoscopes, an assortment of endotracheal tubes, bronchoscopes, and a tracheotomy tray. The infant was intubated at birth, and the tumor was removed electively the next day.

OBSTRUCTION OF THE NOSE AND PHARYNX

Congenital nasal deformities include agenesis of the nose, vestibular atresia, and deviated nasal septum. Birth trauma to the nose also may cause upper airway obstruction. A few neonates have been identified whose nasal airways were occluded by a diffuse swelling of the mucosal lining. Passage of nasal catheters demonstrates patency of the choanae. Administration of a mild vasoconstrictive nasal decongestant, such as 3 percent ephedrine, shrinks the mucosa enough to allow the infant to breathe without difficulty. This cause of airway obstruction is of undetermined etiology. It usually resolves within several days or weeks or ceases to become clinically significant when the child learns to mouth breathe. These infants must be fed with frequent pauses, since they cannot breathe and swallow at the same time. If nose drops do not establish an airway, it may be necessary to insert an oral–esophageal airway and a feeding tube (B. Benjamin, personal communication). If this is unsatisfactory, endotracheal intubation or even a tracheotomy may be necessary.

Bilateral choanal atresia, or congenital atresia of the posterior nares, produces respiratory obstruction in the newborn and requires prompt, effective measures. As with any obstructing lesion above the larynx, opening the patient's mouth and pulling the tongue forward relieves the obstruction. The diagnosis may be established

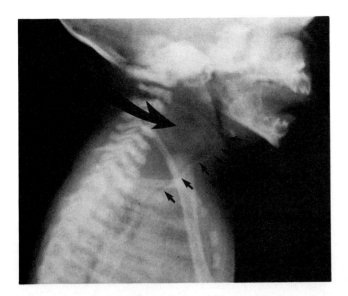

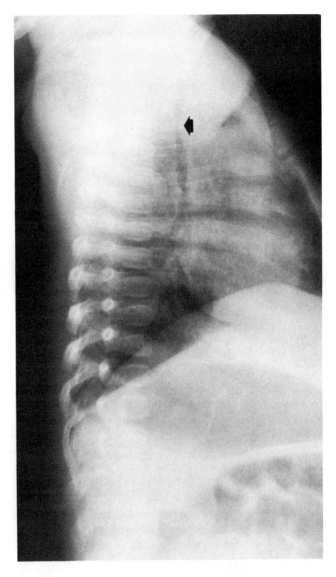

Figure 78–1. Left. An endolateral roentgenogram demonstrating an air–fluid level in a third brachial cyst that was compressing the larynx and trachea. **Right.** Endolateral x-ray of an older infant with tracheomalacia. The trachea is narrow over several centimeters with no definite point of indentation.

by the simple maneuver of passing a catheter through the nose into the nasopharynx. If it cannot be passed beyond 32 mm from the edge of the nostril, atresia is present. If it can be passed 44 mm or more, patency is apparent.[3] If the number 8 or 10 French red rubber catheter will not pass, methylene blue may be dropped into the nostrils; the dye will appear in the pharynx if the choanae are patent. An alternative method involves the instillation of Lipiodol and obtaining a lateral skull film of the infant in a supine position (Fig. 78–2). The definitive study is a coronal computed tomography (CT) scan.

Immediate treatment involves establishing a secure airway for as long as it takes the infant to learn mouth breathing. A McGovern nipple (a rubber nipple with a large hole in it carefully taped in the mouth) frequently is used.[4] Alternatively, an oral airway may be used.

Using the operating microscope, a transnasal approach may be used to correct bony atresia at an early date. If the transpalatal approach is to be used, it is deferred until the infant reaches 6 to 24 months of age.

Pharynx

A large nasopharyngeal mass may completely occlude the nasal airways. As is the case with bilateral choanal atresia, the infant may asphyxiate if an adequate oral airway is not established immediately. Complete obstruction is unusual with these lesions. More often these infants are seen with moderate respiratory distress and an irregular, low-pitched, coarse stridor. Hypertrophied

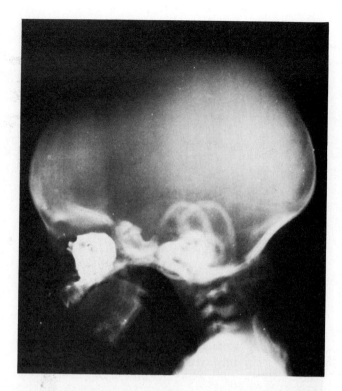

Figure 78–2. Upper airway, choanal atresia. With Lipiodol instilled into the anterior nares, this lateral roentgenogram demonstrates a complete block.

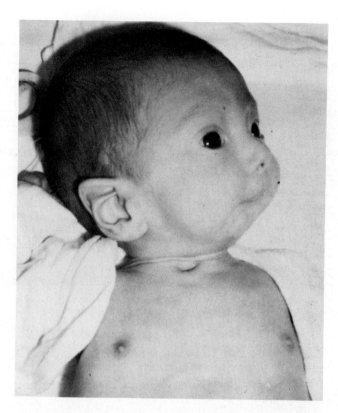

Figure 78–3. The Pierre Robin syndrome is readily recognized by micrognathia, retrodisplaced tongue, and a midline cleft palate.

adenoids may produce partial obstruction, as will cysts, gliomas, and fibromas. Before taking a biopsy or excising such a lesion, one must be certain that there is no communication with the central nervous system, as with an encephalocele or meningocele. A lateral soft tissue radiograph and views of the cervical spine are obtained. CT is the best imaging technique to demonstrate connections with the central nervous system.

Micrognathia when associated with glossoptosis is known as the Pierre Robin syndrome. Over half of afflicted infants have cleft palates, as well (Fig. 78–3). Their difficulty in breathing may be quite severe and is usually associated with dysphagia and failure to gain weight. The characteristic birdlike or Andy Gump appearance of the newborn makes further diagnostic evaluation superfluous. Some infants exhibit only mild respiratory distress and have little difficulty with feeding. These infants usually feed best in a semi-erect position with frequent pauses to breathe. Respiratory distress is minimized by placing the infant in a prone position, allowing gravity to aid in pulling the tongue and mandible forward out of the pharynx to provide an airway. Other infants with Pierre Robin syndrome may be in severe respiratory distress at birth. A towel clip or suture may be placed through the infant's tongue to hold it forward and thus provide an emergency airway until a proper glossopexy can be undertaken. A number 5 silk suture is placed

through the base of the tongue at a depth of 0.5 cm. Each end of the suture is then passed through the cartilaginous portion of the mandible 1 cm lateral to the midline and tied.[5] If respiratory difficulties persist or if the child has continued dysphagia with vomiting and aspiration in spite of good nursing care and gavage feedings, tracheotomy should be undertaken. Monroe demonstrated, with 65 patients at Children's Memorial Hospital in Chicago over a 20-year period, that tracheotomy decreases the time of hospitalization and significantly improves survival in such patients.[6] Eventually, as the mandible grows, the posterior displacement of the tongue is relieved and the child's airway improves.

A mass at the base of the tongue may severely compromise the airway of the newborn. Thyroglassal duct cyst and lingual thyroid are not uncommon, whereas hypertrophy of the lingual tonsils is a most unusual cause of airway obstruction. Diagnosis can be confirmed by palpation of the base of the tongue with an index finger or by lateral soft tissue x-ray of the head and neck. One may temporize by placing a traction suture through the tongue to hold it forward. In some cases, more definitive steps may be necessary to maintain an adequate airway. A thyroid scan should be obtained before any such mass is resected, since there may be no other thyroid tissue present in the normal location in the neck. A cyst may be aspirated and then partially excised and the posterior wall marsupialized.

Bulbar lesions and other causes of paralysis of cranial nerves IX and X, which innervate the pharyngeal musculature, may produce respiratory difficulties because of overflow of secretions into the trachea. Congenital esophageal stenosis and atresia may produce a similar picture.

OBSTRUCTION OF THE LARYNX

The narrowest point in the airway between the nasopharynx and the carina is the larynx. Consequently, it is the most common site of neonatal airway obstruction. The laryngeal aperture of the infant is triangular, approximately 7 mm anteroposteriorly by 4 mm across the posterior commissure. The glottic chink is, therefore, calculated to have an area of 14 mm^2. A single millimeter of edema of the mucosal surfaces of the glottis will reduce the opening to 5 mm^2, only 36 percent of the normal lumen.[7] Similarly, the soft areolar tissue of the subglottic region encased in the rigid cricoid ring rapidly swells with the trauma of intubation or infection at the expense of the airway, producing respiratory obstruction that can be relieved only be reintubation or tracheotomy.

Congenital anomalies of the larynx may produce varying degrees of upper airway obstruction. The infant may have dyspnea, wheezing, stridor, and cyanosis. With laryngeal involvement, there is associated dysphonia, hoarseness, or a weak or absent cry. Dysphagia, aspiration, and other abnormalities of deglutition comprise a third group of symptoms that may be associated with congenital anomalies of the larynx.

Technique of Laryngoscopy

The difficulty of laryngoscopy in infants is due to the small size of the larynx and the curled, short, slippery, omega-shaped epiglottis. The larynx is easily displaced by too deep penetration of the laryngoscope tip into the hypopharynx. The tendency toward laryngospasm as the laryngoscope is introduced often makes visualization of the true cords and glottic airway difficult.

Several types of laryngoscopes are available for use in children, with a range of sizes for each type. The most commonly used laryngoscope is tubular, with a spatulous tip slightly flared at the distal end. A proximal removable section facilitates introduction of a bronchoscope or other instruments. This standard laryngoscope (Jackson) is useful for an overall view of the pharynx, base of tongue, and larynx. It is most useful in the diagnosis of laryngomalacia. The blade of the laryngoscope is placed in the vallecula, and the omega-shaped epiglottis and arytenoids are more easily evaluated with the epiglottis visible under the blade of the laryngoscope. The disad-

vantage of the standard laryngoscope is that visualization of the anterior commissure is difficult, since soft tissue structures usually slide into the field of vision anteriorly. Anterior commissure laryngoscopes that are tubular in shape and somewhat pointed anteriorly overcome this difficulty. In certain instances, an anterior commissure laryngoscope can be passed between the vocal cords to observe the immediate subglottic larynx and proximal trachea. Instrumentation for laryngoscopy of the infant includes a 3 mm × 20 cm ventilating bronchoscope to establish a lumen if obstruction occurs or if laryngospasm cannot be broken. The endoscopist must be accomplished at endotracheal intubation and must have a range of tiny endotracheal tubes available. A tracheotomy set must be in the room for use in an extreme emergency.

The mobility of the true vocal cords is determined either with a small flexible laryngoscope inserted through the nose or with an 8 cm anterior commissure laryngoscope inserted into the vallecula to visualize the glottis and the anterior commissure. Care must be taken to avoid limiting vocal cord mobility with the tip of the laryngoscope, and the initial portion of the examination is done without general anesthesia. The vocal cords are visualized during phonation or a cry. General anesthesia with the insufflation technique is then carried out for more thorough laryngoscopy and bronschoscopy with a 0 degree telescope. If there is severe airway obstruction, a tracheotomy may be necessary.

Laryngomalacia is the most common congenital anomaly of the larynx, comprising 75 percent of all laryngeal anomalies.[7] It produces a transient inspiratory stridor in infants and is caused by an abnormal flaccidity of the supraglottic laryngeal structures: the epiglottis, arytenoids, and aryepiglottic folds, especially the cuneiform cartilages. Typically, the stridor of laryngomalacia is present soon after birth but may first appear as late as 3 months of age. The stridor is low-pitched, may be constant or intermittent, and often varies with the position of the infant. It is louder when the infant is supine and may be absent when the infant is prone. Laryngoscopy is necessary to confirm the diagnosis and to rule out other causes of stridor. The supraglottic structures collapse inward during inspiration and are opened during expiration (Fig. 78–4). Generally, symptoms subside gradually after 12 to 18 months. Tracheotomy has been necessary only in extreme cases when the infant was unable to sleep adequately or when feedings were accompanied by severe cyanosis and the infant failed to gain weight. It has been possible to avoid tracheotomy in some patients with a supraglottoplasty, removing the flaccid obstructing tissue endoscopically.[8]

Bilateral vocal cord paralysis or paresis may produce an alarming degree of respiratory obstruction. It is seen in otherwise normal infants but is found more often in association with other congenital anomalies.[9] Inspiratory

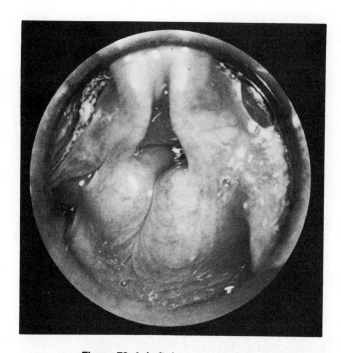 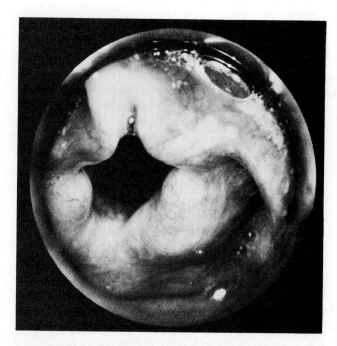

Figure 78–4. Left. Laryngomalacia on inspiration. The arytenoids are seen to collapse inward during inspiration. Only the tip of the photographic speculum prevents the omega-shaped epiglottis from collapsing inward as well. **Right.** Laryngomalacia on expiration. The arytenoids are abducted, and an adequate airway is observed. The larynx appears normal.

stridor is the most prominent symptom of bilateral vocal cord paralysis. The diagnosis of bilateral vocal cord paralysis is obscured by the paradoxical association of a relatively clear cry with varying degrees of respiratory obstruction. This is caused by paralysis of the abductor muscles of the vocal cords, leaving the cords in adduction, the position of phonation (Fig. 78–5). The vocal cords act as a one-way valve, allowing normal cry and expiration but tending to obstruct the larynx and to produce stridor during inspiration. The diagnosis may be overlooked in infants with stridor if the larynx is not examined by direct laryngoscopy without anesthesia. The condition may be overdiagnosed if general anesthesia is used because of the diminished muscular activity produced by the anesthetic. Tracheotomy may be necessary for airway obstruction due to bilateral vocal cord paralysis. The function of the vocal cords is evaluated by laryngoscopy at regular intervals, and the infant is decannulated when abductor function returns and the obstruction resolves.

Congenital subglottic stenosis is the third most common laryngeal anomaly, comprising approximately 6 percent of congenital laryngeal lesions.[10] Congenital subglottic stenosis is a laryngeal stenosis occurring between the glottis (true vocal cords) and the first tracheal ring, within the confines of the cricoid cartilage. The narrowest point is usually 2 to 3 cm below the superior surface of the vocal cords and may be caused by an anterior cartilagenous thickening (Fig. 78–6). The histopathologic clas-

sification of subglottic stenosis is outlined in Table 78–3.

The comprised airway is manifested by inspiratory and expiratory stridor, and tracheotomy is necessary in approximately 40 percent of patients.[11] Less severe stenoses cause recurrent or persistent episodes of croup, which was the presenting problem in 34 percent of 115 consecutive cases of congenital subglottic stenosis seen at the Children's Memorial Hospital in Chicago. Subglottic stenosis is the most common congenital laryngeal lesion that can cause severe respiratory distress. Obstruction may develop with alarming rapidity when an acute respiratory infection is superimposed on the already compromised subglottic airway. Minimal laryngeal inflammation can precipitate a tracheotomy, since the limiting cricoid cartilage does not permit swelling of the tissues in any direction other than inward at the expense of the airway.

The correct diagnosis, suggested by the symptoms and x-rays, is established by direct laryngoscopy. The soft tissue type of stenosis appears as a concentric narrowing or bilateral subglottic swelling that leaves a narrow, oblong lumen. The cartilagenous type of anomaly is diagnosed by palpation of a hard stenosis. The diameter of the subglottic space in a normal newborn is 4.5 mm; if the tip of a 3 mm bronchoscope cannot pass, a subglottic stenosis is present. Mild stenosis resolves with growth of the larynx. Gentle endoscopic dilatation at regular

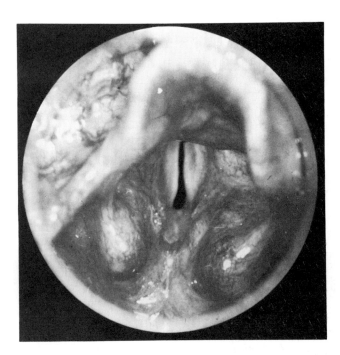

Figure 78–5. Bilateral vocal cord paralysis. The vocal cords are paralyzed in the paramedian position, unable to abduct, producing a marginal airway.

intervals is considered helpful but should not be attempted unless a tracheotomy is already established. Resulting edema can quickly compromise the limited airway.

Acquired subglottic stenosis is most often caused

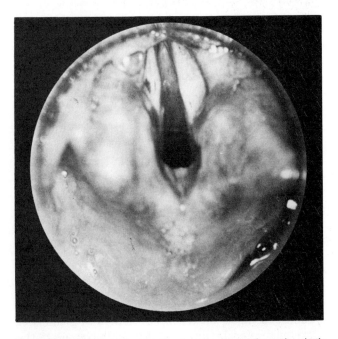

Figure 78–6. Congenital subglottic stenosis. Almost the entire glottic lumen is obliterated by an anterior subglottic stenosis, seen between the vocal cords. Only a small lumen remains posteriorly.

TABLE 78–3. HISTOPATHOLOGIC CLASSIFICATION OF SUBGLOTTIC STENOSIS

Cartilagenous stenosis (usually congenital)
  Cricoid cartilage deformity
    Normal shape, small size
    Abnormal shape
      Large anterior or posterior lamina
      Generalized thickening
      Elliptical shape
      Cleft: partial, occult (submucosal), complete
      Flattened shape
      Other, including acquired lesions
  Trapped first tracheal ring
Soft tissue stenosis (usually acquired)
    Submucosal mucous gland hyperplasia
    Submucosal cysts
    Submucosal fibrosis
    Granulation tissue

by prolonged endotracheal intubation in premature infants with the respiratory distress syndrome. After extubation, there may be an immediate upper airway obstruction that requires reintubation. In some, there is only repeated atelectasis, pneumonia, and progressive symptoms of airway obstruction. In the past, these infants all required a tracheotomy, and the prognosis was more serious than for infants with congenital laryngeal stenosis.[11] Traditionally, after a tracheotomy, these patients were treated with progressive dilatation. The early stenoses responded to this treatment, but many required the tracheotomy for over 2 years.

Alternative methods of management, including surgical reconstruction, are gaining wide acceptance.[12–14] Cotton and Evans reported 101 patients who underwent laryngotracheal reconstruction (LTR) for severe subglottic stenosis. In these patients, it was possible to remove the tracheotomy much earlier than previously, and there was only 1 surgical death.[15]

Ideally, severe subglottic stenosis would be treated without tracheotomy. Cotton and Seid were the first to accomplish this in premature infants by using the anterior cricoid split (ACS).[16] They devised the operation as an alternative to tracheotomy when extubation attempts failed. Johnson and Steward used the infant urethral resectoscope to avoid tracheotomy in 3 children.[17] We have successfully managed 6 infants and children with severe subglottic stenosis with the endoscopic application of the CO_2 laser. A tracheotomy was avoided in all.[18]

Technique of Anterior Cricoid Split

The patient is positioned as for tracheotomy. The thyroid isthmus is divided. The cricoid cartilage and first two tracheal rings are divided in the midline, extending the incision through the mucosa to expose the endotracheal tube (Fig. 78–7). The incision of the thyroid cartilage

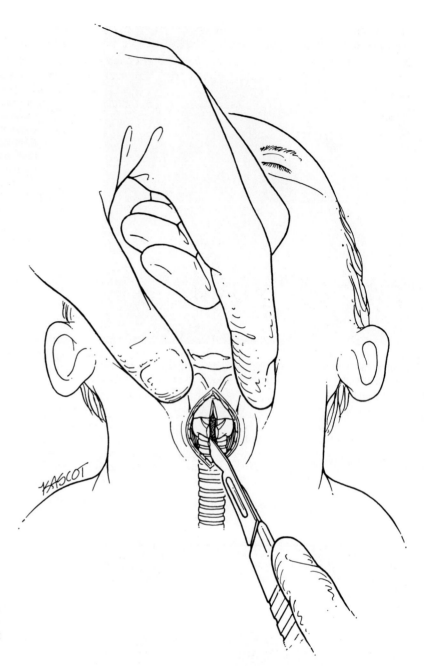

Figure 78–7. Anterior cricoid split incision through the lower two thirds of the thyroid cartilage, the cricoid cartilage, and the first two tracheal rings.

is carried to within 2 mm of the thyroid notch. The soft tissues and skin are loosely approximated, and a small drain is placed. The endotracheal tube is left in place 7 to 14 days. Extreme measures are taken to avoid inadvertent extubation, particularly during the first 5 postoperative days. Heavy sedation and even paralysis with assisted ventilation may be necessary.

Extubation may be carried out in the operating room but more often is accomplished in the neonatal intensive care unit. The patient should be off any ventilator support. Planned extubation is deferred in the presence of pneumonia, atelectasis, fever, or any other acute illness. The presence of a small air leak around the tube at 15

mm of water is a good prognostic sign. Dexamethasone (Decadron, 1 to 1.5 mm/kg) is given as an (IV) bolus several hours before extubation.

Ultrasonic humidity and chest physical therapy are given routinely following extubation. If respiratory distress develops acutely, racemic epinephrine is given by nebulizer. If airway obstruction progresses, the child is returned to the operating room for repeat endoscopic evaluation under general anesthesia. Aspiration of secretions, laryngeal dilatation, or excision of granulation tissue may obviate the need for reintubation. If this fails, repeat ACS or tracheotomy is the only alternative.

The operation has proved to be effective. Of a total

of 138 cases reviewed by Holinger et al., tracheotomy was avoided and extubation was accomplished successfully in 106 (77 percent).[19] In some patients, laryngotracheal stenosis progresses and tracheotomy is unavoidable.

For more than 30 years, various surgical procedures have been advanced for the definitive treatment of severe laryngotracheal stenosis. In 1956, Rethi described techniques by which the anterior and posterior cricoid lamina were divided vertically in the midline then stented.[20] He also stressed the importance of not disturbing scar tissue within the larynx. Grahne also advocated surgical

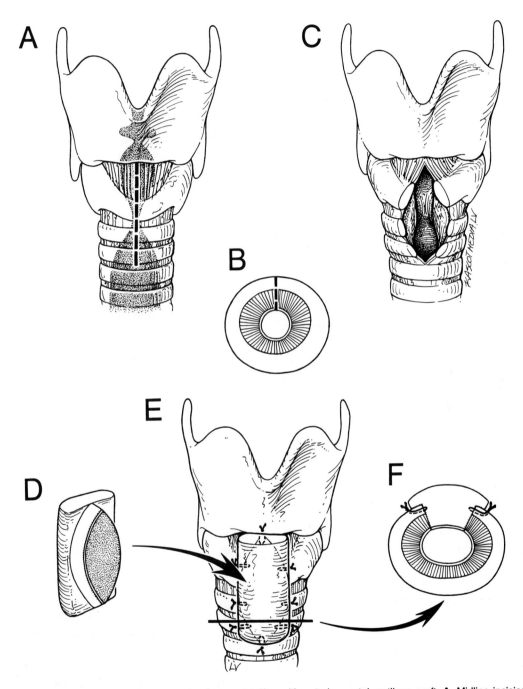

Figure 78–8. Fearon-Cotton laryngotracheal reconstruction with anterior costal cartilage graft. **A.** Midline incision through the involved portions of the larynx and trachea. **B.** Horizontal cross-section of the anterior incision. **C.** Larynx and trachea open anteriorly, revealing the thickened soft tissue subglottic stenosis within the laryngeal lumen. **D.** Fusiform costal cartilage graft with the perichondrium facing toward the laryngeal lumen. **E.** Graft sutured in place. **F.** Horizontal cross-section illustrating the flange that prevents the graft from being displaced into the lumen.

TABLE 78–4. INDICATIONS FOR LARYNGOTRACHEAL RECONSTRUCTION

Severe subglottic stenosis (tracheotomy dependent)
Long-term institutionalization; tenuous home care environment
Severe cricoid cartilage deformity
1 year of age; 8 kg weight
Good pulmonary reserve (no oxygen or ventilator requirement)
Likely failure of conservative (endoscopic) management (Table 78–5)

TABLE 78–5. FACTORS ASSOCIATED WITH FAILURE OF ENDOSCOPIC MANAGEMENT OF SEVERE LARYNGOTRACHEAL STENOSIS

Circumferential cicatricial scarring
Lengthy vertical dimension of stenosis
Significant loss of cartilage
Preceding severe bacterial infection associated with tracheotomy
Posterior commissure stenosis with arytenoid fixation
Refractory to dilation above 12 French × 3
Concomitant mid or lower tracheal pathology[14]

Modified from Simpson et al.[24]

intervention.[21] He modified one of the basic concepts of the procedure by excising scar tissue in cases of cicatricial stenosis. In 1974, Evans and Todd used the term "laryngotracheoplasty" to describe the technique of an anterior casselated incision through the thyroid cartilage, cricoid cartilage, and upper trachea.[22] Scar tissue within the laryngeal lumen was excised, and the larynx was stented. About the same time, Fearon and Cotton proposed a modification of the technique described by Rethi and performed laryngotracheal reconstruction using costal cartilage to expand the laryngeal lumen (Fig. 78–8).[23]

LTR is considered only if the stenosis is so severe that the child is tracheotomy dependent (Table 78–4). Patients are selected for LTR if there is poor response to endoscopic therapy when there is little likelihood of decannulation in the foreseeable future (Table 78–5). Conservative therapy includes serial laryngeal dilatation alone or in conjunction with other modes of therapy, such as (1) endoscopic surgical removal of subglottic or tracheal soft tissue by cupped forceps, CO_2 laser, or resectoscope and (2) rarely, injection of steroids. Before LTR, no attempts are made to treat cartilaginous stenosis by means other than gentle periodic dilatation or by watchful waiting.

Technique of Laryngotracheal Reconstruction

As a prelude to LTR, endoscopic examination of the larynx and tracheobronchial tree is carried out. The mobility of the vocal cords is assessed before induction of general anesthesia. If normal mobility is not seen, the vocal cords and arytenoids are carefully palpated under deep anesthesia or with the patient paralyzed. The precise location and extent of the stenosis are then carefully documented.

When the stenosis is restricted to the confines of the cricoid cartilage, particularly when it is primarily anterior, LTR with an anterior costal cartilage graft is the procedure of choice (Fig. 78–8). The costal cartilage graft also is used when there is loss of cricoid or tracheal cartilages. The graft may be extended from the thyroid cartilage to the superior margin of the tracheostome. A costal cartilage graft also is necessary for certain congenital cricoid cartilage deformities.

With posterior glottic and subglottic stenosis, particularly when associated with ankylosis of the arytenoids, it usually is necessary to divide the cricoid cartilage posteriorly. Often, a cartilage graft will be placed posteriorly to maintain an adequate lumen (Fig. 78–9). An Aboulker polytef prosthesis is used in these cases.[25] The castellated or stepped incision of Evans' laryngotracheoplasty may be used anteriorly (Fig. 78–10). In the most severe cases, anterior and posterior grafts are required (Fig. 78–11).

The anterior neck and right chest are prepared and draped. A 4 cm length of costal cartilage is removed, taking care to leave the perichondrium on the deep side (Fig. 78–11B). Saline is placed in the wound to be sure parietal pleura is intact and the chest has not been entered. The incision is closed, a dressing is applied, and the area is draped out of the surgical field. Lidocaine (0.5 percent) with epinephrine 1:200,000 is injected into a horizontal incision immediately above the stoma. A superior skin flap is raised, and the strap muscles are divided in the midline to expose the larynx and trachea from the thyroid notch to the stoma. The cricoid cartilage is divided precisely in the midline, and the laryngeal lumen is entered through the cricothyroid membrane. The larynx and trachea are carefully inspected. When the stenosis is high and when the posterior plate of the cricoid is to be divided, the incision is carried as far superiorly as the thyroid notch (Fig. 78–9). Likewise, when the stenosis extends inferiorly to the stoma or when a stent must be placed, the incision is carried inferiorly to the superior margin of the stoma.

Great care is taken to divide the structures precisely in the midline. This is done under direct vision using a groove director. A neurosurgical sponge is saturated with 4 percent cocaine and placed in the lumen. A second sponge placed immediately above the cuffed anode endotracheal tube will help prevent leakage of anesthetic gases as well as preventing blood and secretions from entering the lower airway. If the posterior plate of the cricoid cartilage is to be divided, it is done at this point, and the cartilage graft is sutured in place using 5-0 Maxon or Novafil. The perichondrium is placed toward

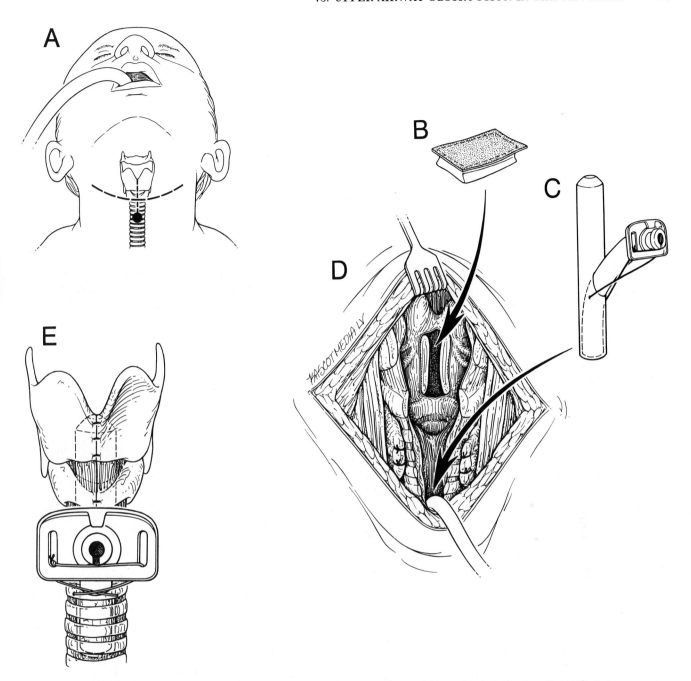

Figure 78–9. Laryngotracheal reconstruction operation for posterior glottic and subglottic stenosis, particularly with ankylosis of the arytenoids. **A.** Horizontal skin incision at the level of the tracheostome. A vertical incision is made through the larynx from the thyroid notch to the superior margin of the tracheostome. **B.** Posterior costal cartilage graft. **C.** Albouker stent with Holinger tracheostomy tube wired into position. The wire usually enters superior to the opening for the tracheostomy tube. **D.** Placement of the graft between the cut margins of the posterior lamina of the cricoid cartilage. **E.** Position of the stent and tracheostomy tube.

the lumen. All sutures are placed before moving the graft into position and securing the knots.

When a stent is used, the proper size is selected at this time. After careful measurement, a hole is cut for the Holinger pediatric tracheostomy tube. The tube is placed through it and wired into position (Fig. 78–9). Sutures are placed through the anterior costal cartilage

graft. The intraluminal side, which is covered with perichondrium, is carved in a fusiform shape, and the external portion is fashioned as a larger rectangle that forms a flange, preventing the graft from slipping or being displaced into the lumen (Fig. 78–8). The position of the stent is checked endoscopically to be certain that it extends well above the vocal cords.

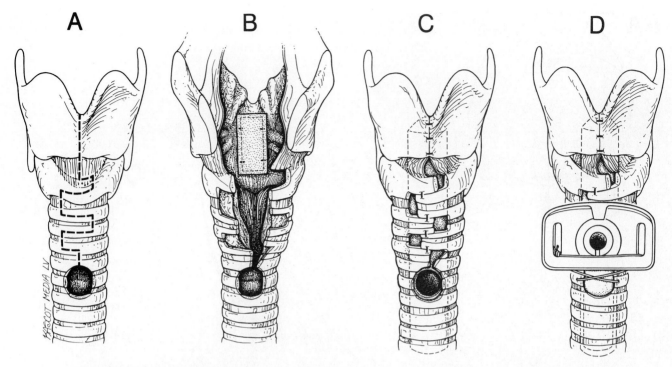

A   **B**   **C**   **D**

Figure 78–10. Posterior costal cartilage graft combined with the casselated anterior incision of Evans' laryngotracheoplasty. The technique combines two operations and is used when only a limited amount of room is needed anteriorly in patients who require more room posteriorly.

The prophylactic antibiotics begun before the procedure are continued for no more than 48 hours postoperatively.

TRACHEOBRONCHIAL OBSTRUCTION

Tracheomalacia and bronchomalacia are frequently observed congenital anomalies of the tracheobronchial tree. Inadequate support of an immature cartilagenous framework of the trachea and bronchi permits collapse on expiration. This produces an expiratory wheeze or stridor with increased respiratory effort similar to that seen with asthma. Fluoroscopy or inspiratory and expiratory lateral x-rays may demonstrate the anteroposterior collapse. The pathology may be overlooked during bronchoscopy if the patient is being actively ventilated by the anesthesiologist. Most of these infants improve spontaneously as they mature. Treatment, therefore, includes supportive care and therapy of recurrent infections and other complications. Secondary tracheomalacia occurs with associated conditions, such as TEF and the anomalous innominate artery.

The correct diagnosis of tracheal webs or stenosis is suggested by x-ray studies and is confirmed by bronchoscopic examination. Careful dilatation may be the only treatment necessary for discrete, thin webs. Longer stenoses may respond to repeated dilatations at regular intervals. Cartilagenous strictures may require resection and end-to-end anastomosis or interposition of autogenous rib cartilage between the cut ends of the narrowed tracheal rings.

Technique of Bronchoscopy

Complete instrumentation and a well-trained pediatric anesthesiologist are of utmost importance for a safe, complete, and detailed endoscopic examination of the tracheobronchial tree. A full range of ventilating bronchoscopes and a Hopkin's rod telescopic system, as well as forceps for foreign body removal, should be available to every pediatric endoscopist. With few exceptions, bronchoscopy is best carried out under general anesthesia. The infant is anesthetized by insufflation of gas anesthetic through a mask, and the larynx is sprayed with 1 to 4 percent lidocaine. The larynx is stabilized with a standard laryngoscope. The bronchoscope is introduced between the vocal cords into the trachea, and the slide of the laryngoscope is withdrawn so that the main portion of the laryngoscope itself can be removed before the bronchoscopic evaluation is begun. Anesthetic gases and oxygen are administered via a closed system through the 15 mm standard adaptor of the bronchoscope. The

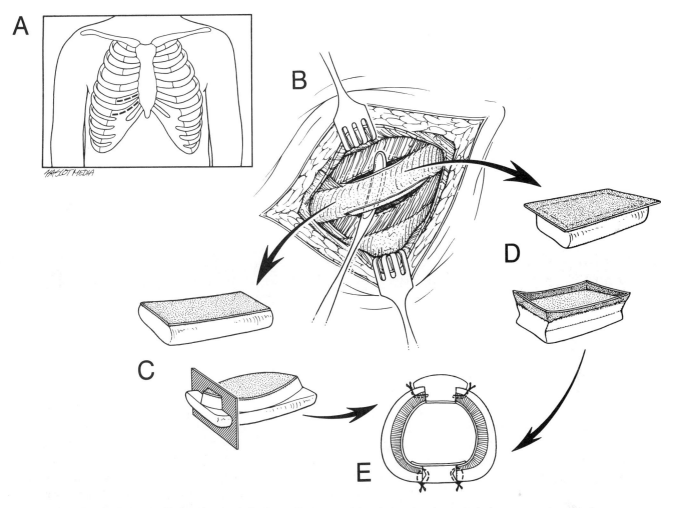

Figure 78–11. Harvesting the costal cartilage grafts for anterior and posterior placement in the most severe stenosis. **E.** Cross-sectional view with grafts sutured into place. A stent is needed in such cases.

anesthetic is maintained at a level that permits the infant to continue to breathe spontaneously. A Hopkin's rod-lens telescope may be passed through the laryngoscope to visualize the trachea and the main bronchi.

The pattern for inspection of the tracheobronchial tree is the same as in the adult. However, there are notable differences in appearance of the various structures in infants and children. The mucous membranes seem slightly pinker and more velvety in appearance, and the movement of the tracheobronchial tree is considerably more noticeable. The carina appears somewhat broader in the infant than in the adult, which is a reflection of the shorter, broader chest of the infant and young child. The configuration of the entire tracheobronchial tree is carefully and systematically examined. The shape and size of the orifices of the major divisions are carefully inspected and noted. Any abnormal compression or motility is noted, as are the color, texture, and secretions of the bronchial mucosa. Proper positioning of the head will allow examination of the orifice of the right upper lobe. To facilitate passage of the bronchoscope into the left main bronchus, the patient's shoulders must remain in the midline, and the head must be brought far to the right in a slightly flexed position.

REFERENCES

1. Raffensperger JG: Surgical management of respiratory problems in the newborn. Contemp Surg 6:81, 1975
2. Leape LL, Holder TM, Franklin JD, et al: Respiratory arrest in infants secondary to gastroesophageal reflux. Pediatrics 60:924, 1977
3. Flake CG, Ferguson CF: Congenital choanal atresia in infants and children. Ann Otol Rhinol Laryngol 73:458, 1964
4. McGovern FH, Fitz-Hugh GS: Surgical management of congenital choanal atresia. Arch Otolaryngol 73:458, 1961
5. Oeconomopholoulos CT: The valve of glossopexy in Pierre Robin syndrome. N Engl J Med 262:1267, 1960

6. Monroe CW: Treatment of micrognathia in the neonatal period. Plast Reconstr Surg 51:317, 1972

7. Holinger PH: Neonatal respiratory tract obstruction. Cardiopulmon Dis 4:285, 1962

8. Kavanagh K, Bobin R: Endoscopic surgical management for laryngomalacia. Ann Otol Rhinol Laryngol 96:550, 1987

9. Holinger LD, Holinger PC, Holinger PH: Etiology of bilateral abductor vocal cord paralysis: a review of 389 cases. Ann Otol Rhinol Laryngol 85:428, 1976

10. Holinger PH, Brown WT: Congenital webs, cysts, laryngoceles and other abnormalities of the larynx. Ann Otol Rhinol Laryngol 76:744, 1967

11. Holinger PH, Kutnick SL, Schild JA, Holinger LD: Subglottic stenosis in infants and children. Ann Otol Rhinol Laryngol 85:559, 1976

12. Calcaterra TC, McClure R, Ward PH: The effect of laryngofissure on the developing canine larynx. Ann Otol Rhinol Laryngol 83:810, 1974

13. Fearon B, Cotton R: Surgical correction of subglottic stenosis of the larynx in infants and children: a progress report. Ann Otol Rhinol Laryngol 83:428, 1974

14. Maddalozzo J, Holinger LD: Laryngotracheal reconstruction for subglottic stenosis in children. Ann Otol 96:86, 1987

15. Cotton RT, Evans JNG: Laryngotracheal reconstruction in children: a five-year follow-up. Ann Otol Rhinol Laryngol 90:515, 1981

16. Cotton RT, Seid AB: Management of the extubation problem in the premature child: anterior cricoid split as an alternative to tracheostomy. Ann Otol Rhinol Laryngol 89:508, 1980

17. Johnson DG, Steward DR: Management of acquired tracheal obstructions in infancy. J Pediatr Surg 10:70, 1975

18. Holinger LD: Treatment of severe subglottic stenosis without tracheotomy: a preliminary report. Ann Otol Rhinol Laryngol 91:407, 1982

19. Holinger LD, Stankiewicz JA, Livingston GL: Anterior cricoid split: the Chicago experience with an alternative to tracheotomy. Laryngoscope 97:19, 1987

20. Rethi A: An operation for cicatricial stenosis of the larynx. J Laryngol Otol 70:283, 1956

21. Grahne B: Operative treatment of severe chronic traumatic laryngeal stenosis in infants up to 3 years old. Acta Otol (Stockh) 72:134, 1971

22. Evans JNG, Todd GB: Laryngotracheoplasty. J Laryngol Otol 88:581, 1974

23. Fearon B, Cotton R: Subglottic stenosis in infants and children: the clinical problem and experimental surgical correction. Can J Otolaryngol 1:281, 1972

24. Simpson GT, Strong MS, Healy GB, et al: Predictive factors of success or failure in the endoscopic management of laryngeal and tracheal stenosis. Ann Otol Rhinol Laryngol 91:384, 1982

25. Aboulker P: Traitement des stenoses tracheales. Probl Actuels d'Oto-rhino-laryngologie Librairie Maloine, 1968, p 273

79
Tracheotomy

Lauren D. Holinger

Fortunately, complete upper airway obstructions are relatively rare. They do occur, often in such situations as automobile accidents and in restaurants, where there are no facilities for an orderly procedure. In these situations, the Heimlich maneuver can be performed to dislodge a foreign body without any special equipment. A cricothyrotomy may be performed at the roadside with only a pocket knife. A tube may be improvised from almost any hollow object, such as the barrel of a pen or a section of tubing from a stethoscope. Fortunately, most of the airway problems that arise in the hospital situation are amenable to careful diagnosis and selection of the optimum procedure. In most cases, the initial choice for airway control is the insertion of an endotracheal tube. A decision may then be made as to whether a tracheotomy is indicated.

The Heimlich maneuver is an emergency technique indicated for relief of complete laryngeal obstruction due to aspiration of a foreign body, usually a solid bolus of food.[1] The child rapidly becomes cyanotic, struggles, and may clutch the throat. He or she is completely aphonic; absolutely no air passes in or out of the lungs through the mouth or nose. The Heimlich maneuver is an abrupt, strong thurst directed posterosuperiorly from the epigastric region. The obstructing foreign body is popped from the larynx and out the mouth. Complete laryngeal obstruction by a foreign body is the only indication for the Heimlich maneuver. If the airway is only partially obstructed, the child is taken immediately to the emergency room or to an area within the hospital that is completely equipped for foreign body extraction. Under no circumstances is the child slapped on the back or a finger inserted in the mouth to try to remove the foreign body. The problem may be compounded, and the child may asphyxiate on the spot.

CRICOTHYROTOMY

The thyroid and the cricoid cartilages of the larynx are joined anteriorly by the fibrous cricothyroid membrane. This is the soft spot that may be palpated approximately 1 cm below the thyroid notch (Adam's apple). It is at this point that the airway is closest to the skin and is most accessible (Fig. 79–1). Traditionally, this has been taught as the location for an emergency tracheotomy. Technically, cricothyrotomy is a laryngotomy not a tracheotomy, since the opening breaks into the airway at the level of the larynx above the trachea. Cricothyrotomy is indicated in emergencies (such as crushing laryngeal trauma) when endotracheal intubation is not possible. The safety and efficacy of the Heimlich maneuver have obviated its use in complete laryngeal obstruction due to a foreign body. Perioral endotracheal intubation is preferable to cricothyrotomy in most patients requiring an emergency airway, after which an orderly tracheotomy is accomplished under controlled conditions in the operating room.

ENDOTRACHEAL INTUBATION/ TRACHEOTOMY

Endotracheal intubation or tracheotomy is indicated for (1) significant obstruction of the upper airway, (2) excessive secretions in the tracheobronchial tree, and (3) alveo-

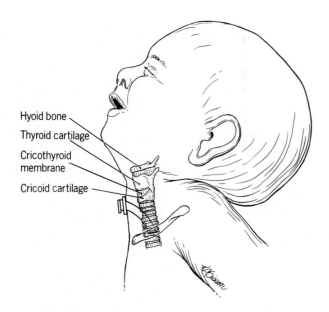

Hyoid bone
Thyroid cartilage
Cricothyroid membrane
Cricoid cartilage

Figure 79–1. Anatomy of the trachea and upper airway.

lar hypoventilation (respiratory insufficiency) requiring mechanical ventilatory assistance. With few exceptions (as with the premature infant or ventilatory pressures exceeding 40 cm H$_2$O), tracheotomy should be considered whenever a tube will be required for more than 4 to 7 days. The decision (intubation or tracheotomy) is based partly on the experience of the physician, the quality of nursing care, and the available equipment. Institutions with well-equipped and well-staffed neonatal and intensive care units have the facilities and experience for atraumatic endotracheal intubation with the appropriate size tube as well as proper care of the tube (adequate stabilization, prevention of extubation, adequate humidification and suctioning). At other institutions, in less optimal circumstances, tracheotomy may offer lower morbidity and mortality for short-term care as well as for periods of more than 4 days. Tracheotomy is better tolerated by the patient, permits normal feedings, and prevents nasal and laryngeal complications, and after parent education, the child may be discharged from the hospital.

Endotracheal intubation is accomplished more readily than tracheotomy, and planned extubation is less difficult. In addition, there are fewer complications with intubation, such as pneumothorax and hemorrhage, and inadvertent extubation is more readily corrected. However, it is difficult to maintain an unobstructed endotracheal tube, and with tracheotomy, the laryngeal complications (ulceration and destruction of the vocal cords and subglottic larynx with resultant glottic and subglottic stenosis) are avoided.

Specific Indications for Tracheotomy or Endotracheal Intubation

Congenital anomalies of the upper airway are the most common indications for a tracheotomy in the neonate, infant, and child. These anomalies include lesions of the pharynx, larynx, and trachea, neoplasms (e.g., lymphangioma and hemangioma), and neurologic conditions (e.g., bilateral vocal cord paralysis).[2] The degree of severity of symptoms and the potential duration determine the need for tracheotomy.

Infectious conditions may require tracheotomy or intubation. Acute supraglottitis (epiglottitis) requires establishment of an airway as soon as the diagnosis is made. The author prefers careful nasotracheal intubation under controlled circumstances in the operating room. It is rarely necessary to establish an airway for the patient with croup (laryngotracheobronchitis, or LTB), since adequate humidification, racemic epinephrine, and steroids usually obviate the need for temporary intubation. Diphtheria, retropharyngeal abscess, and other rare infectious conditions may require temporary tracheotomy or intubation.

External laryngeal trauma, such as the crushing injury frequently suffered in motor vehicle accidents, may produce airway obstruction at the level of the larynx and require tracheotomy. Surgical correction of the laryngeal fracture is indicated as soon as the patient's associated injuries permit. Internal laryngeal trauma, such as that produced by endotracheal intubation or the ingestion of caustic or corrosive agents, may require tracheotomy acutely because of edema or later because of the chronic fibrosis resulting from the healing process.

Tracheotomy rarely is required in children for treatment of papilloma of the larynx. Improved anesthetic and surgical techniques have eliminated its usefulness in treating this disease except in extreme cases.

Tracheotomy is often indicated as a prelude to major surgery of the head and neck, such as the excision of neoplasms of the tongue and neck (e.g., cystic hygroma) or for surgical correction of major craniofacial anomalies.

Neurologic lesions, central or peripheral, may affect cranial nerves IX and X, resulting in chronic aspiration of secretions that can be adequately managed only by tracheostomy. Coma may require intubation or tracheostomy for immediate or long-term airway management. Postoperative thoracotomy patients whose coughing and breathing are restricted by pain require intubation and, infrequently, subsequent tracheotomy for aspiration of retained secretions. Pneumonia, lung abscess, and bronchiectasis also may require temporary intubation or tracheotomy.

Respiratory distress syndrome, specifically hyaline membrane disease, is the most common indication for intubation of the premature infant. Although prolonged intubation may produce significant laryngeal trauma with resulting laryngeal stenosis, the potential complications from tracheotomy probably outweigh the disadvantages of prolonged intubation in this group. When the neonate's lower respiratory problem is resolved and ventilatory support is no longer required, tracheotomy may be unavoidable if extubation is not tolerated.

Other conditions, such as pneumonia, trauma with flail chest or paralysis of the chest wall, bronchiolitis, and allergic small airway disease may require temporary ventilatory assistance. Tracheotomy is considered immediately if it is apparent that the problem will persist for more than 4 to 7 days. If it is anticipated that the problem will resolve in less than 4 days, endotracheal intubation is the preferred alternative.

Technique of Tracheotomy

An orderly tracheotomy is undertaken in the operating room where proper lighting, instrumentation, and ancillary personnel are readily available. The airway is secured by an endotracheal tube or ventilating bronchoscope. The infant's vital signs are monitored by an anesthesiologist who administers an anesthetic or oxygen alone, augmented when necessary by injection of 0.5 percent lidocaine with 1:200,000 epinephrine for local anesthesia. A pulse oximeter is routinely used. A small towel is placed under the infant's shoulders, and the head is extended. The head is held firmly in the midline by the anesthesiologist or the assistant endoscopist, whose gloved middle finger holds the patient's chin in a fixed position and is prepared into the field. Alternatively, the chin may be secured in the midline with adhesive tape.

A vertical midline incision is made in the skin of the anterior neck, beginning immediately below the cricoid cartilage. Care is taken to keep the dissection in the midline, to avoid the apices of the lung, recurrent laryngeal nerves, and the contents of the carotid sheath (carotid artery, internal jugular vein, vagus nerve) encountered laterally. The isthmus of the thyroid gland is identified, routinely clamped, divided, and ligated using a running 3-0 locking suture on each side. Meticulous hemostasis is attained throughout, and the surgeon's index finger is used repeatedly to palpate the trachea, assuring that the dissection is maintained absolutely in the midline. Small forceps are used repeatedly by the surgeon and the first assistant to pick up the soft tissue on each side of the midline before spreading the tissue bluntly in a vertical direction with a tenotomy scissors. Considerable care is taken to identify the cricoid cartilage by the greater thickness and darker color due to the insertion of the cricothyroid muscles. This cartilage is retracted anteriorly and superiorly with a delicate trachea hook or a temporary suture. A vertical incision is made in the trachea, beginning at the second or third tracheal ring and extending through three tracheal rings (Fig. 79–2). At this point, 3-0 nonabsorbable sutures are placed through the tracheal wall on each side of the incision, usually deep to the fourth tracheal ring. These serve as retractors for reinsertion of the tracheostomy tube in the event it becomes displaced during the postoperative period. The sutures are taped to the chest for easy accessibility. The endotracheal tube or bronchoscope is not completely withdrawn until the tracheotomy tape is securely fastened. A square knot is tied, with the infant's head in the flexed position.

The infant is returned to the intensive care unit and stays there until after the first tube change or until the fistulous tract has formed well around the tube (3 to 7 days). A postoperative portable posteroanterior (PA)

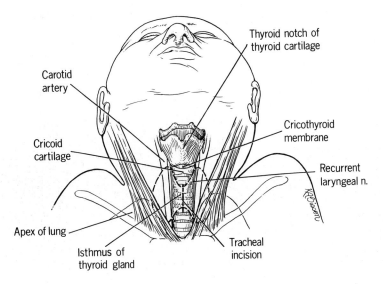

Figure 79–2. Midline vertical incision for a tracheotomy. The isthmus of the thyroid is ligated and divided to expose the tracheal ring. Vertical incision is made in the trachea between two traction sutures.

chest roentgenogram is obtained immediately to rule out intraoperative complications and to evaluate the position of the tube. Particular note should be taken of the position of the distal end of the tracheostomy tube.

Selection of the proper tracheostomy tube is dependent on the indication for the tracheotomy. Tubes with a standard 15 mm adaptor are used in all patients who will require ventilatory assistance or continuous positive airway pressure (CPAP). In cases of upper airway obstruction, a shallow-curve infant tracheostomy tube (Holinger) with an inner cannula is preferred, since it is designed specifically for use in the newborn infant and small child. Appropriate size (diameter and length) is determined by the size of the trachea, which may be estimated from the infant's weight, length, and age.

Postoperative Care

The immediate postoperative period is the most critical time for the infant who has undergone tracheotomy. Inadvertent extubation before the fistulous tract has formed can make reinsertion of the tracheostomy tube quite difficult. Constant observation and care with suctioning, humidity, and position are extremely important. Humidity above 90 percent is necessary to eliminate formation of tenacious secretions and crusting that may occlude the tracheostomy tube or tracheobronchial tree. Three to five drops of 0.5 N saline solution are introduced into the tracheostomy tube at half-hour intervals to liquefy the secretions before vigorous catheter suction. The tube is suctioned more frequently if necessary. The secretions are particularly copious in the immediate postoperative period because of the unaccustomed stimulation from the tube itself. The inner cannula is removed and cleaned as often as secretions adhere to the walls. Nursing personnel are instructed in the most minute details of care before being assigned to the unit caring for these patients. Infants and children under age 5 are constantly monitored for apnea and bradycardia. A nurse or trained family member is always in the immediate vicinity.

Whenever possible, the first tube change is deferred for 4 to 7 days so that adequate tracheocutaneous fistula formation is assured. The tube change is effected in the operating room with a tracheotomy set and bronchoscope available. With a premature infant, a bronchoscope is positioned in the trachea if there is any doubt as to the adequate formation of a fistulous tract.

Complications

Immediate (Operative). Significant hemorrhage may occur during the procedure itself, but this can be managed routinely in the controlled circumstances of the operating room. The laceration of an anomalous major vessel, specifically an aberrant innominate artery, may have disastrous results. Care must be taken to avoid this complication by routinely using careful technique in identification of all structures.

Pneumothorax results from entering the pleural cavities. The apices of the lungs may be extremely high and actually adjacent to the trachea in some children. If the dissection is kept in the midline this complication should be avoided.

Hypoxia and hypothermia may lead to cardiac arrhythmias and death if they are not carefully controlled intraoperatively. This is the responsibility of the anesthesiologist unless the tracheotomy is being done as an emergency procedure in an obstructed child.

Emergency tracheotomy may lead to errors in technique that would otherwise be readily avoided. These include injury to the recurrent laryngeal nerves if the dissection is carried too far laterally or if a horizontal incision in the trachea is used, esophageal perforation if the posterior tracheal wall is lacerated and the esophagus is entered when the tracheal incision is made, and too high or too low a tracheotomy.

Improper size or placement of the tracheostomy tube may produce other complications. If the tracheotomy is too low or the tube is too long, the tip of the tube will rest on the carina or in the right main bronchus. Hypoxia, atelectasis of the left lung (or obstructive emphysema), or erosion of the carina may occur. Selection of a tube that has too great an angle or is too short may lead to its displacement in the chest or to erosion of the anterior tracheal wall.

Delayed. Hemorrhage is to a significant degree the most common delayed complication of tracheotomy.[3] A medium-size vessel may be transected during the tracheotomy when the patient is hypotensive and thus go unrecognized. Later, when a normotensive level is returned, brisk bleeding with aspiration may result. Erosion of a major artery may occur as a result of pressure necrosis. The tip of a poorly fitting or malpositioned tracheostomy tube may erode through the anterior tracheal wall into the innominate artery. If the thyroid isthmus is not completely divided, the midline thyroid artery may be eroded. Infection usually is associated with this complication. In a low tracheotomy, the tube is more likely to erode the innominate artery. A cuffed tube overinflated for too long may produce the same complication. Occasionally, a massive hemorrhage will be preceded by a significant episode of bleeding. In this case, the patient should be taken to the operating room immediately, at which time the tube should be removed under controlled circumstances and the trachea inspected. Preparations for a mediastinotomy should be made if there is a high degree of suspicion. If massive bleeding occurs, it may be tamponaded by inserting a cuffed endotracheal tube and inflating the cuff or, if the child is large enough, using the index finger to compress the bleeding artery from behind against the posterior wall of the sternum.

Infection is a common complication of tracheotomy. Tracheitis occurs in almost all patients, and cultures of tracheotomy wounds routinely grow microorganisms. *Staphylococcus aureus*, *Pseudomonas*, and *Candida* frequently are found. Local care and adequate humidity are usually all that is required. Systemic antibiotics are rarely necessary. Tracheitis can be lessened by meticulous asepsis, adequate humidification, frequent irrigation and suctioning, and careful cleaning of the stoma with peroxide. Pneumonia occasionally complicates tracheotomy. Mediastinitis is quite rare.

Subcutaneous emphysema is a not uncommon complication that may progress rapidly to involve not only the neck but the face, chest, abdomen, groin, and lower extremities in extreme cases. For this reason, one should never apply gauze dressings to a fresh tracheotomy wound. This early complication may occur at any time before an adequate fistulous tract is formed. If air is not allowed to escape through the skin from around the tracheostomy tube, it will dissect in the subcutaneous planes to cause swelling and crepitance. The tracheostomy tube must be repositioned or the skin incision must be enlarged so that this air can readily escape around the tube. The emphysema rapidly resolves.

Pneumothorax, pneumomediastinum, and even pneumoperitoneum may be produced by the same mechanism that produces subcutaneous emphysema. Chest tubes may be necessary to correct the pneumothorax, and one may have to tap the abdomen to relieve the pneumoperitoneum.

Inadvertent decannulation (displacement of the tube) may be disastrous if it occurs within the first 3 or 4 days before formation of a fistulous tract. The structures of the neck rapidly collapse and obliterate the lumen, making reinsertion of the tube extremely difficult even for experienced personnel under ideal circumstances. If the infant is unable to breathe through the mouth and nose, rapid asphyxiation may occur. This complication is prevented by the use of a tube with short flanges, of a proper size, and in the right position, careful securing of the tube tape, adequate sedation or restraint, and proper fixation of appliances, such as CPAP and respirator tubing. The complication is less likely to occur when a vertical incision is used (Fig. 79–3).

Obstruction of the tracheostomy tube is most often the result of a crust or plug of thick mucus. This is prevented by adequate humidity and suctioning. Obstruction also may result from a granuloma, which can develop at the tip of a malpositioned tube.

Atelectasis may result from aspiration of crusts or plugs of mucus. Careful suctioning may resolve the problem. Bronchoscopy for aspiration may be necessary.

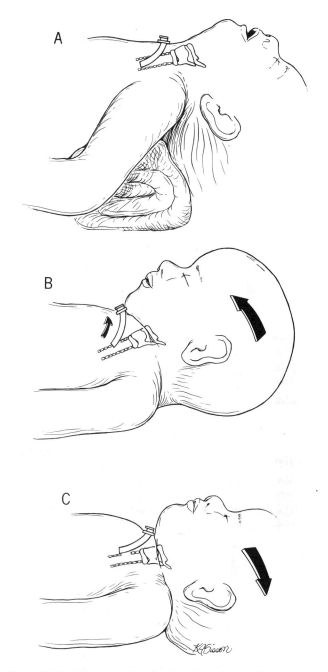

Figure 79–3. This series of drawings demonstrates why the tracheostomy tube must be securely tied to the neck. Otherwise, head motion may cause the tube to be displaced.

Aspiration, dysphagia, and aerophagia are not unusual in association with tracheotomy. These problems usually resolve with time and require symptomatic treatment in the interim. A barium esophagram may delineate a specific problem.

Tracheal stenosis may develop at the site of the tracheostome, at the tip of the tracheostomy tube, or at the level of the cuff. Lower stenoses are the result of poorly fitting tubes or excessive inflation of the cuff.

Stenosis at the level of the tracheostome may result from excision of tracheal cartilage. A horizontal incision in the trachea or a vertical incision that is not sufficiently generous may produce posterior displacement of the anterior tracheal wall immediately above the tracheostome. This may form a granuloma, which can organize to form a fibroma that is extremely difficult to remove endoscopically or through the tracheostome of an infant. The pediatric urethral resectoscope is an excellent instrument for removing these obstructing lesions.

Sudden death for which no cause can be determined occurs in a few infants, either at home or in the hospital. Autopsy discloses no granuloma or mucus plug that might have produced the obstruction and asphyxiation. Reflex apnea, such as that observed with an aberrant innominate artery, may be implicated in some cases. Only constant monitoring of these children can eliminate this complication completely.

A persistent tracheocutaneous fistula is common when the tracheostomy tube has been maintained for a long period of time. It is the result of epithelialization of the tract and is closed by simple dissection and tracheal closure, avoiding endotracheal anesthesia for fear of precipitating another tracheotomy in the postoperative period. A generous cuff of tissue is left, and the fistula is closed horizontally.

Decannulation may be delayed when such complications as tracheal stenosis are overlooked. "Delayed decannulation" is an unfortunate term and does not denote a complication of tracheotomy. Rather this problem is the result of complications of tracheotomy. Some children develop an apparent psychologic dependence on their tracheostomy tubes, which requires special attention. In others, loss of the phasic abductor activity of the vocal cords may be the cause.[4] Progressively smaller tracheostomy tubes and, finally, a 3-0 plug placed over a period of several days facilitates decannulation.

REFERENCES

1. Heimlich HJ: Death from food-choking prevented by a new life-saving maneuver. Heart Lung 5:755, 1976
2. Markus NJ, Schild JA, Holinger PH: Tracheostomy in the first year of life. Am Acad Ophthalmol Otol 82:466, 1976
3. Chew JY, Cantrell RW: Tracheostomy complications and their management. Arch Otolaryngol 96:538, 1972
4. Kirchner JA: Avoiding problems in tracheotomy. Laryngoscope 96:55, 1986

80
Vascular Ring

Farouk S. Idriss

Anomalies of the aortic arch system and pulmonary artery may cause respiratory problems in infancy and at times may be associated with dysphagia in older children. The term "vascular ring" was introduced by Gross in his report of the first successful division of a double aortic arch in 1945.[1] This term describes vascular anomalies that encircle the trachea and esophagus, causing obstructive symptoms (Fig. 80–1). Following the report of Gross, a host of vascular anomalies producing tracheoesophogeal compression were recognized, classified, and surgically treated to alleviate symptoms of obstruction.[2–7] The surgical experience with 204 such anomalies operated at the Children's Memorial Hospital in Chicago formed the basis for this chapter. In general, vascular anomalies that compress the trachea and esophagus can be divided into four groups (numbers indicate breakdown of anomalies at Children's Memorial Hospital).

Group I:	True complete vascular ring	
	a. Double aortic arch	61
	b. Right aortic arch with left ligamentum from descending aorta	52
Group II:	Left arch	82
Group III:	Pulmonary artery sling	9

Understanding of the complex embryonic development of these vascular anomalies was facilitated by Edwards, with a hypothetical schema of a double aortic arch with bilateral ducts in which all embryonic components needed for normal and known abnormal development are left in place[8] (Fig 80–2).

In the double arch subgroup, bilateral embryonic aortic arches remain present without the usual complete resorption of the right-sided arch, thus forming a vascular ring around the trachea and esophagus. The left and right common carotid and subclavian arteries originate, respectively, symmetrically and separately from each arch. The innominate artery is absent. It is uncommon for the right and left aortic arches to be equal (4 patients, or 7 percent). The right, or posterior, arch was larger in 45 patients (73 percent) (Fig. 80–3), and the left, or anterior, arch was dominant in 12 (20 percent) (Fig. 80–4). Segments of the aortic arch may be atretic, represented by a fibrous band and located most often in the posterior or distal end of the nondominant arch. With a dominant right arch, atretic segment of the left occurred in 40 percent of the patients; it occurred in 4 of 12 patients (33 percent) in the dominant left arch group. In our patients, the ligamentum was always noted in the left side, since our surgical approach has been through a left thoracotomy. There are no specific intracardiac anomalies associated with double aortic arch, although ventricular septal defects, atrial septal defects, and transposition of the great arteries were seen in our patients. Tetralogy of Fallot and coarctation of the aorta also have been reported.

Embryologically, in the right arch subgroup, the left arch resorbs and the right persists. There are two variants in this category, the occurrence of which depends on the origin of the left subclavian artery. When the embryonic left fourth arch is absorbed, the left subclavian artery originates from the distal end of the aortic arch as a retroesophogeal or aberrant left subclavian artery (65 percent) (Fig. 80–5). When the posterior end of the embryonic left arch beyond the origin of the sev-

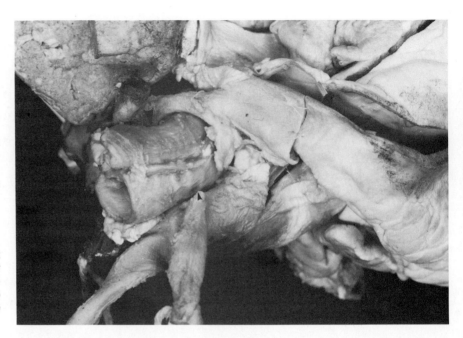

Figure 80–1. Autopsy specimen of a right arch and a ligamentum forming a vascular ring that encircles and compresses the trachea and esophagus. Large arrow points to the esophagus. Small arrow points to the trachea.

enth segmental artery is absorbed, the bracheocephalic vessels will form as a mirror image of the normal branching of a left arch (Fig. 80–6). A vascular ring develops only when the ligamentum arises from the descending aorta. In patients with right arch and a mirror image left innominate artery, the ligamentum may arise from the descending aorta or from the innominate artery. This latter occurrence is uncommon in a surgical series, since this situation does not form a ring and does not produce symptoms. Although a right aortic arch is associated with 25 to 30 percent of patients with tetralogy of Fallot, a vascular ring with right arch and ligamentum

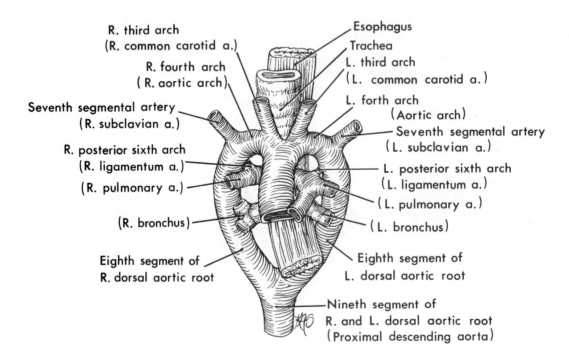

R. third arch
(R. common carotid a.)
R. fourth arch
(R. aortic arch)
Seventh segmental artery
(R. subclavian a.)
R. posterior sixth arch
(R. ligamentum a.)
(R. pulmonary a.)
(R. bronchus)
Eighth segment of
R. dorsal aortic root

Esophagus
Trachea
L. third arch
(L. common carotid a.)
L. forth arch
(Aortic arch)
Seventh segmental artery
(L. subclavian a.)
L. posterior sixth arch
(L. ligamentum a.)
(L. pulmonary a.)
(L. bronchus)
Eighth segment of
L. dorsal aortic root
Nineth segment of
R. and L. dorsal aortic root
(Proximal descending aorta)

Figure 80–2. The embryologic origin of the aortic arch and its major branches. The structures in this diagram are identified by their embryonic names—their eventual anatomic names are included in parentheses. The normal aortic arch develops through the absorption of the structure in the right eighth segment of this diagram. When it is retained, there is a double aortic arch. (*Edwards.*[2])

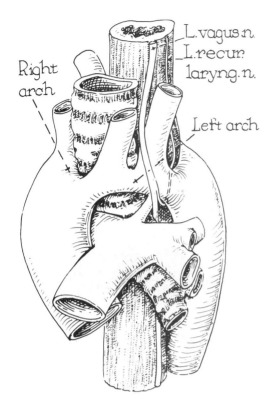

Figure 80–3. Double aortic arch with the right side dominant.

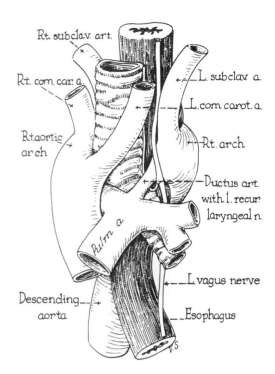

Figure 80–5. Right aortic arch with a retroesophageal left subclavian artery and a left ductus or ligamentum.

was seen occasionally in conjunction with an intracardiac defect, such as tetralogy of Fallot, ventricular septal defect, and patent ductus arteriosus.

Anterior tracheal compression by an innominate artery from a left aortic arch may be due to exaggerated leftward origin and posterior displacement (Fig. 80–7). The incidence of this diagnosis peaked about 10 years ago, resulting in a large number of patients who were operated on. The actual occurrence of respiratory obstruction from innominate artery compression is rather

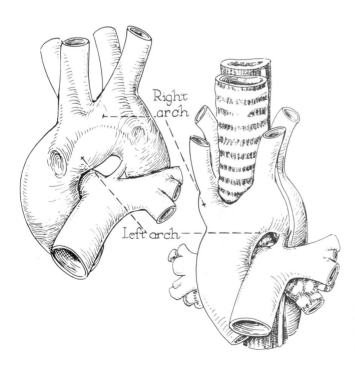

Figure 80–4. Double aortic arch with the left side dominant. **a.** Left anterolateral view. **b.** Anterior view showing compression of trachea and esophagus.

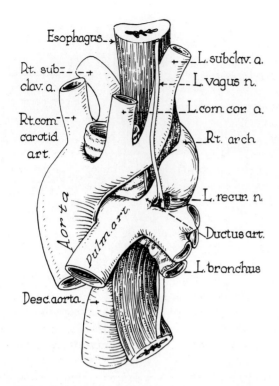

Figure 80–6. Right aortic arch with a left ductus or ligamentum.

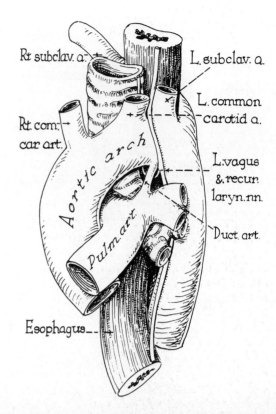

Figure 80–8. Left aortic arch with an aberrant right subclavian artery.

infrequent, especially when a careful and diligent approach is taken to identify other causes of symptoms.

In addition, there is a miscellaneous and uncommon group of anomalies of the left aortic arch or its branches producing compression of the trachea and esophagus.

Seven in our group had an aberrant right subclavian artery originating from the descending aorta and coursing obliquely from left to right behind the esophagus. The innominate artery is absent (Fig. 80–8). Embryologically, this abnormality is secondary to resorption of the right

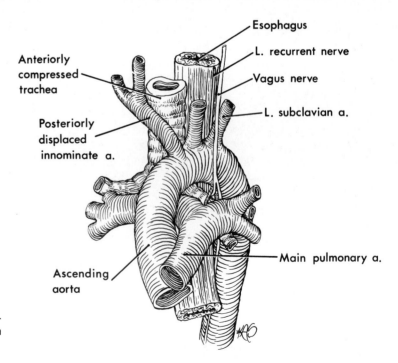

Figure 80–7. The innominate artery originates further to the left than normal and then crosses the anterior tracheal wall.

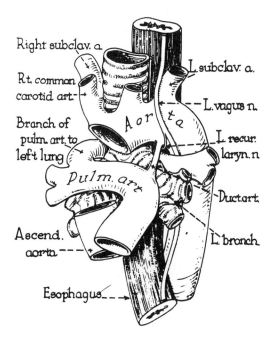

Right subclav. a.
Rt. common carotid art.
Branch of pulm. art. to left lung
L. subclav. a.
L. vagus n.
L. recur. laryn. n.
Aorta
Pulm. art
Duct art.
Ascend. aorta
L. branch.
Esophagus

Figure 80–9. Anomalous left pulmonary artery.

fourth arch, leaving the right subclavian artery attached to the distal aorta. The ligamentum arteriosum is on the left. This abnormality does not form a ring. However, it has been connected with dysphagia. Although 7 patients were operated on in this series early in our experience, we do not believe that an anomalous right subclavian artery causes symptoms in children. The elusive symptoms of dysphagia (dysphagia lusoria) are only a red herring masking the true causes of symptoms.

In group III, the pulmonary artery sling, the aortic arch system usually is normal. In this abnormality, the true main pulmonary artery is not present, and the left pulmonary artery arises from the right pulmonary artery, forming a sling as it circles around the right bronchus passing between the trachea and esophagus toward the left lung (Fig. 80–9). The hypothesis for the embryologic development of this defect is that the left lung loses its connection to the left sixth arch and receives its blood supply subsequently from the right sixth arch, that is, the right pulmonary artery. Associated tracheobronchial anomalies, such as complete tracheal rings and abnormal tracheal branching, are frequent (33 percent) and exaggerate the respiratory obstruction. In 1 patient, a ventricular septal defect was present.

CLINICAL MANIFESTATIONS

The clinical manifestation of patients with compression of the trachea and esophagus may vary with the type of malformation. The clinical symptoms and signs may be so subtle, mimicking various respiratory difficulties, that the diagnosis may be easily missed unless a high degree of vigilance and suspicion is maintained.

Stridor and noisy respiration are very common and develop early in life, especially in the double aortic arch group or in the tight ring from a right arch and a left ligamentum. However, the symptoms in the latter anomaly occur later than those of the double aortic arch. Respiratory distress and labored respiration may be seen and may be severe, especially in the pulmonary artery sling group.

Chronic cough is very common and may have a trumpeting sound quality described as "seal bark" or "brassy cough." Recurrent respiratory infection and pneumonia may be reported. Respiratory distress may become aggravated during or after feeding, especially if an infant is given solid food. This may precipitate episodes of choking and cyanosis, leading to apneic spells and possibly hypoxic seizures. The bolus of food passing through the narrowed area of the esophagus presses on the soft posterior trachea trapped inside the vascular ring, worsening the airway obstruction. Apnea frequently is associated with innominate artery compression and may be due to a reflex initiated by the tracheal compression. The examiner should keep in mind that apneic spells may be caused by other factors rather than being a direct result of tracheal compression.

Vomiting and regurgitation may follow the respiratory difficulties, with accompanying aspiration and pneumonia, and at times may lead to endotracheal intubation or tracheostomy. Often, it is noted that the infant assumes a hyperextended neck or opisthotonic posture. This posture stretches the trachea longitudinally, providing a splinting effect. Generally and in spite of the frequent feeding problems, infants with vascular rings appear to be well fed, since they usually take liquid formula well. When such infants are failing to thrive and in the lower weight percentile, associated cardiac or gastrointestinal anomalies should be suspected.

On examination, one may find only mild stridor. However, in moderate to severe cases, stridor will be associated with tachypnea, increased respiratory effort, nasal flaring, sternal and intercostal retractions with wheezing, and rales. The stridor is both inspiratory and expiratory. Associated pneumonia or atelectasis may be noted on physical examination. Older children with dysphagia may show no significant physical signs, although a history of slow feeding may be elicited. Occasionally, we see an older child 10 or 12 years of age with vascular ring who unconsciously has adapted to the dysphagia by being a slow feeder and chewing food well. Variations in origin and branching of brachiocephalic vessels usually do not produce abnormalities in pulses or blood pressure unless there are other anomalies.

DIAGNOSIS

In addition to the signs and symptoms, diagnostic procedures are needed to confirm a clinical suspicion of tracheoesophageal obstruction by a vascular structure. A
plain roentgenogram of the chest may demonstrate pulmonary infiltrates or atelectasis. Unilateral or bilateral
hyperinflation and air trapping may be seen in patients
with pulmonary artery sling. The location of the aortic
arch on plain chest roentgenogram is extremely helpful.
A right arch with the associated respiratory difficulties
may be an indication of a ring with a left ligamentum.
When the location of the aortic arch is indeterminate,
a double aortic arch may be suspected.

The lateral view may demonstrate an anterior indentation of the tracheal air column, which may be the
only finding of an innominate artery compression. The
barium swallow is the most important single diagnostic
procedure when a vascular ring is suspected (Fig. 80–
10).[9] A double indentation on each side of the esophagus
with the right one higher than the left is diagnostic of
a double aortic arch. A right arch with a left ligamentum
will also produce a double indentation. However, the
left one is usually more oblique or smaller. A posterior
and oblique indentation ascending from left to right on
the esophagogram with a left aortic arch on plain chest
x-ray is indicative of an aberrant right subclavian artery.
An anterior indentation on the esophagogram with a
mass between the esophagus and trachea may be indicative of pulmonary artery sling. Anterior compression of
the trachea by the innominate artery or other branches
of the aortic arch does not produce identifiable abnormalities on barium studies.

Bronchoscopy is not essential in the diagnosis of
vascular rings, although it is often performed in the diagnostic workup because of the insidious and unspecific
respiratory symptoms. However, it is necessary for the
diagnosis of anomalous vessel compressing the trachea
anteriorly. Pulsations are observed at the site of narrowing. Anterior pressure by the tip of the bronchoscope
against the tracheal wall in the narrow area will obliterate
or weaken the affected radial or carotid artery pulses.
Bronchoscopy is helpful in identifying tracheal abnormalities associated with pulmonary artery sling. Although
a bronchogram may be useful in the diagnosis of associated intrinsic anomalies of the airway in pulmonary artery
sling, it could be a dangerous procedure further comprising the narrow airway, and we do not recommend it as
part of the diagnostic studies.

Cineangiography is not necessary in most instances
except for the diagnosis of pulmonary artery sling. However, a cardiac catheterization may be indicated when
associated intracardiac defects are suspected.

Recently, with advances in computed tomography
(CT) scanning and magnetic resonance imaging (MRI),

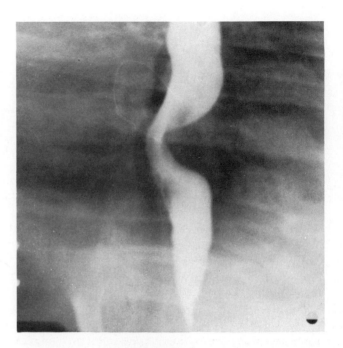

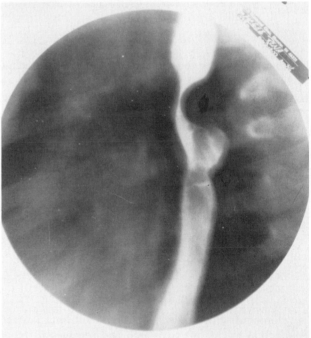

Figure 80–10. Top. Double aortic arch that is displacing both the
esophagus and the trachea anteriorly. **Bottom.** A double aortic arch
that was associated with an esophageal atresia. The black arrow
points to the vascular indentation, and the esophageal anastomosis
just below is marked by the light arrow.

we have been able to make the diagnosis of a double
aortic arch, a right arch with left ligamentum, and a
pulmonary artery sling with complete tracheal rings.
These two diagnostic modalities may eliminate the need
for the usual invasive diagnostic procedures.

When an innominate artery compression is suspected and diagnosed by bronchoscopy, additional studies to clarify the causes of apnea are needed. Sleep studies, complete neurologic evaluation, and radioisotope gastroesophageal reflux studies should be performed before proceeding with surgical treatment.

DIFFERENTIAL DIAGNOSIS

Other causes of respiratory distress should be considered. The commonest of these is tracheobronchomalacia, with which no abnormalities are seen on an esophagogram. Bronchoscopy demonstrates collapse of the trachea with no specific identation. Other cases of extrinsic compression of the tracheobronchial tree include esophageal duplications, bronchogenic cysts, benign and malignant tumors, neurofibromas, and intrinsic tracheobronchial stenosis. Vocal cord paralysis and subglottic stenosis present a distinct inspiratory stridor and are diagnosed easily by endoscopy. Tracheoesophageal fistulas without esophageal atresia or gastroesophageal reflux may cause both respiratory distress and dysphagia.

SURGICAL MANAGEMENT

The indication for operative treatment is the presence of a true and complete vascular ring or a pulmonary artery sling. In the case of a double aortic arch, the symptoms usually are severe and of early onset, and surgical division of the ring should be performed without delay. The infant with pulmonary artery sling with severe respiratory distress may have to be operated on as an emergency procedure. With innominate artery compression, the indication for surgery should be when the tracheal obstruction is over 50 percent of the lumen as judged by bronchoscopy and when other causes of apnea have been ruled out.

A left thoracotomy is the most widely used approach except in cases of innominate artery compression, when a right anterolateral incision is made to suspend the artery to the chest wall. It is helpful to leave some pericardial attachment to the origin of the innominate artery to use for suspension.

A median sternotomy could be used for repair of pulmonary artery sling. It is especially indicated when the repair of the sling is to be performed simultaneously with tracheoplasty for complete tracheal ring.[10]

In preparation for division of a vascular ring, the anesthesiologist should place a blood pressure cuff on both arms of the child and should have access to both carotid and arm pulses. When the components of the aortic arch and vascular rings are exposed and the site for the division of a double aortic arch is clamped, the integrity of the brachiocephalic circulation should be checked. This is especially important when both aortic arches are patent. Most often the ring is divided at the atretic segment.

In a double aortic arch, the ring is divided usually at the posterior end of the lesser arch. The ligamentum arteriosum should always be divided, and careful dissection of any fibrous band that may remain on the trachea or esophagus should be performed. In cases of right arch and a left ligamentum, the ring is released by dividing the ligamentum.

The left pulmonary artery sling is divided between clamps, and the distal end is sutured in front of the trachea to the pulmonary artery. The divided ends of a vascular ring should be sutured rather than tied to avoid dislodgment of a ligature. It is imperative that during the operation, the phrenic, vagus, and recurrent laryngeal nerves be identified and protected.

Diligent and careful postoperative management is of the utmost importance. Humidity, oxygen, chest physiotherapy, and nasotracheal suction may be needed frequently. Postoperative endotracheal intubation should be avoided if possible to decrease the chance of irritation and edema of the tracheal lining.

RESULTS

Relief from respiratory distress usually is apparent immediately after the surgery. However, immediate relief may not occur when there is additional luminal compromise by mucosal edema, deformed tracheal cartilages, or tracheomalacia.[11] Frequent respiratory infection and an unusual cough often persist for several months. We have observed a general trend of continuing improvement over a long period.

Technical problems that contribute to mortality include failure to recognize the pathology, inadequate surgery, and hemorrhage from dislodged ligatures. Postoperative respiratory failure, especially when associated with infection, continues to be a difficult problem. Other major associated anomalies may influence the operative results significantly.

SUMMARY

Tracheoesophageal compression secondary to vascular anomalies requires surgery when it is symptomatic. In cases of respiratory distress in infants and young children, this diagnosis should be considered and proper evaluation should be made, especially with the barium esophagogram. Early diagnosis and surgical repair prevent multiple complications and significant morbidity. Surgeons dealing with these lesions should be familiar with varieties of anatomic anomalies.

REFERENCES

1. Gross RE: Surgical relief for tracheal obstruction from a vascular ring. N Engl J Med 233:586, 1945
2. Edwards JE: Anomalies of the derivatives of the aortic arch. Med Clin North Am 32:925, 1948
3. Gross RE: Arterial malformations which cause compression of the trachea or esophagus. Circulation 11:124, 1955
4. Mustard WT, Trimble AW, Trusler GA: Mediastinal vascular anomalies causing tracheal and esophageal compression and obstruction in childhood. Can Med Assoc J 87:1301, 1962
5. Wychulis AR, Kincaid OW, Weidman WH, Danielson GK: Congenital vascular rings: Surgical considerations and results of operation. Mayo Clin Proc 46:182, 1971
6. Nikaidoh H, Riker WL, Idriss FS: Surgical management of "vascular ring." Arch Surg 105:327, 1972
7. Koopot R, Nikaidoh H, Idriss FS: Surgical management of anomalous left pulmonary artery causing tracheobronchial obstruction. J Thorac Cardiovasc Surg 69:239, 1975
8. Stewart JR, Kincaid OW, Edwards JE: An Atlas of Vascular Rings and Related Malformations of the Aortic Arch Systems. Springfield, IL, Charles C Thomas, 1964
9. Klinkhamer AC: Esophagography in Anomalies of the Aortic Arch System. Baltimore, Williams & Wilkins, 1969
10. Idriss, FS, DeLeon SY, Ilbawi MN, et al: Tracheoplasty with pericardial patch for extensive tracheal stenosis in infants and children. J Thorac Cardiovasc Surg 88:527, 1984
11. Binet JP, Langlois J: Aortic arch anomalies in children and infants. J Thorac Cardiovasc Surg 73:248, 1977

81
Esophageal Atresia and Tracheoesophageal Stenosis

An infant born with an atresia of the esophagus, with or without a tracheoesophageal fistula, presents a challenge that encompasses the gamut of technical, respiratory, nutritional, and ethical problems encountered in pediatric surgery. Perhaps the criterion of real surgical skill should be the ability to successfully manage a 1 kg infant with an esophageal atresia and an imperforate anus. Sporadic attempts were made to correct esophageal atresia and tracheoesophageal fistula during the early part of this century. However, these infants faced a 100 percent mortality prior to 1939. At that time, Ladd and Leven, working separately, divided the fistula and exteriorized the esophagus in the neck.[1,2] Then with multiple operations, they succeeded in bridging the gap between the cervical esophagus and the stomach. In 1941, Haight of the University of Michigan successfully performed a complete primary repair.[3] His work stimulated other surgeons to continue with primary division of the fistula and end-to-end anastomosis of the esophagus.

Each decade since 1940 has seen dramatic improvements in the results of treatment. At the Children's Memorial Hospital in Chicago, 30 percent of 35 patients treated from 1946 to 1950 survived.[4] By 1960 the survival rate was 66 percent, and in the third edition of this text Dr. Swenson reported a survival rate of 78 percent.[5] Since 1970, all infants operated on without other major congenital anomalies have survived, and the overall survival rate, including those who died of other birth defects at a later date, is now 85 percent.

There have been minimal changes in surgical technique, so this dramatic improvement is more related to advancements in anesthesia and in preoperative and postoperative care than to the operative procedure. In addition, efforts to educate nurses and physicians who deal with the neonate have resulted in diagnosis within the first few hours of life.

It is difficult to establish the actual incidence of esophageal atresia, but it is approximately 1 in 3000 live births. This anomaly is found in twins, siblings, and the offspring of adults who themselves had esophageal atresia.[6-12] These reports are suggestive of a genetic etiology, but as yet no definite pattern has been established. David and O'Callaghan could find only that mothers under 20 years of age with no previous offspring and mothers over 35 years of age were more likely to have infants with esophageal anomalies.[13] In their series, there were three times the expected numbers of twins, but in only two cases was esophageal atresia part of a recessively inherited malformation.

PATHOLOGY

The classification of esophageal atresia has become exceedingly complex. Many authors have evolved their own systems, consisting of either numbers or letters, to describe the various defects. These systems are satisfactory for the most common lesions, but even with these, one must have a moderate understanding of the previous literature. The ultimate classification is found in Kluth's "Atlas of Esophageal Atresia," in which all known varieties of these anomalies are illustrated and described.[14] This review is most valuable in pointing out the almost endless variations that exist. It is much simpler to describe the pathology in an individual than to apply any preconceived system of classification.

There are three basic types of esophageal anomalies. The most common, which accounts for 86 percent of these lesions, consists of a proximal esophageal atresia with a fistula between the distal esophagus and the respiratory tract (Fig. 81–1).[15] The proximal esophagus may end in the neck or may overlap the distal esophagus. It becomes dilated and hypertrophied by the efforts of the fetus to swallow amniotic fluid. The dilated proximal

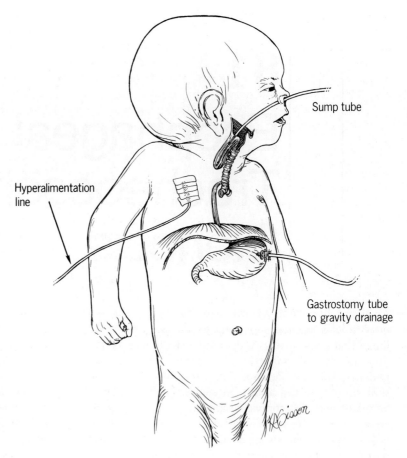

Figure 81–1. Proximal esophageal atresia with distal fistula. This illustration represents our current staging technique for a high-risk infant. The proximal pouch is emptied with a sump tube, the gastrostomy prevents reflux up the esophagus, and nutrition is provided by hyperalimentation.

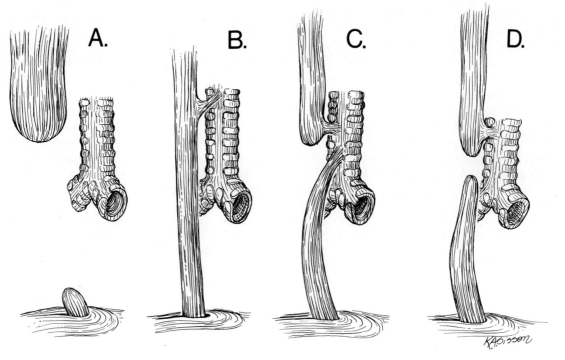

Figure 81–2. A. Esophageal atresia without fistula. **B.** Fistula without atresia. **C.** Both proximal and distal fistulas. **D.** Proximal fistula only.

pouch compresses the trachea and is probably the cause of the tracheomalacia exhibited by many babies. There may even be muscular continuity between the proximal and distal portions of the esophagus. The fistula usually enters the trachea 1 to 1.5 cm above the carina but may join with either mainstem bronchus.

Atresia of the esophagus without fistula is the next most common anomaly (Fig. 81–2A). The proximal pouch ends blindly in the neck or upper thorax, and the distal esophagus is a small nubbin that extends 2 to 3 cm above the diaphragm. There is almost always a long gap between the two esophageal ends, which precludes a primary anastomosis.

Tracheoesophageal fistula without an atresia is the next most common, accounting for about 1 percent of these anomalies (Fig. 81–2B). The fistula usually occurs between the esophagus and the cervical trachea. This is commonly known as the H-type fistula. If the fistula is long and oblique, the symptoms may be minimal and the lesion may remain undiagnosed for many years. Multiple H-type fistulas also have been reported. A fistula between the upper pouch and the trachea, either with or without a distal fistula, occurs in less than 1 percent of reported cases (Fig. 81–2C, D). It is possible, however, that a second fistula overlooked at the first operation may later be considered as a recurrence of the original fistula.

ASSOCIATED DEFECTS

Approximately half of the babies with esophageal malformations have major birth defects in other organ systems. Still more have relatively minor anomalies. Multiple malformations are the most common cause of postoperative complications and death. In reviewing the various series of infants with esophageal anomalies through the years, it would appear that the incidence of multiple defects is increasing. On the other hand, as we have become more aware of multiple defects, greater efforts have been made to study individual infants. Furthermore, in the earlier series of surgical cases, it is possible that infants with major cardiac or central nervous system anomalies died before correction of the esophagus.

The incidence of major cardiovascular anomalies varies from 28 percent in the review of David and O'Callaghan to 14.7 percent in the study by Greenwood and Rosenthal.[16,17] Infants with associated cardiac defects also have lower birth weights and shorter gestations, which factors contribute to an increased mortality. The most common lesions are patent ductus arteriosus, ventricular septal defect, atrial septal defect, and right aortic arch. The cardiac defects are especially severe when there are multiple associated anomalies of the skeletal and gastrointestinal systems. The most common gastroin-

testinal malformation associated with esophageal atresia is the imperforate anus. The rectal defect usually is discovered first. Any infant with an imperforate anus must have a radiopaque catheter passed into the stomach to rule out an esophageal atresia. Other defects include intestinal atresia, malrotation, and pyloric stenosis.[18,19] Diagnosis of these intestinal obstructions may be delayed if the original roentgenograms taken to diagnose the esophageal lesion fail to include the entire abdomen. In addition, when there is only an esophageal atresia without a fistula, it is important to place contrast material in the stomach at the time of gastrostomy to detect distal atresias. Retrospective reviews of the radiographs of infants with esophageal atresia have demonstrated a high incidence of vertebral anomalies. As many as 75 percent of these infants have an extra thoracic or lumbar vertebra.[20,21]

Other musculoskeletal anomalies include hemivertebrae, extra ribs, and extremity defects.[22] The embryonic hypersomatization associated with the extra vertebra may provide a clue to the embryogenesis of esophageal anomalies and in a practical fashion may aid in the radiographic diagnosis of the H-type tracheoesophageal fistula.

As large series of infants with tracheoesophageal anomalies have been accumulated, an association of defects has been noted by several observers.[23,24] The VATER association designates vertebral defects, anal atresia, tracheoesophageal (TE) fistula with esophageal atresia, renal defects, and radial limb dysplasia. This association is random in occurrence, any single infant may not have the complete syndrome. Abnormalities of the external genitalia and chromosomal deletion have also been found in babies with the VATER association.[25,26] The occurrence of tracheoesophageal fistulas in twins, only one of which had the VATER syndrome, further complicates our understanding of the genetic basis for esophageal anomalies.[27]

Tracheobronchial malformations, including tracheal stenosis, bronchobiliary fistula, hypoplasia of the lung, and bronchial stenosis, are rare but will result in severe unexpected pulmonary complications unless they are recognized.[28,29] Difficulties in the original endotracheal intubation may provide a clue to tracheal stenosis. Persistent atelectasis despite vigorous suctioning should prompt bronchoscopy or tracheobronchography to search for these unusual defects.

EMBRYOLOGY

At 20 to 23 days of gestation, when the embryo is 3 mm long, a diverticulum develops in the midline of the ventral wall of the foregut. Initially, this diverticulum occurs between the thyroid primordium and the stomach.

This original single tube separates into the esophagus and trachea by the union of proliferating ridges of the cells composing its endothelial lining. The eventual complete separation of the trachea and esophagus takes place through the proliferation of these cells rather than by external ingrowth of mesenchymal tissue. Coincidental with the separation of the esophagus and trachea, the esophagus must grow at 16 somites to extend from its original site at the thyroid primordium to below the diaphragm. Perhaps a too rapid elongation would diminish the tissue available to the esophagus and cause an imbalance in the growth of the trachea and esophagus. This theory is strengthened by the extra vertebrae or hypersegmentation that frequently accompanies these lesions. Fistulas may be explained by a localized shortage of cells needed to complete the endothelial proliferation essential for complete separation of the two organs.[30] A complete arrest of development of the cephalic end of the septum between the trachea and esophagus leads to a complete laryngoesophageal cleft. This failure to separate may extend from the larynx to the carina.

CLINICAL PRESENTATION

The first sign of an esophageal atresia may be polyhydramnios in the mother. Amniography will demonstrate an obstruction as the fetus swallows amniotic fluid.[31] The infant with an esophageal atresia presents an unforgettable picture, which any alert student nurse can diagnose at a glance. Almost immediately after birth, saliva commences to drip out of the baby's nose and mouth. With each respiration, white, frothy mucus bubbles back and forth out of the nose while a constant stream of saliva drips out of the infant's mouth. After efficient oropharyngeal suctioning, the infant will appear to be perfectly normal, a fact that has misled more than one intern into doubting the nurse's word! In addition to the obvious salivation, there are rhonchi over the lung fields and chest retractions caused by laryngeal obstruction. It is rare now that such an infant is offered a feeding, but if the baby is given water or milk, he or she will cough, choke, and turn cyanotic. If there is no fistula to the lower esophagus, the abdomen is scaphoid, but a tracheoesophageal fistula will force air into the stomach, causing abdominal distention.

Any infant with the slightest hint of respiratory distress, or any other difficulty for that matter, should have a radiopaque tube passed down each nostril and on into the stomach. If there is an esophageal atresia, the tube will stop at 10 to 12 cm. The normal distance to an infant's cardia is about 17 cm. If the tube is soft and flexible, it will curl in the upper pouch and may give one a false sense that it has passed into the stomach.

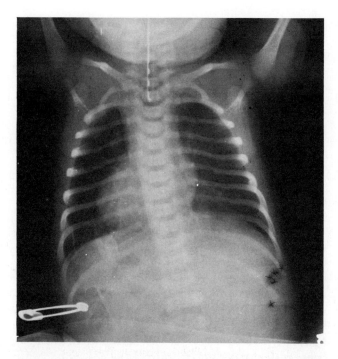

Figure 81–3. Esophageal atresia demonstrated with a radiopaque feeding tube in the proximal pouch.

Consequently, we prefer to use a size 8 French feeding tube that is slightly stiff and also radiopaque (Fig. 81–3). If air is injected into the tube, no bubbles will be heard over the abdomen, but the infant will audibly belch forth the injected air out of the mouth. The tube is taped in place, and anterolateral and posterolateral roentgenograms are obtained. It is important to include the chest and abdomen. In our hospital, the diagnosis was once missed when the catheter went through the larynx, down the trachea, into the fistula, and on into the stomach. The x-rays will demonstrate the catheter coiled in the proximal pouch. If there is a fistula, air will be seen in the stomach and gastrointestinal tract. One simple roentgenogram will make the diagnosis of esophageal atresia and, in most cases, will let us know whether or not there is a distal fistula. The absence of air in the gastrointestinal tract is not an infallible sign that there is no fistula. We observed one baby who had a tiny fistula that had evidently become plugged with mucus. When contrast material was injected into the stomach at the time of gastrostomy, the distal esophagus and fistula were identified. It is important that the entire abdomen be included in the x-ray because this allows one to diagnose other gastrointestinal anomalies. Formerly we did not recommend the use of contrast material in the proximal pouch because of the risk of spilling excess material into the lung (Fig. 81–4). Koop reported a higher mortality rate and an increased incidence of pneumonia in babies who were given contrast

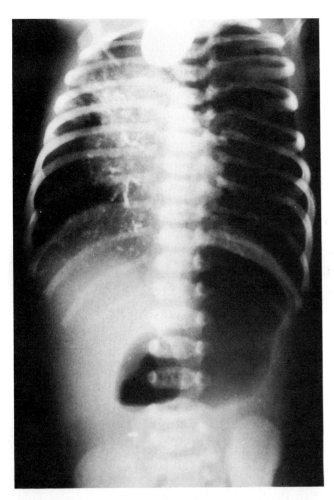

Figure 81–4. Beware of using too much contrast material! One half to one milliliter is enough to outline a proximal fistula without spillage into the lung.

material.[32] After we overlooked three proximal fistulas, we now instill 0.5 to 1 ml of either barium or metrizamide into the upper pouch under fluoroscopic control. A small proximal pouch or immediate spillage of contrast material into the trachea suggests a proximal fistula (Fig. 81–5). The contrast material must be immediately and completely aspirated from the pouch by the radiologist. It is possible to overlook a proximal fistula if the material appears to be aspirated through the larynx.[33,34] If any contrast material enters the trachea, preoperative bronchoscopy is indicated to definitely determine the presence of a proximal fistula. An echocardiogram is a helpful preoperative procedure not only to detect associated cardiac defects but also to determine the side of the aortic arch.

Diagnosis of H-type fistulas is most difficult. These anomalies are exceedingly rare but must be considered in any infant who coughs and chokes with feedings or who has repeated bouts of pneumonia. Some infants cough and choke in the newborn nursery and are suspected of having a typical esophageal atresia, but the catheter will go all the way to the stomach. Gavage feedings will relieve the coughing spells, but as soon as oral feedings are resumed, the infant will cough again. On physical examination, the lungs have coarse rales and rhonchi that clear with coughing. There is also gaseous abdominal distention because of the excess air forced down the fistula. If the diagnosis is not made promptly, the child develops chronic pneumonitis, which responds poorly to antibiotic therapy. Another possibility is an immune deficiency or cystic fibrosis of the pancreas. In several patients, the diagnosis has not been made until adult life.[35] The first step in the diagnosis is very careful cinefluoroscopy of the esophagus by an experienced pediatric radiologist. These fistulas are in the neck. Consequently, the column of barium must be watched very carefully from the mouth down. It is helpful to use thin barium and to place the infant in the prone position (Fig. 81–6). Even then, the contrast material may appear in the fistula and the trachea for only an instant or two before it is coughed out. During the past 16 years, our radiologists have made the diagnosis of all H-type fistulas without the need for more complicated techniques. It may be necessary to repeat the esophagogram if the first try fails to demonstrate a lesion. Sundar et al. believed that a skilled radiologist could make the diagnosis.[36] At the Toronto Children's Hospital, the diagnosis was made radiologically in 14 of 19 babies.[37] On the other hand, others have had so much difficulty making this diagnosis that cervical exploration has been recommended in infants with symptoms of coughing and choking.[38]

Endoscopy has been used in making the diagnosis of tracheoesophageal fistulas since Tucker and Pendergrass successfully passed radiopaque catheters through a standard bronchoscope in 1933.[39] Since then Swenson and others have recommended endoscopic examination of the trachea when an H-type fistula is suspected.[40] Gans and Johnson pioneered the use of modern rod lens telescopic endoscopes in the accurate diagnosis of esophageal anomalies.[41] The fistula can be seen better through the trachea than from the esophagus. By intubating the fistula with a Fogarty balloon catheter, not only is the diagnosis made but the catheter serves also as an accurate guide to the division of the fistula. A simple screening test for an H-type fistula consists of the insufflation of 100 percent oxygen though an endotracheal tube placed just beneath the vocal cords.[42] Gas is then withdrawn from the stomach though a nasogastric tube. If the oxygen concentration in the stomach rises simultaneously with the insufflation of oxygen into the trachea, the diagnosis is practically made. Normally, the intragastric oxygen concentration varies within very narrow limits, from 21 to 23 percent.

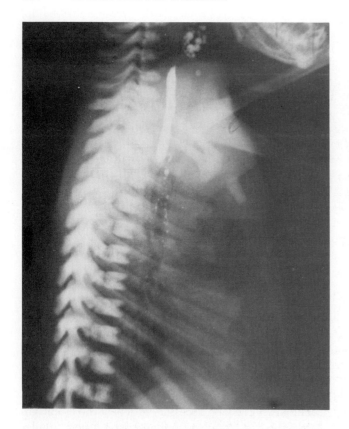
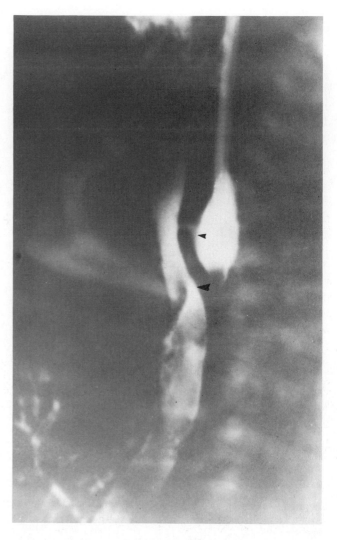

Figure 81–5. Left. The proximal pouch is very narrow because of a small proximal fistula. **Right.** A double fistula—the small arrow points to the proximal fistula and the longer arrow to the distal fistula.

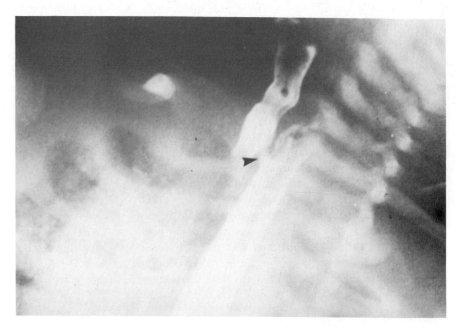

Figure 81–6. An H-type tracheoesophageal fistula in the cervical esophagus.

DIFFERENTIAL DIAGNOSIS

There are few lesions that simulate an esophageal atresia in the newborn infant. The most important is the traumatic perforation of the hypopharynx with a stiff catheter or the obstetrician's finger during a difficult breach delivery.[43–45] These infants are initially depressed or have the respiratory distress syndrome. They are subjected to vigorous attempts at resuscitation, including either the passage of a stiff catheter to aspirate secretions or traumatic efforts to intubate the trachea. Later, they choke and gag on their own saliva. Usually, however, they have either purulent or blood-tinged secretions. Because of hypopharyngeal spasm, it is difficult or impossible to pass a soft catheter into the esophagus. The diagnosis may be made with radiologic studies that demonstrate a pseudodiverticulum commencing at the hypopharynx and extending for varying distances posterior to the esophagus (Fig. 81–7). On laryngoscopic examinaton, there is a tear in the mucosa that is filled with purulent debris. These infants require only respiratory support, antibiotics, and the passage of a soft nasogastric tube under direct vision for feedings. Healing takes place, with closure of the perforation, within 2 or 3 weeks. An operation is required only if there is continued sepsis with evidence of a cervical abscess or mediastinitis. Definite mucosa-lined congenital diverticulae originating from the posterior pharyngeal wall also have been

described.[46–49] Although it is possible that diverticulae could be mistaken for esophageal atresia, in the reported cases the babies were able to swallow but had symptoms of respiratory distress. The diverticulae were easily diagnosed by a barium swallow.

Infants with central nervous system damage often swallow poorly because of cricopharyngeal incoordination.[50] These infants take their feedings poorly and often choke. Radiologic studies demonstrate aspiration of contrast material into the larynx as well as laryngovestibular overflow. These infants should be completely studied, radiologically as well as with endoscopic techniques, to rule out vascular ring and gastroesophageal reflux as well as tracheoesophageal fistula. They usually have fairly obvious neurologic defects that lead to a correct diagnosis.

TREATMENT

As soon as the diagnosis of esophageal atresia is suspected, the mucus and saliva in the nose, throat, and upper blind pouch must be suctioned using sterile technique. If a double lumen sump tube is available, it is inserted into the pouch and attached to suction. Otherwise repeated suctioning is essential to clear the upper airway. The baby's body temperature is maintained by placing him or her in a warm, humidified incubator. Before decompressing the stomach with a gastrostomy, it is probably best to keep the infant in an upright position in an attempt to prevent aspiration of gastric contents into the tracheobronchial tree.

If the infant is to be transferred to a neonatal center, a nurse or physician must accompany him or her to continue suctioning the mouth and upper pouch. On admission to a neonatal surgical unit, pharyngeal secretions are obtained for culture, and antibiotics are administered. Treatment is given for associated problems, such as hyperbilirubinemia, hypoglycemia, and pneumonia, and the baby is evaluated for other congenital defects. A plastic sump tube is passed through the mouth and attached to continuous suction.[51] Usually, several hours are required to evaluate and stabilize the baby. During this time, vigorous suctioning that stimulates a cry or cough will clear the bronchi and open areas of atelectasis. If there is a persistent atelectasis (usually of the right upper lobe), direct laryngoscopic suctioning is indicated. A decision is then made whether to proceed with:

1. Primary esophageal repair, with or without a gastrostomy
2. Gastrostomy with delayed repair
3. Gastrostomy with division of the fistula or other staging procedure
4. No immediate operation

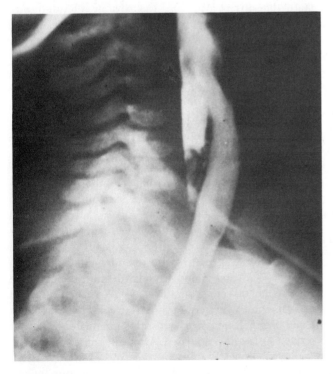

Figure 81–7. Lateral esophagogram demonstrating a hypopharyngeal perforation secondary to the passage of a stiff catheter used to resuscitate the infant at birth.

There are no hard and fast rules as to which is the best course to follow. Many surgeons working in various centers have obtained equally good results with different approaches. Most agree, however, that the poor-risk infant, i.e., the baby with multiple anomalies, prematurity, or pneumonia, will have a better opportunity to survive if the esophageal repair is delayed. The following plan of therapy has evolved at The Children's Memorial Hospital in Chicago.

The open tracheoesophageal fistula allows air to distend the stomach, which elevates the diaphragms and interferes with respirations. In addition, gastric contents regurgitate back through the fistula into the lungs. This chemical pneumonia does more damage than aspiration of saliva. Therefore, a gastrostomy is performed within a few hours after hospital admission. This is done under local anesthesia but with the baby fully monitored and with an anesthesiologist continually observing the infant for signs of airway obstruction (Fig. 81–8). A 2 cm high rectus-splitting incision is made just beneath the left rib margin. This incision must be placed above the transverse colon to prevent evisceration of small bowel through the wound.

The stomach is distended and easily found. A site midway between the greater and lesser curvature is grasped with a mosquito hemostat and encircled with two silk pursestring sutures. The stomach wall is opened with the electrocautery to prevent bleeding, and a size 14 to 16 French Pezzar catheter is inserted and brought out the upper end of the incision. The stomach is sutured to the abdominal wall above and below the tube to prevent separation or leakage. The tube is placed on gravity drainage and secured to the abdominal wall. The general rule for securing gastrostomy tubes is that they must be sutured and taped so securely that the infant can be picked up by the tube! If the baby weighs over 1500 g, is vigorous, cries well, has clear lungs, and has no other obvious birth defects, we proceed with an immediate esophageal repair.

There is some controversy over the routine use of a gastrostomy in babies with TEF. A long series of patients were operated on at the Detroit Children's hospital without using gastrostomies.[52] There was no increase in morbidity or mortality between this group of patients and similar series in which a gastrostomy was employed. There is also some evidence that a gastrostomy may increase the incidence of postoperative gastroesophageal reflux. At this time, we would not perform a gastrostomy in a full-term infant who did not have pneumonia or other major birth defect.

There are some advantages to a brief bronchoscopic examination of the trachea at the time of operation. This study, which can be carried out with either a ventilating bronchoscope or with only a telescopic lens will reveal unexpected fistulas and the location of the takeoff of the esophagus from the trachea. During induction of anesthesia, the endotracheal tube must be carefully positioned. We lost one infant when the endotracheal tube was inserted into the esophagus through the trachea. The bevel of the tube should be anterior, and one can observe for bubbling with the gastrostomy tube underwater to see if there is an air leak down the fistula.

Technique

When the aortic arch is on the left side, the infant is positioned with the right side uppermost, tilted slightly into a prone position (Fig. 81–9A). A single folded towel placed beneath the warming mattress elevates the right chest slightly. The right arm is allowed to drop down, pulling the scapula forward. The incision commences midway between the spine of the scapula and the vertebra and continues around the scapula to the midaxillary line. The needle-tipped electrocautery is used to coagulate all vessels, and with the cutting current, the trapezius, lattissimus dorsi, rhomboid, and paraspinus muscles are divided from the neck of the fourth rib posteriorly to the end of the incision. This allows the scapula to fall forward, exposing the fourth intercostal space. The intercostal muscles are elevated and divided over a curved hemostat layer by layer until the pleura is visible (Fig. 81–9B). At this point it is important to find the extrapleural plane so that the intercostal muscle may be lifted free and divided as far posteriorly as possible.

Small, moistened Kuttner dissectors are used to effect the extrapleural dissection. As soon as space beneath the ribs is available, the ribs are elevated with two small Parker retractors to facilitate the extrapleural dissection (Fig. 81–9C). A small Finochietto retractor is then inserted, and the ribs are slowly spread. The pleura is most adherent posteriorly over the azygos vein (Fig. 81–9D). The Azygos Vein is divided between suture ligatures. These sutures are left long and held with a clamp. By placing this suture over a moistened sponge, the pleural envelope and lung are held away from the operative field. Frequently, no other retraction is necessary to expose the esophagus.

At this point, the trachea and vagus nerve are identified. The distal esophagus usually is found just beneath or slightly distal to the azygos vein. Initially, the distal esophagus is freed from the pleura with the Kuttner dissector, but from then on the esophagus is freed from its surrounding structures by opening the blades of a tenotomy scissors. Blood vessels to the esophagus are seen coming directly from the aorta. These are preserved because they will frequently stretch as the esophagus is mobilized. If necessary, vessels immediately adjacent to the fistula are coagulated. Only the adventitia of the esophagus is picked up with forceps during this dissection. When the esophagus has been freed laterally and posteriorly, a right angle clamp is passed around just

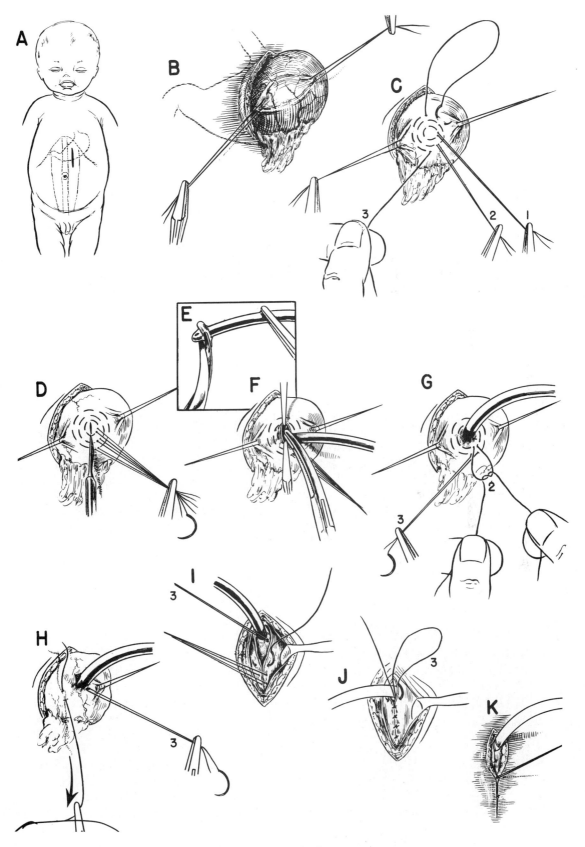

Figure 81–8 Techniques for Stann gastronomy.

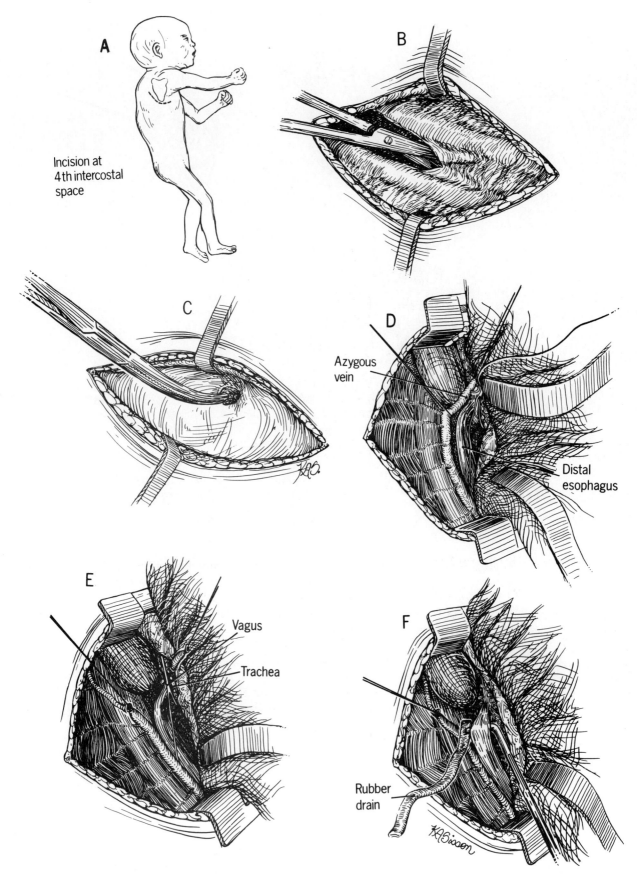

Figure 81–9. Technique for the extrapleural approach to an esophageal atresia and tracheoesophageal fistula, with division of the fistula and end-to-end anastomosis. (Note: especially in the small Parker retractors which elevate and separate the ribs). (Continued)

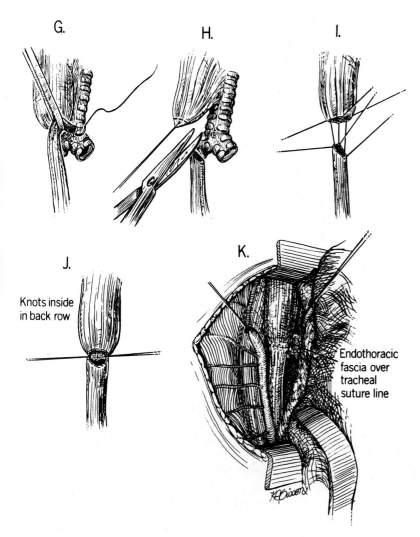

G.

H.

I.

J.

Knots inside
in back row

K.

Endothoracic
fascia over
tracheal
suture line

Figure 81–9 (Cont.)

distal to the fistula (Fig. 81–9F). A slip of rubber drain is used to encircle the esophagus for traction, since this is less traumatic than umbilical cord tape. The esophagus is then elevated and sharply dissected to its junction with the trachea. Before division of the fistula, the anesthesiologist is given an opportunity to expand the lungs and suction any accumulated secretions. The fistula is then divided, leaving 2 mm of esophagus on the trachea. A 6–0 suture is placed, taking a 2 mm bite of tissue on either side of the fistula as soon as the lower end has been divided (Fig. 81–9G). The fistula is completely divided and closed with interrupted sutures. The suture line is then covered with warm saline, and the lungs are again inflated and fully ventilated. If there are no leaks, the tracheal sutures are covered with adjacent fat, areolar tissue, and endothoracic fascia. This step ensures separation of the tracheal and esophageal suture lines and helps prevent a recurrent fistula.

The distal esophagus is covered with a warm, moistened sponge, and exposure is adjusted to the upper mediastinum. The proximal esophagus is definitely iden-

tified by having the anesthesiologist push a firm catheter into the depths of the blind pouch. A 6–0 suture is inserted through all layers of the esophagus precisely at its apex. This suture is then used for traction to facilitate dissection and identifies the site of the anastomosis. The proximal esophagus is freed laterally and posteriorly with a combination of sharp scissors and blunt dissection (Fig. 81–9H). The most difficult part is the separation of the proximal esophagus from the trachea. Sometimes it seems as if the esophagus and trachea share a common fascial or even muscular sheath. This must be very carefully dissected by retracting the esophagus laterally and by opening the plane between the esophagus and trachea by separating the blades of the scissors. This plane seems to open and the separation is easier higher in the mediastinum. The blood supply to the proximal pouch originates from the thyroid arteries, so the pouch may be dissected well up into the neck. Great care must be taken, however, to keep the dissection directly on the esophageal wall so as to prevent injury to the recurrent laryngeal nerves. When the proximal pouch has been completely dissected, it is covered with a moistened gauze and packed to control oozing blood vessels. The distal esophagus is again exposed, and a size 10 catheter is passed down into the stomach to identify a distal congenital stricture. The ends of the distal esophagus are then trimmed so that the opening is oblique. Both ends of the esophagus are exposed, and, with traction on the proximal suture in the blind pouch, the distance between the two ends is evaluated. If there appears to be a considerable gap between the two ends, one is faced with a dilemma. Dissection of the distal esophagus for length must be done at the expense of its blood supply. Consequently, as much length as possible must be obtained by mobilization of the proximal pouch. The vagus nerve should be left undisturbed and attached to the distal esophagus.

In almost every case, an anastomosis is feasible and should be attempted. The proximal pouch is opened transversely just beneath the traction suture, which is left in place to manipulate the upper pouch. We perform a one-layer anastomosis, taking both the muscle and mucosa. Sutures are placed so that the knots are within the lumen on the posterior row and outside the lumen anteriorly. When the first three posterior sutures have been placed, the two closest to the first assistant are held up and crossed to approximate the ends of the esophagus (Fig. 81–9I). The first suture and then the next two are tied. If one 6–0 suture will hold the ends together, the anastomosis will probably hold. Sutures are then placed about the circumference of the anastomosis, taking bites 2 mm back from the cut edges through all layers (Fig. 81–9J, K). The esophagus must not be grasped with forceps! The walls may be manipulated with a nerve hook or with a tissue forceps placed within the lumen to grasp the needle. The success of the anasto-mosis depends on gentleness in handling the tissues, the blood supply, and lack of tension, and not on any particular technique. The sutures are placed 2 mm apart, and an effort is made to invert the mucosa. Care must be taken to include the proximal mucosa, since this has a tendency to retract. It is difficult to gauge the amount of tension that an anastomosis will tolerate. If the upper esophageal pouch is in the neck and the gap between the two ends is 3 to 4 cm, we perform a circular myotomy on the proximal pouch. The procedure described by Livaditis et al. has been studied in labratory animals and has proven effective in bridging gaps of up to 4.5 cm.[53–56] The myotomy is performed by passing a large catheter into the upper pouch (an esophageal stethoscope is perfect) and incising the muscle layers with a scalpel down to the mucosa (Fig. 81–10). Several firm tugs on the traction suture will pull the muscle layers apart to leave exposed mucosa over a distance of 1 to 2 cm. There appears to be no interference with esophageal motility following the myotomy. If there is still too much tension, the distal esophagus is closed, and the anastomosis is delayed. A size 12 or 14 French rubber catheter with extra holes is then inserted through a stab wound below the incision. The tip of this catheter is sutured to the chest wall with a catgut stitch just lateral to the anastomosis. The tube is then connected to an underwater seal. Some surgeons prefer to use a simple soft rubber drain in the retropleural space. If this is done, a dressing must be applied over the drain, and if there is an overlooked perforation of the pleura, there will be a pneumothorax. After the catheter is secured, the ribs are approximated with interrupted catgut and the muscles with continuous 4–0 chromic catgut. The skin edges are closed with Steristrips and no dressing is used.

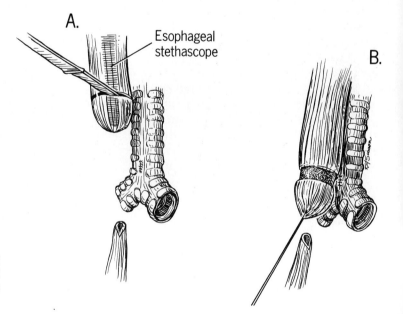

Figure 81–10. Circumferential myotomy of the proximal esophageal pouch, performed to gain the additional length needed for a tension-free anastomosis.

Controversies about the surgical technique center about using the transpleural versus the retropleural approach and the type of anastomosis. In 1964, Holder reported a 28.5 percent mortality for the transpleural route versus a 19 percent mortality for the retropleural approach.[57] An anastomotic leak is less dangerous when it occurs in the retropleural space. Unless there is a complete disruption of the anastomosis, the retropleural drain will handle the leak adequately, and it will then heal. Many surgeons prefer the Haight two-layer anastomosis, in which the proximal mucosa is sutured to the full thickness of the distal esophagus and the proximal muscle layer is then telescoped to cover the first layer. This technique has a lower incidence of reported leaks but a higher incidence of stricture formation.[58] In our experience with 83 patients, there were 3 major leaks and 3 strictures requiring either dilatations or secondary repair. The extra handling required for the Haight anastomosis, with the possibility of damaging the blood supply, would seem to outweigh its advantages. Koop et al. reported only 1 anastomotic leak in 80 cases with the one-layer anastomosis.[59] In our patients, there appears to be no difference in anastomotic complications between silk and synthetic nonabsorbable sutures. Spitz et al., however, found a higher complication rate with silk as compared to either polyglycolic acid or prolene sutures.[60] It is possible that suture granulomas, or stitch abscesses, around nonabsorbable sutures lead to delayed fistulas between the anastomosis and the tracheal suture line.

THE HIGH-RISK INFANT

Infants who weigh less than 1500 g or who have hyaline membrane disease, aspiration pneumonia, or major birth defects tolerate major operations and the possible complications poorly and have a higher mortality rate. Staging procedures that allow the infant to gain weight and recover from respiratory complications before the definitive esophageal repair have been successful in reducing the mortality rate in these high-risk babies. The first staging procedure was retropleural division of the fistula and gastrostomy.[61] In this procedure, the proximal pouch is drained with an indwelling sump tube, and gastrostomy feedings are given until the infant is judged to be sufficiently well to tolerate reexploration and esophageal anastomosis. Emergency ligation of the fistula may be indicated in the premature baby with hyaline membrane disease who requires high ventilatory pressures through an endotracheal tube.[62] An alternative temporizing measure is bronchoscopy with passage of a Fogarty catheter through the trachea and into the esophagus. Inflation of the balloon occludes the fistula, allowing ventilation without the risk of gastric reflux.[63] Early in our current

series, 6 babies were staged, and 3 died, all with associated anomalies. Our current policy is to perform only a gastrostomy under local anesthesia soon after the infant is admitted to the hospital. The tube is left on gravity drainage, and the infant is nourished with IV hyperalimentation until the lungs are clear and the weight is at least 1500 g. At that time, a delayed primary repair is performed. In our relatively small series, we lost only 1 of 9 infants with delayed primary repair. The single death occurred 6 months after the repair, with aspiration secondary to a cleft palate.

We have delayed between 4 and 50 days after admission of the baby to effect primary repair. Our only complication with hyperalimentation in this groups of infants was septic thrombosis of the superior vena cava in a 1000 g infant who survived multiple complications, but is mentally retarded at 10 years of age. Our survival rate in premature infants and those with correctible respiratory disease is no different from that in the full-term, well infant. Abrahamson and Shandling found that with better intensive care for premature infants, the risks of primary repair were less than when staging procedures were used.[64]

The care for an infant with multiple anomalies must be individualized. A colostomy for an imperforate anus is easily performed through the same incision used for the gastrostomy. The correction of an intestinal atresia also may be carried out at the same time if the infant is otherwise in good condition. An upper airway obstruction, such as a choanal atresia or laryngeal stenosis, must either be repaired or bypassed with a tracheotomy before the esophageal operation. Congenital heart lesions usually can be managed medically until the infant has recovered from the esophageal repair. We have also delayed ventriculoperitoneal shunting for hydrocephalus until after recovery from the esophageal operation.

Infants who have both a cleft palate and an esophageal atresia are in a difficult state because they lack the initial swallowing mechanism and have poor peristalsis in the esophagus. They are likely to aspirate at any time. These infants should be fed through a gastrostomy even after the esophageal anastomosis until they have undergone satisfactory palate repair. Babies with an esophageal atresia, a congenital heart defect, skeletal anomalies, or perhaps an imperforate anus have a poor opportunity for long-term survival and an even worse prospect for a normal life. The problem is compounded if there is a chromosomal defect or other evidence of mental retardation. These infants must be completely evaluated and the facts presented to both parents. In Holder's series of 100 infants with TEF, 15 required surgical management of an associated lesion before repair of the esophagus. In 1 baby, a pulmonary–systemic shunt for a severe tetrology of Fallot was performed simultaneously with fistula ligation through a right thoracotomy.[65]

POSTOPERATIVE CARE

The endotracheal tube is removed at the end of the operation if the infant is vigorous and has good respiratory efforts with clear lung fields on auscultation. Most babies are extubated immediately and returned to their warm, humidified incubators in room air or 30 to 40 percent oxygen, depending on blood gas analysis. The nursing staff carries out nasal and oropharyngeal suctioning every 2 to 3 hours or more frequently if necessary. The suction catheters are marked with a piece of tape at about 7 cm so the catheter will not be pushed down to the anastomosis. Positioning of the infant is one of the most important factors in nursing care—no infant should be left flat on the back! In this position, secretions in the throat are aspirated directly into the trachea, where they preferentially drain into the right upper lobe bronchus. The baby should be turned from side to side and should be prone at least part of the time with the head and chest inclined downward 15 to 20 degrees. This position is most important when a staging procedure has been performed and the upper pouch is still obstructed. After 48 hours, chest physiotherapy consisting of percussion and vibration is done three or four times a day. If there are persistent rales or rhonchi or if atelectasis is demonstrated on a chest roentgenogram, a physician directly aspirates the trachea with a laryngoscope. The baby is ventilated with a bag, mask, and 100 percent oxygen before and after this procedure. Cultures are taken of the secretions every other day to guide antibiotic therapy. The poor-risk infant is not extubated until he or she is breathing well and has clear lung fields, a $Paco_2$, below 50, and a Pao_2 in 50 percent oxygen above 50 torr. Either mechanical ventilation or CPAP may be required for varying periods of time. An endotracheal tube should not, in our opinion, be left in place to facilitate the aspiration of secretions from the tracheobronchial tree, since the tube itself is irritating.

Gastrostomy feedings are commenced 2 days after the operation and gradually increased to supply the infant's caloric requirements, depending on how this is tolerated. A barium swallow is performed on the fifth or sixth day, and if there is no anastomotic leak, feedings by mouth are started with a medicine dropper. If these are taken without cough or choking, the baby is given a bottle. The oral feedings are then advanced, and the gastrostomy feedings are decreased. The chest tube is removed on the fifth or sixth day when the x-ray demonstrates an intact anastomosis. Small anastomotic leaks are completely asymptomatic and are noted as a small puddle of contrast material outside the esophageal lumen. When this is seen, we merely delay oral feedings for another week and repeat the roentgenogram. These small leaks heal without complication and require nothing

more than prophylactic dilatations to prevent strictures. An increased respiratory rate, fever, lethargy, or any other change for the worse is an indication to repeat a plain chest x-ray in an attempt to find a pocket of air or fluid in the mediastinum. Usually, however, the first sign of a leak is the appearance of saliva in the chest tube. The diagnosis may be confirmed by giving the baby a few milliliters of dilute methylene blue dye. In addition, we advise a barium swallow to determine the magnitude of the leak and to see if the fluid is being drained well by the chest tube. Cultures are taken of the drainage, and the antibiotics are changed according to sensitivity studies.

Slow-drip gastrostomy feedings usually can be continued, provided the infant is kept upright. If there is reflux of formula and leakage out the tube, the gastrostomy tube is placed on gravity drainage and IV hyperalimentation is given until the anastomosis has healed. We have had little or no success with transduodenal or jejunostomy feedings because the babies with large leaks often are septic and afflicted with a paralytic ileus. If there is a major leak with purulent drainage, the posterior portion of the incision is opened to ensure adequate drainage. When a leak occurs after a transpleural operation, it is often necessary to exteriorize the proximal esophagus in the neck and close off the distal esophagus.

Recurrent tracheoesophageal fistula is suspected when the baby coughs and chokes during feedings in the postoperative period. The same difficulties are encountered in the diagnosis of a recurrent tracheoesophageal fistula as in diagnosis of the primary H variety. A cine-esophagogram is usually successful, but if this fails to make the diagnosis in a suspected case, endoscopy is indicated. When the diagnosis is made in the immediate postoperative period, the infant should be fed by gastrostomy and the repeat operation delayed at least 2 months.

There are differences of opinion regarding routine postoperative esophageal dilatations. We have routinely calibrated the esophagus on about the tenth postoperative day and then continued to pass either mercury or Tucker bougies at intervals of 2 weeks until a size 24 or 26 French bougie could pass with ease. These dilatations must be performed with great gentleness during the first few weeks. The bougie should be no more than one size larger than one that is tight. The technique is simple. The surgeon stands at the baby's head while a nurse or mother holds the infant with his arms at his waist. The index finger of the left hand is passed into the baby's pharynx to guide the bougie and prevent it from kinking. The tapered Tucker bougies will usually pass if they are rotated to find the proper track through the anastomosis. Usually, no more than two or three dilatations are required, but we have continued with intermittent dilatations for as long as 6 months. None of these babies have returned with tight strictures requiring retrograde dilatation or resection.

Older children with neglected strictures are seen occasionally. They may not become symptomatic until they attempt to swallow solid food. If a lumen can be found, these strictures may be dilated with tapered mercury bougies. If not, a guidewire may be passed into the stomach under fluoroscopy, and this may be used to lead a string through the esophagus and out a gastrostomy. The string is then used to pull Tucker dilators through the stricture. An alternative approach is to dilate the stricture with balloon dilatation under fluoroscopy. This technique produces less shearing damage to the surface mucosa. Every infant with a stricture must be carefully studied for gastroesophageal reflux, which contributes to the chronicity. An occasional recalcitrant stricture requires surgical resection.

Some children have a brassy cough and stridor for a year after repair. Their symptoms are aggravated by intercurrent respiratory infections. These infants seem to have softer-than-normal tracheas, which is possibly secondary to the pressure of the enlarged proximal pouch during embryonic development. The parents are warned about this complication and are advised to provide continuous humidity for the baby during the winter months and to seek immediate treatment for the common cold. In our experience, swallowing difficulties have not been a major problem. All of our patients are seen and evaluated with a cine-esophagogram at 1 and 2 years of age. Most are able to tolerate first a soft diet and then table food at the same age as their normal siblings. All of these infants, however, have abnormal motility, especially in the distal esophagus. This observation has been noted by many authors and has been confirmed with esophageal manometric studies.[66–69] The defective motility is probably due in part to division of vagus nerve fibers supplying the distal segment. However, abnormal motility is also seen in babies with the H-type fistula before any operation. The combination of poor motility with an inelastic anastomosis may result in food lodging in the esophagus, even if there is no stricture. The 3- or 4-year-old child tends to bolt food without benefit of chewing. For this reason, we advise parents to cut their child's food, especially hot dogs, into small, bite-size pieces until the child learns to chew.

Gastroesophageal reflux is common in children with esophageal atresia.[70,71] This is due to the decreased lower esophageal sphincter pressure seen in these patients and is aggravated by poor esophageal motility, since the reflux gastric acid is not rapidly cleared from the esophagus. Vomiting, persistent anastomotic strictures, and recurrent episodes of pneumonia result from the reflux. Any child with these symptoms must have a careful cine-esophagogram and endoscopy, since these symptoms are similar to those seen with recurrent fistulas. Persistent minor degrees of dysphagia seen in patients years after repair of the esophagus may be associated with reflux. In one series, 45 percent of 31 patients required a Nissen fundoplication for persistent symptoms.[72] Unfortunately, even the loose wrap used in these patients resulted in continued dysphagia because the poor esophageal motility could not overcome the resistance of the fundoplication. We have had to take down one Nissen fundoplication because of esophageal obstruction. An incomplete fundoplication, such as the Thal procedure, is indicated in these children. Apnea spells have been associated wth gastroesophageal reflux, but these life-threatening spells also have been traced to compression of the trachea between the enlarged esophageal pouch and an abnormal innominate artery.[73] These spells occur up to 20 months of age, commence with stridor and cyanosis, and in some cases progress to apnea, requiring resuscitation. In the reported cases, the trachea was shown to be compressed in an anterior–posterior direction, both on lateral roentgenograms and endoscopically. Suspension of the aorta and innominate artery anteriorly to the sternum relieved the spells.

It is clear that the surgeon's responsibility does not end when the operation is over. An infant who has been successfully operated on must be followed for many years to detect complications related to the defective esophagus. Many such patients continue to rank in the lower percentiles for weight and height and are slightly more prone to respiratory infections.

ESOPHAGEAL ATRESIA WITHOUT A FISTULA

Esophageal atresia without a fistula poses entirely different clinical problems. Primary esophageal anastomosis is rarely possible because the two ends of the esophagus are widely separated. A feeding gastrostomy is performed soon after the diagnosis is made. At that time, contrast material is injected through the tube into the stomach. A portable x-ray is then taken while the infant is still on the operating table. The distance between the two blind pouches is observed as the distance between the contrast material in the distal pouch and the proximal radiopaque catheter. A second film is taken 15 minutes later to observe the flow of contrast material down the small intestine (Fig. 81–11). This step rules out any distal obstructions.

In the past, an immediate cervical esophagostomy was performed to drain saliva away from the trachea. We now leave the proximal pouch intact in the hope that it may be stretched sufficiently to make an anastomo-

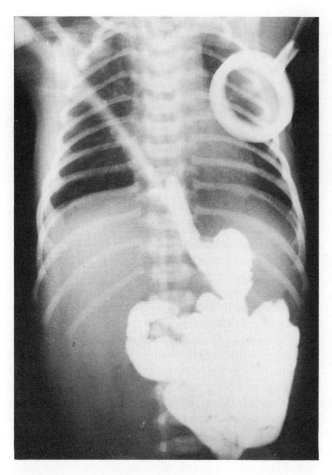

Figure 81–11. Esophageal atresia without a fistula. Contrast material injected into the stomach at the time of gastrostomy will reveal distal atresia for the length of the distal esophagus.

sis to the lower pouch or perhaps to an interposed segment of colon. The intact upper pouch tends to distend with swallowed saliva and may be stretched with mercury bougies.[74,75] We leave a size 14 French mercury bougie at the baby's cribside. The nurses insert the bougie through the infant's mouth and apply pressure to the upper pouch 5 minutes out of every hour. Each time a physician sees the infant, he or she too applies pressure to the upper pouch. The infant must be kept in the prone, head-down position during the time the proximal pouch is intact. This allows saliva to drip out of the mouth and aids the sump tube. Aspiration pneumonia is a continuous threat. Gastrostomy feedings are given, and roentgenograms are obtained at intervals, with contrast material in the stomach and the mercury bougie in the esophagus. When the baby gags, the contrast is regurgitated into the distal pouch (Fig. 81–12). Unfortunately, up to 3 months may be necessary to elongate the esophagus to the extent that an anastomosis can be made. Furthermore, in the reported cases in which an anastomosis was "successfully" made under tension,

there was a high incidence of anastomotic leak, stricture, hiatus hernia, and motility disorders. In addition, the prolonged hospitalization cannot help but have an effect on the bonding between the baby and the parents.

Infants who spend long periods in high-risk newborn nurseries are always at risk of developing serious nosocomial infections. One of our patients died with an overwhelming *Pseudomonas* pneumonia during the stretching process.

The objections to early esophagostomy and delayed interposition have centered about the morbidity and functional problems associated with any form of intestinal interposition. If definite progress is being made during the first 2 weeks, we continue the stretching for another 2 weeks. By this time, most infants have gained considerable weight and are strong enough to tolerate a major operation. At this point, we explore the baby through a right retropleural approach and mobilize the two esophageal pouches. The addition of a circular myotomy has allowed us to perform a tension-free anastomosis. If this is not possible, we go ahead with an immediate colon interposition between the proximal and distal portions of the esophagus. When one is operating through the right chest, this procedure requires an additional abdominal incision. The colon is brought up through the enlarged esophageal hiatus. White performed a similar procedure through the left chest.[76]

Our treatment of ten infants with isolated atresia can be summarized as follows.

Treatment	Number of Patients
Cervical esophagostomy, delayed colon bypass	3
Bougie, colon interposition	1
Bougie, esophageal anastomosis	5 (1 died after cardiac surgery)
Bougie, no anastomosis	1 death, *Pseudomonas* sepsis

TRACHEOESOPHAGEAL FISTULA WITHOUT ATRESIA

The main difficulty with an isolated tracheoesophageal fistula lies in making the diagnosis. These infants frequently have aspiration pneumonia and are poorly nourished. Preliminary gavage or gastrostomy feedings with antibiotics and chest physiotherapy are needed to prepare these infants for the operation.

Precise localization of the fistula before surgery is essential. Most fistulas are above or at the level of the

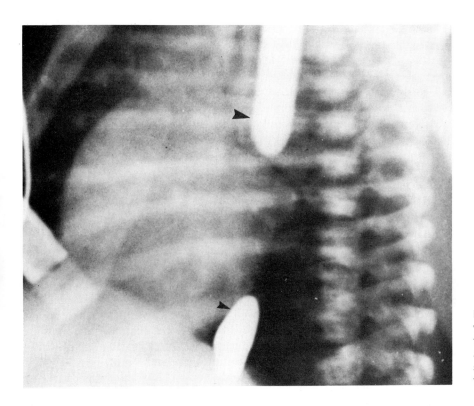

Figure 81–12. Esophageal atresia after 2 weeks of bougienage. The two ends are still too far apart for an anastomosis. The large arrow points to the proximal pouch, and the small arrow points to contrasting material in the distal pouch.

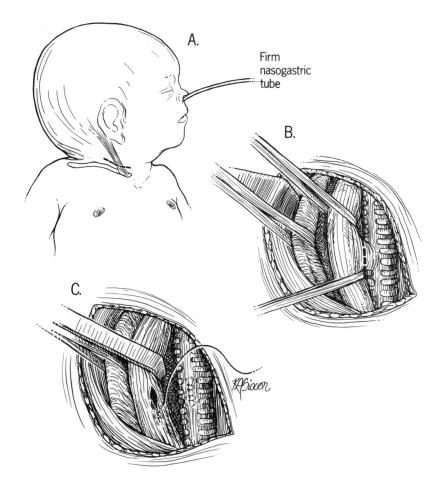

Figure 81–13. Closure of an H-type fistula. A cervical incision is made with retraction of the carotid sheath laterally. The esophagus is isolated between two soft rubber tubes, and the fistula is divided. The best protection for the recurrent nerves is to keep the dissection immediately on the esophageal wall.

clavicle and can be most easily reached through a right cervical incision. A few, however, occur lower in the trachea, but all are well proximal to the carina. If he or she has not done so before, the surgeon should, after induction of anesthesia, inspect the vocal cords with direct laryngoscopy and visualize the trachea with a bronchoscope. A catheter is passed though the fistula into the esophagus. A complete laryngotracheal cleft may simulate a small H-type fistula, and this is the only way to evaluate the infant with this lesion. More than one fistula may be present. A right transcervical incision with lateral retraction of the carotid sheath will expose the trachea, the esophagus, and the fistula without much difficulty. The fistula may then be divided and oversewn (Fig. 81–13). The recurrent laryngeal nerves lie in the esophagotracheal groove at the low point in this dissection and are extremly vulnerable to injury. In a newborn infant, they are no larger than 6–0 and 5–0 suture material. The left nerve is particularly at risk because it cannot be seen from the right.

We have treated 12 infants with isolated tracheoesophageal fistulas. One patient had a temporary bilateral nerve paralysis.

LARYNGOTRACHEOESOPHAGEAL CLEFT

A complete lack of closure of the tracheoesophageal septum results in failure of separation of the embryonic foregut into trachea and esophagus. This defect may be limited to a cleft between the posterior wall of the larynx and the upper esophagus, or there may be a common channel between the posterior wall of the larynx, cricoid cartilages, the trachea, and the esophagus. The defect may be associated with an esophageal atresia and distal fistulas. In one successfully treated case, there was an esophageal atresia and two separate fistulas in addition to a cleft that extended from the larynx to the third tracheal ring.[77,78]

These infants start to choke and aspirate at birth. They have an excessive amount of saliva. Some have stridor and either an abnormal cry or no cry at all. An esophagogram demonstrates spillage of contrast material into the trachea. A lateral esophagogram that demonstrates an anteriorly displaced nasogastric tube certainly suggests the diagnosis. The diagnosis should also be suspected when an endotracheal tube passed for ventilatory support persists in slipping into the esophagus. Any infant with these symptoms, especially one with spill of contrast material into the trachea, must be subjected to careful endoscopic examination. The cleft may close during quiet breathing, but Hendren has observed that the defect will open and may be observed when air is blown into a plastic catheter placed in the pharynx.[79] A slightly larger than usual endotracheal tube will separate the posterior cleft when passed under direct laryngoscopic view.

In 1983, there were 85 cases of complete larnygotracheal cleft reported, with only 46 survivors.[80] Partial clefts limited to the larynx or the esophagus and trachea in the neck may be repaired through a cervical incision. A preliminary gastrostomy and tracheotomy are performed, and the infant's pneumonia is treated until the lungs are clear. A long incision anterior to the sternocleidomastoid muscle is performed on the right side. The thyroid, larynx, and hyoid are mobilized and retracted laterally to expose the posterior wall of the larynx and trachea. Every effort must be made to divide the cleft exactly between the esophagus and the trachea. If too much trachea is taken, there will be a tracheal stenosis. On the other hand, incorporation of the esophagus into the back wall of the trachea will result in a floppy trachea that is obstructed on inspiration. Hendren advises dividing no more than 2 mm at a time, after which the trachea is precisely closed with interrupted Tevdek sutures.[79] the esophagus is closed, and a pedicle flap consisting of the sternohyoid muscle is interposed between the two suture lines. Hendren reported two long-term survivors with this technique. If the proximal esophagus is atretic, it is separated away from the cleft, closed, and exteriorized as a split fistula. Later, the esophagus is reconstructed with a segment of colon.

Donahoe and Gee's report of a patient with a type III cleft extending from the larynx to the carina presents a detailed account of the surgical and intensive care required for the survival of an infant with this defect.[81] During the first 24 hours of life, a gastrostomy and tracheotomy were performed, but the tracheotomy slipped into the esophagus. A bifurcation tube was made that allowed intubation of each bronchi and ventilation of the patient. This tube was held in place by a suture passed around the tube and tied over a bolster in the anterior neck. Repair of the defect was delayed until the baby's pneumonia had cleared with antibiotics and suctioning through the bifurcation tube. The trachea and esophagus were separated through a combined cervical and right thoracotomy incision. On the right side, the esophagus and trachea were separated exactly at their junction, but 1 cm of esophagus was left attached to the left side of the trachea. This flap of esophagus was used as a membranous posterior tracheal wall, and the esophagus was closed with a continuous suture. After this operation, the infant was kept intubated, paralyzed, and ventilated for 2 weeks. Both anastomoses healed. This infant later required a fundoplication so he could be fed without reflux. He survived but required intense care and long-term attention to tracheotomy care and education in oral feeding. This article as well as the other references should be read in detail by anyone planning to repair these complex defects.

RESULTS

The hospital survival rates of four large series of patients with esophageal anomalies operated on during the past 15 years vary from 85 percent to 93 percent.[52,60,65,82] The only important cause of death in these series is the presence of severe associated birth defects or major chromosomal anomalies. Such factors as prematurity and whether the operation was done by the transpleural or retropleural route no longer influence immediate mortality. The 1-year survival rate in patients operated on at our hospital is 87 percent. One infant died before surgery could be performed during induction of anesthesia because the endotracheal tube slipped into the distal esophagus. One other child died at 3 years of age after dilatation of a stricture. All other deaths in our patients have resulted from severe associated cardiac or neurologic abnormalities.

Recurrent pneumonia plagues some children during the first postoperative years. Some continue to have wheezing and bronchitis with decreased pulmonary function in later years.[83] Both the initial episodes and the long-term loss of pulmonary volume appear to be related to poor esophageal motility and aspiration.[84,85] Koop et al. studied the social and emotional problems found in 31 families 10 to 25 years after their children's esophageal repairs.[86] In retrospect, the mothers seem to have felt left out of the babies' early problems because of their own hospital confinement. Some 21 mothers felt that the experience of rearing a child with an anomaly was no different from rearing a normal child. Fourteen thought it was more difficult, and 4 were quite frustrated. The surgeons' relationships with the families were reported to be most helpful in alleviating guilt feelings, but intrafamily conflicts might have been avoided if the surgeons had insisted on seeing both parents during follow-up visits so that each could hear the same explanation.

REFERENCES

1. Ladd WE: Surgical treatment of esophageal atresia and tracheoesophageal fistula. N Engl J Med 230:625, 1944
2. Leven NL: Congenital atresia of the esophagus with tracheoesophageal fistula. J Thorac Surg 10:648, 1941
3. Haight C: Congenital atresia of the esophagus with tracheoesophageal fistula. Ann Surg 120:623, 1944
4. Potts WJ: Congenital atresia of the esophagus with tracheoesophageal fistula and congenital atresia of the esophagus. J Thorac Surg 20:671, 1950
5. Potts WJ, Idriss F: Review of our experience with atresia of the esophagus with and without complicating fistulae. Md State Med J 9:528, 1960
6. David TJ, O'Callagan SE: Twinning and oesophageal atresia. Arch Dis Child 49:660, 1974
7. Copleman B, Cannata BV, London W: Tracheoesophageal anomaly in siblings. J Med Soc NJ 47:415, 1950
8. Dennis NR, Nicholas JC, Kuvar I: Oesophageal atresia: Three cases in two generations. Arch Dis Child 48:980, 1970
9. Engel PM, Vos LJ, Devries JA, Kuijer PJ: Esophageal atresia with tracheoesophageal fistula in mother and child. J Pediatr Surg 5:564, 1970
10. Forrester RM, Cohen SJ: Esophageal atresia with an anorectal anomaly and probably laryngeal fissure in three siblings. J Pediatr Surg 5:674, 1970
11. Griere JG, McDermott JG: Congenital atresia of the esophagus in two brothers. Can Med Assoc J 41:180, 1936
12. Hausmann PF, Close AS, Williams LP: Occurrence of tracheoesophageal fistula in three consecutive siblings. Surgery 41:542, 1957
13. David TJ, O'Callaghan SE: Oesophageal atresia in the southwest of England. J Med Genet 12:1, 1975
14. Kluth D: Atlas of esophageal atresia. J Pediatr Surg 11:901, 1976
15. Holder TM, Cloud DT, Lewis EJ Jr, Pilling GP IV: Esophageal atresia and tracheoesophageal fistula. Pediatrics 34:542, 1964
16. David TJ, O'Callaghan SE: Cardiovascular malformations and oesophageal atresia. Br Heart J 36:559, 1974
17. Greenwood RD, Rosenthal A: Cardiovascular malformation associated with tracheoesophageal fistula and esophageal atresia. Pediatrics 57:87, 1976
18. Boston VE, Wagget J: An unusual case of tracheoesophageal fistula and esophageal atresia complicated by malrotation and a partial duodenal diaphragm. J Pediatr Surg 10:835, 1975
19. Glasson MJ, Bandrevics V, Cohen DH: Hypertrophic pyloric stenosis complicating esophageal atresia. Surgery 74:530, 1973
20. Bond-Taylor W, Starer F, Atwell JD: Vertebral anomalies associated with esophageal atresia and tracheoesophageal fistula with reference to the initial operative mortality. J Pediatr Surg 8:9, 1973
21. Stevenson RE: Extra vertebrae associated with esophageal atresias and tracheoesophageal fistulas. J Pediatr 81:1123, 1972
22. Hodson CJ, Shaw DG: Congenital atresia of the oesophagus and thirteen pairs of ribs. Pediatr Radiol 1:248, 1973
23. Quan L, Smith DW: The VATER association—Vertebral defects, Anal atresia, T-E fistula with esophageal atresia, Radial and renal dysplasia: a spectrum of associated defects. J Pediatr 82:104, 1973
24. Barry JE, Auldist AW: The VATER association. Am J Dis Child 128:769, 1974
25. Apold J, Dahl E, Aarskog D: The VATER association: malformations of the male external genitalia. Acta Paediatr Scand 65:150, 1976
26. McNeal RM, Skoglund RR, Francke U: Congenital anomalies including the VATER association in a patient with a del(6)q deletion. J Pediatr 91:957, 1977

27. King SL, Ladda RL, Shochat SJ: Case report: monozygotic twins concordant for tracheo-esophageal fistula and discordant for the VATER association. Acta Paediatr Scand 66:783, 1977

28. Toyama WM: Esophageal atresia and tracheoesophageal fistula in association with bronchial and pulmonary anomalies. J Pediatr Surg 7:302, 1972

29. Kalayoglu M, Olcay I: Congenital bronchobiliary fistula associated with esophageal atresia and tracheoesophageal fistula. J Pediatr Surg 11:463, 1976

30. Smith EI: The early development of the trachea and esophagus in relation to atresia of the esophagus and tracheoesophageal fistula. Carnegie Institute of Washington Publication 611:41, 1957

31. Queenan JT, Gadow E: Amniography for detection of congenital malformations. Obstet Gynecol 35:648, 1970

32. Koop CE: Recent advances in the surgery of oesophageal atresia. Progr Pediatr Surg 2:41, 1971

33. Dudgeon DL, Morrison CW, Woolley MM: Congenital proximal tracheoesophageal fistula. J Pediatr Surg 7:614, 1972

34. Berdon WE, Baker DH: Radiographic findings in esophageal atresia with proximal pouch fistula (type B). Pediatr Radiol 3:70, 1975

35. Ferguson CC, Schoemperlen CB: Congenital tracheoesophageal fistula in an adult. Ann Surg 149:582, 1959

36. Sundar B, Guiney EJ, O'Donnell B: Congenital H-type tracheo-oesophageal fistula. Arch Dis Child 50:862, 1975

37. Bedard P, Girvan DP, Shanding B: Congenital H-type tracheoesophageal fistula. J Pediatr Surg 9:663, 1974

38. Moncrief JA, Randolph JG: Congenital tracheoesophageal fistula without atresia of the esophagus. J Thorac Cardiovasc Surg 51:434, 1966

39. Tucker G, Pendergrass EP: Congenital atresia of the esophagus: a new diagnostic technic. JAMA 101:1726, 1933

40. Winslow PR, Bryant LR, Hasbrouck JD: Cystoscope endoscopy in the H-type tracheoesophageal fistula. Arch Surg 93:520, 1966

41. Gans SL, Johnson RO: Diagnosis and surgical management of H-type tracheoesophageal fistula in infants and children. J Pediatr Surg 12:223, 1977

42. Korones SB, Evans LJ: Measurement of intragastric oxygen concentration for the diagnosis of H-type tracheoesophageal fistula. Pediatrics 60:450, 1977

43. Lynch FP, Coran AG, Cohen SR, Lee FA: Traumatic esophageal pseudodiverticula in the newborn. J Pediatr Surg 9:675, 1974

44. Wells SD, Leonidas JC, Conkle D, et al: Traumatic prevertebral pharyngoesophageal pseudodiverticulum in the newborn infant. J Pediatr Surg 9:217, 1974

45. Eklof O, Lohr G, Okmian L: Submucosal perforation of the esophagus in the neonates. Acta Radiol 8:187, 1969

46. Brintnall EJ, Kridelbaugh WW: Congenital diverticulum of the posterior hypopharynx stimulating atresia of the esophagus. Ann Surg 131:564, 1950

47. Grant JC, Arneil C: Congenital diverticulum of the esophagus. Surgery 46:966, 1959

48. Theander G: Congenital posterior midline pharyngoesophageal diverticula. Pediatr Radiol 1:153, 1973

49. MacKellar A, Kennedy JC: Congenital diverticulum of the pharynx simulating esophageal atresia. J Pediatr Surg 7:408, 1972

50. Utian HL, Thomas RC: Cricopharyngeal incoordination in infancy. Pediatrics 43:402, 1969

51. Replogle RL: Esophageal atresia: plastic sump catheter for drainage of the proximal pouch. Surgery 54:296, 1963

52. Bishop P, Klein M, Philippart A, Hertzler J: Transpleural repair of esophageal atresia without primary gastrostomy: 240 patients treated between 1951 and 1983. J Pediatr Surg 20:823, 1985

53. Livaditis A, Radberg L, Odensjo G: Esophageal end-to-end anastomosis: reduction of anastomotic tension by circular myotomy. Scand J Thorac Cardiovasc Surg 6:206, 1972

54. Muangosombat J, Hankins JR, Mason GR, McLaughlin JS: The use of circular myotomy to facilitate resection and end-to-end anastomosis of the esophagus. J Thorac Cardiovasc Surg 68:522, 1974

55. Eraklis AJ, Rossello PJ, Ballantine TVN: Circular esophagomyotomy of upper pouch in primary repair of long-segment esophageal atresia. J Pediatr Surg 11:709, 1976

56. Lindahl H, Louhimo I: Livaditis myotomy in long-gap esophageal atresia. J Pediatr Surg 22:109, 1987

57. Holder TM: Transpleural versus retropleural approach for repair of tracheoesophageal fistula. Surg Clin North Am 44:1433, 1964

58. Ashcraft KW, Holder TM: Esophageal atresia and tracheoesophageal fistula malformations. Surg Clin North Am 56:299, 1976

59. Koop CE, Schnaufer L, Broennie AM: Esophageal atresia and tracheoesophageal fistula: supportive measures that affect survival. Pediatrics 54:558, 1974

60. Spitz L, Kiely E, Brereton R: Esophageal atresia: five-year experience with 148 cases. J Pediatr Surg 22:103, 1987

61. Holder TM, McDonald VG Jr, Woolley MM, Gross RE: The premature or critically ill infant with esophageal atresia: increased success with a staged approach. J Thorac Cardiovasc Surg 44:344, 1962

62. Templeton JM, Templeton J, Schnaufer L, et al: Management of esophageal atresia and tracheoesophageal fistula in the neonate with severe respiratory distress syndrome. J Pediatr Surg 20:394, 1985

63. Filston H, Chitwood W, Schkolne B, et al: The Fogarty balloon catheter as an aid to management of the infant with esophageal atresia and tracheoesophageal fistula complicated by severe RDS or pneumonia. J Pediatr Surg 17:149, 1982

64. Abrahamson J, Shandling B: Esophageal atresia in the underweight baby: a challenge. J Pediatr Surg 7:608, 1972

65. Holder T, Ashcraft K, Sharp R, Amoury R: Care of infants with esophageal atresia, tracheoesophageal fistula and associated anomalies. J Thorac Cardiovasc Surg 94:828, 1987

66. Lind JF, Blanchard RJ, Guyda H: Esophageal motility in tracheoesophageal fistula and esophageal atresia. Surg Gynecol Obstet 153:557, 1966

67. Orringer MB, Kirsh MM, Sloan H: Long-term esophageal function following repair of esophageal atresia. Ann Surg 186:436, 1977

68. Duranceau A, Fisher SR, Flye MW, et al: Motor function of the esophagus after repair of esophageal atresia and tracheoesophageal fistula. Surgery 82:116, 1977

69. Laks H, Wilkinson RH, Schuster SR: Long-term results following correction of esophageal atresia with tracheoesophageal fistula: a clinical and cinefluorographic study. J Pediatr Surg 7:591, 1972

70. Shermeta DW, Whittington BF, Seto DS, Haller JA: Lower esophageal sphincter dysfunction in esophageal atresia: nocturnal regurgitation and aspiration pneumonia. J Pediatr Surg 12:871, 1977

71. Ashcraft KW, Goodwin C, Amoury RA, Holder TM: Early recognition and aggressive treatment of gastroesophageal reflux following repair of esophageal atresia. J Pediatr Surg 12:317, 1977

72. Curci M, Dibbins A: Problems associated with a Nissen fundoplication following tracheoesophageal fistula and esophageal atresia repair. Arch Surg 123:618, 1988

73. Filler RM, Rossello PJ, Lebowitz RL: Life-threatening anoxic spells caused by tracheal compression after repair of esophageal atresia: correction by surgery. J Pediatr Surg 11:739, 1976

74. Howard R, Myers NA: Esophageal atresia: a technique for elongating the upper pouch. Surgery 58:725, 1965

75. Mahour GH, Wooley MM, Gwin JL: Elongation of the upper pouch and delayed anatomic reconstruction in esophageal atresia. J Pediatr Surg 9:373, 1974

76. White JJ: Early short segment left colon interposition for esophageal atresia. J Pediatr Surg 11:735, 1976

77. Mahour GH, Cohen SR, Woolley MM: Laryngotracheoe-sophageal cleft associated with esophageal atresia and multiple tracheoesophageal fistulas in a twin. J Thorac Cardiovasc Surg 65:223, 1973

78. Donahoe PK, Hendren WH: The surgical management of laryngo-tracheoesophageal cleft with tracheoesophageal fistula and esophageal atresia. Surgery 71:363, 1972

79. Hendren WH: Repair of laryngo-tracheoesophageal cleft using interposition of a strap muscle. J Pediatr Surg 11:425, 1976

80. Roth B, Rose K-G, Benz-Bohm G, et al: Laryngotracheoesophageal cleft: clinical features, diagnosis and therapy. Eur J Pediatr 140:41, 1983

81. Donahoe P, Gee P: Complete laryngotracheoesophageal cleft: management and repair. J Pediatr Surg 19:143, 1984

82. Louhimo I, Lindahl H: Esophageal atresia: primary results in 500 consecutively treated patients. J Pediatr Surg 18:217, 1983

83. Couriel J, Hibbert M, Olinsky A, et al: Long-term pulmonary consequences of oesophageal atresia with tracheoesophageal fistula. Acta Paediatr Scand 71:973, 1982

84. LeSouef P, Myers N, Landau L: Etiologic factors in long-term respiratory function abnormalities following esophageal atresia repair. J Pediatr Surg 22:918, 1987

85. Myers NA: Oesophageal atresia with distal tracheoesophageal fistula: a long-term follow-up. Prog Pediatr Surg 10:5, 1977

86. Koop CE, Schnaufer L, Thompson G: The social, psychological and economic problems of a patient's family after successful repair of esophageal atresia. Z Kinderchir [Suppl] 17:125, 1975

82
Congenital Esophageal Stenosis

Esophageal stenosis may cause symptoms indistinguishable from those of an atresia during the first day or so of life, if the stricture is very narrow. More often, the baby will be able to swallow and will later regurgitate, causing poor weight gain and aspiration pneumonia. Symptoms may not appear until solid foods are offered.

An esophagogram that demonstrates a narrow segment above the cardia is diagnostic for a congenital stricture when found during the neonatal period. Strictures found later may be secondary to reflux esophagitis. An obstruction at the cardia is more likely to be achalasia. A simple diaphragm or fibromuscular stenosis is most common, and stenoses secondary to retained tracheobronchial remnants are the next most common lesion.[1] Stenosis has been described in association with a congenital deficiency in the submucosa.[2] Strictures secondary to ectopic gastric mucosa are indistinguishable from congenital strictures unless a biopsy of the gastric mucosa is obtained by esophagoscopy.[3,4] Two patients with ectopic gastric mucosa and stricture were operated on at the Children's Memorial Hospital. One had symptoms of choking from birth. The second suddenly developed dysphagia at 5 years of age (Fig. 82–1). In addition to the esophagogram, which will demonstrate the location, degree, and length of the stricture, esophagoscopy and biopsy should be performed in an attempt to diagnose one of these lesions.

TREATMENT

Peroral dilatations with tapered rubber or mercury dilators are sufficient for mild, short congenital strictures. If there is a long, narrow stricture, it is far safer to perform a gastrostomy and pass a string in order to dilate the esophagus with Tucker dilators (Fig. 82–2). A single dilatation will rupture a simple fibromucosal diaphragm,

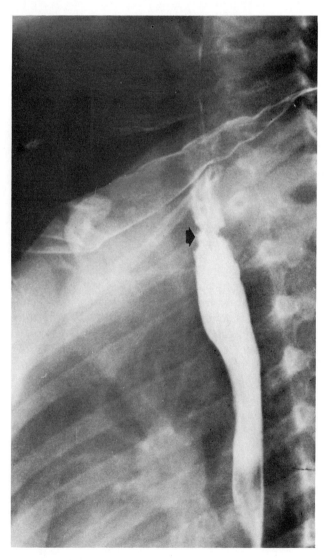

Figure 82–1. Esophageal stricture secondary to ectopic gastric mucosa in the cervical esophagus.

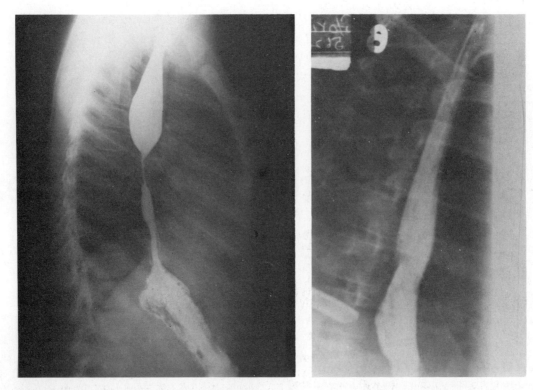

Figure 82–2. A long, congenital stricture that was dilated successfully via retrograde application of Tucker dilators through a gastrostomy.

but if there is recurrence of symptoms and roentgenographic findings after a series of six to eight dilatations, an operation is necessary. Further, if the biopsy demonstrates ectopic gastric mucosa or tracheobronchial remnants, dilatation will offer only temporary relief.

Surgery

A stricture above the thoracic inlet is best approached through a cervical incision. Hence, it is necessary to accurately localize the stricture by roentgenograms and endoscopy. It is helpful if an assistant positions a flexible fiberoptic endoscope just at the stricture. In a darkened room, the light can be seen if the stricture is in the neck. The esophagoscope is kept in place until the surgeon has accurately located the stricture because the esophagus may appear to be perfectly normal externally. A stricture in the middle third of the esophagus is approached through the right chest, whereas the left side provides a more convenient exposure of a lower third lesion. As much as 1 to 2 cm of esophagus can be resected,

and an end-to-end anastomosis can be constructed if the entire esophagus is mobilized. This is not true of strictures secondary to caustic ingestion because of the periesophaeal scar and mucosal damage above and below a caustic stricture. After the resection, a one-layer anastomosis is made as described for an esophageal atresia.

REFERENCES

1. Ohkawa H, Takahashi H, Hoshino Y, Sato H: Lower esophageal stenosis in association with tracheobronchial remnants. J Pediatr Surg. 10:453, 1975
2. Takayanagi K, Komi N: Congenital esophageal stenosis with lack of submucosa. J Pediatr Surg 10:425, 1975
3. Hanson EL, Daly JF, Davis DA: Ulceration associated with an islet of columnar epithelium in the midesophagus: new evidence for an acquired etiology of Barrett's syndrome. J Pediatr Surg 5:370, 1970
4. Rector LE, Connerley ML: Aberrant mucosa in that esophagus in infants and in children. Arch Pathol 31:285, 1941

83
Diaphragmatic Anomalies

_____ *Marleta Reynolds*

Anomalies of diaphragmatic formation include the posterolateral foramen of Bochdalek hernia, the substernal Morgagni hernia, and varying degrees of eventration or paralysis of the diaphragm. A Bochdalek hernia is one of the most important surgically correctable causes of respiratory distress in the newborn. Despite advances in the diagnosis and treatment of birth defects, there remains an appalling mortality in babies born with this defect.

BOCHDALEK HERNIA

Pathology

The foramen of Bochdalek is usually a 2 by 3 cm posterior slit in the diaphragm just superior to the adrenal gland (Fig. 83–1). On occasion, this defect may extend from the lateral chest wall to the esophageal hiatus. A rim of muscle is almost always folded against the posterior abdominal wall underneath the peritoneum. The entire diaphragm may be absent.[1,2] In most series, including our own, 80 percent of Bochdalek hernias occur on the left side.

Bilateral hernias are extremely rare. They are usually found at autopsy and are associated with multiple other congenital defects.[3] In 20 percent of left-sided hernias, there is a sac that represents the pleuroperitoneal membrane. The entire small bowel with portions of the colon, stomach, spleen, and kidney may fill the left pleural cavity.

On the right side, we have observed a defect posterior to the liver that allowed bowel to slip into the chest. Most often, however, the right lobe of the liver herniates upward, whereas the medial portion of the liver remains attached to the inferior vena cava by the hepatic veins.[4]

Associated Defects

The most important secondary effect of a Bochdalek hernia is compression and inhibition of lung growth. In experimental animals, production of an intrauterine diaphragmatic hernia results in hypoplastic lungs whose weights are only 23 to 75 percent of normal, with abnormally low air capacity and poor compliance.[5–7]

Infants who develop symptoms of respiratory compromise in the first day of life exhibit a spectrum of pulmonary hypoplasia ranging from minimal hypoplasia on the side of the hernia to severe bilateral hypoplasia. The degree of hypoplasia directly affects the early survival of these infants.[8,9] The pulmonary hypoplasia appears to result from an arrest in bronchial branching, with a decrease in the number of bronchial generations. There are an appropriate number of alveoli for each bronchiole.[10,11] Thickening of the walls of medium-sized pulmonary aterioles, as well as a decrease in the size of the entire pulmonary vascular bed, in autopsy specimens of infants with Bochdalek hernias has been identified.[12,13] Infants who are adequately oxygenated in the early postoperative period (demonstrating a honeymoon period) have less pulmonary hypoplasia than those who have persistent hypoxemia. In addition, the no-honeymoon infants have been found to have more severe structural remodeling of the pulmonary arteries.

Infants with no honeymoon period have abnormal muscularization of intraacinar arterioles and no increase in compliance in small preacinar arteries. These changes markedly affect the pulmonary vascular resistance in the newborn period.[14]

Twenty-three percent of infants with congenital diaphragmatic hernia treated at Children's Memorial Hospital from 1962 to 1983 had major associated anomalies. An extralobar sequestration was found in the left periaor-

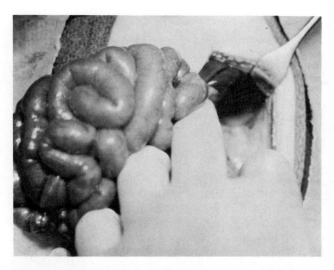

Figure 83–1. Operative view of a left foramen of Bochdalek hernia. The entire visible bowel was in the chest.

tic region in 9 of our infants. Cardiac defects were found in 11 of 146.[9] Since the adominal viscera have resided in the chest, the abdomen is small and underdeveloped. In left-sided hernias, there is always an associated nonrotation of the midgut. The duodenum may be kinked and partially obstructed by Ladd's bands.

David and Illingworth reported an extensive epidemiologic and pathologic study of 143 infants with diaphragmatic hernia in southwest England treated from 1943 to 1974.[15] Since 39 of these infants were stillborn, it is not surprising that 50 percent had associated congenital defects. Anomalies of the nervous, gastrointestinal, genitourinary, and cardiovascular systems were most frequent. This extensive review confirmed the 75 to 90 percent incidence of left-sided hernias, the preponderance of the anomaly in girls, and the lack of familial occurrence. David and Illingworth estimated the incidence of diaphragmatic hernia as 0.45 per 1000 total births. A smaller but more recent report from Puri and Gorman in Ireland identified 36 cases of congenital diaphragmatic hernia in 75,512 births from 1973 to 1982, an incidence of 1 per 2097 births. Twenty infants (11 stillborn and 9 live born) had lethal nonpulmonary associated anomalies.[16] Forty percent of babies with diaphragmatic hernia diagnosed with prenatal ultrasonography had associated anomalies or chromosomal abnormalities.[17]

Embryology

The diaphragm is formed from four components: the transverse septum, the mediastinum, the pleuroperitoneal membranes, and the body wall musculature derived from cervical myotomes. During the first 3 to 4 weeks of embryonic development, the transverse septum, a condensation of mesenchyme, provides an early, incom-

plete division of the extraembryonic coelom from the pericardial cavity. At 5 to 6 weeks, the mediastinal component results from fusion of two lateral ridges of mesenchyme with the mediastinum in the midline dorsally. The pleuroperitoneal canal, located posterolaterally, remains as an opening between the pleural and peritoneal cavities. These canals are finally closed by the pleuroperitoneal membranes at 8 weeks.[18]

Once the canals are closed, the enlarging pleural cavities burrow under the innermost layers of the thoracic wall musculature, adding this layer to the posterior and lateral aspects of the diaphragm. The junction of these two muscular groups, the lumbocostal trigone, was originally described by Bochdalek and bears his name. In a patient with congenital diaphragmatic hernia, rotation and fixation of the intestine are incomplete. When the midgut returns from the umbilical stalk at 10 weeks, loops of bowel may enter the left pleural cavity so that there is no opportunity for the normal counterclockwise rotation and mesenteric fixation.

Diagnosis

In the past, the diagnosis of congenital diaphragmatic hernia occasionally was made antenatally by fetography.[19] Prenatal ultrasonography has now replaced fetography. In a detailed survey of obstetricians and surgeons in North America, Adzick et al. obtained important information about the natural history of congenital diaphragmatic hernia. The diagnosis was made by prenatal ultrasonography in 88 of 94 infants born with congenital diaphragmatic hernia. In the majority of cases (66 percent) the ultrasound study was obtained because the mother is large for date and is found to have polyhydramnios.[20] A smaller number of ultrasound diagnoses were made as part of a routine obstetric evaluation. Several cystic adenomatoid malformations, a cystic teratoma, and a primary lung sarcoma were misdiagnosed as a diaphragmatic hernia. In a different study, abnormally low amniotic fluid lecithin–sphingomyelin ratios have been found in association with congenital diaphragmatic hernia.[21] Prenatal diagnosis and the advantages of excellent prenatal care and maternal transport to a tertiary neonatal center have not improved the survival of infants with congenital diaphragmatic hernia.[17]

Because of the poor prognosis of many of these infants, Harrison et al. have undertaken elaborate studies to create an experimental model to determine if in utero correction of the hernia would improve outcome. They have successfully created a fetal lamb model of congenital diaphragmatic hernia, corrected the defect in utero, and documented reversal of the pulmonary changes associated with the hernia.[22–25] They have now performed several unsuccessful in-utero human repairs.

In the infant who has not been previously diagnosed, respiratory distress appears during the first 24 to 48 hours of life. In fact, many infants will have low Apgar scores, with symptoms at birth. Strangely, there have been a number of reports of typical congenital postero-lateral hernias occurring in older children and even in adults.[26–32] We have observed two infants who had normal chest roentgenograms at 1 month but at 3 months had typical, though small, Bochdalek hernias. Older children and adults are more likely to have gastrointestinal symptoms.

The typical infant will be tachypneic, with grunting respirations and pallor or cyanosis. All symptoms become progressively more severe as the baby swallows air, distending the intrathoracic bowel with further pulmonary compression and mediastinal shift. The most prominent physical findings are a scaphoid abdomen and an increased anteroposterior diameter of the chest. The PMI is displaced away from the side of the defect, usually to the right (Fig. 83–2). Breath sounds are difficult to hear on either side of the chest because these infants have a very small tidal volume.

Any infant with respiratory distress must have an immediate chest roentgenogram. The diagnosis is easily made when the chest x-ray demonstrates air-filled and fluid-filled loops of bowel in the chest, with a paucity of intestinal gas in the abdomen (Fig. 83–3). The picture is less typical with right-sided lesions. A smooth elevation of the liver may appear to be an eventration, a lobar consolidation, or fluid. It is possible to mistake the solid mass of liver in the pleural cavity for a tumor. We have observed two neonates with congenital cystic disease of the lung who at first were thought to have diaphragmatic hernias.[33] The intraabdominal gas pattern was normal on x-ray, and a normal barium enema ruled out a diaphragmatic hernia. In older children, the correct diagnosis has been confused with staphylococcal pneumonia.[34]

Other studies can facilitate diagnosis in unusual cases (Fig. 83–4). Umbilical arteriography, contrast peritoneography, and liver scintography have now been replaced by ultrasonography and computed tomography (CT).[35–37] These ancillary procedures rarely are indicated in newborns and are contraindicated if they will delay immediate treatment.

Treatment

As soon as the diagnosis of Bochdalek diaphragmatic hernia is made, a gastric tube is passed to release swallowed air and to prevent further intestinal distention.

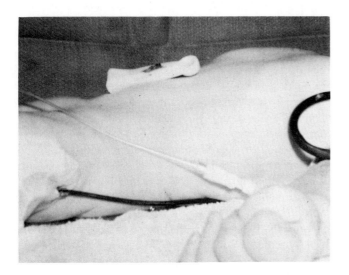
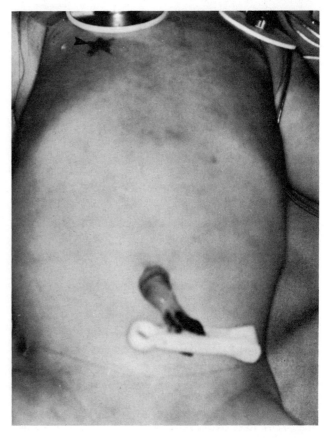

Figure 83–2. The physical findings in a newborn infant with a Bochdalek hernia. **Left.** The scaphoid abdomen. **Right.** The cardiac impulse is shifted to the right (**arrow**).

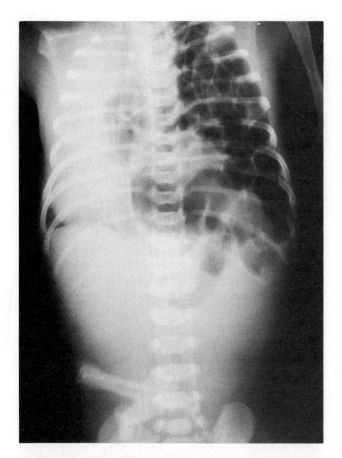

Figure 83–3. Plain film of a 3-hour-old baby that demonstrates the presence of all of the bowel in the left pleural cavity via a Bochdalek hernia. Note the absence of gas in the abdomen.

The infant is placed in a warmed isolette with the side of the hernia in a dependent position. The infant should be given oxygen by a head hood. Pulse oximetry is now routinely used to monitor oxygen saturation during resuscitation of the infant and transport to a pediatric surgical center. Manipulations should be held to a minimum during initial evaluation and transport. Personnel trained in endotracheal intubation must accompany the baby. Intubation and gentle bag ventilation are indicated if the infant deteriorates despite oxygen therapy. Resuscitation by bag and face mask is absolutely contraindicated, since more air will be forced into the intrathoracic intestine.

The infant is moved to the operating room as rapidly as possible. Temperature is monitored, and the infant is warmed with infrared heat lamps and a water mattress. A right radial arterial cannula is inserted while the operating team is being organized. Simultaneously, the anesthesiologist places an endotracheal tube for efficient ventilation. Initial blood gas samples will reveal varying degrees of both respiratory and metabolic acidosis with retention of CO_2 and hypoxia.[38,39] A pH below 7 and a Pco_2 above 100 imply a poor prognosis.[40] If the infant

is warm and improves with endotracheal intubation and ventilation with oxygen, we proceed immediately with operation. On the other hand, if the baby is moribund, with severe acidosis, he or she is supported with ventilation and given dilute sodium bicarbonate. It is difficult to know how long these resuscitative efforts should be carried out. As long as the lung is compressed, the infant is unable to exchange CO_2 and O_2. Nevertheless, an immediate operation on a cold, moribund baby is doomed to fail. Most infants will achieve maximum preoperative improvement with vigorous resuscitation within 1 or 2 hours.

An air–oxygen mixture is all that is given until the bowel is brought down from the chest. The skin can be infiltrated with a local anesthetic, and fentanyl can be given IV. Some babies will tolerate halothane, and all are given a muscle relaxant. Gentle hand ventilation with a minimal amount of pressure is effective for some infants. For those babies who do not respond to gentle ventilation, we bring the neonatal ventilator into the operating room. Low pressure (<30 cm H_2O) and high-frequency ventilation (80 to 130 breaths/minute) are instituted. The goal of therapy is to raise the pH above 7.5 by creating a combined respiratory and metabolic alkalosis with Pco_2s less than 30. Hyperventilation and a continuous infusion of sodium bicarbonate help to accomplish this goal.

Surgical Technique. An abdominal incision is indicated for left-sided hernias for several reasons: it is easier to pull bowel down from the chest than to push the viscera into a small abdominal cavity, abnormal rotation of the bowel may require division of Ladd's bands, and on occasion the peritoneum and fascia must be left open to relieve diaphragmatic pressure (Fig. 83–5). A left subcostal incision allows excellent exposure of the defect, but a vertical left rectus incision allows easier construction of a ventral hernia. We prefer the vertical incision. When the peritoneal cavity is opened, the defect is visualized by upward retraction on the abdominal wall. It is helpful but not necessary to pass a soft red rubber catheter into the chest to break the negative pressure around the viscera. The loops of bowel, spleen, and other viscera are withdrawn into the abdomen with gentle traction and covered with warm, moist pads. Sometimes, adhesions must be severed between the defect and the splenic flexure of the colon to completely free the bowel. After the hernia has been reduced, a curved retractor is inserted into the defect to visualize the thoracic cavity. Often, there is nothing to see but a disappointingly small nubbin of lung at the apex. One must always search for a sac and for an extralobar sequestration lying in the left posterior gutter. A sac can be easily overlooked because it is thin and membranous.[41]

Ordinarily, the edges of the defect are sharp and

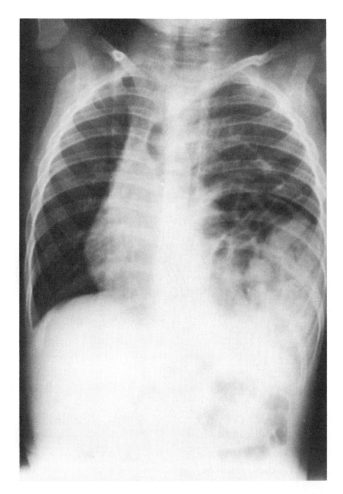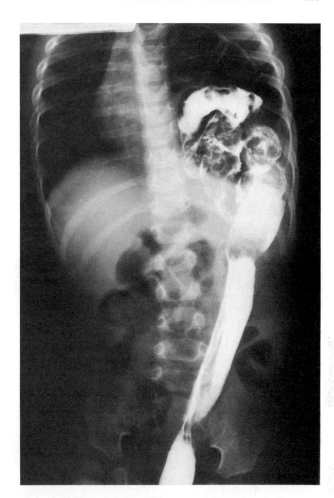

Figure 83–4. Foramen of Bochdalek hernia in a 6-year-old boy whose symptoms consisted of a failure to grow and poor appetite. **Left.** Plain film. **Right.** Diagnosis confirmed with a barium enema.

obvious. With a sac, they are indistinct and pulled up into the chest. A long curved hemostat is used to grasp the posterior pleura and identify the sac. It is then pulled down into the abdomen and excised. A small chest tube is inserted into the chest through a separate stab wound and attached to a stop cock and 5 ml syringe. The bowel is placed on the right side of the abdomen and retracted with moist pads. The posterior rim of the defect is mobilized by incising the overlying peritoneum. The defect is closed with interrupted nonabsorbable sutures, buttressed with Teflon felt pledgets. Careful dissection often is needed to accurately define the medial portion of the defect where the left crus of the esophageal hiatus may be involved. The kidney may be in the thoracic cavity and should be placed in its usual retroperitoneal position before the defect is closed. This closure may be further secured by a second layer of tissue developed from Gerota's fascia. If there is no posterior rim, sutures may be passed around a rib. Intercostal muscle alone will not hold. A large defect may be closed by developing a flap of peritoneum, posterior fascia, and transversalis

muscle from the left upper abdominal wall. The flap is detached inferiorly but left as a pedicle based on the costal margin.[42,43] Agenesis of the diaphragm will require the insertion of Marlex mesh or Gortex membrane.[44] Regardless of the technique, care must be taken to recreate the contour of the diaphragm as closely as possible to normal. Meticulous hemostasis will reduce postoperative bleeding. If extracorporeal support becomes necessary, the hemostasis will be of paramount importance.

After reduction of the hernia and closure of the defect, ventilation should improve, and intraoperative blood gases will demonstrate an increase in Po_2 and a decrease in Pco_2. The duodenum is traced from the pylorus to the jejunum, releasing all overlying folds of peritoneum. With the abdomen open, a size 3.5 French argyle umbilical artery catheter is placed to monitor the postductal blood gases. In an infant who is more than 24 hours old, the abdomen may be closed after stretching the abdominal wall muscles. We will not close the peritoneum and fascia in high-risk infants, that is, those who are operated on when under 24 hours of age, those with

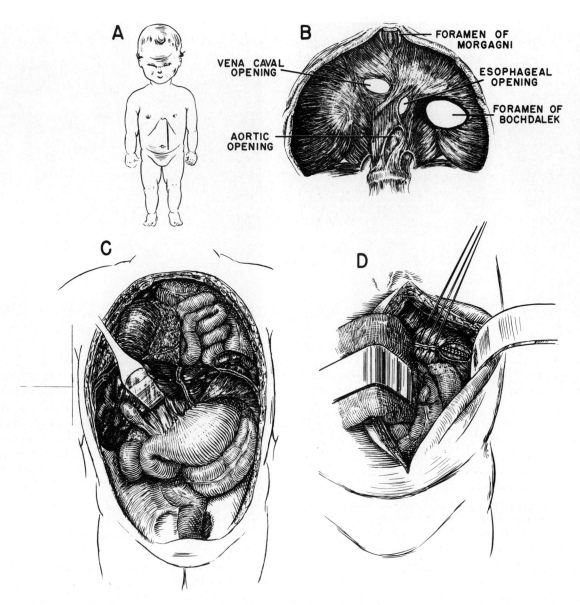

Figure 83–5. Operative treatment for a foramen of Bochdalek hernia. **A.** We prefer a left rectus muscle-splitting incision for rapid access and for greater ease in creating a ventral hernia. **B.** The foramina of the diaphragm. **C.** This illustrates the bowel within the chest with mediastinal shift. **D.** The bowel is pulled down from the abdomen and held to the right with a refractor over a warm, moist pad for exposure of the defect. After dissecting the posterior rim, the defect is closed with two layers of nonabsorbable suture.

an initial Apgar score below 5, or those with persistent, uncorrectable acidosis. If we do attempt a fascial closure and the anesthesiologist observes decreasing lung compliance, we remove the sutures and close only the skin. By undermining skin and subcutaneous fat for 1 or 2 cm on each side of the incision, a ventral hernia can be formed that is sufficent to relieve pressure on the diaphragm. An alternative technique is the use of a Silon pouch similar to that used for infants with a gastroschisis.[45,46] Repair of the ventral hernia can be delayed until the patient is 1 year of age.

Postoperative Care

While the infant is still on the operating table, a portable roentgenogram is obtained to determine the position of the umbilical artery catheter and the mediastinum. Swenson advocated aspirating enough air from the pleural cavity to leave the mediastinum in the midline, allowing the hypoplastic lung to expand gradually as the residual air was absorbed (Fig. 83–6). Others attach a chest tube to waterseal drainage. Unfortunately, as the baby cries and strains, air is rapidly expelled from the pleural cavity. In some babies, the mediastinum

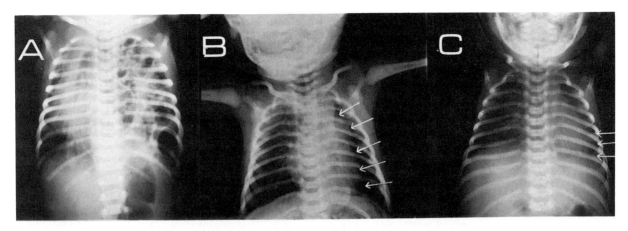

Figure 83–6. A,B,C. This series of roentgenograms demonstrates the gradual absorption of air with lung expansion over 10 days. Note the left hypoplastic lung with gradual mediastinal shift from right to left.

shifts too quickly to the left, with overdistention of the right lung. Removal of air from the pleural cavity on the side of the hernia will fail to expand a hypoplastic left lung but may permit the contralateral right lung to overexpand. We believe that this overexpansion contributes to the pneumothorax occasionally seen on the contralateral side.

In two independent animal experiments, we have demonstrated that if the mediastinum is kept stable in the midline, puppies tolerate removal of one lung with no change in blood gases. If air is removed from the empty pleural cavity with mediastinal shift, there is an immediate rise in the alveolar CO_2 with arterial hypoxemia. All animals in whom the mediastinum was allowed to shift died within 24 hours; others survived indefinitely. As a result of these studies and clinical observations, we believe strongly that the mediastinum should be stabilized in the midline. Air is aspirated in 10 ml increments while following the point of maximal cardiac impulse and monitoring with repeated chest roentgenograms. The chest catheter is left clamped when the mediastinum is in the midline and when the anesthesiologist notes an improvement in lung compliance. Further air is either aspirated or injected as necessary to maintain optimum expansion of the contralateral lung. If mechanical ventilation is needed, positive inspiratory pressures increase the risk of pneumothorax in an overdistended lung.

Infants who are more than 24 hours old at the time of diagnosis are extubated in the operating room if they are breathing vigorously and have normal blood gases. They are placed in a head hood and given supplemental oxygen as required. The endotracheal tube is left in place in poor-risk babies even if they have improved after operation. If they are breathing spontaneously and have normal blood gas determinations, they are maintained on CPAP. The Po_2 of the right radial artery determines the Fio_2 delivered. The infant who remains stable

may be extubated and placed in a head hood with supplemental oxygen and humidity within 12 to 24 hours.

The poorest-risk infants will require assisted ventilation and maximum medical support (Fig. 83–7). Initially, these infants are given 100 percent oxygen and ventilated with low pressures and rapid rates. We routinely ventilate these infants with rates from 80 to 130. High-frequency oscillatory ventilators (375 to 100 cycles/minute) available in a few centers in North America have been used to support these babies,[47] but there has been only minimal improvement in outcome.[48] Unlike other clinical situations, there should be no hurry to reduce the oxygen concentration, even if the Po_2 levels are extremely high. The reduction of the oxygen concentration by as little as 10 percent may trigger intense pulmonary vasospasm, acidosis, and death. The oxygen concentration is decreased in increments of 2 percent at intervals of 2 to 3 hours. In these extremely ill infants, one must knowingly run the risk of retrolental fibroplasia with high arterial O_2 level. Since most of these infants are full-term babies, the risk of death from hypoxia far outweighs the possibility of retinal injury.

Refinements in monitoring and in mechanical ventilators have not increased the survival rates of these high-risk infants. Raphaely and Downes observed a decrease in survival from 47 percent to 28 percent among infants diagnosed during the first 24 hours when comparing results of two 5-year periods.[49] During the first period, with the highest survival rate, neither ventilation nor blood gas analysis was available. A persistently high mortality rate in this group of infants has been noted by others.[50,51] Ventilatory insufficiency cannot be the only cause for this mortality, since some babies show remarkable improvement after reduction of the hernia, with delayed but progressive deterioration beginning 2 to 24 hours later.

Several sophisticated studies have shed light on this

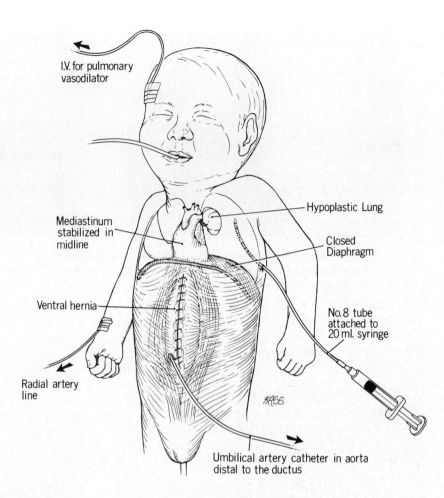

Figure 83–7. Illustration of the total postoperative management of a poor-risk infant. The mediastinum is stabilized by the aspiration or injection of air through the pleural catheter, blood gases are monitored above, and the ductus and the scalp vein IV line are used for the administration of pulmonary vasodilator drugs.

I.V. for pulmonary vasodilator

Hypoplastic Lung

Mediastinum stabilized in midline

Closed Diaphragm

Ventral hernia

No.8 tube attached to 20 ml. syringe

Radial artery line

Umbilical artery catheter in aorta distal to the ductus

enigma. Murdock et al. observed right-to-left shunting across the foramen ovale and the ductus arteriosus in infants with diaphragmatic hernias by simultaneous measurements of the Pao$_2$ in the radial artery and in the aorta below the ductus.[52] The persistence of fetal circulation with a right-to-left shunt and with pulmonary artery hypertension has been further confirmed by cardiac catheterization. The right ventricular end-diastolic pressure is increased with elevation of both right and left atrial pressures. Angiography demonstrates minimal pulmonary artery flow with a right-to-left shunt at the ductus.[53] Pulmonary artery pressure is increased by acidosis, positive end-expiratory pressure, and sudden increases in pulmonary blood volume. Hypoxemia and acidosis cause pulmonary arterial vasoconstriction and delayed closure of the ductus.[54,55]

Infants with diaphragmatic hernia and hypoplastic lungs appear to have a decrease in total capacitance of the pulmonary vascular bed as well as hyperreactive vessels. Experimental investigations have confirmed these findings.[56,57] Medical support is directed at preventing or relieving this pulmonary hypertension and shunting. Every effort is made to maintain a normal Pao$_2$. Oxygen (100 percent) is delivered for as long as

necessary, and the Fio$_2$ is only gradually lowered. Sodium bicarbonate is given to correct acidosis, generate a metabolic alkalosis, and help lower pulmonary vascular resistance.

Vasodilating drugs are used to treat the pulmonary arterial hypertension, with a resulting decrease in the right-to-left shunt and improved oxygenation. Tolazoline (Priscoline) is primarily an alpha-adrenergic blocking agent that has a direct nonadrenergic relaxing effect on smooth muscle as well as direct cardiotonic action.[58] The continuous infusion of tolazoline has dramatically relieved hypoxia in some infants with diaphragmatic hernias, persistent fetal circulation, and a variety of other pulmonary disorders.[59–61] This improvement has been attributed to relaxation of pulmonary arterial vasospasm. An increase in the infraductal Po$_2$ indicates a decrease in right-to-left shunting through the ductus with a fall in pulmonary pressure and increased capacitance of the pulmonary bed. The degree of shunting can be estimated by comparing the preductal and postductal arterial oxygenation. The effectiveness of tolazoline on pulmonary vasodilation is best determined by following the degree of shunt. The infusion of 0.5 to 2 mg/kg/hour may be effective. Good results have been obtained by infusing the drug into a vein that drains into the superior vena cava and is directed to the right ventricle and pulmonary artery. Systemic vasodilatation and relative hypovolemia can cause hypotension and reduce renal blood flow. In additon, tolazoline increases gastric acid secretion and may result in gastrointestinal bleeding. Cimetidine should not be used to prevent this side effect because it reduces the action of tolazoline. Gastric irrigation with sodium bicarbonate solutions or antacids is usually sufficient to prevent bleeding. In conjunction with tolazoline, dopamine or dolbutamine infusion may improve cardiac output without the need for large fluid infusion and overload. Other drugs have been used to lower pulmonary vascular resistance and support cardiac output. Methylprednisolone, chlorpromazine, digitalis, nitroglycerine, and sodium nitroprusside have had inconsistent and poorly sustained results.[62] Vacanti et al. have recommended the use of a continuous infusion of fentanyl during the postoperative period (3 µg/kg/hour).[63] We have also adopted this practice.

Collins et al. saved three infants who appeared to be dying by combining the use of pulmonary vasodilators with ligation of the patent ductus.[64] However, we cannot at this time recommend ductus ligation. If pulmonary arterial hypertension can be reduced, the ductus will no longer be significant; otherwise, the ductus is necessary for pulmonary artery decompression, minimizing right ventricular strain. In addition, high pulmonary vascular resistance results in additional shunting across the foramen ovale as well as within the microcirculation of the lung.

Extracorporeal membrane oxygenation (ECMO) has been used in infants with congenital diaphragmatic hernia who do not respond to maximal medical management and who meet institutional criteria for ECMO (see Chapter 12). Only those infants who appear to have adequate lung parenchyma (as indicated by the presence of a honeymoon period or any documented $Po_2 > 100$) are considered ECMO candidates at some institutions.[65] Other centers do not restrict the use of ECMO on these grounds.[66] Results differ depending on selection criteria and range from 70 to 86 percent survival.[65–67] The ECMO Registry 1988 data with 221 cases of infants with congenital diaphragmatic hernia reports a 65 percent overall survival (Neonatal–ECMO Registry, Ann Arbor, MI, personal communication). Bleeding complications are the highest in this group of ECMO patients.

Clearly, there are some infants with bilateral pulmonary hypoplasia who will die regardless of therapy. Others will survive only with intense, devoted attention to every detail of management. Survival may very well depend more on a physician and a team of nurses who remain at the bedside to continuously monitor the infant, responding appropriately to small changes, than on any specific drug or therapeutic maneuver.

Right-sided Bochdalek Hernia

The right-sided Bochdalek lesion, although embryologically and anatomically similar, is clinically different from the hernia on the left. The symptoms usually are less severe, so most are diagnosed after 72 hours of age. Seventy-six percent of the cases reviewed by Ban and Moore revealed tamponading of the defect by the liver, preventing bowel herniation.[68] The main problem is in deciding whether to repair the hernia through a thoracic or an abdominal incision. When only the liver is above the diaphragm, it is simpler to make a seventh intercostal space incision, push the liver down into the abdomen, and close the defect. If there is bowel or stomach in the chest, it is best to use an abdominal approach, as previously described. When there are both liver and bowel, a thoracic incision can be extended across the costal margin into the abdomen. With this approach, it is possible to pull the bowel and liver down into the abdomen and protect the viscera during closure of the diaphragm.

Postoperatively, the lung expands promptly, and there are few if any complications. The survival rate is nearly 100 percent if the defect is small.

Results

McNamara et al. reported an 80 percent survival rate of 114 infants treated at the Boston Children's Hospital from 1940 to 1966.[69] There was no mortality in 36 patients over 24 hours of age treated between 1950 and 1966. The excellent results with these infants have been typical of those in most pediatric surgical centers. Paradoxically, the mortality rate in babies under 24 hours appears to have remained the same over the last 20 years. Harrison et al. identified 37 babies born with diaphragmatic hernias in Norway during a 6-year period who died without operation or referral to a children's center.[70] This previously hidden mortality represented babies with severely hypoplastic lungs who died shortly after birth. Many of these extremely high-risk infants are now being diagnosed during their first few hours of life, resuscitated, and then transported to major centers. This is quite likely the main factor in the continued reported mortality rate of approximately 50 percent in the very young infants.

We operated on 144 patients with Bochdalek hernias at Children's Memorial Hospital between 1962 and 1983. Of these, 32 developed symptoms after the first 24 hours of life. All of these children survived. One hundred twelve babies developed symptoms during the first 24 hours of life and were transferred immediately to our hospital. Of these, 73 (65 percent) survived. We identified a subset of 27 critical infants who became symptomatic immediately after birth and required aggressive resuscitation. Ten of these 27 infants survived. There

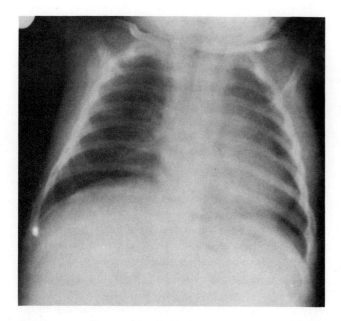
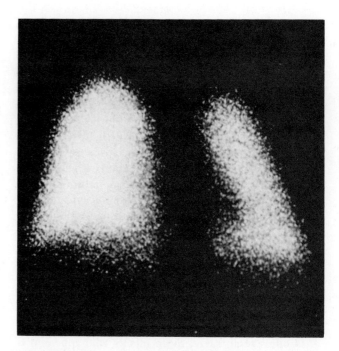

Figure 83–8. This infant had severely hypoplastic lungs and required priscoline for resuscitation. **Left.** Chest x-ray at 3 months, demonstrating continued hypoplasia of the left lung. **Right.** Lung scan that verifies continued subnormal perfusion on the left.

has been no operative mortality outside of this critical group since 1979.

Very small steps have been made in reducing mortality in infants with congenital diaphragmatic hernia over the past 20 years. A few drugs, high-frequency conventional ventilation, high-frequency oscillatory ventilation, and finally ECMO have improved the outcome for some babies. We believe there is still a small group of infants with congenital diaphragmatic hernia whose pulmonary hypoplasia is so severe that survival is impossible. We are at present unable to determine which babies will not benefit from any of these heroic measures.

Long-term evaluations of infants who have been treated successfully for posterolateral diaphragmatic hernia indicate that approximately half have normal chest roentgenograms and normal pulmonary function. The remainder have varying degrees of emphysema of the left-sided hypoplastic lung, indicating that the lung expanded to fill the pleural cavity not by generation of new lung tissue but by overexpansion.[71,72] Lung scans demonstrate hypoperfusion of the lung of the affected side, but in general, there are no overt functional complaints or increased respiratory infections among the observed patients[73,74] (Fig. 83–8).

FORAMEN OF MORGAGNI HERNIA

The failure of fusion between the central and lateral portions of the diaphragm leaves a gap immediately behind the xiphoid. The superior epigastric artery lies at the lateral margin of the hernia, which usually has a sac.[75,76] Approximately 3 to 5 percent of diaphragmatic defects, excluding hiatus hernias, occur through the foramen of Morgagni. Most often, the transverse colon or omentum is in the sac, but the presence of the small bowel, liver, and stomach has also been observed.

Diagnosis

Most of these lesions are asymptomatic and have been found incidentally on chest roentgenograms taken for respiratory infections. Very rarely, a newborn infant will have respiratory distress because of herniation of small bowel into the chest.[77] One of our patients was initially thought to have congenital heart disease because the left lobe of the liver had herniated into the pericardium and gave the appearance of an enlarged heart. A barium enema demonstrated the hernia, which contained transverse colon.

Treatment

Even though a foramen of Morgagni hernia is asymptomatic, repair is indicated because intestinal contents may become incarcerated. We strongly prefer an abdominal incision over a thoracic approach because, although the lesion is immediately beneath the sternum, it can extend laterally to either the right or the left. After reduction, the posterior rim of the hernia is sutured to the undersurface of the xiphoid. It is helpful to buttress each mattress suture with a pledget of Teflon felt to prevent the suture from tearing through the muscular diaphragm. Postoperative pneumopericardium is a potentially lethal complication after repair. If the pericardium is entered during the dissection of the sac, it should be drained with a small tube connected to an underwater seal.[78] We had to reoperate on one child who developed an adhesive obstruction. Otherwise, the results of surgery have been excellent.

EVENTRATION OF THE DIAPHRAGM

Small eventrations of the diaphragm are areas of congenital localized muscular aplasia. The defect is often no more than 3 or 4 cm in diameter and may occur on either side, although it is most commonly on the right (Fig. 83–9). Congenital eventration may be associated with lung hypoplasia or a variety of other birth defects.[79,80] Small eventrations are asymptomatic incidental findings on chest roentgenograms. A hernia containing liver tissue may be differentiated from a tumor by a liver scan or CT.

Small eventrations must be clearly differentiated from those involving an entire hemidiaphragm. It is difficult or impossible to determine whether an eventration of a hemidiaphreagm is primarily due to lack of muscle development or is secondary to phrenic nerve paralysis. With either lesion, the diaphragm is thin, fibrotic, and functionless. A phrenic nerve paralysis may result from birth trauma when it is associated with a brachial plexus palsy or from surgical damage. Cardiac procedures and the removal of mediastinal tumors can be complicated by phrenic nerve injury. A paralyzed or atrophic hemidiaphragm rises to the fourth or fifth interspace and seriously hampers ventilation, especially in a newborn, who depends primarily on diaphragmatic respiration. The pathophysiology is easily appreciated by observing the chest during fluoroscopy. With inspiration, the affected hemidiaphragm rises and the mediastinum shifts to the opposite side. Thus, neither lung can expand properly.

Diagnosis

A newborn infant with an eventration (or paralysis) of a hemidiaphragm will have a respiratory rate of 80 to 100 breaths/minute and will be dusky but not cyanotic. There is often a history of a difficult delivery and an associated brachial plexus palsy. On examination, the affected chest is dull to percussion, and the heart is shifted. The breath sounds are heard poorly in both hemithoraces. In addition to their respiratory distress, these infants suck poorly, become tired during feedings, and fail to gain weight. We have observed infants at 3 months of age who were still at birth weight. The diagnosis is made by a plain chest roentgenogram that demonstrates the elevated diaphragm (Fig. 83–10). It is sometimes difficult to differentiate a right-sided eventration

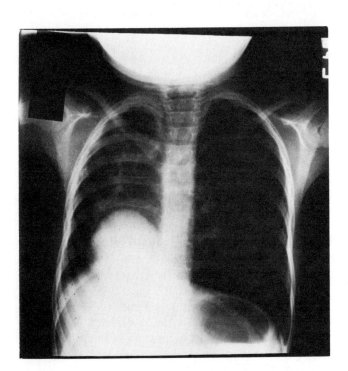
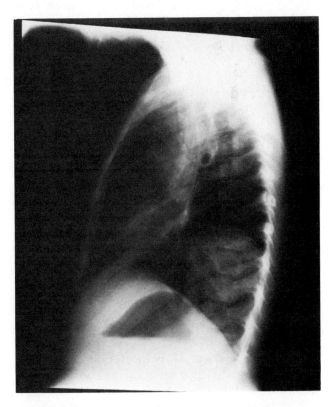

Figure 83–9. Asymptomatic posterior right eventration of the diaphragm. A liver scan proved the mass to be liver. **Left.** Posteroanterior view of the chest. **Right.** Lateral view of the chest.

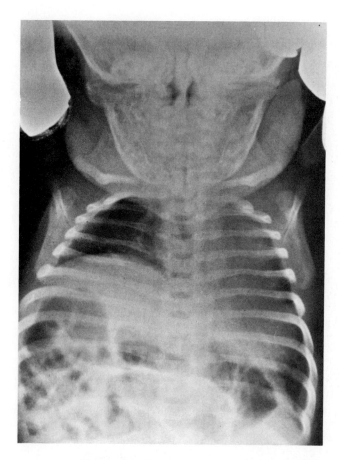 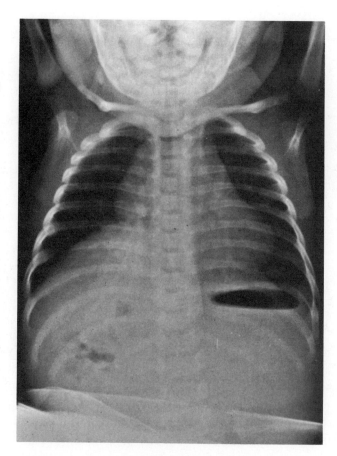

Figure 83–10. Left. A 1-week-old infant with a brachial plexus palsy and severe respiratory distress secondary to paralysis of the diaphragm. Note the severe mediastinal shift. **Right.** Postoperative film. There was immediate relief from the respiratory distress.

from a Bochdalek hernia with a sac. Fluoroscopy will demonstrate the swinging mediastinum, with absence of diaphragmatic motion. The diagnosis can be completely obscured in the infant who is on positive pressure ventilation, which expands the lungs and flattens the diaphragm. This diagnosis must always be considered when it is difficult to wean a baby from a respirator. One x-ray should always be obtained with the infant off the machine and breathing on his or her own. Occasionally, a child with an eventration of the diaphragm at several months of age has pneumonia. There is almost always a history of rapid breathing from birth. Others, particularly those with left-sided lesions, have a history of vomiting because the stomach rises up with the diaphragm (Fig. 83–11).

Treatment

Initially, the infant with an eventration is treated in the upright position. Nutrition can be supplemented by tube drip feedings. If the resting respiratory rate does not promptly fall to less than 80 breaths/minute, an operation should be considered. We do not agree with authors who advise a prolonged period of conserva-

tive support.[81] Babies who are treated conservatively suffer needless respiratory insufficiency, fail to grow, and are susceptible to repeated lung infections. Several authors have reported deaths in conservatively treated patients.[82,83] Simple plication of the diaphragm offers immediate relief from respiratory symptoms, and most infants can be discharged from the hospital within 5 to 7 days. Operative therapy carries far fewer risks than mechanical ventilation or expectant observation.

On the right side, the operation is performed through a seventh intercostal space incision. The relaxed, bulging diaphragm is above the level of the incision but is readily pushed down. A row of nonabsorbable sutures is placed parallel to the branches of the phrenic nerve in the center of the anterolateral third of the diaphragm, which is pulled upward with tissue forceps or Babcock clamps to protect the underlying liver. Each suture picks up several centimeters of tissue in two or three bites. When the row of sutures has been placed and tied, the diaphragm is imbricated and lowered. A second row of sutures also may be placed in the center of the posterior third of the diaphragm.[84,85] By imbricating in this fashion, the branches of the phrenic nerve

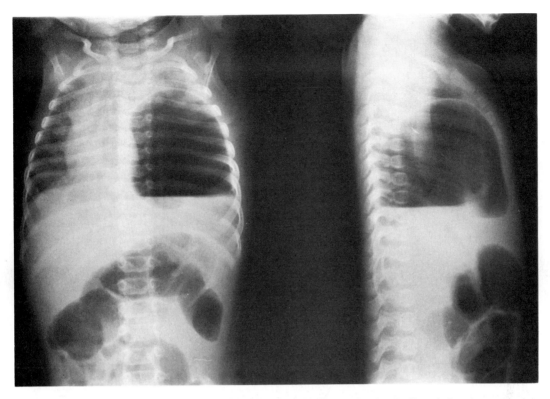

Figure 83–11. Eventration of the left diaphragm. The stomach was tremendously distended and caused acute respiratory distress in a 3-month-old child. Her initial symptom was episodic vomiting.

are avoided, and if regeneration does occur, nerve fibers will not have been injured by the sutures. It is never necessary to resect any portion of the diaphragm.

A left-sided eventration is best repaired through a subcostal abdominal incision in order to better visualize the stomach and esophageal hiatus. If the phrenic nerve is knowingly injured during a mediastinal operation, the diaphragm should be plicated immediately to avoid postoperative problems. In our experience, there has been no postoperative mortality, and both immediate and long-term results have been excellent.

Stone et al. reported a 1 to 7 year follow-up of 6 of 11 patients who underwent diaphragmatic plication for eventration secondary to phrenic nerve injury. Fluoroscopic evaluation revealed complete return of diaphragmatic function in these patients. Early plication resulted in a shorter duration of endotracheal intubation and a shorter stay in the intensive care unit.[86]

REFERENCES

1. Koontz AR, Levin MB: Agenesis of the right half of the diaphragm. Am Surg 34:657, 1968
2. Benjamin B: Agenesis of the left hemidiaphragm. J Thorac Cardiovasc Surg 46:265, 1963
3. Nicolisi CR, Leaf D, Schulenberg R: Bilateral congenital posterolateral diaphragmatic hernia. Minn Med 60:791, 1977
4. Blank E, Campbell JR: Congenital posterolateral defect in the right side of the diaphragm. Pediatrics 57:807, 1976
5. DeLorimier AA, Tierney DF, Parker HR: Hypoplastic lungs in fetal lambs with surgically produced congenital diaphragmatic hernia. Surgery 62:12, 1967
6. Ohi R, Suzuki H, Kato T, Kasai M: Development of the lung in fetal rabbits with experimental diaphragmatic hernia. J Pediatr Surg 11:955, 1976
7. Starrett RW, deLorimier AA: Congenital diaphragmatic hernia in lambs: hemodynamic and ventilatory changes with breathing. J Pediatr Surg 10:575, 1975
8. Berdon WE, Baker DH, Amoury R: The role of pulmonary hypoplasia in the prognosis of newborn infants with diaphragmatic hernia and eventration. Am J Roentgenol Radium Ther Nucl Med 103:413, 1968
9. Reynolds M, Luck SR, Lappen R: The "critical" neonate with diaphragmatic hernia: a 21-year perspective. J Pediatr Surg 19:364, 1984
10. Areechon W, Reid L: Hypoplasia of lung with congenital diaphragmatic hernia. Br Med J 1:230, 1963
11. Boyden EA: The structure of compressed lungs in congenital diaphragmatic hernia. Am J Anat 134:497, 1972
12. Naeye RL, Shochat SJ, Whitman V, Maisels MJ: Unsuspected pulmonary vascular abnormalities associated with diaphragmatic hernia. Pediatrics 58:902, 1976
13. Levin DL: Morphologic analysis of the pulmonary vascular

bed in congenital left-sided diaphragmatic hernia. J Pediatr 92:805, 1978

14. Geggel RL, Murphy JD, Langleben D, et al: Congenital diaphragmatic hernia: arterial structural changes and persistent pulmonary hypertension after surgical repair. J Pediatr 107:457, 1985

15. David TJ, Illingworth CA: Diaphragmatic hernia in the southwest of England. J Med Genet 13:253, 1976

16. Puri P, Gorman F: Lethal nonpulmonary anomalies associated with congenital diaphragmatic hernia: implications for early intrauterine surgery. J Pediatr Surg 19:29, 1984

17. Nakayama DK, Harrison MR, Chinn DH, et al: Prenatal diagnosis and natural history of the fetus with a congenital diaphragmatic hernia: initial clinical experience. J Pediatr Surg 20:118, 1985

18. Weils LJ: Development of the human diaphragm and pleural sacs. Contrib Embryol 35:107, 1954

19. Bell MJ, Ternberg JL: Antenatal diagnosis of diaphragmatic hernia. Pediatrics 60:738, 1977

20. Adzick NS, Harrison MR, Glick PL, et al: Diaphragmatic hernia in the fetus: prenatal diagnosis and outcome in 94 cases. J Pediatr Surg 20:357, 1985

21. Berk C, Grundy M: "High-risk" lecithin/spingomyelin ratios associated with neonatal diaphragmatic hernia: case reports. Br J Obstet Gynecol 89:250, 1982

22. Harrison MR, Jester JA, Ross NA: Correction of congenital diaphragmatic hernia in utero: I. The Model: intrathoracic balloon produces fatal pulmonary hypoplasia. Surgery 88:174, 1980

23. Harrison MR, Bressack MA, Chung AM, de Lorimier AA: Correction of congenital diaphragmatic hernia in utero: II. Simulated correction permits fetal lung growth with survival at birth. Surgery 88:260, 1980

24. Harrison MR, Ross NA, deLorimier AA: Correction of congenital diaphragmatic hernia in utero: III. Development of a successful surgical technique using abdominoplasty to avoid compromise of umbilical blood flow. J Pediatr Surg 16:934, 1981

25. Adzick NS, Outwater KM, Harrison MR, et al: Correction of congenital diaphragmatic hernia in utero: IV. An early gestational fetal lamb model for pulmonary vascular morphometric analysis. J Pediatr Surg 20:673, 1985

26. Wiseman NE, MacPherson RI: "Acquired" congenital diaphragmatic hernia. J Pediatr Surg 12:657, 1977

27. Hurdiss LW, Taybi H, Johnson LM: Delayed appearance of left-sided diaphragmatic hernia in infancy. J Pediatr 88:990, 1976

28. Kirchner SG, Burko H, O'Neill JA, Stahlman M: Delayed radiographic presentation of congenital right diaphragmatic hernia. Radiology 115:155, 1975

29. Raichoudhury RC, Patnaik SC, Sahoo M, et al: Foramen of Bochdalek hernia in adults. Chest 64:259, 1973

30. Woolley MM: Delayed appearance of a left posterolateral diaphragmatic hernia resuting in significant small bowel necrosis. J Pediatr Surg 12:673, 1977

31. Brill PW, Gershwind ME, Krasna IH: Massive gastric enlargement with delayed presentation of congenital diaphragmatic hernia: report of three cases and review of the literature. J Pediatr Surg 12:667, 1977

32. Fingerhut A, Pourcher J, Pelletier JM, et al: Duex observa-

tions de hernie diaphragmatique posterolaterale congenitale (dite de Bochdalek) revele `es a l'age adulte par des complications severes. J Chir (Paris) 115:135, 1978

33. Campbell D, Raffensperger J: Congenital cystic disease of the lung masquerading as diaphragmatic hernia. J Thorac Cardiovasc Surg 64:592, 1972

34. Welch FT, Reynolds SA: Diaphragmatic hernia simulating staphylococcal pneumonia. Rocky Mt Med J 69:37, 1972

35. Miller FJ, Varan LA, Shocat SJ: Umbilical arteriography for the rapid diagnosis of congenital diaphragmatic hernia in the newborn infant. J Pediatr 90:993, 1977

36. Yeung WC, Haines JE, Larson SM: Diagnosis of posterolateral congenital diaphragmatic (Bochdalek) hernia by liver scintigram: case report. J Nucl Med 17:110, 1976

37. White JJ, Oh KS, Haller JA: Positive-contrast peritoneography for accurate delineation of diaphragmatic abnormalities. Surgery 76:398, 1974

38. Rowe MI, Uribe FL: Diaphragmatic hernia in the newborn infant: blood gas and pH considerations. Surgery 70:758, 1971

39. Boles ET, Schiller M, Weinberger M: Improved management of neonates with congenital diaphragmatic hernia. Arch Surg 103:344, 1971

40. Boix-Ochoa J, Peguero G, Seijo G, et al: Acid-base balance and blood gases in prognosis and therapy of congenital diaphragmatic hernia. J Pediatr Surg 9:49, 1974

41. Kenigsberg K, Gwinn JL: The retained sac in repair of posterolateral diaphragmatic hernia in the newborn. Surgery 57:894, 1965

42. Rosenkrantz JG, Cotton EK: Replacement of left hemidiaphragm by a pedicled abdominal muscular flap. J Thorac Cardiovasc Surg 48:912, 1964

43. Simpson JS, Gossage JD: Use of abdominal wall muscle flap in repair of large congenital diaphragmatic hernia. J Pediatr Surg 6:42, 1971

44. Geisler I, Gotlieb A, Fried D: Agenesis of the right diaphragm repaired with Marlex. J Pediatr Surg 12:587, 1977

45. Priebe CJ, Wichern WA: Ventral hernia with a skin-covered Silastic sheet for newborn infants with a diaphragmatic hernia. Surgery 82:569, 1977

46. Simpson JS: Ventral Silon pouch: method of repairing congenital diaphragmatic hernias in neonates without increasing intraabdominal pressure. Surgery 66:798, 1969

47. Karl SR, Ballantine TVN, Snider MT: High-frequency ventilation at rates of 375 to 1800 cycles per minute in four neonates with congenital diaphragmatic hernia. J Pediatr Surg 18:822, 1983

48. Bohn D, Tamura M, Perrin D, et al: Ventilatory predicators of pulmonary hypoplasia in congenital diaphragmatic hernia, confirmed by morphologic assessment. J Pediatr Surg 111:423, 1987

49. Raphaely RC, Downes JJ Jr: Congenital diaphragmatic hernia: prediction of survival. J Pediatr Surg 8:815, 1973

50. Adelman S, Benson CD: Bochdalek hernias in infants: factors determining mortality. J Pediatr Surg 11:569, 1976

51. Ehrlich FE, Salzberg AM: Pathophysiology and management of congenital posterolateral diaphragmatic hernias. Am Surg 44:26, 1978

52. Murdock A, Burrington JB, Sawyer P: Alveolar to arterial oxygen tension difference and venous admixture in newly

born infants with congenital herniation through the foramen Bochdalek. Biol Neonate 17:161, 1971

53. Dibbins AW, Wiener ES: Mortality from neonatal diaphragmatic hernia. J Pediatr Surg 9:653, 1974

54. Rudolph AM, Yvons AM: Response of the pulmonary vasculature to hypoxia and H^+ ion changes. J Clin Invest 45:399, 1966

55. Naeye R, Letts H: The effects of prolonged neonatal hypoxemia on the pulmonary vascular bed and heart. Pediatrics 30:902, 1962

56. Gersony WM, Morishima HO, Daniel SS, et al: The hemodynamic effects of intrauterine hypoxia: an experimental model in newborn lambs. J Pediatr 89:631, 1976

57. Haller JA, Signer RD, Golladay ES, et al: Pulmonary and ductal hemodynamics in studies of simulated diaphragmatic hernia of fetal and newborn lambs. J Pediatr Surg 11:675, 1976

58. Ahlquist RP, Huggins RA, Woodbury RA: The pharmacology of benzyl-imidazoline (Priscol). J Pharmacol Exp Ther 89:271, 1947

59. Goetzman BW, Sunshine P, Johnson JD, et al: Neonatal hypoxia and pulmonary vasospasm: response to tolazoline. J Pediatr 89:617, 1976

60. Moodie DS, Telander RL, Kleinberg F, Feldt RH: Use of tolazoline in newborn infants with diaphragmatic hernia and severe cardiopulmonary disease. J Thoracic Cardiovasc Surg 75:725, 1978

61. Levy RJ, Rosenthal A, Freed MD, et al: Persistent pulmonary hypertension in a newborn with congenital diaphragmatic hernia: successful management with tolazoline. Pediatrics 60:740, 1977

62. Dibbins AW: Neonatal diaphragmatic hernia: a physiologic challenge. Am J Surg 131:408, 1976

63. Vacanti JP, Crone RK, Murphy JD, et al: The pulmonary hemodynamic response to perioperative anesthesia in the treatment of high-risk infants with congenital diaphragmatic hernia. J Pediatr Surg 19:672, 1984

64. Collins DL, Pomerance JJ, Travis KW, et al: A new approach to congenital posterolateral diaphragmatic hernia. J Pediatr Surg 12:149, 1977

65. Stolar C, Dillon P, Reyes C: Selective use of ECMO in the management of congenital diaphragmatic hernia. J Pediatr Surg 23:207, 1988

66. Langham MR, Krummer TM, Greenfield LJ, et al: ECMO following repair of congenital diaphragmatic hernia. Ann Thorac Surg 44:247, 1987

67. Hardesty RL, Griffith BP, Debski RF, et al: ECMO: successful treatment of persistent fetal circulation following repair of congenital diaphragmatic hernia. J Thorac Cardiovasc Surg 81:556, 1981

68. Ban JL, Moore TC: Intrathoracic tension incarceration of stomach and liver through right-sided congenital posterolateral diaphragmatic hernias. J Thorac Cardiovasc Surg 66:969, 1973

69. McNamara JJ, Eraklis AJ, Gross RE: Congenital posterolateral diaphragmatic hernia in the newborn. J Thorac Cardiovasc Surg 55:55, 1968

70. Harrison MR, Bjordal R, Longmark F, Knutrud O: Congenital diaphragmatic hernia: the hidden mortality. J Pediatr Surg 13:227, 1978

71. Chatrath RR, El Shafie M, Jones RS: Fate of hypoplastic lungs after repair of congenital diaphragmatic hernia. Arch Dis Child 46:633, 1971

72. Hislop A, Reid L: Persistent hypoplasia of the lung after repair of congenital diaphragmatic hernia. Thorax 31:450, 1976

73. Wohl MEB, Griscom NT, Strieder DJ, et al: The lung following repair of congenital diaphragmatic hernia. J Pediatr 90:405, 1977

74. Reid IS, Hutcherson RJ: Long-term follow-up of patients with congenital diaphragmatic hernia. J Pediatr Surg 11:939, 1976

75. Baran EM, Houston HE, Lynn HB, O'Connell EJ: Foramen of Morgagni hernias in children. Surgery 62:1076, 1967

76. Bentley G, Lister J: Retrosternal hernia. Surgery 57:567, 1964

77. Pokorny WJ, McGill CW, Harberg FJ: Morgagni hernias during infancy: presentation and associated anomalies. J Pediatr Surg 19:394, 1984

78. Thomas GG, Clitherow NR: Herniation through the foramen of Morgagni in children. Br. J Surg 64:215, 1977

79. Michelson E: Eventration of the diaphragm. Surgery 49:410, 1961

80. Laxdal O, McDougall H, Mellin G: Congenital eventration of the diaphragm. N Engl J Med 250:401, 1954

81. Wayne E, Campbell J, Burrington JD, et al: Eventration of the diaphragm. J Pediatr Surg 9:643, 1974

82. Stauffer UG: Diaphragmatic paralysis due to birth trauma. Helv Paediatr Acta 27:253, 1972

83. Bishop HC, Koop C: Acquired eventration of the diaphragm in infancy. Pediatrics 22:1088, 1958

84. Paris R, Glasco E, Canto A, et al: Diaphragmatic eventration in infants. Thorax 28:66, 1973

85. Swartz M, Filler R: Plication of the diaphragm for symptomatic phrenic nerve paralysis. J Pediatr Surg 13:259, 1978

86. Stone KS, Brown JW, Canal DF, et al: Long-term fate of the diaphragm surgically plicated during infancy and early childhood. Ann Thorac Surg 44:62, 1987

84
Diseases of the Pleura

PNEUMOTHORAX

Spontaneous pneumothorax may occur in otherwise normal babies after a difficult delivery. The degree of distress is directly related to the amount of air in the pleural cavity. Physical diagnosis is helpful only when there is a large amount of air, with collapse of the lung and shift of the mediastinum. Transillumination of the chest with a high intensity fiberoptic light source is a rapid means of detecting air in the pleura.[1] The light source is placed on the infant's chest, and the halo of transilluminated light is compared with the opposite side. A chest roentgenogram is the best diagnostic tool, however.

Treatment

A pneumothorax that occupies no more than 25 percent of the pleural cavity, with no shift of the mediastinum, will in all probability quickly reabsorb without treatment. Nothing is done if the infant has only mild distress and is improving. A baby who is restless or tachypneic or who has pneumothorax that is increasing in severity should be treated with an intercostal tube connected to a waterseal (Fig. 84–1).

In the newborn, it is important to tunnel the tube over one or two ribs in order to diminish the chances of air entering the chest during removal. Pneumothorax is a frequent complication of ventilator therapy in neonates with hyaline membrane disease. It also occurs following the vigorous resuscitation of infants who have had a respiratory or cardiac arrest. These babies have areas of overinflated alveoli that rupture and allow air to escape into the pleural cavity and also into the mediastinum, abdomen, and pericardium.[2,3] Any detectable pneumothorax in an infant with the respiratory distress syndrome or who requires respiratory therapy must be treated with an intercostal waterseal drain. A tube of at least size 10 or 12 is used. Needle aspiration or the insertion of plastic IV cannulas are unsatisfactory.

Pneumomediastinum may require the insertion of a second tube adjacent to the xiphoid process up into the mediastinum. A waterseal drain is sufficient for infants with simple pneumothorax. The lung will reexpand, and when the tube has ceased to bubble for 24 hours, it may be removed. Unfortunately, when a pneumothorax develops in an infant requiring positive pressure respiration, there is likely to be a persistent or recurrent leak of air. The chest tube must be completely inspected every day because one cause of persistent pneumothorax

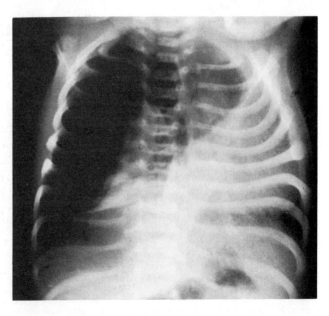

Figure 84–1. Severe tension pneumothorax in a newborn infant. The classic signs are shift of the mediastinum, widening of the interspaces, and depression of the diaphragm.

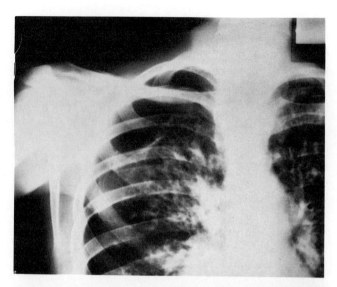

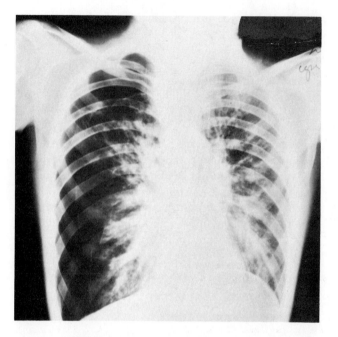

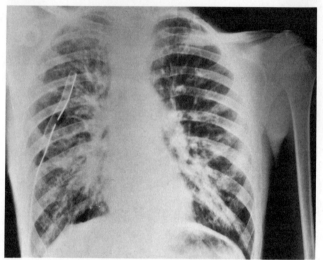

Figure 84–2. A 12-year-old boy with cystic fibrosis of the pancreas who required bilateral thoracotomy and pleurodesis for control of recurrent pneumothorax. **Left.** Left pneumothorax with extensive bilateral lung disease. **Top right.** Apical bullae that were eventually resected. **Bottom.** Full expansion of the lung with a properly placed chest tube, inserted laterally at the 6th ICS and directed toward the apex.

is the presence of a hole in the tube outside the chest or a leak around the site of chest tube insertion. If the lung fails to reexpand with a waterseal drain, as much as 20 cm of water suction may be added to the system. Grosfeld et al. successfully performed an emergency thoracotomy on 10 infants with pneumothorax that resisted tube drainage. A large lung tear was found and sutured in every case. Nine of these severely ill babies survived.[4]

In older children, pneumothorax may occur secondary to trauma or as a complication of chronic lung disease, especially cystic fibrosis of the pancreas. In these children, the presence of a persistent or recurrent pneumothorax is an indication for thoracotomy, excision of lung blebs, and pleurodesis[5] (Fig. 84–2).

CHYLOTHORAX

Chylothorax is the most common cause of pleural fluid in the neonate. Yancy and Spock found that most infants with apparently spontaneous chylothorax were full-term and had no associated anomalies.[6] The effusion may occur on either side or bilaterally. Approximately half appear during the first 24 hours of life, and another quarter appear by the end of the first week. There is a gradual onset of respiratory distress with shift of the mediastinum away from the affected side and dullness to percussion. Chest roentgenograms demonstrate an opacity on the affected side, with layering of the fluid on a decubitus film. The diagnosis is made by a thoracentesis, which will reveal a milky, opaque fluid after the infant has begun to take feedings. A Sudan III stain will reveal fat globules. If the thoracentesis is performed before feedings, the fluid will be clear yellow. Repeated aspirations after milk feedings will prove the diagnosis. Chylothorax also can follow thoracic operations, especially for coarctation of the aorta, and has been seen after repair of a Bochdalek diaphragmatic hernia. We once encountered this complication after repair of an esophageal atresia with a right aortic arch.[7] Chylothorax has been known to follow thrombosis of the superior vena cava and the left subclavian veins. In each case, the thrombosis was a complication associated with a central hyperalimentation catheter. In older children, chylothorax may occur with extensive mediastinal lymphangiomas.

Treatment

Persistent drainage of chyle from the chest results in rapid development of malnutrition. Consequently, the fluid must be replaced, initially with plasma, in order to maintain a normal blood volume. The basal rate for flow in the thoracic duct is 1.38 ml/kg/hour, but fat feeding significantly increases the rate of chyle production.[8] Although multiple aspirations of the chest may be performed, we much prefer to establish continuous pleural drainage with a tube and waterseal drainage. Medium-chain triglycerides are absorbed into the portal system rather than into the thoracic duct, and several authors have reported success with formulas that use triglycerides in place of fat.[9,10] In our experience, these formulas have resulted in a continuous flow of chyle, especially in infants with thrombosis of a major vein. We prefer to insert a chest tube and replace the initial volume of chyle with IV plasma and then give the infant nothing by mouth and feed by IV hyperalimentation until the chyle flow from the tube has completely stopped for several days. The next step is a continuous intragastric drip of an elemental diet (Vivonex). During this period, older children are given clear liquids and carbohydrates, although their nutrition comes mainly from the elemental diet. When this has been tolerated without reaccumulation of chyle, the diet is advanced to include a medium-chain triglyceride formula, such as Portagen or Pregestimil. Older children are given a fat-free diet. Later, fat is introduced, and the chest is watched closely. We operated on only one child for a persistent and recurrent chylothorax. This was a 3-year-old boy with an extensive mediastinal and retroperitoneal lymphangioma. After excision of the lymphangioma, suture of all oozing points in his mediastinum, and a pleurodesis, he stopped reaccumulating fluid. He eventually died 4 years later with recurring chylothoraces, ascites, and diffuse lymphangiomatosis.

Hemothorax

Intrapleural bleeding may occur spontaneously in infants who have a coagulation disorder, particularly hypoprothrombinemia and particularly following a difficult delivery.[11] Treatment consists of evacuation of the blood by needle aspiration, transfusion to replace the lost blood, and correction of the coagulation disorder.

EMPYEMA

The incidence of empyema and pyopneumothorax has decreased sharply since the staphyloccocal epidemic of the 1950s, when over 70 infants and children were treated for empyema in a 1-year period at the Cook County Children's Hospital. Staphylococcal pneumonia continues to account for most empyemas seen in children, although other organisms (such as *Escherichia coli* and other enteric organisms) are found in neonatal empyema.[12,13]

Staphylococcal pneumonia occurs as a primary respiratory tract infection in infants, or it may complicate measles, chickenpox, or influenza. The illness occurs with nonspecific signs, such as fever, nasal discharge, and cough. When it is untreated, there is a rapid progression to tachypnea, dyspnea, and cyanosis. Antibiotic therapy, especially a shot or two of penicillin, will diminish the initial symptoms but will allow the disease to progress with a more indolent course until there is a thick pleural exudate.

The staphylococcus causes a purulent interstitial peribronchial inflammation that results in abscess formation within the lung parenchyma. These small abscesses coalesce to form a cavity, or they can break through the pleura and cause an acute pyopneumothorax. An abscess within the lung will resolve with antibiotic therapy, leaving a pneumatocele that resembles a congenital cyst. These pneumatoceles, however, have no endothelial lining and will obliterate and disappear completely without further therapy (Fig. 84–3).

Diagnosis

An infant with pneumonia who rapidly worsens must have an immediate x-ray. If there is an air–fluid level in the pleural cavity, the infant has an acute pyopneumothorax secondary to rupture of a small bronchus. If there is opacification of the pleural cavity with obliteration of the costophrenic sinus, there is only fluid. Cultures of the nasopharynx, the sputum, and the pleural fluid are necessary to plan antibiotic therapy.

Treatment

A chest tube must be inserted immediately into the pleural cavity of an infant with a pyopneumothorax. The site of insertion is determined by careful study of the

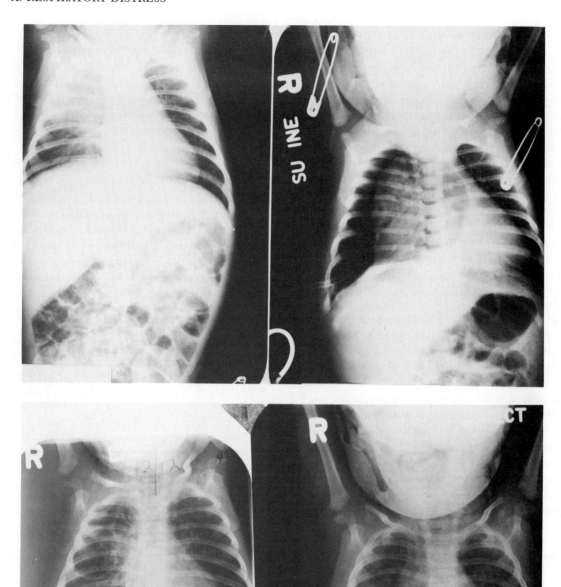

Figure 84–3. Staphylococcal pneumonia with progression to a pneumothorax, pneumatocele, and complete clearing. **Top left.** Consolidation of the right upper lobe. **Top right.** Pneumothorax, treated with a waterseal drain. **Bottom left.** Pneumatoceles—if these were seen without the prior history of a staphylococcal pneumonia, it would be impossible to differentiate the pneumatocele from a lung cyst. **Bottom right.** Complete clearing within 6 months.

x-rays, physical examination, and preliminary needle aspiration. The tube must be as large as can be inserted between an interspace—usually a size 14 or 16 French tube is the largest that can be used in an infant under 1 year of age. Needle aspiration alone with intensive antibiotic therapy may be sufficient for the child with pneumonia and a cloudy, thin pleural effusion. If the postaspiration roentgenogram demonstrates a completely expanded lung, a chest tube need not be inserted unless the fluid recurs.

Chronic empyema with multiple loculated pockets of thick pus is seen in children who have been treated only with antibiotics and no chest drainage. Inadequate drainage through a small or poorly placed tube also will result in a chronic empyema. If the lung is reasonably well expanded and the child is getting along well clinically, the pus will absorb and leave no long-term problems. However, if the child continues to have a low-grade fever with partial collapse of the lung and loculated pockets of pus, we prefer to perform a modified open drainage.

The loculated pus is localized with skin markers and chest roentgenograms. The child is given a general anesthetic, and the affected chest is completely prepared and draped. An incision is made over a rib adjacent to the pus. A 3 to 4 cm segment of rib is resected, and the pleural cavity is entered through the bed of the resected rib. Adhesions between the lung and pleura are taken down with finger dissection to open pockets of loculated pus. Fibrinous material and the thick exudate are removed with suction and irrigation. (See Fig. 104-2.)

The thickest exudate will be found posteriorly and in the costodiaphragmatic angle. The anesthesiologist will be able at this point to inflate collapsed segments of lung. This procedure is not a formal decortication but merely a simple technique for removing fibrinous material and thick pus from the chest through a small incision while the child is under anesthesia. This is far less traumatic than the insertion of multiple chest tubes in a conscious child. A large tube with multiple holes is then accurately placed in the pleural cavity to establish dependent drainage. The incision is closed tightly about the tube, which is connected to a waterseal with 20 mm of water suction.

Formal decortication is never required in infants and small children. Thickened pleura resolves over a period of several months, leaving no residual disability. On the other hand, teenagers may require decortication of thickened pleura, especially when an infected hemothorax has followed trauma.

REFERENCES

1. Kuhns LR, Bedmarek FJ, Wyman ML, et al: Diagnosis of pneumothorax or pneumomediastinum in the neonate by transillumination. Pediatrics 56:355, 1975
2. Grosfeld JC, Kilman JW, Frye TR: Spontaneous pneumopericardium in the newborn period. J Pediatr 76:614, 1970
3. Mansfield PB, Graham CB, Beckwith JB, et al: Pneumopericardium and pneumomediastinum in infants and children. J Pediatr Surg 8:691, 1973
4. Grosfeld JL, Lemons J, Ballantine T, Schreiner R: Emergency thoracotomy for acquired bronchopleural fistula in the premature infant with respiratory distress. Presented at the 28th annual meeting of Surg Sec of Am Acad of Pediatr, San Francisco, 1979
5. Luck SR, Raffensperger JC, Sullivan HJ, Gibson LE: Management of pneumothorax in children with chronic pulmonary disease. J Thorac Cardiovasc Surg 74:834, 1977
6. Yancy WS, Spock A: Spontaneous neonatal pleural effusion. J Pediatr Surg 2:313, 1967
7. Wiener ES, Owens L, Salzberg AM: Chylothorax after Bochdalek hernioraphy in a neonate treatment with intravenous hyperalimentation. J Thorac Cardiovasc Surg 65:200, 1973
8. Bessone LN, Ferguson TB, Burford TH: Chylothorax: review. Ann Thorac Surg 12:537, 1971
9. Kosloske AM, Martin LW, Schubert WK: Management of chylothorax in children by thoracentesis and medium-chain triglycerides feeding. J Pediatr Surg 9:365, 1974
10. Gershank JJ, Jonsson HT Jr, Riopel DA, Packer RM: Dietary management of neonatal chylothorax. Pediatrics 53:400, 1974
11. Mazzi E, White JJ, Nishida H, Risenberg H: Neonatal respiratory distress from hemothorax. Pediatrics [Suppl] 59:1059, 1977
12. Bechamps GJ, Lynn HB, Wenzl JE: Empyema in children: review of Mayo Clinic experience. Mayo Clin Proc 54:43, 1970
13. Turner JAP: Staphylococcal pneumonia, a contemporary rarity. Clin Pediatr 11:69, 1972

85
Congenital Malformations of the Lung

Congenital pulmonary defects, including lung cysts, sequestration, and lobar emphysema, may cause respiratory distress by overinflation and compression of normal lung tissue or by secondary infection. Although these lesions share a common pathologic spectrum, they can be readily differentiated on the basis of clinical presentation and radiologic appearance. Consequently, they should be considered separately even though they may be interrelated and share a common origin.[1,2] These are relatively rare. From 1962 through 1984, at the Children's Memorial Hospital, we operated on 25 cases of lobar emphysema, 23 pulmonary sequestrations and 25 cystic lesions of the lung.

EMBRYOLOGY

Following separation of the trachea and esophagus, the trachea bifurcates while it is still in the cervical region of the 4 mm embryo. The trachea and bronchi descend into the thorax and form bronchial buds during the sixth week. All major bronchial budding is complete in the 23 mm embryo. Until 16 weeks of gestational age, lung development is in a glandular stage while bronchial budding is taking place in solid pulmonary mesenchyme. From 24 weeks to birth, the distal ends of the bronchial buds open, and alveoli are formed. New alevoli continue to develop after birth.[3] Alveolarization of terminal bronchioles continues to 4 years of age, and the number of alveoli increases during the first 8 years.[4,5] Unilateral agenesis or hypoplasia of the lung represents a failure of development beyond the fourth week. Sequestrations have their origin during the sixth to eighth weeks and lung cysts as late as the 24th week.[6] These lesions represent abnormal budding or diverticulae from the bronchus.

CONGENITAL LUNG CYSTS

Congenital lung cysts are lined by ciliated pseudostratified columnar epithelium. The wall of the cyst contains smooth muscle, elastic tissue, and varying amounts of cartilage (Fig. 85–1). The cysts may appear to be unilocular on roentgenograms, but when the cyst is opened, it is usually found to be multilocular (Fig. 85–2). These features should clearly differentiate a congenital cyst from the acquired pneumatoceles that follow staphylococcal pneumonia. The infectious cysts may become lined with respiratory epithelium, but there will be fibrous tissue in the wall rather than smooth muscle.[7] The differentiation can be made clinically, since postinfection cysts or pneumatoceles follow severe pulmonary infections. The problem of differential diagnosis is further confused by the fact that a congenital lung cyst may become infected and lose its ciliated epithelium. The differentiation between a lung cyst and a bronchogenic cyst is made by the location. Lung cysts are definitely within pulmonary parenchyma, whereas bronchogenic cysts are either paratracheal or in the mediastinum. Cystic adenomatoid malformation is a related yet separate entity that is differentiated from the simple, solitary or multilocular cyst by the following features: (1) absence of bronchial cartilage, (2) absence of bronchial tubular glands, (3) presence of tall columnar, mucinous epithelium, (4) overproduction of terminal bronchiolar structures without alveolar differentiation, and (5) massive enlargement of the affected lobe, causing displacement of other thoracic structures.[8] After reviewing the material from the Armed Forces Institute of Pathology, Stocker et al. described three types of cystic adenomatoid malformations.[9] Type one is composed of large cysts with thick, smooth walls. This type may actually represent the solitary or multilocular cysts described previously. The second type has multiple

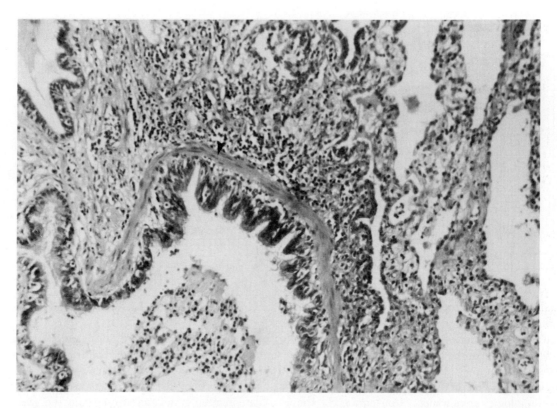

Figure 85–1. This lung cyst contains ciliated epithelium and connective tissue. The arrow points to a layer of smooth muscle, which is never found in pneumatoceles.

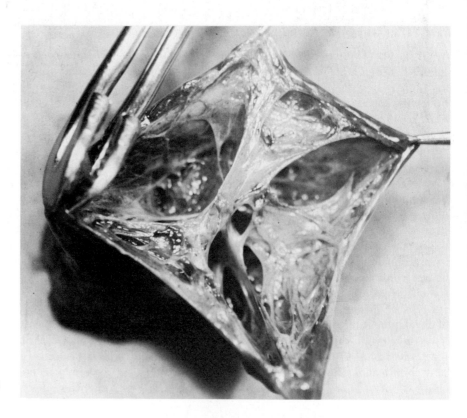

Figure 85–2. Congenital lung cyst with a smooth lining and multiple loculations.

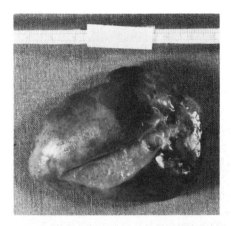

Figure 85–3. Cystic adenomatoid malformation of the entire lung. There are multiple small cysts throughout the lung.

small cysts less than 1 cm in diameter that blend with normal parenchyma. The third type occupies an entire lobe or lung and is composed of multiple bronchiole-like structures with masses of cuboidal, epithelium-lined, alveolar structures (Fig. 85–3). Many of the infants in this series were stillborn, and 10 of the 38 infants studied had severe associated congenital anomalies. Cystic adenomatoid malformation has been reported to be associated with an anomalous systemic artery. However, it

would be more reasonable to classify this as a sequestration.[10] Rhabdomyosarcoma has been found arising from a congenital cystic adenomatoid malformation, providing yet another example of the relationship of congenital defects and malignant childhood tumors.[11]

Diagnosis

There was an even distribution of boys and girls with congenital lung cysts among patients reviewed from our own files, and all lobes of the lung were involved. Two lobes were involved in six patients. Two patients had involvement of an entire lung, and one child had cysts throughout her right lung and in the upper segment of her left lung. The apical segment of the right upper lobe was all that was involved in one child. Respiratory distress with cyanosis and shift of the mediastinum due to an expanding cyst occurred in patients under 3 months of age. Children older than 3 months had infected cysts. Their symptoms were primarily the result of lung suppuration. These patients showed their cysts on the initial roentgenograms. Some partially cleared with antibiotic therapy, but all of the patients were eventually proven to have infected cysts. In the neonatal period, multiple lung cysts may be mistaken for a diaphragmatic hernia.[12,13] In such cases, there were densities in the left pleural cavity that later became air-filled cysts resem-

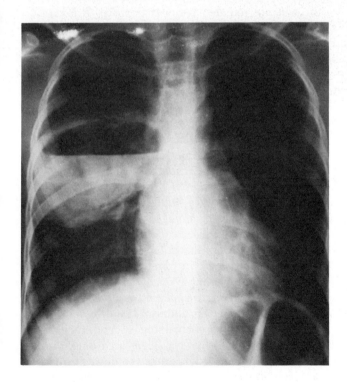

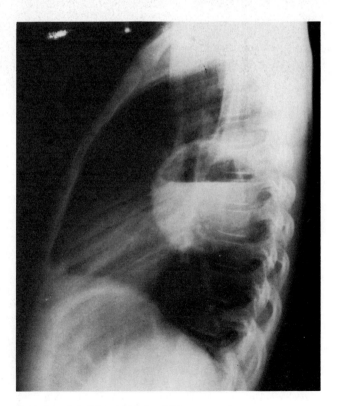

Figure 85–4. Congenital lung cyst of the apical segment of the right lower lobe.

bling loops of intestine. The presence of loops of intestine below the diaphragm or use of a barium enema should make this differential diagnosis.

Radiographically, a solitary cyst may be filled with fluid or completely air-filled, or there may be an air–fluid level (Fig. 85–4). The lesion is rounded and is clearly within lung tissue. Cystic adenomatoid malformation either may have multiple small cysts or be relatively solid with small radiolucencies (Fig. 85–5). Two of our children with lung cysts were initially thought to have lobar emphysema, and in four patients the initial diagnosis was lung abscess. Few of these cysts have bronchial communications large enough to fill with contrast material. Bronchoscopy has demonstrated only distortion of the major bronchi. These studies are contraindicated in neonates with respiratory disease due to lung cysts.

Treatment

Excision of the cyst is indicated, by either segmental resection or lobectomy. This may be required as an emergency procedure when there is respiratory distress in

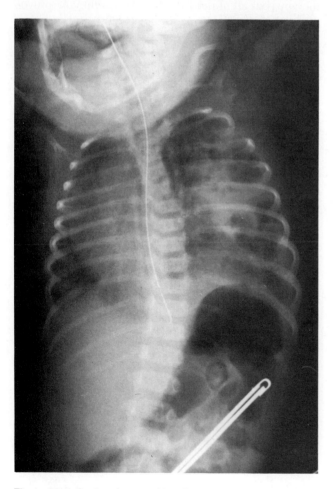

Figure 85–5. Cystic adenomatoid malformation of the left lung. This could easily be confused with a diaphragmatic hernia, except that there is air below the diaphragm.

infants under 3 months of age. In older children, associated infections are treated with antibiotics, bronchial drainage, and, if indicated, bronchoscopic aspiration of secretions. Two of our patients required pneumonectomy because of the involvement of the entire lung. Another survived pneumonectomy and a later contralateral segmental resection.

CONGENITAL LOBAR EMPHYSEMA

Lobar emphysema is an important cause of respiratory distress in young infants. It is best described as overinflation or severe distention of one lobe with compression atelectasis of adjacent lobes, shift of the mediastinum, and herniation of the lung across the midline. The left upper lobe is involved in 47 percent of reported cases, the right middle lobe in 28 percent, the right upper lobe in 20 percent, and the lower lobes in only 5 percent.[14,15]

Pathology

Grossly, the involved lobe almost fills the pleural cavity. When the chest is opened, the lobe herniates out of the wound, but unlike normal lung tissue, it does not inflate and deflate in response to pressure changes. The tissue has the consistency of sponge rubber and springs back to shape after it has been indented, and the edges of the lobe are rounded rather than sharp. It is rare to find a specific abnormality of the lobar bronchus, and even after the bronchus has been transected, the lobe remains inflated (Fig. 85–6). In most cases, no specific etiology is found. However, some authors have found folds of mucosa or abnormal bronchial cartilage.[16,17] We have never observed gross bronchial abnormalities in the lobar or segmental bronchi. Very careful dissection of the segmental bronchi after the injection of formalin into the lung has demonstrated abnormal orientation and a disordered distribution of the bronchial cartilage.[18–20] There is also an increase in fibrous tissue about the distended alveoli that may hinder their collapse.[21] Regardless of the specific etiology, it would appear that lobar emphysema is a disease involving both the small bronchi and the alveoli that interferes with the normal static recoil of the lung on expiration.

The term "lobar emphysema" also has been used to describe pulmonary overinflation secondary to partial bronchial obstruction from aberrant blood vessels, bronchial cysts, congenital bronchial stenosis, and atresia.[22–27] These lesions should be classified according to the specific obstruction in order to avoid confusing terminology. A condition closely resembling lobar emphysema occurs in the right lower lobe of premature infants who have required long-term ventilatory support.[28] Bronchial obstruction secondary to the effects of intubation and

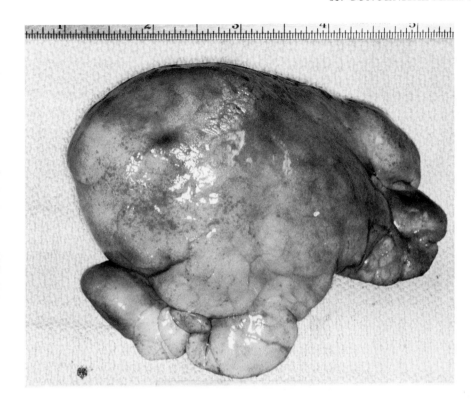

Figure 85–6. Lobar emphysema of the middle lobe. The lung remains inflated even after the bronchus is transected.

repeated suctioning usually accounts for the overinflation. On the other hand, we operated on one infant with a left upper lobe emphysema, which at first was thought to be caused by the ventilator but, in all probability, represented lobar emphysema that had been treated as the respiratory distress syndrome. The Swyer–James or unilateral hyperlucent lung syndrome also must be differentiated from lobar emphysema.[29,30] Here one entire lung is radiolucent because of decreased pulmonary blood flow and alveolar overdistention.

Congenital heart lesions are associated with lobar emphysema. The most common among these have been ventricular septal defect, coarctation of the aorta, and patent ductus.[31,32]

Diagnosis

Approximately half of infants with lobar emphysema have varying degrees of respiratory distress (such as tachypnea and noisy respirations) from birth. Some have severe dyspnea, and the diagnosis is made during the first few days of life. Others have minimal symptoms until they develop an intercurrent respiratory tract infection and appreciably deteriorate over a period of few hours. Most of our patients and those reported in the literature were not diagnosed until they developed severe dyspnea when between 1 and 4 months of age, even though they had some respiratory difficulty earlier.

Physical findings consist of mediastinal shift, hyperresonance to percussion, and diminished breath sounds on the affected side. Roentgenograms demonstrate over-

distention of the affected lobe (Fig. 85–7). Within the radiolucent zone, there are faint bronchovascular markings. It is necessary to examine the x-ray before a spotlight to differentiate severe lobar emphysema from pneumothorax. When the left upper lobe is involved, the left lower lobe is compressed into a small atelectatic pancake against the lower heart border. The distended lobe not only displaces the mediastinum but also herniates across to the opposite side. An x-ray taken in the newborn period may demonstrate an opaque lobe rather than one that is radiolucent.[33,34] This finding may lead to a mistaken diagnosis of pleural effusion or thoracic tumor, but within a few days, the opacity will clear and the typical picture will emerge. It would appear that the lung retains fetal fluid via the same mechanism that prevents it from expelling air. In older children with milder symptoms, there may only be a segment of a lobe involved, or the overexpansion may be less severe than that seen in infants.

The diagnosis in most cases can be made from the clinical picture and plain roentgenograms. Other studies, particularly bronchoscopy and bronchography, are contraindicated in babies with severe respiratory distress. These studies are useful, however, in older children with milder symptoms in whom there is a greater opportunity for finding a specific obstruction. We prefer to bronchoscope older children to rule out a foreign body or other lesions. If nothing specific is found, the operation is performed under the same anesthetic. Radiosotope perfusion scanning and pulmonary angiography are valu-

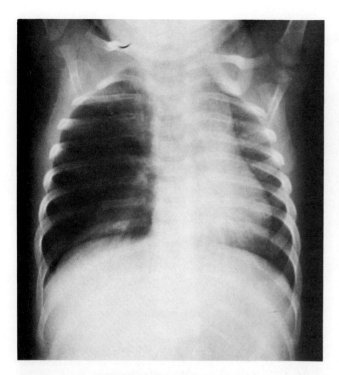

Figure 85–7. Lobar emphysema of the right middle lobe. There is a shift of the mediastinum with compression of the upper and lower lobes.

able tools for evaluation of the degree of function in the affected lobe as well as the effect of the abnormal lobe on normal lung tissue.[35] The involved lobe has a diminished perfusion, and the pulmonary vessels are spread so that vessels in the adjacent lobes are crowded. These studies are particularly valuable in determining if the overexpansion of the lobe is secondary to collapse of the lung on the opposite side.

Treatment

Emergency thoracotomy with lobectomy is necessary for infants with severe respiratory distress. While preparations for the operation are being carried out, the infant is kept in an oxygen-enriched, humidified atmosphere. Positive pressure ventilation might do more harm than good, and in our experience, it has always been possible to relieve the symptoms by prompt operation. Everything must be ready to immediately open the chest after induction of anesthesia. As soon as the affected lung has herniated out of the incision, the anesthetist will notice improved pulmonary compliance and easier control of ventilation.

The proper therapy for older infants and children who have minimal symptoms with lobar emphysema is less clear. Eigen et al. followed five children with lobar emphysema in whom the diagnosis was first made when the patients were between 3 months and 9 years of age.[36] At the time of examination, from several months to years

after diagnosis, Eigen et al. found continued overinflation of the lobe on physical examination and roentgenograms, although pulmonary function tests revealed little difference when compared to patients who had undergone lobectomies in the neonatal period. Both groups of patients had reduced forced vital capacities, large volumes of trapped intrapulmonary gas, and delay in forced expiration. Demuth and Sloan also found long-term respiratory problems in children who had undergone surgery for lobar emphysema in infancy.[37]

Other authors have gone even further and have recommended "expectant treatment," including ventilatory support, for infants with lobar emphysema. They would reserve lobectomy for infants with repeated pneumothorax, failure to improve with mechanical ventilation, or respiratory or cardiac failure.[38] We agree with this advice only in the cases of infants whose lobar inflation is clearly secondary to ventilator treatment or follows a reversible infectious bronchiolitis. Infants who are operated on for lobar emphysema are immediately relieved of their symptoms and in our institution have a 100 percent survival rate. On the other hand, two children who are followed to 4 and 9 years of age had persistent wheezing and multiple episodes of pneumonia in the adjacent compressed lung until the emphysematous lobe was removed.

PULMONARY SEQUESTRATION

Pulmonary tissue that has no connection with the normal bronchial tree and that receives its blood supply from a systemic artery is separated from the normal lung is sequestrated.[39] The sequestered lung is extralobar when it has no connection with the lung and intralobar when it is within the lung. Several clinical series of bronchopulmonary sequestration have clearly defined these two conditions as separate clincial and pathologic entities even though they are developmentally related.[40–49]

Pathology

Extralobar pulmonary sequestration involves development of a completely separate lung with its own pleural envelope. It is usually found in the left posterior costodiaphragmatic angle adjacent to the esophagus and the aorta. The blood supply to this portion of lung originates from the thoracic or abdominal aorta. Aberrant pulmonary tissue also has been found within the abdomen.[50] Extralobar sequestrations are small and flattened, with a liverlike consistency. There is no identifiable bronchus, but microscopically one finds tertiary bronchial structures with alveoli. There may be cystic changes, but since there is no connection with the lung, there is no inflammation. Extralobar sequestrations often are found incidentally during repair of left Bochdalek diaphragmatic hernias or at thoracotomy for other congenital malformations.

Intralobar sequestration occurs within the lung, most often within the posterior basal segment of the lower lobe. Here too the sequestered lung has no connection with the bronchus, although it may be inflated through adjacent alveoli. The blood supply to this portion of the lung is from a systemic artery that may originate from the thoracic or abdominal aorta or from intercostal vessels. When the blood supply is from the abdominal aorta, the anomalous vessel pierces the posterior portion of the diaphragm and enters the lower lobe through the inferior pulmonary ligament. The venous drainage of either the extralobar or the intralobar sequestration may be into either the left atrium, the azygos vein, or the vena cava. Cystic changes and secondary inflammation are common in intralobar sequestrations. The cystic changes are most likely congenital, although in older patients they may be secondary to infection.

An entire lung may be sequestered, in which case the lung is hypoplastic and has no bronchial connection. In our patients with this problem, there was no definite pleural cavity. The blood supply to the lung arose from multiple infradiaphragmatic vessels.

Hypoplasia of the right lung with a normal systemic, arterial supply and a pulmonary vein draining into the inferior vena cava produces a radiologic picture of dextrocardia, with a scimitar shape to the right rear border. Whereas sequestration occurs on either side, the scimitar syndrome is a right-sided lesion.[51,52] The bronchial tree is normal in the scimitar syndrome. Bronchiectasis may develop in later life, but in childhood the symptoms of the scimitar syndrome are related to the vascular shunting of blood and to associated intracardiac defects.

Related lesions include communications between the lung and the esophagus. In such patients the vascular supply is normal but the bronchus originates from the esophagus (Fig. 85–8).[53–55] Sequestrations have been associated with gastric and colon duplications.[56–57] These

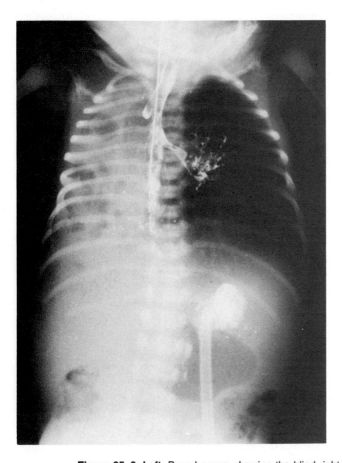 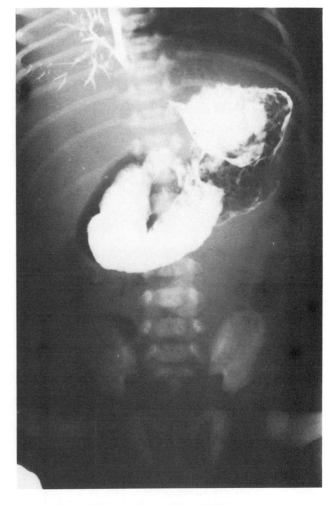

Figure 85–8. Left. Bronchogram showing the blind right bronchus. **Right.** Esophagogram with the right bronchus originating from the lower esophagus.

factors, plus the coexistence of classic intralobar and extralobar sequestrations, would suggest a developmental origin from an anomaly of foregut budding.[58,59]

Iwai et al. carefully constructed three-dimensional figures of specimens of sequestrations from serial microscopic sections.[60] In one of their patients, there was a fibrous stalk connecting the esophagus with the sequestration, and in another, there were coexisting intralobar and extralobar sequestrations. In all cases, the malformed lung developed from the posterior, medial, basal part of the lower lobe in an upward and lateral direction to fuse with the normal lung. These studies lend further support to the view that sequestrations arise from an accessory bronchopulmonary bud on the foregut. The accessory bronchial bud with its malformed bronchoalveolar tree may or may not be enveloped by the normal lung tissue. The anomalous blood supply represents remnants of the early splanchnic plexus that envelops the developing foregut.

Diagnosis

Extralobar sequestrations usually are asymptomatic and are discovered either at autopsy in infants with multiple congenital abnormalities or during repair of a left Bochdalek diaphragmatic hernia. Some extralobar sequestrations are sufficiently large, however, to cause respiratory distress in a newborn infant.[61,62]

Intralobar sequestrations classically cause recurrent infections. Afflicted children may only have bouts of pneumonia in the affected lobe, or they may have what appear to be lung abscesses. In older patients, hemoptysis secondary to chronic infection and erosion of the systemic vessels becomes a serious problem. In our patients with total sequestration of one lung, the primary problem was shunting of blood through unoxygenated tissue.

The diagnosis is most often made on plain rotentgenograms of the chest. Extralobar sequestration appears as a posterior mediastinal tumor. Intralobar sequestration must be suspected any time there are cystic changes or signs of persistent pneumonia in a lower lobe.

In the past, the definitive diagnosis was made with angiography, which demonstrated the anomalous blood vessel (Fig. 85–9). Computed tomography (CT) scans of the lungs provide all the information necessary for preoperative diagnosis, including demonstration of the abnormal blood supply. Aortography is no longer necessary. However, every surgeon must be continually aware of the possibility of a systemic vessel supplying any congenital abnormality of the lung. Radionuclide scans following the bolus IV injection of ^{99m}TC as pertechnetate has demonstrated the anomalous blood supply.[63]

Treatment

Extralobar sequestrations are removed easily by ligating and dividing the systemic blood supply to the lung. Intralobar sequestrations require lobectomy because it is difficult if not impossible to remove only the involved seg-

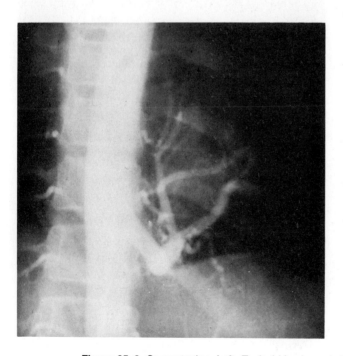 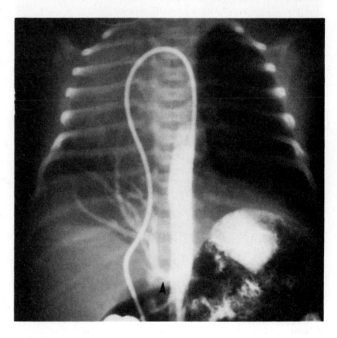

Figure 85–9. Sequestration. **Left.** Typical blood supply to the left lower lobe by means of a vessel arising from the abdominal aorta. **Right.** Bronchogram demonstrating an intralobar sequestration in the left lower lobe. Total sequestration of the right lung; the blood supply comes from the abdominal aorta.

ment. By the time these patients are operated on, the entire lobe is involved with an inflammatory process. The only important technical aspect is the careful observation, palpation, and identification of every structure in the inferior pulmonary ligament. The anomalous vessel must be doubly suture-ligated before its division. Surgical disasters have occurred in which an artery originating from below the diaphragm was divided and allowed to retrace into the abdomen.

Results

The prognosis of infants with extralobar sequestrations is dependent on their associated anomalies. The bronchopulmonary suppuration caused by an intralobar sequestration is cured by lobectomy.

AGENESIS AND HYPOPLASIA OF THE LUNG

Agenesis of one lung consists of the complete absence of a bronchus, parenchyma, and vessels. Hypoplasia consists of varying degrees of underdevelopment of one lung. Perhaps the most common etiology for pulmonary hypoplasia is a congenital posterolateral diaphragmatic hernia.

This group of developmental defects is frequently associated with other congenital malformations—primarily of the heart and great vessels, although tracheoesophageal fistula and imperforate anus also are seen. Agenesis, or complete absence of one lung, is compatible with survival, but associated congenital anomalies account for a 33 percent mortality rate during the first year of life and a 50 percent mortality during the first 5 years.[64,65] Patients who survive childhood are prone to chronic respiratory infections, wheezing, and dyspnea. Pulmonary function studies have demonstrated obstructive emphysema of the remaining lung, probably on the basis of elongation and distortion of the tracheobroncheal tree, since the remaining lung expands to fill both thoracic cavities.[66]

Most infants with agenesis of one lung are dyspneic and cyanotic during the newborn period. Physical examination reveals minimal asymmetry of the chest. With right lung agenesis, the heart sounds are heard next to the right chest wall. Breath sounds may be heard anteriorly on the right but are absent in the axillary area. A chest roentgenogram will reveal a completely opaque hemithorax with shift of the mediastinum to the lateral chest wall. The heart border is obscured, and the lung may be visible above the heart on the affected side because of the herniation of the remaining lung. The differential diagnosis includes atelectasis of one lung as well as a tension disorder of the opposite side that is pushing the mediastinum to the right. An angiocardiogram is the preferred first study when agenesis of a lung is sus-

pected (Fig. 85–10). With agenesis of the right lung and dextroposition of the heart, superior and inferior vena cavae are displaced to the right. The right ventricular outflow tract arches cranially to the left, forming a wide arch with the left pulmonary artery, which tends to be angled toward the horizontal plane. The absence of a right pulmonary artery confirms the absence of a functioning lung. The greatest value of the angiocardiogram is the ease with which associated intracardiac defects are diagnosed. Atrial and ventricular septal defects, patent ductus arteriosus, and infantile coarctation are most frequent. Furthermore, by observing the aorta, it is possible to make the diagnosis of an anomalous systemic vessel, which may feed a hypoplastic sequestered lobe on the affected side. When there is only hypoplasia of the right lung, there may be anomalous venous drainage into the inferior vena cava with a partial systemic blood supply to the lung. This constellation of findings has been termed the "scimitar syndrome" because the anomalous pulmonary vein follows a curving course, giving the right heart border a convex (or scimitar) appearance. The electrocardiogram may indicate that the heart has shifted its position and has rotated, but it is otherwise of little value in diagnosing specific lesions.

The treatment of children with agenesis or hypoplasia of the lung is directed to correction of associated defects. The elongated, distorted trachea and bronchus may be obstructed by the aortic arch and ductus.[67] Unfortunately, direct attempts to relieve the pressure by aortic or bronchial resection have not been successful. We placed a Silastic tube within a narrowed left main bronchus as a splint for 2 weeks. The child was eventually weaned away from a ventilator, but it appeared that the long-term ventilatory support and growth were more responsible for overcoming the collapsed bronchus than

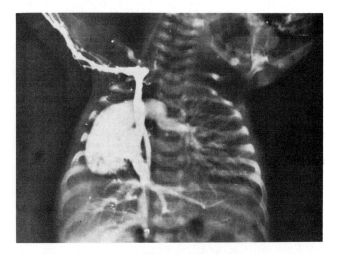

Figure 85–10. Angiocardiogram illustrating complete shift of the heart to the right with the pulmonary artery arching to the left.

the operation. There is a higher incidence of associated anomalies and more severe mediastinal shift and distortion of the great vessels and remaining lung with agenesis of the right lung. For this reason, the prognosis is worse when this lung is affected.[68]

Hypoplasia of a lung or agenesis of one lobe, particularly on the left, is associated with fewer symptoms and carries a lower incidence of serious associated malformations. There are more pulmonary infections and more occasions in which chest roentgenograms may initially be interpreted as diagnostic of atelectasis. CT scans and ventilation-perfusion nuclear studies will make the diagnosis. Treatment consists of antibiotic therapy for intercurrent infections and pulmonary resection of a hypoplastic lobe when it has an anomalous blood supply or bronchiectasis.

REFERENCES

1. Demos NH, Teresi A: Congenital lung malformations. J Thorac Cardiovasc Surg 70:260, 1975
2. Buntain WL, Isaacs H, Payne VC, et al: Lobar emphysema, cystic adenomaloid malformation, pulmonary sequestration, and bronchogenic cyst in infancy and childhood: a clinical group. J Pediatr Surg 9:85, 1974
3. Buchner V, Reid L: Development of the intrasegmental bronchial tree: the pattern of branching and development of cartilage at various stages of intrauterine life. Thorax 16:207, 1961
4. Boyden EA: Differentiation of the lung between infancy and childhood. Anat Rec 160:320, 1968
5. Dunnil MS: Postnatal growth of the lung. Thorax 17:329, 1962
6. Gray SW, Skandelakis JE: Embryology for Surgeons. Philadelphia, Saunders, 1972, pp 299, 313
7. Pryce DM: The lining of healed but persistent abscess cavities in the lung with epithelium of the ciliated columnar type. J Pathol Bacteriol 60:259, 1948
8. Bain GO: Congenital cystic adenomatoid malformation of the lung. Dis Chest 36:430, 1959
9. Stocker JT, Madewell JE, Drake RM: Congenital cystic adenomatoid malformation of the lung. Hum Pathol 8:155, 1977
10. Hutchin P, Friedman PJ, Saltzstein SL: Congenital cystic adenomatoid malformation with anomalous blood supply. J Thorac Cardiovasc Surg 62:220, 1971
11. Ueda K, Gruppo R, Unger F, et al: Rhabdomyosarcoma of lung arising in congenital cystic adenomatoid malformation. Cancer 40:383, 1977
12. Campbell DP, Raffensperger JG: Congenital cystic disease of the lung masquerading as diaphragmatic hernia. J Thorac Cardiovasc Surg 64:592, 1972
13. Monclair T, Schistad G: Congenital pulmonary cysts versus a differential diagnosis in the newborn. Diaphragmatic hernia. J Pediatr Surg 9:417, 1974
14. Keith HH: Congenital lobar emphysema. Pediatr Ann 6:7, 1977
15. Miller CG, Woo-Ming MO, Carpenter RA: Lobar emphysema of infancy: case report of bilateral involvement with congenital heart disease. West Indian Med J 17:35, 1968
16. Raynor AC, Capp P, Sealy WC: Lobar emphysema of infancy. Ann Thorac Surg 4:374, 1967
17. Murray G: Congenital lobar emphysema. Surg Gynecol Obstet 124:611, 1967
18. Stovin P: Congenital lobar emphysema. Thorax 14:254, 1959
19. Whimster W: Techniques for the examination of excised lungs. Hum Pathol 1:305, 1970
20. Powel HC, Elliott ML: Congenital lobar emphysema. Virchows Arch [Pathol Anat] 374:197, 1977
21. Bolande RB, Scheider AF, Boggs JD: Infantile lobar emphysema. Arch Pathol 61:289, 1956
22. Fischer HJ, Potts WJ, Hollinger PH: Lobar emphysema in infants and children. J Pediatr 41:403, 1952
23. Potts WJ, Hollinger PH, Rosenblum AH: Anomalous left pulmonary artery causing obstruction to right main bronchus. JAMA 155:1409, 1954
24. Sherman FE: Anomalous course of left pulmonary artery: a cause of obstructive emphysema in infants. J Pediatr 54:93, 1959
25. Hanna EA, Vattanapat S, Derrick JR: Congenital lobar emphysema with bronchial atresia. Ann Thorac Surg 7:357, 1969
26. Wilson EB, Jones RJ: Segmental bronchial atresia of the left upper lobe with resultant bronchial mucocele. J Thorac Cardiovasc Surg 63:486, 1972
27. Iancu T, Boyanover Y, Eilam N, et al: Infantile sublobar emphysema and tracheal bronchus. Acta Paediatr Scand 64:551, 1975
28. Cooney DR, Menke JA, Allen JE: "Acquired" lobar emphysema: a complication of respiratory distress in premature infants. J Pediatr Surg 12:897, 1977
29. Cumming GR, Macpherson RI, Chernick V: Unilateral hyperlucent lung syndrome in children. J Pediatr 78:250, 1971
30. Swyer PR, James G: A case of unilateral pulmonary emphysema. Thorax 8:133, 1953
31. Kluge T, Eek S, Sorland S, Semb G: Infantile lobar emphysema associated with cardiovascular anomalies. Scand J Thorac Cardiovasc Surg 5:75, 1971
32. Strunge P: Infantile lobar emphysema with lobar agenesis and congenital heart disease. Acta Paediatr Scand 61:209, 1972
33. Fagan CJ, Swischuk LE: The opaque lung in lobar emphysema. Am J Roentgenol Radium Ther Nucl Med 114:300, 1972
34. DeLuca FG, Wesselhoeft CW, Frates R: Congenital lobar emphysema documented by serial roentgenograms. J Pediatr 82:859, 1973
35. Mauney FM, Sabiston DC: The role of pulmonary scanning in the diagnosis of congenital lobar emphysema. Am Surgeon 36:20, 1970
36. Eigen H, Leman RJ, Waring WW: Congenital lobar emphysema: long-term evaluation of surgically and conservatively treated children. Am Rev Respir Dis 113:823, 1976
37. Demuth GR, Sloan H: Congenital lobar emphysema: long-term effects and sequelae in treated cases. Surgery 59:601, 1966

38. Shannon DC, Todres ID, Moylan FMB. Infantile lobar hyperinflation: expectant treatment. Pediatrics 59:1012, 1977

39. Pryce DM: Lower accessory pulmonary artery with intralobar sequestration of the lung. J Pathol 58:457, 1946

40. Holstein P, Hjelms E: Bronchopulmonary sequestration. J Thorac Cardiovasc Surg 65:462, 1973

41. deParedes CG, Pierce WS, Johnson DG, Waldhausen JA: Pulmonary sequestration in infants and children: a 20-year experience and review of the literature. J Pediatr Surg 5:136, 1970

42. Khalil KG, Kilman JW: Pulmonary sequestration. J Thorac Cardiovasc Surg 70:928, 1975

43. Sade RM, Clouse M, Ellis FH: The spectrum of pulmonary sequestration. Ann Thorac Surg 18:644, 1974

44. Buntain WL, Woolley MM, Mahour GH, et al: Pulmonary sequestration in children: A twenty-five year experience. Surgery 81:413, 1977

45. Flye MW, Conley M, Silver D: Spectrum of pulmonary sequestration. Ann Thorac Surg 22:478, 1976

46. Saegesser F, Besson A: Extralobar and intralobar pulmonary sequestrations of the upper and lower lobes: report of eleven cases, including one case of the scimitar syndrome. Chest 63:69, 1973

47. Telander RL, Lennox C, Sieber W: Sequestration of the lung in children. Mayo Clin Proc 51:578, 1976

48. Brasfield DM, Longino LA, Hicks GM, Tiller RE: Sequestration of the lung in children. South Med J 69:1572, 1976

49. Krishnan M, Snelling MRJ: Lobar pulmonary sequestration. Aust NZ J Surg 39:362, 1970

50. Valle AR, White ML: Subdiaphragmatic aberrant pulmonary tissue. Dis Chest 13:63, 1947

51. Kittle LF, Crackett JE: Vena cava bronchovascular syndrome: a triad of anomalies involving the right lung. Ann Surg 156:222, 1962

52. Derksen OS: Scimitar syndrome and pulmonary sequestration. Radiol Clin 46:81, 1977

53. Nikaidoh H, Swenson O: The ectopic origin of the right main bronchus from the esophagus. J Thorac Cardiovasc Surg 62:151, 1971

54. Mukai S, Kikuchi H, Akiyama H, Morio M: Management of anesthesia in an infant with an anomalous lung arising from the oesophagus. Br J Anaesth 49:379, 1977

55. Flye MW, Izant RJ: Extralobar pulmonary sequestration with esophageal communication and complete duplication of the colon. Surgery 71:744, 1972

56. McClelland RR, Kapsner AL, Uecker JH: Pulmonary sequestration associated with a gastric duplication cyst. Radiology 124:13, 1977

57. Lewis JE, Murray RE: Pulmonary sequestration with bronchoesophageal fistula. J Pediatr Surg 3:575, 1968

58. Pendse P, Alexander J, Khademi M, Groff DB: Pulmonary sequestration: coexisting classic intralobar and extralobar types in a child. J Thorac Cardiovasc Surg 64:127, 1972

59. Albrechtsen D: Pulmonary sequestration. Scand J Thorac Cardiovasc Surg 8:64, 1974

60. Iwai K, Shindo G, Hajikano H, et al: Intralobar pulmonary sequestration, with special reference to developmental pathology. Am Rev Respir Dis 107:911, 1973

61. Robertson S: Extralobar lung sequestration in a newborn infant: an unusual cause of respiratory distress. Centr Afr J Med 19:74, 1973

62. Pearl M: Sequestration of the lung. Am J Dis Child 124:706, 1972

63. Gooneratne N, Conway JJ: Radionuclide angiographic diagnosis of bronchopulmonary sequestration. J Nucl Med 17:1035, 1976

64. Nicks R: Agenesis of the lung with persistent ductus arteriosis. Thorax 12:140, 1956

65. Wexels P: Agenesis of the lung. Thorax 6:171, 1951

66. Messumi R, Teleghani M, Ellis I: Cardiorespiratory studies in congenital absence of one lung. J Thorac Cardiovasc Surg 51:561, 1961

67. Harrison MR, Hendren A: Agenesis of the lung complicated by vascular compression and bronchomalacia. J Pediatr Surg 10:813, 1975

68. Sbokos C, McMillan I: Agenesis of the lung. Br J Dis Chest 71:183, 1977

86
Pulmonary Resection

The principles of pulmonary resection are the same in children as they are in adults. If anything, the resilient chest wall of a child allows for easier intrathoracic exposure through smaller incisions, and since the hilar structures of children are rarely involved in an inflammatory process, their identification and dissection are easier than with adults. With the exception of pneumonectomy in young infants, which we will discuss in detail, children tolerate pulmonary resections extremely well. The accepted indications for lung resection have changed considerably over the past few years. When Baffes and Potts reported on 47 cases of pulmonary resection treated at the Children's Memorial Hospital prior to 1954, the primary indication for lobectomy was bronchiectasis.[1] Currently, most major lung resections are performed for congenital malformations and metastatic tumors.

SUBSEGMENTAL RESECTION OR LUNG BIOPSY

Most metastatic tumors, especially Wilms' tumors and rhabdomyosarcomas, are on the lung surface. Single, multiple, and even bilateral lesions may be removed at one operation by wedge resection. Immunosuppressed children, especially those who are receiving cancer chemotherapy, frequently develop undiagnosed lung infiltrates. Open lung biopsy has proved to be a rapid route to diagnosis of this disease.

Technique
The metastatic lesion or site of maximum pulmonary infiltrate is localized on the roentgenogram. A short intercostal incision is made over the pathologic site. A Satinsky vascular clamp is applied beneath the lung lesion, and a specimen is removed for immediate smear, culture, and microscopic examination.

A 5–0 nonabsorbable suture is placed beneath the clamp as a running horizontal mattress stitch. It is tied and the clamp is removed. A second over-and-over running suture is placed over the first to obtain a firm, airtight suture line. A metastatic lesion may be removed in the same fashion, or two clamps may be used to remove a V-shaped wedge of tissue in order to obtain a 1 cm margin of normal tissue around the lesion. It is absolutely necessary to suture the lung with silk or some other nonabsorbable material. These lungs are often stiff as a result of radiation or infection, and the child may require ventilatory support with positive pressure. If the excision site is not carefully closed, absorbable sutures will cause a delayed leak, with pneumothorax. The wound is closed tightly around a waterseal tube that is removed as soon as the lung has expanded and there is no air leak.

SEGMENTAL RESECTION

Segmental resection is rarely indicated in childhood. Congenital malformation usually involve an entire lobe, although we were able to perform left apical segmental resections in two older children with localized emphysema and one right apical segmental resection for a congenital lung cyst. Lilly et al. reported on 5 infants—4 with congenital cystic disease and 1 with lobar emphysema—in whom they were able to preserve lung tissue with segmental resection.[2] Of their 5 patients, 3 had bronchovascular anomalies that required careful dissection for identification. Buntain et al. reported a 100 percent incidence of major complications, including a prolonged air leak that required another thoracotomy and lobectomy after segmental resection.[3] Bronchiectasis has become a rare disease, but when it does occur, basal segmental resection is sometimes sufficient for a localized lesion that has been carefully mapped with bronchography or computed tomography (CT).

Technique

The segmental arteries are dissected outward from the hilum of the lung but are not ligated until the entire segment has been localized. Intersegmental veins must be left to drain the adjacent retained lung. The line of segmental separation is found by clamping the segmental bronchus. This causes atelectasis of the lung tissue about to be resected. The division of lung tissue across segmental planes and the division of incompletely formed tissue between lobes are the sources of most postoperative air leaks. The most effective technique of controlling both air leaks and bleeding is to divide the lung tissue between straight mosquito hemostats. The lung that is to be retained is then suture-ligated with figure-eight sutures placed beneath each hemostat. The multiple small bites of tissue do not distort the remaining lung and effectively close the alveoli and small bronchioles that cause postoperative air leaks.

LOBECTOMY

During recent years, congenital malformations and large metastatic tumors have become the most common indications for lobectomy. Chest physical therapy, effective postural drainage, and intermittent antibiotic therapy will control the symptoms of the occasional case of bronchiectasis and will clear almost every case of chronic pneumonia with atelectasis. Children with immune diseases are the exceptions. Lobectomy may be indicated for chronic pneumonia with recalcitrant lung abscess or for specific infections, such as aspergillosis.

Technique

A posterolateral incision through the fifth interspace provides access to all lobes of the lung. Care must be taken not to extend the incision too far anteriorly, injuring the developing breast bud in little girls. It is never necessary to resect a rib in a child merely to provide exposure. All adhesions are sharply dissected until the entire lung has been mobilized.

The surgical anatomy and techniques for individual ligation of lobar vessels at the hilum are beautifully illustrated in *Surgery of the Chest*.[4] We prefer to suture-ligate all vessels proximally and to leave a small mosquito hemostat on the distal vessel. Small vessels, especially those encountered in adhesions and about the bronchus, are electrocoagulated. There are several pitfalls in arterial ligation that may be avoided by carefully identifying every single vessel before it is ligated. The blood supply to the left upper lobe is quite variable. Great care must be taken to leave the segmental artery to the apical

segment of the lower lobe and to avoid injury to the main pulmonary artery to the lower lobe. The same observations are important when performing either a right middle lobectomy or a superior segmental resection on the right. The artery to the superior segment may originate at the same level as the arteries to the middle lobe. Alternate retraction of the lung posteriorly and anteriorly provides positive identification of hilar strictures. Sharp dissection within the sheath of the vessel provides greater safety and more rapid identification of vessels than the blunt pushing away of adventitia and lymph nodes. One must never pass a clamp around a vessel until it has been cleanly dissected from surrounding tissue and any branches from its back wall have been identified.

The lobar bronchus is found posteriorly. It is first occluded with a noncrushing vascular clamp for positive identification, then divided a few millimeters away from the mainstem bronchus. It should be sutured with a nonabsorbable suture as it is being divided in order to decrease the air leak. The bronchial closure and any severed lung tissue are checked for air leaks under saline while the anesthesiologist applies pressure to the airway. Every air leak must be controlled before the chest is closed. The bronchial stump is then securely covered with an adjacent flap of pleura or adventitia. We prefer to leave a single chest tube in the pleural space connected to a simple waterseal drain. The wound is closed in layers with continuous absorbable sutures through the muscle layers and the skin is Steristripped. No dressing is applied so that the chest may be auscultated during the immediate postoperative period.

Results

The most important and immediate complication has been atelectasis of a remaining lobe or segment. This may be prevented by vigorous early tracheal suctioning, humidity, encouraging the child to cough, intercostal local anesthetic blocks, mild analgesics, and early ambulation. One advantage of securing all air leaks at the time of operation is early removal of the chest tube, which is painful and prevents deep breathing and coughing. There has been one operative death following pulmonary lobectomy at the Children's Memorial Hospital since the report of Baffes and Potts, who performed 47 pulmonary resections with no mortality between 1942 and 1953.[1] The long-term results are dependent on the lesion resected. About half of our children operated on for lobar emphysema have had minimal problems, mainly occasional wheezing and apparently increased susceptibility to respiratory infections. Children operated on for bronchiectasis have had continued cough and frequent infections from residual disease. Part of this is due to the child's failure to persist with postural drainage and chest physiotherapy. These observations are supported by long-term studies of children who have undergone pulmonary resection. A lobectomy results in minimal if any chest wall deformity and no decrease in exercise tolerance and is compatible with normal growth and development.[5-7]

Pulmonary function studies have demonstrated normal values for the vital capacity and forced expiratory volume. However, an occasional patient has an increase in the residual volume, which reflects emphysematous expansion of the remaining lung.

PNEUMONECTOMY

Profound physiologic changes follow the removal of an entire lung. The empty pleural cavity is obliterated by shift of the mediastinum with overexpansion of the opposite lung, elevation of the diaphragm, and an effusion that becomes fibrotic. Contraction of the chest also leads to variable degrees of scoliosis. Experimentally, immature animals tolerate pneumonectomy better than do mature animals. There appears to be an increase in the number of alveoli, which results in compensatory hypertrophy of the contralateral lung.[8-10] Puppies tolerate exercise stress better and have better pulmonary function and less alveolar overdistention than adult dogs following pneumonectomy.[11]

Long-term follow-up of children who survived pneumonectomy demonstrates that they can lead healthy, normal lives.[12] Cardiopulmonary function studies have demonstrated only moderate overinflation of the remaining lung, with a reduced vital capacity and an increase in residual volume. Mean pulmonary arterial pressures rose with exercise.[13-15] These long-term studies suggest that hyperplasia of remaining lung tissue occurs as an adaptive mechanism.

The patients in these long-term studies underwent pneumonectomy when they were over 1 year of age. Most had bronchiectasis and were operated on at between 5 and 10 years of age. Gross has performed at least two successful pneumonectomies in newborn infants with cystic disease[16] (S.R. Schuster, personal communication, 1975). One of these patients has been followed into adulthood and has no significant difficulties. On the other hand, there were four infants in the series of Pierce et al. who died following pneumonectomy.[17]

Our own experience with pneumonectomy in infancy and childhood with 21 patients over a 25-year period is shown in Table 86-1. Two infants died during the immediate postoperative period. Each had other severe defects. A third infant died 6 months after the pneumonectomy with tracheal obstruction secondary to severe mediastinal shift (Fig. 86-1). As a result of this experience, we have since stabilized the mediastinum with Silastic prostheses.

Severe airway obstruction and respiratory arrest also followed a pneumonectomy in a patient reported by Adams et al.[18] This patient recovered after the placement of lucite balls in the pleural cavity. Experiments with puppies in our laboratory have demonstrated significant increases in alveolar and arterial P_{CO_2} and depressed oxygenation with rapid removal of air from the pleural cavity following pneumonectomy. This experience has led us to believe that prosthetic stabilization of the mediastinum may be helpful in preventing the tracheal obstruction and alveolar overdistention that result from a rapid shift of the mediastinum in small infants (Fig. 86-2). This technique may also diminish chest wall collapse and scoliosis.

In older children, particularly those with a contracted lung secondary to bronchiectasis, some degree of compensation has already taken place, and the mediastinum is relatively fixed. In these older patients, the long-term prognosis depends on disease in the opposite lung. One of our "long-term" deaths was secondary to cystic fibrosis and progressive pulmonary suppuration. Another was caused by radiation of the contralateral lung. Three more children have shown significantly reduced pulmonary function.

Three pneumonectomies in our series were performed for compression of the left mainstem bronchus with atelectasis of the entire lung. Currently, we would attempt to either correct the underlying cardiac anomaly or stent the bronchus in an attempt to preserve the lung.

Technique
Pneumonectomy for congenital lesions is easily performed through an anterolateral incision with the operated side slightly elevated. This position allows the anesthetist to ventilate the child with greater ease during the operation. All the hilar structures are dissected and individually suture-ligated. The bronchus is closed with interrupted sutures and securely covered with a flap of pleura. When it is necessary to perform a pneumonectomy for extensive inflammatory disease or for tumor, it is easier to isolate the major vessels within the pericardium. Topical antibiotics are left in the pleural cavity at the completion of the operation. Either Silastic-filled testicular or breast prostheses are placed in the pleural cavity to stabilize the mediastinum. We have now followed patients with these prostheses for over 12 years and have yet to see complications with their use.

BRONCHOPLASTY

Lung resections may be minimized or avoided in children who have benign tumors or congenital defects of the bronchus. We have removed one obstructing hemangioma at the carina with a local resection and reanastomosis of the right mainstem bronchus to the trachea (Fig. 86–3). In another 2-month-old baby with a hemangioma in the right bronchus intermedius, a sleeve resection with reanastomosis was carried out. The carinal resection required the use of a sterile endotracheal tube, which was placed in the open left bronchus through the open chest for intraoperative ventilation. Each of these patients has now been followed for over a year with repeat endoscopy. Neither developed a bronchial stricture. A pneumonectomy was avoided in a boy with a bronchial adenoma that originated in his left upper bronchus and extended into the mainstem by lobectomy with repair of the mainstem bronchus with a flap. A similar procedure was used to avoid a pneumonectomy in a teenage girl with a carcinoid tumor of the left lower lobe bronchus, which extended to the lateral wall of the upper lobe. In each of these patients, accurate localization of the tumor was possible by CT and endoscopic study. Intraoperative frozen sections of the bronchial wall are essential to ensure tumor-free margins while maximizing the conservation of available bronchial tissue (Fig. 86–4).

TABLE 86–1. PNEUMONECTOMIES AT CHILDREN'S MEMORIAL HOSPITAL, 1958–1981

	Age at Operation	Diagnosis	Comments	Results
Patients with tumors				
CK	3 years	Wilms' tumor (metastatic), right pneumonectomy	Severe scoliosis—Rx: radiation	Seven postoperative years vital capacity; ⅓ predicted emphysema, mixed restrictive and obstructed disease present, unable to attend school, died of respiratory insufficiency, 1978
MW	14 years	Leomyosarcoma, left main bronchus	Did well immediately postoperation	
KZ	8 years	Metastatic rhabdomyosarcoma, right lung	Immediately postoperation, well	CNS metastasis, died
Patients with congenital lesions				
JG	1 day	Left lung—cystic adenomatoid lung	Agenesis, right kidney—4 lb 4 oz	Died 2 days after operation, hyaline membrane disease on right
EA	3 days	Total sequestration, right lung	Kinked trachea, mediastinum shifted, to right—respirator, 3 months Rx	Died 6 months after operation
LH	1 month	Cystic neuroectodermal right lung	Pierre Robin syndrome, wedge resection on cysts of left upper lobe; 1 year later, mediastinum with Silastic	Full physical activity 12 years after operation
DM	11 weeks	Pulmonary artery with obstructed left bronchus	Tetralogy	Died 10 hours after operation
TM	9 days	Right main bronchus from esophagus	Hypospadius, duodenal stenosis	Living, well
VF	1 month	Right main bronchus from esophagus		Requires O₂ at night, episodes of pneumonia in left lung
DW	6 months	Dysplastic left lung with pneumonia		Well after 2 years
W		Collapsed left mainstem bronchus, atelectasis, chronic infection	Omphalocele	Tracheotomy, requires positive pressure, 10 years after operation
RP	4 months	VSD, large pulmonary artery with collapse of left bronchus		Survived closure of VSD 1 year later

TABLE 86–1 (cont'd).

	Age at Operation	Diagnosis	Comments	Results
Patients with inflammatory lesions				
PP	9 years	Right atelectasis, bronchiectasis	Cleft palate	Has done well at 15 years, mediastinal shift
TW	4 years	Left bronchiectasis, atelectasis		Age 12, marked mediastinal shift, rotated tracheobronchial tree, carina transverse on bronchoscopy
JP	4 years	Right pneumonectomy, previous right upper lobe lobectomy	Bronchiectasis on left, cystic fibrosis	Died 3 years after operation
TM	11 years	Left saccular bronchiectasis		Tracheal deviation, lung herniation 1 year after operation
HH	3 years	Lung abscess, bronchiectasis, left pneumonectomy		Singer with a band, 21 yrs.
WD	9 years	Tuberculosis, destroyed left lung		Amateur boxer at age 18, scoliosis (see x-ray)
CD	18 months	Abscess in left upper lobe, then left lower lobe	Immune deficiency	Severely restricted pulmonary function
WM	6 years	Previous right upper lobartoma completed, middle and lower pulmonary function since May 1	Aspergillosis	Lost to follow-up
Patients suffering from trauma				
BJ	5 years	Fracture, left mainstem bronchus with complete atelectasis	Auto accident with hemothorax 3 years prior to operation	Normal activity 5 years later

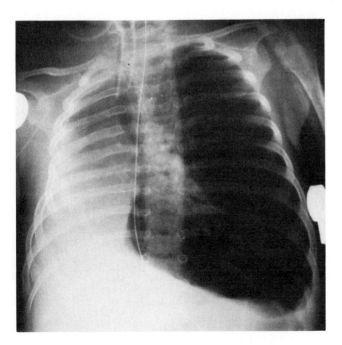 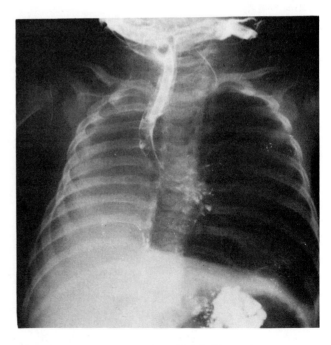

Figure 86–1. Severe mediastinal shift following a right pneumonectomy for sequestration. The child died 6 months after surgery. **Left.** Severe overdistention of the left lung. **Right.** Bronchogram demonstrating tracheal shift.

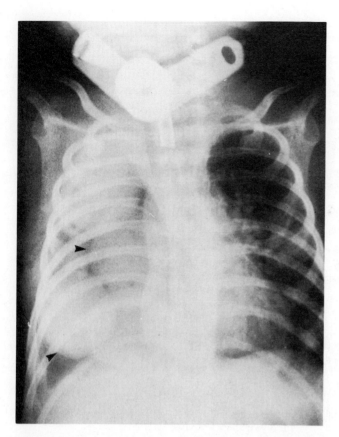

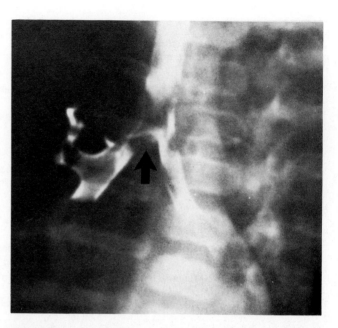

Figure 86–3. Hemangioma of carina in 3-month-old child. The hemangioma was resected, and the carina was repaired.

Figure 86–2. Silastic prostheses inserted into the pleural cavity to stabilize the mediastinum following pneumonectomy for cystic disease of the entire lung. The cystic disease seen here in the apical segment of the left lobe was resected 6 months later.

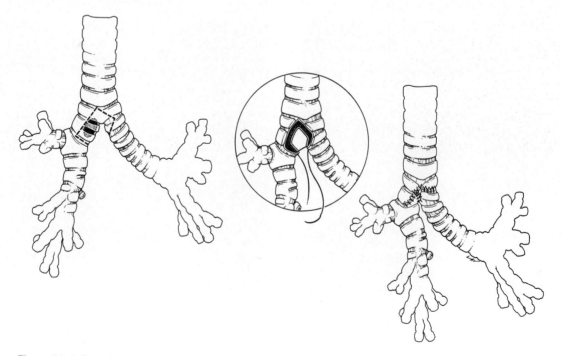

Figure 86–4. Bronchoplasty techniques. Resection of the carina for an obstructing hemangioma. Ventilation maintained during the operation with a sterile endotracheal tube passed into the left mainstem bronchus and secured with an umbilical cord tape. A second anesthetic machine was used to ventilate each lung separately.

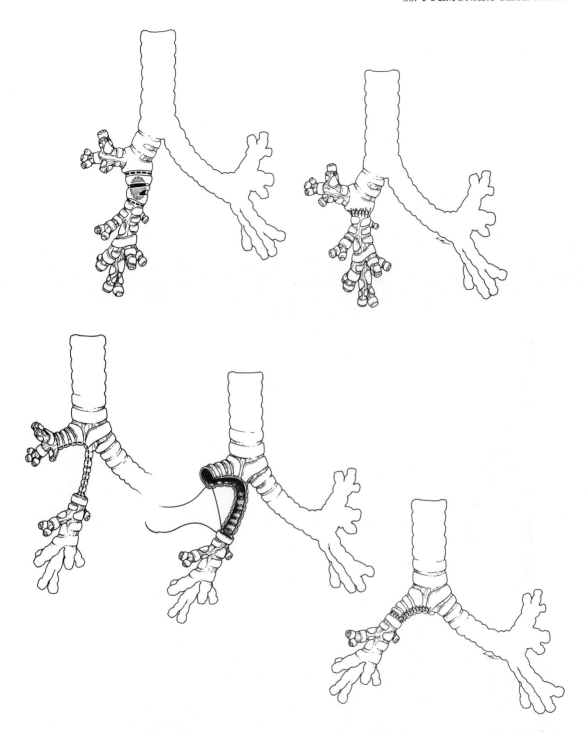

Figure 86–4. cont. Top. Hemangioma of the bronchus intermedius, resected with reanastomosis of the bronchus. **Bottom.** There was lobar emphysema of the right upper lobe with atelectasis of the lower lobe because the lower lobe bronchus which originated from the carina was stenotic. The upper lobe was resected, but its bronchus was used to patch the opened lower lobe bronchus.

REFERENCES

1. Baffes TG, Potts WJ: Pulmonary resection in infants and children. Pediatr Clin North Am 1:709, 1954
2. Lilly JR, Wesenberg RL, Shikes RH: Segmental lung resection in the first year of life. Ann Thorac Surg 22:16, 1976
3. Buntain WI, Isaac H, Payne UC, et al: Lobar emphysema, cystic adenomatoid malformation, pulmonary sequestration, and bronchogenic cysts in infancy and childhood: a clinical group. J Pediatr Surg 9:85, 1974
4. Johnson J, MacVaugh H, Waldhausen JA: Surgery of the Chest, 4th ed. Chicago, Year Book, 1970
5. Brandesky G: Long-term results of pulmonary resections in childhood. Prog Pediatr Surg 20:297, 1977
6. Zdenek S: Pumonary resection in children. Pediatr Surg 54:810, 1963
7. Peters RM, Wilcox BR, Schultz EH Jr: Pulmonary resection in children: long-term effect on function and lung growth. Ann Surg 159:652, 1964
8. Tartter PI, Goss RJ: Compensatory pulmonary hypertrophy after incapacitation of one lung in the rat. J Thorac Cardiovasc Surg 66:147, 1973
9. Bremer JL: The fate of the remaining lung tissue after lobectomy or pneumonectomy. J Thorac Surg 6:336, 1937
10. Edwards FR: Studies in pneumonectomy and the development of a two-stage operation for the removal of a whole lung. Brit J Surg 27:392, 1939
11. Longacre JJ, Johansmann W: An experimental study of the fate of the remaining lung following total pneumonectomy. J Thorac Surg 10:131, 1940
12. Laros C, Westerman C: Dilatation, compensatory growth, or both after pneumonectomy during childhood and adolescence. Cardiovasc Surg 93:570, 1987
13. Stiles QR, Meyer BW, Lindesmith GG, Jones JC: The effects of pneumonectomy in children. J Thorac Cardiovasc Surg 58:394, 1969
14. Giammona St, Mandelbaum I, Battersby JS, Daly WJ: The late cardiopulmonary effects of childhood pneumonectomy. Pediatrics 37:79, 1966
15. Sery ZD, Ressl J, Vyhnalek J: Some late sequels of childhood pneumonectomy. Surgery 65:343, 1969
16. Gross RE: Congenital cystic lung, successful pneumonectomy in a three-week-old baby. Ann Surg 123:229, 1946
17. Pierce WS, deParedes CG, Raphaely RC, Waldhausen JA: Pulmonary resection in infants younger than one year of age. J Thorac Cardiovasc Surg 61:875, 1971
18. Adams HD, Junod FL, Aberdeen E, Johnson J: Severe airway obstruction caused by mediastinal displacement after right pneumonectomy in a child: a case report. J Thorac Cardiovasc Surg 63:534, 1972

87
Foreign Bodies in the Air Passages and Esophagus

_____ *Gabriel F. Tucker, Jr.*

There is a wide range of clinical problems associated with foreign bodies in the airways. Larger objects that lodge in the larynx may cause suffocation and, often, death. Other material may lodge in a peripheral bronchus to cause atelectasis and chronic pulmonary suppuration. The problems are compounded in children because there may be no specific history of ingestion. Furthermore, the technical problems associated with the removal of objects from the tracheobronchial tree are increased because the relatively smaller airway requires miniaturized instruments. Edema produced by either the object or its manipulation may produce more obstruction. The same 1 or 2 mm of laryngeal edema that produces hoarseness in an adult may cause severe obstruction in a 2-year-old child.

DIAGNOSIS

A child, usually a toddler, may be seen to place a toy or other object in the mouth and then choke or gag. The symptoms may continue or subside if the object drops down into the bronchi. A larger object that obstructs the larynx may not cause spluttering or choking sounds because the child may be unable to move enough air to produce a sound.[1] Following the initial suspicious incident, there often will be a symptom-free interval. Chest pain is unusual, but dysphagia may occur when objects are lodged in the hypopharynx or esophagus. Wheezing or croupy stridor may continue after the initial incident but also may appear later and will be diagnosed as asthma or bronchitis. Antibiotic or steroid therapy will temporarily relieve the symptoms and will delay the diagnosis. The sudden onset of wheezing should arouse suspicion of foreign body inhalation. One must be particularly concerned when the symptoms occur while eating popcorn or peanuts, which could be inhaled during a particularly exciting episode on television. The physical examination may reveal poor air exchange and retractions when the object is lodged in the larynx or trachea. Partial obstruction causes an expiratory wheeze or stridor, but a complete bronchial obstruction results in a collapsed lung with shift of the mediastinum, dullness to percussion, and absence of breath sound on the affected side. As a general rule, if there is any suspicion that a child has inhaled a foreign body, the child should have roentgenographic studies. Some may require bronchoscopy to settle the question.

X-Ray Studies

Some foreign bodies are readily visible on plain chest roentgenograms (Fig. 87–1). Fortunately, radiolucent objects still provide clues with proper study. The endoscopic lateral film of the neck and upper chest is especially useful in detecting tracheal, hypopharyngeal, or laryngeal objects because the entire upper airway is seen in profile.[2] The child's arms are held backward, and the neck is extended for this view. In addition to the routine posterioranterior and lateral chest films, x-rays must be obtained in both deep inspiration and expiration. The usual film taken in full inspiration may be completely normal. However, an object that partially obstructs a bronchus will allow air to pass distally, while during expiration, the bronchus will collapse about the object, trapping air distally (Fig. 87–2). Localized emphysema is diagnostic for partial bronchial obstruction. An even more dynamic demonstration of this air trapping is seen during fluoroscopy of the chest. A completely obstructing

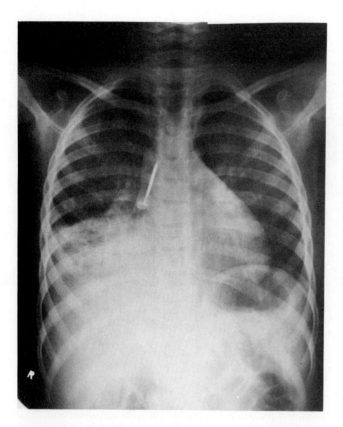

Figure 87–1. Nail in right main bronchus with atelectasis and infiltrate in the right lower lobe.

object will produce atelectasis of a lobe or even collapse of an entire lung (Fig. 87–3). Contrast studies are rarely indicated in the localization or diagnosis of a bronchial foreign body, but a bronchogram may be helpful in determining the etiology of an atelectasis secondary to long-retained objects.[3] When roentgenographic studies are negative, clinical judgment is required to determine the need for endoscopy. If the child's symptoms were of sudden onset and are unrelieved by medical measures, such as humidity, decongestants, and bronchodilators, bronchoscopy is indicated. This is particularly important, since fewer than half of the children with a foreign body in the bronchi have a positive history. If there is no history of cystic fibrosis of the pancreas, asthma, or allergy to explain the symptoms or the picture of a localized emphysema or atelectasis, endoscopy must be performed.

TREATMENT

Although foreign bodies in the tracheobronchial tree may be expelled spontaneously or by the aid of postural drainage and bronchodilators, in our opinion, endoscopic removal is safer and more reliable. A foreign body in the trachea, which is allowing air exchange, could become lodged in the larynx if it is encouraged to move upward.

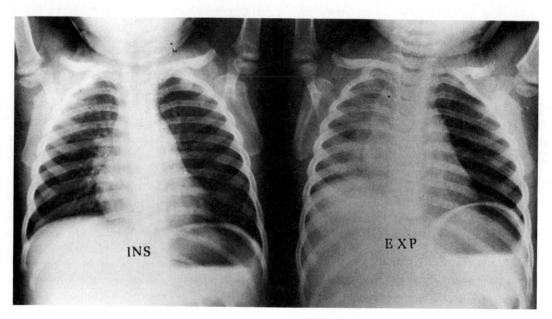

Figure 87–2. Inspiratory and expiratory films demonstrating air trapping in a partially occluded bronchus during expiration. There is a shift of the mediastinum away from the side of the foreign body.

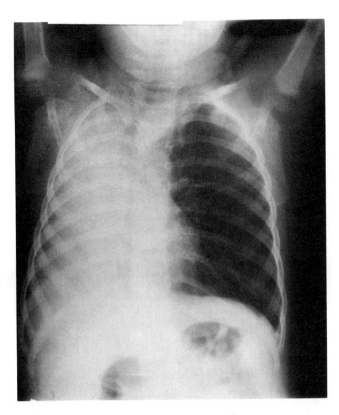

Figure 87–3. A bean was lodged in the right mainstem bronchus, with complete collapse of the lung. Note shift of the trachea and mediastinum and herniation of the left lung.

Ideally, removal of foreign bodies in the tracheobronchial tree or esophagus should be performed by a well-trained endoscopist who has at his or her disposal facilities for pediatric anesthesia and biplane fluoroscopy. It may be necessary, however, to remove obstructing hypopharyngeal objects at the scene or in a hospital emergency room. Otherwise, preparation should be made in advance to have a complete armamentarium of pediatric instruments and experienced assistants. In most instances, it is preferable to transfer a child to a well-equipped center rather than to attempt the removal of an object in suboptimal circumstances. Large objects in the trachea or larynx constitute true emergencies and must be removed immediately. Smaller foreign bodies, particularly such vegetable matter as peanuts or beans, swell when exposed to moisture in the tracheobronchial tree. These should all be removed as soon as possible. Small metallic or plastic objects in the bronchi present no immediate respiratory threat, and their removal may be postponed until the child is in optimum condition and the endoscopic team is in complete readiness. In general, 2 or 3 hours is sufficient time for preparation and is time well spent, since it is better to spend 2 hours in preparation and remove the object in 2 minutes than to rush into the procedure poorly equipped and spend more time with poorly functioning or inadequate instruments. The condition of the patient also dictates the timing of the procedure. If the material, such as a nut or bean, has been in the bronchus long enough to set up edema and a chemical reaction and has swelled to occlude the bronchus, the child may be febrile with pneumonia and have considerable airway edema. The child's condition may be improved with antibiotics, humidity, and bronchodilators. In addition, such drugs as an aerosol of racemic epinephrine will reduce the mucosal edema and simplify removal of the object.

Anesthesia

Larnyngeal and hypopharyngeal foreign bodies are best removed in an awake, restrained child who retains cough and gag reflexes. With very small or poor-risk infants, endoscopy should be performed with the patient awake because the object may be coughed into the bronchoscope, thereby shortening the procedure.[4] It is also an advantage to have an awake, coughing patient at the end of the procedure. On the other hand, anesthesia ensures a quieter working field, allows longer working time, and allows one to employ a larger bronchoscope. Furthermore, the child's respirations are completely controlled under anesthesia. The child must have complete temperature and cardiac monitoring with IV fluids running before induction of anesthesia. It is also helpful to perform laryngoscopy on the child before anesthetic induction to make sure that the bronchoscope may be easily introduced.

The choice of agents is left to the anesthesiologist, but in general induction is effected with halothane and IV succinylcholine. The bronchoscope is then inserted under laryngoscopic guidance. Our preference is for the Sanders ventilating attachment or the Holinger ventilating bronchoscope. Oxygen and anesthetic gases are insufflated into the sidearm while the proximal end of the instrument is sealed with a glass window. When it is necessary to remove the glass window for instrumentation, ventilation is carried out at intervals by covering the end of the bronchoscope with a thumb. It is preferable to have the child continue to breathe during the procedure rather than to induce apnea.

A plan for the actual removal of the object is made in advance. If possible, a sample of the object is obtained so the proper forceps may be selected. Firm, smooth plastic objects are difficult to grasp. On the other hand, vegetable products (such as a bean) incite surrounding edema and may disintegrate during removal. The specific mechanical problem can be worked out with the duplicate foreign body on a practice board.

The bronchoscope is advanced to inspect the object and to determine again the proper choice of forceps.

The instrument is then withdrawn to create a space for opening the forceps around the object. Care must be taken not to push the foreign body further down into the bronchus. The forceps is advanced beyond the bronchoscope in a closed position, but is opened widely before it approaches the object. The forceps is then advanced until the blades are around the object. Since the bronchus is distensible, it is safe to keep the blades open against the wall of the airway during the maneuver. The cylinder of the forceps is advanced, which closes the blades about the object. This must be done by touch because often the bronchoscope is so small that one cannot visualize both the object and the forceps. Once one has a firm grasp on the object, it is held tightly and withdrawn into the bronchoscope. If the object and forceps are small enough, they are withdrawn through the bronchoscope. Otherwise, the scope, forceps, and foreign body are withdrawn as a unit while the thumb of the scope hand locks the forceps and scope together. If the object cannot be removed, repeated instrumentation may be undertaken again in several days. Treatment with humidity, bronchodilators, and corticosteroids may reduce edema, making removal possible at a second attempt. A nut or bean that fragments may require several attempts for complete removal. Saline irrigation and suction will also remove small, retained bits of vegetable matter.

POSTOPERATIVE CARE

The child is observed in a recovery unit and given humidity for 24 hours. If there is stridor secondary to laryngeal edema, racemic epinephrine is given. A chest roentgenogram is obtained routinely. Complications include pneumothorax, mediastinal air, and minimal hemoptysis. It should rarely if ever be necessary to resort to a thoracotomy for removal of a bronchial foreign object. Biplane fluoroscopy will allow the passage of forceps into segmental bronchi for the removal of distal objects.[5] Timothy grass, however, will penetrate deep into pulmonary parenchyma because of its barblike action. The resultant atelectasis and pulmonary suppuration may eventually require bronchotomy or even a pulmonary resection.

ESOPHAGEAL FOREIGN BODIES

Though many ingested objects pass through the entire gastrointestinal tract without difficulty, congenital or acquired esophageal strictures may arrest the passage of a foreign body that otherwise would have passed with ease. Sharp objects, such as open safety pins, bones, and toys, tend to become lodged either in the hypopharynx or at one of the sites of physiologic narrowing: the

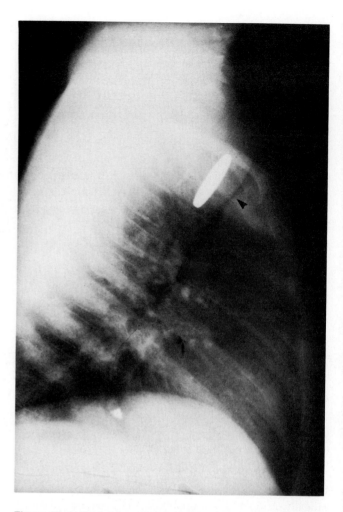

Figure 87–4. Tracheal narrowing from a nickel in the esophagus. Many objects that lodge in the upper esophagus cause respiratory symptoms rather than dysphagia.

cricopharyngeus, the aortic arch, or the cardioesophageal sphincter. Most children will complain of dysphagia and will have a choking spell when they swallow the object. Compression of membranous trachea by objects in the esophagus produces respiratory symptoms (Fig. 87–4). Strangely, some objects (such as coins) may remain in place for prolonged periods of time without causing symptoms. If there is doubt and plain roentgenograms are normal, a barium swallow will make the diagnosis.

Treatment
All esophageal foreign bodies below the cricopharyngeus muscle are best removed while the child is under general anesthesia. This usually is a straightforward procedure. The endoscope and forceps are advanced, and the object is grasped as described for bronchial objects. An open safety pin offers a particularly difficult problem. If the spring is toward the operator, it may be grasped and the open pin drawn into the scope. If the point is embedded in the wall of the esophagus and the spring is distal,

the pin must be grasped with a rotating forceps and carried into the stomach with the point trailing. Then, with fluoroscopic guidance, the pin is turned and regrasped so that the point is trailing. Then the pin may be safely drawn into the esophagoscope and removed. Another difficult problem is that of a coin lodged just below the cricopharyngeus muscle. There is normally a dangerous weak spot that is perforated easily just proximal to this muscle. This danger is compounded when a coin is lodged in such a manner that the endoscope pushes the mucosa over the object. It is possible to advance the scope the length of the esophagus without seeing the coin. The problem is avoided by rotating the bevel of the tip upward as the cricopharyngeus is approached. This will stretch the muscle and flatten the mucosa so the coin may be seen and grasped.

REFERENCES

1. Tucker GF Jr: Foreign bodies in the esophagus or respiratory tract. In Paparella M, Shumway (eds): Otolaryngology. Philadelphia, Saunders 1973, vol 3, p 753
2. Holinger PH: Foreign bodies in the air and food passages. Trans Am Acad Ophthalmol Otolaryngol 66:210, 1962
3. Tucker GF Jr: Laryngeal and tracheobronchial foreign bodies. Trans Pa Acad Ophthalmol Otolaryngol 19:12, 1966
4. Tucker GF Jr, Adriani J, Atkins J, et al: Symposium: Anesthesia in peroral endoscopy. Trans Am Bronch Esoph Assoc 49:116, 1969
5. Norris CM, Tucker GF Jr, Woloshin JH: Bronchoesophagogic application of recent advances in fluoroscopy. Ann Otol 80:528, 1971

88
Congenital Deformities of the Chest Wall

Pectus excavatum, the most common defect of the chest wall, varies in severity from a mild, scarcely noticeable depression to a deep, funnel-shaped defect that nearly touches the vertebrae. Other chest wall deformities include the protruding sternum, pectus carinatum, failure of fusion of portions of the sternum, absence of ribs, and dystrophy of the entire chest wall.

EMBRYOLOGY

The development of the sternum or anterior thorax is closely related to that of the anterior abdominal wall. Lower sternal clefts may be in continuity with an omphalocele. The human embryo commences with the development of the posterior body wall and spinal column and ends with formation of the anterior body wall by progressive fusion from the cranial, caudal, and lateral directions. The thoracic and upper abdominal wall form from the ventral portion of the embryonic head fold, with the caudal limits of the thorax demarcated by the transverse septum. The early thoracic wall consists only of somatopleure covering the pericardial cavity. Skin forms from this layer, but other components of the body wall arise from the dorsal mesoderm. Ribs and the lateral vertebral processes form from extension of the posterior mesoderm during the sixth fetal week. The sternum arises independently of the ribs as a pair of midline mesenchymal bands. The uppermost portion of the sternum, or presternum, which will eventually become the manubrium, arises from mesenchyme associated with the developing shoulder girdle. The paired sternal bands fuse with the presternum cranially, and then during the seventh week fusion takes place from this cephalic end in a caudal direction toward the xiphoid.[1-3] Failure of the cephalic fold to close results in sternal defects. Any teratogenic insult that would produce defects in the ster-num or thoracic wall would have to take place during or before the seventh week of fetal life. There is a familial tendency to chest wall defects, especially with pectus excavatum. It is not uncommon to see siblings or a parent and child with this defect. We have observed one child with a congenital absence of several ribs and a portion of the pectoral muscle whose grandmother had an identical defect.

FUSION DEFECTS OF THE STERNUM

Simple failure of fusion of the sternum results in a soft, skin-covered defect between the two sternal halves. Either the entire sternum or only the upper one third is involved (Fig. 88–1). The diagnosis is made by observation and palpation of the defect at birth. There is paradoxical respiration but surprisingly little respiratory distress. Despite the fact that an infant with a sternal cleft has little or no distress, the defect should be corrected in the newborn period. When the ribs are soft and elastic, it is possible to bring the two halves of the sternum together with direct sutures. In older children, attempts to close sternal clefts have resulted in cardiac compression, and various prostheses have been inserted to bridge the gap.[4-10]

Technique

The child must be monitored for central venous pressure, intra-arterial pressure, and skin oxygen saturation, since the most serious complication of sternal defect closure is cardiac compression.

In the neonate, a midline incision is made over the defect, and flaps of skin are created to expose the sternal edges. The entire sternal edge is exposed from the thoracic inlet in the neck to either the junction of normally fused sternum or the xiphoid. The dissection

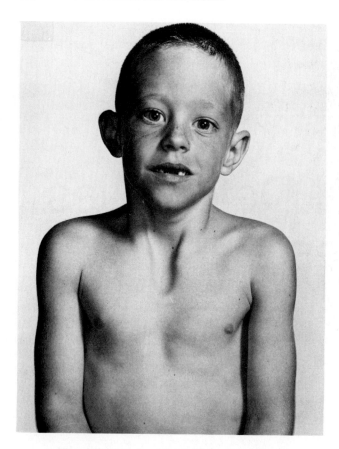

Figure 88–1. Fusion defect of the upper sternum.

is performed anterior to the thymus. If there is a complete sternal cleft, the two halves of the sternum are encircled with nonabsorbable sutures. When all sutures have been placed, they are snugged up and tied while cardiac action is carefully monitored. If this is tolerated, the procedure is completed by suturing the upper rectus and the pectoral muscles in the midline. If return of the heart to the chest causes problems, the bone defect is covered with a Silastic prosthesis, which is then closed in stages. The sternocleidomastoid muscles should also be approximated to prevent a suprasternal defect. If there is a V-shaped defect in the upper sternum, it is necessary to transect the lateral sternal bars just above their junction and to continue this incision through an intercostal space. This incision will allow the upper sternal cleft to be closed by sliding only the upper chest wall together. It may be necessary to divide several costal cartilages lateral to the sternal halves in order to relax the chest wall. In older children with upper incomplete sternal clefts, the chest is sufficiently rigid that it is difficult to obtain primary approximation. A variety of prosthetic devices have been used to close these defects, but an autologous rib graft removed through a second lateral incision has provided excellent stability and a good cosmetic result. Each rib is split longitudinally and placed across the

defect. These rib struts may then be reinforced with adjacent flaps of pectoral fascia.

PECTUS EXCAVATUM

Depression deformities of the sternum consist primarily of a downslope of the sternum that commences just distal to the manubrium. The upper sternum and the first two or three costal cartilages are normal, but the cartilages are bent inward. The concavity may be an abrupt, deep depression with an otherwise normal thorax, or the entire anterior wall of the chest may be sunken and flattened in an anterior–posterior direction (Fig. 88–2). Lesions occur in which one side of the chest is normal in size and the sternum tips downward to the other

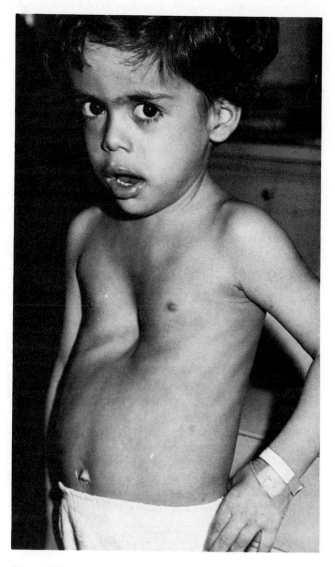

Figure 88–2. A typical patient with deep pectus excavatum. Note the rounded shoulders and protuberant abdomen.

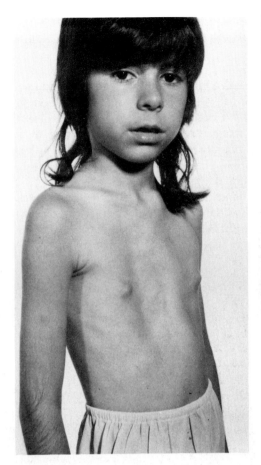
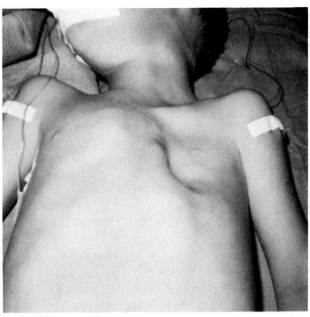

Figure 88–3. Left. There is a deep, right-sided depression extending out to the nipple. The sternum is tilted downward toward the right. **Right.** Severe left-sided depression.

side, which is smaller. These defects are most prominent in girls, who show asymmetrical breast development (Fig. 88–3). During infancy, the defect may not be as noticeable as it is in later years, but some infants who later develop pectus excavatum have a paradoxical movement of the sternum during inspiration. In these infants, there appears to be an upper airway obstruction, but roentgenographic studies and endoscopy are negative. The clinical picture of a pectus excavatum becomes increasingly noticeable and is full-blown in most children by the time they are 3 years of age. There appears to be another increase in the deformity at 8 to 10 years of age and still another during puberty. The child with a moderate or severe pectus excavatum will have very poor posture. He or she stands with sagging shoulders and a protuberant abdomen. Examination of the spine reveals a kyphosis and often a mild degree of scoliosis. In addition to scoliosis, pectus excavatum is associated with other birth defects, including congenital heart disease, lung cysts, Marfan's syndrome, Ehler-Danlos syndrome, and a number of other musculoskeletal anomalies. Although there is no embryologic relationship between the respective developments of the ribs and sternum, we observed one child with a pectus excavatum with absence of the pectoralis major muscle and underlying ribs on the right side.

Symptoms

There has been considerable controversy about the physiologic effects of a pectus excavatum. We are indebted to Dr. Mark Ravitch for his lifelong interest and study of this problem. He has summarized the world's literature on the effects of this deformity on cardiorespiratory function.[11] It has become quite clear from his review that a moderate to severe pectus excavatum causes respiratory and cardiac symptoms that become increasingly severe as the patient grows older. Exertional dyspnea and tachycardia commence during the late teen years and become progressively worse, with decrease in exercise tolerance and eventual congestive heart failure and atrial fibrillation. Despite these dire observations, some children with a pectus excavatum are top notch athletes, fully able to compete with their peers. Are these supermotivated individuals who have worked to overcome a handicap, or have we exaggerated the problem? We must be careful not to attribute nonspecific symptoms, such as chest pain or asthma, to a pectus excavatum, although we have observed wheezing to improve after the operation. Complaints of chest pain may be the child's method of drawing the parents' attention to the defect. One little boy said "I have to get it fixed so I can be a policeman."

A pectus excavatum will exaggerate any other heart or lung defect, especially the normal degenerative effects of aging. Physiologic studies in children generally demonstrate a minimal decrease in pulmonary function. Later, there are decreases in the vital capacity, total lung volume, and maximum breathing capacity.[12–14] We have observed low normal ranges in all aspects of pulmonary function. Primarily, there is a decrease in the maximum breathing capacity. Some patients will have a mild

to moderate restrictive defect. Some have an increase in airway resistance. The only other children who had changes in pulmonary function were those who had concomitant lung disease, such as asthma or a lung cyst. In these children, however, lung function was depressed more than one would suspect from their lung diseases alone. In young chidren, the electrocardiogram is normal or at most demonstrates rotation and displacement of the heart to the left. Others have found inverted T waves, changes in the QRS complex, and conduction abnormalities, mainly right bundle branch block.[15–20] Angiograms demonstrate displacement of the heart as well as pressure on the right atrium and ventricle.[21] Computed tomography (CT) clearly demonstrates cardiac displacement and compression. This is currently the best technique to

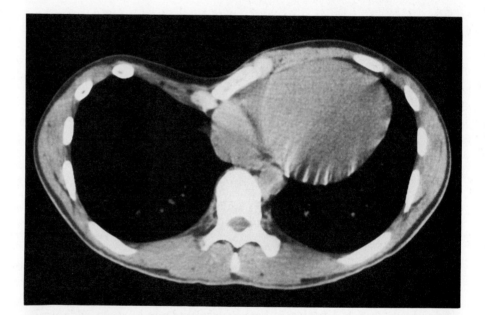

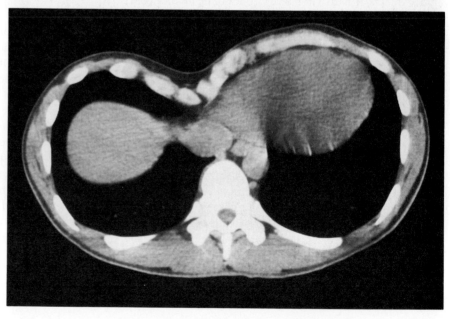

Figure 88–4. Top. CT scan demonstrating Tilt of sternum with compression of heart and decreased volume in right thorax. **Bottom.** Same patient with a CT cut at depth of depression.

demonstrate the full extent of the lesion (Fig. 88–4). Recent data derived from cardiac catheterization indicate a normal cardiac output at rest but impaired output during exercise.[22,23]

Many have stated that pectus excavatum is merely a cosmetic deformity that is in itself no indication for an operation. We cannot agree with this point of view. Although there are few children who have objective evidence of cardiorespiratory embarrassment, this is certainly a problem in the older patient. Furthermore, the cosmetic problem is serious. Anyone who has had experience with adolescents understands the emotional problems encountered with even minor cosmetic deformities. Boys with a pectus excavatum become more and more reluctant to participate in sports as they grow older. Smaller children will swim and take part in activities, but when their peers begin to tease them about their sunken chests, they tend to avoid the locker room and swimming pool. By avoiding sports and other physical activities, the child's muscular tone and physique suffer even more. Asymmetrical lesions in girls are serious cosmetic problems.

Management and Indications for Surgery

At the first interview with the child's parents, a complete history is obtained, which includes specific inquiries about respiratory problems, associated illness, and the child's physical activities. The physical examination is performed by watching the child walk using normal posture. The spine is specifically examined for scoliosis. The child also is examined for the stigmata of Marfan's and Ehler-Danlos syndromes. With the child lying supine, the depth of the defect is determined by measuring from a tongue blade placed across the chest to the deepest portion of the sternum (Fig. 88–5). Finally, the child is asked to stand erect with the abdomen sucked in and shoulders drawn back. This posture makes the defect less prominent and is demonstrated to the family. At this point, one can differentiate the obvious deep, narrow cleft that will require an operation from a minimal defect that will never cause distress. We tend to advise an operation when the sternum is depressed more than 3 cm below the rib cage. When the defect is 2 to 2.5 cm depressed, we recommend that the family return in 1 year for further evaluation and measurement. Depressions less than 2 cm do not require an operation; the child and his family are reassured, and follow-up in a year or so is suggested. In an effort to obtain a more objective measurement of the depression, Haller et al. have used a single CT scan, taken at the point of maximum depression.[24] The anterior–posterior and the transverse measurements of the chest are then compared as a ratio. The pectus index is the transverse measurement of the chest divided by the measurement from the sternum to the anterior edge of a vertebral body. In their patients, an operation was performed when the ratio was greater than 3.25.

The decision to operate on moderate lesions depends somewhat on the wishes of the child and the parents. Historically, the surgeons in the Children's Memorial Hospital have been conservative in their indications for surgery in pectus excavatum. The child and parents should ask for the operation; they should never be talked into it. If after hearing the pros and cons, which include information concerning the controversial

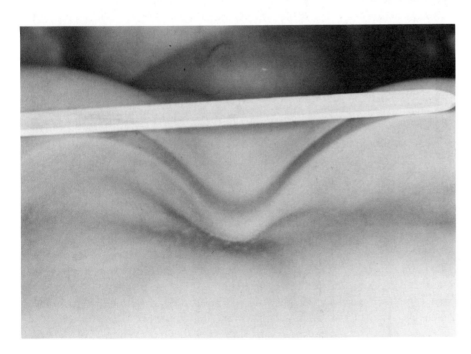

Figure 88–5. A tongue blade placed across the defect allows one to measure the depth of the depression. One can thereby make an objective measurement for comparison in follow-up examinations.

nature of the indications for an operation, some children definitely want to get rid of the "hole in their chest." If the family is undecided, a program of shoulder girdle-strengthening exercises is advised, and the child is seen again in 1 year. Exercises consisting of weight lifting, calisthenics, and swimming are advised for all patients. If one can improve the child's posture and muscular development, mild defects become less noticeable, and those that require an operation are less likely to recur following an operation. Although Randolph et al. reported on 50 children who were successfully operated on before 3 years of age, we prefer to wait until the child is at least 5 years.[25] One of our recurrences occurred when the operation was performed at 3 years of age, and since there appear to be few if any physiologic abnormalities in younger children, we prefer to wait. The operation is more tedious but not more difficult in teenagers.

Each child with a moderate to severe defect should have a chest roentgenogram and echocardiography. This test has demonstrated a prolapsed mitral valve in approximately 25 percent of our patients who have had this test. Furthermore, this is an excellent screening test for Marfan's syndrome if the aortic root is found to be dilated. Pulmonary function tests are ordered on older children, more out of curiosity than scientific necessity. There is only moderate correlation between changes in these tests and the indications for surgery.

Preoperative Care

These patients are admitted to the hospital one day before the operation. This allows completion of the preoperative evaluation and provides an opportunity to teach the child to cough and breathe deeply on command. In addition, the child is taught to use "blow bottles." These measures simplify postoperative care and reduce the incidence of atelectasis.

Technique

The basic operation for pectus excavatum consists of subperichondrial resection of the deformed costal cartilages and an osteotomy of the sternum, which allows it to move forward in a normal position. The operation may be performed with equal facility through either a vertical midline or a transverse submammary incision. Controversy stems from the type of fixation used to maintain a satisfactory position of the sternum.

Since 1965, Ravitch performed a posterior transverse osteotomy on the sternum at the point where it commences to turn inward.[26] A wedge of rib is sutured into this defect. In addition, the costal cartilages on either side are cut at an angle so they may be sutured in an overlapped position. Other authors have used this technique, sometimes with slight modifications, and have obtained excellent results.[27,28]

Others claim superior results using internal fixation with steel struts or bars that are sutured to the ribs and pass behind the sternum or are inserted into the ends of the ribs and pass over the sternum, which is then sutured to the strut.[29-32] External traction is contraindicated because any suture or foreign body that penetrates the skin is a portal of entry for bacteria to contaminate the large area of dissection.

The details of the operation as we are currently performing it at the Children's Memorial Hospital are as follows (Fig. 88–6).

A folded sheet is placed beneath the child's shoulders, and the entire chest, including the lateral thoracic wall, is included in the sterile field. A vertical midline incision is made only in boys with long, deep defects. Otherwise, a submammary incision that is curved upward at the midpoint is made over the deepest portion of the sternal defect (Fig. 88–6A). This incision is carried down to the costal cartilages and through the pectoralis fascia and the upper attachments of the rectus muscle. Sharp rake retractors are inserted to elevate flaps consisting of skin, subcutaneous tissue, and muscle in one layer (Fig. 88–6C). This is carried out by inserting the flat blades of the scissors along the costal cartilages and ribs. As the scissors are spread, the pectoral muscle is easily elevated from the cartilage. An alert assistant coagulates each strand of tissue that does not separate easily with the scissors. In this way, perforating vessels to the pectorals are controlled. On occasion, it is easier to perform this dissection with the needle-tipped cautery. The skin and musculofascial flap are raised as a unit to expose the sternum and costal cartilages. With this modification, the transverse incision offers as rapid exposure and is as bloodless as the vertical incision.

When the deformed costal cartilages have been completely exposed, the perichondrium is incised with the needle-tipped cautery in the form of an H. This step is performed on all the costal cartilages on one side (Fig. 88–6D). The edges of the perichondrium are then grasped with multiple blunt-nosed hemostats, which are used to scrape the perichondrium away from the underlying cartilage. The remainder of the subperichondrial dissection is carried out with a small, sharp periosteal elevator. It is difficult to stay in the correct plane because the perichondrium is densely adherent, especially on the lowermost cartilages. Further difficulties are encountered because the lower cartilages often are fused. It is helpful to divide the cartilage as soon as the perichondrium has been removed from the midportion. The cartilage is then elevated with a Kocher hemostat, allowing dissection of the cartilage from the posterior perichondrium. The cartilage is removed from its junction with the rib to within 1 cm of the sternum. The uppermost normal cartilages are left intact on either side, but all deformed cartilages are resected. When this has been accomplished, the xiphoid is disarticulated from the sternum (Fig. 88–6E). At this point, one or two large vessels will require ligation. When the lower end of the sternum is free from the xiphoid, it is elevated with an Allis forceps and dissected free from the anterior mediastinal tissues. After the sternum has been completely freed, the lower three intercostal bundles, with the perichondrial envelopes, are divided close to the sternum. Care must be taken not to injure the internal mammary artery during this step. When the sternum can be held well forward, its back wall is deeply scored at the point where it angles backward with the edge of a sharp osteotome. This cuts through the posterior periosteum and allows one to fracture through the cortex until the sternum is hinged by its anterior periosteum. With this accomplished, the perichondrium of the upper normal cartilage, usually the second or third, is opened. When the cartilage is completely free from the perichondrium, it is cut obliquely from within outward in such a way that the inner cartilage may be overlapped and sutured (Fig. 88–6F). This step, plus the insertion of a wedge of rib into the posterior osteotomy, holds the sternum firmly forward (Fig. 88–6G). Heavy sutures mounted on a trocar needle are necessary to penetrate the sternum in order to pass a suture around the wedge of bone. On occasion, in older children, it has been necessary to first drill holes before passing the needle.

Technically, it is simpler and the results seem to be no different if one makes an anterior osteotomy in the sternum and removes a wedge of bone. Heavy sutures, then angle the sternum forward, based on the intact posterior periosteum. Observations of the results through the years are convincing that a posterior bar or strut is desirable to hold the sternum in its elevated position. Steinman pins are difficult to hold in place and tend to migrate beneath the skin. We have used perforated stainless steel bars that are used to stabilize fractures, but these plates tend to break at either edge of the sternum because of metal fatigue. The best results I have seen in the surgery of pectus excavatum are those of Ellis in Fort Worth, Texas (R. Ellis, personal communication). Ellis has operated on nearly 200 children using a solid metal bar obtainable from the V. Mueller Division of the Baxter Healthcare Corporation, Morton Grove, Ill. Certainly, a strut or support is indicated in any child with a connective tissue disease, such as Marfan's syndrome or the Ehler-Danlos syndrome. My recurrences severe enough to require reoperation have all been in children in whom a strut was not used. Furthermore, the chests of children who have not had a strut are always slightly flatter than when a strut is used. The stainless steel plates available from V. Mueller can be ordered in various sizes, but each must be further fashioned at the operating table to fit the child. The ends are bent down to conform with the anterior rib cage,

then placed beneath the sternum, with the ends resting on the ribs beneath the pectoral muscles. The operation is completed by suturing the intercostal bundles back to the sternum. The pectoral muscles and rectus fascia are closed, and a Silastic catheter is left under the sternum, brought out a separate stab wound, and placed on suction. The skin is closed with subcuticular absorbable sutures and Steristrips. At the end of the operation, an intercostal block is performed on both sides with 0.5 percent bupivacaine. An Elastoplast dressing is applied to provide wound compression for 3 or 4 days.

Postoperative Care

Antibiotics are given during the operation and for 48 hours afterward. The child is encouraged to cough as soon as he or she awakens. We remove the suction tube within 24 to 48 hours depending on the amount of drainage. Most children are able to tolerate oral liquids and then a general diet a day or so after the operation. Almost all have considerable pain, requiring narcotics during the first 24 hours. After that time, they are given acetophenamin every 6 hours for the next 2 or 3 days and only occasional doses of a narcotic. They are allowed to go home when they are ambulatory without help, usually within 3 to 5 days. At home, they are encouraged to commence walking and riding a bicycle and then to gradually increase their activities to running, swimming, and noncontact sports. These aerobic exercises are designed to improve cardiopulmonary fitness. By 6 weeks postsurgery, upper extremity and shoulder girdle exercises with weights are recommened to strengthen these groups of muscles. These patients should carry their books and other burdens in a knapsack to encourage better posture. These measures may not prevent a recurrence of the deformity, but they contribute to the overall well-being and body image of the child.

Results

It is difficult to determine long range results in many series of patients because the evaluation is often subjective or based on parental satisfaction. Furthermore, since recurrences can occur years after the operation, it is necessary to follow these patients through their adolescent growth spurt. Welch reported his objective results in 862 patients operated on from 1952 to 1981. Most immediate complications were minor wound problems or atelectasis, but there were 16 recurrences that required reoperation.[33] Cahil et al. studied patients before and after repair and found small improvements in total lung capacity but significant improvement in voluntary ventilation. Their work supports the thesis that an operation results in physiologic improvement in cardiac stroke volume as well as ventilation parameters.[34] Another objective method of postoperative study used CT scans.[35] These authors found better results when a metal strut

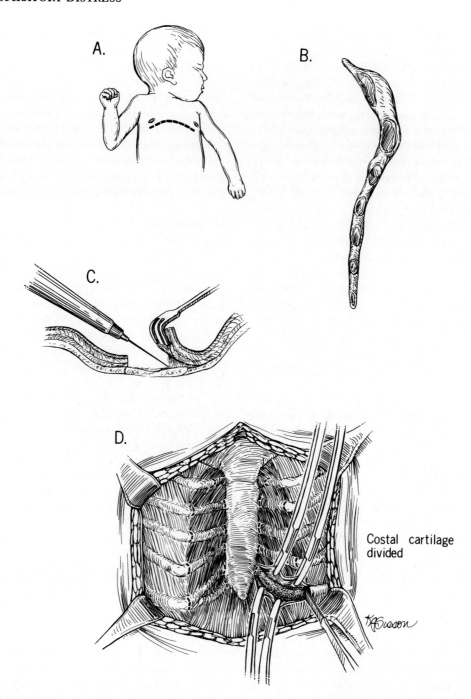

Figure 88–6. This technique for repair of a pectus excavatum was modified from Ravitch's procedure. **A.** A curved submammary incision is carried down to the sternum and costal cartilages. **B.** Side view of the defective sternum. **C.** The skin, subcutaneous tissue, and muscles are all elevated from the sternum and costal cartilages as one flap. This is performed with a scissors dissection and generous use of the electrocoagulation unit. **D.** The perichondrium is opened over each costal cartilage and grasped with hemostats in such a way that the perichondrium is freed from the underlying cartilage. The underside of the costal cartilage is dissected with a sharp periosteal elevator. (Continued)

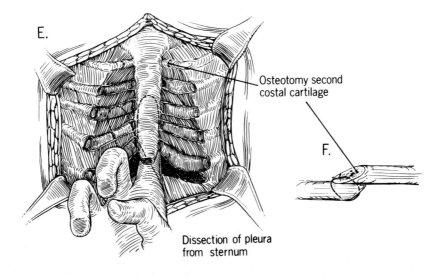

Osteotomy second
costal cartilage

Dissection of pleura
from sternum

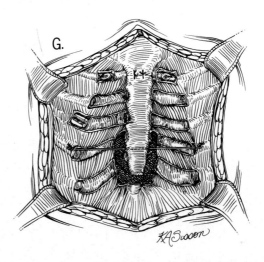

Figure 88–6. (Cont.) E. The xiphoid is first elevated with an Allis forceps and separated from the diaphragm with scissors; then a finger is inserted to completely free the back wall of the sternum. This figure also illustrates the oblique incision of the uppermost normal costal cartilages. **F.** Overlap of the costal cartilages. **G.** Completion of the operation, with a steel bar inserted beneath the sternum.

had been used in the repair, and the poorest results were in patients with flat rib cages in addition to the pectus deformity.

There have been 150 children with pectus excavatum operated on at our hospital by a group of surgeons from 1970 to 1986. There was one postoperative hematoma that required drainage, and in another, it was necessary to drain a serum collection several weeks after the operation. There were two staphylococcal infections that necessitated reopening the wound. In one of these, we eventually had to remove a bit of sequestered cartilage. It has been necessary to remove 10 Steinman pins because of pain or migration under the skin and two fenestrated steel plates fractured beneath the sternum. The removal of these pins and plates was carried out on an outpatient basis.

Our best long-term results have been in boys who were well muscled and vigorous and who had deep, symmetrical depressions. It is impossible to completely restore symmetry to a chest when one entire thorax is smaller than the other. We have now observed four known recurrences that have required reoperation. All recurrences became obvious within a year after the operation. In one, there was too much cartilage left laterally, which bent inward. One recurrence was blamed on performing the operation at 3 years of age. The other two recurrences are inexplicable. It is necessary to follow these patients for years; one patient operated on in 1963 had an excellent result until his pubertal growth spurt, when his entire repair caved in. It is possible that some recurrences are on the basis of connective tissue disorders, since there seems to be a group of children who are asthenic, have a pectus excavatum, mitral valve prolapse, and some scoliosis. Possibly, they have a forme fruste Marfan's syndrome. There was one death from a ruptured aortic aneurysm in a boy with the Ehler-Danlos syndrome 3 years after his operation. Aside from the four severe recurrences and the one death, parents and children alike express almost 100 percent satisfaction with the operation.

PROTRUSION DEFORMITIES

Pectus carinatum is far less common than pectus excavatum. From 1970 to 1986, only 18 carinatum defects were repaired in our hospital. In this deformity, the sternum itself may be normal, but the costal cartilages bend inward in such a way that the lower sternum is excessively prominent. In the second type, the sternum itself protrudes forward at the junction of the second costal cartilage (Fig. 88–7). There are many variations of these two types of defects, with both forms occurring in the same patient.

There have been fewer physiologic studies performed on patients with pectus carinatum. With this anomaly, the chest eventually becomes locked in expansion, with gradual loss of compliance of the lung.[36] Surgical correction in children usually is requested because of the unsightly deformity, which increases during growth spurts.[37] It is a particularly important cosmetic problem in girls.

Treatment

The operation is similar to that used for pectus excavatum in that the costal cartilages are resected through a transverse submammary incision. An anterior osteotomy is performed at the site of greatest sternal protrusion. By removal of a generous wedge, the sternum can be brought into line with the rest of the chest. If necessary, portions of the anterior sternum may be chiseled away to remove bony protrusions. The intercostal muscle bundles are left attached to the sternum and are reefed up with multiple interrupted sutures to increase the backward pull on the sternum. The upper rectus fascia is sutured to the front of the sternum to bring the anterior chest and abdominal walls into alignment.

A common minor defect is the protrusion of one costal cartilage, which simulates a tumor. These are smooth, regular defects with no roentgenographic changes. No treatment is necessary.

RIB DEFECTS

Congenital absence of the lateral ribs results in a bulging hernia of the lung. Symptoms depend on the size of the defect. If there is considerable paradoxical respiration, the defect may be covered with adhesive strapping. The split rib grafts may be inserted to stabilize the rib cage.[38]

Poland's deformity consists of congenital absence of the sternocostal head of the pectoralis muscle, absence deformity of the ribs underlying the absent muscle, and syndactyly or absence of fingers on the same side (Fig. 88–8).[39] The breast is hypoplastic. There are many variations of these associated defects. Absence of the pectoralis muscle, hypoplasia of the breast, and absence of the ribs may occur without the hand deformity. One of our patients had an associated pectus excavatum, and another had a congenital hydronephrosis. Even though these children have had paradoxical respirations, none have had respiratory symptoms.

In girls, treatment is indicated primarily for cosmetic reasons. Another reason for treatment is that if the defect is sufficiently large, there is an increased likelihood that trauma will injure the heart and great vessels.

With this anomaly, the skin is very thin and is separated from the pleural cavity only by the pleura. For this reason, the incision is made very carefully by going through the skin over the normal chest and then separating the skin and pleura by spreading the tips of scissors

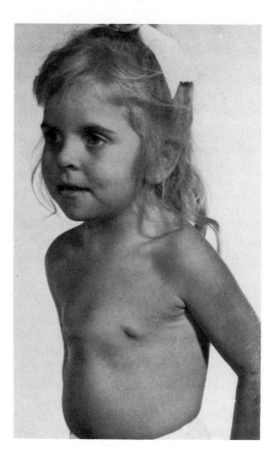

Figure 88–7. Pectus carinatum with a marked protrusion defect.

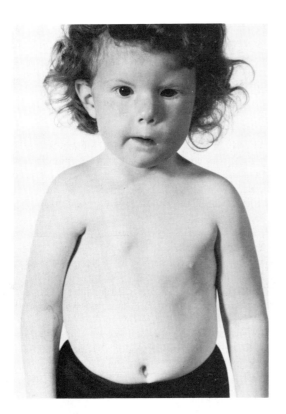

Figure 88–8. Poland's anomaly. There is an absence of the right breast and pectoral muscle as well as the 3rd, 4th, and 5th ribs from the sternum to the posteroaxillary line.

before the skin over the defect is opened. When the rib margins have been exposed and separated from the pleura, a second incision is made laterally and segments of two ribs are removed. These are split longitudinally with heavy scissors and then sutured to the rib edges. Ravitch advocates reinforcing this repair with a sheet of Teflon felt, but our patients have had a strong repair without this addition.[40] Later, a Silastic breast prosthesis may be inserted on the rib graft base to complete the chest wall reconstruction. Haller et al. have proposed reconstruction of the Poland defect with rib grafts and a flap of the latissimus dorsi muscle.[41]

THORACIC DYSTROPHY

Defective growth at the costochondral junctions results in a small thorax with a fetal or bell-shape chest that flares out at the lower ribs. The "asphyxiating" thoracic dystrophy was described by Jeune et al., but there are many other syndromes that include thoracic growth failure.[42,43] In addition to the small thoracic cage, the lungs are hypoplastic, with reduction in the number of alveoli and alveolar ducts. The pattern is similar to the hypoplastic lung seen in infants with Bochdalek diaphragmatic hernias.[44]

Most of these infants die with respiratory failure during the first few days of life. Those who survive lead a precarious existence, since they must breathe entirely with their diaphragms. Several efforts have been made to extend the size of the chest. Perhaps the most successful was that of Karjoo et al.[45] They split the infant's sternum, which was then held apart with steel struts. The defect was further covered with a sheet of Marlex mesh. If an operation is performed, long-term respiratory support is indicated for the postoperative period.

REFERENCES

1. Chen JM: Studies of the morphogenesis of the mouse sternum, II: Experiments on the origin of the sternum and its capacity for self-differentiation in vitro. J Anat 86:387, 1952
2. Chen JM: Studies on the mouse sternum and its capacity for self-differentiation in vitro. J Anat 87:130, 1953
3. Hanson FB: The ontogeny and phylogeny of the sternum. Am J Anat 26:41, 1919
4. Sabiston DC Jr: The surgical management of congenital bifid sternum with partial ectopic cordis. J Thorac Surg 35:118, 1958
5. Billig DM, Immordino PA: Congenital upper sternal cleft: a case with successful surgical repair. J Pediatr Surg 5:257, 1970
6. Verska JJ: Surgical repair of total cleft sternum. J Thorac Cardiovasc Surg 69:301, 1975
7. Ravitch MM: Congenital Deformities of the Chest Wall and Their Operative Correction. Philadelphia, Saunders, 1977, p 39
8. Jewett TC Jr, Butsch WL, Hug HR: Congenital bifid sternum. Surgery 52:932, 1962
9. Maier HC, Bortone F: Complete failure of sternal fusion with herniation of pericardium. J Thorac Surg 18:851, 1949
10. Roccaforte DS, Mehnert JH, Peniche A: Repair of bifid sternum with autogenous cartilage: a case report. Ann Surg 149:448, 1959
11. Ravitch MM: Congenital Deformities of the Chest Wall and Their Operative Correction. Philadelphia, Saunders, 1977, pp 113–44
12. Brown AL, Cook O: Cardio-respiratory studies in pre- and post-operative funnel chest (pectus excavatum). Dis Chest 20:378, 1951
13. Orzalesi MM, Cook CD: Pulmonary function in children with pectus excavatum. J Pediatr 66:898, 1965
14. Weg JG, Krumholz RA, Harkleroad LE: Pulmonary dysfunction in pectus excavatum. Am Rev Respir Dis 96:936, 1967
15. Dressler W, Roesler H: Electrocardiographic changes in funnel chest. Am Heart J 40:877, 1950
16. Elisberg EI: Electrocardiographic changes associated with pectus excavatum. Ann Intern Med 49:130, 1958
17. Fabricus J, Davidsen HG, Hansen AT: Cardiac function in funnel chest: twenty-six patients investigated by cardiac catheterization. Dan Med Bull 4:251, 1957
18. Gahrton G: ECG changes in pectus excavatum (funnel

chest): a pre- and post-operative study. Acta Med Scand 170:431, 1961

19. Landtman B: The heart in funnel chest: pre- and post-operative studies of 70 cases. Ann Paediatr Fenniae 4:181, 1958

20. Wachtel FW, Ravitch MM, Grishman A: The relation of pectus excavatum to heart disease. Am Heart J 52:121, 1956

21. Howard R: Funnel chest: its effect on cardiac function. Arch Dis Child 34:5, 1959

22. Bevegard S: Postural circulatory changes at rest and during exercise in patients with funnel chests, with special reference to factors affecting the stroke volume. Acta Med Scand 171:695, 1962

23. Beiser GD, Epstein SE, Stampfer M, et al: Impairment of cardiac function in patients with pectus excavatum, with improvement after operative correction. N Engl J Med 287:267, 1972

24. Haller J, Kramer S, Lietman S: Use of CT scans in selection of patients for pectus excavatum surgery: a preliminary report. J Pediatr Surg 22:904, 1987

25. Randolph JG, Tunnell WP, Morton D Jr: Repair of pectus excavatum in children under three years of age: a 12-year experience. Ann Thorac Surg 23:364, 1977

26. Ravitch MM: Technical problems in the operative correction of pectus excavatum. Ann Surg 162:29, 1965

27. Welch KJ: Satisfactory surgical correction of pectus excavatum deformity in childhood. J Thorac Surg 36:724, 1958

28. Haller JA Jr, Katlic M, Shermeta D, et al: Operative correction of pectus excavatum: an evolving perspective. Ann Surg 184:554, 1976

29. Sbokos CG, McMillan IK, Akins CW: Surgical correction of pectus excavatum using a retrosternal bar. Thorax 30:40, 1975

30. Rehbein F: The use of internal steel struts in the operative correction of funnel chest. J Pediatr Surg 1:80, 1966

31. Heydorn WH, Zajtchuk R, Schuchmann GF, Strevey TE: Surgical management of pectus deformities. Ann Thorac Surg 23:417, 1977

32. Holcomb GW Jr: Surgical correction of pectus excavatum. J Pediatr Surg 12:295, 1977

33. Welch K: In Welch K (ed): Complications of Pediatric Surgery, Prevention and Management. Philadelphia, Saunders, 1982, chap 14, p 170

34. Cahill J, Lees G, Robertson H: A summary of preoperative and postoperative cardiorespiratory performance in patients undergoing pectus excavatum and carinatum repair. J Pediatr Surg 19:430, 1984

35. Nakahara K, Ohno K, Miyoshi S, et al: An evaluation of operative outcome in patients with funnel chest diagnosed by means of computed tomogram. J Thorac Cardiovasc Surg 93:577, 1987

36. Sanger PW, Taylor FH, Robicsek F: Deformities of the anterior wall of the chest. Surg Gynecol Obstet 116:515, 1963

37. Welch KJ, Vos A: Surgical correction of pectus carinatum. J Pediatr Surg 8:659, 1973

38. Rickham PP, Lester J, Irving I: Neonatal Surgery, 2nd ed. London, Butterworths, 1978, pp 157–159

39. Mace JW, Kaplan JM, Schanberger J, et al: Poland's syndrome: report of seven cases and review of the literature. Clin Pediatr 11:98, 1972

40. Ravitch MM: Congenital Deformities of the Chest Wall and Their Operative Correction. Philadelphia, Saunders, 1977, pp 260–261

41. Haller J, Colombani P, Miller D, Manson P: Early reconstruction of Poland's syndrome using autologous rib grafts combined with a latissimus muscle flap. Journal of Ped Surgery 19:423, 1984

42. Jeune M, Berard C, Curron R: Dystrophie thoracique asphyxiante de caractère familial. Arch Fr Pediatr 12:886, 1955

43. Hull D, Barnes ND: Children with small chests. Arch Dis Child 47:12, 1972

44. Finegold MJ, Katzew H, Genieser NB, Becker MH: Lung structure in thoracic dystrophy: case reports. Am J Dis Child 122:153, 1971

45. Karjoo M, Koop CE, Cornfield D, Holtzapple P: Pancreatic exocrine enzyme deficiency associated with asphyxiating thoracic dystrophy. Arch Dis Child 48:143, 1973

SECTION XI

Abdominal Wall Defects

The abdominal wall is a beautifully constructed housing for the viscera, although it is usually regarded as a barrier to be gotten through in the performance of abdominal operations. This remarkable structure of muscle, fascia, peritoneum, and skin not only holds in the viscera but also aids in breathing, sitting up, having a bowel movement, and urinating. Disturbances in the closure of the body of the embryo result in a continuous series of interrelated defects that center at the umbilicus. They may extend upward to involve the chest wall and inferiorly to the bladder and hindgut structures. At 2 weeks, the embryo is a mere disk of ectoderm apposed to entoderm. The third germ layer, the mesoderm, grows between these layers, splitting them into an outer somatic layer, the somatopleure, and an inner visceral layer, the splanchnopleure. When one visualizes a cross-section of the embryo, the body wall is like a sandwich of parietal entoderm, which will become the peritoneum or pleura, the mesoderm, which will become the body wall musculature, and the ectoderm or skin. Until the 12th week, the anterior body wall is open at the umbilical ring. This defect is closed by four folds of splanchnic wall that grow out from the lateral portion of the embryo to form the ventral body wall.

The cephalic fold closes the foregut and forms the anterior thoracic and upper abdominal wall with the septum transversum or anterior portion of the diaphragm. This portion of the anterior body wall forms first to provide coverage for the heart. Next, the caudal fold migrates inward to close the hindgut and the somatic layer of the allantois, which forms the hypogastrium. Finally, the third and fourth lateral folds close the midgut and form the lateral and anterior abdominal wall. All of these folds converge on the umbilical ring as the intestine returns to the abdominal cavity at about the 10th week.[1,2] Midabdominal defects, omphalocele, and gastroschisis are most common. Infraumbilical lesions, including exstrophy of the bladder and vesicointestinal fissure, are next most common, whereas supraumbilical lesions of the abdomen and anterior chest wall with ectopia cordis and diaphragmatic defects are quite uncommon.

It is unknown why these folds fail to obliterate the umbilical cord. Does failure of the intestine to return to the abdominal cavity prevent the four folds from meeting in the midline? Or does failure of the folds to meet allow the intestine to remain outside? Since the heart, liver, and bladder do not normally occur outside their respective body cavities but are rather exposed by failure of the body wall to develop, one would think that the defect lies in some failure of mesodermal development.

The prenatal diagnosis of abdominal wall defects is being made with increasing frequency in many perinatal centers. It is difficult to accurately differentiate between gastroschisis and omphalocele and between simple omphalocele and complex lesions, such as cloacal exstrophy. These distinctions are critical, since we must counsel families on an appropriate course of action when these prenatal diagnoses are made. We have seen no advantage to cesarean section over vaginal delivery of these infants. In fact, the only instance of intestinal damage seen in our series of 122 babies with gastroschisis was in one delivered by cesarean section. It is desirable, however, to have the infant delivered in a center with immediate access to a team of pediatric surgeons.

REFERENCES

1. Duhamel B: Embryology of exomphalos and allied malformations. Arch Dis Child 38:142, 1963
2. Hutchin P: Somatic anomalies of the umbilicus and anterior abdominal wall. Surg Gynecol Obstet 170:1075, 1965

89
Omphalocele and Gastroschisis

OMPHALOCELE

An omphalocele is a translucent avascular sac consisting of peritoneum and amniotic membrane at the base of the umbilical cord. It varies in size from a few centimeters in diameter, containing only a few loops of small intestine, to a huge sac containing the entire midgut, stomach, and liver. There are many variations in the size and configuration of an omphalocele. It may be mushroom-shaped, with a narrow neck that opens into a large sac, with as much as half of the wall covered with skin. The umbilical cord emerges from the apex of the sac (Fig. 89–1). The rectus muscles and the rest of the abdominal wall are intact, but when the intestine and liver are herniated into the sac, the true abdominal cavity is extremely small. When the liver is involved, it is broadly attached to the upper portion of the sac rather than to the undersurface of the diaphragm. In these cases, it seems that the muscular portion of the anterior diaphragm also is missing. The incidence of omphalocele varies from 1 in 3200 to 1 in 10,000 live births.[1] Genetic factors may play a role in the development of omphaloceles because in every published series, as well as in our own experience, there is a high incidence of congenital defects. Omphaloceles have been found with greater than the expected frequency in the families of affected children.[2]

Associated Anomalies
Nonrotation of the intestine is always present in infants with large omphaloceles, but aside from Meckel's diverticulum and an occasional persistent omphalomesenteric duct, other intestinal anomalies are rare. Greenwald et al. carefully studied 159 infants treated at the Boston Children's Hospital for associated congenital defects.[3] Of the 159, 31 (or 19.5 percent) had congenital heart disease. The most common lesion was tetralogy of Fallot,

and the secundum type atrial septal defect was next most common. Other significant defects included diaphragmatic hernias, meningocele, trisomy syndromes, and microcephaly.[3] In our series of 92 omphaloceles seen over the past 17 years, 14 (15 percent) had chromosomal abnormalities, 32 (35 percent) had cardiac defects, and 7, or 7 percent, had the Beckwith-Wiedemann syndrome. A similar high rate of associated anomalies has been reported in other series.[4–6]

The Beckwith-Wiedemann syndrome consists of umbilical anomalies, macroglossia, gigantism, and hypoglycemia (Fig. 89–2).[7,8] The enlarged tongue may present anesthetic problems or postoperative spells of apnea. The blood sugar must be carefully monitored, and these children must be carefully followed because they are at risk to develop Wilms' tumors. One of our infants with the Beckwith-Wiedemann syndrome also had a cleft palate. Prematurity is unusual in babies born with omphaloceles.

Diagnosis
The diagnosis of an omphalocele is simple, but time should be spent before operative treatment to perform a careful, complete physical examination and to obtain a chest roentgenogram and echocardiogram. Patency of the esophagus and gastrointestinal tract is proven by a nasogastric tube and the passage of large amounts of meconium stool after a digital rectal examination. Even if other congenital lesions are not discovered before treatment, they must be suspected when the baby has respiratory or other complications in the postoperative period.

Treatment
At birth, a single layer of povidone-iodine-soaked gauze is placed over the sac. The entire abdomen and lower chest are wrapped with multiple layers of gauze bandage. A sterile plastic bag is drawn up over the baby's lower

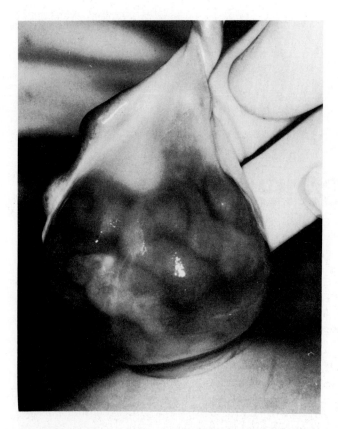

Figure 89–1. A typical moderate-size omphalocele with a translucent membrane covering loops of small bowel. There is no liver and the umbilical cord emerges at the apex.

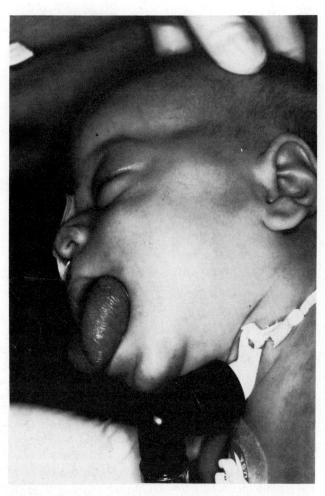

Figure 89–2. Enlarged tongue seen in Beckwith-Wiedemann syndrome.

body to the chest, where it is tied or taped to the skin. Intestinal bags hold moisture and allow examination of the sac or eviscerated bowel.[9] The infant must be in a heated incubator with additional oxygen provided as required during all phases of transport.

Preoperative care consists of administering IV 10 percent glucose, a nasogastric tube, and rectal irrigations to decompress the intestine and antibiotics. All IV fluids are administered through the upper extremity.

The size of the defect and its contents dictate treatment. Sacs that measure up to 5 cm in diameter and contain only small intestine are easily treated by removal of the sac, ligation of the umbilical vessels, and closure of the peritoneum and fascia in one layer. The skin is then closed with sterile tapes. It is not necessary to explore the abdomen if patency of the gastrointestinal tract has been proven by the passage of meconium and roentgenographic studies before operation.

Omphaloceles up to 6 cm in diameter also may be closed primarily, although with more difficulty. The infant is transported to the operating room with the povidone-iodine dressing in place. First, rectal irrigations are given until meconium has been completely removed from the bowel. The infant is anesthetized and paralyzed.

The dressings are removed while the baby is under infrared lights to avoid heat loss. A preliminary indication of the difficulty of closure is obtained by twisting the apex of the sac, forcing viscera into the abdomen. If this maneuver causes an increase in airway pressure, the twisted sac is tied with several heavy sutures, and complete closure of the defect is postponed for 2 or 3 days. When the viscera can be replaced, the sac is excised and the abdominal wall is enlarged by manual stretching. The skin is dissected free, and mattress sutures are placed 0.5 cm back from the fascial edge. When all sutures are in place, they are pulled down and tied. Closure of the skin with a subcuticular pursestring suture eventually puckers down to an almost normal appearing umbilicus.[10] It is essential to maintain these infants on complete muscular paralysis and mechanical ventilation until the abdomen softens and spontaneous respiration is possible.

A giant omphalocele may be defined as one that contains almost all the liver and bowel, with a circumference of 5 cm or greater. Infants with giant omphalocele are more likely to have associated anomalies, but more importantly, they have a narrow thoracic cage with relative pulmonary hypoplasia (Fig. 89–3). We found a 41 percent incidence of prolonged respiratory insufficiency in 22 infants with giant omphalocele.[11] These infants have narrow chests, with their posterior ribs angled inferiorly so they appear more vertical than normal. The calculated lung volumes and lung volume found at autopsy indicated significant pulmonary hypoplasia. It is possible that the failure of the liver to return to the abdominal cavity leaves the lower chest cage underdeveloped. The diaphragmatic contractions appeared to be inefficient in several of these infants. Since these babies are already in a precarious respiratory state, general anesthesia with endotracheal intubation should be avoided whenever possible. Anything that will further impair respiratory function, such as increased intraabdominal pressure, barotrauma or oxygen toxicity, might lead to the need for long-term ventilator support. It is important to achieve gradual closure of the giant omphalocele while maintaining the sac intact. We have used two types of conservative approach to these infants. With

each, the infant is left in the isolette. With sterile technique, a heavy ligature is tied to the end of the umbilical cord above the omphalocele and then to the top of the incubator. This suspends the bowel and liver. The sac and surrounding skin are painted with povidone-iodine and dressed with a sterile gauze bandage. Rectal irrigations are given, and an orogastric tube is placed to empty the bowel. Nutrition is maintained with IV alimentation until the infant can take formula by mouth. If nothing further is done, the sac will gradually contract, and over a period of several weeks, the sac is covered with epithelium. This requires prolonged hospitalization, and there is the risk of premature separation of the sac from the skin. The omphalocele sac is a tough membrane that will hold sutures, even if it is torn during delivery.[12] The process of reduction of the sac's contents may be hastened by either infolding the sac with sutures or the application of progressive ligatures to the apex of the sac over the course of several days (Fig. 89–4). After a week or 10 days, when the contents are reduced, the infant may be operated on, the sac removed, and the defect closed. The omphalocele sac may also be reduced

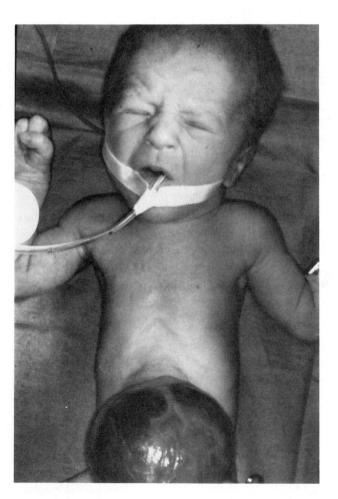

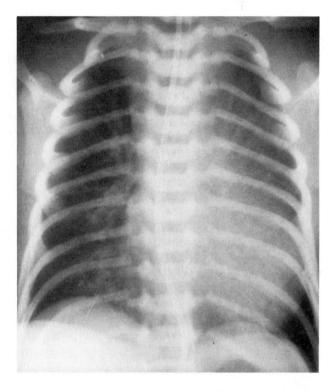

Figure 89–3. Giant omphalocele with narrow thorax.

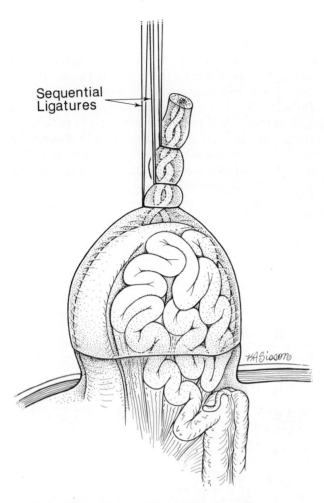

Figure 89–4. Large omphalocele with liver and small bowel in the sac. Ligatures are placed on the cord to elevate the sac. More ligatures are tied about the sac every day to gradually squeeze the contents into the abdominal cavity.

in size by wrapping the sac first with an antiseptic dressing and then a pressure bandage. With each dressing change, the contents of the sac are gradually reduced until the defect is closed.[13]

There are many surgeons who advocate immediate operation for all infants with omphalocele, with excision of the sac and staged closure after suture of Silastic sheets to the abdominal wall. This procedure was popularized by Schuster in 1967.[14] His operation was first designed to close gigantic ventral hernias created in older children by the closure of large omphaloceles with widely mobilized skin flaps. The technique was later applied to newborns with omphalocele and gastroschisis. As it is currently carried out, the sac is excised, and a sheet of Silastic is sutured first to either side of the defect and then the two sheets are sutured to each other (Fig. 89–5). It is then necessary to return the child to the operating room at intervals to tighten the Silastic until the material can be removed and the abdominal wall closed. In our hands, excision of the sac from the liver results in unnec-

essary blood loss. Other complications of the Silastic membrane include premature separation from the abdominal wall, wound infection, and sepsis.[15] It is preferable, in difficult cases, to stretch the abdominal wall as much as possible. If it is impossible to close the fascia, close only flaps of skin over the liver; then at 1 year of age, repair the ventral hernia.

Results

From 1970 through 1987 we treated 92 infants with omphaloceles. In 47, the diameter of the defect was less than 5 cm. Thirty-seven of these babies recovered after primary closure. Nine others had associated lethal anomalies, and all died in the hospital or at home. The defect was closed in 5 of these infants, 1 dehisced, and 4 had no operation. Seven of 45 infants with giant omphaloceles had lethal chromosome defects or extreme prematurity and were treated nonoperatively without expectation of survival. Twenty-eight infants with giant omphaloceles were closed surgically, by the use of either skin flaps or Silastic. One died with cardiac disease and 6 died with respiratory insufficiency, although only 1 had required preoperative ventilation. Two survivors remain on partial ventilatory support at 3 and 14 years of age. The majority of long-term survivors have small to moderate ventral hernias. Ten with giant omphalocele have been treated by ligation or painting of the sac. Six required preoperative ventilation, but only 2 had postoperative respiratory insufficiency, both of whom died at 6 months with cardiac disease. The remaining 8 patients are well at 1 to 6 years. All have had uneventful repair of ventral hernias.

Our overall mortality rate is 35 percent in giant omphaloceles and 17 percent in small omphaloceles. Nonoperative techniques would appear to have kept some infants alive who might have died in surgery, without any increase in duration of hospitalization. In most other services, low birth weight and associated malformations are the most common cause of death.[16–18]

Supraumbilical Defects

When the body wall fails to close, one finds a midline supraumbilical abdominal defect with a sac covering the liver, a defect in the sternum, a deficiency in the anterior diaphragm, and cardiac anomalies.[19,20] There are minor variations in the degree to which these defects are involved, but in the typical case, the heart rests on top of the liver and is palpable just beneath the junction of the skin and the omphalocele sac. In addition to these local defects, Toyama found associated cranial and facial anomalies in 11 of 61 reported cases.[21]

The preoperative evaluation of these infants must include a chest roentgenogram and an electrocardiogram. Since there is a known high incidence of intracardiac anomalies, it might be good to perform an angiocardiogram and cardiac catheterization through the intact um-

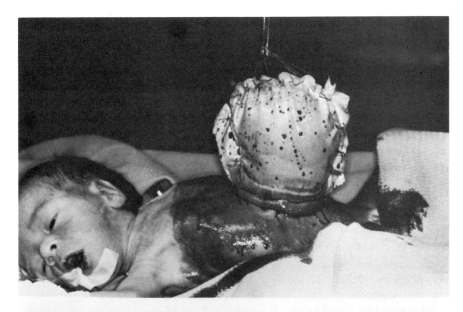

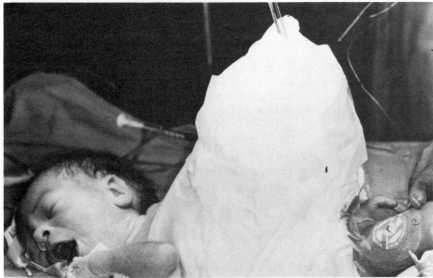

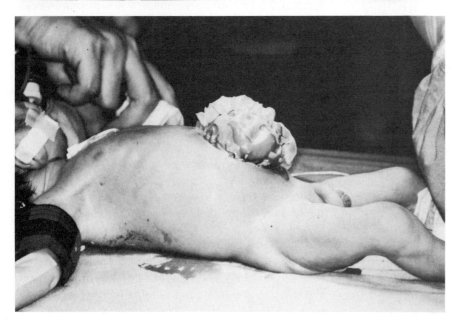

Figure 89–5. Top. Two sheets of Silastic were sutured to the abdominal wall and then to each other to form a sac for the intestine. **Middle.** The sac and the skin were cleansed with povidone-iodine and encased in a large sterile dressing that was suspended from the isolette. **Bottom.** The sac was reduced about halfway by the fourth postoperative day.

bilical vein before an operation. Although correction of major intracardiac defects should not necessarily be performed at the time of body wall repair in the neonatal period, it would be good to excise a ventricular diverticulum at that time.[22]

Treatment

Obviously, repair must be individualized, but at the end of any such operation, the heart must have sufficient room or there will be tamponade. In addition, the abdomen must be separate from the thoracic cavity and pericardium. Prosthetic material is required to meet these goals when there is a major defect. Excision of the sac, taking care to avoid injury to the liver, is the first step. The abdomen is enlarged by splitting the fascia down the midline beneath the skin to create a lower abdominal ventral hernia. In addition, the abdomen is manually stretched. If the heart can be replaced into the pericardium without creating tamponade, the diaphragm and pericardial edge are sutured together to the undersurface of the sternum. The anterior portion of the pericardium is left open. If this procedure puts too much pressure on the heart, the diaphragm and pericardium must be reconstructed with a Silastic sheet. Closure of the upper abdomen by direct suture of the fascia pulls the lower rib cage together and in our hands has caused intolerable tension on the suture line. It is far preferable to allow relaxation of the lower abdomen by dividing the fascia, after which the large upper abdominal defect is closed with plastic mesh. We have found it perfectly satisfactory to suture Silastic sheeting directly to the fascia, despite the fact that tissue does not grow into the Silastic as it does with other types of mesh. Every effort should then be made to obtain skin closure over the Silastic. If the defect is too large for skin closure, the Silastic is removed in successive stages during the following two weeks.

GASTROSCHISIS

In gastroschisis, bowel protrudes through a full-thickness defect in the abdominal wall adjacent to the umbilical cord. The defect is invariably to the right of the umbilicus, and the bowel has no covering other than a pseudomembrane of thickened, inflamed peritoneum (Fig. 89–6). There are several important differences between gastroschisis and omphalocele. The bowel in gastroschisis has been exposed to amniotic fluid. It is nonrotated, and the thick, edematous loops of bowel adhere to one another in an inflammatory mass. The second important difference is the fact that although the entire midgut, stomach, ovaries and fallopian tubes are eviscerated in gastroschisis, the liver is always in the abdomen. Moore and Khalid surveyed 16 pediatric surgical centers from all over the world to compare gastroschisis with omphalo-

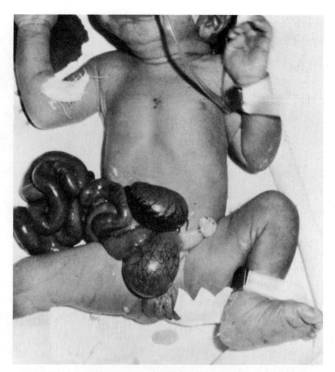

Figure 89–6. Gastroschisis. The bowel, stomach, and bladder are outside the abdomen and completely uncovered. The umbilical cord is lateral to the small defect. Note that the liver is never outside the abdominal cavity in an infant with gastroschisis.

cele. Their most striking finding was the rarity of associated congenital birth defects in the 203 cases of gastroschisis. Only 12 of these infants had minor defects outside the gastrointestinal tract, whereas 74 percent of babies with omphalocele had serious cardiac or neuromuscular anomalies. Moore and Khalid also noted a worldwide increase in reports of gastroschisis commencing in the early 1970s. Their evidence points strongly to an environmental etiology for gastroschisis, whereas omphalocele appears to have a genetic basis.[23] In our series of 126 infants with gastroschisis, the incidence of birth defects in organs outside the gastrointestinal tract was very low. One infant had trisomy 18, one had hepatic hemangiomatosis, five had Meckel's diverticulum, three had minor extremity anomalies, and five had small ventricular septal defect. Thus, the scarcity of anomalies of the cardiovascular system in babies with gastroschisis is significantly different from those with omphalocele.

There is a vigorous controversy concerning the embryologic origin of gastroschisis.[2,24] Although we do not agree with Shaw when he calls gastroschisis a myth, he has pointed out the most obvious embryologic explanation, stated as follows. Originally, there are paired right and left umbilical veins. The right vein disappears, leaving a weakened area on the right side of the cord through which the bowel herniates. This theory explains the fact that gastroschisis invariably appears to the right of the cord and also explains the juxtaposition of the defect with the base of the cord.

Associated Intestinal Defects

Although defects in other organ systems are unusual, Moore and Khalid found a 16 percent incidence of gastrointestinal malformations.[23] In our series of 126 infants with gastroschisis, 7 had intestinal atresia or stenosis. In 3, the entire intestine was infarcted, and 1 other had a 6 inch segment of intestinal gangrene. Three had intestinal perforation. All these intestinal complications are caused by the volvulus, or the herniation of intestine through a very small defect in the abdominal wall, which constricts the blood supply. The left colon was avulsed from its mesentery by a cesarean section delivery. Thus 14, or 12 percent, of our patients had major intestinal problems.

Treatment

The initial treatment of an infant with gastroschisis consists of keeping the exposed intestine moist and the infant warm. Hypothermia is a common problem because the exposed intestine acts as a heat exchanger. This leads to acidosis and hypoglycemia. Antibiotics and vitamin K are given while the infant is being stabilized in preparation for surgery. Phillipart et al. noted an excessive fluid loss in babies with gastroschisis, but we have found that it is rarely necesary to give more than the usual maintenance fluid requirements during the first 24 hours.[25] If there are clinical signs of hypovolemia, lactated Ringer's solution or serum albumin (20 ml/kg) sufficient to restore the vital signs to normal is given.

With gastroschisis, the abdominal cavity is small and underdeveloped, but the liver is always within the abdomen, unlike cases involving large omphaloceles. Thus only the bowel, which is compressible, must be placed within the abdominal cavity. Each infant's treatment must be individualized—in some the viscera is easily replaced after stretching the abdominal wall, and the fascia may be closed without creating undue tension. When it would appear that fascial closure cannot be accomplished, simple skin closure is far safer. The alternative in babies who will not tolerate skin closure is the application of Silastic prosthesis.[26]

Technique

The baby is placed on the operating table under warming lights and given an endotracheal halothane anesthetic. One physician gently washes the eviscerated intestine and abdominal wall with povidone-iodine and then applies temporary sterile drapes about the abdomen. An assistant irrigates the rectum with a large catheter and a warm solution of 1 percent acetylcysteine. The catheter is guided up into the bowel until all meconium has been removed. This procedure, along with decompression of

the stomach and duodenum with an orogastric tube, diminishes the size of the intestine, which must be placed within the abdominal cavity. The bowel and abdominal wall are again prepared with povidone-iodine, and new sterile drapes are applied. The umbilical vessels and the urachus are individually tied beneath the skin away from the defect. If the abdominal defect is small, it is enlarged with incisions upward toward the xiphoid and downward toward the pubis. The skin must not be separated from the edges of the defect at this point, in case it becomes necessary to apply a Silon sac. The abdominal wall is then forcibly stretched. The fingers of one hand are placed against the posterior abdominal wall while the fingers of the other hand apply constant pressure with a kneading or massaging motion to the anterior and lateral abdominal wall. This procedure requires application of considerable force. Further relaxation may be obtained by incision of the fascia in the midline beneath the skin up to the xiphoid and down to the pubis. Then, with meticulous sharp dissection, the loops of intestine are separated from one another and any loose gelatinous exudate is removed. This procedure will release sharp kinks in the shortened intestine, but no effort should be made to remove the adherent thickened peel. This is actually the thickened, edematous seromuscular layer of the bowel, and its removal results in severe hemorrhage. The entire intestine is then examined for anomalies. Areas of gangrenous, perforated, or atretric bowel are resected, and a single-layer end-to-end anastomosis is performed. The abdominal wall is again stretched in all directions, and at this time a short-acting muscle relaxant is given by the anesthesiologist. The intestine is placed in the abdomen, commencing with the duodenojejunal loop on the right side. The cecum and colon are placed on the left so that the nonrotated position of the bowel is maintained.

Occasionally, the left testicle is outside the abdominal cavity. It may be passed easily through the external ring and secured with a suture in the scrotum. When all the bowel has been placed in the stretched abdominal cavity, an attempt may be made to close the fascia. In many cases, a complete fascial closure is possible, using 3-0 absorbable monofilament sutures. If the fascial closure is too tight, the skin is dissected back from the edge of the defect for 1 or 2 cm, and the fascia is divided in the midline down to the pubis and up to the xiphoid. After more stretching of the skin, it is closed with subcuticular sutures and strips of sterile tape (Fig. 89–7). This does not leave a large ventral hernia but only a midline diastasis that relaxes the abdomen and is easily closed at 1 year of age. If the baby is vigorous, endotracheal extubation is performed at the end of the operation. If airway pressures increase to 30 cm of water and the infant does not have a satisfactory tidal volume, he or she is left intubated and is placed on mechanical ventila-

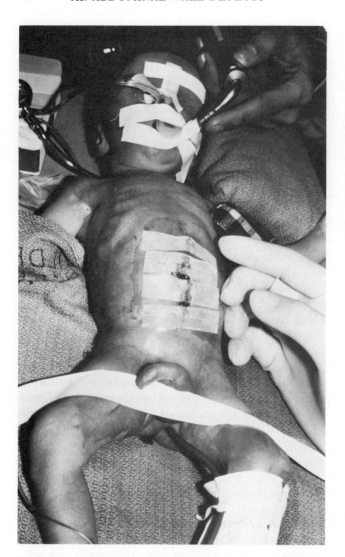

Figure 89–7. Gastroschisis closed primarily. Large Steristrips support the skin closure.

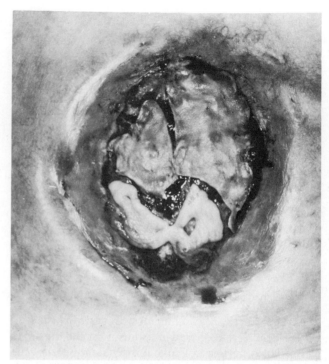

Figure 89–8. Split-thickness skin grafts applied to the granulating surface of the bowel after the Silastic sheet had pulled away.

tion. Observation of the skin oxygen saturation and arterial blood gases may help in this decision. If compression within the abdominal cavity produces intestinal cyanosis, bowel is released and a Silastic prosthesis is used.

When it is not possible to place the bowel into the abdominal cavity, a sheet of Silastic, 0.007-inch thick, is sutured to each side of the defect with interrupted figure-eight or mattress sutures, taking large bites of the skin, fascia, and peritoneum. The Silastic sheeting is everted to leave a smooth surface facing the bowel. The two sheets of Silastic are then closed with running sutures of the same material (Fig. 89–5). A large dressing soaked in povidone-iodine solution is then applied to the Silastic sheets and wrapped around the abdomen. A suture at the apex of the sac is tied to the top of the incubator to hold the bowel upright. The infant is then returned to the operating room at intervals of 2 to 3 days, where, under sterile conditions but without anesthesia, the bowel is squeezed back into the abdominal cavity. The final stage of closing the abdominal wall is performed under general anesthesia. Once again, it often is possible to close the full thickness of the abdominal wall, but since the edges of the wound are often friable and infected, it is best to simply close the skin.

If the Silastic pulls away from the abdominal wall or if the abdomen simply cannot be closed at the final stage, the defect may be temporarily covered with wet dressings, porcine skin, or amniotic membrane.[27] By the time separation of the prosthesis has occurred, there is a pseudomembrane over the bowel, and adhesions will prevent a gross evisceration. We prefer to continue with antibiotic dressings on the wound surface and, after 2 or 3 days, apply a split-thickness skin graft taken from the baby's buttock. This has been successful in two patients. Remarkably, 1 year later, when the ventral hernia was repaired, the bowel had separated from the skin graft, leaving a pseudoperitoneum on the underside of the skin (Fig. 89–8).

Postoperative Care

Peripheral hyperalimentation is commenced on the second or third postoperative day, or if skin closure was achieved, a central hyperalimentation line is inserted. The risks of sepsis are increased when a central catheter is inserted in an infant who has a Silastic prosthesis.

Consequently, with these babies, there is no alternative to peripheral alimentation. A gastrostomy increases the risk of infection. Consequently, the stomach is drained with a small plastic catheter. Bowel function in these babies is delayed. It is rare for them to tolerate full oral feedings in less than 2 weeks after a primary closure. The delay in bowel function is even more pronounced when a Silastic prosthesis is required. We have had to maintain babies with hyperalimentation for as long as 3 months before they would tolerate sufficient calories by mouth. This prolonged intestinal dysfunction is not caused by any identifiable point of obstruction, and repeat operations searching for an obstructing lesion have been fruitless. Roentgenographic studies demonstrate slow peristalsis with intestinal dilatation.[28]

Results

Thirty-six of our 113 surviving babies with gastroschisis were discharged from the hospital within 28 days. Twenty-one patients required a Silastic pouch because of our inability to safely close the abdomen with available tissue. These infants required IV alimentation for prolonged periods before they could be fed by mouth and were hospitalized for considerably longer than babies who could be closed primarily.[29] Associated intestinal atresia or stenosis also required more prolonged nutritional support and a longer hospitalization. There was no difference in babies whose intestinal anomaly was repaired with an immediate primary anastomosis and those who first had a stoma with a later repair. There were 13 deaths, for a mortality rate of 10 percent among our 122 patients. The mortality rate was higher in infants of very low birth weight, but it was not affected by mode of delivery. Specifically, in our series there was no advantage to cesarean section delivery. One infant died with trisomy 18 and another with hepatic hemangiomatosis. Three deaths were due to gangrenous midgut volvulus and 1 to extreme prematurity. Thus, six deaths were unavoidable. Three deaths were caused by delayed central line sepsis, and 4 were due to surgical technique. Tight closure of the abdomen resulted in intestinal gangrene and early death in 2; 1 infant was extubated during the operation and never recovered from hypoxia. During the early years of this series, one baby closed with large undermined skin flaps succumbed to skin necrosis and sepsis.

Most authors who have reported large series of gastroschisis individualize their method of repair. Most now use primary fascial closure or minimal skin flaps when possible, saving closure with a Silastic prosthesis for severe visceroabdominal disproportion.[30] There is a tendency, however, to favor closure without a prosthesis, since there is an earlier return of gastrointestinal function with earlier discharge from the hospital.[31–34] The management of associated intestinal defects is controversial, perhaps because there are so few patients with these problems. Total intestinal infarction with gangrene is incompatible with life, and we have advised discontinuation of treatment. Atretic intestine may be resected and anastomosed at the time of primary treatment, with good results. However, there will be a prolonged period of intestinal dysfunction. We have exteriorized distal atresias, especially those in the colon, then carried out an anastomosis months later. Pokorny et al. recommend leaving the atretic intestine in place, then reoperating several weeks later, when the bowel edema has diminished, to carry out the resection and anastomosis.[35] There is no definitive answer to this question. Each surgeon must decide what he or she perceives to be the best course of action at the time.

Ventral Hernia Repair

Following skin closure of gastroschisis, there often is a small diastasis that requires no repair. In others, however, the ventral hernia enlarges to an extent sufficient to require secondary repair. We have not seen the huge ventral hernias that occurred following the mobilization of skin flaps to the flanks for closure of large defects.

We delay secondary repair of the ventral hernia until the child is at least 1 year of age. At that time the child is brought into the hospital and prepared for operation with a clear liquid diet, rectal irrigations, and placement of a nasogastric tube the evening before surgery. In all of our current patients, this preparation has been sufficient to allow primary fascial repair. No attempt is made to separate the abdominal wall layer, but the peritoneum and fascia are closed in one layer with interrupted figure-8 polyglyconate sutures.

An important part of the operation is the construction of a deep umbilicus at the exact center of the abdomen. A single, inferiorly based skin flap is sutured into a tube and then anchored to the deep fascia. The resultant umbilicus will hold a jewel and will be a suitable receptacle for salt while drinking tequila on Mexican beaches.

REFERENCES

1. Mahour GH: Omphalocele. Surg Gynecol Obstet 143:821, 1976
2. Noordijk JA, Bloemsma-Jonkman F: Gastroschisis: no myth. J Pediatr Surg 13:47, 1978
3. Greenwald RD, Rosenthal A, Nada AS: Cardiovascular malfunctions associated with omphalocele. J Pediatr Surg 85:181, 1974
4. Jones PG: Exomphalos: a review of 45 cases. Arch Dis Child 39:180, 1963
5. Mahour GH, Weitzman JJ, Rosenkrantz JG: Omphalocele and gastroschisis. Ann Surg 177:478, 1973
6. Girvan DP, Webster DM, Shandling B: The treatment of omphalocele and gastroschisis. Surg Gynecol Obstet 139:222, 1974

7. Irving J: Exomphalos with macroglossia: a study of 11 cases. J Pediatr Surg 2:499, 1967

8. Roe TF, Kershnar AK, Weitzman JJ, Madrigal LS: Beckwith's syndrome with extreme organ hyperplasia. Pediatrics 52:372, 1973

9. Sheldon RE: The bowel bags, a sterile transportable method for warming infants with skin defects. Pediatrics 53:267, 1974

10. Canty T, Collins D: Primary fascial closure in infants with gastroschisis and omphalocele: a superior approach. J Pediatr Surg 18:707, 1983

11. Hershenson M, Brouillette R, Klemka L, et al: Respiratory insufficiency in newborns with abdominal wall defects. J Pediatr Surg 20:348, 1985

12. Sli M: Combined treatment of omphalocele. Surgery 61:314, 1967

13. Barlow B, Cooper A, Gandhi R, et al: External silo reduction of the unruptured giant omphalocele. J Pediatr Surg 22:75, 1987

14. Schuster S: A new method for the staged repair of large omphaloceles. Surg Gynecol Obstet 125:837, 1967

15. Schwartz M, Tyson K, Milliorn K, Lobe T: Staged reduction using a Silastic sac is the treatment of choice for large congenital abdominal wall defects. J Pediatr Surg 18:713, 1983

16. Schwartzberg S, Pokorny W, McGill C, Hasberg F: Gastroschisis and omphalocele. Am J Surg 144:650, 1982

17. Stringel G, Filler R: Prognostic factors in omphalocele and gastroschisis. J Pediatr Surg 14:515, 1979

18. Mayer T, Black R, Matlak M, Johnson D: Gastroschisis and omphalocele. Ann Surg 192:783, 1980

19. Spitz L, Bloom KR, Milner S, Levin SE: Combined anterior abdominal wall, sternal, diaphragmatic, pericardial, and intracardiac defects: a report of five cases and their management. J Pediatr Surg 10:491, 1975

20. Cantrell JR, Haller JA, Ravitch MM: A syndrome of congenital defects involving the abdominal wall, sternum, diaphragm, pericardium, and heart. Surg Gynecol Obstet 107:602, 1958

21. Toyama WM: Combined congenital defects of the anterior abdominal wall, sternum, diaphragm, pericardium, and heart: a case report and review of the syndrome. Pediatrics 50:778, 1972

22. Symbas PN, Ware RE: A syndrome of defects of the thoracoabdominal wall, diaphragm, pericardium, and heart: one-stage surgical repair and analysis of the syndrome. J Thorac Cardiovasc Surg 65:914, 1973

23. Moore T, Khalid N: An international survey of gastroschisis and omphalocele (490 cases). 1. Nature and distribution of additional malformations. 2. Relative incidence, pregnancy and environmental factors. Pediatr Surg Int 1:46, 109, 1986

24. Shaw A: The myth of gastroschisis. J Pediatr Surg 10:235, 1975

25. Phillipart AI, Canty TG, Filler RM: Acute fluid volume requirements in infants with anterior abdominal wall defects. J Pediatr Surg 7:553, 1972

26. Allen RG, Wrenn EL Jr: Silon as a sac in the treatment of omphalocele and gastroschisis. J Pediatr Surg 4:3, 1969

27. Seashore JH, MacNaughton RJ, Talbert JL: Treatment of gastroschisis and omphalocele with biological dressings. J Pediatr Surg 10:9, 1975

28. Touloukian RJ, Spackman TJ: Gastrointestinal function and radiographic appearance following gastroschisis repair. J Pediatr Surg 6:427, 1971

29. Luck S, Sherman J, Raffensperger J, Goldstein I: Gastroschisis in 106 consecutive newborn infants. Surgery 98:677, 1985

30. Fonkalsrud E: Selective repair of neonatal gastroschisis based on degree of visceroabdominal disproportion. Ann Surg 191:139, 1980

31. Bower R, Bell M, Ternberg J, Cobb M: Ventilatory support and primary closure of gastroschisis. Surgery 91:52, 1982

32. Ein S, Rubin S: Gastroschisis: primary closure or silo pouch. J Pediatr Surg 15:549, 1980

33. Filston H: Gastroschisis—primary fascial closure the goal for optimum management. Ann Surg 194:260, 1983

34. DiLorenzo M, Yazbeck S, Ducharme J: Gastroschisis: a 15-year experience. J Pediatr Surg 22:710, 1987

35. Pokorny W, Harberg F, McGill C: Gastroschisis complicated by intestinal atresia. J Pediatr Surg 16:261, 1981

90
Prune-Belly Syndrome

The prune-belly syndrome, or absence of the musculature of the abdominal wall, is associated in the male with undescended testicles and varying degrees of urinary tract malformation. This syndrome is easily recognized in the neonatal period by the flaccid, wrinkled appearance of the abdominal wall; hence the term "prune-belly" (Fig. 90–1). The abdominal wall is easily picked up between two fingers—there is only skin and peritoneum, perhaps with some fibrous tissue. Loops of intestine are visible and palpable, and the bladder can be felt in the lower abdomen. There is a spectrum of malformations, varying from the infant who has a wrinkled flaccid abdominal wall with severely dysplastic kidneys to children with minimal urinary tract dysfunction whose abdominal walls improve with age (Fig. 90–2). The complete syndrome does not exist in girls, but we have observed the flaccid abdominal wall as a separate entity and also have seen it in association with an omphalocele. In severe cases, the rectus abdominus, the oblique muscles, and the transversus abdominus are absent or rudimentary, bilaterally. More often, the infraumbilical rectus muscles are absent, and the obliques are deficient. The urinary abnormality consists of dilated tortuous ureters and an enlarged, thick-walled bladder, often with a patent urachus and a dilated urethra. The kidneys are hydronephrotic, with varying degrees of renal dysplasia. The severity of the urinary tract abnormality is related to the appearance of the abdominal wall, in that the infants with the most severe degree of abdominal wall deficiency will have the poorest functioning of the urinary tract.

PATHOLOGY

Nunn and Stephens carefully studied children who had survived the prune-belly syndrome as well as several who died in infancy.[1] In surviving patients, urinary pressure and radiologic studies demonstrated no evidence of mechanical urinary tract obstruction. The bladder capacity was greatly increased, but voiding pressures were normal. There was no peristaltic activity within the dilated tortuous ureters. These findings correlated with their microscopic studies, which demonstrated the patchy or total absence of muscle fibers in the abdominal wall, bladder, and ureters. The prostatic urethra was also dilated, with a reduction of smooth muscle and an increase of connective tissue in its wall. The testes were most often found within the abdominal cavity at or near the ureterovesical junction. The testes were small, but the germinal epithelium, epididymis, and vas deferens appeared to be normal for their age. Nunn and Stephens proposed that the explanation for these anomalies lay not in urinary obstruction but in a failure of the musculature of the abdominal wall and urinary tract to develop from the mesenchyme during the sixth to the tenth weeks of fetal development.[1] Occasionally, there are associated defects, such as dysplastic hips and talipes equinovaris or an imperforate anus. A patent urachus is associated with the more severe forms of the anomaly and allows free drainage of urine from an otherwise nearly functionless bladder.

DIAGNOSIS

When the diagnosis of the syndrome is made by physical examination, special studies to determine urinary tract function are indicated. A voiding cystourethrogram and intravenous pyelogram will provide information concerning the size and shape of the bladder, ureters, and kidney. Cinefluoroscopy and manometry will determine the degree of impairment of ureteral peristalsis and bladder emptying. The blood urea nitrogen, creatinine, and creatinine clearance tests are performed as baseline studies and also to follow the course of renal function. Initial

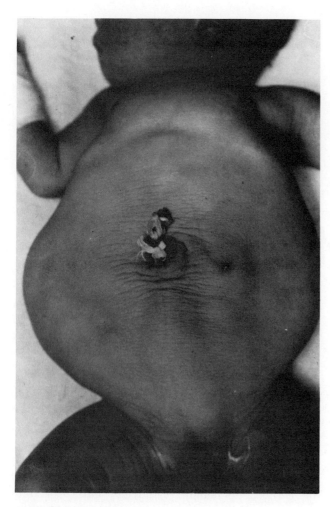

Figure 90–1. The wrinkled skin and flaccid abdominal wall, which protrudes laterally, are typical of the prune-belly syndrome.

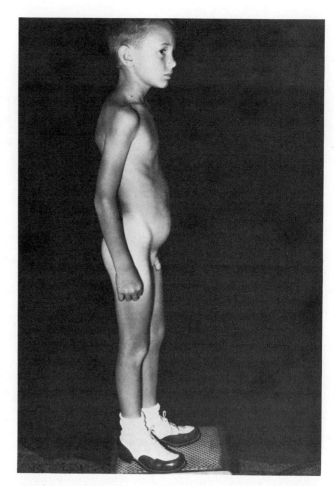

Figure 90–2. This boy continues to have a protuberant abdomen, but it is much better than it was at birth.

and frequent urine cultures are essential to the management of these patients, since stagnation of urine invites infection.

MANAGEMENT

Treatment is directed primarily at the urinary tract. Opinion is divided as to whether these children should have an immediate high urinary diversion via a pyelostomy with later reconstruction of the urinary tract or conservative therapy. Duckett is of the opinion that these children should be given antibacterial agents to suppress infection and at the most a vesicostomy to decompress the urinary tract if infection is a problem.[2] He doubts that adominal wall plication or reconstruction of the urinary tract will improve the prognosis. This opinion is also shared by Nunn and Stephens and others, who point out that the natural history of these chidren is one of improvement. We have observed children whose abdom-

inal walls have developed substance and who have improved with exercise as they have grown older. On the other hand, Randolph has advocated pyelostomy in the neonate with complete reconstruction by resection and reimplantation of the ureters, orchiopexy, and resection of the lower abdominal wall when the child is 1 year old.[3] Kim and Hendren prefer primary reconstruction of the urinary tract without pyelostomy.[4] At this time, there is little evidence to suggest that surgical drainage of the urinary tract offers a better long-term prognosis than mere observation.[5] An orchiopexy is indicated in all of these children. The testicle is easily brought down to the scrotum by extraperitoneal mobilization of the testicular vessels and the vas.

REFERENCES

1. Nunn IN, Stephens FD: The triad syndrome: a complete anomaly of the abdominal wall, urinary system and testes. J Urol 86:782, 1961

2. Duckett JS: The prune belly syndrome. In Kelalis PP, King LR, Belman AB (eds): Clinical Pediatric Urology. Philadelphia, Saunders, p 615
3. Randolph JG: Total surgical reconstruction for patients with abdominal muscular deficiency (prune belly syndrome). J Pediat Surg 12:1033, 1977
4. Kim S: Discussion. J Pediatr Surg 12:1042, 1977
5. Duckett J: Prune belly syndrome. In Welch K, Randolph J, Ravitch M, et al. (eds): Pediatric Surgery. Chicago, Year Book, 1986, p 1195

91
Exstrophy

A complete exstrophy of the bladder represents a failure of closure of the infraumbilical anterior abdominal wall. Fortunately, exstrophy occurs in only 1 in 30,000 to 40,000 live births. Males are affected three to four times as frequently as girls.

PATHOLOGY

The posterior wall of the bladder bulges forward as the infant cries, and usually the ureteral orifices are plainly visible with a continuous dribble of urine covering the exposed epithelium. The umbilicus is at the upper edge of the bladder, and the medial edges of the rectus sheaths blend with the lateral bladder margins (Fig. 91–1). Grossly, the bladder varies in size from a tiny vestigial organ to 5 or 6 cm in diameter at the time of birth. The penis is short, broad, and angulated upward in a reverse chordee. Since the corpora cavernosa are attached to the undersurface of the separated inferior pubic rami, much of the penile length is dissipated as the corpora cavernosa. One or both corpora may be hypoplastic. In girls, the labia do not meet in the midline and the clitoris is separated into paired structures on either side of the open urethra. The pubic bones fail to meet in the midline. This results in a weakened pelvic floor and, occasionally, in rectal prolapse. The outward rotation of the hips causes a waddling gait, but the pelvis is stable and older children are capable of strenuous physical activity. The bladder mucosa may appear to be normal, but more often the surface is edematous and becomes covered with friable, polypoid structures. Histologically, the bladder muscle is deficient and is interspersed with loose, edematous, fibrous tissue.[1] Thus, the intravesicle ureter is insufficiently supported, and ureterovesical reflux is the rule following bladder repair. The kidneys and ureters usually are normal but may become secondarily dilated by reflux and infection. The most frequently associated anomalies are inguinal hernias and prolapse of the rectum.

EMBRYOLOGY

Exstrophy results from a continuation of the cloacal cleft onto the infraumbilical body wall. A 1 mm plastic wedge placed just above the cloacal membrane in a 2- or 3-day-old chick embryo prevents formation of the anterior cloaca and produces the avian equivalent of an exstrophy.[2] Injury to the cloaca in a 3- to 5-week-old human embryo may have the same result. Exstrophic lesions are sporadic, with no known genetic or environmental predisposition.

TREATMENT

The goals of treatment in a baby born with bladder exstrophy are to achieve closure of the bladder, reconstruction of the abdominal wall, genital reconstruction, and eventual urinary continence. It is highly desirable to commence treatment during the neonatal period. Initially, it was thought that a bladder less than 2.5 cm in diameter was unsuitable for closure. However, if the bladder bulges forward with crying or if it can be indented into the abdominal cavity with finger pressure, it may have a greater volume than meets the eye and will distend with time. Furthermore, closure of even a very tiny bladder will conserve tissue, and later bladder augmentation with a segment of intestine may be feasible. A further advantage of immediate closure of the bladder is the flexibility of the iliac bones, which allows closure of the pubis without resorting to iliac osteotomy. One can deter-

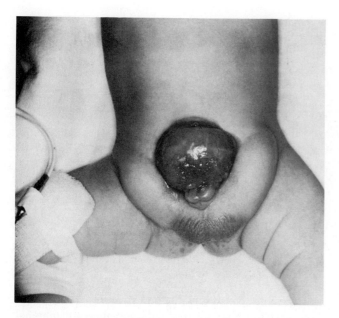

Figure 91–1. Typical exstrophy of the bladder, with short, epispadic penis.

mine flexibility of the pelvis by applying manual pressure to the lateral sides of the pelvis. Often it is possible to close the pelvic ring anteriorly with only moderate pressure.

Technique of Bladder Closure

The infant's entire lower body from nipples to knees is prepared and draped into the sterile field. The umbilicus is ligated and divided flush with the skin at the apex of the bladder mucosa. Size 5 French plastic catheters are placed in the ureters and sutured to the mucosa with fine catgut. The bladder mucosa is next separated from the skin of the abdominal wall with sharp dissection. Bleeding is minimized by using the electrocautery after the initial incision. If the bladder is small, 2 to 3 mm of skin is left attached to the bladder mucosa for traction and inclusion in the eventual closure (Fig. 91–2A). Bladder muscle fuses with the rectus muscles, and additional tissue may be gained by separating the full thickness of bladder together with peritoneum a bit laterally. As the dissection of the bladder proceeds inferiorly to the pubic bone, several blood vessels are encountered that must be coagulated. Sphincter muscle lying between the separated pubic bones is preserved by taking perichondrium from the bone, thus preserving every bit of tissue that can be wrapped around the bladder neck. The mucosa on the dorsum of the penis is then divided below the veru, extending the incision rostrally and laterally to outline paired flaps of thin skin from either side of the exstrophy, which will eventually be used to resurface the lengthened penis (Fig. 91–2B,C). The corpora

cavernosa are identified proximally and are followed laterally, detaching the erectile bodies from the inferior pubic rami to gain penile length (Fig. 91–2D,E). This dissection can be carried quite far laterally, as the corpora receive their blood supply and innervation via Alcock's canal. After the corpora have been mobilized satisfactorily, a row of 4-0 absorbable sutures are placed on the dorsal and ventral aspects to approximate the distal mobilized corpora in the midline, thus lengthening the penile portion of the corpora cavernosa. The flaps of mobilized skin attached to the penis are rotated to the midline to close the skin defect on the dorsal aspect of the lengthened penis.

The bladder has been dissected free from all surrounding tissue to at least 1 cm below the pubis. It now is folded in and the mucosa closed with interrupted chromic catgut or polyglycolate sutures. A Silastic mushroom catheter is placed at the apex of the bladder as a suprapubic tube, and the previously placed ureteral catheters are brought out the urethra. The bladder neck is closed and the splayed out external sphincter dissected from the pubic bones is wrapped around the bladder neck. The bladder muscle is closed with monofilament polyglyconate interrupted sutures. The neourethra is left widely patent, and the penis in a boy is left open as an epispadias. This will allow free drainage of urine until the second-stage operation. The bladder should have been separated enough from the pelvic ring to drop back into the pelvis. Several different types of sutures, including wire and nonabsorbable sutures, have been advocated for closure of the pubis. These often cut through the bladder neck or spit out. A heavy, size 0 plastic absorbable suture, such as monofilament polyglyconate, will hold the pubis together for 6 weeks, when there should be a solid fibrous union. Two of these heavy sutures are passed through or around the bone and tied down while an assistant applies manual pressure to the trochanters, pushing the pubis together. Closure of the pubis can be easily performed during the neonatal period without a pelvic osteotomy. This facilitates closure of the abdominal wall and brings together the separated puborectalis muscle. This step may contribute to the ultimate development of urinary continence, and by supporting the puborectalis, rectal prolapse is avoided. The rectus fascia and skin are closed, and both the ureteral catheters and suprapubic tubes are anchored to the skin with sutures and tape.

Postoperatively, the baby's legs are suspended in Bryant's traction because apposition of the legs will maintain position of the pubis. This traction is continued for 3 weeks, and even after the baby goes home, the legs are kept together with a soft bandage for a total of 6 weeks after the operation. The ureteral catheters are removed within a week or 10 days.

A cystogram is performed through the suprapubic catheter at 2 or 3 weeks after the operation to make sure there is free flow of urine from the neourethra and to determine if there is vesicoureteral reflux. Urine cultures, nuclear reflux scans, and either pyelograms or ultrasound examinations of the kidneys are carried out at intervals to follow the upper urinary tracts.

Antibiotics are continued for at least 6 months, and thereafter their use is based on cultures of the urine. Bladder capacity should increase over the first 2 or 3 years, but because of the abnormal entry of the ureters into the bladder wall, there is almost universal vesicoureteral reflux. At the second operation, the ureters are reimplanted, the bladder neck is tightened, and the penis is reconstructed. If a pubic closure was not done at the first operation, it should be done at this time.

Technique for Bladder Closure and Iliac Osteotomy

The baby is anesthetized and placed in the prone position. The sciatic notches are palpated. An incision is made 1 cm lateral to the sacroiliac joint. The gluteal muscles are divided in the line of the incision, exposing the periosteum and the outer table of the iliac bone. Just lateral to the joint, the periosteum is incised from the sciatic notch to the upper border of the ileac wing. An osteotome is then used to divide both the inner and outer tables. When working inferiorly, a blunt periosteal elevator is wedged into the sciatic notch to prevent the osteotome from cutting the gluteal artery. The cranial rim of growing cartilage is divided with the knife. The bony edges are then separated to ascertain that both bony tables are completely divided. The incision is closed, and the procedure is repeated on the opposite side.

Technique for Second-stage Bladder Neck Repair

The bladder is evaluated cystoscopically just before operation to determine the position of the ureters and the condition of the mucosa and the bladder neck. The bladder is opened by a midline incision, and the ureters are cannulated. The ureteric orifices will be too close to the bladder neck to permit tubularization to form a sphincter. Consequently, the ureters are reimplanted by the Cohen technique.[3] The ureters are detached and led through a new muscular hiatus about 2 cm above the original position. The ureters cross the midline on the posterior wall of the bladder so that an adequate ratio of intravesical ureteral length to width may be achieved to reliably prevent reflux. In exstrophy, because of weakness in the detrusor, a 7: or 8:1 ratio is preferred to the usual 5:1. The ureter is sutured to the underlying

muscle and overlying mucosa with fine chromic catgut to form the new meatus, which faces laterally.

In order to form the new bladder neck, designed to produce continence, a 3 cm strip of mucosa, 18 to 20 mm wide, extending from just distal to the new ureteric orifices to the urethra is outlined (Fig. 91-3D,E). Parallel incisions are made, and the mucosa is separated from the bladder muscle and rolled into a tube, which is sutured with fine catgut. A catheter or sound is passed from time to time to avoid making too narrow a tube. The detrusor is then incised on either side just lateral to the new bladder neck, and the outlined flaps of inferior bladder muscle are denuded of mucosa. These flaps are snugly interdigitated above the new trigonal urethra to provide needed outlet resistance (Fig. 91-3F). The newly formed sphincter can be tested by measuring the intravesical pressure through a suprapubic tube. An opening pressure of 30 to 34 cm of water is optional. Resistance above 35 cm of water is usually accompanied by postoperative hydronephrosis.

Attention is next turned to the epispadias repair (Fig. 91-4). A midline strip of dorsal penile skin 14 to 16 mm in width is outlined by parallel longitudinal skin incisions extending from the prostatic urethra through the glans to the tip of the penis. This strip is rolled into a tube and sutured. The corpora cavernosa lateral to the new urethra are approximated in the dorsal midline, giving the penis a more normal cylindrical appearance (Fig. 91-4), and the lateral edges of the glans are approximated over the distal portion of the urethra for a pleasing cosmetic effect. The ventral hood of foreskin is then detached just behind the corona and the foreskin is unrolled (Fig. 91-4E). This skin is transposed to the dorsal aspect of the penis by dividing the prepuce in the midline and transposing a flap along either side of the glans. The skin edges are tailored to conform with the contour of the penis as the more proximal dorsal skin edges are approximated to correct most of the reverse chordee.

Cystostomy drainage is maintained for 2 weeks, after which the cystostomy tube is clamped. If postoperative edema prevents urination, cystostomy drainage is maintained for another week, after which the tube is again clamped. If voiding occurs, the cystostomy is removed. If the child is unable to void, cystoscopy is performed to rule out a stricture. Adhesions obstructing the urethra can generally be lysed at this time by urethral dilatation. Eventually, edema will subside and the child will be able to urinate. Voiding may be difficult, with overflow incontinence, or the child may seem to leak from an empty bladder. Several months may pass before the child may begin to have dry periods with urinary control. An intravenous pyelogram is obtained in this interval. If upper tract dilatation becomes marked, interval neph-

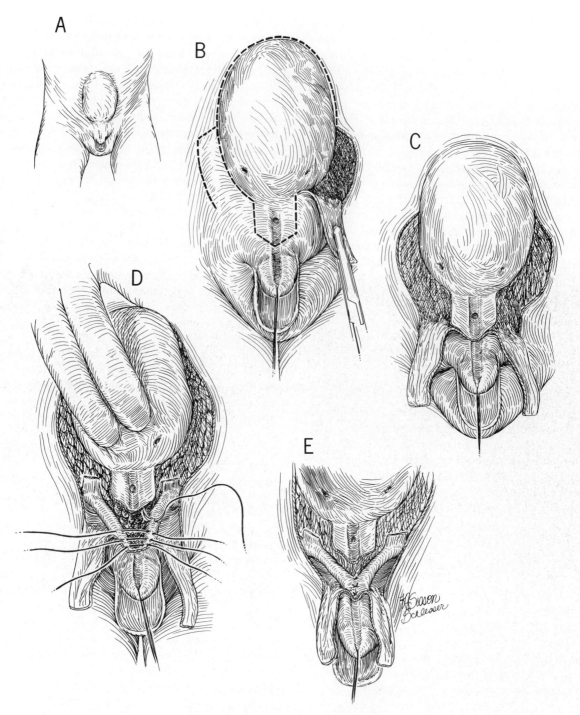

Figure 91–2. A. The technique of bladder closure with penile lengthening which is done in the neonatal period after posterior iliac osteotomies (after Jeffs). The infant is placed on his back, and the bladder is circumscribed. **B.** Flaps of mucosalike skin are raised on either side at the inferior margin of the exstrophy. **C.** The corpora cavernosa are partially detached from the underside of the inferior pubic rami and sewn together in the midline to lengthen the penile shaft (**D** and **E**).

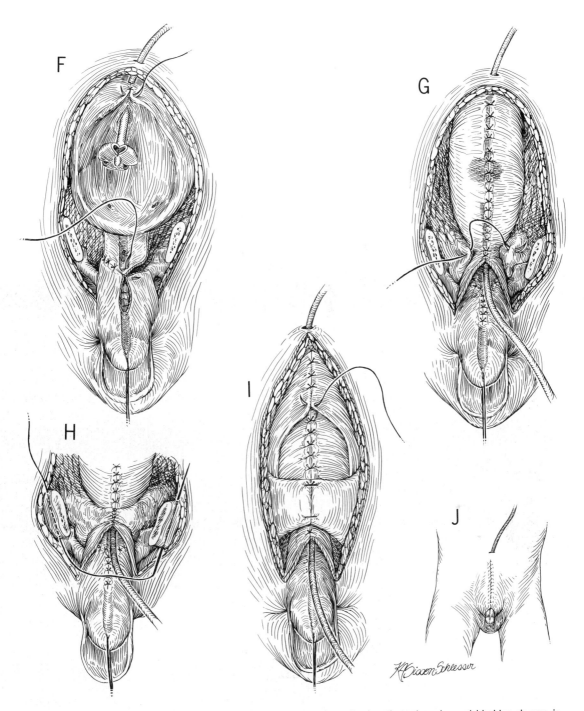

Figure 91–2 (Cont.). F. The flaps of skin are used to resurface the lengthened penis, and bladder closure is begun around a suprapubic tube. Ureteral catheters may be employed to keep the wound as dry as possible during healing. **G.** The bladder neck is closed, but not tightly, since no attempt is made to produce urinary continence at this stage. Paravesical connective tissue is closed over the bladder neck (**H**), and the pubic bones are approximated, which helps displace the bladder posteriorly into a more normal anatomic position. **J.** The epispadias repair is deferred until the second stage.

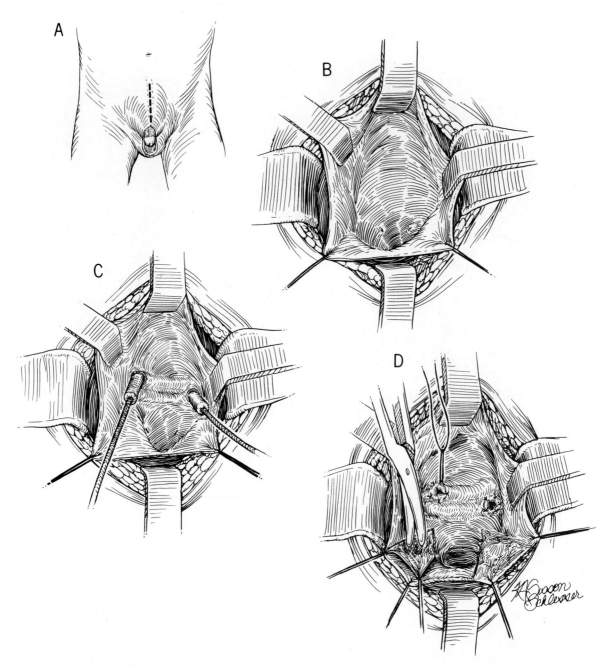

Figure 91–3. The second stage of exstrophy repair, usually performed when the child is 3 or 4 years of age. **A.** A midline incision is employed. **B.** The opened bladder. Since the trigone will be used to form a muscular urethral sphincter, the ureters must be reimplanted higher on the back of the bladder. **C.** The ureters are drawn through a new hiatus, and a crossed Cohen type of reimplant is performed (**D**).

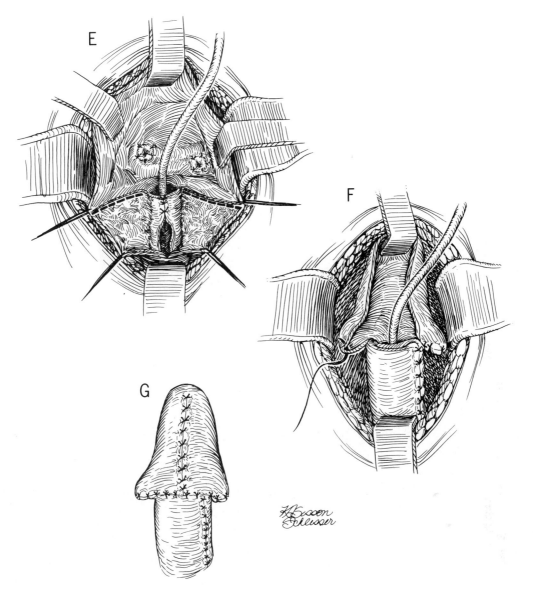

Figure 91–3 (Cont.). E. A strip of trigonal mucosa 18 mm wide and 3 cm long is rolled into a tube. The denuded trigonal muscle lateral to the tube is incised so that the muscle can be imbricated over the cylinder of mucosa forming a sphincter (**F**), and the bladder is then closed with a suprapubic tube in place (**G**). In males, the epispadias repair is then completed as shown in Figure 91–4.

rostomy should be considered to prevent ureterectasis or loss of kidney function, since these changes make secondary ureterosigmoidostomy more difficult and more hazardous.

If a fistula occurs in the epispadias repair, closure should be deferred for at least 6 months to allow full healing. This delay maximizes the possibility that secondary closure will be successful. While the child is anesthetized, a Z-plasty of the skin at the base of the penis usually is advisable to release residual dorsal chordee. In boys without fistula, skin contractures may necessitate further procedures to rotate more skin onto the dorsum of the penis. It is difficult to provide totally adequate dorsal penile skin coverage concomitant with the initial repair of the epispadias.

In girls, the epispadias repair consists only of approximating the paired clitoris and the labia in the anterior midline.

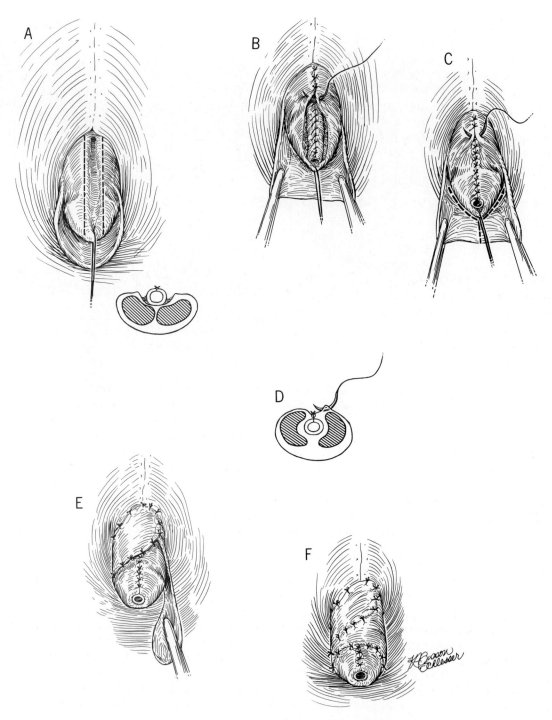

Figure 91–4. Epispadias repair. The penis was previously lengthened, as depicted in Figure 91–3, diagramming the first stage of exstrophy closure. **A.** Paired dorsal incisions free a strip of skin about 12 mm in width, which is rolled into a tube to provide needed urethral length. Lateral tissues are then approximated over the new urethra in two layers. (**B–D**). **C.** The ventral foreskin is then detached and unrolled and the skin transposed to the dorsum of the penis to provide needed skin coverage (**E,F**).

RESULTS

Early bladder closure results in an anatomically restored abdominal wall and prevents the complication of rectal prolapse. Early closure also protects the bladder mucosa and makes care of the infant much easier. The final measure of success is whether or not the child can remain dry long enough to participate in school and social affairs and is able to achieve sexual function. An average daytime dry interval exceeding 3 hours is considered an excellent result. Bladder continence after closure varies from 20 to 86 percent in various recent series of patients.[4–7] In a long-term follow-up of patients from the Mayo Clinic, the cosmetic appearance of the genitalia was considered satisfactory in 55 percent.[8] All patients had normal erectile function, and 61 percent of postpubertal patients had satisfactory intercourse. Twelve were married, and 5 had fathered children. Successful pregnancy is possible, but Cesarean section is advised for women who have undergone bladder closure.[9] Overall, most patients who have been followed for a prolonged period appear to be well adjusted socially.[10]

Urinary diversion may become necessary when bladder closure fails or if complications, such as hydronephrosis or persistent incontinence, develop.

CLOACAL EXSTROPHY

Cloacal exstrophy is far more complex than simple bladder exstrophy. The umbilical stalk is displaced inferiorly toward the tail end of the body, and there is an omphalocele of variable size, beneath which is the open bladder. Between the two bladder halves, there is a strip of intestinal mucosa, with an orifice in its center where meconium drains (Fig. 91–5). The strip of intestine represents the terminal ileum, with another orifice for the colon, which ends blindly. At the lower end of the mucosa, there are the two halves of either a small deformed penis or a divided clitoris. There may be a small vagina visible in a girl, but there is no anus, and the anal dimple seems to be displaced forward. There is practically no perineal body. The colon is often a short stub of cecum attached to the open mucosa, with perhaps a 3 or 4 cm segment of ascending colon. In addition, almost all the babies with this defect will have either an overt myelomeningocele or a tethered spinal cord. Thus, simple physical examination will reveal a constellation of defects of the genitourinary, gastrointestinal, and nervous systems. This constellation of defects has been termed "vesicointestinal fissure," "extrophia splanchnica," or even "turned-out organs." The early reports of this severe anomaly were pessimistic to the point that some authors recommended either no treatment or delayed urinary diversion and an ileostomy.[11–15] These

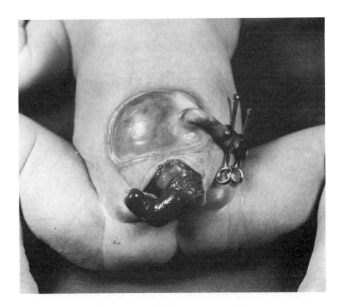

Figure 91–5. Cloacal exstrophy, or vesicointestinal fissure. There is a small omphalocele superiorly with prolapsed ileum between the two halves of the bladder.

babies often have a malrotation of the midgut with a shortened small intestine. There are so many variations of the anomaly that each must be described in detail, rather than giving them names or fitting them into a classification. In one variation, a partial cloacal exstrophy, there is a small omphalocele, with the bladder open only at its apex. The ileum enters the back wall of the bladder, and there is only a short stump of cecum and colon beyond the bladder. The diagnosis may be made by injecting contrast material into the bladder and visualizing the bladder and bowel (Fig. 91–6).

Complete functional reconstruction of an infant born with this severe defect is difficult or impossible. The complete repair of this anomaly may take several operations over the course of years, and even then the child may still be incontinent of stool and urine. The family members must be given complete information concerning their baby's condition and long-term prognosis. They should be given the opportunity to discuss the situation with other family members, their clergyman, and, perhaps, a lawyer if they decide against therapy. When there were severe associated defects, we have supported the family if they chose not to have an operation performed. These infants will often succumb to diarrhea and infection. We currently advise an attempt at repair of the bladder, with a pullthrough of the colon to the perineum in the neonatal period. If the infant is a boy, the diminutive size of the separated corpora cavernosa precludes reconstruction of male genitalia. Consequently, these infants are assigned female gender.[16,17] Complete repair of the bladder and bowel in the newborn period accomplishes several worthwhile goals. From a

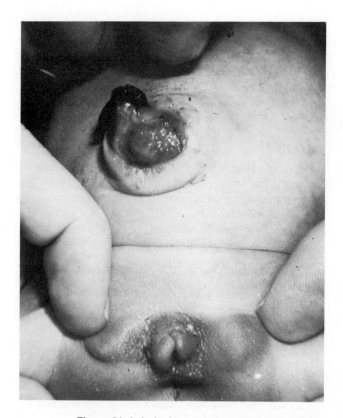 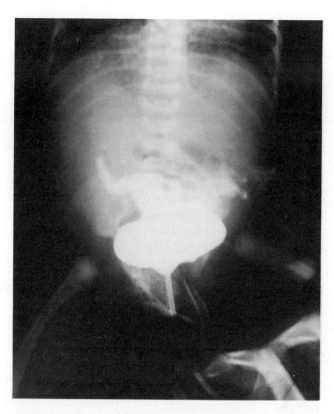

Figure 91–6. Left. A partial cloacal exstrophy. There is a small omphalocele, an imperforate anus, and a single opening on the perineum for stool and urine. **Right.** Contrast material injected into the perineal orifice outlines the bladder with attached ileum and a short segment of cecum. In this case, the bowel was detached from the bladder and pulled through to the perineum.

cosmetic standpoint, the abdominal wall can be made to look almost normal. Closure of the bladder protects its mucosa so it may distend and be reconstructed later in an attempt to achieve continence. By saving every bit of colon and pulling it through to the perineum, the absorptive surface of the bowel is maximized, and by closing the pubis, the levator sling is closed around the bowel, providing some chance for eventual fecal control. The problem of gender assignment is settled in the neonatal period before the infant goes home.

Preoperative studies include ultrasonography of the kidneys and spine with appropriate cardiac and neurosurgery consultation to determine the extent of associated anomalies. A major chromosomal defect is a contraindication to surgical correction.

Technique

The lower abdomen, perineum, back, and upper thighs are prepared and draped into a single sterile field. Excision of the omphalocele sac allows abdominal exploration and identification of internal genitalia, ureters, and the various segments of intestine. Each ureter is catheterized, and the catheters are sutured to the bladder mu-

cosa. The prolapsed ileum is replaced, and with traction on both the ileum and the stump of colon, the strip of mucosa with its blood supply is separated from the two lateral halves of the bladder with careful sharp dissection. This open bowel is now sutured into a tube, so the ileum is in continuity through the rolled tube with the stump of colon. The two halves of the bladder are sutured together, so the bladder is a simple exstrophy. It is separated from the abdominal wall and the separated pubis and rolled into a tube (Fig. 91–2). The testicles are removed from a boy, but the separated corpora are preserved to eventually form a clitoris and the vaginal vestibule. Since the pelvis is wide open, the puborectalis muscle is opened like a V, with its apex posterior on the perineum. With a nerve stimulator, it is possible to identify external sphincter muscle so the tip of the colon may be pulled through to the perineum within these fibers as well as within the levator complex. The pelvis may be so crowded with bowel and the bladder that it is difficult to completely close the pubis anteriorly. This step of the operation should be attempted, however. Two size 0 polyglyconate absorbable sutures are passed through the pubic bones, and with manual pressure on the trochanters by an assistant, the pubis is pulled together as far as possible. Closure of the rectus fascia then places the bladder beneath the abdominal wall, and the reconstructed urethra will be beneath the pubis. A suprapubic tube is left in place, and the ureteral catheters are brought out through the neourethra. The baby is placed in Bryant's traction to maintain apposition of the pubis for at least 3 weeks, and then at home, the legs are kept bandaged together. There is likely to be considerable edema and ureteral obstruction for several weeks. Therefore, contrast material should be injected into the ureteral catheters to ensure that there is good drainage of the kidneys before the catheters are removed (Fig. 91–7).

After the infant has recovered from this procedure, the myelodysplasia is reevaluated and repaired if indicated. The early removal of a lipomeningocele and release of a tethered cord may improve neurologic function.

We have examined these infants under anesthesia at intervals in order to dilate the neourethra and the anal openings. The bladder should have free drainage to avoid hydronephrosis, but we have tended to keep the anal opening small, making daily irrigations necessary to stimulate a bowel movement. With salvage of the colon, the short gut syndrome and diarrhea have not been problems. A complete evaluation is carried out at 3 to 4 years of age. At that time, a second-stage bladder repair is performed as described for bladder exstrophy.

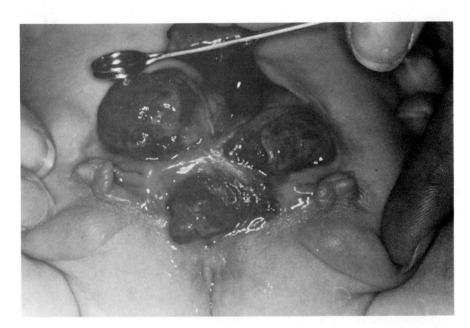

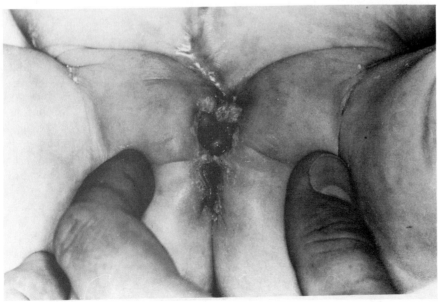

Figure 91–7. Cloacal exstrophy. **Top.** The umbilicus with a small omphalocele is at the top. The bladder halves protrude laterally and just inferior to the omphalocele. Lateral to the bladder there are duplicate vaginas and a separated clitoris. The bowel mucosa is beneath the bladder but between the duplicate vaginas. **Bottom.** Postoperative view. The rectal mucosa is slightly prolapsed. The orifice between the abdominal scar and the anus is the combined urethral opening and vagina. At 18 months, this child had partial rectal control.

One of our patients had ureteral reimplantation and a bladder augmentation with vaginal reconstruction with segments of intestine at another institution.

Results

There have been 11 infants with cloacal exstrophy treated at our hospital during the past 12 years. Two with severe chromosomal defects were given no active treatment and died. We have closed the bladder and pulled the colon through to the perineum in 6 infants, and the remaining 3 had bladder closure with an intestinal stoma. One child, a girl, who was operated on 12 years ago had a longer than usual length of colon, no myelodysplasia, and good perineal musculature. She is socially continent of both stool and urine. The bladder and abdominal wall separated completely in another child, who now has a ureterostomy and a colostomy. She has had multiple hospitalizations for recurrent urinary infections and diarrhea. She is our worst result. The remaining 4 children with pulled-through bowel are alive and do not have diarrhea, and 1 is socially continent of stool with daily irrigations. None are continent of urine, but only 1 had had a second-stage bladder operation. This experience is small, but it would appear that complete repair of both the bladder and bowel in one stage offers several advantages, including the conservation of all tissue, better intestinal absorption, and a reconstructed abdominal wall.

Howell et al. at the Philadelphia Children's Hospital have treated 15 patients, with an 85 percent long-term survival rate.[17] Their current recommendation is to remove the omphalocele, close the bladder, create an end colostomy, and assign the female gender. This is perhaps a safer and more conservative course of treatment than ours, which also leaves the door open to future anorectal reconstruction as well as secondary operations on the bladder in the hope of achieving continence. There is clearly no best treatment and no way, as yet, to compare the results of treatment.

REFERENCES

1. Culp DA: The histology of the exstophied bladder. J Urol 91:538, 1964
2. Muecke EC: The role of the cloacal membrane in exstrophy: The first successful experimental study. J Urol 92:659, 1964
3. Cohen SJ: Ureterozystoneostomie: Eine neue Antireflux-technik. Akt Urol 6:1, 1975
4. O'Donnell B: The lessons of 40 bladder exstrophies in 20 years. J Pediatr Surg 19:547, 1984
5. Ansell J: Exstrophy and epispadias. In Glenn J (ed): Urologic Surgery. Philadelphia, Lippincott, 1983, p 647
6. Mollard P: Bladder reconstruction in exstrophy. J Urol 124:523, 1980
7. Lepar H, Jeffs R: Primary bladder closure and bladder neck reconstruction in classical bladder exstrophy. J Urol 130:1142, 1983
8. Mesrobian H, Kelalis P, Kramer S: Long-term follow-up of cosmetic appearance and genital function in boys with exstrophy: Review of 53 patients. J Urol 136:256, 1986
9. Krisiloff M, Puchner P, Tretter W, et al: Pregnancy in women with bladder exstrophy. J Urol 119:478, 1978
10. Woodhouse C, Ransley P, Williams D: The exstrophy patient in adult life. Br J Urol 55:632, 1983
11. Spencer R: Estrophia splanchnica cloaca (exstrophy of the cloaca). Surgery 57:751, 1965
12. Markland C, Fraley EE: Management of infants with cloaca exstrophy. J Urol 109:740, 1973
13. Rickham PP: Vesoco-intestinal fissure. Arch Dis Child 35:97, 1960
14. Hayden PW, Chapman WH, Stevenson JK: Exstrophy of the cloaca. Am J Dis Child 125:879, 1973
15. Potts W: The Surgeon and the Child. Philadelphia, Saunders, 1959, pp 6–7
16. Tank E, Lindenauer S: Principles of management of exstrophy of the cloaca. Am J Surg 119:95, 1970
17. Howell C, Caldamone A, Snyder H, et al: Optimal management of cloacal exstrophy. J Pediatr Surg 18:365, 1983

SECTION XII

Functional and Acquired Disorders of the Esophagus

The ability to swallow normally, like many other bodily functions, is a gift that is taken for granted. The barium esophagogram, nuclear scanning, pH monitoring, and motility and pressure studies have contributed to our knowledge of esophageal function. These studies have been especially helpful in the diagnosis of gastroesophageal reflux. This was once thought to be a benign, self-limiting disorder but is now recognized as a major problem in pediatric practice. The more we learn about this particular problem, the more we realize that gastroesophageal incompetence may represent only one facet of an underlying central nervous system lesion.

Although a wave of enthusiasm has swept many pediatric surgical centers for the surgical treatment of reflux, the indications for operation are continuing to evolve. Furthermore, there would appear to be several different surgical procedures that are effective in the treatment of reflux. More time is needed to evaluate these operations.

Esophageal substitution still is occasionally necessary for children with congenital esophageal atresia, but for the most part, bypass of the esophagus is now most often performed for recalcitrant strictures of the esophagus secondary to caustic ingestion.

SECTION XI

Functional and Acquired Disorders of the Esophagus

92
Gastroesophageal Reflux

A normal esophagogastric junction that allows the passage of food yet prevents regurgitation of gastric contents back into the esophagus is critical for normal growth and development of children. Defects in this area lead to vomiting, failure to grow, esophagitis, pulmonary complications, and even sudden death. It is a difficult, complex area to understand, and there is tremendous controversy among investigators concerning the normal function of the gastroesophageal junction. There is also poor correlation between anatomic and physiologic findings with individual symptoms. Gastroesophageal reflux occurs relatively frequently in all age groups. All of us have suffered heartburn after a late evening spicy meal. Some degree of spitting up and vomiting is considered normal in infants up to 6 or 8 weeks of age. Thus, we commence with the premise that some reflux is normal. What are the limits of normal and how do we correlate our patient's symptoms with the findings of reflux? To make matters more complex, reflux is associated with many other diseases, particularly those of the central nervous system. It is sometimes difficult to know whether reflux is the cause of a problem, such as cough or wheezing, or merely a component of the basic disease. Some anatomic defects—hiatus hernia and esophageal atresia—predispose to reflux. Long-standing severe gastroesophageal reflux, by injuring the esophagus, sets up a vicious self-perpetuating cycle that will defy any treatment but surgical correction of the reflux.

NORMAL PHYSIOLOGY

In the newborn infant, swallowing-induced peristaltic waves cause a momentary relaxation of the distal end of the esophagus to allow food to pass into the esophagus. The distal, or intraabdominal, portion of the esophagus is the critical point in preventing the regurgitation of food and gastric juice into the thoracic esophagus. In older children and adults, there is a high pressure zone in the abdominal esophagus that contributes to the valve-like mechanism in this area.

Anatomically, the intraabdominal esophagus is no more than 3 to 4 cm in length, but it is 1.5 cm in young children.[1] Physiologically, manometric studies have demonstrated that the intraabdominal esophagus is actually longer, approximately 1 cm at birth and up to 3 cm by 6 months of age. Boix-Ochoa has performed 4000 manometric esophageal measurements in 680 normal infants from 1 day to 6 months of age, which have elegantly demonstrated the importance of the intraabdominal esophagus.[2] A pressure of between 5 and 7 mm Hg in this segment is necessary to prevent significant reflux. Maturation of this sphincter mechanism is achieved by 6 or 7 weeks of age, or about the time when normal infants cease to spit up. The differential between positive intraabdominal pressure and the negative intrathoracic pressure contributes to the antireflux mechanism by a sucking effect, which collapses the intraabdominal esophagus. An acute angle of His also is important; when fluid is injected into the stomach of dogs under pressure, the fundus fills first and compresses the esophagus, closing it off. Finally, mucosal folds at the esophagogastric junction act as a choke valve, further preventing reflux.[3] When the stomach is above the diaphragm, as in a hiatal hernia, none of these mechanisms are in force, and there is no obstacle to the free reflux of gastric contents into the esophagus.[4]

In attempting to explain the mechanisms involved in gastroesophageal reflux, most investigators concentrate on measuring the lower esophageal sphincter pressure (LESP). Some have found higher LESP pressures in the newborn and young infant than Boix-Ochoa found.[5,6] Differences in the actual pressures are probably of no importance, since the measurements depend on the type of catheter, whether or not the child is fed, the child's position, and whether he or she is asleep or awake. Most studies agree, however, that children with reflux have a lower LESP than normal.[7-9] A delay in gastric emptying also may contribute to gastroesophageal reflux. Is this a cause of reflux, or is it merely a part of delayed neuromuscular development?[10-13]

Local anatomic defects, such as a hiatus hernia (Fig. 92–1) or a paralyzed diaphragm, completely alter all the normal mechanisms against reflux. In particular, the angle of His becomes more obtuse, and with even a small portion of the stomach above the diaphragm, there is no pressure differential to collapse the distal esophagus, and the mucosal folds will not coapt to close off the junction. Perhaps the most important factor is neuromuscular development. Delay in maturation may account for reflux in the infant. Most likely, there is some abnormality in neurologic development that may not be detect-

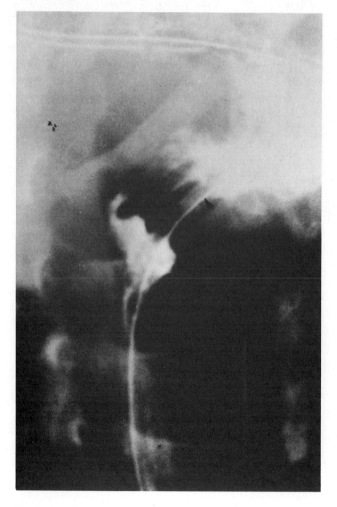

Figure 92–1. The rugal folds above the diaphragm are diagnostic of a hiatus hernia. Abdominal pressure was required to demonstrate this finding.

able during infancy. Certainly in older children, brain damage from any cause is associated with not only gastroesophageal reflux but abnormalities of oropharyngeal function as well. Control of the gastroesophageal junction and esophageal junction is in the midbrain. Increased intraabdominal pressure can overcome the defense mechanisms against reflux in the hypertonic child with cerebral palsy and perhaps in the child with asthma or cystic fibrosis who tenses the abdominal muscles to cough. This also may be a factor in the premature infant who struggles against a ventilator, tensing the abdominal muscles.

Small amounts of refluxed gastric contents are removed rapidly by normal esophageal peristalsis. Twenty-four hour pH monitoring has demonstrated that the severity of esophagitis is in proportion to the quantity of refluxed material and the duration of time it is in contact with the esophageal mucosa.[14,15] The duration of each reflux episode is correlated also with respiratory complications.[16] Thus, a small amount of reflux will cause more problems if there is poor esophageal motility. This is often seen in infants who have been operated on for esophageal atresia, and may be a factor in some neurologically impaired children. Even when poor esophageal motility persists, if the reflux is controlled, symptoms are relieved.[17]

SYMPTOMS OF REFLUX

The first and most common symptom of gastroesophageal reflux is vomiting. This often commences during the first days of life. At first, the vomiting is thought to be normal because the vomitus consists only of the baby's formula, is not stained with bile, and regurgitation is usually effortless. The vomiting may take place during the feeding but most often occurs just after the infant has taken the bottle. Bloody or coffee-ground emesis occurs in children who have esophagitis. We observed massive hematemesis in two children—one had severe peptic esophagitis and another had a single esophageal ulcer just above a hiatus hernia. Mild anemia is a frequent finding, which may reflect malnutrition as well as chronic blood loss from esophagitis.

Failure to gain weight, with retardation in the attainment of developmental milestones, occurs in direct proportion to the degree of vomiting and malnutrition. Infants with gastroesophageal reflux frequently are referred with the diagnosis of pyloric stenosis. When the typical olive cannot be felt, gastroesophageal reflux is a likely diagnosis.

Pulmonary complications consisting of episodic aspiration pneumonia, chronic nocturnal wheezing, and cough are the next most common symptoms. Chronic aspiration may occur without vomiting, causing wheezing that simulates allergic asthma.[18,19] These symptoms commence during the first few months of life, but the diagnosis is often delayed while the child is treated with antibiotics, bronchodilators, and even steroids. Close questioning may reveal a history of nocturnal regurgitation, with food particles found in the child's bed. There must be a clear history of aspiration before reflux is accepted as a cause of asthma. In one patient sample, 47 percent of steroid-dependent asthmatic children had reflux, but medical therapy made no difference in symptoms.[20] Nighttime continuous pH studies have demonstrated that nighttime apnea, coughing, and choking are more likely than wheezing to result from reflux.[21,22] Massive aspiration of gastric contents has resulted in the deaths of children with hiatus hernias and gastroesophageal reflux.[23,24] Leape et al. clearly documented the association between gastroesophageal reflux and episodes of respiratory arrest in 10 infants under 6 months of age. Five of their patients had no previous history of vomiting or other sign of reflux. They proposed that occult reflux causes laryngospasm and may initiate the sudden infant death syndrome.[25] Similar observations were made by Herbst et al.[26] We observed an episode of respiratory arrest while one of our patients was lying supine during a nuclear scan, which demonstrated reflux, and a 4-month-old infant had several apneic episodes in the hospital while she was being treated for asthma. Unfortunately, although reflux occurs in many infants with apnea, there is not always a clear-cut causal relationship. Simultaneous polysomnographic and esophageal pH recordings suggest that apnea and episodic reflux are not always related, but both may represent developmental delay.[27,28]

Strictures secondary to chronic peptic esophagitis are more likely to occur in older children (Fig. 92–2), but we saw a stricture in a 6-month-old infant with chronic, severe reflux. Of 28 cases of stenosis reported by Monereo et al., 20 had a history of vomiting since birth.[29]

Reflux is associated with a variety of neurologic diseases, including Down's syndrome, cerebral palsy, the Riley-Day syndrome, hydrocephalus, and head injury.[30] Frequently, the vomiting is blamed on a central nervous system problem when the child actually has severe reflux. The rumination syndrome, in which a child will regurgitate, chew, and reswallow previously ingested food, has been found in babies with hiatus hernia.[31] Perhaps the most bizarre clinical picture is the Sandifer syndrome. This involves children with a history of vomiting soon after birth who commence to assume bizarre torsion spasms of the neck and abnormal posturing.[32] Apparently, these maneuvers help the child to swallow. In our practice, many children with gastroesophageal reflux

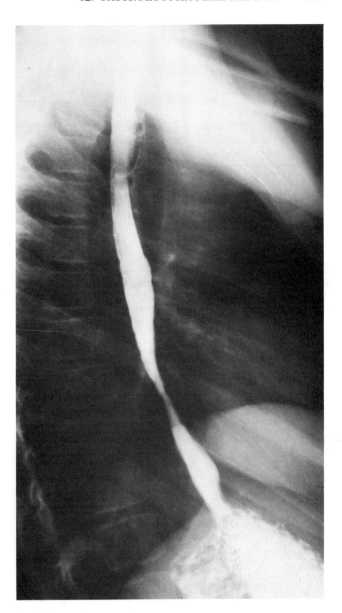

Figure 92–2. Esophageal stricture secondary to reflux esophagitis in an 8-year-old boy. He had persistent vomiting as an infant, then was asymptomatic until he developed dysphagia at 6 years of age. He was cured with a Nissen fundoplication and dilatation with mercury bougies.

that requires treatment during the early months of life have some form of neurologic damage. This may not be evident until the child is older and fails to meet developmental milestones. There also appears to be a correlation between infants who have apneic spells and subclinical neurologic deficits.

Associated medical problems in our series of 121 patients treated from 1980 to 1987 included 46 with neuromuscular diseases, 12 with esophageal atresia, 4 with diaphragmatic hernia, and 49 with multiple assorted congenital anomalies or severe prematurity. Only 10 of our patients were normal aside from their reflux.

DIAGNOSIS

The history must include a complete documentation of the onset and character of the child's vomiting or respiratory symptoms. Frequently, the mother will observe that the child vomits less when held upright than when in the supine position. It is helpful to observe the mother while she feeds the baby and to actually see the child vomit. Frequently what the mother considers vomiting is really normal spitting up. A history of weight loss or failure to gain weight is significant in differentiating true organic lesions from normal regurgitation. The physical examination must include auscultation of the chest and a neurologic examination. The usual laboratory determinations are nonspecific, but one should check the blood count for anemia and the serum electrolytes if there has been persistent vomiting.

An esophagogram with an upper gastrointestinal follow-through is essential for any infant with unexplained vomiting or respiratory symptoms. If the examination is to be of any value in the detection of esophageal reflux or a hiatal hernia, the radiologist must have considerable experience with children. Cinefluoroscopy with recording of the study on film or tape also is essential. It is helpful if the clinician tells the radiologist that he or she suspects gastroesophageal reflux. Fluoroscopy commences with the infant in the supine position, drinking barium from a bottle. An esophagus that is flaccid with shallow and inadequate peristaltic waves is often seen with reflux. After the barium has passed through into the stomach, it is observed during crying and deep inspiration as well as with abdominal pressure. Reflux is more likely to occur when barium is in the antrum of the stomach (Fig 92–3). After this initial examination, the infant is examined in the prone and the Trendelenburg positions. Reflux may be transitory and only momentarily visible.[33] It is often difficult to determine if there is stomach above the diaphragm. The criteria used by British roentgenologists for the diagnosis of a hiatus hernia include finding of wormlike rugal folds above the diaphragm, an intrathoracic pouch that lacks peristalsis, and a vestibule that is almost closed between the barium-filled esophagus and the diaphragm[34](Figs. 92–1 and 92–2). Unfortunately, roentgenograms may demonstrate reflux in normal infants, and on occasion reflux is discovered with other techniques that was not demonstrable on x-rays.

Gastroesophageal scintiscanning, using technetium-99m-sulfur colloid, is a convenient, noninvasive technique that accurately demonstrates reflux.[35] This test is particularly useful in children because unlike x-rays,

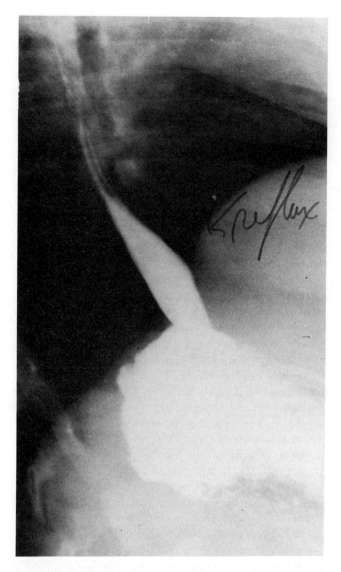

Figure 92–3. Reflux of barium into the esophagus without any evidence of a hiatus hernia. This must be documented with cinefluoroscopy.

which require considerable manipulation, once the isotope has been swallowed or infused into the stomach via a tube, the infant may rest in any position and often will go to sleep. Thus, the test is performed under more normal conditions. In our hospital, the scintiscan has demonstrated reflux when roentgenograms were normal. pH monitoring of the distal esophagus has proven to be a sensitive diagnostic test for reflux.[36,37] A pH probe is passed through the nose and positioned in the distal esophagus, monitoring either by x-ray or by manometery. Gastric pH must be between 1 and 3. A continuous recording is made over a 24-hour period, during sleep, in various positions, and after eating. An episode of reflux is defined as a drop in esophageal pH below 4 for at least 15 seconds. The 24-hour monitoring of upper esophageal pH is particularly important in the evaluation of patients with pneumonia and apnea.[38] The most sensitive study yet devised for continuous esophageal pH monitoring consists of a computerized teletransmission system that records pH data at 15-second intervals from four levels within the esophagus.[39] By comparing the results of this study against other tests and patient outcome, extended pH monitoring was 92 percent accurate in detecting clinically important gastroesophageal reflux. It has the further advantage of allowing outpatient studies during the patient's normal activities. According to esophageal pH studies, asymptomatic individuals have about one episode of reflux per hour. Patients with severe esophagitis have the most severe and prolonged reflux, with the poorest acid clearance from the esophagus. pH studies document reflux but fail to pinpoint the cause of the abnormality. Furthermore, it is still necessary to prove that the symptom under study correlates with the pH findings. Esophagoscopy with the flexible endoscope is the best method to evaluate the effects of reflux on the esophageal mucosa. One can observe gradations in the severity of esophagitis from mild hyperemia to severe inflammation and even ulcer formation. Mild esophagitis can be detected only with a mucosal biopsy.[40] By observing the esophagogastric junction, one can determine whether or not it is continually open and patulous, as in a hiatus hernia, or closes normally. Periodic esophagoscopy also is useful to follow the course of therapy for esophagitis.

It is not necessary to perform all tests in every child. The barium esophagogram, in most cases, will provide all the information necessary to plan a course of treatment. When the symptoms suggest reflux and the esophagogram demonstrates massive repeated reflux, there is no doubt about the diagnosis. If x-rays are equivocal, our next test is the scintiscan. If this is positive, one can assume that the diagnosis is correct. pH studies are required only in difficult diagnostic situations, such as to determine if reflux is the cause of respiratory problems.

TREATMENT

The treatment of a child with gastroesophageal reflux depends on age and severity of symptoms. Almost all otherwise well infants who vomit as a result of reflux will commence to have symptoms by 6 weeks of age. If nothing is done, most will become symptom free, by 8 months. It is an extremely rare infant who will not respond promptly to medical therapy. We have not operated on an infant solely for vomiting in our hospital for over 10 years. Conservative therapy begins with reducing the volume while increasing the frequency of feedings. Although there is controversy about the value of thickened feedings, we advise the addition of at least 2 or 3 teaspoons of rice cereal to each bottle. In the past, infants were placed upright in an infant seat. This position produces more episodes of reflux than if the patient is placed prone in a 30 degree upright position.[41,42]

The prone, upright position is maintained by placing extra cushions beneath the head end of the crib mattress, then placing a small pillow or sandbag at the baby's feet to prevent sliding. This position is maintained all the time the baby is out of the mother's arms. Attempts to keep babies upright in special chairs fail, partly because they slump forward, pushing up their diaphragms. The prone upright position places the esophagogastric junction above the pool of fluid in the stomach. These simple measures can be carried out at home. When successful, vomiting promptly improves, and success is noted by satisfactory weight gain. Babies with more severe vomiting who fail this therapy or others in whom the diagnosis is delayed and there is either weight loss or failure to thrive require more vigorous therapy. Intravenous fluids and even hyperalimentation may be required initially to correct dehydration and malnutrition. Bethanechol is a parasympathomimetic drug that increases peristaltic activity in both the esophagus and stomach. It has proven effective in controlling symptoms and decreasing the number of episodes of reflux as measured by pH studies.[43–45] Some of the improvement may have resulted from an increase in the lower esophageal sphincter pressure. The 24-hour dose of bethanechol is 8.7 mg/m^2 per day given in three divided doses. Domperidone, a benzimidazole derivative, another drug that promotes gastric emptying and improves esophageal motility, has also proved to be helpful in treating reflux. Up to 0.6 mg/kg dose of this drug has been given four times daily without side effects.[46] Some babies with reflux appear to be in pain, probably because of esophagitis. They seem to feel better when given small doses of antacids several times a day.

This intense medical therapy is commenced in the hospital. When vomiting stops and the baby gains weight, the parents are taught the importance of postural therapy and thickened feedings. When they understand how to care for their baby, he or she is allowed to go home but must be followed carefully to see that weight gain is maintained. Plotting weight on growth charts is an excellent way to follow these infants. Surgical therapy is practically never required in uncomplicated gastroesophageal reflux. Only 4.2 percent of 1525 patients in Boix-Ochoa et al.'s series who were under 1 year of age required an operation.[47] The successful conservative therapy in these younger patients most likely represents normal maturation of the lower esophageal sphincter. They must be followed for prolonged periods of time because esophagitis and stricture formation can develop insidiously.

An operation is indicated when reflux is shown definitely to produce apneic spells or when there are repeated episodes of aspiration pneumonia. Often, infants with recurrent pneumonia are poorly nourished and neglected and fail to respond to conservative management. Sometimes, the only way to overcome the aspiration is to put them on nothing by mouth and intravenous nutrition in preparation for an operation. Some infants have choking or gagging spells that are difficult to correlate with reflux. Occasionally, these symptoms are refractory to medical therapy, and there is great parental anxiety. One must be extremely careful in operating on infants with these unusual symptoms. Reflux that occurs after repair of an esophageal atresia is a special problem that is likely to require an operation.[48,49] The disordered peristalsis in the distal esophagus prevents clearing of gastric acid and contributes to recalcitrant anastomotic strictures. Infants and children with neurologic problems due to birth asphyxia or congenital brain abnormalities have multiple problems in addition to gastroesophageal reflux. These pitiful infants often are unable to eat or to swallow their own saliva. They not only have reflux, but also suffer from oropharyngeal discoordination and require tube feedings. They have aspiration pneumonia and are malnourished. Some are referred for a gastrostomy for "easier nursing care." This is hardly an indication for major surgery, and an operation should be undertaken only after long discussions with the family and referring physicians. A soft, plastic feeding tube is no more difficult to care for than a gastrostomy tube. If, on the other hand, there is some hope of recovery or if a nasogastric tube interferes with speech development and the family clearly understands the risks and benefits, one may offer a gastrostomy. Tube gastrostomies have been implicated in the development of reflux by interfering with the lower esophageal sphincter.[50-53] It is far more likely that either reflux was overlooked before the gastrostomy or there was progression of the neurologic disease. It is also possible that the larger feedings given through the gastrostomy tube resulted in overdistention of the stomach and reflux. These infants should have an antireflux procedure carried out at the same time a feeding gastrostomy is performed if there is the slightest suspicion of reflux. An antireflux procedure will not change the oropharyngeal discoordination nor stop the aspiration of saliva.

Severely retarded or brain-damaged older children also are referred for gastrostomy or an antireflux procedure. They may have suffered from chronic vomiting for years and have severe esophagitis and chronic aspiration pneumonia.[54] This group of patients has a high incidence of postoperative complications, including death from pneumonia and poor wound healing. Spastic patients have a high incidence of breakdown of the repair.

For these reasons, an operation should be approached cautiously. These complications can be reduced by a period of continuous tube feeding, hyperalimentation, and drug therapy to improve peristalsis and reduce gastric acidity. Every effort should be made to control seizures and spasticity with anticonvulsant medications. Medical measures will control symptoms in about one fourth of these patients.[55] They are, however, less responsive to medical management than nonbrain-damaged patients, but a period of intensive care will improve their general condition.

Surgical Management

There are a number of procedures that will control gastroesophageal reflux with a minimum of complications. They have in common the placement of the gastroesophageal junction well below the diaphragm to lengthen the intraabdominal esophagus, recreation of an acute angle of His, and the creation of a valvelike mechanism to force the fundus of the stomach against the esophagus. At this time, the Nissen fundoplication and the anterior fundoplication of Thal are the most popular operations in the United States.[56,57]

Nissen Fundoplication. A size 22 to 38 mercury bougie is passed through the child's mouth and into his stomach after the induction of anesthesia. A left subcostal incision is made, providing excellent exposure (Fig. 92–4). The falciform ligament and the left triangular ligament are divided, and the liver is rolled under and held out of the way with a moist laparotomy pad and a retractor. The superior three or four short gastric vessels are carefully suture-ligated and divided to provide complete mobility of the greater curvature of the stomach. The spleen is then covered with a moist pad and retracted inferiorly. This allows excellent exposure of the esophagogastric junction. The peritoneum overlying the esophagus is opened, and the esophagus is mobilized with scissors dissection. A soft Penrose drain is then passed about the esophagus, which is elevated. Further peritoneal attachments of the stomach to the diaphragm and the posterior abdominal wall are divided, and the diaphragmatic crura are cleared of fatty tissue. During this dissection, small vessels are electrocoagulated. Regardless of whether or not a hiatus hernia has been radiologically identified, the crura are sutured together. Since the diaphragmatic crura are muscular, sutures are likely to pull out. In the past, a loose hiatus has allowed the entire fundoplication to retract up into the chest. Consequently, we now use 2-0 or 3-0 mattress sutures that are threaded through Teflon felt pledgets. These sutures are tied relatively loosely. The addition of the pledgets provides greater security in holding the crura together during postoperative coughing and straining. Three to four cm of esophagus is mobilized into the abdomen in infants and 5 to 6 cm in older children.

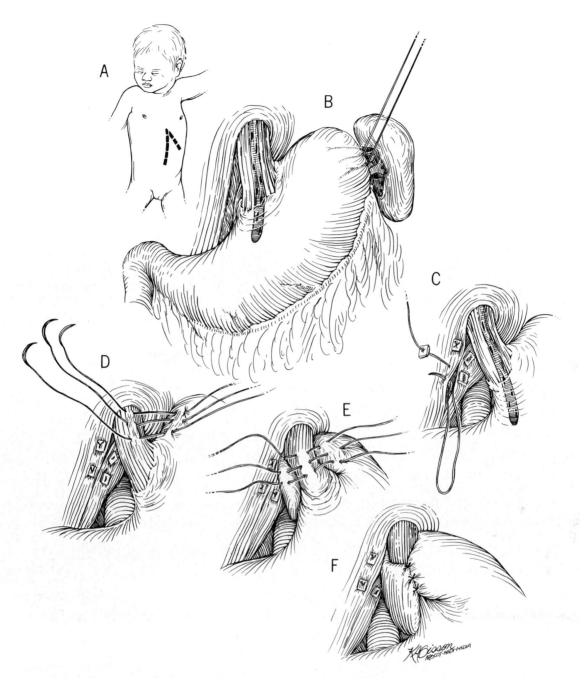

Figure 92–4. Nissen fundoplication. **A.** The operation may be performed through either a vertical or a left subcostal incision. **B.** A large catheter (from size 22 in infants to size 38 in older children) is placed in the esophagus. The short gastric vessels are ligated and divided to mobilize the upper one third of the greater curvature. **C.** The hiatus is closed with silk sutures, which are passed through Teflon felt pledgets. Large bites of tissue are taken. **D.** The apex of the greater curvature is then sutured to the intraabdominal esophagus. All of these sutures are placed and then tied. **E.** The sutures placed for the wrap are also passed through the esophageal wall. **F.** A second row of sutures is then placed to create a fundoplication 1 or 2 inches in length.

We have observed recurrences when the esophagus pulled completely out of its "wrap." This is prevented by suturing the greater curvature to the esophagus with three or four sutures (Fig. 92–4D). The first is placed just at the esophagogastric junction, and all are inserted before they are tied. With this accomplished, a Babcock forceps is used to grasp the posterior portion of the greater curvature, which is brought to the right side of the esophagus. The first row of sutures is placed through the anterior fold of the stomach, taking a bite of esophagus and then passing through the posterior fold of the stomach. The first row of sutures determines the tightness of the fundoplication. The plication should be loose even around the mercury dilator. With this accomplished, a few sutures are taken between the fundus of the stomach and the undersurface of the diaphragm. We perform a gastrostomy on poorly nourished infants, on brain-damaged children, and whenever it seems necessary to dilate an esophageal stricture during the postoperative period. A pyloroplasty is performed if there has been any evidence of pyloric obstruction.

Postoperative Care. The gastrostomy tube or a soft nasogastric tube is kept on gravity drainage until there are good bowel sounds and no evidence of distention. The tube is clamped for 24 hours before oral liquids are allowed. When the child can tolerate liquids by mouth, the diet is advanced to include the foods that are usual for the age group. Strictures associated with reflux will not resolve until after the reflux is corrected. Dilatations are commenced at the time of the fundoplication and are continued at intervals until the esophagus is of normal caliber. O'Neill et al. found that 3 of 18 patients required only intraoperative dilatations, and the rest had from 1 to 10 more dilatations over the course of 8 months after surgery.[58] All their patients were cured or symptomatically improved. Nine of our 121 patients required reoperation because the Nissen fundoplication slipped into the chest. One Nissen fundoplication was converted to a Thal fundoplication. Most of these occurred early in our series and have been eliminated by using sutures with pledgets to close the crura and a second row of sutures in the fundoplication. We now perform a Thal partial fundoplication if there is poor esophageal peristalsis.

Paraesophageal hiatus hernia requiring reoperation has been observed in from 8 to 15 percent of patients.[59,60] In these patients, as well as ours, it appeared at reoperation that the crural repair had disrupted to allow the fundic wrap to retract into the chest. All authors stress the importance of careful suture repair of the hiatus at the time of the original operation. The problem of a Nissen wrap that is too tight is rarely mentioned, but in our experience, it has been a concern, especially when esophageal motility is poor. Postoperative dilatations may help the patient's symptoms of dysphagia, but one of our patients required complete release of the fundoplication. In almost all series, the Nissen fundoplication has provided almost 100 percent effective relief for vomiting, failure to thrive, aspiration pneumonia, and strictures.[61,62]

It is difficult to estimate the incidence of minor annoying symptoms, such as slow eating, minor dysphagia, or occasional choking spells, that are attributed to the operation. In 25 children recalled for long-term follow-up after 5 years by the group in Salt Lake City, 36 percent had mild to moderate symptoms of gas bloat, 28 percent were unable to burp or vomit, 32 percent were described as being slow eaters, and 25 percent choked on solid foods. Since 17 patients in this group had a Boerema anterior gastropexy, which does not disturb the gastroesophageal junction, it is difficult to relate these symptoms to the operation.[63] Children who are operated on for reflux who have major neurologic problems will continue to experience symptoms related to their primary disease. Thus, in patients with familial dysautonomia, vomiting, aspiration pneumonia, and esophageal bleeding were controlled by an operation, but the dysautonomic crises were unaffected.[64]

Thal Fundoplication. The long-term annoying complications of the Nissen fundoplication have increased interest in operations that will control reflux yet interfere less with the gastroesophageal junction. The Thal operation, popularized in children by Ashcraft et al., increases the length of the intraabdominal esophagus, restores an acute angle of His, and creates a valvelike effect by applying a patch of the gastric fundus to the esophagus.[65] Since the wrap is incomplete, the child can still burp and vomit postoperatively, thus eliminating the problems associated with the gas bloat syndrome and dysphagia associated with poor esophageal peristalsis. Ashcraft's long-term results have answered earlier criticism that the partial fundoplication would not control reflux as efficiently as the Nissen operation.

The esophagus is mobilized as described for the Nissen operation, taking care to include the posterior vagus nerve with the esophagus in the encircling tape (Fig. 92–5). The esophageal crura are closed with a figure-8 suture, which is also passed through the back wall of the esophagus to fix the intraabdominal segment of the esophagus. From 2 to 4 cm of esophagus is exposed below the diaphragm, depending on the age of the child. Traction applied to the encircling tape at the esophagogastric junction exposes both the esophagus and the stomach. A 2-0 suture is started at the gastroesophageal junction on the greater curvature side. This is tied and then is run up the left side of the esophagus, taking bites through the greater curvature. At the top of the esophagus, this suture incorporates bites of stomach, the diaphragmatic hiatus, and the esophagus. The suture is then continued down the right side of the esophagus, again taking bites through the esophageal muscularis and the stomach (Fig. 92–5B). This suture applies the anterior wall of the stomach to the esophagus as a patch over more than 180 degrees of its circumference.

The incidence of postoperative reflux appears to be no more with this operation than with the Nissen fundoplication, and Ashcraft et al. had only 14 patients in 605 who required reoperation because of breakdown of the fundoplication or the development of a hiatus hernia.[65]

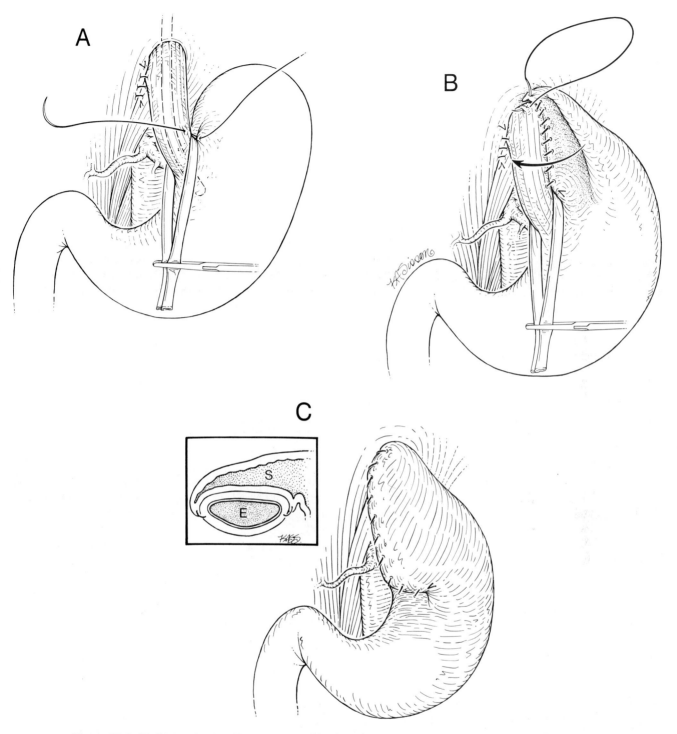

Figure 92–5. Thal fundoplication. The exposure of the esophagus and hiatus is similar to that described for the Nissen operation. It is not necessary to ligate the short gastric arteries to the spleen because only the anterior wall of the stomach is mobilized for the fundoplication. A suture closes the hiatus, and is used to anchor the esophagus in the abdomen. **A.** A tape is passed around the esophagus, exactly at its junction with the stomach. A continuous suture is commenced to the left of the esophagus. **B.** The suture is continued up the esophagus and takes bites of stomach, diaphragmatic hiatus, and esophagus. **C.** The suture continues down the right side of the esophagus to achieve approximately a 180 to 210 degree partial wrap around the anterior wall of the esophagus. (*After Ashcraft.*)

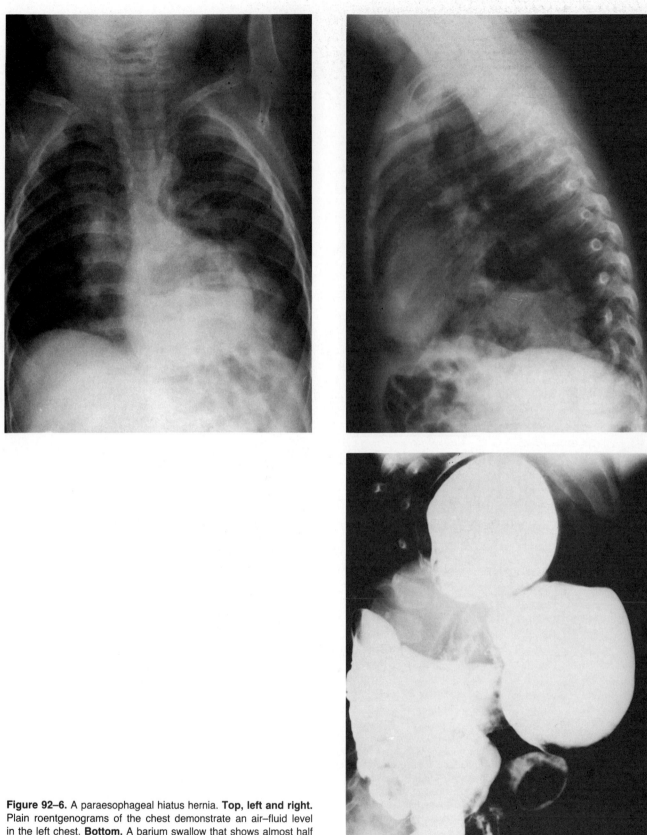

Figure 92–6. A paraesophageal hiatus hernia. **Top, left and right.** Plain roentgenograms of the chest demonstrate an air–fluid level in the left chest. **Bottom.** A barium swallow that shows almost half the stomach above the diaphragm. This type of hernia is not associated with reflux, but the stomach may twist to form a volvulus.

PARAESOPHAGEAL HIATUS HERNIA

The esophagogastric junction is normally below the diaphragm in a paraesophageal hernia. There is a peritoneal sac extending through the hiatus alongside the esophagus that allows the greater curvature of the stomach to extend up into the chest. Three children at the Children's Memorial Hospital with paraesophageal hiatus hernia vomited during the newborn period. Another was asymptomatic until 4 weeks of age, when she commenced to vomit. This child had both a pyloric stenosis and a large hernia. Afflicted children may be asymptomatic, but volvulus and strangulation of the stomach can occur.

Diagnosis

Plain chest roentgenograms will demonstrate an air–fluid level in the lower chest behind the heart. An upper gastrointestinal examination readily makes the diagnosis (Fig. 92–6).

Treatment

An operation is indicated when the diagnosis is made. A symptomatic child is operated on as an emergency procedure because of the danger of volvulus of the stomach. The operation is performed through the abdomen. After mobilization of the left lobe of the liver, the stomach is pulled down into the abdomen. The peritoneal sac is removed, and the edges of the defect are carefully outlined. In some cases, the diaphragmatic crura may be intact, with a defect lateral to the true hiatus. In either case, the defect is closed with mattress sutures and reinforced with pledgets of Teflon felt to prevent the sutures from cutting through the muscle tissue.

REFERENCES

1. Botha CS: The gastroesophageal region of infants. Arch Dis Child 33:78, 1958
2. Boix-Ochoa J: The physiologic approach to the management of gastric-esophageal reflux. J Pediatr Surg 21:1032, 1986
3. Edward DA: The raspberry or "flutter" valve in the antireflux mechanism. In Smith AN (ed): Surgical Physiology of the Gastrointestinal Tract: Proceedings of a Symposium. Edinburgh, Royal Coll. Surgeons of Edinburgh, 1962, pp 24–28
4. Chrispin AP, Freidland GW: Functional disturbances in hiatal hernia in infants and children. Thorax 22:422, 1967
5. Moroz S, Beiko P: Relationship between lower esophageal sphincter pressure and serum gastrin concentration in the newborn infant. J Pediatr 99:725, 1981
6. Vanderloof J, Rapaport P, Paxson C: Manometric diagnosis of lower esophageal sphincter incompetence in infants: Use of a small single-lumen perfused catheter. Pediatrics 62:805, 1978
7. Moroz SP, Espinoza J, Cumming W, et al: Lower esophageal sphincter function in children with and without gastroesophageal reflux. Gastroenterology 71:236, 1976
8. Euler A, Ament M: Value of esophageal manometric studies of the gastroesophageal reflux of infancy. Pediatrics 59:58, 1977
9. Werlin S, Dodds W, Hogan W, Arndorfer R: Mechanisms of gastroesophageal reflux in children. J Pediatr 97:244, 1980
10. Tornwall L, Lind J, Peltonen A, et al: The gastrointestinal tract of the newborn. Ann Paediatr Finn 4:219, 1958
11. Hillemeier A, Lange R, McCallum R, et al: Delayed gastric emptying in infants with gastroesophageal reflux. J Pediatr 98:190, 1981
12. Bryne W, Kangorloo H, Ament M, et al: "Antral dysmotility," an unrecognized cause of chronic vomiting during infancy. Ann Surg 193:521, 1981
13. Jolley S, Leonard J, Tunnell, W: Gastric emptying in children with gastroesophageal reflux with an estimate of effective gastric emptying. J Pediatr Surg 22:923, 1987
14. Boix-Ochoa J, Lafuente J, Gil-Vernet J: 24-hour esophageal pH monitoring in gastroesophageal reflux. J Pediatr Surg 15:74, 1980
15. Little O, DeMeester T, Kirchner P: Pathogenesis of esophagitis in patients with gastroesophageal reflux. Surgery 88:101, 1980
16. Jolley S, Herbst J, Johnson D, Book L: Mean duration of gastroesophageal reflux identifies children with reflux-induced respiratory symptoms. Gastroenterology 78:1189, 1980
17. Arona J, Tovar J, Garay J: Abnormal preoperative and postoperative esophageal peristalsis in gastroesophageal reflux. J Pediatr Surg 21:711, 1986
18. Berquist W, Rachelefsky G, Kadden M, et al: Gastroesophageal reflux—associated recurrent pneumonia and chronic asthma in children. Pediatrics 68:29, 1981
19. Davis O, Casar C, Larrain A, Pope CE: Esophageal reflux—an unrecognized cause of recurrent obstructive bronchitis in children. J Pediatr 89:220, 1976
20. Shapira G, Christie D: Gastroesophageal reflux in steroid-dependent children. Pediatrics 63:207, 1979
21. Hughes D, Spier S, Rivlin J, Levison H: Gastroesophageal reflux during sleep in asthmatic patients. J Pediatr 102:666, 1983
22. Jolley SG, Herbst J, Johnson D, et al: Esophageal pH monitoring during sleep identifies children with respiratory symptoms from gastroesophageal reflux. Gastroenterology 80:1501, 1981
23. Lilly JR, Randolph JG: Hiatal hernia and gastroesophageal reflux in infants and children. J Thorac Cardiovasc Surg 55:42, 1968
24. Forshall I: The cardio-esophageal syndrome in childhood. Arch Dis Child 30:46, 1955
25. Leape LL, Holder TM, Franklin JD, et al: Respiratory arrest in infants secondary to gastroesophageal reflux. Pediatrics 60, 1977
26. Herbst JJ, Book L, Bray PF: Gastroesophageal reflux in the "near miss sudden infant death syndrome." J Pediatr 92:73, 1978
27. Walsh J, Farrell M, Keenan W, Lucas M: Gastroesophageal

reflux in infants: relationship to apnea. J Pediatr 99:197, 1981

28. Ariagno R, Guilleminault C, Baldwin R, et al: Movement and gastroesophageal reflux in awake term infants with "near miss" SIDS, unrelated to apnea. J Pediatr 100:894, 1982

29. Monereo J, Cortes L, Blesa E: Peptic esophageal stenosis in children. J Pediatr Surg 8:475, 1973

30. Abrahams P, Burkett B: Hiatal hernia and gastroesophageal reflux in children and adolescents with cerebral palsy. Aust Paediatr J 6:41, 1970

31. Herbst J, Friedland GW, Zboralske FF: Hiatal hernia and "rumination" in infants and children. J Pediatr 78:261, 1971

32. Sutcliff J: Torsion spasms and abnormal postures in children with hiatus hernia, Sandifers syndrome. Prog Pediatr Rad 2:190, 1960

33. Singleton ER, Wagner ML, Ditton J: Radiology of the alimentary tract in infants and children. Philadelphia, Saunders, 1977, pp 38–40

34. Chrispin AR, Friedland GW: Fractional disturbances in hiatal hernia in infants and children. Thorax 22:422, 1967

35. Fisher RS, Malmud LS, Roberts GS, Lobis IF: Gastroesophageal (GE) scintiscanning to detect and quantitate GE reflux. Gastroenterology 70:301, 1976

36. Jolley SG, Johnson DG, Herbst JJ, et al: An assessment of gastroesophageal reflux in children by extended pH monitoring of the distal esophagus. Surgery 84:16, 1978

37. Hill JL, Pelligrini CA, Burrington JD, et al: Technique and experience with 24-hour esophageal pH monitoring in children. J Pediatr Surg 12:877, 1977

38. Ramenofsky M, Leape L: Continuous upper esophageal pH monitoring in infants and children with gastroesophageal reflux, pneumonia and apnea spells. J Pediatr Surg 16:374, 1981

39. Hasse G, Meagher D, Goldson E, Falor W: A unique teletransmission system for extended four channel esophageal pH monitoring in infants and children. J Pediatr Surg 22:68, 1981

40. Leape L, Bhan L, Ramenofsky M: Esophageal biopsy in the diagnosis of reflux esophagitis. J Pediatr Surg 12:379, 1981

41. Orenstein S, Whitington R, Orenstein D: The infant seat as treatment for gastroesophageal reflux. N Eng J Med 309:760, 1983

42. Meyers W, Herbst J: Effectiveness of positioning therapy for gastroesophageal reflux. Pediatrics 69:555, 1982

43. Euler A: Use of bethanechol for the treatment of gastroesophageal reflux. J Pediatr 96:321, 1980

44. Sondheimer J, Mintz H, Michaels M: Bethanechol treatment of gastroesophageal reflux in infants: effects on continuous esophageal pH records. J Pediatr 104:128, 1984

45. Strickland A, Chang J: Results of treatment of gastroesophageal reflux with bethanechol. J Pediatr 103:311, 1983

46. Grill B, Hillemeir A, Semeravo L, et al: Effectiveness of domperidone therapy on symptoms and upper gastrointestinal motility in infants with gastroesophageal reflux. J Pediatr 106:311, 1985

47. Boix-Ochoa J, Casasa J, Gil-Vernet J: Esophageal Disorders in Pathophysiology and Therapy. New York, Raven, 1985, pp 459–468

48. Pieretti R, Shandling B, Stephens CA: Resistant esophageal stenosis associated with reflux after repair of esophageal atresia: A therapeutic approach. J Pediatr Surg 9:355, 1974

49. Ashcraft KW, Goodwin C, Amoury RA, Holder TM: Early recognition and aggressive treatment of gastroesophageal reflux following repair of esophageal atresia. J Pediatr Surg 12:317, 1977

50. Wesley J, Coran A, Sarahan T, et al: The need for evaluation of gastroesophageal reflux in brain-damaged children referred for feeding gastrostomy. J Pediatr Surg 16:866, 1981

51. Mollit D, Golladay E, Seibert J: Symptomatic gastroesophageal reflux following gastrostomy in neurologically impaired patients. Pediatrics 75:1124, 1985

52. Jolley S, Tunell W, Hoelzer D, Thomas S: Lower esophageal pressure changes with tube gastrostomy: a causative factor of gastroesophageal reflux in children? J Pediatr Surg 21:624, 1986

53. Canel D, Vane D, Goto S, et al: Reduction of lower esophageal sphincter pressure with Stamm gastrostomy. J Pediatr Surg 22:54, 1987

54. Byrne W, Euler A, Ashcraft E, et al: Gastroesophageal reflux in the severely retarded who vomit: Criteria for and results of surgical intervention in twenty-two patients. Surgery 91:95, 1982

55. Wilkinson J, Dudgeon D, Sondheimer J: A comparison of medical and surgical treatment of gastroesophageal reflux in severely retarded children. J Pediatr 99:202, 1981

56. Nissen R: Gastropexy and fundoplication in surgical treatment of hiatal hernia. Am J Dig Dis 6:954, 1961

57. Thal A: A unified approach to surgical problems of the esophagogastric junction. Ann Surg 168:542, 1968

58. O'Neill J, Betts J, Ziegler M, et al: Surgical management of reflux strictures of the esophagus in childhood. Ann Surg 196:453, 1982

59. Tunell W, Smith I, Carson J: Gastroesophageal reflux in childhood: the dilemma of surgical success. Ann Surg 197:560, 1987

60. Fester C: Paraesophageal hernia: a major complication of Nissen's fundoplication. J Pediatr Surg 16:496, 1981

61. Fonkelsrud E, Ament M, Berquist W: Surgical management of the gastroesophageal reflux syndrome in childhood. Surgery 97:42, 1985

62. Spitz L, Kirtane J: Results and complications for gastroesophageal reflux. Arch Dis Child 60:943, 1985

63. Hornsberger J, Covey J, Johnson D, Herbst J: Long-term follow-up of surgery for gastroesophageal reflux in infants and children. J Pediatr 102:505, 1983

64. Axelrod F, Schneider K, Ament M, et al: Gastroesophageal fundoplication and gastrostomy in familial dysautonomia. Ann Surg 195:253, 1982

65. Ashcraft K, Holder T, Amoury R, et al: The Thal fundoplication for gastroesophageal reflux. J Pediatr Surg 19:480, 1984

93
Achalasia

Achalasia of the esophagus is a functional disorder in which the lower esophageal sphincter fails to relax with swallowing. With progression of the disease, the entire esophagus loses its motility and becomes progressively more dilated. Of 287 patients with achalasia seen at the Mayo clinic, 15 experienced the onset of symptoms before they were 15 years of age.[1] The mean age of onset in that series was 8.5 years. The diagnosis has, however, been made in infancy, and the disease has been reported in siblings.[2–4]

PATHOLOGY

There is no true stricture in achalasia because an esophagascope or dilators will pass easily into the stomach with minimal resistance. At one time there was thought to be a defect in the ganglion cells in Auerbach's plexus, but this has not been proven in children. Electron microscopic studies have demonstrated degeneration of the vagus nerve. Evidence thus far points to a central nervous system lesion in the dorsal motor nucleus of the vagus.[5]

DIAGNOSIS

The primary symptom is difficulty in swallowing. Some children are able to take liquids but are unable to swallow solid foods. As the disease progresses and the proximal esophagus becomes distended, they will vomit the retained food and liquid. These symptoms are insidious, and because the disease is so unusual in children, the diagnosis is often delayed and and the symptoms are attributed to psychologic problems. Younger children fail to gain weight, whereas teenagers tend to lose weight over a period of several months. Nocturnal aspiration results in recurrent bouts of pneumonia. The diagnosis often can be made by observing a dilated esophagus with an air–fluid level on the chest roentgenogram. A

barium swallow outlines a dilated esophagus that narrows concentrically at the cardioesophageal junction. Fluoroscopy demonstrates disordered or poor peristalsis in the dilated proximal esophagus. Esophagoscopy under anesthesia demonstrates the concentric narrowing without

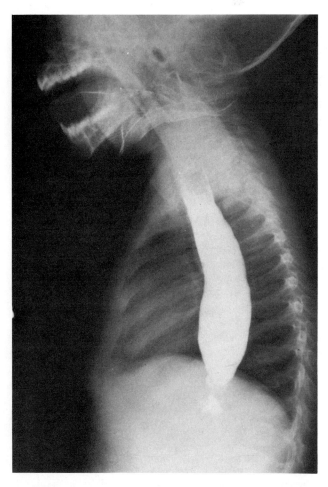

Figure 93–1. Esophagogram illustrating achalasia of the esophagus in an infant.

signs of esophagitis. The sphincter will relax to allow passage of the instrument into the stomach. This rules out congenital stricture and stenosis secondary to reflux (Fig. 93–1).

TREATMENT

Dilatation with the esophagoscope and mercury dilators offers temporary relief, but the long-term results with pneumatic dilatation have been unsatisfactory in children.

The Heller myotomy has provided excellent long-term results in all reported childhood series. In the series of Cloud et al. of 7 patients who had a Heller operation, 6 had an excellent result and 1 required postoperative dilatation.[6] The proximal esophageal dilatation returned to normal within 2 years. Cineradiograms also demonstrated return of peristalsis. Unfortunately, gastroesophageal reflux is a postoperative complication of the Heller myotomy.

Several authors have recommended the addition of an antireflux operation to the myotomy.[7,8] Lemmer et al. have recommended a transthoracic Heller operation with a modified Belsey fundoplication if it is necessary to carry the myotomy across the gastroesophageal junction.[9] A 360 degree Nissen fundoplication should not be performed in these patients because the poor peristalsis in the esophagus could not overcome any degree of obstruction imposed by a 360 degree wrap.

Technique
Although the standard Heller operation is carried out through the 7th intercostal space of the left chest, there are advantages to using the same upper abdominal approach used with antireflux operations. We now believe that this is the preferred approach because the exposure of the distal esophagus and the gastroesophageal junction is just as good, if not better, than through the chest, and it is easier to perform an adequate antireflux operation.

Figure 93–2 illustrates the transabdominal myotomy

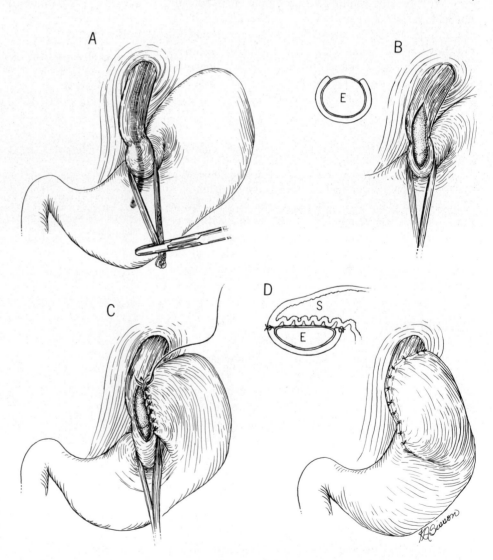

Figure 93–2. Technique for the Gavrilu transabdominal esophageal myotomy with an antireflux flap. E, esophagus; S, stomach.

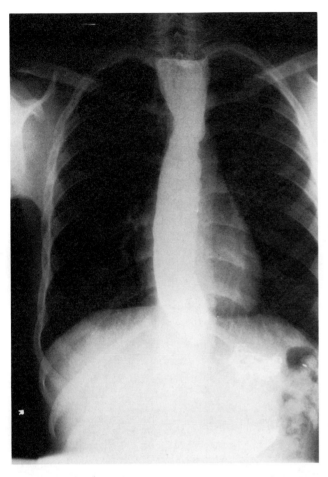 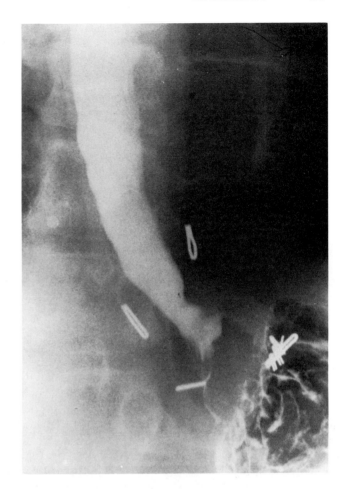

Figure 93–3. Left. Preoperative esophagogram. **Right.** Esophagogram after a Gavrilu myotomy and antireflux operation.

and antireflux procedure advocated by Gavrilu.[10] After the abdomen is opened through a left subcostal incision, a large bougie is passed down the esophagus into the stomach under direct vision. The esophagus is then mobilized, encircled with a tape, and dissected through the hiatus until the dilated portion has been brought down into the abdomen. The initial surface incision through the muscle is started with a scalpel. The muscle fibers are separated just as for a Ramstedt pyloromyotomy down to the mucosa. Then, by dissecting with scissors, the muscle is progressively divided and further separated from the mucosa until mucosa pouches out into the incision. The incision must be carried down onto the stomach. Great care is taken to divide every strand of fibrous tissue overlying the mucosa. This ensures a complete myotomy. A flap of greater curvature is then sutured over the esophageal mucosa. This flap is similar to a Thal fundoplication, but it not only acts as an antireflux valve but also keeps the muscular edges of the esophagus apart and enhances the myotomy. Figure 93–3 illustrates the preoperative and postoperative appearance of the esophagogastric junction with the Gavrilu operation.

We have performed seven of these operations. A follow-up during the past 10 years has shown that all but one boy is asymptomatic. This young man, now 20 years old, claims he cannot work because of his swallowing problems, but his esophagogram demonstrates no obstruction or reflux. A review of 78 reported modified Heller operations in children indicated an overall 95 percent success rate, yet reoperation has been required because of reflux or recurrent obstruction.[11]

REFERENCES

1. Tachovsky TJ, Lynn HB, Ellis FH: The surgical approach to esophageal achalasia in children. J Pediatr Surg 3:226, 1968
2. Asch MJ, Liebman W, Lochman R, Moore TC: Esophageal achalasia: diagnosis and cardiomyotomy in a newborn infant. J Pediatr Surg 9:911, 1974
3. Vaughan W, Hunter J, Williams L: Familial achalasia and pulmonary complications in children. Pediatr Radiol 1:407, 1973

4. Moazam F, Rodgers BM: Infantile achalasia: brief clinical report. J Thorac Cardiovasc Surg 72:809, 1976

5. Caselle RR, Brown AC, Sayre CP, Ellis FH: Achalasia of the esophagus: pathologic and etiologic considerations. Ann Surg 110:474, 1964

6. Cloud DT, White RF, Linkner IM, Taylor LC: Surgical treatment of esophageal achalasia in children. J Pediatr Surg 1:137, 1966

7. Murray G, Battaglini J, Keogy N: Selective application of fundoplication in achalasia. Ann Thorac Surg 37:185, 1984

8. Ballantyne T, Fitzgerald J, Grosfeld J: Transabdominal esophagomyotomy for achalasia in children. J Pediatr Surg 15:457, 1980

9. Lemmer J, Coran A, Wesley J, et al: Achalasia in children: Treatment by anterior esophageal myotomy (modified Heller operation) J Pediatr Surg 20:333, 1985

10. Gavrilu D: Aspects of esophageal surgery. Curr Probl Surg 12:29, 1975

11. Azizkhan R, Tapper D, Eroklis A: Achalasia in childhood: A 20-year experience. J Pediatr Surg 15:452, 1980

94
Caustic Esophageal Burns

_____ *Lauren D. Holinger*

A variety of corrosive substances continues to find its way into the hands and mouths of children. Much of this is the result of parental negligence, ignorance, or even child abuse. As the patient age increases, the possibility of suicidal intent also must be considered. High family stress, especially marital conflict, mental and physical illness, and loss of a family member, are associated with caustic ingestions.[1]

In the past, lye and Drano ingestions were the most common, but the heavy liquid drain cleaners were the most dangerous, since they burned both the esophagus and the stomach.[2]

The Poison Prevention Packaging Act, which mandated child-resistant containers and warning labels, has reduced the incidence of ingestion of these substances. However, farm children are still at risk because of their exposure to highly caustic dairy pipeline cleaners.[3,4]

PATHOLOGY

Injuries caused by chemical burns of the esophagus were classified by Holinger with a system similer to that used to describe thermal burns of the skin.[5] A first-degree burn signifies minimal involvement, characterized by superficial mucosal hyperemia, mucosal edema, and superficial sloughing. A second-degree burn is transmucosal, involving the entire wall of the esophagus, with exudate, ulceration, loss of mucosa, and extension into muscle. A third-degree burn is one that has eroded through the esophagus into the periesophageal tissues, including the mediastinum, or has perforated into the pleural or peritoneal cavities.

These injuries begin with an acute inflammatory phase during the first 4 days. This is followed by a subacute phase that lasts up to 15 days, toward the end of which the necrotic tissue sloughs away and leaves a denuded, ulcerated surface. Granulations appear as fibroblasts, and new blood vessels develop. The esophagus is considered weakest during this time, from the end of the first week through the second week. Swelling subsides, and often swallowing begins to return to normal, leading to the false conclusion that whatever therapy has been used was effective and need not be continued.

Cicatrization, the third phase, begins during the third and fourth weeks as the inflammatory reaction subsides and connective tissue contractures begin. Submucosa and muscularis are replaced by dense fibrous tissue, and adhesions involving the esophageal wall as well as surrounding structures cause bands with circular or spiral strictures that may result in the segmental obliteration of the lumen. Reepithelialization is complete by the sixth week, but in deep burns, the normal physiology of secretion, elasticity, and peristalsis is lost to varying degrees.

LOCATION

The child who merely dabbles in a powdered corrosive or crystals and then puts fingers into the mouth will have only superficial burns of the lips or tongue and surrounding skin. In the usual case, the burn is most severe at the anatomic areas of normal narrowing of the esophagus. The patient who deliberately gulps a large amount of a caustic agent, especially a liquid, will burn the mouth, the hypopharynx, the entire esophagus, and even the stomach.[6,7]

DIAGNOSIS

Any history of a child playing with a container that contained a caustic solution is suspicion enough for study to rule out an esophageal burn. In most cases of actual caustic ingestion, the child will drool and refuse food. He or she may complain of pain in the mouth or during attempts to swallow. If the burn is severe, the child may have a hoarse cry and respiratory distress. The history should include the type, amount, and if possible the brand name of the material ingested. The container should be brought to the hospital. It is helpful to know what home or other emergency treatment was given.

The child must be restrained for a careful examination of the mouth and pharynx—a good light and suction are necessary. There may be excessive secretions with obvious edema or even ulceration in the mouth and the surrounding skin with a severe burn (Fig. 94–1). The abdomen is examined for evidence of peritonitis, which would follow a severe gastric burn. If there is no evidence of an oropharyngeal burn, esophagoscopy and gastroscopy are performed under general anesthesia within 48 hours. The esophagus is examined for its full length or until a burn is encountered. Initially, the area of the cricopharyngeus and cervical esophagus is examined with a rigid esophagoscope. Then the flexible fiberoptic instrument is passed to continue the examination of the esophagus and stomach.

A barium esophagogram is of little value during the acute phase, since it will not detect mild injury and will delay the esophagoscopy. A later esophagogram may demonstrate an atonic or dilated esophagus.

TREATMENT

In the usual patient with a first- and second-degree burn, the child is given maintenance intravenous fluids and

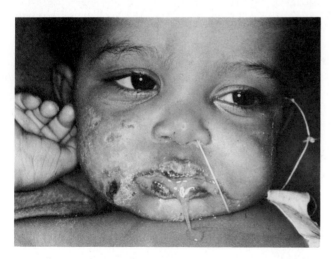

Figure 94–1. Extensive lye burns of the face and mouth. The child is unable to swallow her own saliva.

kept on nothing by mouth until he or she can swallow the saliva without difficulty. No attempt is made to induce vomiting or to gavage the stomach. The patient is then started on clear liquids and advanced to a soft diet. Steroid therapy, consisting of dexamethasone at 0.3 mg/kg/per day divided into six-hourly doses, is commenced as soon as possible, preferably within the first 48 hours after the burn. Both clinical and experimental evidence suggests that steroid therapy, when begun early and continued throughout the period of healing, will diminish the amount of scar tissue. Antibiotics are given simultaneously to diminish potential infection. With this regimen, Haller et al. found that of 69 children with proven burns, only 8 developed strictures, all of which responded to esophageal dilatation.[8] None of these patients required esophageal substitution.

At Children's Memorial Hospital in Chicago, the child is reexamined endoscopically in approximately 1 week to 10 days. If the mucosa has healed, the steroid therapy is tapered off and discontinued in another week. If there is continuing evidence for ulceration, the steroids are continued. If at any point there is a definite evidence of increasing dysphagia, a repeat esophagogram is performed. If there is a stricture in spite of steroid therapy, a gastrostomy is performed for feeding and in order to pass a string for future dilatations. In our experience, the string can be easily brought out the stomach at the time of gastrostomy if the endoscopist will simultaneously pass a small esophagoscope and then advance either a Fogarty catheter or a feeding tube into the stomach. The string is tied to the catheter and pulled back into the mouth. A gastrostomy for a lye stricture must be performed with extreme care to prevent leakage of gastric contents. The tube is placed between the usual purse-string sutures, after which more stomach is sutured about the tube to create a long tunnel that will prevent leakage.

If the child remains asymptomatic and the esophagogram is normal after the steroid therapy, he or she is discharged from the hospital but is followed with repeated esophagograms in 3 weeks and 3 and 6 months. The follow-up should continue for a least 1 year. It is unsafe to combine steroid therapy with mechanical dilatation because of the increased incidence of esophageal perforation. For this reason, if a stricture develops, dilatation is postponed until the child is off medication, and even then the stricture is dilated with extreme care. Although mild strictures may be dilated with peroral bougies, Tucker pointed out 65 years ago that the safest dilatation was accomplished by traction of the dilator through the stricture instead of pulsion.[9] Prograde dilatation is preferred to the retrograde approach. The string is brought out the mouth and tied to successively larger dilators, which are drawn through the stricture by traction on the string from the stomach. The dilator is never brought out the gastrostomy, since this has a tendency to enlarge the gastrostomy and cause leakage. Considerable judgment is required to choose the largest dilator that may be drawn safely through a stricture. In general, if blood appears on a dilator that required considerable traction, it is best to stop. Otherwise, it is safe to use one size larger than that which passed through the stricture with resistance. Initially, it may be necessary to dilate an established stricture two to three times each week for 1 to 2 weeks, until larger dilators pass through the esophagus with minimal resistance. The intervals between dilatations are then lengthened, and the dilatations are eventually discontinued. The persistence of a severe stricture for a year or more with little progress with dilatations is an esophageal bypass (Fig. 94–2).

The gastrostomy is valuable early after a severe burn or stricture to maintain nutrition with tube feedings. Later, the tube is removed, and only the string is left exiting through a small fistulous tract. The opening closes spontaneously after removal of the string.

Management of a Severe Caustic Burn

Children who have ingested large amounts of liquid caustic material may have severe respiratory distress from laryngeal burns as well as deep ulcers of the mouth and lips. These patients are admitted directly to the intensive care ward for close monitoring. They are given antibiotics, maintenance intravenous fluids, and, if necessary, serum albumin or whole blood for hypovolemia and shock.

Milder degrees of respiratory distress are treated with a mist tent and an oxygen-enriched atmosphere. Chest roentgenograms and endolateral films of the neck are obtained to determine the extent of tracheal edema, mediastinal widening, and other signs of esophageal perforation. A tracheotomy is indicated if there is an increasing degree of stridor. Shock and signs of peritonitis are indications of extensive necrosis with perforation of the stomach as well as extensive esophageal injury. Steroids must not be given to patients with evidence of severe injury, since these drugs mask the signs of perforation and infection and will fail to prevent stricture formation when the entire esophagus has been denuded.[10] Although some authors have advocated total esophagogastrectomy when there is coagulation necrosis of the stomach, in our experience exteriorization of the esophagus in the neck with excision of the stomach is sufficient.[6,11] Perforation of the esophagus may occur within a few days after a severe burn or following dilatation in a child who has been given steroids. Early perforations are an indication of almost total destruction of the esophagus. Our efforts to salvage the severely damaged esophagus

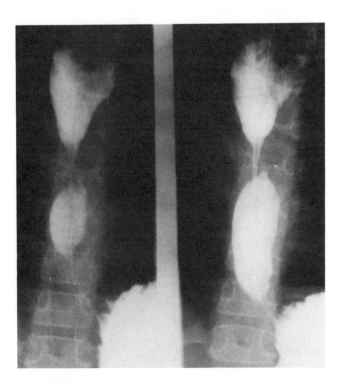

Figure 94–2. A 2-year-old esophageal stricture caused by ingestion of Liquid Plumber. There is a persistent, severe stricture in the mid-esophagus with gastroesophageal reflux due to shortening of the esophagus. A substernal colon bypass was performed in this patient.

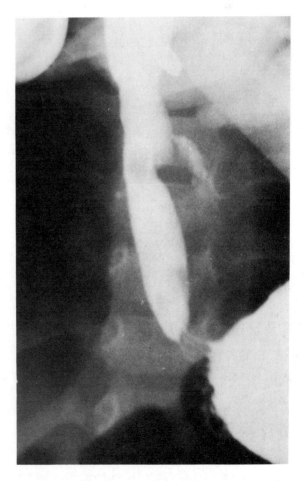

Figure 94–3. A small esophageal perforation following esophagoscopy and dilatation in a child with an old lye stricture. This healed with conservative, nonoperative treatment.

by closure of the perforation and subsequent dilatations have resulted in prolonged morbidity and eventual esophageal substitution. Consequently, we now believe that these children should be treated with immediate cervical esophagostomy, with division of the esophagus in the abdomen and a feeding gastrostomy. Continuity is restored later with an esophageal bypass. On the other hand, a delayed or instrumental esophageal perforation in a child may be handled by allowing nothing by mouth and administering supportive IV fluids and antibiotics (Fig. 94–3).[12,13] If there is persistent fever or signs of mediastinal widening, drainage is indicated.

Coughing, choking, and the appearance of food or fluid given by gastrostomy in a tracheotomy are indications of a tracheoesophageal fistula secondary to erosion through the esophagus into the trachea. The diagnosis is made by instilling aqueous dionosil or other contrast material suitable for bronchography into the esophagus (Fig. 94–4). We attempt to separate and repair three of these acquired fistulas by thoracotomy. One of our patients died with failure of healing of the trachea, and the fistula recurred in a second child. Burrington and Raffensperger have successfully treated three fistulas by performing cervical esophagostomy, gastrostomy, and division of the esophagus in the abdomen (Fig. 94–5).[14] The esophagus becomes a fibrotic scar that closes the fistula. The child is fed via gastrostomy until there is

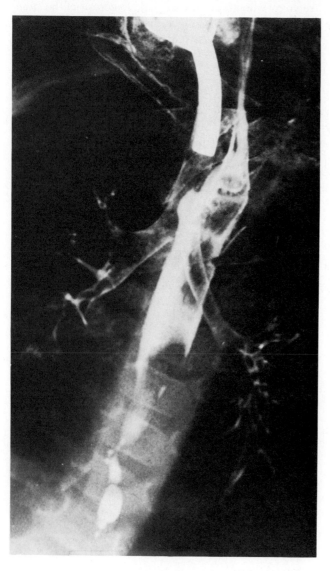

Figure 94–4. This 4-year-old boy swallowed a slurry of crystalline lye mixed with water. He required a tracheotomy soon after admission to the hospital and then a gastrostomy. Three days later, milk given by gastrostomy was suctioned from his tracheostomy after a bout of coughing. Contrast material admitted into the upper esophagus here demonstrates a fistula at the carina.

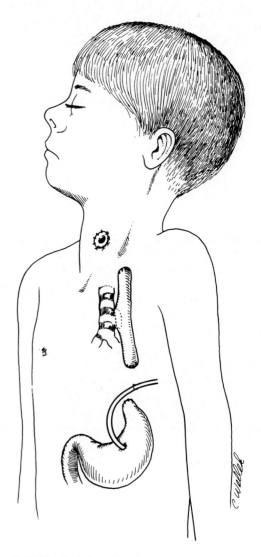

Figure 94–5. The technique developed by Burrington for dealing with a caustic fistula between the esophagus and trachea. The esophagus is left in situ but is diverted in the neck and divided in the abdomen. The child is then fed via a gastrostomy tube until there has been sufficient healing in the pharynx for an esophageal substitution.

swallowing but eventually learn to handle food and liquids almost normally.

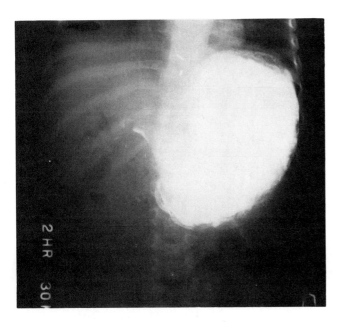

Figure 94–6. Gastric outlet obstruction in a 4-year-old boy who also had a caustic tracheoesophageal fistula. Symptoms were relieved by a gastroduodenostomy.

complete healing of the pharynx, and then an esophageal bypass is performed. Shaw et al. reported on a similar successfully treated patient in whom the necrotic esophagus was left in place.[15] They later bypassed the stomach as well as the esophagus with a segment of right colon, which was anastomosed to the esophagus in the neck and to the duodenum. One of our patients developed a gastric outlet obstruction 2 months after lye ingestion and required a gastroduodenostomy (Fig. 94–6).

Our current most difficult problems are with those children with severe burns of the hypopharynx and larynx. Frequently, even the cervical esophagus is so badly contracted that it is useless for an anastomosis. If the child has a tracheotomy, an esophageal bypass should not even be attempted until the hypopharynx has been dilated sufficiently to relieve the airway obstruction. It often is necessary to make the anastomosis of proximal bowel to the lateral pharynx because there is no usable esophagus. Such children have prolonged difficulty with

REFERENCES

1. Friedman E: Caustic ingestions and foreign body aspirations: An overlooked form of child abuse. Ann Otol 96:709, 1987
2. Leape L, Ashcraft K, Scarpelli D, et al: Hazard to health: Liquid lye. N Engl J Med 284:578, 1971
3. Walton W: An evaluation of the Poison Prevention Packaging Act. Pediatrics 69:363, 1982
4. Edmonson M: Caustic alkali ingestion by farm children. Pediatrics 79:413, 1987
5. Holinger P: Management of lesions caused by chemical burns. Ann Otol Rhinol Laryngol 71:819, 1968
6. David LL, Raffensperger J, Novak G: Necrosis of the stomach secondary to ingestion of corrosive agents. Chest 62:48, 1972
7. Ritter F, Newman M, Newman D: A clinical and experimental study of corrosive burns of the stomach. Ann Otol Rhinol Laryngol 77:819, 1968
8. Haller J, Andrew H, White J, et al: Pathophysiology and management of acute corrosive burns of the esophagus: Results of treatment in 285 children. J Pediatr Surg 6:578, 1971
9. Tucker GF Sr: Cicatricial stenosis of the esophagus with particular reference to treatment by continuous string retrograde bougienage with the author's bougie. Ann Otol Rhinol Laryngol 3:1180, 1924
10. Kirsh M, Peterson A, Brown J, et al: Treatment of caustic injuries of the esophagus: a ten-year experience. Ann Surg 188:675, 1978
11. Gago O, Ritter FN, Martel W, et al: Aggressive surgical treatment for caustic injury of the esophagus and stomach. Ann Thorac Surg 13:243, 1972
12. Shephard R, Raffensperger J, Goldstein IR: Pediatric esophageal perforation. J Thorac Cardiovasc Surg 74:261, 1977
13. Van de Zee D, Festen C, Severijnen R, Vand der Stook F: Management of pediatric esophageal perforation. J Thorac Cardiovasc Surg 95:692, 1988
14. Burrington JD, Raffensperger JG: Surgical management of tracheoesophageal fistula complicating caustic ingestion. Surgery 84:329, 1978
15. Shaw A, Garvey J, Miller B: Lye burn requiring total gastrectomy and colon substitution for esophagus and stomach in a two-year-old child. Surgery 65:837, 1969

95
Esophageal Substitution

Extensive caustic burns that are resistant to dilatations are the most common indication for esophageal bypass. Replacement is now practically never necessary for esophageal atresia because one can make an esophageal anastomosis after stretching and circular myotomy of the upper pouch. Partial replacement of the lower one third of the esophagus is now rarely necessary when there is a severe stricture due to recalcitrant peptic esophagitis.

Various segments of the colon and a tube formed from the greater curvature of the stomach are currently the most satisfactory substitutes for the esophagus. Each of the various operations has its own advantages. None is perfect; all are technically demanding. Great care must be taken to guard the blood supply to the segment of intestine or stomach. The substitute must reach the proximal esophagus without compression or kinking, and the anastomoses must be made with scrupulous care to avoid leaks and strictures. For the best long-term results, the segment chosen should resist reflux of gastric contents and be relatively insensitive to peptic ulceration. Each surgeon will choose the operation with which he or she has had the most experience, but it is helpful to be familiar with alternate techniques so that the best procedure may be chosen for any particular child. Although esophageal bypass can be performed in infants, it is best to wait until the child is 1 year old.

SUBSTERNAL COLON BYPASS

The colon is resistant to peptic ulceration because of its mucus production.[1,2] Evaluations of the blood supplies of the various colon segments demonstrate a higher incidence of marginal venous deficiencies in the right colon than in the left.[3,4] Despite these observations, the right colon, usually with an attached segment of ileum based on the middle colic artery, has become the most widely used esophageal substitute since this procedure was introduced 35 years ago.[5-10] True peristalsis does not occur in the intact colon, and emptying of the transplanted colon is effected primarily by gravity or strong mass peristalsis. We leave the ileum attached to the cecum to preserve the ileocecal valve, which prevents reflux.

Preoperative Preparation

All children who require an esophageal bypass have had a gastrostomy, and many have had a cervical esophagostomy. They are admitted to the hospital 3 days in advance of the operation for a program of mechanical bowel preparation consisting of an elemental diet, rectal irrigations, and laxatives administered through the gastrostomy tube. They are given neomycin (a total of 100 mg/kg) 24 hours before surgery in four separate doses. It is helpful to reduce the bacterial flora of the mouth with peroxide mouth washes and sips of 1 percent neomycin.

Technique

The child is placed supine on the operating table with a folded towel beneath the shoulders to hyperextend the head, which is turned away from the esophagostomy. If there is no esophagostomy, the head is turned to the right, exposing the left neck. The entire neck, chest, and abdomen are prepared and draped. The gastrostomy tube is removed. There need be only one scrub nurse, but it is helpful to have two suction and electrocoagulation units. The teams work simultaneously. The surgeon working in the neck isolates and mobilizes the cervical esophagus and prepares the cervical end of the substernal tunnel while the abdominal team mobilizes a segment of bowel.

A paraxiphoid incision commencing at the sternum and extending below the unbilicus is made either in the midline or just to the right, avoiding the gastrostomy site. The falciform ligament is divided, and if necessary the gastrostomy site is mobilized so that the cologastric anastomosis may be made high on the anterior wall of the stomach. The terminal ileum, cecum, right colon, and transverse colon are then mobilized (Fig. 95–1). The blood supply to the right colon and terminal ileum is carefully inspected. If one finds a long marginal artery and vein with good arcades to the right colic and ileocolic artery, the transplant may be based on the midcolic artery. We have found frequently that the ileocolic artery has better arcades to the ascending colon and terminal ileum. The ideal transplant should consist mainly of the terminal ileum with a short segment of cecum and ascending colon. This may not be possible, however, if the midcolic artery is chosen. The segments of blood supply are further verified by isolating the right colic artery and branches from the superior mesenteric artery to the terminal ileum and temporarily clamping them with noncrushing bulldog clamps. At the same time, Potts clamps are placed across the bowel and adjacent marginal arteries. This completely isolates the chosen segment of bowel. Pulsations should continue in the marginal vessels, and the bowel must remain pink. The blood supply to the cecum is further evaluated by removing the appendix and observing blood flow from the appendiceal artery while the bulldog clamps are in place. If the blood supply from one vessel appears to be inadequate, another may be used. Either the ileocolic or middle colic artery should be satisfactory. All vessels must be carefully cleared of fat and lymph nodes in order to preserve not only the marginal artery and vein but also the arcuate vessels, which provide additional collateral flow. All vessels that are to be divided are first cleaned and isolated and then ligated in continuity with 5-0 silk. Hemostats are not used, since they may accidentally

damage a collateral vessel. The bowel is then divided between Potts clamps, and the ileum, which is to be anastomosed to the esophagus, is closed with inverting sutures that are cut long.

The cervical portion of the operation is commenced with a transverse incision that encircles the esophagostomy and extends down over the sternal notch. The skin, subcutaneous tissues, and cervical fascia are divided to expose the sternocleidomastoid muscle, and the carotid sheath is then retracted laterally to expose the esophagus. If there is a cervical esophagostomy, it is closed with interrupted sutures, which are used for traction. The esophagus is then dissected as high as necessary to get above any strictures. A segment of esophagus at least 4 cm long is necessary to make a satisfactory anastomosis. If the esophagus is intact, it is dissected down into the mediastinum as far as is convenient. Interrupted sutures are inserted into its wall, and it is divided for a short distance, after which more sutures are placed. In this way the esophagus is divided and closed securely without any danger of its retracting down into the mediastinum.

The upper border of the sternum is exposed by dividing the cervical fascia and the origin of the sternocleidomastoid muscle at the sternum with electrocoagulation. The sternoclavicular joint also is exposed by removing all fascial and muscular attachments with a periosteal elevator. Tissues posterior to the sternum are then bluntly dissected until the entire upper 2 or 3 cm of sternum is free of attachments. The upper sternum, which curves backward, is then removed with a rongeur (Fig. 95–1B). This is an essential part of the operation and must be carried out in order to create a large tunnel for the transplanted bowel. Failure to remove a portion of the upper sternum and the adjacent sternoclavicular

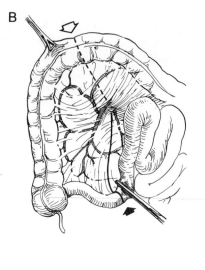

Figure 95–1. A. Simultaneous incisions are made in the neck and abdomen by two teams of surgeons. **B.** The terminal ileum and cecum are mobilized, and the mesenteric vessels are identified, then temporarily occluded with bulldog clamps. If possible, the transplant is based on the ileocal artery. (Continued)

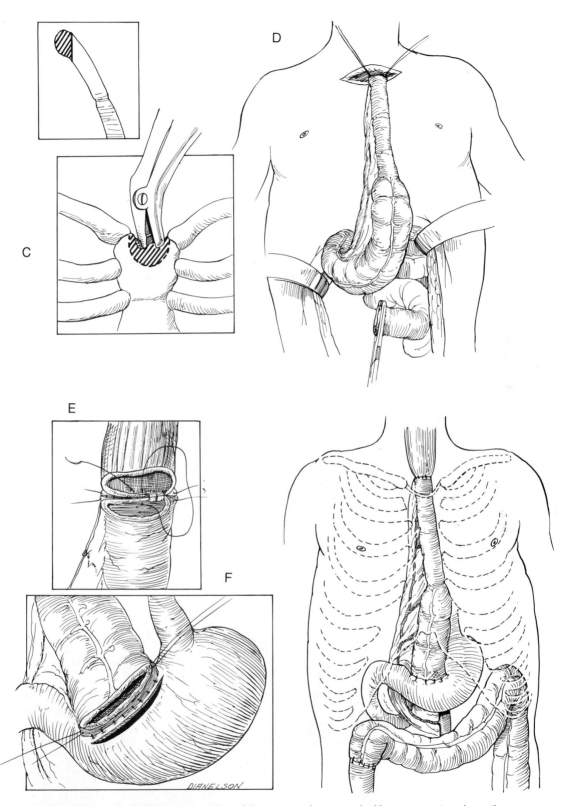

Figure 95–1 (Cont.). C, D. The upper portion of the sternum is resected with a rongeur to enlarge the upper mediastinal portion of the tunnel. **E.** The transplant is tested for length by placing it on the anterior chest wall before it is passed up the substernal tunnel. **D.** The esophagoileal anastomosis is effected with one layer of 5-0 nonabsorbable suture material. **E.** The cologastric anastomosis is performed with two layers of sutures, primarily to achieve hemostasis on the gastric side. **F.** The completed transplant must be as short as possible and free from redundancy.

joint will either obstruct the venous return from the anastomosis or possibly at a later date obstruct the passage of solid food. Bleeding from the cut sternum is controlled with bone wax and electrocoagulation. The substernal tunnel is continued with blunt finger dissection from the cervical incision. Meanwhile, the abdominal team has mobilized and isolated the bowel segment. The xiphoid is then elevated, and attachments between the diaphragm and sternum are severed. The tunnel is continued with further blunt finger dissection from below. The final tunnel must be wide enough to easily accommodate three fingers from above and below. Before the bowel is passed through the substernal tunnel, it is tested for length by bringing it up to the neck on the anterior chest wall (Fig. 95–2). The vessel chosen to supply the transplant is dissected to its origin with the superior mesenteric artery, and the bowel with its blood supply is passed behind the stomach. A long, curved clamp is passed down from the cervical incision to grasp the sutures on the ileum. The transplant is then led through the substernal tunnel with gentle traction while the abdominal surgeon prevents twists and kinking. It is frequently necessary to resect ileum in the neck to prevent a redundant loop of bowel just below the esophageal anastomosis. Three 5-0 sutures are inserted between the wall of the esophagus and the ileum in order to line up the anastomosis. These are tied, bringing together the angles and the midportion of the anastomosis. The remaining sutures are placed through the full thickness of bowel and esophagus. The mucosa in the esophagus, which may retract, must be carefully picked up with each stitch. Knots are placed on the inside on the back row and on the outside anteriorly. A drain is then placed

in the anterior mediastinum, and the cervical incision is loosely closed. While the cervical esophageal anastomosis is being performed, the abdominal team divides the colon after ligating marginal vessels close to the wall of the bowel. The bowel must lie straight, with no redundancy, and the anastomosis must leave 5 to 6 cm of colon within the abdomen. When the ileocolic vessels are used, there is often only a few centimeters of cecum with the ileocecal valve within the abdomen. The cologastric anastomosis is completed with two layers of sutures, and the terminal ileum is anastomosed to the colon. A new gastrostomy is fashioned, if necessary.

Postoperative Care

The gastrostomy tube is left on gravity drainage until there is evidence of peristalsis, at which time it is elevated and feedings are commenced by gravity. The tube is never clamped until it is obvious that the intestinal tract is functioning properly and there is no reflux up the transplanted bowel. The cervical drain is removed after 48 hours, and if there is no drainage from the neck wound, a barium swallow is obtained 1 week after the operation. If there are no leaks or strictures, the child is allowed to take food and fluid by mouth. The gastrostomy tube is left in place for several weeks, however, as a safeguard against delayed anastomotic problems. A barium swallow is indicated about 6 weeks later and again 1 year after the operation (Figs. 95–3 and 95–4).

COLON BYPASS

An alternative approach to right colon bypass is the interposition of a segment of transverse colon between the

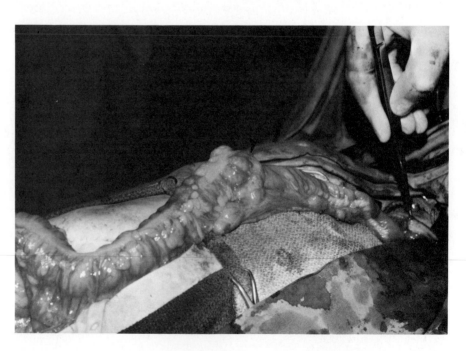

Figure 95–2. Intraoperative picture of the right colon and ileum lying on the surface of the chest; there is more than enough length. An arrow marks the cecum.

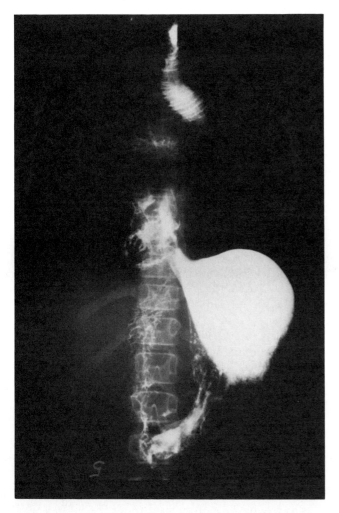

Figure 95–3. An ileocecal substernal transplant performed in an 8-year-old girl for a recalcitrating lye stricture. The transplant is minimally redundant.

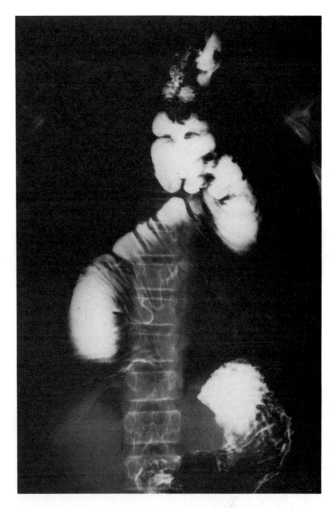

Figure 95–4. This is a typical right colon transplant, seen here in a 15-year-old boy. This operation was performed when the boy was 1½ years old. Although the colon is somewhat redundant, the boy swallows normally.

proximal esophagus and either the distal stump of an esophageal atresia or the stomach. Waterston et al. have described this technique in several publications.[11–13] The transverse colon based on the ascending branch of the left colic artery provides an isoperistaltic conduit that is less bulky and less apt to become redundant than the right colon. In addition, the transplant is in the posterior mediastinum, so the esophagocolic anastomosis pursues a more direct course than the anastomosis made anterior and lateral to the trachea.

Technique

A left thoracotomy or thoracoabdominal incision allows excellent access to the upper abdomen once a portion of the diaphragm has been detached from the rib margin. The colon is mobilized and its blood supply is evaluated as described for the right colon operation. The transverse colon based on the middle colic artery is used to replace the lower portion of the esophagus for peptic esophagitis or varices, but the transverse and descending colon are required if the entire esophagus is to be bypassed. Waterston passes the vascular pedicle posterior to the tail of the pancreas through an opening in the posterior reflection of the left leaf of the diaphragm and thence up the paravertebral gutter posterior to the hilum of the lung.[11–13] A second incision in the neck mobilizes the cervical esophagus, after which the colon is passed through the apex of the pleural cavity, where it is anastomosed to the esophagus in the neck. The cologastric anastomosis is made low on the anterior wall of the stomach. The resultant long, intraabdominal colonic segment with its sharp angle of entry into the stomach prevents reflux. When it is necessary to resect the distal esophagus for varices or peptic esophagitis, the Waterston technique is modified by bringing the colonic transplant with its vascular pedicle through the esophageal hiatus.

GASTRIC TUBE

The greater curvature of the stomach receives its blood supply from the right and left gastroepiploic vessels, which communicate freely through both extramural and intramural collaterals. A very long tube may be fashioned from the curvature, commencing at the pyloric end of the stomach. Gavrilu has even included a portion of the duodenum and pylorus with the gastric tube to reach the pharynx.[14] He performed 580 gastric tube bypasses of the esophagus between 1951 and 1975 with the following technique, which is here modified for use in children.

The abdomen is opened through a midline incision. After inspection of the greater curvature of the stomach, the spleen and pancreas are mobilized by dividing the peritoneum between these organs and the posterior abdominal wall. Although Gavrilu recommended splenectomy, this is not necessary or desirable in children.[14] The fundus of the stomach is, however, separated from the diaphragm. The greater omentum is then detached from the transverse colon. Sufficient omentum is taken along with the stomach to form a flap that will be wrapped around the completed anastomosis.

The right gastroepiploic artery is then ligated and divided 2 or 3 cm from the pylorus. This point will become the proximal end of the gastric tube. Potts clamps are applied at right angles to the greater curvature, and the stomach is incised to a depth of 3 or 4 cm. The tube itself is cut wide enough to be sutured about a size 24 to 28 French catheter (depending on the size of the child). The gastric incision may be made freehand by cutting for a few centimeters and then suturing the cut edges immediately to control bleeding. The catheter may also be held between large Babcock clamps while a curved bowel clamp is applied to the stomach side. The tube and stomach are then closed with a continuous layer of 4-0 chromic catgut and interrupted silk. An alternate technique is to divide the tube from the stomach between rows of staples.[15] The completed suture line is then wrapped with the omental flap and passed through a substernal tunnel for anastomosis to the cervical esophagus. The completed tube must be no more than 2 cm in diameter.

A gastric tube is not our operation of choice. Even when the initial operation with an ileocolic segment has failed, we prefer to use another segment of colon. Recently, esophageal replacement by total gastric transposition has been revived. The authors report a 9 percent mortality rate among 34 patients operated on from 1981 to 1986.[16] We have had no deaths from a colon transposition since 1963. Furthermore, the recent experience with gastric transposition has had a minimum followup. This operation was attempted in our hospital many years ago but was given up by Potts because distention of the stomach resulted in respiratory distress.

RESULTS

All of the operations described have provided satisfactory results when properly performed. The most common complications have been leaks and strictures at the proximal anastomosis. A leak developed at the cervical esophagocolic anastomosis in 30 percent of 20 cases of substernal colon transplant reported by Schiller et al. All of these closed spontaneously, but late strictures developed in 25 percent of those with leaks.[17] Of the 7 patients with stricture, 5 responded to dilatations. German and Waterston reported a 20 percent incidence of anastomotic leak and a 16 percent incidence of stricture.[13] On the other hand, Anderson and Randolph reported a 50 percent incidence of anastomotic leakage in 15 children with gastric tubes.[18] Another of their patients died after dilatation of a stricture, and 1 patient developed an ulcer in the tube.[18] Anastomotic leakage was reported in 70 percent and stricture in 50 percent of children who had gastric tubes constructed at the Toronto Children's Hospital.[19] The anastomosis was delayed in these patients. During the interval between construction of the tube and the anastomosis, the authors noted free reflux of gastric contents out the cervical opening of the stomach. Groves and Silver noted a higher incidence of proximal stricture and reflux with the gastric tube in comparison with colonic interposition.[20]

Long-term results following colon interposition have demonstrated an early growth delay.[21] This is seen primarily in children with an esophageal atresia. These children catch up in their growth, and 80 percent are classified as having a very good result.[22] Children who have had a bypass performed for a caustic stricture appear to grow and develop at a normal rate. Rodgers et al. performed detailed functional and metabolic studies on eight children.[23] These studies further demonstrated growth retardation in children with esophageal atresias, and particularly in those with other birth defects. Rodgers et al. also found abnormal vitamin B_{12} absorption in children in whom segments of ileum longer than 10 cm in length were used for the transplant. However, these children did show peristaltic activity in the ileal segment. Despite the problems of slow peristalsis in the transposed colonic segment, a large number of children with colonic transposition have now been followed for periods of more than 20 years. The long-term results in these patients justify the continued use of this operation.[24,25]

In our experience with esophageal replacement in 40 patients, there have been 2 deaths, both more than 25 years ago. The first was due to immediate postoperative respiratory depression before the introduction of ventilator support. The second child had an extensive lye burn of his pharynx that required a tracheostomy and an anastomosis of his colon to the pharynx. He died of aspiration pneumonia 6 months after the operation. Two patients developed necrosis of the transplanted bowel. Each of these patients later had a successful transverse colon bypass. Four (13 percent) developed immediate postoperative fistulas; all of these healed. Only 2 patients (6 percent) have required treatment for anastomotic strictures, but both are able to eat. Each of these children had pharyngeal caustic burns that required an anastomosis between the bowel and the scarred esophagus or pharynx. One child required reoperation because of short segment of ileum herniated through a pleural defect into the left chest and became obstructed (Fig. 95–5). He has swallowed normally since the hernia was reduced and a redundant segment of ileum was resected. One child developed a colonic ulcer adjacent to the gastric anastomosis 12 years after her original operation. This was resected, and she is now well. Two of our patients had failed substernal bypasses performed in other hospitals. We were unable to elongate the re-

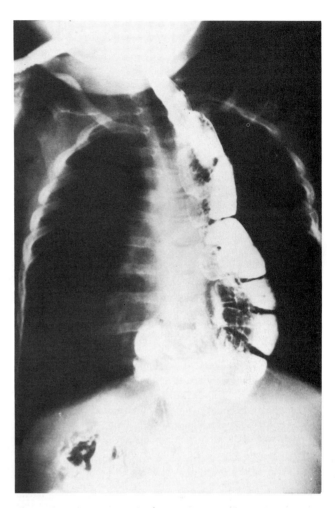

Figure 95–6. There are two alternatives when an esophageal substitution has failed. If there is sufficient transverse colon, as there is in this patient, the mid and proximal left colon may be used. It is best to bring the new transplant through a pleural cavity because the mediastinum will be obliterated.

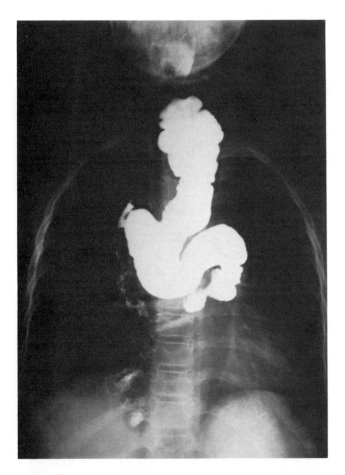

Figure 95–5. A freak complication. There were two problems: (1) the ileum was too long and redundant, and (2) there was a perforation in the pleura. The ileum than herniated into perforation and became obstructed. This was corrected by splitting the sternum and resecting the bowel within the mediastinum. This is a perfectly feasible solution to difficulty caused by a redundant intestinal conduit.

maining bowel in either patient. One now has a satisfactorily functioning gastric tube, and the other has an isoperistaltic segment of transverse colon that was brought anterior to the hilum through the left chest (Fig. 95–6).

One of our patients has now been followed for 30 years, and another has been followed for 27 years. The oldest patient reports that she must chew and swallow her food slowly; the other is normal. Both are leading normal lives. After reviewing our own experience, as well as that of others, it seems that the substernal ileocolic transplant has fewer immediate postoperative complications than the gastric tube, and the long-term results of the former are satisfactory. In our hands, proximal anastomotic leaks and strictures have been related to scarring in the esophagus from previous caustic ingestion. Our greatest problems have occurred in cases involving a scarred pharynx and respiratory problems. Even children with these hindrances eventually learn to swallow with minimal difficulty.

REFERENCES

1. Schechter JJ, Sequitz RH: The colon as replacement for the esophagus: Its resistance to reflux or gastric juice. Wis Med J 38:677, 1959

2. Sirak HD, Clatworthy HW, Elliott DW: An evolution of jejunal and colonic transplants in experimental esophagitis. Surgery 36:399, 1954

3. Rooney B: The blood supply of the colon in esophageal replacement. Ir J Med Sci 2:301, 1969

4. Nicks R: Colonic replacement of the oesophagus: Some observations on infarction and wound leakage. Br J Surg 54:124, 1967

5. Longino LA, Wooley MJ, Gross RE: Esophageal replacement in infants and children with the use of a segment of colon. JAMA 171:1187, 1959

6. Dale WA, Sherman CD: Late reconstruction of congenital esophageal atresia by intrathoracic colon transplantation. J Thorac Surg 29:344, 1955

7. Javid H: Esophageal reconstruction using colon and terminal ileum. Surgery 36:132, 1954

8. Neville WE, Clowes GH: Colon replacement of the esophagus in children for congenital and acquired disease. J Thorac Cardiovasc Surg 40:507, 1960

9. Battersby JD, Moore TC: Esophageal replacement and bypass with the ascending and right half of the transverse colon for the treatment of congenital atresia of the esophagus. Surg Gynecol Obstet 21:207, 1959

10. Martin LW, Flege JB Jr: Use of colon as a substitute for the esophagus in children. Am J Surg 108:69, 1964

11. Waterston DJ: Colonic replacement of esophagus (intrathoracic). Surg Clin North Am 44:1441, 1964

12. Azar H, Chrispin AR, Waterston DJ: Esophageal replacement with transverse colon in infants and children. J Pediatr Surg 6:3, 1971

13. German JC, Waterston DJ: Colon interposition for the replacement of the esophagus in children. J Pediatr Surg 11:227, 1976

14. Gavrilu D: Aspects of esophageal surgery. Curr Probl Surg 12:40, 1975

15. Heimlich HJ: Esophagoplasty with reversed gastric tube: Review of 53 cases. Am J Surg 123:80, 1972

16. Spitz L, Kiely E, Sparnon T: Gastric transposition for esophageal replacement in children. Ann Surg 206:73, 1987

17. Schiller M, Frye TR, Boles ET: Evaluation of colonic replacement of the esophagus in children. J Pediatr Surg 6:753, 1971

18. Anderson KD, Randolph JG: Gastric tube interposition: A satisfactory alternative to the colon for esophageal replacement in children. Ann Thorac Surg 6:521, 1978

19. Vizas D, Ein S, Shandling B: Thirteen years of gastric tubes. J Pediatr Surg 3:638, 1978

20. Groves LK, Silver GM: Esophagoplasty with bowel segments and reversed gastric tubes. Surgery 74:381, 1973

21. Louhimo L, Pasilo M, Visakorpi JK: Late gastrointestinal complications in patients with colonic replacement of the esophagus. J Pediatr Surg 4:663, 1969

22. Schiller M, Frye TR, Boles ET: Evaluation of colonic replacement of the esophagus in children. J Pediatr Surg 6:753, 1971

23. Rodgers B, Talbert JL, Moazam F, Felman AH: Functional and metabolic evaluation of colon replacement of the esophagus in children. J Pediatr Surg 1:35, 1978

24. Postlethwaite R: Colonic interposition for esophageal substitution. Surg Gynecol Obstet 156:377, 1983

25. Hendren WH, Hendren WG: Colon interposition in children. J Pediatr Surg 20:829, 1985

SECTION XIII

Gastrointestinal Diseases of the Older Child

It is usually possible to discover an etiology and offer specific treatment to the child who has acute abdominal pain. This is particularly true if there are other significant symptoms or signs, such as vomiting, abdominal distention, localized tenderness, or a palpable mass, which points to a definite organic problem. Chapters in this section deal with some of the diseases that have a primary symptom of abdominal pain. Other diseases of the gastrointestinal and genitourinary tracts show bleeding, a mass, or other readily observable findings and are discussed elsewhere in this text.

Some children with recurrent or chronic abdominal pain defy diagnosis. They may be referred to a surgeon after the usual diagnostic studies are all found to be negative. The referral is often prompted by a questionable finding on a roentgenogram or in a laboratory test in the physician's relentless search for an organic lesion. A surgeon can do a great deal of harm to an emotionally disturbed child with abdominal pain by advising an operation. An appendectomy for chronic abdominal pain may well be the beginning of a series of needless abdominal operations that leave the patient even more convinced that there is an organic lesion. On the other hand, a careful surgeon who without hesitation makes the diagnosis of psychogenic abdominal pain can do a great deal of good by simply explaining why an operation is not indicated.

Approximately 10 percent of 1000 British school children gave a history of chronic abdominal pain and were subjected to a detailed history and physical examination.[1] They ranged in age from 5 to 10 years, and girls were affected slightly more often than boys. The pain itself is best characterized as vague. When a careful history is obtained, one finds no relationship between the pain and eating, urinating, defecating, sleep, or medication. Specifically, the pain is rarely described as colicky but is rather periumbilical or occurs throughout the entire abdomen and is unrelieved by anything, except perhaps staying home from school and resting. Headaches and lethargy are the most common associated symptoms. There are no positive findings on physical examination, and these children are in normal percentiles for height and weight.

There often is a family history of migraine, epilepsy, or a chronic illness, which seems to focus the family members' thoughts on problems of health. Although there are well over 100 organic lesions that may cause abdominal pain, most of them fall into clearly recognized syndromes that will be suspected from the history and physical examination. Some organic lesions that must be considered in unusual situations are milk or lactose intolerance, which causes abdominal pain, bloating, and loose stools, kidney problems, especially hydronephrosis, peptic ulcer, and intestinal parasites. In teenagers one must not forget porphyria. One specific clue to psychogenic abdominal pain is a prolonged absence from school. Both the child and the family will assert that the child likes school and wants to go to school more than anything else in the world, but the pain is just too severe. Once the child is at school, he or she complains and is sent home.

The child might actually have performed well academically and is often able to keep up with classmates with homework or a tutor, while all attempts to send the child back to school fail. Frequently, at the onset there is a flu-like syndrome or an upper respiratory infection, and as soon as the child goes back to school after the cessation of the original illness, the abdominal pain commences.

The only laboratory tests required in the children

are complete blood count, urinalysis, stool for occult blood, and an abdominal ultrasound study.

Treatment of these difficult problems proceeds simultaneously with the examination. If the history brings out emotional problems and if the family and child are allowed to express their feelings about the abdominal pain, therapy will be more readily accepted.

First, one can point out that if the pain has been going on for several months or a year, it is unlikely to be caused by a progressive lesion (such as malignancy). Next, one can explain that despite the illness, the child appears to be healthy and has not lost weight. Third, one can discuss the usual causes for organic abdominal pain and make the observation that the child's symptoms do not fit into any specific pattern. As a clincher, one might make the following statement, "As a surgeon, I earn my living operating on children with diseases that respond to an operation. Your child does not need an operation." It is helpful to further state that although there is no organic cause for the child's pain, the exact cause of the symptoms remains unknown. This leads into a discussion of the subjective nature of pain and how a minor ache to one person may seem to be a major problem to another. It is useful to use the analogy of a headache, which, as everyone knows, does not necessarily occur secondary to an organic problem. Finally, an attempt should be made to find out if the child and the mother are achieving secondary gains. It is possible that the child really wants to avoid contact with classmates who may be causing problems. The mother may take the opportunity to remain home from her work to take care of her "sick" child. The following advice is often curative: "If he is too sick to go to school, he must stay home in bed with no books or television and must have a diet of only clear liquids." This simple advice has produced an occasional miraculous cure. Fortunately, most of these problems are self-limiting, although some require psychologic counseling.

The surgeon must not lightly brush off children who have no demonstrable cause for abdominal pain. Occasionally, an obscure organic problem will be found that will respond to an operation. It is just as bad to pursue a psychologic problem with endless laboratory tests and roentgenographic examinations, or even an operation, as it is to overlook an organic lesion. The conscientious surgeon who actively aids in the diagnosis and treatment of psychogenic abdominal pain will gain stature among colleagues and occasionally will win the gratitude of patients who do not require surgery.

REFERENCE

1. Apley J, Naish: Recurrent abdominal pains: a field survey of 1000 school children. Arch Dis Child 33:165, 1958

96
Appendicitis

Abdominal pain is a ubiquitous complaint in the pediatric age group. Even though the pain is most often caused by dietary indiscretion or simple enteric infections, the physician must always consider appendicitis. This is the most common acute surgical emergency in childhood. An appreciation of its many vagaries and complications depends on an accurate knowledge of many diseases that can cause abdominal pain in childhood. Complicated appendicitis may lead to generalized peritonitis, subphrenic and pelvic abscess, empyema, and intestinal obstruction. The prevention and proper management of these problems require the knowledge and application of the full range of surgical principles. Errors in diagnosis and surgical technique continue to result in approximately 100 childhood deaths from appendicitis annually.[1] Even more children suffer prolonged morbidity from intraabdominal sepsis, stress ulcers, and leakage of the appendiceal stump. These complications are avoidable.

INCIDENCE

Acute appendicitis occurs in all age groups but is most common during later childhood and early adult life. The mean age range in the pediatric population is 6 to 10 years, but appendicitis is encountered in newborns and infants as well as older children.

PATHOLOGY

In almost every case, the base of the appendix is at the convergence of the taenia of the colon in the right lower quadrant of the abdomen, beneath McBurney's point.[2] In about 5 percent of patients, the appendix turns behind the cecum and ascends in a retroperitoneal position behind the ascending colon.[3] When the cecum has failed to undergo normal rotation, the appendix may be anywhere in the peritoneal cavity. In children, it is relatively longer and thinner than in adults. Hence, it is more likely to perforate at an earlier stage in the disease. The greater omentum remains thin, short, and flimsy until approximately 10 years of age. Thus it is less likely to wall off a perforation, so generalized peritonitis is more common in children than in adults.

Appendicitis is caused by obstruction of the lumen. This results in edema, venous engorgement, and increased intraluminal pressure distal to the obstruction. Ultimately, there is bacterial invasion through the wall, ulceration of the mucosa, and perforation.

The base of the appendix in the newborn infant is broad and funnel-shaped and is thus rarely obstructed. Hirschsprung's disease in the distal colon may be the obstructing mechanism that accounts for appendicitis in newborn infants.[4,5] A fecalith is the obstructing mechanism in approximately one third or more of children with appendicitis, and calcified fecaliths are not unusual. Fecal concretions may be related to the low-residue western-type diet, since acute appendicitis is practically unknown in Africans who eat high-residue foods.[6] Submucosal lymphoid follicles increase in frequency and reach a peak incidence in adolescence, after which the occurrence decreases. Edema or hypertrophy of this lymphoid tissue, occurring during intercurrent viral infections, accounts for most cases of appendicitis. Intestinal parasites also obstruct the appendix. Pinworms are sometimes found in normal-appearing appendices.[7] Foreign bodies may lodge in the appendix for prolonged periods of time without causing symptoms, but the risk of perforation is sufficient that when diagnosed radiographically the foreign bodies should be removed.[8]

Bacterial Flora

When the appendix perforates or becomes gangrenous, the peritoneal cavity is rapidly inoculated with colonic organisms. *Escherichia coli* is the most common aerobic organism found. As symptoms progress, multiple organisms, including *Proteus*, *Klebsiella*, *Streptococcus*, and *Pseudomonas*, are found. Improved techniques for obtaining cultures of the peritoneal fluid have revealed the importance of anaerobic organisms, especially *Bacteriodes*, in appendiceal infections.[9] In a very careful study, Stone found a definite correlation between the duration of symptoms and the bacterial flora encountered at operation.[10] Anaerobic organisms were found in the peritoneal fluid of a third of patients with simple appendicitis and in all those with suppurative appendicitis. Anaerobes appeared with appendiceal gangrene, and multiple bacterial species were found with frank perforation and peritonitis. When the child had diffuse abdominal tenderness, a fever of 38C or over and a leukocytosis of over 13,000 were found, and anaerobic organisms were found in all cultures. Furthermore, anaerobes, especially *Bacteriodes*, were found in all children with postoperative infections.

DIAGNOSIS OF APPENDICITIS

The appendix has the same innervation as the small intestine, the 9th to the 11th thoracic nerves. Consequently, in the typical patient, crampy periumbilical pain coincides with obstruction of the lumen of the appendix. After several hours, the pain shifts to the site of peritoneal inflammation—most often the right lower quadrant of the abdomen. It is the change in location of the pain that is important, regardless of whether it is to the flank, pelvis, or left lower quadrant. After the pain shifts, it is steady and described as an ache rather than a cramp. In small children, it is difficult to get a definite history of the type and onset of the pain. Consequently, one must rely on physical findings. Anorexia and vomiting almost invariably follow shortly after the onset of pain. During the first few hours of the illness, the child may continue to take and retain liquids. Usually, however, he or she will vomit all recently ingested food during the first 12 hours of the illness. Later, there is a paralytic ileus secondary to peritonitis and persistent, bilious vomiting. The child will not have had a bowel movement after the onset of pain unless the appendix is in the pelvis, where it irritates the rectum and produces tenesmus and diarrhea. During the first 12 to 24 hours a fever of 38.1 to 38.3C is usual. The fever then rises in direct proportion to the duration of symptoms. A dehydrated child with peritonitis will have a fever of 40C. However, if the fever is much over 38.3C and the child does not have signs of a definite peritonitis, it is wise to look elsewhere for the cause of the fever.

The History

Older children will readily tell the time of the onset of symptoms and are fairly accurate in localizing the pain. The questions must be clearly phrased and the child's abdomen must be uncovered so that he or she can point to where the pain first started and where it has localized. After the child and parents have given their versions of the illness, it is important to find out when the child was last perfectly well. Did the pain keep him out of school the day before? Could he sleep the night before? Did he eat breakfast that morning? Few children have any real concept of time. Consequently, the initial onset of pain must be related to a specific event. One should show the child how to point with one finger to indicate where the pain started and where it is at the time of examination. Sometimes parents are helpful, but they can also be vague and contradictory. Younger children localize pain poorly, and it is difficult to evaluate the severity of pain in overly emotional teenage girls and in stoic little boys. You may get some idea of this factor by observing the patient's reaction to an intravenous needle. You can help the child understand the concept of a cramp or intermittent pain by alternately squeezing and relaxing his or her arm with your hand. Intermittent pain suggests gastroenteritis or a "green apple bellyache." Vague fleeting pains that are difficult to describe are more likely to exist on a functional basis. A steady pain that has its onset in the flank or bladder area is likely to be of urinary tract origin. The pain of appendicitis is gradual in onset, whereas a twisted ovarian cyst, a ruptured graafian follicle, or a testicular torsion will cause an abrupt onset of pain. The history of anorexia, nausea, and vomiting must also be obtained with care. Find out when the child last ate a normal meal. Does he normally eat well or is he picky? Healthy boys will claim to be hungry almost by reflex, but if they have appendicitis they will turn pale at the mention of a hot dog. If a child is really hungry or has recently eaten a meal, it is unwise to make the diagnosis of appendicitis. In children under 3 years of age, the only symptoms may be refusal to eat and fussiness. Appendicitis usually is accompanied by mild constipation or no change in bowel habits. Diarrhea occurs more often in infants. A pelvic appendicitis rarely causes true diarrhea—there will be tenesmus with the passage of small amounts of loose stool rather than the copious watery discharge associated with enteritis. A laxative can alter this picture. An inflamed appendix in the pelvis will also cause a frequent and urgent need to urinate. This is an important point in the history that is easy to overlook, since it does not fit our preconceived notion of appendicitis.

A girl's first few menstrual periods may be associated with discomfort and lower quadrant pain. Ovulatory pain (Mittelschmerz) is a sudden sharp twinge that leaves a dull ache. Its relationship to the intermenstrual cycle and its sudden onset should make this diagnosis.

One should note in detail any other information pertinent to a complete history, especially concerning recent travel with possible exposure to intestinal parasites, previous episodes of abdominal pain, respiratory infections, skin rashes, allergies, and headaches.

The Physical Examination

Observe how the child lies on the examination table. If the child has an unhappy expression and is lying on the side with knees drawn up, there is real abdominal pain. The child who jumps about and asks to go home probably has a worried mother but a normal appendix. Rapid respiration with flaring of the nostrils is indicative of either pneumonia or advanced peritonitis. Observation of the abdomen from the side will determine if there is distention. The normal abdomen is scaphoid. In fact, the umbilicus of a skinny boy nearly touches his backbone. A flat abdomen is really slightly distended. Look at the conjunctivae for pallor or jaundice, palpate the neck for enlarged tender nodes, and check for meningitis, leaving the throat and ear examination until the last. Count the pulse to accustom the child to your touch. Examine the abdomen with warm, freshly washed hands and a warmed stethoscope. Parents expect this and one should not surprise the child with cold hands or an icy instrument. Abdominal palpation is commenced by lightly touching the abdomen well away from the area of pain. The left flank or left iliac crest is a good starting point. Gently palpate the entire abdomen away from the area of pain. Gentle palpation of the entire abdomen with only the fingertips will give considerable information about tenderness, muscular rigidity, and superficial masses. During the entire abdominal examination, divert the child's attention with a toy or conversation, but watch the facial expression for a grimace of pain. Avoid rough, rapid motions, since these will frighten the child, making it quite impossible to evaluate for tenderness. After the initial superficial examination of the entire abdomen, commence again the left lower quadrant with deep palpation. If the child winces, find out if the pain occurred at the site of palpation or in a remote area. Rovsing's sign, or pain in the right lower quadrant in response to left-sided palpation, is one of the more certain signs of appendicitis. The key to the diagnosis of acute appendicitis is the finding of point tenderness in the right lower quadrant. The area of tenderness is localized to the parietal peritoneum overlying the inflamed appendix and is usually no more than 1 or 2 cm in diameter. The muscles in the right lower quadrant will be in spasm while the remainder of the abdomen is soft. A retrocecal appendix will produce few abdominal findings, but there will be flank tenderness midway between the iliac crest and the costal margin. Abdominal tenderness in pelvic appendicitis is mild and occurs just above the pubis. Testing for rebound tenderness or pain on sudden release of pressure on the abdomen is frightening and unnecessarily painful. Similarly, the psoas and obturator tests are of little value in children. However, one will often observe a positive cremasteric reflex with gentle palpation over the right lower quadrant. This is presumably due to irritation of the ilioinguinal nerve.

Generalized tenderness may be difficult to evaluate, especially in a very ill, young child with a perforated appendix. The child will cry and complain of pain no matter where the abdomen is palpated. Crying produces abdominal rigidity, which makes the problem even more difficult. The fact that the child keeps pushing the doctor's hand away is significant and means that the abdomen hurts. It is helpful to sit down, distract the child, and tell him or her that you are going to listen to the "tummy," then apply gentle pressure with a stethoscope. If the child winces or cries, there is definite tenderness. The character of peristaltic sounds is not especially helpful, but a silent abdomen suggests generalized peritonitis.

A careful rectal examination may make the diagnosis of a pelvic appendicitis, if there is definite tenderness, or an enlarged appendix is palpable. Take time with the rectal examination. Ask the child to strain down as if he or she is going to "poop" as you insert your finger. Wait until the child settles down and then palpate the sacrum and the left and right sides of the pelvis in that order. The uterus and adnexa can be palpated as well or better rectally as vaginally. A formal pelvic examination is rarely necessary except in older girls in whom there is a strong suspicion of pelvic inflammatory disease.

Very young or irritable children are sometimes impossible to evaluate. These children are admitted to the hospital and given a mild nonnarcotic sedative, such as pentobarbital (2.5 mg/kg) by a rectal suppository. After 45 minutes or 1 hour, the child will be drowsy and can be examined. If he awakens and cries during abdominal palpation, he almost certainly has peritonitis. Sedation is helpful also in relaxing the child so that the mass of an appendiceal abscess can be appreciated.

Pitfalls in Diagnosis

Errors in the diagnosis of appendicitis are most likely to occur when the appendix is in an unusual location, as well as in preschool children who have an atypical history and are difficult to examine. Appendicitis in newborn infants is associated with nonspecific signs and symptoms consisting of fever, abdominal distention, bile-stained vomitus, and diarrhea.[11,12] Abdominal distention has occurred 67 percent of reported cases, and some infants will develop cellulitis of the abdominal wall in the right lower quadrant. Roentgenographic findings of an ileus with a right lower quadrant mass or intraperitoneal fluid are helpful in arriving at a decision to operate on an ill newborn infant. The cecum should be exteriorized when a perforated appendix is found in this age group because of possible associated Hirschsprung's disease. We have observed two neonates with total colon aganglionosis and appendicitis.

Over 80 percent of appendices in children under 4 years of age are perforated by the time a diagnosis is made, and the mortality rate in children under 36 months of age is higher than in older children. However, 40 infants under 2 years of age with appendicitis were treated at the Boston Children's Hospital, with no deaths.[13] The interval from the onset of symptoms to diagnosis averaged 4 days. All of these infants were severely ill, with dehydration and abdominal distention. Abdominal tenderness or a mass in the right lower quadrant was appreciated in these infants only after proper sedation. Roentgenographic studies were helpful in establishing or confirming the diagnosis of 18 of 21 patients studied.

Children with any other illness may develop appendicitis. The problem of diagnosis is particularly difficult when they are being given corticosteroids or chemotherapy or when the original lesion, such as leukemia or cystic fibrosis of the pancreas, may cause abdominal symptoms. The proper diagnosis will be made only by taking the time to evaluate each new symptom and sign and by appreciating the significance of localized abdominal tenderness.

Aids to Diagnosis

Laboratory help is rarely necessary when the history and physical examination are typical. A mild leukocytosis of 11,000 to 14,000 is usually associated with acute appendicitis. It is unusual to find white blood counts above 18,000 in the absence of perforation. There is considerable variability in the white count, but a shift to the left with increased numbers of polymorphonuclear leukocytes increases the probability of a bacterial rather than a viral infection. If one is undecided about the diagnosis, a normal or only slightly elevated white count provides an excellent excuse to postpone the operation.

A carefully performed urinalysis gives valuable information. The specific gravity and acetone content are guides to dehydration and acidosis. Pus cells and bacteria in the urine indicate an acute pyelonephritis, but an acutely inflamed appendix resting on the ureter or bladder can produce 10 to 15 white blood cells per high power field in the urine.

Roentgenographic studies, including plain films of the chest and abdomen, the IV pyelogram, and the bar-ium enema, have improved our ability to diagnose the atypical case. These studies are also valuable in aiding in the diagnosis of lesions that mimic appendicitis, such as a right-sided hydronephrosis or acute regional enteritis. The only specific radiologic finding in early appendicitis is a calcified fecalith (Fig 96–1). These are present in about 12 percent of patients. They are characteristically laminated and oval or rounded in shape. Other less specific findings include dilatation of the cecum with air–fluid levels and edema of the bowel wall, scoliosis with a tilt of the lumbar spine to the right, and obliteration of the preperitoneal fat line or the psoas shadow.[14–16] Disproportionate distention of the jejunum also has been seen in children with perforated appendicitis with peritonitis.[17] This finding may be either a reflex phenomenon or a representation of an intestinal obstruction due to fibrinous adhesions.

The IV pyelogram is most useful in making a differential diagnosis between a retrocecal appendicitis and renal pathology. If one finds a definite kidney lesion, the child should be treated and observed rather than operated on immediately. On the other hand, an inflamed appendix resting on the ureter produces a moderate dilatation of the upper two thirds of the ureter with a fusiform narrowing below. This finding also has been noted with terminal ileitis.

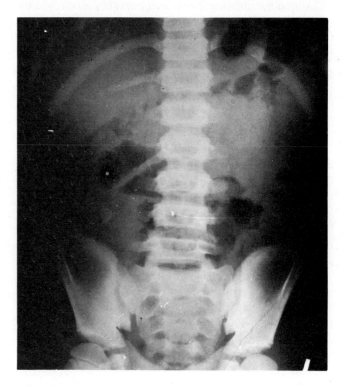

Figure 96–1. There is a large calcified fecalith above the anterior–superior iliac spine. Note also the dilatation of the small bowel and the absence of gas in the right lower quadrant, both due to an abscess.

The barium enema is another useful radiologic tool, particularly in excluding the diagnosis of appendicitis in doubtful cases or when there is a serious preexisting disease that would make anesthesia and surgical exploration hazardous. This test will also locate the cecum when the pain and tenderness suggest the diagnosis but are in the wrong place. If the appendix fills with barium, the diagnosis can be pretty well ruled out, but we have all seen distal obstruction of the appendix with a perforation at the tip. For this reason, the barium enema must not be regarded as 100 percent accurate.

In the Soter technique, the cecum and terminal ileum are filled with barium in an attempt to visualize the lumen of the appendix.[18] No more than 90 cm of water pressure is applied to the column of barium. Signs of appendicitis on the barium enema include partial filling of the appendix, mucosal irregularity, and indentation of the cecum by an abscess. Jona et al. reported on a series of 58 children in whom barium enemas were used as a diagnostic aid in abdominal pain.[19] None of the 27 children whose appendices filled completely had appendicitis. Acute appendicitis was found in 18 of 29 patients in whom the appendix failed to fill with barium. The barium enema has been most useful in ruling out appendicitis by demonstrating a perfectly normal cecum and appendix in the child who has had atypical or recurrent abdominal pain. Some of these children have undoubtedly been spared an unnecessary operation.

We now use ultrasonography in every child with abdominal pain in whom the diagnosis is not immediately obvious. This test reliably makes the diagnosis of ovarian cysts, gallstones, pancreatitis, and renal disease, all problems that enter in the differential diagnosis. With increasing experience, our ultrasonographers have identified noncalcified fecaliths, distended, nonperforated appendices, and appendiceal abscesses with almost 100 percent reliability. In other series of patients, ultrasonography excluded the diagnosis when findings were perfectly normal and made the diagnosis in 39 of 52 patients later shown to have the disease.[20]

Differential Diagnosis

There are a few rare surgical conditions that closely mimic appendicitis. These include a perforated Meckel's diverticulum, a foreign body perforation of the ileum or colon, and omental torsion. In girls, a twisted ovarian cyst or torsion of a normal adnexa causes lower abdominal pain and tenderness, but the onset of pain is sudden, and often one can palpate a mass on rectal examination. An operation is indicated for all these conditions, and the usual muscle-splitting incision is adequate for exposure in all. Consequently, no harm is done when the preoperative diagnosis of appendicitis is erroneous. When a normal appendix is found and there are clear preoperative indications for an operation, the abdomen should be explored for one of these other lesions. There are a number of other pediatric diseases that do not require an operation. Simple constipation may cause cecal distention and pain in the right side. There are no signs of peritonitis, and a small enema or suppository is curative. A ruptured ovarian follicle causes sudden abdominal pain, followed by a dull ache. Ultrasonography will demonstrate free pelvic fluid and an enlarged ovary. Pelvic inflammatory disease usually commences with lower abdominal pain, a high fever, and a purulent vaginal discharge following a menstrual period. Dysuria is common, but gastrointestinal symptoms are not as prominent with this ailment as with appendicitis. Both salpingitis and pelvic appendicitis cause severe pain when the cervix is moved. If gram stains of the vaginal discharge demonstrate a gram-negative intracellular diplococcus a period of observation, with intravenous antibiotics, is in order. Observation and frequent reexamination will usually lead to the correct diagnosis, but in some cases the diagnosis can be made only at operation. Primary peritonitis is now rarely seen, but it should be considered when a child with nephrosis develops abdominal pain. An abdominal paracentesis may be performed. If gram-positive cocci are obtained, the child is treated with the appropriate intravenous antibiotics. There should be a prompt response, with decrease in the fever, pain, and tenderness. In recent years, there has been a decrease in pneumococcal primary peritonitis, with a relative rise in the number of gram-negative organisms. In most series of children with primary peritonitis, the diagnosis was made at operation.[21,22] The pain of primary peritonitis is diffuse throughout the abdomen, the fever is higher at the onset, and tenderness is more diffuse. These findings should make one consider primary peritonitis. If a barium enema rules out appendicitis, the child may be safely observed and given antibiotics.

The abdominal pain associated with diabetic acidosis is generalized, but there is little if any tenderness. There will be a history of polyuria, polydipsia, and weight loss. The abdominal pain clears promptly as the disease is treated with insulin and intravenous fluids.

Henoch-Schoenlein purpura is a diffuse vasculitis that often commences with diffuse colicky pain. There can be right lower quadrant tenderness. We operated on one child with this diagnosis before the onset of his skin rash and found edema with ecchymotic spots on the cecum. Typically, there is a flat, sharply defined purplish skin rash several millimeters in size that does not blanch on pressure. It is located predominantly on the buttocks and lower extremities. Edema of the dorsum of the feet, arthralgia, and microscopic hematuria complete the clinical picture. There may be grossly bloody stools, and one must remember that an intussusception complicates the cases of 2 to 3 percent of children with purpura.

Children with sickle cell anemia have abdominal crises with severe pain. They appear chronically ill, are obviously anemic and listless, and lie on their sides with their hips and knees flexed. The pain is more severe than that associated with nonperforated appendicitis, and there is abdominal distention and tenderness and diminished intestinal sounds. In young children, the spleen is palpable. A positive sickle cell test will make one think of the diagnosis. The white blood count is of no help, since the asymptomatic child with sickle cell disease normally has a white blood count of 15,000 to 20,000 with 80 percent polymorphonuclear leukocytes.

Sufficient intravenous fluids are given to the child with a suspected sickle cell crisis to induce a brisk diuresis with reduction of the urine specific gravity to 1.002. The abdominal pain should subside within 8 to 12 hours after commencement of therapy. If the diagnosis is still in doubt, a barium enema may be helpful.

Pancreatitis caused an abrupt onset of upper abdominal pain, vomiting, and distention. The pain remains in the upper abdomen and radiates through to the back. Children with pancreatitis often sit up in bed and lean forward. A serum amylase determination is performed at the slightest suspicion of the disease. Plain roentgenograms of the abdomen may demonstrate a localized ileus, or sentinal loop, in the upper abdomen. Ultrasound studies have been most helpful in diagnosing pancreatitis. Therapy for the acute episode consists of nasogastric suction, intravenous fluids, and sedation. After the acute episode, the child is studied for a specific etiology for the pancreatitis.

Lead poisoning is one of the facts of life in large cities where children live in substandard housing. Attacks of abdominal pain that lead to hospitalization occur more frequently in the summer months. There is colicky abdominal pain, constipation, and vomiting. Physical examination reveals an irritable child with diffuse intermittent abdominal pain; there are no localized findings. Abdominal roentgenograms may demonstrate flecks of plaster. The child will be anemic with basophilic stippling of the red blood cells and will have lead lines in the long bones and an elevated blood lead level.

Enteric infections, especially shigellosis and salmonella infections, may cause severe abdominal pain, fever, and marked toxicity. The diarrhea associated with these diseases is profuse and watery, completely unlike that seen with pelvic appendicitis. A history of recent exposure to contaminated food or water is helpful, but stool cultures will make the diagnosis. Appendicitis has been associated with shigellosis. In the reported cases, there was localized tenderness with guarding in the right lower quadrant and failure to improve after a course of antibiotics.[23] *Yersinia enterocolitica* is a human pathogen that causes a syndrome characterized by right lower quadrant abdominal pain, fever, and diarrhea.[24] Diarrhea

precedes the onset of pain, but many of these patients have been operated on. The appendix is normal, but the terminal ileum is infected and turgid, and the mesenteric lymph nodes are enlarged. The diagnosis may be made by stool cultures and by serum antibody studies. Patients who appear to have acute regional enteritis or Crohn's disease should have cultures and serum titers for *Yersinia*.[25]

Upper respiratory infections, especially streptococcal pharyngitis, are often associated with considerable abdominal pain. The fever is higher than is found with simple appendicitis, and the lymph nodes in the neck are tender. Headache, muscular pains, and a lack of persistent gastrointestinal symptoms are further evidence of a systemic disease, often of viral origin, rather than a surgical problem.

Children who are receiving chemotherapy, corticosteroids, or immunosuppressive drugs for malignant tumors or following renal transplantation suffer a wide variety of gastrointestinal complications.[26–30] Many of these lesions simulate appendicitis, but making the problem more difficult, acute gangrenous appendicitis also is found in this group of patients. In transplant recipients, large doses of corticosteroids appear to be an important etiologic factor. Most of the patients who have developed colon lesions have had cadaver transplants and have been treated with a variety of antibiotics in addition to the immunosuppressive drugs. The colon lesion is that of ischemic colitis, often with a superimposed staphylococcal infection. There may be ulcers of the colon, infarction, and gangrene or perforation. Three patients in our hospital developed right lower quadrant pain indistinguishable from that of appendicitis. The barium enema revealed edema of the cecum with no filling of the appendix. At operation, the appendix was normal, but the cecum was edematous, thickened, and inflamed. These patients recovered after prolonged supportive therapy. A similar necrotizing lesion of the cecum, or typhlitis, is seen in leukemic children who have been on drug therapy. In one autopsy series of 191 children with leukemia, 9.9 percent had typhlitis and 5.8 percent had appendiceal involvement.[31]

With this group of very ill patients, every diagnostic effort should be made, including a reasonable period of observation and supportive treatment. However, surgery may be the only way to diagnose gangrenous areas of bowel or appendicitis. After the aforementioned intellectual review of diseases that mimic appendicitis has been combined with the indicated diagnostic aids, there will remain a number of children in whom the diagnosis is still in doubt. Former teaching was "better safe than sorry," or "when in doubt, cut it out." We no longer believe that one must have a certain percentage of operations on patients with normal appendices to avoid missing the diagnosis. All patients with whom there is any consideration of appendicitis are admitted to the hospital, given intravenous fluids, and observed. Within 4 to 8 hours, the child who has simple abdominal pain associated with an intestinal upset or systemic illness will improve. The usual rapid progression of appendicitis will make the diagnosis obvious after this interval. If the child does have appendicitis, the general condition will have been improved by the intravenous fluids. In our hospital, this plan has resulted in a 4 percent incidence of surgery on patients with normal appendices, with no increase in the incidence of perforation. Similar intensive in-hospital observation has reduced the incidence of operations on patients with normal appendices to less than 10 percent in other institutions.[32,33] Our goal should be to make an accurate diagnosis in every patient in order to eliminate unnecessary abdominal surgery with the potential complication of postoperative adhesive intestinal obstruction.

TREATMENT

Uncomplicated Appendicitis

A child with simple acute appendicitis requires intravenous fluids to correct mild dehydration, and a nasogastric tube is inserted if there is vomiting. Antibiotics are given before operation in all children with appendicitis. They are discontinued after surgery if there is no perforation. Perioperative antibiotics reduce the incidence of wound infection and appear to shorten the average length of hospital stay.[34]

Operation. The muscle-splitting or gridiron incision is ideal when the point of maximal tenderness is just medial to the anterior iliac spine of the ileum. The skin incision commences slightly above this point and extends in an oblique direction for approximately 2 inches. (Fig. 96–2). The incision is continued through the skin, the subcutaneous tissues, and the aponeurosis of the external oblique while assistants maintain firm pressure to control skin bleeding (Fig. 96–3). It is then necessary to coagulate only the larger vessels. Retraction of the external oblique aponeurosis exposes the internal oblique fascia, which is sharply incised before blunt separation of its fibers. There is almost always a sizable blood vessel that requries coagulation in the lateral part of the internal oblique muscle. The transverse abdominus muscle is then divided and held apart with Parker retracters to allow the peritoneum to bulge into the operative field. Both aerobic and anaerobic cultures are obtained of peritoneal exudate as soon as the abdomen is opened. With luck, the appendix will pop into the incision. Otherwise, it is necessary to digitally explore the right lower quadrant. The appendix is palpated and then freed with blunt finger dissection lateral and inferior to the appendix and deliv-

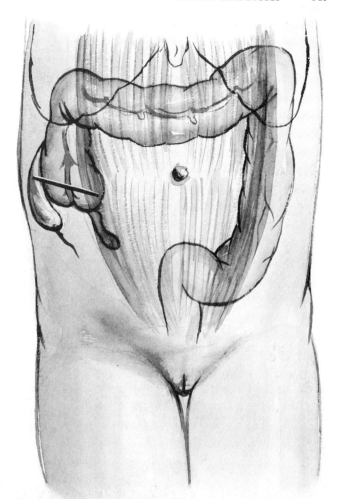

Figure 96–2. The incision for the appendectomy should be higher and more lateral in young children.

ered into the incision. This blind dissection must not be performed medial to the appendix because of the danger of injuring the mesoappendix and causing hemorrhage deep in the wound. If the appendix is not found immediately, the cecum is identified, and the base of the appendix is found by tracing the taenia to their confluence at the tip of the cecum. It is occasionally necessary to mobilize the cecum laterally to find the appendix. If there is difficulty, the wound should be extended, the loops of small intestine packed away, and more of the cecum mobilized. When the appendix has been delivered into the wound, it is surrounded by moist pads. The mesoappendix is clamped and divided by taking small bites of mesentery and is then ligated. It is easier to tie around a right-angled clamp, especially if the mesoappendix is short and difficult to deliver. The appendix must be freed all the way to the cecal wall. At times, it is held tightly against the muscularis by a fold of peritoneum. Unless this is carefully dissected, it is possible to leave a 2 to 3 cm stump of appendix, which would invite a recurrent attack of appendicitis. The appendix

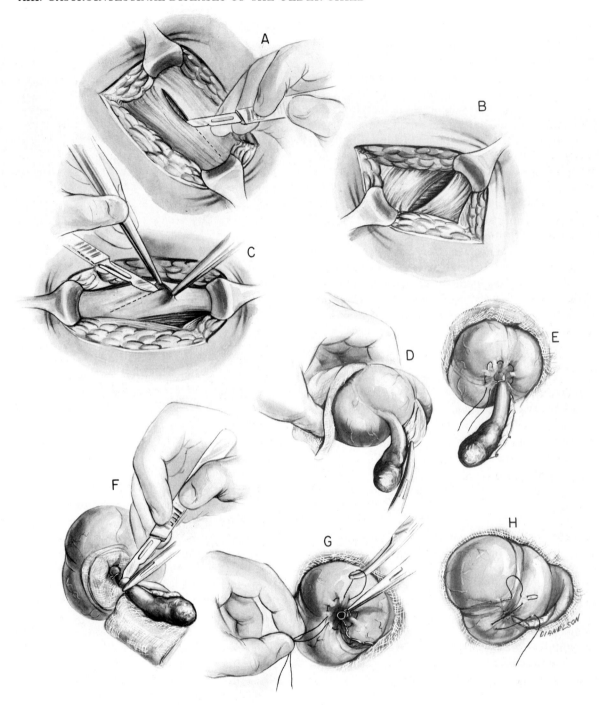

Figure 96–3. Technique of appendectomy.

is then crushed with a clamp flush with the cecum. The crushed area is ligated with catgut. The appendix is held by an assistant while a pursestring suture is applied 0.5 to 1 cm away from the appendix. The mucosa is electrocoagulated, and the stump is inverted. A second simple, or Z, stitch is then applied across the top of the first suture to ensure inversion of the stump. Some surgeons merely ligate the appendiceal stump. The au-

thor has observed approximately 2000 appendectomies at the Cook County Children's Hospital and the Children's Memorial Hospital in Chicago. There has never been a blown stump in any of the children with inverted stumps. On the other hand, three patients were referred to The Children's Memorial Hospital with extensive intraperitoneal sepsis and a fecal fistula after mere ligation of the appendiceal stump. A perforation near the base of the appendix or severe cecal induration may make inversion difficult or impossible. In this situation, a tube is inserted through the base of the appendix and brought out the wound as a cecostomy tube.

APPENDICITIS WITH PERFORATION

The incidence of peritonitis with perforation or gangrene of the appendix varies from 17 to 66 percent in reported series.[35-38] The highest incidence of perforation is in younger children and in series reported from large charity hospitals.

The child with generalized peritonitis secondary to a perforated appendix is dehydrated, febrile, and often septic. Large volumes of plasma-rich fluid are sequestered in the peritoneal cavity. These children require an intensive 4- to 6-hour period of fluid therapy, fever control, and gastric drainage before appendectomy. An initial bolus of lactated Ringer's solution (20 ml/kg) in 5 percent dextrose is given to the child in the emergency room. This is followed by 20 ml plasma or 5 percent albumin per kilogram if the patient is severely hypovolemic. Otherwise, the child is given more lactated Ringer's solution at twice the usual maintenance rate in order to obtain a urine output of 1 ml/kg per hour. A nasogastric tube is inserted and placed on gravity drainage. Acetaminophen suppositories (60 mg/year of age) are given to reduce the child's fever. If the temperature is above 102F on admission to the hospital, alcohol sponges and sedation are indicated for fever control. The goal is to reduce the fever to below 101F and the pulse to below 110. In addition, before the operation, the child should have a urine output of 1 ml/kg per hour with a falling urine specific gravity.

A combination of antibiotics that will be effective against a broad spectrum of aerobic and anaerobic bacteria is given before and after the operation. The combination of ampicillin (100 mg/kg), amikacin (15 mg/kg), and clindamycin (40 mg/kg) in divided doses over 24 hours has been effective in treating sepsis and eliminating the major complications of perforated appendicitis. Metronidazole is active against gram-negative anaerobic bacteria and is well distributed in body fluids and tissues. It is less expensive and may be substituted for clindamycin.[39,40] Eventually, single-drug therapy with the newer cephalosporins may prove to be as effective as multiple drug treatment.[41]

Operation for Perforated Appendicitis
An appendectomy is performed as described previously through a lateral, muscle-splitting incision. All purulent fluid is suctioned from the abdominal cavity, which is then irrigated with copious amounts of saline with 4g cephalothin per liter. If the appendix has perforated, a search must be made for a fecalith, which may be free within the cavity.

In the last edition of this text, I fervently advocated the placement of drains in all children with perforated appendices. We have since abandoned drainage and close all skin wounds primarily. We now leave a small plastic tube, such as an umbilical artery catheter, in the peritoneal cavity. This is brought out the edge of the incision, and 1 day's dosage of amikacin in instilled into this tube in divided amounts, every 6 hours for 5 days. This practice, plus the addition of clindamycin or metronidazole to our antibiotic regimen, has remarkably decreased the incidence of complications and has allowed earlier discharge from the hospital.

Postoperative Care
The child is maintained in the Fowler position during the first 24 hours. Gastric drainage, intravenous fluids, and antibiotics are continued. Gastrointestinal function usually commences within 2 or 3 days, at which time oral feedings are started cautiously. Both systemic and intraperitoneal antibiotic therapy is continued for at least 5 days or until the child has been afebrile for 48 hours.

Appendiceal Abscess
A child who has a well-walled-off appendiceal abscess when first seen will have a palpable abdominal mass with no tenderness in the remainder of the abdomen. If the child improves rapidly with a decrease in fever and pain during a brief period of treatment with antibiotics and intravenous fluids, he or she should be treated conservatively. The abscess will resolve, but an interval appendectomy should be performed within 3 to 6 months to prevent another attack. If the tenderness spreads or if the child remains febrile, the abscess should be drained. The appendix may be removed at that time only if the surgeon can find it easily without dissection. Otherwise, it is left in the patient and removed at a later date.

Complications of Appendicitis with Peritonitis
Prolonged abdominal distention with a high output of green material from the nasogastric tube is caused by severe paralytic ileus. The intestinal sounds remain quiet and repeated roentgenograms demonstrate air–fluid levels in loops of dilated intestine. If the ileus fails to resolve after 2 or 3 days, peripheral hyperalimentation is commenced, and the fluid and electrolytes lost from the stomach must be measured and replaced at 8-hour intervals. When the ileus is associated with a fever, there usually are pockets of purulent material between loops of intestine. Prolonged conservative therapy is indicated

unless there is definite evidence of an intraabdominal abscess that requires drainage. We have seen only two mechanical intestinal obstructions that required an operation during the first month after an appendectomy. Persistent fever is associated with a wound infection or an intraabdominal abscess. Wound infections respond to warm, moist dressings. If the skin was closed at operation, it must be opened. All wound drainage is cultured and antibiotic sensitivities are determined. If the organisms are sensitive, the original antibiotics are continued for 7 days. If the child has a persistent fever, the abdomen, chest, and rectum must be examined repeatedly. A pelvic abscess will cause diarrhea and is palpable rectally. An ultrasound examination will readily demonstrate a pelvic abscess. The abscess is drained only if it becomes fluctuant or shows no sign of resolution. We prefer to drain a pelvic abscess through the original appendectomy wound rather than via the rectum or vagina. A subphrenic or subhepatic abscess will only cause prolonged fever, anorexia, and malaise. There is rarely localized tenderness, but roentgenograms often will demonstrate localized atelectasis or a pleural effusion on the side of the abscess. Occasionally, there is a definite air–fluid level beneath the diaphragm. Gallium scans and ultrasonography have been helpful in localizing residual pockets of pus. One must resist the temptation of trying one antibiotic after another, since this practice only allows the abscess to smolder and become larger while the child wastes away. The abscess must be localized and drained through an extraperitoneal route.

REFERENCES

1. Vital Statistics of the United States. Washington DC, DHEW, 1950–1973
2. McBurney C: Experience with early operative interference in cases of disease of the vermiform appendix. NY State J Med 50:676, 1889
3. Wakeley CP: Position of the vermiform appendix as ascertained by an analysis of 10,000 cases. J Anat 67:277, 1933
4. Soper RT, Opitz JM: Neonatal pneumoperitoneum and Hirschsprung's disease. Surgery 51:527, 1962
5. Martin LW, Perrin EV: Neonatal perforation of the appendix in association with Hirschsprung's disease. Ann Surg 166:779, 1967
6. Burkitt DP: The etiology of appendicitis. Br J Surg 58:695, 1971
7. Boulos PB, Cowie AGA: Pinworm infestation of the appendix. Br J Surg 60:975, 1973
8. Kassner EG, Mutchler RW, Klotz DH, Rose JS: Uncomplicated foreign bodies of the appendix in children: Radiologic observations. J Pediatr Surg 9:207, 1974
9. Leigh DA, Simmons K, Norman E: Bacterial flora of the appendix fossa in appendicitis and postoperative wound infection. J Clin Pathol 27:997, 1974
10. Stone HH: Bacterial flora of appendicitis in children. J Pediatr Surg 11:37, 1976
11. Neve R, Quenville N: Appendicitis with perforation in a 12-day-old infant. J Can Med Assoc 94:447, 1966
12. Hardman RP, Bowerman D: Appendicitis in the newborn. Am J Dis Child 105:99, 1963
13. Bartlett RH, Eraklis AJ, Wilkinson RH: Appendicitis in infancy. Surg Gynecol Obstet 130:99, 1970
14. Jenkins D, Lee P: Radiology in acute appendicitis. J Coll Surg Edinburgh 15:34, 1970
15. Soter CS: The contribution of the radiologist to the diagnosis of acute appendicitis. Semin Roentgenol 8:375, 1973
16. Hatten LW, Miller RC, Hester CL, Moynihan PC: Appendicitis and the abdominal roentgenogram in children. South Med J 66:803, 1973
17. Riggs W Jr, Parvey LS: Perforated appendix presenting with disproportionate jejunal distention. Pediatr Radiol 5:47, 1976
18. Soter SC: The use of barium in the diagnosis of acute appendiceal disease: A new radiological sign. Clin Radiol 19:410, 1968
19. Jona JZ, Belin RP, Selke HC: Barium enema as a diagnostic aid in children with abdominal pain. Surg Gynecol Obstet 144:351, 1977
20. Puylaert J, Rutgers P, Lalisang R, et al: A prospective study of ultrasonography in the diagnosis of appendicitis. N Engl J Med 317:666, 1987
21. Fowler R: Primary peritonitis: Changing aspects, 1956–1970. Aust Paediatr J 7:73, 1971
22. Golden GT, Shaw A: Primary peritonitis. Surg Gynecol Obstet 135:513, 1972
23. Sanders DV, Cort CR, Stubbs AJ: Shigellosis associated with appendicitis. J Pediatr Surg 7:315, 1972
24. Rodgers B, Karn G. Yersinia enterocolitis. J Pediatr Surg 10:497, 1975
25. Saebo A: Some surgical manifestations of mesenterial lymphadenitis, associated with infection of yersinia enterocolitica. Acta Chir Scand 140:655, 1974
26. Libertion JA, Zinman L, Dowd JB, Braasch JW: Gastrointestinal complications related to human renal homotransplantation. Surg Clin North Am 51:733, 1971
27. Demling RH, Salvatierra O Jr, Belzer FO: Intestinal necrosis and perforation after renal transplantation. Arch Surg 110:251, 1975
28. Bernstein WC, Nivatvongs S, Tallent MB: Colonic and rectal complications of kidney transplantation in man. Dis Colon Rectum 16:255, 1973
29. Arvanitakis C, Malek G, Uehling D, Morrissey JF: Colonic complications after renal transplantation. Gastroenterology 64:533, 1973
30. Perloff LJ, Chon H, Petrella EJ, et al: Acute colitis in the renal allograft recipient. Am Surg 183:77, 1976
31. Wagner ML, Rosenberg HS, Fernbach DJ, Singleton EB: Typhlitis: A complication of leukemia in childhood. Pediatrics 129:341, 1970
32. Jones PF: Emergency Abdominal Surgery. London, Blackwell Scientific, 1974, p 142
33. White JJ, Santillana M, Haller JA: Intensive in hospital observation: A safe way to decrease unnecessary appendectomy. Am Surg 41:793, 1975

34. Winslow R, Dean R, et al: Acute nonperforating appendicitis. Efficacy of brief antibiotic prophylaxis. Arch Surg 118:651, 1983

35. Marchildon MB, Dudgeon DL: Perforated appendicitis: current experience in a children's hospital. Ann Surg 185:84, 1977

36. Brickman IS, Leon W: Acute appendicitis in childhood. Pediatr Surg 60:1083, 1966

37. Stone HH, Sanders SL, Martin JD Jr: Perforated appendicitis in children. Surgery 69:673, 1971

38. Button L, Gillis DA: Acute appendicitis in children. Nova Scotia Med Bull 52:117, 1973

39. Kirkpatrick J, Anderson B, Louie J, et al: Double-blind comparison of metronidazole plus gentamicin and clindamycin plus gentamicin in intraabdominal infection. Surgery 93:215, 1983

40. Smith J, Forward A, Skidmore A: Metronidazole in the treatment of intraabdominal sepsis. Surgery 93:217, 1983

41. Gutierrez C, Garcia-Sala C, Villa J, et al: Study of appendicitis in children with four different antibiotic regimens. J Pediatr Surg 22:865, 1987

97
Adhesive Intestinal Obstruction

In older children, intestinal obstruction may occur secondary to congenital lesions as well as intussusception, tumors, and even *Ascaris* infestation. Unfortunately, intestinal obstruction in older children is almost always secondary to adhesions from a previous abdominal operation. However, an obstruction that occurs within a few days after another operation is more likely to be caused by an intussusception than by adhesions.[1-3] The exception to this rule is the child who has recently undergone surgery for a perforated appendix. In this situation, an early postoperative obstruction is most likely the result of inflammatory adhesions.

The symptoms and signs of the early postoperative intussusception are insidious and are often thought to be signs of a prolonged paralytic ileus. Intestinal bleeding and a palpable mass, the two most important signs of intussusception, are rarely present in the postoperative period.[4] Thus, the diagnosis rests upon careful, daily observations of the abdomen. Initial improvement after an abdominal operation, with passage of flatus and a diminished return from the nasogastric tube, followed by a worsening condition, with distention and a resumption of bilious drainage from the tube, must lead one to suspect an intussusception. Roentgenograms demonstrate dilated loops of intestine with air–fluid levels and an absence of gas in the colon. The postoperative intussusception is either jejunojenunal or ileoileal. Two of the intussusceptions we encountered were gangrenous because of delayed diagnosis. With an increased realization that intussusception is the most common cause for postoperative intestinal obstruction, we have come to operate on such children before vascular compromise. Simple manual reduction is all that is necessary. Recovery is prompt, and we have not seen any recurrences.

An adhesive intestinal obstruction may develop at any time after an abdominal operation. Children operated on for ruptured appendices and those with anomalies of intestinal rotation are more likely to develop adhesive obstructions. Any serosal injury, whether from peritonitis, drying, rough handling with gauze, or glove powder, will incite adhesion formation. The mechanism of obstruction may be simple kinking, internal hernia between adherent loops of intestine, or volvulus about adhesions.

DIAGNOSIS

The child with adhesive intestinal obstruction will have cramping abdominal pain. It is difficult to elicit this type of pain in an infant, but if there is cramping, the baby will at first be relatively comfortable and then cry and pull up the legs. The vomitus initially consists of recently ingested food but becomes bile stained within a few hours. Abdominal distention is never as prominent in children, especially in muscular boys, as it is in adults. In addition, there will be little if any distention with a high intestinal obstruction. At first, there may be a few loose bowel movements, but if the obstruction is complete, the child will then pass neither stool nor gas. These are all classic symptoms of obstruction in an adult. Unfortunately, the symptoms may be masked by an intercurrent respiratory illness or a recent gastrointestinal upset. Furthermore, if the child is receiving radiation of chemotherapy, it is too easy to ascribe the symptoms to treatment. The key symptom of an intestinal obstruction in the older child, as in the newborn infant, is bilious vomiting. Inspection of the abdomen may reveal obviously dilated loops of bowel or some degree of distention. Gentle palpation is carried out to evaluate for tenderness, since this is the only indication for an immediate operation in an adhesive obstruction.

One must sit at the bedside listening for intestinal sounds for no less than 10 minutes to be sure that bowel sounds are present and to learn their character. The total absence of bowel sounds indicates a paralytic ileus, either from peritonitis or, possibly, from a gangrenous loop of intestine. The sounds of obstruction vary from frequent, high-pitched tinkles to infrequent, low-pitched borborygmi.

As the obstruction continues and the proximal bowel becomes dilated and decompensated, the intestinal sounds become more infrequent and low-pitched, demonstrating the need to listen for a prolonged period of time before deciding that the bowel sounds are absent. The well-known rotengenographic signs include dilated loops if intestine with air–fluid levels and, in a complete obstruction, an absence of gas in the colon. Actually, there may still be a bit of gas in the colon, which confuses the diagnosis, but repeated films usually demonstrate the passage of this gas and give the picture of a complete obstruction.

In the emergency room situation, if a child has an abdominal scar, it is wise to ascribe any abdominal symptom to adhesive obstruction and admit the child for observation.

TREATMENT

Initial treatment consists of insertion of a nasogastric tube to decompress the stomach and to prevent vomiting. The tube also has diagnostic value, since if bile-stained material is returned, one is probably dealing with an obstruction. It is folly, however, to believe that a nasogastric tube will decompress dilated loops of small intestine. The child's fluid and electrolyte losses are estimated and replaced with lactated Ringer's solution and, if necessary, 5 percent serum albumin. These fluids are given in boluses of 20 ml/kg until the tongue is moist, the pulse is normal, and the urine output is 1 ml/kg per hour. Further fluid therapy is guided by determination of the serum electrolytes. Reevaluation at frequent intervals may elicit tenderness, tachycardia, or other signs that would suggest gangrenous bowel. If distention diminishes, some stool or gas is passed, and the dilated loops of intestine are reduced in size on repeated roentgenographic examination, this form of therapy is continued. If there is no improvement after 12 hours, an operation is indicated.

Operation

A transverse supraumbilical incision provides excellent exposure of the entire small intestine and is the incision of choice unless it would intersect the previous incision. In this situation, we would use the old scar but would commence the incision 1 or 2 inches above the scar, entering the peritoneal cavity away from the bowel, which may be adherent to the previous incision. Injury

to the bowel is avoided by carefully entering the abdomen at one point. The peritoneum is then elevated with rake retractors while adhesions between the bowel and peritoneum are separated with sharp scissors or scalpel dissection.

With the abdomen opened, dilated loops of intestine are eviscerated onto warm, moist pads as adhesions are severed. The bowel is then followed distally until the obstruction is found and relieved. The entire small bowel from the ligament of Treitz to the cecum is followed, and all adhesions are severed. Failure to perform this maneuver may well result in a continued obstruction in the early postoperative period. Hugely dilated loops of intestine are difficult to replace into the peritoneal cavity and regain their function slowly. For this reason the bowel should be decompressed, either by the passage of a tube from the stomach into the dilated intestine or with a large needle. With the latter technique, a size 14 needle is attached to suction and inserted through the bowel within a pursestring suture. The needle is directed at an angle through the bowel wall; as it enters the lumen, the pursestring suture is snugged down. Air and fluid are aspirated by continually moving the needle to prevent it from becoming occluded by the intestinal mucosa. The entire bowel may be emptied by milking air and fluid toward the aspirating needle. Intubation of the entire small intestine may be performed for both decompression and plication to prevent recurrence of an obstruction.[5,6]

Grosfeld et al. intubated the entire small bowel

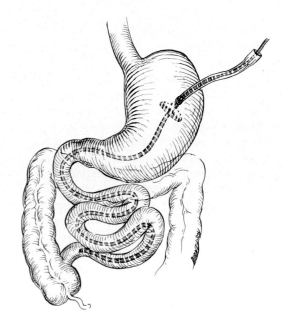

Figure 97–1. Intubation of the entire small bowel through a gastrostomy provides complete decompression and splints the bowel to prevent constrictions.

through a gastrostomy by using a long, balloon-tipped, size 12 to 16 tube (Fig. 97–1).[7] The balloon is inflated after the tip of the tube has been manipulated past the pylorus. Then, with traction on the balloon, the tube is pulled the length of the small bowel and on into the cecum. The tube must be sufficiently long to allow the loops of bowel to lie in gentle curves, so as to prevent future kinks as new adhesions form. The bowel is splinted for 10 days. During this time, the stomach is decompressed with a nasogastric tube, and the child is given hyperalimentation.

There were no recurrent obstructions in the original 20 patients reported by Grosfeld et al. (5-year follow-up) (J. Grosfeld, personal communication). This procedure is advisable in children with recurrent adhesive obstructions, particularly if the first operation was for malrotation.

REFERENCES

1. Raffensperger JG, Baker RJ: Postoperative intestinal obstruction in children. Arch Surg 94:450, 1967
2. Hays DM: Intussusception as a postoperative complication in pediatric surgery. Surg Gynecol Obstet 112:583, 1961
3. Guttman FM, Durchar JC, Collin PP: Intussusception after major abdominal operations in children. Can J Surg 13:427, 1970
4. Cox JA, Martin LW: Postoperative intussusception. Arch Surg 106:263, 1973
5. Baker JW: Stitchless plication for recurring obstruction of the small bowel. Ann J Surg 116:316, 1968
6. Moore T, Salzberg A, Talman E: Jejunoiliocolic intubation and plication for intestinal obstruction caused by massive adhesions in infancy. Surgery 67:363, 1970
7. Grosfeld J, Cooney D, Csiciko J: Gastrointestinal tube start plication in infants and children. Arch Surg 110:594, 1975

98
Gallbladder Disease in Childhood

_____ *Jessie L. Ternberg*

The gallbladder functions as a reservoir for bile storage and concentration. With meals, the gallbladder contracts as the sphincter of Oddi relaxes in response to the hormone cholecystokinin and related peptides. Following cholecystectomy, the flow of bile depends on the sphincter of Oddi. Absence of the gallbladder is rarely of physiologic significance in the child or adult. Although congenital anomalies of the gallbladder are rare, acquired conditions of the gallbladder are of clinical importance in a significant number of infants and children. These conditions are usually related to (1) gallstones and their complications, (2) inflammation of the gallbladder with or without stones, and (3) dilatation (hydrops) of the gallbladder in response to a systemic ailment.

CONGENITAL ANOMALIES

The gallbladder develops between 30 to 35 days of gestation as an outgrowth of the developing common bile duct (CBD) that connects the hepatic cords to the foregut. When first recognizable, the gallbladder is hollow, but subsequent epithelial growth obliterates the lumen. The lumen is reestablished by the process of vacuolization. Abnormal vacuolization can lead to the anomalies of agenesis, hypoplasia, multiseptation, or diverticulum of the gallbladder. These malformations are rare and, in general, cause no symptoms and have no surgical significance. Double gallbladders can develop if two outgrowths bud from the common duct. Multiple gallbladders are not associated with an increase in the incidence of cholelithiasis or cholecystitis. Gallstones are not usually considered a congenital problem but have been demonstrated on antenatal ultrasonography.[1]

CHOLELITHIASIS AND ITS COMPLICATIONS

The gallbladder's major clinical problem results from the development of gallstones. Graham, in 1932, was quoted as being of the opinion that many cases of cholelithiasis first recognized later in life had their origin in childhood, when they were regarded as catarrhal jaundice, gastroenteritis, or mild cases of indigestion. Now, as then, many surgeons consider cholelithiasis and cholecystitis a rarity in children. This traditional misconception accounts for a part of the difficulty in diagnosing gallbladder disease in children.

Etiology of Gallstones

Gallstones are composed of calcium bilirubinate, cholesterol, or a mixture of calcium, proteins, and fatty acids. Pigment stone formation results from the precipitation of calcium bilirubinate in the gallbladder. Bilirubin stones are responsible for between 10 and 15 percent of the gallstones in recently reported series of pediatric age patients.[2,3] Recent studies of bilirubin stones suggest that bacteria may be a part of the etiology of bilirubin stones because, on electron microscopy, most bilirubin stones have microcolonies of bacteria, but bacteria are absent in cholesterol stones.[4] Acute hemolytic episodes, especially when caused by sepsis, can be complicated by the development of stones. The chronic hemolysis that may occur after heart valve replacement has been implicated as a cause of pigment stones.[5] Parasite infestation also can cause pigment stone formation.[6,7] The presence of *Escherichia coli* in the biliary system can cause a sufficient increase in beta-glucuronidase activity to hydrolyze conjugated bilirubin.[8] Nonconjugated bilirubin is insoluble, and pigment stone formation may result.

Any patient with a chronic hemolytic disease may develop pigment stones. The most common hemoglobinopathy leading to stone formation is sickle cell anemia. About 25 percent of patients with sickle cell (SC) disease develop stones by 15 years of age, and the incidence increases to 70 percent in adults.[9–11] A 12-year review of our recent cases of cholelithiasis show that 36 of 88 patients had either sickle cell anemia or hereditary spherocytosis as a contributing factor in stone formation (Fig. 98–1). Pigment stones occur (but with a lesser incidence) with hemoglobin SC disease or hemoglobin S-thalassemia. In hereditary spherocytosis (HS), an autosomal dominant condition, stones are often found in the pediatric age range.[12] Our youngest HS patient with gallstones was 5 years old. All patients having a splenectomy for HS should have preoperative ultrasound evaluation of their gallbladder. If gallstones are found, cholecystectomy should be performed at the time of splenectomy.

Other reported predisposing factors for cholelithiasis include obesity, pregnancy, ileal resection, ileal disease, total parenteral nutrition (TPN), genetic factors, cystic fibrosis, duodenal surgery, oral contraceptives, diuretics, and chronic sepsis. The role of stasis is not clear, but it appears to be a factor in stone production. Stones, for example, are frequently found in choledochal cysts, a congenital anomaly associated with partial biliary tract obstruction. Congenital anomalies, such as stenosis or a splitting of the distal cystic duct, have been cited as a cause of cholecystitis and cholelithiasis in children.[13] The increased incidence of gallstones in female patients at puberty has been attributed to hormone-induced alteration of gallbladder motility.[14] These various factors may be additive in their pathophysiology, since they may lead to both gallbladder stasis and a change in the bile composition. Any aberration of the balance of cholesterol, bilirubin, and lecithin within the bile is likely to precipitate crystals that lead to stone formation.

The ileum is important in bile salt metabolism because it is the site of bile salt absorption and is part of the enterohepatic circulation. Ileal resection for necrotizing enterocolitis and ileal involvement by Crohn's disease are two examples of pediatric surgical settings with great risk of stone formation.[15] These same patients may receive a course of TPN that will put them at an even greater risk of gallstone formation.[16,17] Part of the propensity for stones in TPN patients may be the lack of frequent emptying of the gallbladder because the primary underlying condition prevents oral intake.[18,19] Premature infants on prolonged intravenous nutrition or diuretics may develop stones (almost always pigmented).[20] There are reports on cholecystitis, biliary tract obstruction, and CBD perforation in neonates.[21,22] Our youngest patient (17 days) suffered a perforated CBD with choledocholithiasis.

The female preponderance reported for adult series of cholethiasis has been substantiated in some pediatric reviews. The male/female ratio for patients with hemolytic disease was 1:1 in our series compared to 1.6:1 for patients with a nonhemolytic cause. When the two groups are combined, a slight female preponderance persists.

Diagnosis

The child with calculous cholecystitis most often has right upper quadrant pain. Vomiting is frequent (80 percent), and the pain often is colicky. Localization may be difficult in the anxious child with pain. It is apparent in reviewing the literature that neither the localization of the pain nor the nature of the pain can be regarded as typical in about half of the patients.[23–25] It is the younger child who presents the most difficulty in diagnosis and in whom the localization of pain is more difficult and less consistent. The pain may resolve over several hours or may persist as the gallbladder becomes more edematous and inflamed. Fever and jaundice may be evidence of cholangitis or common duct obstruction. Ap-

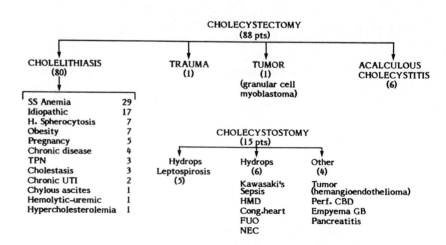

Figure 98–1. Gallbladder operations at the Children's Hospital of Washington University Medical Center, St. Louis, Missouri, 1973–1986.

pendicitis is often the first diagnosis considered in the younger child with poorly localized pain. The danger in operating on these patients for the wrong diagnosis lies in the failure to recognize the error and establish the correct diagnosis. In one series of reported cases of cholecystitis,[24] 10 of the children were operated on for a diagnosis of appendicitis, and in only 1 child was the gallbladder disease correctly diagnosed at operation. Hepatitis, pyelonephritis, and sickle cell crisis are three of the more frequent nonsurgical diagnoses that can cause a delay in treatment. The delay in the diagnosis of cholelithiasis has varied from 1 year to as many as 10 years in some of the larger series of cases.[24] The single most important factor leading to the diagnosis is awareness that cholelithiasis and cholecystitis can occur in children.

The diagnosis of gallstones can usually be made by real-time ultrasonography. The size of the gallbladder, the mobility of the stones, the thickness of the gallbladder wall, the size of the common bile duct, and any enlargement of the intrahepatic ducts can all be determined accurately and noninvasively (Fig. 98–2). The use of oral cholecystography has nearly been eliminated by the accuracy and availability of ultrasonography. The diagnosis of cholecystitis is facilitated by a radioactive isotope test, the DISIDA (diisopropyl iminodiacetic acid) scan, which depends on liver function and excretion. Cholecystitis causes edema of the gallbladder and cystic duct, preventing the entrance of isotope and resulting in nonvisualization of the gallbladder.

The potential for common duct stones exists in all patients with gallstones. The problem can be one of acute obstruction associated with jaundice and pain or chronic obstruction damaging the liver and ducts with or without intermittent jaundice. The question of common duct stones must be considered at the time of cholecystectomy for cholelithiasis and in the differential diagnosis of obstructive jaundice. Computed tomography (CT) can be useful in visualizing common duct stones, especially when duodenal gas overlies the distal common duct. Common duct stones also can be imaged by ultrasonography (Fig. 98–3). At operation, a cystic duct cholangiogram is indicated when clinical findings (small stones, jaundice, enlarged common duct, or pancreatitis) suggest the possibility of common duct stones.

Treatment

Once the diagnosis of cholecystitis is established, attempts to alleviate the symptoms are instituted. Hydration, nasogastric decompression, and antibiotics are started. If the symptoms subside with this conservative management, elective cholecystectomy during the primary hospital stay is recommended to obviate the problem of recurrence, which is likely to happen if the patient is discharged with plans for elective surgery some months later. If fever, pain, and right upper quadrant tenderness persist or worsen, the emergency cholecystectomy occasionally is necessary.

Symptomatic gallstones should be treated by cholecystectomy. Stones found incidentally in patients with an underlying etiologic factor also should be managed by elective cholecystectomy. This latter recommendation is regarded as controversial in the patient with sickle

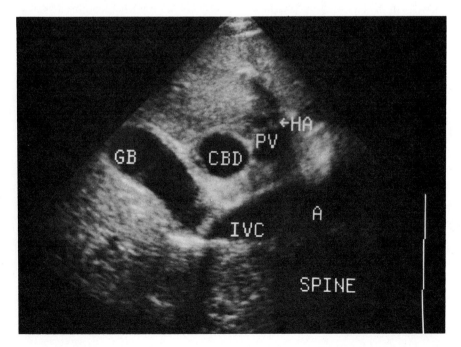

Figure 98–2. Ultrasonography, transverse view at level of gallbladder showing anatomy.

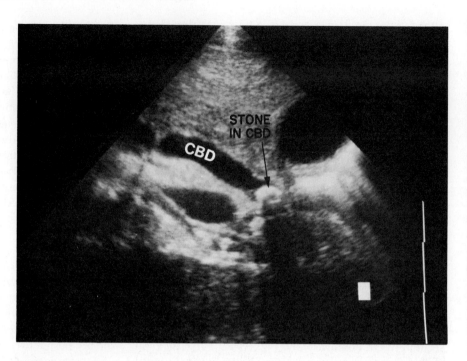

Figure 98–3. Ultrasonography showing stone in common bile duct.

cell anemia, for whom some pediatricians advise chole- cystectomy only when symptoms have appeared. Our recent experience with 29 symptomatic SC patients in- cluded 8 patients with common duct stones (27 percent). This small experience would support a more aggressive approach to asymptomatic stones in SC patients to pre- vent this complication. The risk of cholecystectomy in SC patients can be minimized by adequate hydration and the prevention of hypoxia. We have not used preop- erative transfusions to decrease hemoglobin levels, al- though others consider this to be a valuable part of man- agement.

There is a high incidence of echogenic sludge and actual gallstone formation in infants on TPN. Although these stones can cause cholecystitis and obstructive jaundice, recent reports suggest that some of these stones can undergo spontaneous resolution.[26,27] Observation by ultrasonography rather than immediate cholecystectomy, therefore, seems justifiable until more experience is gained by surgeons and radiologists.

ACALCULOUS GALLBLADDER DISEASE

Most cases of inflammation of the gallbladder are caused by stones, but inflammation can occur in the absence of stones. Acalculous cholecystitis most frequently devel- ops as a complication of another ongoing problem, such as an injury, a burn, an infection, or the postoperative state. Clinically, acalculous cholecystitis overlaps with

what has been called "hydrops" of the gallbladder. Those who distinguish between hydrops and acalculous chole- cystitis do so on the basis that histologic examination shows less inflammation of the mucosa in the case of hydrops. It is possible that rather than considering these as separate clinical entities, acalculous cholecystitis rep- resents a complication of hydrops.

Diagnosis

The signs and symptoms of acalculous cholecystitis and hydrops may be similar, with abdominal pain and tender- ness, a palpable mass, and possibly fever, leukocytosis, and jaundice. Abdominal pain, fever, and jaundice may already be present as part of the primary illness. Ultraso- nography is an important diagnostic method of demon- strating the presence of a grossly enlarged gallbladder (Fig. 98–4). Cholecystitis is suggested by the presence of edema or thickening of the gallbladder wall and by nonfilling of the gallbladder on DISIDA scan. Hydrops implies an enlarged gallbladder, but cholecystitis can be present in a normal-sized gallbladder. Nonrecognition or delay of the diagnosis because of the tendency to regard gallbladder disease as rare in children can result in increased morbidity and mortality.

Treatment

Once other diagnoses (such as appendicitis) are dis- counted, management of the patients with acalculous cholecystitis or hydrops depends on the clinical course. Fever, tenderness, or progressive enlargement of the

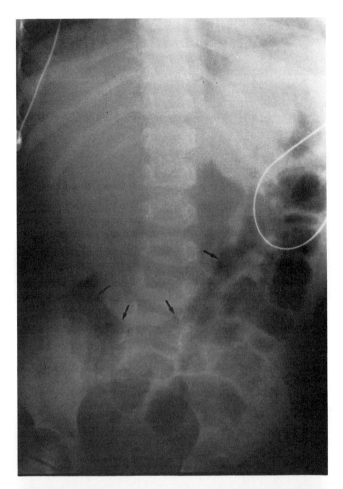

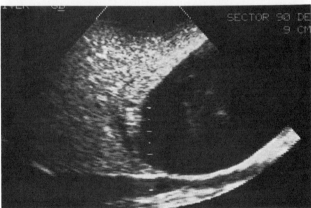

Figure 98–4. Top. Plain film of abdomen showing enlarged gallbladder. **Bottom.** Ultrasound view of same patient showing the enlarged gallbladder.

gallbladder (determined by ultrasonography or physical examination of the abdomen) may necessitate exploration. Most patients with hydrops or cholecystitis will recover with nonoperative management with nasogastric decompression, hydration, and possibly antibiotics.

When an operative approach for acalculous cholecystitis or hydrops is necessary, cholecystectomy is the recommended treatment for adults, based on experience that indicates an unacceptably high rate of recurrence of cholecystitis after treatment by drainage and nonremoval of the gallbladder. There may be exceptions to this principle in the treatment of children, but the information available at this time is insufficient to warrant any definitive statement. Treatment must be tempered by the patient's condition. When the underlying condition is serious and ongoing, placement of a cholecystostomy tube decompresses the gallbladder, allows direct inspection of the gallbladder, and gives access to the biliary tree for further radiologic evaluation. If a gallbladder of questionable viability is found on exploration, cholecystectomy is mandatory. When a cholecystostomy instead of cholecystectomy has been performed as an expeditious procedure in the severely ill child and follow-up studies show a normal gallbladder, we favor removing the tube and not automatically proceeding with cholecystectomy.

A spectrum of disease exists from hydrops to histologic changes of acalculous cholecystitis to gangrene of the gallbladder. Clinical judgment and repeated examinations are much more important in determining treatment than they are in the patient with calculous cholecystitis, for whom cholecystectomy is the indicated treatment.

SUMMARY

A scheme of pathogenesis is shown in Figure 98–5, in which hydrops is considered to represent a first stage of the pathology after the development of biliary tract obstruction. There is no proof for this, but from a practical point of view, the concept is useful in considering the diagnosis and the treatment of gallbladder disease. Obstruction can result from a variety of causes. Once stasis is present, susceptibility to infection is increased. The potential for irritation by chemical or mechanical means also is greater.

The gallbladder response is limited and can be remarkably typical regardless of the initial cause of obstruction. As in all situations involving the possibility of the acute surgical abdomen, many factors are involved, and each patient must be evaluated initially. Although resolution of the problem without an operation is possible, close observation is essential, and complications often can be avoided by earlier surgical treatment. It must be remembered that childhood cholecystitis can be a cause of abdominal pain, either de novo or as a complication of trauma or a prior illness.

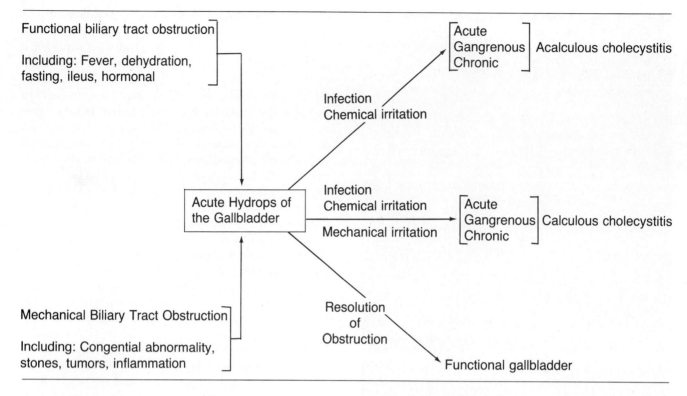

Figure 98–5. A scheme of pathogenesis for childhood cholecystitis.

REFERENCES

1. Heijne L, Ednay D: The development of fetal gallstones demonstrated by ultrasound. Radiography 51:155, 1985
2. Pokorny WJ, Saleem M, O'Gorman RB, et al: Cholelithiasis and cholecystitis in childhood. Am J Surg 148:742, 1984
3. Holcomb GW Jr, O'Neill JA, Holcomb GW III: Cholecystitis, cholelithiasis and common duct stenosis in children and adolescents. Ann Surg 191:626, 1980
4. Stewart L, Smith AL, Pellegrini CA, et al: Pigment gallstones form as a composite of bacterial microcolonies and pigment solids. Ann Surg 206:242, 1987
5. Williams HJ, Johnson KW: Cholelithiasis: a complication of cardiac valve surgery in children. Pediatr Radiol 14:146, 1984
6. Lorvenburg H, Mitchell A: Cholecystitis in childhood. J Pediatr 12:203, 1938
7. Mendoza-Tapia HR: Abdominal surgical emergencies in children caused by *Ascaris*. Rev Esp Pediatr 15:353, 1959
8. Maki T: Pathogenesis of calcium bilirubinate gallstone: Role of *E. coli*, B-glucuronidase and coagulation by inorganic ions, polyelectrolytes and agitation. Ann Surg 164:90, 1966
9. Sarnaik S, Slovis TL, Corbett DP, et al: Incidence of cholelithiasis in sickle cell anemia using the ultrasonic gray-scale technique. J Pediatr 96:1005, 1980
10. Lachman BS, Lazerson J, Starshak RJ, et al: The prevalence of cholelithiasis in sickle cell disease as diagnosed by ultrasound and cholecystography. Pediatrics 64:601, 1979
11. Rutledge R, Croom RD, Davis JW Jr, et al: Cholelithiasis in sickle cell anemia: surgical considerations. South Med J 79:28, 1986
12. Croom RD III, McMillan CW, Sheldon GF, et al: Hereditary spherocysosis. Ann Surg 203:34, 1986
13. Forshall I, Rickham PP: Cholecystitis and cholelithiasis in childhood. Br J Surg 42:161, 1954
14. Nilsson S: Gallbladder disease and sex hormones: A statistical study. Acta Chir Scand 132:275, 1977
15. Kurchin A, Ray JE, Bluth EI, et al: Cholelithiasis in ileostomy patients. Dis Colon Rectum 27:585, 1984
16. Roslyn JJ, Berquist WE, Pitt HA, et al: Increased risk of gallstones in children receiving total parenteral nutrition. Pediatrics 71:784, 1983
17. Pellerin D, Bertin P, Nihoul-Fekete CL, et al: Cholelithiasis and ileal pathology in childhood. J Pediatr Surg 10:35, 1975
18. Benjamin DR: Hepatobiliary dysfunction in infants and children associated with long-term total parenteral nutrition. A clinico-pathologic study. Am J Clin Pathol 76:276, 1981
19. Matos G, Avni F, Van Gansbeke D, et al: Total parenteral nutrition (TPN) and gallbladder disease in neonates. Sonographic assessment. J Ultrasound Med 6:243, 1987
20. Ramey SL, Williams JL: Nephrolithiasis and cholelithiasis in a premature infant. J Clin Ultrasound 14:203, 1986
21. Man DWK, Spitz L: Choledocholithiasis in infancy. J Pediatr Surg 20:65, 1985
22. Descos B, Bernard L, Brunelle F, et al: Pigment gallstones of the common bile duct in infancy. Hepatology 4:678, 1984

23. Brenner RW, Stewart CF: Cholecystitis in children. Rev Surg 21:327, 1964

24. Soderlund S, Zetterstrom B: Cholecystitis and cholelithiasis in children. Arch Dis Child 37:174, 1962

25. Leo WA: Acute calculous cholecystitis in childhood. Mo Med 588:564, 1961

26. Keller MS, Markle BM, Laffey PA, et al: Spontaneous resolution of cholethiasis in infants. Radiology 157:345, 1985

27. Jacir N, Anderson KD, Eichelberger M, et al: Cholelithiasis in infancy: resolution of gallstones in three of four infants. J Pediatr Surg 21:567, 1986

99
Superior Mesenteric Artery Syndrome

John D. Burrington

Extrinsic compression by the superior mesenteric artery or the root of the mesentery can cause partial or complete duodenal obstruction. This obstruction occurs in the third portion of the duodenum as it passes behind the mesenteric root and is usually referred to as the superior mesenteric artery syndrome (SMA). This is an unfortunate designation, since it is often confused with midgut ischemia resulting from partial or complete obstruction of the superior mesenteric artery.[1]

SYMPTOMS

Most patients with SMA are children or young adults who have lost weight from dieting or illness. Some children who have not lost weight but have grown rapidly without concomitant weight gain have also developed SMA. Patients of any age who undergo correction of kyphosis and immobilization of the spine in extension may develop extrinsic duodenal compression, but in this special instance the syndrome is called the "cast" syndrome.[2]

Initial symptoms usually include epigastric pain and vomiting. After several weeks, however, these distressing symptoms often subside, not because the obstruction has been relieved but because the patient begins to eat several small meals a day consisting mainly of liquid.

ANATOMY

The duodenum normally crosses the vertebral column and aorta at the level of the third lumbar vertebra or slightly above. Since the superior mesenteric artery arises at an angle of 45 to 60 degrees from the aorta opposite the level of the first lumbar vertebra, it normally produces no extrinsic compression of the duodenum. With weight loss and reabsorption of retroperitoneal fat, extension of the spine in a cast, or rapid axial growth, the angle between the superior mesenteric artery and the aorta decreases to 15 degrees or less. The resulting nutcracker analogy is undoubtedly simplistic, but it provides a conceptual model of how and where the duodenum is compressed. Since only a small proportion of patients will develop SMA after weight loss, there are undoubtedly some predisposing anatomic factors. In my patients, the duodenum crosses the vertebral column at a higher level than normal, and the ligament of Treitz also is high, with a well-developed muscular component.[3,4]

DIAGNOSIS

Although a careful history is very important to separate children with SMA from those with anorexia nervosa and a variety of causes of vomiting and abdominal pain, fluoroscopy of the stomach and duodenum is the only way to confirm the diagnosis. Initial x-ray studies of the abdomen may show a double bubble characteristic of duodenal obstruction (Fig. 99–1). If this is present, the stomach and duodenum must be emptied before beginning the contrast study.

Typically, the stomach is quite elongated and assumes an exaggerated J-shape. The heavy barium will accentuate this trait (Fig. 99–2). Barium passes freely through the pylorus and fills the first and second portions of the duodenum, which also are dilated and may be

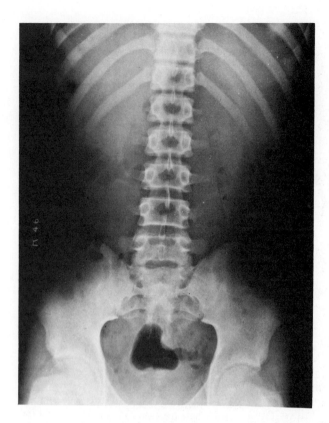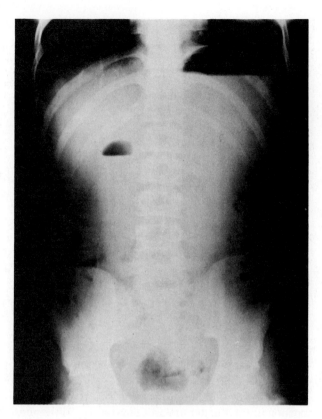

Figure 99–1. Upright (**right**) and supine (**left**) x-rays of 14-year-old boy with SMA. Note dilated duodenum filled with air on supine view and double bubble on upright x-ray.

transiently atonic. The duodenum has vigorous churning without orderly peristalsis or passage of the barium beyond an area just to the right of the vertebral column. There is periodic, vigorous retrograde peristalsis with ejection of barium from the dilated duodenum back into the stomach. The patient frequently complains of nausea each time this occurs.

If the patient is turned to the left lateral decubitus position or is even slightly prone, the barium may pass rapidly across the spine, and in this position, the obstruction may be difficult to demonstrate.

TREATMENT

A majority of children with SMA who are diagnosed early can be treated at home with frequent small, highly caloric, liquid feedings. The child may benefit from lying in the left-lateral position or even by staying on hands and knees for a short time after eating. Both positions relieve the tension on the mesenteric root and seem to relieve the extrinsic duodenal compression. Once the child has begun to gain weight, the symptoms will rapidly abate, and the child can resume more normal eating habits.

Obviously, if the SMA has developed in a child with ulcerative colitis, burns, or other debilitating disease, control of the underlying problem is important.[5,6] Gavage feeding of 50 to 75 cal/kg per day by constant infusion occasionally will establish a weight gain and eventually relieve the duodenal compression. During gavage, the stomach must be aspirated at regular intervals to check residual volumes and to prevent vomiting and aspiration.

On rare occasions, full intravenous nutrition may be required, especially if the gastrointestinal tract is obstructed distally or is not functioning normally. It also has been used in treatment of uncomplicated SMA syndrome, but the risks and cost must be carefully balanced against other forms of treatment. Shandling has reported success in treating children with metoclopramide.[7]

Indications for Surgery

My indications are perhaps more liberal than some, but I have seen many children who have spent weeks or months enduring a variety of unsuccessful medical regimens.[8] In general, if no weight gain can be established at home on frequent, high-calorie feedings, the child should be admitted to the hospital for a trial of gavage feedings. If these are not successful in 5 to 7

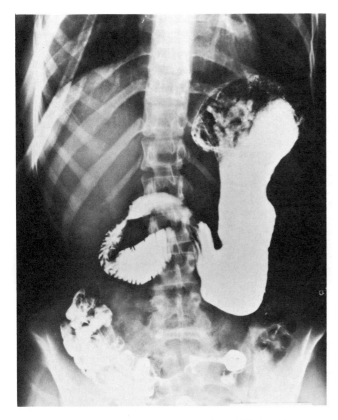

Figure 99–2. Typical radiographic appearance of SMA, with J-shape stomach and dilated duodenum compressed as it crosses the spine at the level of the second lumbar vertebra.

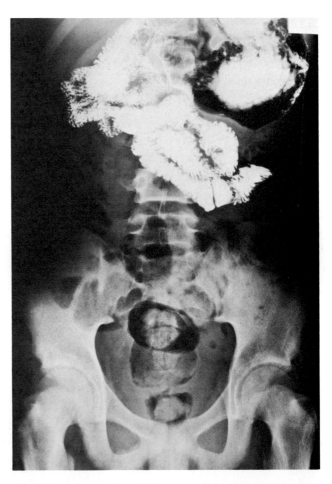

Figure 99–3. Contrast study obtained 4 weeks after operative relief of SMA, as described in text. Note that the entire duodenum and proximal jejunum appear to the right of the mesenteric root.

days, the child should be considered for surgery. Too often, unsuccessful therapy is unduly prolonged, so that when surgery is decided on, the child is emaciated and the family is hostile.

Technique

My own preference for operation involves mobilization of the second and third portions of the duodenum, lysis of the ligament of Treitz, and completely freeing the duodenum from beneath the root of the mesentery. The opening behind the mesentery is enlarged sufficiently to permit passage of the surgeon's entire hand from left to right beneath the mesentery. The entire duodenum and proximal jejunum are then passed beneath the mesentery so that they lie in the right gutter just as they do after a Ladd procedure (Fig. 99–3). The cecum and ileocecal region are left attached to the retroperitoneum so that there is no risk of midgut volvulus. This operation effectively displaces caudally the portion of small bowel that crosses beneath the mesentery and completely relieves the extrinsic compression. It has the advantage of quick return of bowel function. It is a clean operation, since the bowel is not entered, and there is minimal derangement of bowel function suffered.

ANOREXIA NERVOSA

Many adolescent girls have been diagnosed as having anorexia nervosa without benefit of an upper gastrointestinal examination to exclude SMA. Consequently, in any group of patients with anorexia, there is likely to be at least one who has a mechanical cause for her vomiting. More confusing, however, is the child who originally suffers from anorexia nervosa, becomes emaciated, and then develops SMA as a result of the anorexia, so that all efforts at psychiatric rehabilitation are doomed until the mechanical obstruction is recognized and relieved. Such patients obviously require careful screening and close cooperation among the psychiatrist, the pediatrician, and the surgeon.

REFERENCES

1. Akin JT, Gray SW, Skandalakis JE: Vascular compression of the duodenum: Presentation of ten cases and review of the literature. Surgery 79:515, 1976

2. BunchW, Delaney J: Scoliosis and acute vascular compression of the duodenum. Surgery 67:901, 1970

3. Burrington JD: Superior mesenteric artery syndrome in children. Am J Dis Child 130:1367, 1976

4. Burrington JD, Wayne ER: Obstruction of the duodenum by the superior mesenteric artery: Does it exist in children? J Pediatr Surg 9:733, 1974

5. Ogbuokiri CG, Law EJ, MacMillan BG: Superior mesenteric artery syndrome in burned children. Am J Surg 124:75, 1972

6. Ray JF, Lawton BR, Myers WO, Sautter RD: Wilkie's syndrome: A true clinical disease entity. Wis Med J 73:S71, 1974

7. Shandling B: The so-called superior mesenteric artery syndrome. Am J Dis Child 130:1371, 1976

8. Wayne ER, Burrington JD: Duodenal obstruction by the superior mesenteric artery in children. Surgery 73:762, 1972

100

Inflammatory Bowel Disease

Bruce H. Kaufman

In their classic forms, ulcerative colitis and Crohn's disease are distinct clinical entities. By analyzing clinical, radiologic, and pathologic features, one can distinguish between the two entities in 80 to 90 percent of patients.[1] Typically, ulcerative colitis is limited to the mucosa of the large intestine. There is a penetration through the wall of the colon only in fulminant cases of toxic megacolon. Regional enteritis usually involves the terminal ileum. The mucosa is involved, but the pathology extends through the thickness of the bowel wall and may penetrate into adjacent viscera.

In making a correct histologic diagnosis, the pathologist remains dependent on the gross impressions of the endoscopist and the surgeon. A pattern of injury often will emerge suggesting a specific diagnosis. Regional enteritis sometimes involves other segments of the small intestine, with skip areas of intervening normal intestine. Ulcerative colitis, on the other hand, may involve only the rectum (ulcerative proctitis), but there is never a normal area of bowel between diseased segments. Many of the older series of patients were described before Crohn's disease of the colon (granulomatous colitis) could be differentiated from ulcerative colitis.[2] Granulomatous colitis is more likely to involve the right side of the colon along with the terminal ileum, although the entire colon may be involved. Segmental granulomatous colitis is suspected when the rectum appears normal but there is involvement of the remaining colon. Unfortunately, one can make no clear differentiation between the two diseases in about 20 percent of the patients with inflammatory bowel disease.[3] Since we have specific operations for curatively treating chronic ulcerative colitis, this gray area remains a source of frustration. Indeed, some authorities believe that ulcerative colitis and Crohn's disease may be the same and prefer to use the term "chronic inflammatory bowel disease" to describe both disorders.

ETIOLOGY

The etiology of inflammatory bowel disease remains unknown. Attempts to implicate specific bacterial, viral, psychologic, or dietary factors have been inconclusive. There are probably several etiologic factors. There is some evidence for a genetic predisposition, since both ulcerative colitis and Crohn's disease may occur in families.[4] Identical twins have been affected.[5–7] The higher incidence in patients of Jewish extraction has been cited,[8,9] although recently reported data suggest that this information has been exaggerated.[10]

The lymphatic tissue in the intestine is important in the immune homeostasis of the body and produces immunoglobulin.[11,12] Increased levels of IgA are found during quiescent periods in the course of regional enteritis.[13] The immune factors in inflammatory bowel disease may be an antigen-antibody reaction to bacteria or food, or there may be an autoimmune response to intestinal mucosa. Experimentally, instillation of carrageen, a sulfated polysaccharide, into the intestines of experimental animals has produced mucosal changes resembling ulcerative colitis.[14] Lymphocytes obtained from patients with either ulcerative colitis or Crohn's disease are cytotoxic for colonic cells in tissue culture. Circulating antigen-antibody complexes have been demonstrated in these diseases.[15] Experimental models for ulcerative colitis have been described in which T cells play prominent pathogenic roles.[16] Antibodies against a dietary protein, bovine serum albumin, have been found in a high proportion of patients with ulcerative colitis or Crohn's disease.[17] There is also a higher than usual incidence of personal and familial allergic diseases in patients with inflammatory bowel disease.[18-20] The success of the steroid drugs is thought to be the result of an alteration or suppression of the patient's immune mechanism. Moreover, the rationale for the use of immunosuppressive agents in the treatment of both ulcerative colitis and Crohn's disease is that these diseases are thought to affect the immune response.[21]

Successful attempts to transmit to experimental animals a condition similar to Crohn's disease by inserting filtrates of human ileum have given support to the viral hypothesis.[22-24] Mycobacteria, *pseudomonas*-like bacteria, and *Chlamydia* organisms recently have been incriminated as infectious agents in Crohn's disease, but these reports remain unconfirmed.

Inflammatory bowel disease (IBD) in the pediatric population must be regarded differently from the disease in adults for four major reasons.

1. IBD in the infant or very young child has an atypical course, being relatively more severe in the pediatric age group.
2. Growth failure is a major problem in prepubertal children.
3. Chronic disease accentuates the usual emotional problems of the adolescent.
4. The chance of developing cancer of the colon is increased after long-standing colitis in childhood.

Growth retardation and delay in sexual maturation complicate the childhood onset of Crohn's disease in nearly 20 percent of patients, with a somewhat lower rate for ulcerative colitis.[25] Surgical procedures for the management of growth failure in children with IBD have been recommended by several authorities.[26-29] In order to understand the role of surgical therapy in the management of growth failure, it is necessary to consider the underlying process responsible for this lack of growth. Kelts et al. studied 7 children, 9 to 17 years old, with Crohn's disease and growth failure, as defined by a cessation of linear growth for at least 1 year, a decrease of one standard deviation in height percentile, and/or bone age delay greater than 2 years.[30] The nutritional status of all patients was evaluated, and endocrinologic and metabolic balance studies were performed in 5 of the 7 patients. These studies clearly demonstrated that growth failure resulted solely from low calorie intake. There was no evidence of endocrine dysfunction. Even in the face of continued disease, these patients resumed normal and even accelerated growth when given 75 calories/kg per day by a combined oral and parenteral route. Their growth rate was maintained for up to 1 year with no change in associated therapy. Four of the 7 patients

remained on constant doses of prednisone during their growth spurt. Thus, any alteration in growth induced by steroid therapy may be reversed by adequate nutrition. Furthermore, many patients with Crohn's disease begin to grow after adequate steroid therapy.[31]

The anorexia that is a prominent feature of IBD is a factor in the failure of these children to ingest adequate calories. Any therapy, either medical or surgical, that will control the disease and allow sufficient caloric and protein intake will thereby allow normal growth and maturation.

In the patient with remaining growth potential, control of the child's Crohn's disease remains a relatively urgent matter. Be it produced by surgical or medical means, remission of symptoms permitting improved nutrition remains essential to avoid permanent growth failure. Bone age films and objective developmental assessment help the clinician in this regard. Alperstein et al. have shown that reversal of growth failure remains poor once the patient has reached the Tanner IV or V stage of development.[32]

Patients beset by ulcerative colitis in childhood are at greater risk of developing carcinoma of the large bowel than the general population. Moreover, the longer the children with ulcerative colitis are followed, the more colon cancers are seen to occur. Actuarial analysis of the long-term survival of 396 children suffering from ulcerative colitis showed that survival rates were 78, 58, 39, and 27 percent at 10, 20, 30, and 43 years, respectively.[33] The death rate was 20 percent/decade. The risk of development of cancer was also 20 percent/decade for those at risk, but this began after the first 10 years of ulcerative colitis.

In addition to the length of follow-up, the extent of the colitis has been found to correlate with a higher percentage of neoplastic disease. In Sweden, 234 patients with "extensive" colitis or involvement of the large bowel to at least the right flexure were observed for a mean period of 8.5 years.[34] The cumulative incidence of carcinoma 25 years after the onset of colitis for the whole group of patients was 34 percent, and for those who developed the disease before 25 years of age, it was 43 percent. Although the incidence of carcinoma complicating Crohn's disease is less than in ulcerative colitis, the risk of colorectal carcinoma is still 20 times greater than in the general population.[35] With this kind of data, it is hardly surprising that many surgeons have advocated proctocolectomy and ileostomy in all patients who have had ulcerative colitis for 10 or more years.[36] However, care must be taken with this approach. Ulcerative colitis may be mimicked by Crohn's disease or other types of colitis, which carry a much lower risk of cancer. Moreover, the potential risk of colon cancer is minimal in patients with colitis limited to the rectum and sigmoid.[37]

The risk of developing colon cancer has been altered

by three developments. Removal of the colon has become the accepted treatment for severe, acute colitis unresponsive to medical measures and for chronic disabling disease. Thus, many patients at particularly high risk for developing carcinoma are removed from the high-risk group. The observation of cellular dysplasia, which predisposes to cancer, might indicate an individual prone to developing carcinoma.[38] Repeated colonoscopy with biopsies from all areas of the colon may help one detect patients who have developed precancerous epithelial lesions. Importantly, the presence of dysplasia or frank neoplastic change correlates poorly with the clinical status of these patients.[39] Thus, routine pancolonoscopy should be part of the overall management of the individual whose colon remains in situ. If one identifies dysplastic changes on histologic analysis, one should strongly consider removal of the patient's colon. Colonoscopy can circumvent the necessity of performing routine colectomy on all patients merely because of the length of time they have had the disease.[40,41]

EVALUATION

It would be convenient if we had a universally accepted scoring system for evaluation of the severity of disease in comparing the results of different therapeutic regimens. Truelove and Witts classified attacks of ulcerative colitis into mild, moderate, and severe.[42] Diagnostic criteria for these classifications are simple to perform and have been applied widely. Werlin and Grand have enlarged on the definition of severe attacks of colitis in childhood.[43] The National Cooperative Crohn's Disease Study Group has developed a Crohn's Disease Activity Index that uses eight selected variables in assessing the activity of the disease.[44] Unfortunately, this index results in lower scores in the pediatric age group and does not take into account growth curves or the serum albumin, which is a simple measure of nutritional deficiency. The physician's subjective impression of the patient's well-being is useful in grading the severity of illness in adolescents with IBD.[31] Lloyd-Still and Green have devised a clinical scoring system for patients with Crohn's disease and ulcerative colitis.[45] In our experience, this clinical score is easy to use and has been helpful in the initial evaluation of follow-up of these patients (Table 100-1). The score is divided into five sections with a point system that adds up to a total of 100 points. The various subdivisions include physical activity (10 points), physical examination and complications (30 points), nutrition (20 points), x-rays (15 points), and laboratory (25 points). A normal, healthy patient has a maximum score of 100 points, and patients with scores in the 20s and 30s have severe disease. This score can be used in the evaluation of patients for comparison of different therapeutic modalities.

Table 100-2 lists some of the other investigative procedures that are important in the initial evaluation of these patients. The complete blood count enables one to assess the degree of anemia. The erythrocyte sedimentation rate is raised in the majority of patients with Crohn's disease, but it may be normal in patients with severe ulcerative colitis. A raised reticulocyte count will indicate a response to bleeding or administration of oral iron. The stools should be cultured for the presence of pathogenic organisms, ova, and parasites. It is advisable to send a specimen of serum to the Communicable Disease Center for an indirect hemagglutination fixation test, which is positive in about 98 percent of patients with severe amebic colitis.

Assessment of the protein status, especially of the level of serum albumin, is one of the most important initial evaluations and correlates well with the severity of disease. The iron status of the child can be measured by the serum ferritin or serum iron and by total iron-binding capacity. Marked ileal disease may result in low folic acid levels. Serum levels of vitamin B_{12} are almost always normal. However, results of measurement of vitamin B_{12} malabsorption by the Schilling test frequently are abnormal and can be used as a test of terminal ileal function. In patients with persistent fever, measurement of febrile agglutinins (especially against *Salmonella*) is advisable. A xylose absorption test is a sensitive test of upper intestinal function, and a 72-hour fecal fat excretion test will document the degree of steatorrhea.

ULCERATIVE COLITIS

Pathology

The appearance of the colon at operation or through a proctoscope depends on the stage of the disease. Initially, there is only edema with increased friability, granularity, and bleeding of the mucosa. It is extremely difficult to make a definitive diagnosis until there is mucosal ulceration. Small ulcers remain discrete at first and later coalesce. The intervening mucosa becomes thickened and undermined and develops a pseudopolypoid appearance. After treatment, the mucosa is smooth and atrophic but is still friable and bleeds when touched with an instrument. The dull red serosal surface, often partially covered with fat in resected specimens, reflects chronic severe disease. In long-standing cases, the entire colon is shortened, thickened, and scarred. A striking feature of ulcerative colitis is the abrupt transition to normal tissue at the terminal ileum. The earliest histologic findings consist of nondescript infiltration of the mucosa with inflammatory cells.[46] Later, there is a decrease in the goblet cells and the appearance of crypt abscesses, which are microscopic collections of pus within the glandular

TABLE 100–1. CLINICAL SCORING SYSTEM FOR PATIENTS WITH CROHN'S DISEASE AND ULCERATIVE COLITIS

General activity (10)	
10	Normal school attendance, < 3 BM/day
5	Lacks endurance, 3–5 BM/day, misses < 4 weeks school/year
1	Fever, home tutor, > 5 BM/day, severely restricted activity
Physical examination and complications (30)	
Abdomen	
10	Normal
5	Mass
1	Distention, tenderness
Proctoscopy/perianal	
10	Normal, no fissures
5	Friability, 1 fissure
1	Ulcers, pseudopolyps, bleeding, multiple fissures, fistulas
Arthritis	
5	Nil
3	One joint/arthralgia
1	Multiple joints
Skin/stomatitis/eyes	
5	Normal
3	Mild stomatitis
1	Erythema nodosum, pyoderma, severe stomatitis, uveitis
Nutrition (20)	
Height	
10	> 2 in/year
5	< optimal %
1	No growth
Weight	
10	Normal
5	No gain
1	Weight loss
X-rays (15)	
15	Normal
10	Ileitis, colitis to splenic flexure
5	Total colon or ileocolic involvement
1	Toxic megacolon, obstruction
Laboratory (25)	
Hematocrit	
5	> 40
3	25–35
1	< 25
Erythrocyte sedimentation rate	
5	Normal
3	20–40
1	> 40
White blood cells	
5	Normal
3	< 20,000
1	> 20,000
Albumin	
10	Normal
5	3.0 g/dl
1	< 2.5 g/dl

crypts.[47] The microscopic changes involve the mucosa and submucosa, but the muscularis is usually unaffected.

Signs and Symptoms

Although most cases of ulcerative colitis are first diagnosed in patients between 15 and 30 years of age, the onset of symptoms often occurs earlier, and cases have been described in babies under 1 year of age.[48]

The most common early presenting symptom is rectal bleeding. This may be streaking of the stool with mucus and blood, or there may be an episode of brisk, bright red bleeding. Diarrhea, colicky abdominal pain, and tenesmus usually occur initially or may follow the rectal bleeding by weeks or months. Nocturnal diarrhea that awakens the child at night particularly requires investigation. Incontinence with diarrhea also is a sign of

TABLE 100–2. PERTINENT INVESTIGATIVE PROCEDURES IN CHILDREN WITH INFLAMMATORY BOWEL DISEASE

History and physical examination
Laboratory work
  Complete blood count, reticulocyte count, erythrocyte sedimentation rate
  Stool cultures for pathogens, ova, and parasites
  Amebiasis—indirect hemagglutination titer (>1:125 positive)
  Yersinia—complement-fixation test
  Salmonella—febrile agglutins
  Total protein, albumin
  Serum iron, ferritin, total iron-binding capacity
  Folate, vitamin B$_{12}$
  Xylose absorption test
  72-hour fecal fat
Radiology
  Upper gastrointestinal series and follow-through
  Barium enema, IV pyelogram
Sigmoidoscopy and rectal biopsy
Other
  Psychologic evaluation
  Colonoscopy

organic pathology. The stool contains blood and mucus and is foul-smelling. Stringy bits of mucosa may be seen on examination. Additional symptoms include arthritis, signs of anemia, stomatitis, erythema nodosum, and iritis. There is often a familial history of IBD. In untreated patients or during relapses, the physical examination will reveal pallor of the skin and mucus membranes, weight loss, mild dehydration, and fever, with tachycardia. These are signs of hypovolemia and toxicity. These children often are quiet, withdrawn, and fearful, especially when they have had a prolonged illness with multiple hospitalizations. The child's apathetic emotional response improves with successful treatment. The height and weight percentiles should be plotted on a growth chart as part of the physical examination. During acute episodes, the abdomen is tender, especially over the sigmoid colon. There may be mild distention, but severe distention with tenderness and rigidity is seen only when there is a perforation or toxic megacolon. The liver is occasionally enlarged to palpation. If proctoscopic examination is planned, the rectal examination is sometimes deferred, since this is extremely uncomfortable because of sphincter spasm and rectal tenderness.

Proctosigmoidoscopy is the most valuable initial diagnostic tool and is useful in following the course of the disease. Older, cooperative patients may be examined with mild sedation, but younger children often require a general anesthetic. After the child feels better and has established rapport with the physician, proctoscopy can be carried out without sedation in the outpatient department. One should specifically observe for ramifying blood vessels, friability of the mucosa, patchy or diffuse mucosal involvement, and whether or not the mucosal changes are in the distal rectum. The presence

of pseudopolyps and ulcers is a sign of more advanced disease. In addition to observation, a mucosal biopsy and specimens of mucus are obtained for bacteriologic study and immediate examination for ova and parasites. In young infants, it may be difficult to differentiate early ulcerative colitis from milk colitis, and at any age, common diarrheal diseases may simulate ulcerative colitis. Repeated examinations may be indicated before making a definitive diagnosis. Mucosal flattening and pallor are often seen after successful treatment and relief of symptoms. The typical undermined ulcers with pseudopolyps are clearly diagnostic of long-standing, chronic disease. When the diagnosis of ulcerative colitis has been made or is suspected because of proctoscopy and biopsy, a barium enema is indicated to determine the severity and extent of the disease. A barium enema must not be performed until 2 days after a proctoscopy and biopsy to avoid perforating the colon. Further, a barium enema is contraindicated when a child clearly has severe ulcerative colitis on clinical and proctoscopic examination, since it may precipitate an acute toxic megacolon. In the severely ill child, plain films of the abdomen are valuable. A colon more than 6 cm in diameter is diagnostic for toxic megacolon, and upright films may reveal free air from a perforation. As the disease progresses, a barium enema is useful to detect strictures, fibrosis, and carcinoma. Colonoscopy has, however, provided more detailed information on the extent and severity of the disease than the radiologic examination. A fairly well child in whom the diagnosis is only suspected may have cleansing enemas to prepare the colon for a barium enema. If there is diarrhea and bleeding, no special preparation is given before the x-ray examination. The barium enema results may be completely normal during the early phases of the disease.[49] Later, one finds loss of the mucosal pattern and fine spicule formation, indicating superficial ulcers. As the disease progresses, one sees mucosal granularity, obvious ulceration, rigidity, and loss of the haustral markings (Fig. 100–1). Postevacuation films and air contrast studies provide the best mucosal detail.

It may be difficult to diagnose ulcerative colitis when the first attack is mild or atypical and there are normal radiologic findings. When the proctoscopic examination reveals only mild inflammation, we are reluctant to make the diagnosis and prefer to follow the child carefully for the development of more positive findings. The disease may be mild and limited to the rectum. These children with ulcerative proctitis have bleeding, diarrhea, and tenesmus. The rectum is involved, but the sigmoid mucosa is normal, and there are normal x-ray findings. These children may have a more benign course with few complications.[50,51] An occasional child, especially among those under 10 years of age, will have an acute severe onset with fulminating bloody diarrhea, abdominal pain, distention, and tenderness. There is a considerable risk of acute colon distention (toxic megaco-

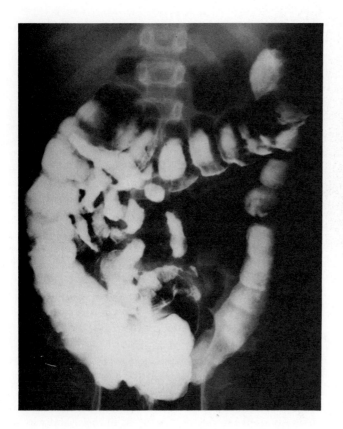

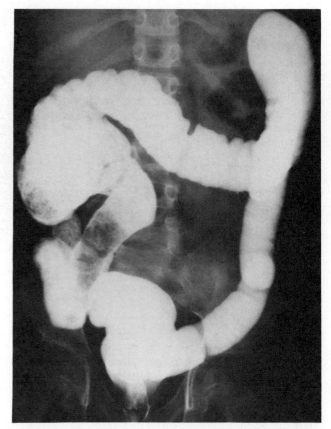

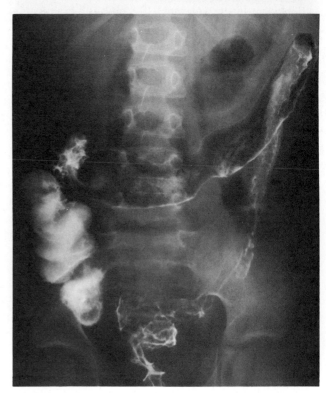

Figure 100–1. Barium enema examinations in children with ulcerative colitis. **Top left.** This barium enema was performed 6 months after the child began to have symptoms. The only significant changes seen here are in the sigmoid colon, which has lost its haustral markings. **Top right.** The same child 1 year later. Here the entire colon is involved. The descending and sigmoid sections of the colon have a lead pipe appearance, and the transverse colon has lost almost all its haustral markings. **Bottom right.** Far-advanced ulcerative colitis. The arrow points to deep longitudinal ulcerations. The sigmoid is narrow and fibrotic.

lon) and intestinal perforation in these children unless they undergo prompt, vigorous treatment.[52] Anticholinergic drugs and opiates may precipitate toxic megacolon in children with established disease. Ulcerative colitis that develops in infancy is particularly likely to run a fulminant course, with severe bloody diarrhea, weight loss, and dehydration.[53] The disease is so severe in infants under 1 year of age that an ileostomy or possibly a colectomy is indicated more often than in older children.[49,54]

Differential Diagnosis

Parasitic and bacterial infections, such as amebiasis or shigellosis, may mimic ulcerative colitis. The diagnosis of a bacterial infection is easily made with stool cultures, but the diagnosis of amebiasis is more difficult. Fulminant amebic colitis mimics severe ulcerative colitis and can result in a toxic megacolon.[55,56] Microscopic examination of multiple fresh stool specimens for ova and parasites must be performed on every patient suspected of having ulcerative colitis, especially before the administration of steroids. Fresh specimens of mucus obtained during proctoscopy on an unprepared colon are most likely to be positive for parasites. In addition, the indirect hemagglutination tests are positive in 98 percent of patients with active amebiasis.[57] The Serameba test, produced in kit form by Ames, is simple and rapidly performed and is reasonably accurate.

Granulomatous colitis must always be considered in the differential diagnosis of ulcerative colitis. The diagnosis may be suspected when there are perianal disease and skip lesions in the bowel. Fortunately, a biopsy will differentiate between the two diseases in most cases.

Medical Therapy

Medical therapy consists of physical rest, restoration of nutrition, control of infection, resolution of the inflammation, and adjustment of associated emotional disturbances. Each patient presents an individual problem, although certain principles can be applied. Treatment should attempt to control the acute attack and prevent relapses.

Mild Attacks. Patients with mild attacks have diarrhea with minimal rectal bleeding or mucus and occasional tenesmus. Weight loss is not severe, and anemia is not present. There is no associated fever, and the patients remain normally active. There is no evidence that dietary restrictions are beneficial, and indeed, these may lead to reduction of caloric intake. Corticosteroids are not required, although some authorities give 1 to 2 week courses of corticosteroid enemas if tenesmus is severe. These enemas are effective in alleviating symptoms, but it must be remembered that 40 percent of the rectal dose of corticosteroid is absorbed. Azulfidine (2 to 4 g/day) is the basis of therapy and is usually given

for at least a year, if tolerated. Added multivitamins and folic acid (1 mg/day) are prescribed. Iron will be necessary if there is evidence of iron deficiency anemia. These patients have a good prognosis.

Moderate Attacks. These patients have more severe diarrhea, usually with associated bleeding and tenesmus. Malnutrition and anemia may be present, but fever is unusual. Abdominal pain is common. Extraintestinal symptoms, such as stomatitis and arthritis, often are present. Hospitalization may be required, especially with the first attack. Anorexia is frequently marked, and the diet should encourage a high-caloric, high-protein intake. In practice, this is often difficult to achieve until the attack is controlled. Lactose-free milk may lessen abdominal symptoms if lactose intolerance is present. Corticosteroids, such as prednisone (1 to 2 mg/kg per day, up to a maximum of 60 mg/day), are given for 2 to 4 weeks until the index of disease activity as determined by clinical symptoms and the serum albumin is improved. Prednisone is tapered by 5 mg/week until a maintenance dose of 5 to 10 mg/day is reached. After the child is symptomatic for another month or longer, daily prednisone is slowly discontinued. Azulfidine (2 to 4 g/day) is given at the onset of the attack and is continued after the steroids are discontinued. Maintenance is usually continued for at least 2 years, providing the drug is tolerated. There are no controlled trials to ascertain this drug's benefit in children, but adults will continue to benefit from maintenance. Azulfidine treatment is continued for several years after the last relapse.

Multivitamins and folic acid (1 mg/day) are prescribed. Anticholinergics are contraindicated. Associated psychogenic problems must be dealt with if medical therapy is to be successful.

Severe Attacks. These patients are characterized by having more than five grossly bloody stools per day, fever greater than 100°F, tachycardia, and hematocrit less than 30, an erythrocyte sedimentation rate over 30 mm/hour, and serum albumin less than 3 g/100 ml.[58] They frequently have severe nutritional and electrolyte imbalance, as well as hypomagnesia.[59] In recent years, an intensive therapeutic program has been used in adults with severe attacks of ulcerative colitis, and this has been adapted to children by Werlin and Grand.[43] This regimen consists of intravenous fluids and electrolytes, blood and albumin transfusions, and intravenous hydrocortisone (10 mg/kg per day). Most patients have been treated with antibiotics and hyperalimentation. Nasogastric suction is required if a toxic megacolon is present. Anticholinergic drugs are contraindicated. Of the 19 children with severe colitis in the series of Werlin and Grand, 32 percent had a rapid response to medical therapy. However, the remission was short-lived, and the majority of these patients with severe colitis required surgery within 3 years of the onset of the attack.

Surgical Management

Since massive hemorrhage will respond to medical therapy, and toxic megacolon and intestinal perforation are rarely seen, there is essentially little reason for an emergency colectomy in children. Thus, the indication for an operation is usually failure to respond to medical treatment. When there is chronic or recurrent disease that prevents the child from attending school and taking part in the usual activities and that causes repeated hospitalizations, one must consider an operation. The patients who fail to respond to medical therapy demonstrate progressive roentgenographic and proctoscopic changes and have usually had symptoms for 3 or more years. Growth retardation, poor nutrition, and extracolonic symptoms are further indications that must be considered in the decision to operate. An initial severe attack that progresses to chronic symptoms without a definite remission suggests a poor prognosis and the eventual need for colectomy.

The increased risk of cancer is another relative indication for surgery; this must be weighed in each individual case. Schneider et al. recommended surgery in children who continue to demonstrate major symptoms after 2 years of steroid therapy,[60] whereas Ehrenpreis and Ericsson recommended an operation after 1 year of total disability or after 5 years of intermittent disability.[61] The evaluation of need for operation must be carefully individualized and fully discussed with the family.

Preoperative Care. The standard operation for treatment of chronic ulcerative colitis used to be a one-stage total colectomy with a permanent ileostomy. In rare cases, this procedure may still be appropriate. Two teams should be used for simultaneous perineal excision of the anus and rectum with the abdominal colectomy. The perineum is closed over a suction tube to eliminate dead space below the reperitonealized pelvic floor.[62] Endorectal stripping of the mucosa without removal of the rectal muscle lessens the prolonged perineal drainage and reduces the chances for bladder or sexual dysfunction.[63] The ileostomy site must be marked before the operation. It is best placed slightly below the midpoint of a line drawn from the umbilicus to the anterior–superior iliac crest. The incision must be placed to the left of the midline so it will not interfere with placement of the appliance. After removal of the colon, the mesentery of the ileum is divided proximal to the arcuate vessels for approximately 10 cm. A 2 cm button of skin is removed, and the abdominal wall is cut in a cruciate fashion to allow unobstructed passage of the ileum through the abdominal wall. The parietal peritoneum is carefully sutured to the seromuscular layer of the ileum, and the

mesentery is fixed to the abdominal wall to prevent an internal hernia. From 3 to 4 cm of ileum must be brought through the abdominal wall so that there will be a nipple-like everted stoma protruding for at least 2 cm. The ileum is turned back on itself, and the mucosa is sutured to the skin (Fig. 100–2). A temporary plastic bag is fitted about the ileostomy while the child is still in the operating room, and after the edema has subsided, the child is fitted with a permanent bag.

Any operation designed to cure chronic ulcerative colitis should include removal of the entire colon or, at least, its mucosal lining. The gold standard remains a total proctocolectomy with creation of a permanent Brooke end-ileostomy. While this operation eradicates the disease, it does so with appreciable morbidity. The procedure compels the patient to wear a stomal appliance, and it deprives him or her of the ability to voluntarily control bowel movements. In 1969, Koch addressed these problems by describing a technique for construction of a continent ileostomy.[64] Koch reconstructed the terminal ileum, creating an ileal reservoir proximal to an intussuscepted nipple valve. Patients were then taught to periodically intubate the reservoir in order to empty the pouch of retained feces. In some centers, the so-called Koch pouch enjoyed considerable success.[65] Other surgeons, however, became disenchanted with the procedure. Clearly, the procedure was more appealing than the standard proctocolectomy. No longer did the patient require an ostomy appliance, and a well-functioning continent ileostomy eliminated the social embarrassment of uncontrolled flatus. Still, the patient could not defecate per anum. Furthermore, in comparison to the Brooke ileostomy, the more complicated construction of the Koch pouch demanded even greater attention to detail. Potential complications included difficulty in intubating the pouch and pouch incontinence. The complication rate remained so high that the technique became relegated to certain centers where the procedure could be done only with relatively great frequency.[66] Today, the Koch pouch remains a reasonable alternative for the patient with ulcerative colitis in whom relatively normal anorectal function cannot be expected, no matter how the rectum may be reconstructed.

The most attractive operation for the treatment of chronic ulcerative colitis currently combines near-total colectomy, rectal mucosectomy, and anastomosis of the terminal ileum to the anus. With this procedure, the patient may have controlled and anatomically normal bowel movements. This so-called ileoanal anastomosis (IAA), first theorized by Ravitch and Sabiston in 1947,[67] was initially fraught with numerous complications when applied clinically.[68] Encouraged by the success of the Soave endorectal pullthrough for Hirschsprung's disease, however, Martin et al., in 1977, reintroduced the IAA for the treatment of chronic ulcerative colitis.[69] Modifica-

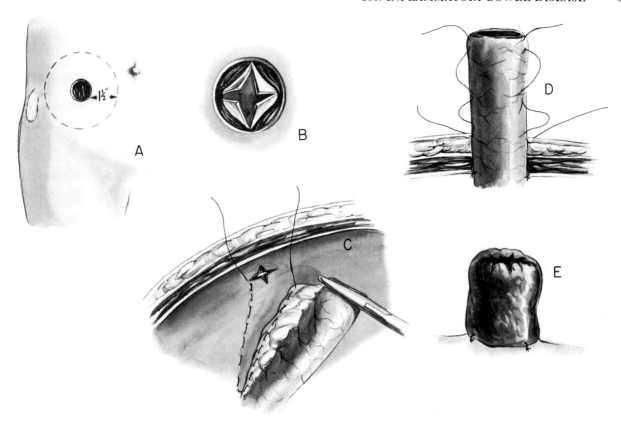

Figure 100–2. Ileostomy technique for ulcerative colitis. **A.** The ileostomy site is marked on the skin before the operation, and the child is fitted with a temporary bag for use after the operation. **B.** Either the abdominal wall is cored out or cruciate incisions are made through the peritoneum and fascia so that there will be no obstruction. **C.** The mesentery is sutured to the posterior and anterior abdominal wall so that there will be no space for an internal hernia. **D.** Catgut sutures are taken through the protruding stoma and the skin in order to evert the mucosa. The seromuscular layers of the bowel are sutured to the abdominal wall. **E.** The completed ileostomy should have a stoma that protrudes for 2 or 3 cm.

tions of the technique, particularly those in which one creates an ileal reservoir similar to the Koch pouch, have further enhanced the popularity and applicability of the IAA. The operation has evolved through the present time so that today's patient afflicted with chronic ulcerative colitis can look forward to a curative procedure that is neither disfiguring nor socially incapacitating.

Most patients with chronic ulcerative colitis face fluctuating degrees of debilitation as well as the potential development of toxic megacolon or colorectal cancer. Thus, IAA remains appropriate for any but the patient with the mildest form of ulcerative colitis or the individual in whom anorectal continence is already impossible. The operation has no place in emergency situations, such as toxic megacolon or life-threatening hemorrhage. If a patient requires an emergency procedure, however, a subtotal colectomy does not prevent the surgeon from later performing an IAA.

Patient selection can affect one's results with the IAA. Not all patients are candidates for this procedure. The operation requires a commitment on the part of the patient as well as the surgeon. Although most children

undergoing this procedure are satisfied with the results, approximately one fourth of these patients will have a major complication. Furthermore, all patients must be willing to have a temporary ileostomy, and the parents must accept the responsibility for daily postoperative anal dilatations. Still, despite these complications and commitments, results over the last 10 years remain positive with respect to patient acceptance and cure of the disease.[70]

Preoperative Preparation. Preoperative preparation includes careful nutritional assessment. Most patients undergoing this procedure are steroid dependent. Additionally, severe protein-calorie malnutrition may be sufficient cause for staging the IAA. Martin has suggested that the operation be routinely staged unless the rectal mucosa is free of ulceration or significant inflammation.[14] In the latter situation, he restricts the first operation to a subtotal colectomy, leaving the entire rectum in place. Having removed the bulk of the nutritionally depleting organ, he then supports the patient with TPN as he treats the defunctionalized rectum with steroid enemas. Following nutritional recovery, an IAA is performed. In selected patients, this approach may be warranted, but, in the vast majority of patients, the entire resection and IAA can be done in one stage.

Bowel preparation, emphasizing the mechanical aspects of the regimen, can usually be accomplished beginning the day before surgery. The absence of formed stools makes cleansing of the colon a relatively easy task. Using a polyethylene glycol electrolyte regimen solution will usually suffice.[71] At the time of surgery, one may further irrigate the rectum with a providone-iodine solution.

Operative Technique. After general anesthetic induction, one should insert a urinary catheter into the bladder. The closed-system drainage tubing should be placed anterior to the leg in a groin crease so that it does not obstruct either the abdominal or perineal operative field. Subsequent placement of the patient in the lithotomy position requires fastidious attention. One should exercise extreme care in cushioning the calves and in elevating the legs to minimize postoperative neurologic complications. Comfortable padding, such as foam eggshell mattress material, may relieve pressure at anatomically vulnerable sites. The individuals responsible for positioning the patient should avoid stretching the hamstring muscles, since prolonged tension along the posterior aspect of the thigh may contribute to postoperative sciatic nerve dysfunction.

Skin preparation and sterile draping of the operative field are similar to that for an abdominoperineal resection of the colon and rectum. Two teams can work simultaneously during the latter aspects of the IAA in order to minimize operative time. The respective operating fields should, however, be separated by sterile drapes. An arrangement that works well employs one instrument stand over the patient's head and chest while a separate stand for the perineal surgery remains just past the foot of the table and immediately to the perineal surgeon's left side. (The left-handed surgeon may choose to have instruments delivered and retrieved from the right side.) Finally, an extension tray attached to the foot of the operating table provides a convenient work table during the perineal aspect of the procedure.

A lower midline incision provides good exposure for the laparotomy. If necessary, one can extend the incision in a cephalad direction to more safely mobilize the splenic flexure. In performing the subtotal colectomy, the surgeon should preserve as much of terminal ileum as possible for creation of the J-pouch reservoir. Likewise, he or she should protect the collateral branches of the ileocecal artery, since he or she may later need to interrupt this vessel more proximally in order to alleviate tension at the IAA.

Careful inspection of the terminal ileum at this time in the operation enables the surgeon to rule out findings suggestive of Crohn's disease. Although the final decision to do an IAA rests on the histologic examination of the subtotal colonic specimen, the surgeon shares the diagnostic responsibility in this setting. He or she is obligated to inform the pathologist of his or her clinical impression as well as the gross findings, particularly with respect to the unsubmitted specimen of terminal ileum. If one identifies creeping mesenteric fat, abnormal thickening, or mesenteric engorgement despite the microscopic findings of chronic ulcerative colitis, the pathologist should be invited to inspect these gross findings as well. The surgeon may opt to avoid doing an IAA after considering his or her opinion and that of the pathologist.

Despite favorable gross findings, the pathologist may only be able to provide a diagnosis of indeterminate colitis. Although one may be tempted to abandon the notion of an IAA in this case, recent data in adult patients suggest that the procedure may still be feasible.[72] In cases of indeterminate colitis, an ileoproctostomy or end-ileostomy leaving the oversewn rectum in place may provide a reasonable compromise between an IAA and an abdominoperineal resection. Depending on the patient's future course, an IAA may be performed at a later date.

One may begin constructing the ileal reservoir (Fig. 100–3) after receiving a diagnosis of chronic ulcerative colitis. Creation of a J-pouch begins with selection of a convenient site on the antimesenteric approximately 12 to 15 cm from the distal end of the terminal ileum. With this point serving as an apex, the bowel is folded onto itself, apposing the antimesenteric border of the most distal terminal ileum to that of the immediately more proximal bowel. One may then use a GIA stapler to accomplish a side-to-side anastomosis between these two portions of bowel. The anastomosis requires three separate stapling cartridges so that nearly the entire length of each limb of the J is used. If one uses a stapler to create the J-pouch, a bridge of tissue will remain within the pouch near the apex. (Handsewing this anastomosis does not produce this bridge.) In order to avoid disturbing confusion on subsequent neorectal examinations, the surgeon should transect this bridge with a fourth cartridge. Finally, one should carefully and completely close the insertion site of the stapler into the pouch using individually placed inverting sutures.

After the J-pouch is made, one may complete the abdominal aspect of the colon resection. As the surgeon nears the proximal end of the rectum, he or she should maintain the dissection on the bowel wall much as in a Swenson procedure for Hirschsprung's disease. Posteriorly, one may develop the plane down to the levator musculature. Anteriorly, in order to reduce injury to the nervi erigentes, one's dissection should remain proximal to the common wall between the rectum and prostatic urethra.

In beginning the perineal aspect of the procedure,

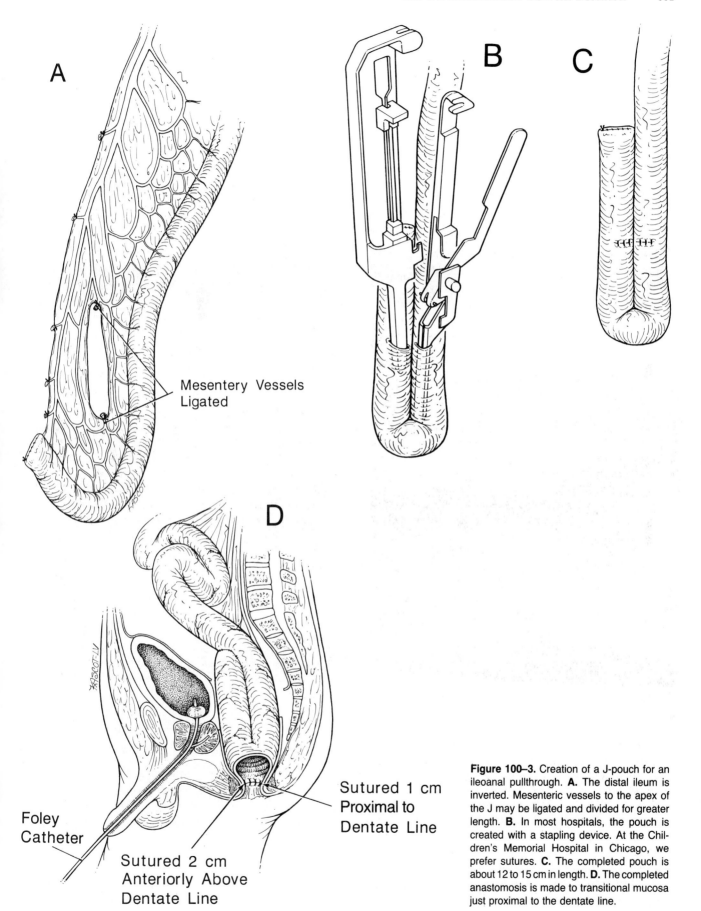

A

Mesentery Vessels
Ligated

B

C

D

Foley
Catheter

Sutured 2 cm
Anteriorly Above
Dentate Line

Sutured 1 cm
Proximal to
Dentate Line

Figure 100–3. Creation of a J-pouch for an ileoanal pullthrough. **A.** The distal ileum is inverted. Mesenteric vessels to the apex of the J may be ligated and divided for greater length. **B.** In most hospitals, the pouch is created with a stapling device. At the Children's Memorial Hospital in Chicago, we prefer sutures. **C.** The completed pouch is about 12 to 15 cm in length. **D.** The completed anastomosis is made to transitional mucosa just proximal to the dentate line.

one can appreciate the convenience and excellent exposure afforded by Gelpi retractors and a head lamp. Placement of the prongs at the dentate line allows the surgeon to begin stripping the most distal rectal mucosa from the underlying musculature. One can then adjust these retractors at various angles to enhance exposure throughout all 360 degrees of the initial dissection. A 1:1000 epinephrine in normal saline solution infused submucosally enables the surgeon to identify the appropriate tissue plane, and the epinephrine helps to maintain hemostasis. The needlepoint cautery is an excellent instrument for doing this dissection, and one should preferentially use the cutting current, reserving the coagulation mode for actively bleeding sites. In keeping the resultant mucosal tube thin, the surgeon may ensure maximal preservation of the muscularis. It is necessary to strip no more than 5 cm of the mucosal lining. In fact, a longer residual muscular tube may limit adequate drainage and actually increase the incidence of postoperative pelvic infections.

When the endorectal dissection is near its completion, the full thickness of the rectum is incised circumferentially so that what remains of the large intestine may be extracted en bloc with the mucosal tube. After removing the diseased bowel, the surgeon and assistants should irrigate the pelvis extensively with normal saline solution. With care being taken to avoid twisting the mesentery, an assistant now feeds the J-pouch through the pelvis into the muscular canal. The apex of the J-pouch should lay comfortably at the dentate line so that the future anastomosis will be under no undue tension. This latter concept remains crucial to avoid an anastomotic dehiscence and its associated complications. Careful inspection of the mesenteric vascular pattern usually indicates that the limiting length of mesentery lies parallel to a medium-sized branch of the ileocecal artery. Preserving the mesenteric arcades on either side of this vessel, one may sever the latter structure without compromising the viability of the pouch. Another 3 to 4 cm of mesenteric length may be comfortably gained with this maneuver.

In beginning the anastomosis of the J-pouch to the anus, one should first place Silastic drains alongside the pouch and bring them out through the anterior abdominal wall. Then anchor the pouch to the anal canal with several absorbable sutures, approximating the seromuscularis to the adjacent sphincteric musculature. The apex of the pouch is then incised perpendicular to and away from the staple lines. A small incision, barely enough to admit one's index finger, suffices and precludes further technical difficulties. One may then handsew the full-thickness edge of bowel to the edge of the anoderm with interrupted absorbable suture material (Fig. 100-3D).

Finally, during creation of the IAA, assistants may close the resultant posterior mesenteric defect and create a diverting loop ileostomy in the right lower quadrant.

Eversion of the afferent limb of this stoma in a Brooke fashion prevents troublesome serositis.[73]

Unless there are extenuating circumstances, one may first examine the ileoanal suture line 2 weeks postoperatively. At this time, parents are instructed on a safe technique for daily digital dilatation of the anastomosis. Although closure of the protective diverting ileostomy may take place 2 months from the date of the original operation, dilatation should be continued for a total of 6 months. Faithful adherence to this regimen usually results in a nonstenotic anastomosis. Before closure of the ileostomy, the surgeon should obtain a limited lower gastrointestinal x-ray to rule out the presence of an anastomotic leak. Rarely, one may note a small paraintestinal sinus tract extending from the posterior aspect of the suture line. This tract will usually heal spontaneously, but some surgeons may choose to unroof this space in a separate operation before closure of the ileostomy. Regardless, complete healing should be confirmed before one reestablishes intestinal continuity.

Postoperative Management. After stomal closure, most patients will experience approximately 2 days of bowel inactivity. Thereafter, these children can expect to begin having as many as 12 or more bowel movements per day. As the patient learns to use the neorectum, previously unused ileum adapts, and initial diarrhea begins to decrease in a relatively rapid fashion. The patient should be warned that he or she will probably have at least one bowel movement at night with very little warning, soiling the bed linens.

Once the surgeon is sure that the patient has no bowel obstruction, he or she may begin administering psyllium hydrophilic mucilloid (for teenagers, 1 tablespoon three times a day with minimal amounts of water) to help improve the consistency of the patient's stool. One may subsequently add loperamide hydrochloride to the regimen if uncontrolled diarrhea persists.

Before discharge from the hospital, the patient should be having approximately six to eight bowel movements per day. Over the next 6 months, most patients can expect six or fewer bowel movements per day, depending on the judiciousness with which they control their diets. Similarly, minor nocturnal soiling (less than 5 ml) may be controlled in large measure by abstinence from nighttime snacks.

Complications. The numerous complications associated with IAA create a discouraging tone as one evaluates the results of this operation. Although nearly 25 percent of these children experience some major complication related to the procedure, these problems usually can be managed quite successfully.

One may categorize these complications into those that occur in the early postoperative period and those that manifest themselves during long-term follow-up.

The former group includes neurologic impairment of the lower extremities, small bowel obstruction, and infectious complications. Potential problems during long-term follow-up include pouchitis and the development of Crohn's disease. Sciatic neuropraxia may develop as a result of placing the patient in the lithotomy position. One should take care to stretch the sciatic nerve roots as little as possible to reduce the incidence of this problem. In one series, neurologic complications occurred in 6 percent of patients.[70] Up to 33 percent of these children will develop a small bowel obstruction after IAA.[70] Approximately half will require an additional laparotomy to correct the problem. Careful replacement of the bowel into the peritoneal cavity and complete closure of the mesenteric defect may lessen the frequency of this complication.

In a recent series of adult patients, cuff abscesses occurred in approximately 5 percent.[74] Fortunately, timely drainage prevented these infections from impairing future continence. The creation of a relatively short cuff in comparison to that used for a Soave pullthrough may lessen the incidence of this problem.

Patients afflicted with pouchitis will complain of watery, foul-smelling diarrhea (often containing blood) associated with fever, malaise, abdominal cramping, urgency, and incontinence. Pouchitis probably results from bacterial overgrowth within the J-pouch, and one may easily treat the problem with oral metronidazole given four times a day for 1 to 2 weeks. Adherence to the prescribed regimen for dilatation will reduce the incidence of anal stricture formation and, possibly, the incidence of bacterial overgrowth.

Finally, a rare patient returns with anorectal findings reminiscent of Crohn's disease. Whether these patients had Crohn's disease all along or whether they have developed the problem since undergoing IAA remains unknown. Unfortunately, treatment usually requires removal of the pouch and creation of a permanent endostomy.

Results. Results of the IAA with respect to patient satisfaction remain excellent. With careful patient selection, more than 95 percent of these children consider the use of their neorectums preferable to that of the temporary ileostomy.[70] Most patients have approximately four to six controlled bowel movements per day, and even minimal nocturnal soiling is rarely a problem. Most of these children enthusiastically return to school without the formerly debilitating aspects of their disease.

CROHN'S DISEASE

Crohn's disease may involve any portion of the alimentary tract, from the esophagus to the anus. It is a disease of unknown etiology that is relentlessly progressive and for which there is no specific medical or surgical therapy. When the disease occurs in the colon, some prefer the term "granulomatous colitis," although granulomas are not always present on histologic examination. Therefore, from a historic and pathologic standpoint, the eponym "Crohn's disease" may be applied to the disease when it appears in any portion of the gastrointestinal tract.[75]

Pathology

There is an inflammatory thickening of the entire wall of the affected bowel. This usually involves the terminal ileum, but skip areas are commonly observed in other portions of the small bowel, as in the colon. At operation, the bowel is firm, the mesentery is thickened and edematous, and there are enlarged mesenteric lymph nodes. The serosal surface is dull, granular, and hyperemic. Typically, the mesenteric fat grows over the serosa toward the antimesenteric surface of the bowel. Bowel loops may be matted together by adhesions that surround abscess cavities and fistulas between loops of bowel. Fistulas may connect with the ureter or bladder, and there may be sinus tracts to the abdominal wall. The mucosa is edematous and red. In advanced disease, there are deep, longitudinal ulcers.

Histologic examination of surgical specimens will reveal granulomas consisting of epithelioid and giant cells in about 60 percent of patients. These granulomas are found in all layers of the intestinal wall, in the regional lymph nodes, and in the liver. There is no caseation, and some resemble the granulomas seen in sarcoidosis. Small linear ulcers or fissures through the mucosa are surrounded by necrotic tissue, macrophages, and lymphocytes. The ulcers become intramural abscesses that may penetrate the bowel and eventually form fistulas with surrounding viscera. The scattering of foci of lymphocytes through all layers of the bowel is probably the only consistent feature of Crohn's disease.[76] This lymphoid hyperplasia and lymphedema, which contribute to the submucosal thickening, are perhaps the earliest signs of Crohn's disease. The intestinal lumen may be obstructed by edema of the bowel wall early in the disease, but later there will be narrowing of the lumen secondary to irreversible fibrosis.

Clinical Manifestations

The onset of Crohn's disease is very rare before 7 years of age. Most cases are seen in adolescents. Children affected with Crohn's disease have recurrent abdominal pain, poor weight gain, chronic diarrhea, and anemia. Children are more likely than adults to have fever, pallor, and nutritional disturbances. The diarrhea is usually mild, with no tenesmus, and is only occasionally marked by mucus or blood in the stool. Children may complain of nonspecific postprandial pain before other symptoms develop, or the pain may simulate an acute appendicitis. Colicky pain results from intestinal obstruction and is a late symptom. Weight loss is the result of anorexia and malabsorption. Failure to grow and mature sexually is one of the most prominent symptoms of untreated or poorly treated Crohn's disease. Anal lesions consisting of fissures, ulcers, and fistulas may occur at any time during the course of the disease. In about a quarter of afflicted patients, the anal complication is the first sign.[77] Extraintestinal symptoms, such as monarticular arthritis, recurrent iridocyclitis, and clubbing of nails, are also symptomatic of Crohn's disease.[78] The most important physical finding is a tender right lower quadrant mass that mimics an appendiceal abscess. The mass consists of edematous adherent loops of intestine and sometimes includes an abscess. Abdominal distention is a late complication caused by an intestinal obstruction. A careful rectal examination may reveal indolent ulcers with edematous skin and undermined edges. These ulcers are surprisingly painless. Anal lesions may occur with disease of the small intestine, but more commonly they accompany colonic lesions. A proctoscopic examination will reveal edema of the mucosa, longitudinal ulcers, and considerable bleeding when the colon is involved. Even when the rectum is grossly normal at sigmoidoscopy, there is almost always microscopic evidence of lymphocytic infiltration of the submucosa. Occasionally, a granuloma is seen.[79] Complete gastrointestinal roentgenograms are indicated to aid in making the diagnosis and to determine the extent of the disease. A barium enema is performed first. Barium is often refluxed into the terminal ileum, demonstrating small bowel disease. After complete evacuation of the colon, an upper gastrointestinal examination and small bowel followthrough are performed. The mucosal folds are thickened and irregular, with straightening of the valvulae conniventes. Longitudinal ulcers appear as linear streaks of barium. Later, the ulcers fuse, and there is a cobblestone appearance to the mucosa. Edema separates the loops of bowel, which eventually become rigid and fixed. The string sign is the result of edema and thickening of the bowel wall and must be distinguished from stenosis which is accompanied by proximal dilatation of the bowel (Fig. 100–4). The involved intestine is sharply demarcated from normal bowel, but skip areas may occur anywhere in the small bowel or colon. Early filling of remote loops of intestine may indicate fistulas from diseased proximal intestine (Fig. 100–5). An IV pyelogram and cystogram are indicated to detect fistulas to the urinary tract and ureteral obstruction (Fig. 100–6).

Differential Diagnosis

Acute ileitis must be clearly differentiated from Crohn's disease. Occasionally, when a normal appendix is found at laparotomy, the terminal ileum is found to be inflamed and thickened, and the mesentery is indurated with enlarged lymph nodes. This acute ileitis of childhood is most often caused by *Yersinia enterocolitica* or *Y. pseudotuberculosis*. It is difficult to culture these organisms, but they can be found in lymph nodes, and specific antibodies are found in a high percentage of these patients.[80] The disease is self-limiting. When it is found, it is safe to perform an appendectomy because there is no concern about an intestinal fistula.[81]

Ileocecal tuberculosis is exceedingly rare in the Western world, but there are still sporadic case reports of this disease occurring in children even in the United States.[82] A familial history of tuberculosis, a positive chest x-ray, and sputum positive for acid-fast organisms will clearly make the diagnosis when there is intestinal involvement. In a recent large series reported from India, however, the diagnosis was only made by finding caseating granulomas in the bowel and mesenteric lymph nodes. Only 14 percent of these patients had positive tissue cultures for mycobacteria, but guinea pig inoculation was positive in 76 percent.[83]

Lymphosarcoma of the small intestine may commence with a fever of undetermined origin and nonspecific abdominal complaints. In addition, the radiologic features may be indistinguishable from those of Crohn's disease.[84] If a rectal biopsy does not aid in distinguishing between these two diseases, an exploratory laparotomy and biopsy may be indicated. It may not always be possible to distinguish between ulcerative colitis and Crohn's disease. Involvement of the ileum and skip areas are more likely in Crohn's disease, and complete radiologic studies, proctoscopy, and biopsy should differentiate between the two conditions. Occasionally, a period of observation is necessary before the diagnosis is apparent.

Miller has described a form of transmural inflammatory disease that affects segments of both the small and large bowel in infants under 1 year of age.[85] Although there were deep penetrating ulcers that histologically resembled Crohn's disease, these infants recovered after a proximal diverting enterostomy and TPN. The bowel healed, and these infants remained well after closure of the enterostomy. This appears to be a separate entity that should not be considered to be Crohn's disease.

Medical Therapy

Mild Attack. The patient complains of abdominal pain, mild diarrhea, and weight loss. Perianal disease may be associated, but there is rarely fever or anemia. Many of these patients respond to treatment with 2 to 4 g of Azulfidine daily, but there are no controlled data as to its efficiency in children. No special diet is advisable, but multivitamins and attention to adequate nutrition are important. Most patients with mild Crohn's disease have good prognoses.

Moderate Attack. The majority of children with Crohn's disease fit into this group. There is usually ileo-

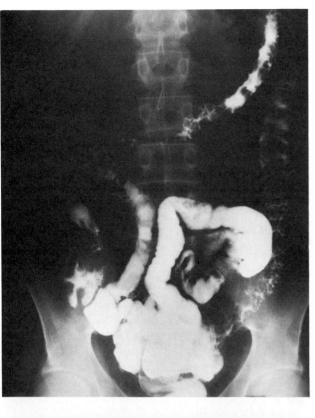
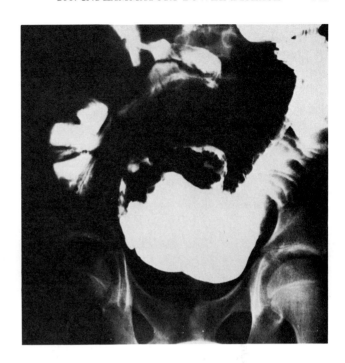
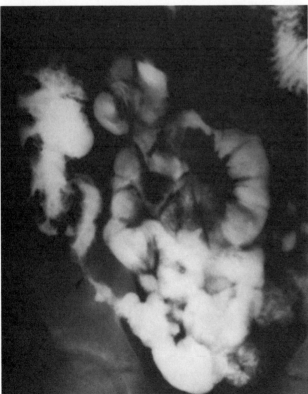
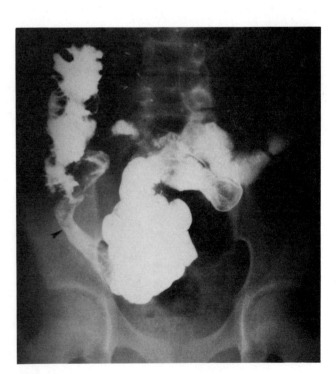

Figure 100–4. Crohn's disease involving the terminal ileum. **Top left.** The bowel is rigid and fixed, and there is an indentation on the ileum from a mass of lymph nodes and edematous mesentery. **Top right.** Obstruction of the jejunum, with proximal dilatation of bowel. **Bottom left.** Minimal narrowing of the ileum with a ragged appearance, or cobblestoning, of the mucosa. **Bottom right.** Fibrosis of the terminal ileum with loss of the mucosal pattern.

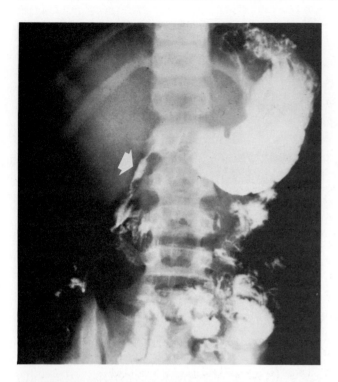

Figure 100–5. Upper gastrointestinal examination demonstrating early filling of the transverse colon (arrow), indicating a duodenocolic fistula in a 10-year-old boy with severe Crohn's disease.

colic involvement, often with skip areas. More rarely, there may be widespread involvement of the small intestine. Abdominal pain, diarrhea, and extraintestinal complications (such as perianal disease, arthritis, and stomatitis) are common. Psychologic disturbances may be present. If multiple systemic or obstructive symptoms are present, corticosteroids are indicated in the same dosages given for ulcerative colitis. In contrast to patients with ulcerative colitis, many of these patients require continuous low-dose corticosteroid therapy to maintain control of their disease. Azulfidine (2 to 4 mg/day) is given with multivitamins and folic acid (1 mg/day). Iron is often required, owing to the associated iron deficiency anemia. Lactose-free milks are advisable, but the most important dietary recommendation is the administration of an adequate caloric intake, including elemental dietary supplements, if necessary.

Severe Attack. These children are toxic, have considerable rectal bleeding, poor nutrition, and, if there is extensive disease in the small intestine, obstruction. These are the patients who develop fistulas to adjacent viscera and who are most likely to have extensive colonic involvement. Immediate treatment consists of steroid therapy, TPN, replacement of trace element deficiencies,

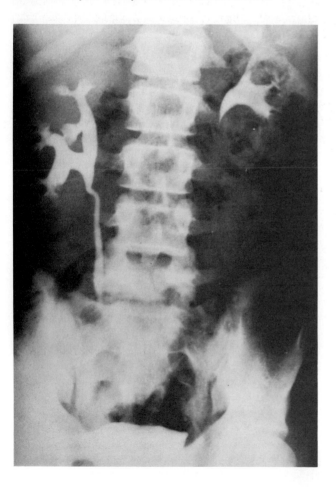

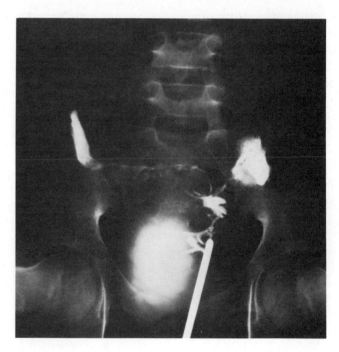

Figure 100–6. Urologic complications of Crohn's disease. **Left.** Ureteral obstruction from disease of the terminal ileum and retroperitoneal edema. **Right.** Fistula from the terminal ileum to the bladder as demonstrated by cystoscopy and a cystogram.

transfusions, and perhaps nasogastric or long-tube drainage of the small bowel to relieve distention. These patients often require surgery to control complications.

Despite numerous uncontrolled, anecdotal reports on the use of immunosuppressive agents in the treatment of inflammatory bowel disease, the status of these drugs remains unclear. It is difficult to sort out the multiple variables, since Azulfidine and corticosteroids usually have been given at the same time as the immunosuppressive agents. A national cooperative trial for the therapy of Crohn's disease has been in progress for the last 2 years. No conclusions can be drawn yet. Several groups have reported improvement with the immunosuppressive agents in addition to conventional therapy.[86] There was a 50 percent relapse rate in some of these series when the drug was discontinued. Definitive recommendations on the use of immunosuppressive agents must await further clinical trials. In the pediatric age group, the side effects of immunosuppressive agents on the reproductive system necessitate caution in their use.

Recent data published by Wellman et al. support the use of whole gut lavage with a solution of S-aminosalicylic acid.[87] They contend that severe Crohn's disease attacks are associated with endotoxemia, and whole gut irrigation will treat the more severe of these endotoxins.

Surgical Management
The indications for surgical treatment of Crohn's disease include fistulas to other viscera or to the abdominal wall, abscess formation, recurrent intestinal obstruction, chronic debility, and severe anorectal disease that fails to respond to intensive medical management.[88] Growth arrest and retardation of sexual maturation are relative and perhaps controversial indications for surgery in the prepubertal child. The best results are obtained in those with fibrotic obstruction. The indications for operation in each individual child must be carefully weighed against the risk of recurrence following operation. This risk is worth taking if the pubertal child can be given a relatively symptom-free interval to mature and grow during the critical adolescent years.

TPN and continued steroid treatment will reduce intestinal inflammation and may relieve an inflammatory intestinal obstruction, aside from improving the child's general condition. Transfusions of whole blood and plasma are indicated to correct anemia and hypovolemia. These measures will bring the child into a positive nitrogen balance and will improve postoperative wound healing. Immediately before operation, the levels of serum electrolytes, including magnesium and calcium, must be determined.

Despite extensive fissures and anal ulcers, many patients experience surprisingly little rectal discomfort. We have avoided direct surgical excision of anal disease whenever possible. Currently, we are giving patients

with fissures and fistulas Bactrim and Flagyl in addition to maximum medical therapy for their primary disease. Careful anal cleansing is recommended in addition to warm sitz baths. Specific antibiotics are given when bacteria are cultured from fistulas and abscess cavities. Severe anorectal disease, particularly when associated with colonic Crohn's disease, is a relative indication for excision of the primary involved bowel.

Resection of the involved bowel with an end-to-end anastomosis is indicated when there is disease of the jejunum or ileum. Commonly, Crohn's disease is grossly confined to the terminal ileum. In these cases, it is often necessary to remove a portion of the ascending colon as well. Recurrence in the colon is unusual when the primary disease is on the ileum. Therefore, a margin of 5 to 7 cm of normal colon beyond the gross disease is sufficient. Since it is necessary to weigh the risk of recurrent disease against the known complications of the short gut syndrome, which results from an extensive ileal resection, it is wisest to remove no more than 10 cm of grossly normal intestine proximal to the diseased bowel. Removal of excessive amounts of normal bowel beyond grossly involved margins probably has little effect on the recurrence rate. In addition, asymptomatic proximal skip areas without obstruction or fistula formation may be left in place and treated medically. In widespread disease with many obstructing strictures, one may consider doing multiple enteroplasties by incising the stricture longitudinally and then closing the enterotomy in a transverse fashion.

The surgical management of colonic disease is more difficult. If the rectum is normal, the proximal colon may be resected and an ileorectal anastomosis performed. Total colonic involvement may require a proctocolectomy with permanent ileostomy, but many cases can be managed by leaving the rectum in place as a Hartmann's pouch. Diversion of intestinal contents seems to quell the disease of the previously used bowel, and preservation of the rectum affords the child the possibility of some day defecating normally.

Recurrence of Crohn's disease requiring reoperation varies among institutions. This variance is most likely secondary to one's threshold for surgically treating recurrent disease. Certainly, early recurrences are more likely to be treated medically, and these patients may be erroneously considered surgical successes. Rutgeerts et al. found that routine endoscopic evaluation of the ileocolonic anastomosis after curative surgery showed a recurrence rate of 72 percent at 1 year.[89]

In postoperative treatment of small intestinal disease, gastric decompression is continued for several days after the onset of bowel function, since intestinal healing might be delayed by steroid administration. Central TPN is continued until the child clearly can tolerate a satisfactory oral diet. The steroid dosage is gradually tapered over several days. Levine et al. observed postoperative seizures in 5 of 21 children operated on for inflammatory bowel disease.[90] All of these patients had significant fluid retention and hypertension before the seizure activity. This was thought to be due to an exaggerated antidiuretic hormone response and a lower threshold of convulsive activity being triggered by chronic steroid administration. Thus, it is extremely important to maintain an accurate record of fluid intake and output and to maintain normal serum electrolytes in the postoperative period.

Since surgical resection removes only bowel that is involved with the complications and does not cure the disease itself, it is logical to continue long-term medical follow-up and treatment after an operation. The incidence of reoperation continues to rise as the patients are followed for longer periods of time. Still, when an operation allows the child to eat an adequate diet, there will be prompt weight gain and resumption of growth following surgery. In one long-term series of 19 children, all reached their ideal body weights within 6 months after the operation.[91]

REFERENCES

1. Rickert RR: The important "imposters" in the differential diagnosis of inflammatory bowel disease. J Clin Gastro 6:153, 1984
2. Marshak RH, Wolf BS, Eliasoph J: Segmental colitis. Radiology 73:706, 1959
3. Schahchter H, Goldstein MJ, Rappaport H, et al: Ulcerative and granulomatous colitis validity of differential and diagnostic criteria: A study of 100 patients treated by total colectomy. Ann Intern Med 72:841, 1970
4. Lewkonia RM, McConnell RB: Familial inflammatory bowel disease: Hereditary or environment? Gut 17:235, 1976
5. Singer HC, Anderson JG, Frischer H, et al: Familial aspects of inflammatory bowel disease. Gastroenterology 61:423, 1971
6. Slight DR, Galpin JE, Condon RE: Ulcerative colitis in female monozygotic twins and a female sibling. Gastroenterology 61:507, 1971
7. Sachar DB, Janomitz HD: Inflammatory bowel disease. DM 1:44, 1974
8. Monk M, Mendeloff AI, Siegel CL, et al: An epidemiological study of ulcerative colitis and regional enteritis among adults in Baltimore. III: Psychological and possible stress participating factors. J Chronic Dis 22:565, 1970
9. Evans JG: The epidemiology of Crohn's disease. Clin Gastroenterol 1:335, 1972
10. Mayberry JF, Rhodes J: Epidemiological aspects of Crohn's Disease: a review of the literature. Gut 25:886, 1984
11. Henry C, Faulk WP, Kuhn L, et al: Immune responses of Peyer's patches. J Exp Med 131:1200, 1970
12. Crabbe PA, Corbonava AO, Heremans JF: The normal human intestinal mucosa as a major source of plasma cells containing A immune globulin. Lab Invest 14:235, 1965
13. Bolton PM, James SL, Newcombe RG, et al: The immune competence of patients with inflammatory bowel disease. Gut 15:213, 1974
14. Martin LW. In Welch KJ, Randolph JG, Ravitch MM, et al. (eds): Pediatric Surgery, 4th ed. Chicago, Year Book, 1986, p 972
15. Thayer WR: Are the inflammatory bowel diseases immune complex diseases? Gastroenterology 70:136, 1976
16. Streilein TW: Inflammatory bowel disease: T lymphocytes may be the culprits. Gastroenterology 75:150, 1978
17. Falchuk KR, Isselbacher KT: Circulative antibodies to bovine albumin in ulcerative colitis and Crohn's disease. Gastroenterology 70:5, 1976
18. Broberger O, Perlman P: In vitro studies of patient serum with human fetal colon cells in tissue cultures. J Exp Med 117:705, 1963
19. Kroft SC: Cellular immunity in Crohn's disease. Gastroenterology 61:545, 1971
20. Watson DW: Immune responses and the gut. Gastroenterology 56:944, 1969
21. Wall AJ, Kirsner JB: The management of ulcerative colitis and granulomatous colitis. Mod Treatment 8:944, 1971
22. Cave DR, Mitchell DN, Brooke BN: Induction of granulomas in mice by Crohn's disease tissues. Gastroenterology 75:632, 1978
23. Sachar DB, Auslander MO: Missing pieces in the puzzle of Crohn's disease. Gastroenterology 75:745, 1978
24. Gitnick GL, Arthur MH, Shibata I: Cultivation of viral agents from Crohn's disease. Lancet 2:215, 1976
25. Kirschner BS, Voinchet O, Rosenberg IH: Growth retardation in inflammatory bowel disease. Gastroenterology 75:504, 1978
26. Ehrenpreis TH: Surgical treatment of ulcerative colitis in childhood. Arch Dis Child 41:137, 1966
27. Berger M, Gribetz D, Korelitz BI: Growth retardation in children with ulcerative colitis: The effect of medical and surgical therapy. Pediatrics 55:459, 1975
28. Foglia R, Ament ME, Fleisher D, Fonkalsrud EW: Surgical management of ulcerative colitis in childhood. Am J Surg 134:58, 1977
29. Block GE, Moossa AR, Simonowitz D: The operative treatment of Crohn's disease in childhood. Surg Gynecol Obstet 144:713, 1977
30. Kelts DG, Grand RJ, Shen G, et al: Nutritional basis of growth failure in children and adolescents with Crohn's disease. Gastroenterology 76:720, 1979
31. Whittington PF, Barnes HV, Bayless TM: Medical management of Crohn's disease in adolescence. Gastroenterology 72:1338, 1977
32. Alperstein G, Daum F, Fisher SE, et al: Linear growth following surgery in children and adolescents with Crohn's disease: relationship to pubertal status. J Pediatr Surg 20:129, 1985
33. Devroede GJ, Taylor WF, Sauer WG, et al: Cancer risk and life expectancy of children with ulcerative colitis. N Engl J Med 285:17, 1971
34. Kewenter J, Ahlman H, Hulten L: Cancer risk in extensive ulcerative colitis. Ann Surg 188:824, 1978
35. Weedon DD, Shorter RG, Ilstrup DM, et al: Crohn's disease and cancer. N Engl J Med 289:1099, 1973

36. Devroede G, Taylor WF: On calculating cancer risk and survival of ulcerative colitis patients with the life table method. Gastroenterology 71:505, 1976

37. Kirsner JB: Ulcerative colitis 1970—Recent Developments. Scand J Gastroenterol [Suppl] 6:63, 1970

38. Nugent FW, Haggitt RC, Colcher H, Kutteruf GC: Malignant potential of chronic ulcerative colitis. Gastroenterology 76:1, 1979

39. Brostron O, Lofberg R, Ost A, et al: Cancer surveillance of patient with long-standing ulcerative colitis: A clinical endoscopical and histologic study. Gut 27:1408, 1968

40. Lennard-Jones JE, Morson BC, Ritchie JK, et al: Cancer in colitis: assessment of the individual risk by clinical and histological criteria. Gastroenterology 73:1280, 1977

41. Yardley JH, Bayless TM, Diamond MP: Cancer in ulcerative colitis. Gastroenterology 76:221, 1979

42. Truelove SC, Witts LJ: Cortisone in ulcerative colitis: Final report on a therapeutic trial. Br Med J 2:1041, 1955

43. Werlin SL, Grand RJ: Severe colitis in children and adolescents: Diagnosis, course and treatment. Gastroenterology 73:828, 1977

44. Best WR, Becktel JM, Singleton JW, Kern F: Development of a Crohn's disease activity index. National Cooperative Crohn's Disease Study. Gastroenterology 70:439, 1976

45. Lloyd-Still JD, Green O: A clinical score for inflammatory bowel disease in childhood. Dig Dis Sci 24:620, 1979

46. Price AB, Morson BC: Inflammatory bowel disease: The surgical pathology of Crohn's disease and ulcerative colitis. Hum Pathol 6:7, 1975

47. Warren S, Sommers SC: Pathogenesis of ulcerative colitis. Am J Pathol 26:657, 1949

48. Ein SH, Lynch MJ, Stephens C: Ulcerative colitis in children under one year: A 20-year review. Pediatr Surg 6:264, 1971

49. Stein G, Roy R, Finkelstein A: Roentgen changes in ulcerative colitis. Semin Roentgenol 3:3, 1968

50. Davidson M, Blood AA, Lugler MM: Chronic ulcerative colitis in childhood. J Pediatr 67:471, 1965

51. Nugent FW, Veidenheimer MC, Zuberi S, et al: Clinical course of ulcerative proctosigmoiditis. Am J Dig Dis 15:321, 1970

52. Broberger O, Langercrantz R: Ulcerative colitis in childhood and adolescence. Adv Pediatr 14:9, 1966

53. Euzer NB, Hymans JC: Ulcerative colitis beginning in infancy. J Pediatr 63:437, 1963

54. Fonkalsrud EW, Barker WF: Ulcerative colitis in infancy. Surgery 54:9, 1963

55. Stein D, Bank S, Louw J: Fulminating amoebic colitis. Surgery 85:349, 1979

56. Giacchino JL, Pickleman J, Bartizal J, Banich F: The therapeutic dilemma of acute amebic and ulcerative colitis. Surg Gynecol Obstet 146:599, 1978

57. Kessel JR, Lewis WP, Pasquel CM, Turner JA: Indirect hemagglutination and complement fixation test for amoebiasis. Am Trop Med Hyg 14:540, 1965

58. Misdiagnosis of amoebiasis (Editorial). Br Med J 2:379, 1979

59. Grand RJ, Homer DR: Approaches to inflammatory bowel disease in childhood and adolescence. Pediatr Clin North Am 22:835, 1975

60. Schneider K, Becker J, Korelitz B, et al: The surgical treatment of ulcerative colitis in childhood: A study of 38 cases. Pediatr Surg 3:12, 1968

61. Ehrenpreis T, Ericsson NO: Surgical treatment of ulcerative colitis in childhood. Surg Clin North Am 44:1521, 1964

62. Silen W, Glotzer DJ: The prevention and treatment of persistent perineal sinus. Surgery 75:535, 1974

63. Fonkalsrud EW, Ament M: Endorectal mucosal resection without proctectomy as an adjunct to abdominoperineal resection for non-malignant conditions: Clinical experience with five patients. Ann Surg 188:245, 1978

64. Koch NG: Intra-abdominal "reservoir" in patients with permanent ileostomy; preliminary observations on a procedure resulting in fecal "continence" in five ileostomy patients. Arch Surg 99:223, 1969

65. Beahrs OH, Kelly KA, Adson MA, Chong GC: Ileostomy with ileal reservoir rather than ileostomy along. Ann Surg 179:634, 1974

66. Dozois RR, Kelly KA, Beart RW Jr, Beahrs OH: Improved results with continent ileostomy. Ann Surg 192:319, 1980

67. Ravitch MM, Sabiston DC Jr: Anal ileostomy with preservation of the sphincter; a proposed operation in patients requiring total colectomy for benign lesions. Surg Gynecol Obstet 84:1095, 1947

68. Pemberton JH, Heppell J, Beart RW Jr, et al: Endorectal ileoanal anastomosis. Surg Gynecol Obstet 155:417, 1982

69. Martin LW, LeCoultre C, Schubert WK: Total colectomy and mucosal protectomy with preservation of continence in ulcerative colitis. Ann Surg 477, 1977

70. Perrault J, Telander RL, Zinsmeister AR, Kaufman BH: The endorectal pull-through procedure in children and young adults: a follow-up study. J Pediatr Gastroenterol (in press)

71. Tuggle DW, Hoelzer DJ, Tunnell WP, Smith EI: The safety and cost effectiveness of polyethylene glycol electrolyte solution bowel preparation in infants and children. J Pediatr Surg 22:513, 1987

72. Relationship of "indetermineant" colitis to outcome after ileal pouch–anal anastomosis. Submitted for paper preservation, American Society of Colon and Rectal Surgeons, Washington, D.C., 1987

73. Corman ML, Veidenheimer MC, Coller JA: Loop ileostomy as an alternative to end stoma. Surg Gynecol Obstet 149:585, 1979

74. Pemberton JH, Kelley KA, Beart RW Jr, et al: Ileal pouch–anal anastomosis for chronic ulcerative colitis: long-term results. Ann Surg 206:504, 1987

75. Crohn BB, Ginzberg H, Oppenheimer G: Regional ileitis: a pathological entity. JAMA 99:1323, 1932

76. Morson BC: Pathology of Crohn's disease. Clin Gastroenterol 2:270, 1972

77. Lockhart-Mummery HE: Anal lesions of Crohn's disease. Clin Gastroenterol 2:377, 1972

78. Burbige EJ, Hsang S, Bayless TM: Clinical manifestations of Crohn's disease in children and adolescents. Pediatrics 55:866, 1975

79. Dyer NH, Stansfield AG, Dawson AM: The valve of rectal biopsy in the diagnosis of Crohn's disease. Scand J Gastroenterol 5:491, 1970

80. Weber J, Finalyson NB, Mark JDB: Mesenteric lymph-adenitis and terminal ileitis due to *Yersinia pseudotuberculosis.* N Engl J Med 283:172, 1970

81. Gump FE, Lapore M, Barker HG: A revised concept of acute regional enteritis. Ann Surg 166:942, 1967

82. Porter JM, Snowe RJ, Silver D: Tuberculosis enteritis with perforation and abscess formation in childhood. Surgery 71:254, 1972

83. Singh HN, Vaidya MP, Roy SK: The laboratory diagnosis of intestinal tuberculosis: A study of 50 cases. Aust NZ J Surg 42:411, 1973

84. Marshak RH, Wolf BS, Eliasoph J: The roentgen findings of lymphosarcoma of the small intestine. Am J Roentgenol 86:682, 1961

85. Miller R: Surgical management of infantile ulcerative enteritis. J Pediatr Surg 10:367, 1975

86. Rosenberg JL, Levin B, Wall AJ, Kirsner JB: A controlled trial of azathioprine in Crohn's disease. Am J Dig Dis 20:721, 1975

87. Wellman W, Fink PC, Benner F, et al. Endotoxemia in active Crohn's disease. Treatment with whole gut irrigation as 5-aminosalicylic acid. Gut 27:814, 1986

88. Farmer RG, Hawk WA, Turnbull RB: Indications for surgery in Crohn's disease: Analysis of 500 cases. Gastroenterology 71:245, 1976

89. Rutgeerts P, Cehoes K, Vantrappen G, et al. Natural history of recurrent Crohn's disease at the ileocolonic anastomosis after curative surgery. Gut 25:665, 1984

90. Levine AM, Pickett L, Touloukian RJ: Steroids, hypertension and fluid retention in the genesis of postoperative seizures with inflammatory bowel disease in childhood. J Pediatr Surg 9:715, 1974

91. Henrikson B, Hulten L, Filipson S, Rademark C: Long-term study of Crohn's disease. Prog Pediatr Surg 11:61, 1978

101
Pancreatitis

Pancreatitis is one of the least common causes of abdominal pain in the pediatric age group, yet this diagnosis must be considered in every child with unexplained abdominal symptoms.[1]

Trauma and congenital dilatation of the bile duct, two causes for pancreatitis, are discussed in other chapters. In childhood, pancreatitis may be associated with a common viral illness, such as mumps or chickenpox.[2] Anomalies of the pancreatic duct and those cases of hereditary origin have recurrent attacks. Some of the most severe cases are associated with drug therapy and other serious illnesses. The corticosteroids seem to be the worst offenders. Other unusual etiologies for pancreatitis include metabolic problems, such as diabetes, hyperparathyroidism, and hyperlipemia.

In the tropics, scorpion bites and *Ascaris* obstruction of the duct are etiologies for pancreatitis.[3,4]

PATHOGENESIS

Anything that causes vagal stimulation will increase the flow of pancreatic enzymes. This may be the result of central nervous system stimulation, such as intracranial pressure or a scorpion bite.[5] Some drugs, such as L-asparaginase used to treat leukemia and valproic acid, an anticonvulsant, are associated with pancreatitis. Both have central nervous system side effects and may stimulate the vagus nerve.[6,7] Teenage boys who fast before wrestling and then eat a gargantuan meal will have an increased flow of pancreatic juice and pancreatitis. At autopsy, patients who have been treated with steroids have inspissated secretions and rupture of ductules. Obstruction of the pancreatic duct itself is not necessarily a cause of pancreatitis, since many patients with stenosis of a duct associated with pancreas divisum do not have symptoms until they are adults. Possibly, a relative obstruction becomes symptomatic during periods of increased secretion. Morphine, which causes spasm of the sphincter of Oddi, is a contributing factor. Hypovolemia with decreased arterial perfusion of the pancreas is necessary for the necrosis seen in severe forms of the disease.

Regardless of etiology, there is only edema of the gland in mild forms of pancreatitis. When there is disruption of a main duct or diffuse leakage of enzymes from ductules, there is more severe inflammation and a collection of enzyme-rich fluid in the lesser sac. In the most severe cases, the pancreas and surrounding tissue undergo necrosis, with retroperitoneal hemorrhage and fluid leakage into the general peritoneal cavity.

Acute collections of fluid in the lesser sac should not be termed "pseudocysts." To avoid confusion in diagnosis and treatment, the term "pseudocyst" should be reserved for chronic fluid collections encased in a thick fibrous wall. Fluid from the lesser sac may escape into the peritoneal cavity, the left pleural space, or the mediastinum.

DIAGNOSIS

The pain associated with pancreatitis is poorly localized in the upper or midabdomen. Unlike adults, a child rarely complains of pain radiating to the back. There is nausea, vomiting and anorexia, and often fever. In mild cases, with a viral illness such as mumps, there is minimal, nonspecific upper abdominal tenderness. Unlike appendicitis, the pain does not shift and is constant, and there is minimal, if any, tenderness in the lower abdomen. One should always inquire about a history of trauma. Often, the child has forgotten or does not want his or her parents to know about a fall from a bicycle. In young children, it is most important to maintain a high index of suspicion for child abuse. When abdominal pain commences in a child who is ill with another disease requiring drug treatment, especially with corticosteroids, pancreatitis should be one's first thought. A serum amylase is determined in any child with unexplained abdominal pain. The serum lipase test is also useful, and if these studies are nondiagnostic, urine should be saved for amylase determination. Abdominal pain associated with a history of jaundice should alert one to the possibility of pancreatitis secondary to congenital dilatation of the bile duct.

We now obtain an abdominal ultrasound study on every child with undiagnosed abdominal pain. This test will reveal dilatation of the bile duct, edema of the pancreas, and fluid collections in the lesser sac. An abdominal computed tomography (CT) scan is an excellent tool to determine the size of the pancreas, duct dilatation, the presence of intestinal duplications within the gland, and abnormal fluid collections. Whenever fluid is aspirated from the peritoneum or a pleural cavity, a sample should be sent for amylase determination. CT scanning provides sufficient detail to determine the need for an operation if the pancreatic duct is dilated or if there is a pseudocyst. Endoscopic retrograde cholangiopancreatography (ERCP) may be useful, especially in older children, in diagnosing ductal stenosis.[8] We have missed the diagnosis in a child with pancreatic divisum because we failed to perform an ERCP. We now feel that the study is essential in any child with pancreatitis in whom the etiology is not clear. A pancreaticogram may be performed at the operating table by transecting the tail of the pancreas and catheterizing the duct.

TREATMENT

Regardless of etiology, the initial treatment for pancreatitis is to give the child nothing by mouth, insert a gastric tube to keep the stomach empty and provide intravenous fluids. If there is hypovolemia, third-space fluid losses are replaced with albumin, plasma, or lactated Ringer's solution while monitoring the vital signs and urinary output. Pain should be relieved with Demerol rather than morphine, and although its value has never been proven, it makes sense to give a vagal blocking agent, such as atropine. These simple measures are all that are necessary in the majority of cases, particularly those due to minor trauma or mumps or for individual attacks associated with anomalies of the bile or pancreatic ducts. If the symptoms are prolonged, total intravenous nutrition may be necessary. The course of the disease is followed with serum amylase determinations and abdominal ultrasonography to detect or to follow fluid collections in the lesser sac. When all symptoms have been relieved for a day or more, the gastric tube is removed, and small, frequent, low-fat feedings are started.

Collections of fluid in the lesser sac suggest a more

serious illness that may prolong pain and vomiting. Some of these collections will spontaneously reabsorb, and if the symptoms abate, the child is followed with abdominal ultrasonography. If there are continued symptoms for a week or more, the fluid should be drained externally. Although this may be accomplished percutaneously with ultrasound guidance, an operation will allow more complete drainage and inspection of the pancreas. A short left subcostal incision will allow mobilization of the greater curvature of the stomach away from the spleen and transverse colon and entrance into the lesser omental sac. The fluid is drained, and the pancreas is inspected for disruption. Soft Silastic suction tubes are left along the pancreas and brought out the lateral edge of the wound. The child's symptoms are promptly relieved. There is often minimal drainage for several days to 2 weeks, but the child may go home with the drains in place. They are gradually shortened and then removed. Although an established pancreatic pseudocyst is expeditiously drained with a cystogastrostomy, this operation is best reserved for adult alcoholics. I prefer to drain an established thick-walled cyst into an isolated roux-en-Y loop of jejunum to avoid exposing the pancreas to gastric juice.

Although several drugs are associated with pancreatitis, corticosteroid used for children with nephrosis, malignancy, or collagen disease is the main culprit.[9] When the diagnosis of pancreatitis is made in these children, they are often critically ill with renal or respiratory failure. Initially, they were resuscitated with colloid and lactated Ringer's solution. If there is ascites, a paracentesis may relieve abdominal distention and help breathing. Conservative therapy with total intravenous nutrition, treatment of the underlying disease, and support for multiple organ failure is indicated. Many of these patients are already ventilator dependent and have central nervous system complications. When imaging studies demonstrate persistent fluid collections and necrotic tissue within the abdomen, simple drainage is not sufficient.

The tissue destruction associated with hypoperfusion and the continued release of enzymes are an ongoing process. Repeated surgical drainage and debridement are necessary. We have treated three patients by packing open the abdominal wound. These children were supported with prolonged intravenous nutrition and assisted ventilation. They were taken to the operating room every day for dressing changes and further debridement of necrotic tissue until the wound was clean and granulating (Fig. 101–1). In one patient, the open wound was covered with skin grafts, and in two, it was partially closed after several weeks of daily dressing changes. All three survived the pancreatitis, but one girl died a year later with lupus erythematosus, and another required prolonged renal dialysis, nephrectomy, and renal transplantation for severe nephrosis.

Chronic relapsing pancreatitis may be caused by

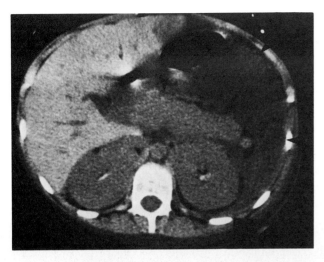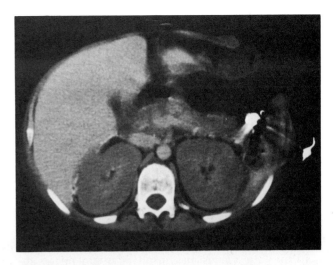

Figure 101-1. Left. CT scan of extensive pancreatitis with surrounding debris and necrosis in a 7-year-old boy with end-stage nephrosis. Small arrow points to the edematous pancreas. Large arrows indicate necrotic, injected debris. **Right.** Postoperative CT with the wound debrided and packed open. Arrows point to an abdominal wall defect.

an underlying ductal anomaly or inherited as an autosomal dominant disease.[10–12] Tudor has now reviewed 371 cases, including 80 kindreds from the world's literature of this fascinating problem.[13] Formerly, many of these patients were thought to have idiopathic pancreatitis. Now, with modern diagnostic techniques, some are found to have ductal stenosis, and others have an associated hyperlipidemia, aminoaciduria, or hyperparathyroidism. Many in the past were subjected to a series of useless operations, including cholecystectomy and gastric resection. Some have a dilated pancreatic duct with pancreatic calculi easily observed with CT scans (Fig. 101–2). The exact anatomy of the pancreatic duct may be further studied either with ERCP or a pancreaticogram obtained at operation after removal of the tail of the pancreas and cannulation of the duct. The symptoms are relieved by opening the duct lengthwise and draining it into an isolated Roux-en-Y jejunal loop.[14]

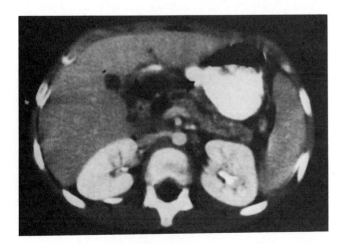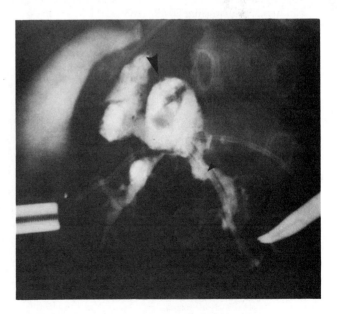

Figure 101-2. Left. CT scan of pancreas demonstrating a dilated pancreatic duct (small arrow) and a small pseudocyst (large arrow) in a 7-year-old girl with recurrent episodes of pain. **Right.** Pancreatogram performed at operation after transecting the tail of the pancreas and catheterizing the duct. A Roux-en-Y drainage of the distal pancreas was performed, and the symptoms were relieved.

Pancreas divisum, or the separate drainage of the ducts of Wirsung and Santorini into the duodenum, is found in approximately 4 percent of patients studied with ERCP. When there is stenosis of the duct of Santorini, a sphincteroplasty may relieve the patient's symptoms of abdominal pain.[15] The diagnosis is usually made in adults who may have had symptoms since childhood but usually have other causes for their pain.

Intrapancreatic intestinal duplications may cause pain by obstruction of the pancreatic duct and may be mistaken for a small pseudocyst when observed by CT scan or ERCP.[16] At operation, the wall of the cyst is examined by frozen section. If intestinal or gastric mucosa is found, the cyst is excised, and the pancreatic duct is drained into an isolated loop of jejunum.

Pancreatic ascites may result in asymptomatic abdominal distention. A paracentesis reveals fluid with a high amylase level, indicating a problem with the pancreas. Most often, there is leakage from the main duct or from a pseudocyst.[8,17] Trauma caused by child abuse was eventually suspected in the one case of pancreatic ascites that I have treated. These children should have complete studies, including CT scans and visualization of the pancreatic duct either by ERCP or at operation. Drainage of the transected pancreas into an isolated loop of jejunum is curative.

REFERENCES

1. Eichelberg M, Hoelzer D, Koop C: Acute pancreatitis: the difficulties of diagnosis and therapy. J Pediatr Surg 17:244, 1982
2. Tam P, Saing H, Irving I, Lister J: Acute pancreatitis in children. J Pediatr Surg 20:58, 1985
3. Millar A, Rode H, Stunden R, Cywes S: Management of pancreatic pseudocysts in children. J Pediatr Surg 23:122, 1988
4. Bartholomew C: Acute scorpion pancreatitis in Trinidad. Br Med J 1:666, 1970
5. Eichelberger M, Chatten J, Bruce D, et al: Acute pancreatitis and increased intracranial pressure. J Pediatr Surg 16:562, 1981
6. Caniano D, Browne A, Boles D: Pancreatic pseudocyst complicating treatment of acute lymphoblastic leukemia. J Pediatr Surg 20:452, 1985
7. Williams L, Reynolds R, Emery J: Pancreatitis during sodium valproate treatment. Arch Dis Child 58:543, 1983
8. Filston H, McLeod M, Bolman R, Jones R: Improved management of pancreatic lesions in children aided by ERLP. J Pediatr Surg 15:121, 1980
9. Reimenschneider T, Wilson J, Vernier R: Glucocorticoid-induced pancreatitis in children. Pediatrics 41:428, 1968
10. Crane L, Amoury R, Hellerstein S: Hereditary pancreatitis: Report of a kindred. J Pediatr Surg 8:893, 1973
11. Forbes A, Leung J, Cotton P: Relapsing acute and chronic pancreatitis. Arch Dis Child 59:927, 1984
12. Dean R, Scott H, Law D: Chronic relapsing pancreatitis in childhood: Case report and review of the literature. Ann Surg 173:443, 1971
13. Collected and published by R. B. Tudor. Quain and Ramstedt Clinic, 222 North 7th Street, Bismark, ND 58501. April 1, 1988
14. Puestow CB, Gillesby WJ: Retrograde drainage of pancreas for chronic relapsing pancreatitis. Arch Surg 76:898, 1958
15. Warshaw A, Richter J, Schapiro R: The cause and treatment of pancreatitis associated with pancreas divisum. Ann Surg 198:443, 1983
16. Black P, Welch J, Eraklis A: Juxtapancreatic intestinal duplications with pancreatic ductal communication: A cause of pancreatitis and recurrent abdominal pain in childhood. J Pediatr Surg 21:257, 1986
17. Coupland G: Pancreatic ascites in childhood. J Pediatr Surg 5:570, 1970

SECTION XIV
Surgical Infections

Formerly, the bulk of pediatric surgical practice consisted of caring for children with osteomyelitis, empyema, cervical adenitis, and the complications of tuberculosis. Antibiotics have drastically reduced the incidence of these diseases. They continue to be major problems in areas where medical care is suboptimal, and we must all be aware of infections due to unusual organisms, such as the atypical mycobacteria, fungi, and resistant strains of common bacteria.

Even though antibiotic therapy is extremely effective, inadequate treatment may only mask the signs and symptoms of infection so that now one rarely observes a typical surgical infection. The diagnosis is difficult when there is no fluctuation and only minimal signs of inflammation.

A localized infection must be considered in many differential diagnoses. Clues often will be found in the child's history. A boil or furuncle may lead to a suppurative mediastinitis or an extradural abscess. Tonsillitis, otitis, pyoderma of the scalp, or a dental infection almost invariably precedes bacterial cervical adenitis. A detailed history of the child's antibiotic therapy is important. All too frequently, a hospital chart merely states that antibiotics were given, without any indication of the dose, the duration of therapy, or the name of the drug. A further integral part of the history concerns the child's exposure to pets and other animals and travel to areas of the country endemic for the various fungal diseases.

A family history is a must, especially for tuberculosis. Finally, a child who develops recurrent infections must be studied for immune deficiency.

102
Infections of the Head and Neck

CERVICAL LYMPHADENITIS

Cervical lymphadenitis typically follows a bout of pharyngitis or tonsillitis. Initially, there is enlargement of the submandibular and anterior triangle nodes associated with the primary infection. Increasing cervical pain, a high fever, and cellulitis of the surrounding tissues follow within a few days. The overlying skin becomes reddened, and the node softens and becomes fluctuant. Proper antibiotic therapy will abort the disease before the node suppurates. Frequently, however, inadequate treatment produces an initial drop in the fever while the infection smolders within the node. The child then has fever and an enlarged, indurated, tender node. Only the history of the preceding infection distinguishes this clinical picture from tuberculous adenitis, cat-scratch fever, or a lymphoma.

At this point, vigorous antibiotic therapy and warm compresses may still effect a cure. However, it is far better to aspirate the node under local anesthesia because if there is a small pocket of pus, antibiotic therapy is unlikely to succeed. Needle aspiration will at least provide material for culture and sensitivity and may be sufficient to drain the pus. The most common organisms are the group A streptococcus, beta-hemolytic streptococcus, and staphylococcus. Anaerobic organisms are associated with dental infections.[1,2]

Diagnosis
The diagnosis of bacterial adenitis is usually made by the history and needle aspiration of the lymph node. A blood count will demonstrate leukocytosis with a shift to the left. A tuberculin skin test is always performed, especially if no pus is recovered on needle aspiration. The continued unexplained presence of an enlarged tender lymph node is indication for an excisional biopsy.

Treatment
Antibiotics are continued, and warm, wet dressings are applied for an hour four times a day. Needle aspiration is carried out in the outpatient department with the child sedated if necessary. The affected area is painted with povidone-iodine, and the skin is infiltrated with 1 percent lidocaine. A 16-gauge needle connected to a 10 ml syringe is inserted into the node. If pus is obtained, specimens are taken for smears, aerobic and anaerobic cultures, and studies for fungi and tuberculosis. All the pus is aspirated, after which a second syringe filled with saline is attached to the needle, and the abscess cavity is irrigated and again aspirated. Warm compresses are continued. Usually one aspiration results in an immediate decrease in the child's fever and clinical improvement. A second aspiration may be carried out in 24 to 48 hours. If there is recurrence, surgical drainage under general anesthesia is indicated. A transverse skin incision is made over the fluctuant area. High in the neck, there is some risk of injuring the mandibular branch of the facial nerve. Thus all dissection is carried out with a hemostat after the initial skin incision. All loculations are broken down and the cavity is packed with ¼-inch gauze. Antibiotics are of little value once the abscess has been drained. A wet dressing is applied, and the entire neck is wrapped with Kerlix or Kling. Tape should never be applied to the skin near an infected area! The gauze packing is removed in the course of 4 or 5 days to allow the cavity to contract while the skin edges are kept open.

The presence of a skin pustule or failure to respond to usual antibiotic therapy should alert one to the diagnosis of a rare infection, such as nocardiosis, tularemia, or actinomycosis.

TUBERCULOUS ADENITIS

Enlarged cervical lymph nodes that persist for several weeks without an antecedent history of a primary infection should not be blindly treated with antibiotics but require an orderly diagnostic approach. Tuberculosis remains a health problem in the inner city, in some rural areas, and in American Indians. In these groups of patients, *Mycobacterium tuberculosis* and *Mycobacterium bovis* continue to infect the cervical lymph nodes.[3] Skin testing with intermediate strength PPD-S is indicated in every child with inexplicably large cervical lymph nodes. Children infected with *M. tuberculosis* will have a strongly positive reaction. However, most children with tuberculous adenitis in this country are infected with one of the atypical mycobacteria.[4-6] They will have a negative or doubtfully positive reaction to the usual screening Tine test or the PPD-S. The atypical organisms were classified by Runyon into four groups, depending on their pigmentation on exposure to light and the rapidity of their growth.[7]

Runyon's Classification of Atypical Mycobacterium
Group I: Photochromogens: colonies become pigmented in light.
Group II: Scotochromogens: colonies are pigmented when grown in the dark.
Group III: Nonchromogens: faintly colored organisms not influenced by light.
Group IV: Rapid growers: these form well-developed colonies after 1 or 2 weeks.

To save time in arriving at a diagnosis, skin testing for the atypical organisms should be carried out simultaneously with the routine PPD. There will be a positive reaction to at least one of these antigens if the child has tuberculous adenitis.

The human tubercle bacillus, which is passed from human to human, may enter through the tonsils and infect the submandibular or upper jugular lymph nodes. Bovine tuberculosis, on the other hand, enters through the gastrointestinal tract, and the left supraclavicular or Virchow's node is the first to be involved. The atypical organisms do not appear to spread from human to animal or from animal to human but are picked up from the environment. Any group of cervical nodes may be involved, but the submandibular group is most frequently infected.

Initially, there is only a granulomatous reaction within the lymph node—the center breaks down and liquefies. The pus is contained within the fibrous envelope of the node but then bursts through to occupy the space limited by the deep cervical fascia of the neck. Later, this fascial sheath gives way, and the pus ruptures through to involve the compartment beneath the superficial cervical fascia. From here, it is only a matter of time before the pus burrows its way to the skin, which becomes reddened and indurated. This is the start of the collar button abscess, in which the superficial large abscess connects through a tortuous tract to a deeper

affected lymph node.[8] Ruptures of the abscess result in the typical draining, scrofulous sinus tract.

Clinical Course
A child of any age may be affected with cervical tuberculosis, but almost all are under 5 years of age. Initially, there are only painless enlarged cervical lymph nodes. Signs of systemic illness are rare. Only a few patients have fever, anorexia, or weight loss. Cervical adenitis may, however, be a sign of disseminated tuberculosis in very ill children. This is particularly true for patients under 1 year of age who have been in close contact with an adult who harbors this disease. We observed a child with pulmonary tuberculosis who developed huge mediastinal lymph nodes that obstructed the trachea. After these were drained, he suddenly developed a tuberculous abscess of the neck while on isoniazid therapy.

Physical Signs
The dimensions of the involved node may be as large as 3 by 5 cm. There are matted adherent lymph nodes adjacent to the main mass, which may be fluctuant in the center (Fig. 102–1). In addition to skin tests, a chest x-ray is indicated. Excisional biopsy of the node, with histologic and bacteriologic study, is the most important diagnostic measure.

Treatment
Surgical excision is the preferred treatment for tuberculous lymph nodes. A transverse incision is made in a skin crease. Thin, reddened skin or sinus tracts are excised with the initial incision. If the abscess has broken through the deep cervical fascia, pus may be encountered early in the operation. All caseating material is irrigated from the wound if this occurs. It is much nicer to excise the affected skin, abscess, and lymph nodes with an en bloc dissection.

Most often, there are one or more large caseating nodes, with other adjacent nodes matted together in a dense mass of fibrous tissue. Distortion of the anatomy requires careful dissection and a nerve stimulator to locate the mandibular branch of the facial and spinal accessory nerve. The spinal accessory nerve is large and is identified by dissection along the upper third of the anterior border of the sternocleidomastoid muscle. It is superficial to the internal jugular vein and descends obliquely behind the digastric and stylohyoid muscles to enter the upper part of the sternocleidomastoid muscle. As the carotid sheath is exposed, the lymph nodes are seen to be smaller, less adherent, and more easily removed. The nodes deeper than the spinal accessory nerve and between this structure and the tip of the mastoid should be removed to prevent recurrence. The hypoglossal nerve is identified as it emerges from between the internal carotid artery and the jugular vein.

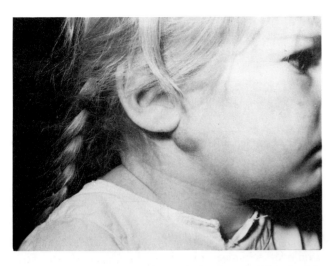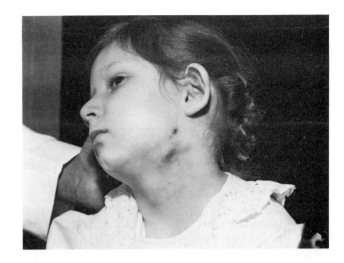

Figure 102–1. Tuberculosis of cervical lymph nodes. **Left.** A fluctuant red node just below the ear. There is minimal tenderness but considerable induration. **Right.** Chronic induration and drainage following incision.

It then swings downward and forward to become superficial below the digastric muscle. It is necessary to remove all caseating nodes, but it is safe to leave smaller nodes behind even if they are hypertrophied. The wound is irrigated, and all vessels are either ligated with fine catgut or coagulated. The wound is closed with subcuticular sutures and Steristrips, after which a pressure dressing is applied.

The removed nodes must be carefully handled. In the operating room, tissue as well as caseating material is placed on saline-soaked gauze in covered Petri dishes for immediate transfer to the microbiology laboratory, where specimens are taken to be checked for fungi as well as tuberculosis. Several nodes are placed in formalin and sent for pathologic study.

The postoperative results are excellent when all the involved nodes have been removed. Therapy with isoniazid is indicated only in children infected with *M. tuberculosis*, but antibiotics are of no value in atypical disease.[9]

BCG vaccination may produce a typical granulomatous reaction in the axillary lymph nodes that goes on to fibrous formation and sinus tracts. The pathologic and clinical picture is identical to that seen with tuberculous adenitis in the neck, except that there are no viable organisms found on culture. The history of BCG vaccination is sufficient to make the diagnosis. Treatment consists of an axillary dissection to remove all the involved lymph nodes.

CAT-SCRATCH DISEASE

Kittens are not ordinarily looked on as dangerous animals, or even as vectors of disease. In fact, however, one should always inquire about a past history of a cat

scratch when evaluating a child with lymphadenopathy (Fig. 102–2). Carithers has reviewed 1200 personally followed patients.[10] All had lymphadenopathy, 99.1 percent reported contact with a cat, and in 92.6 percent

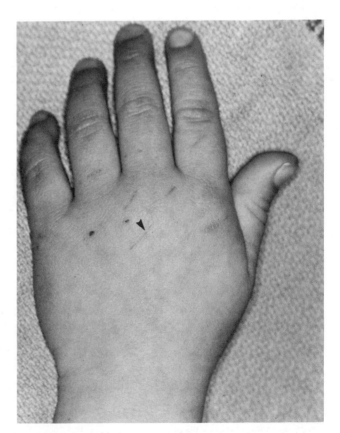

Figure 102–2. This child had numerous scratches on her hand from playing with a kitten. One aspiration of a fluctuant axillary node led to a cure.

there was a definite inoculation site or pustule where the patient was scratched. The skin papule appears 3 to 5 days after exposure to the cat, but the papule usually has long disappeared and has been forgotten by the time the child appears with an enlarged lymph node. The oculoglandular syndrome of Parinaud, or preauricular adenopathy, associated with conjunctivitis occurs when the scratch is on the face. Fever and suppuration of the node occurs in as many as 25 percent of affected patients. Before pus formation, the nodes are firm, movable, and nontender. When suppuration does occur, the node becomes fluctuant and the overlying skin may be red, but there is not the degree of pain and tenderness usually associated with a bacterial lymphadenitis. According to Carithers, the diagnosis can be made with certainty when there is a positive history of contact with a cat, lymphadenopathy, and a positive skin test. He has prepared the skin test antigen from pus obtained from suppurating nodes. One tenth of 1 milliliter of the antigen is injected intradermally, just as with a tuberculin skin test. If there is doubt about the diagnosis or if the node suppurates, it may be excised for diagnosis or merely aspirated. Unfortunately, excised nodes demonstrate a nonspecific granulomatous reaction that may be confused with tuberculosis or fungal infections. Material from lymph nodes should be cultured, since a small, gram-negative, pleomorphic organism has been found in the primary inoculation site and involved lymph nodes.[11,12] The Warthin-Starry silver impregnation stain provides the best method of identification. Although cat-scratch disease usually is benign and self-limiting, convulsions due to central nervous system involvement have been observed.[13]

PAROTITIS

The differential diagnosis of recurrent parotitis includes tumors and is discussed in Chapter 55. Suppurative parotitis is exceedingly rare, but adjacent lymph node infections may appear to involve the parotid gland.

INFECTION IN A THYROGLOSSAL DUCT CYST

A preexisting thyroglossal duct cyst may become tender and more swollen after an upper respiratory infection. Warm soaks and antibiotics relieve the child's symptoms, but it is almost necessary to aspirate the pus with a needle or to incise and drain the infected cyst (Fig. 102–3). The parents are always warned that this procedure will result in a draining sinus tract. In our experience, a previous infection is the most frequent single factor in recurrent sinus tracts. A wider than usual excision is required to remove all bits of epithelial tissue.

SUPPURATIVE THYROIDITIS

Suppurative thyroiditis is extremely rare, presumably because of the gland's excellent blood supply.[14] We observed only one definite case, which occurred in a 9-year-old girl. The left lobe of her thyroid gland was enlarged and tender and became fluctuant. Tests showed her thyroid function to be elevated, presumably secondary to the inflammation. Therapy with antibiotics over a period of several weeks resulted in only minimal im-

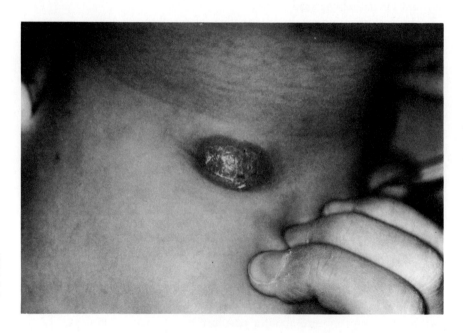

Figure 102–3. An infected thyroglossal duct cyst. This was aspirated with a syringe and needle and treated with soaks and antibiotics. Surgical excision should be delayed for several months in such patients.

provement. There was prompt relief of symptoms and a drop in her fever after the pus was aspirated with a needle and syringe. It was not necessary to incise and drain the abscess.

REFERENCES

1. Dajiui A, Garcia R, Wolinsky E: Etiology of cervical lymphadenitis in children. N Engl J Med 268:1329, 1963
2. Barton L, Feiqui R: Childhood cervical lymphadenitis: A reappraisal. J Pediatr 84:846, 1974
3. Lampe R, Baker C, Septimus E, Wallace R: Cervicofacial nocardiosis in children. J Pediatr 99:593, 1981
4. Mazzei E, Fonkalsrud E: Cervical lymphadenitis in children due to atypical mycobacteria. Am Surg 34:798, 1968
5. Altman R, Margileth A: Cervical lymphadenopathy from atypical mycobacteria: Diagnosis and surgical treatment. J Pediatr Surg 10:419, 1975
6. Belin R, Richardson J, Richardson D, et al: Diagnosis and management of scrofula in children. J Pediatr Surg 9:103, 1974
7. Runyon E: Anonymous bacteria in pulmonary disease. Med Clin North Am 43:273, 1959
8. Bailey H: Tuberculous cervical adenitis. Lancet 1:313, 1948
9. White M, Bangash H, Goel K, Jenkins P: Nontuberculous mycobacterial lymphadenitis. Arch Dis Child 61:368, 1986
10. Carithers H: Cat-scratch disease: An overview based on a study of 1200 patients. Am J Dis Child 139:1124, 1985
11. Wear D, Margileth A, Hadfield T, et al: Cat-scratch disease: A bacterial infection. Science 221:1403, 1983
12. Margileth A, Wear D, Hadfield T: Cat-scratch disease: Bacteria in skin at the primary inoculation site. JAMA 252:928, 1984
13. Lewis D, Tucker S: Central nervous system involvement in cat-scratch disease. Pediatrics 77:714, 1986
14. Ford R, Sanders D, Myers R: Thyroid abscess in a 14-month-old child. J Pediatr Surg 8:943,1973

103
Infections of the Hand

A fingertip infection or felon is dangerous because of the extensive fibrous compartmentation of the palmar surface of the fingertip. This prevents external swelling, and the infection produces sufficient pressure to compromise the blood supply to the terminal phalangeal bone. This may result in a chronic osteomyelitis. There may be a history of a minor injury to the finger, which has commenced to throb and is exquisitely tender. The tip is red and only slightly swollen.

The offending organism is usually a staphylococcus, but some rapidly progressive infections are caused by a streptococcus.

The initial treatment consists of elevating the hand and the continuous application of warm, wet dressings. A large, bulky bandage will immobilize the finger and offer some relief from the pain. If this treatment together with systemic antibiotic therapy does not promptly relieve the pain and swelling, the finger must be drained. This requires a general anesthetic. A lateral incision is made over the distal phalanx a third of the distance from the nail to the palmar surface. When pus is encountered, a wick of gauze is inserted, and a large, moist dressing is again applied. When a felon has become chronic, an x-ray is taken to detect an osteomyelitis. This must be treated by a wide incision with debridement and curettage of the bone. Antibiotics are then given until the wound is healed.

A paronychia is an infection lateral to the nail that may result from a hangnail or trauma. The finger is painful, and on examination, there is a white line of pus visible just under the skin at the junction of the nail. If a paronychia is neglected, the infection will extend around to the base of the nail, which becomes loosened and elevated by a subungual pocket of pus. Early on, it is possible to release the pus without anesthesia with the tip of a number 11 scalpel blade. Later, a general anesthetic is required, and often it is necessary to remove all or a portion of the nail. Antibiotics are not required for this superficial infection, but a moist dressing is left on the wound for at least 24 hours.

Occasionally, one sees a child who appears to have a fingertip infection, but on close examination, the epidermis is elevated and appears blistered. If there is a history of a herpetic lesion in the mouth or if the mother has had herpes, the child may have a herpetic whitlow. When the blister is opened, there is no underlying abscess but only a cloudy, watery fluid. Cultures are usually negative. Incision and drainage are of little help. The only satisfactory treatment is to protect the finger from trauma with a dressing until the blister is healed. There may be residual parenthesias or numbness in the affected area.

Deep infections in the palm of the hand are serious. These children should be admitted to the hospital and placed at bedrest with elevation of the hand, which is encased in a bulky, warm, moist dressing. A systemic antibiotic—either penicillin or erythromycin—is administered. If there is only a cellulitis, the symptoms of pain and swelling will rapidly improve. On the other hand, if passive movement of a finger causes pain in the palm, there is likely to be a tendon space infection. This must be drained in the operating room under general anesthesia through an incision that follows the transverse creases of the palm.

Every surgeon should be familiar with Kanavel's classic textbook on infections of the hand, which describes the anatomy of tendon space infections.[1]

REFERENCE

1. Kanavel A: Infections of the Hand, 5th ed. Philadelphia, Lea & Febiger, 1925

104
Chest Infections

MEDIASTINITIS

Suppurative mediastinitis may occur secondary to foreign body perforations of the pharynx or esophageal perforation or in association with staphylococcal abscesses in other areas of the body. A seemingly minor injury inflicted by a wooden candy stick or a pencil to the back of the throat can result in a severe infection.[1] The retropharyngeal space is in direct continuity via the periesophageal tissues with the posterior mediastinum (Fig. 104–1). Thus, purulent material can rapidly find its way from the neck to the mediastinum. In this situation, there will be a mixed flora reflecting the variety of organisms found in the oral cavity. Children with this type of infection deteriorate rapidly. They have a high fever, tachycardia, dysphagia, and respiratory distress. Initial treatment consists of the administration of large doses of broad-spectrum antibiotics. If there is not a prompt response or if subcutaneous emphysema develops, the entire retropharyngeal and paraesophageal spaces are opened through a low cervical incision. The carotid sheath is retracted laterally, and with blunt finger dissection both up and down along the esophagus, pus will be found.[2] The space is irrigated and liberally drained. Infections secondary to a perforation in the distal portion of the esophagus are approached by resecting a rib over the abscess. The mediastinum is then entered through an extrapleural dissection, and the pus is drained. In recent years it has been possible to accurately localize the purulent collection with an ultrasound examination combined with needle aspiration. With accurate localization, the pus is drained by the percutaneous insertion of a tube.

Hematogenous spread from a staphylococcal abscess or pneumonia may cause mediastinitis.[3] In these cases, the pus must be localized by x-ray or ultrasonography because an anterior extrapleural incision through the fifth intercostal space is indicated rather than a posterior incision. We have drained an upper mediastinal abscess secondary to a staphylococcal infection through a cervical incision.

LUNG INFECTION

During the past 16 years, the only children with lung abscesses who required an operation in our hospital had an underlying immunodeficiency. The others in whom this diagnosis was initially made actually had infected lung cysts. In the past, lung abscesses in children were secondary to staphylococcal pneumonia and aspirated foreign bodies.[4] Currently, antibiotic therapy, together with postural drainage and bronchodilator treatment, will result in drainage of the pus and obliteration of the cavity. Groff and Marquis have demonstrated the effectiveness of transbronchial drainage.[5] In this technique, the child is bronchoscoped under general anesthesia to rule out a foreign body. The bronchoscope is then withdrawn, and an endotracheal tube with a right-angled connector is inserted. Under fluoroscopic control, the endotracheal tube is positioned near the involved segmental orifice, and an angiographic catheter is passed through the tube and segmental bronchus to puncture the abscess. Pus may be aspirated with this technique, after which the cavity is irrigated with saline or an antibiotic solution. This procedure was successful in three patients.

EMPYEMA

Empyema in children most often is secondary to an acute pneumonia. However, chronic lung disease, such as bronchiectasis, cystic fibrosis, and chronic aspiration, also may lead to this disease. Empyema may occur in a poorly drained hemothorax after trauma or after surgery

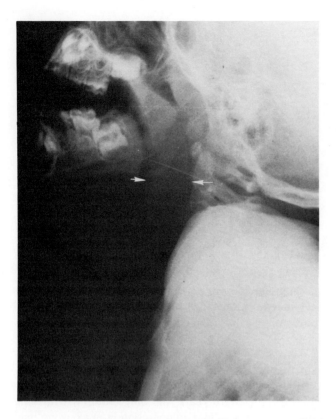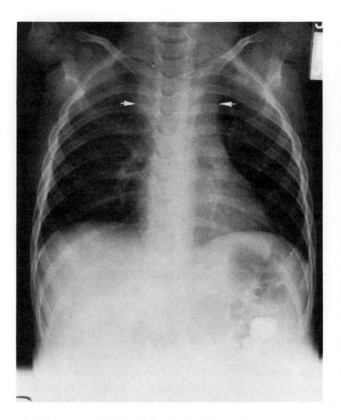

Figure 104–1. Retropharyngeal abscess extending into the mediastinum. **Left.** Widened retropharyngeal spore. **Right.** Superior mediastinal widening.

on the lungs or esophagus. Postpneumonic empyema may be caused by infection with *Staphylococcus aureus, Haemophilus influenzae, Streptococcus pneumoniae,* and a variety of other organisms, including anaerobes.

The clinical picture of a child with an acute empyema is one of serious respiratory distress and high fever. Physical examination and roentgenographic studies demonstrate an opacified pleural cavity with mediastinal shift or an air–fluid level diagnostic of a tension pyopneumothorax. When an empyema develops acutely, the pus is thin and easily aspirated with a syringe and a needle and can be effectively drained by the insertion of an intercostal catheter connected to a waterseal. Unfortunately, an empyema is often treated only with antibiotics. When these children are seen later, the chest roentgenogram may demonstrate an opacity, and it is difficult to determine how much of the child's problem is due to pneumonia and how much is due to pleural involvement. Computed tomography (CT) scans of the chest have been extremely helpful in resolving this issue. These studies have demonstrated considerably more pleural fluid than one would expect from x-rays. The CT scan allows very accurate location of the empyema cavity. When the diagnosis of an empyema is delayed, the pus is thick and loculated and will not drain well through a simple intercostal tube. Furthermore, the insertion of an intercostal

drainage tube under local anesthesia is very painful. For these reasons, we adopted a minithoracotomy to drain the thick, loculated fluid usually found in subacute empyemas.[6] Kosloske et al. have recommended aggressive early operation for children with empyema who do not respond to conventional therapy.[7]

The minithoracotomy is performed under general anesthesia, with the child in the lateral position. It is essential to have the empyema cavity well localized before the operation because we make only a 2 to 3 inch incision over the empyema (Fig. 104–2). A segment of rib is resected, and the cavity is entered. All loose fibrinous material and liquid pus are aspirated with suction, and loculations are broken with finger dissection. Any thick fibrinous peel over the lung or parietal pleura that comes away easily is removed. No attempt is made to perform a formal decortication because it is unwise to tear the lung and produce a postoperative air leak. The cavity is then copiously irrigated, and the anesthesiologist inflates the collapsed lung. One chest tube is placed through a skin incision below the primary incision, but the tube is brought through the bed of the resected rib. The incision is then closed, leaving the tube on waterseal suction. There is usually prompt expansion of the lung, but pleural thickening will remain visible on an x-ray for several months. The tube is left in place

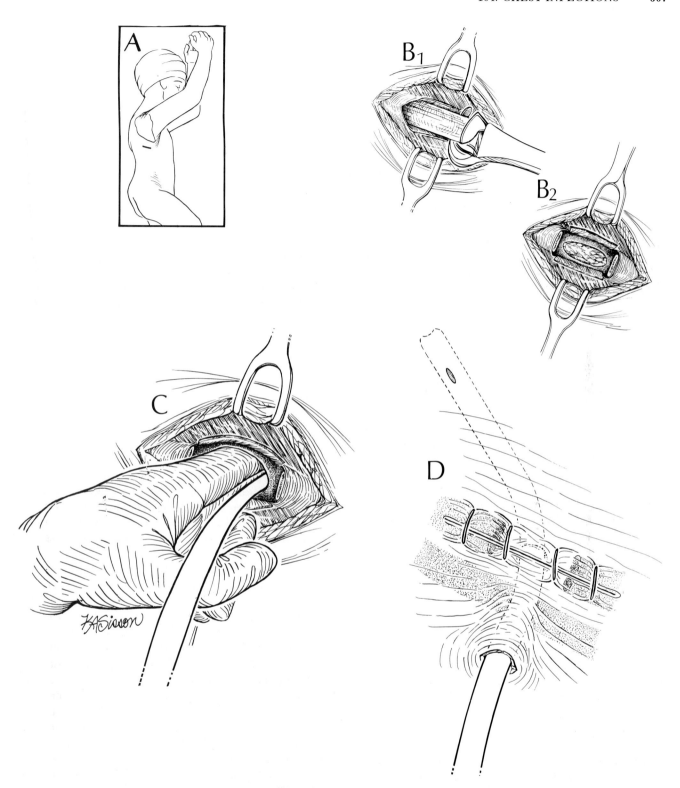

Figure 104–2. Minithoractomy for empyema drainage. A 2-inch segment of rib is resected, and all fibrous debris and exudate are removed with suction and finger dissection. A large chest tube is placed through the chest wall incision but is brought out through a separate skin wound.

until the lung has expanded and drainage has ceased. In our hands, the duration of the fever and the length of hospitalization are shorter after the minithoracotomy than after simple chest tube drainage.

Two complications have occurred in 22 patients. One child required reoperation when a new empyema accumulated after the first chest tube was removed, and one girl was reoperated on for bleeding.

PURULENT PERICARDITIS

The diagnosis of pericarditis should be suspected in any febrile child who is acutely ill and who has an enlarged cardiac shadow on a chest x-ray. The major differential diagnosis is between myocarditis with cardiac dilatation and pericarditis. Both can produce muffled heart tones, a globular-shaped heart, diminished cardiac pulsations, and dilated jugular veins. An echocardiogram will differentiate between these two diagnoses and can reliably demonstrate as little as 10 to 20 ml. of pericardial fluid. When the diagnosis is made, a pericardiocentesis should be performed, and the fluid should be gram-stained and cultured. Pericarditis caused by *S. pneumoniae* or *S. aureus*, the two most commonly found organisms, may be managed with pericardiocentesis and antibiotic therapy. Garvin et al. recommended drainage through an upper abdominal extraperitoneal incision extended up to the pericardium.[8] A segment of the pericardium is removed, and the cavity is irrigated and drained.

H. influenzae, which is the causative agent in 7 to 11 percent of children with pyogenic pericarditis creates a thick, fibrinous pericardial exudate. Four children with pericarditis caused by this organism at our hospital required a complete anterior pericardiectomy to achieve adequate drainage.[9]

BRONCHIECTASIS

The elimination of measles, pertussis, and tuberculosis has practically made bronchiectasis "extinct" in the United States. In addition, the improved medical therapy for pneumonia, together with chest physiotherapy, postural drainage, bronchodilators, and humidity, has essentially done away with chronic atelectasis. In the past, these were the underlying diseases that produced chronic pulmonary suppuration and bronchiectasis.

This diagnosis should still be suspected, however, in a child who has a chronic productive cough or episodes of pneumonia with wheezing and a persistent pulmonary infiltrate in one area of the lung. If there are persistent symptoms, bronchoscopy is indicated to rule out a foreign body, and at the same time a bronchogram may be obtained. When the diagnosis is made, it is worthwhile

to outline a course of medical therapy that will result at least in symptomatic improvement. Postural drainage three times a day is the most important aspect of treatment. In addition, cultures of sputum obtained at bronchoscopy form the basis for vigorous antibiotic therapy. A member of the family may be taught how to administer chest physiotherapy. In our experience, there is almost always some degree of bilateral disease. Consequently, this medical therapy must be continued for the rest of the patient's life, even if an operation is performed. For this reason, an operation is indicated only if there is sputum production that is recalcitrant to medical therapy. Complete mapping of the entire tracheobronchial tree is indicated before an operation. In most instances, the disease will predominate in one lower lobe. Bronchiectasis may also be associated with immune deficiency diseases and cystic fibrosis of the pancreas. An operation is indicated for bronchiectasis in these situations only when medical therapy has clearly failed.

There is a congenital form of bronchiectasis. The history of recurrent pneumonia goes back to the newborn period, and one usually finds chronic wheezing, clubbing of the nails, and poor growth and development. Small children do not have a productive cough because they swallow their sputum, but on physical examination, one finds sticky rales and rhonchi over the affected area. Chest roentgenograms demonstrate recurrent infiltrates in one region of the lung, and often the affected lung is either hypoplastic or contracted secondary to chronic infection. A bronchogram or CT scan makes the diagnosis—one will see extensive sacular bronchiectasis with nearly complete loss of normal lung parenchyma (Fig. 104–3). Medical therapy is used only to prepare the

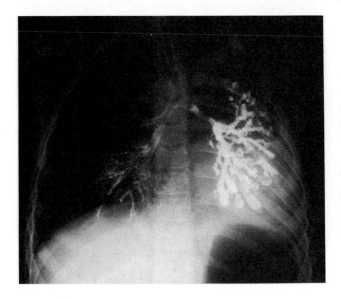

Figure 104–3. Congenital bronchiectasis in an 8-year-old girl: a preoperative bronchogram.

child for an operation because this type of disease is well localized and amenable to surgical cure.

REFERENCES

1. North J, Emanuel B: Mediastinitis in a child caused by perforation of pharynx. Am J Dis Child 129:962, 1975
2. Payne S, Larson R: Acute mediastinitis. Surg Clin North Am 49:999, 1969
3. Slim M, Rizk G, Uwaydah M: Mediastinal complications of staphylococcal infection in childhood: Experience with six consecutive cases. Surgery 69:755, 1971
4. Mark P, Turner J: Lung abscess in childhood. Thorax 23:216, 1968
5. Groff D, Marquis J: Transtracheal drainage of lung abscesses in children. J Pediat Surg 12:303, 1977
6. Raffensperger JG, Luck S, Sckolnick A, Ricketts R: Minithorectomy and chest tube insertion for children with empyema. J Thoracic Surg 84:497, 1982
7. Kosloske A, Cushing A, Shuck J: Early decortication for anerobic empyema in children. Pediatr Surg 15:422, 1980
8. Garvin P, Danis R, Lewis E, Willman V: Purulent pericarditis in children. Surgery 84:471, 1978
9. Ricketts R, Ilbawi M, Idriss F: Management of *Haemophilus influenzae* pericarditis. J Pediatr Surg 17:285, 1982

105
Subphrenic Abscess

In children, a subphrenic or subhepatic abscess is almost always the sequela of a perforated appendicitis with generalized peritonitis. The second most common etiology is upper abdominal trauma, particularly when there has been a liver injury combined with a perforation of the gastrointestinal tract. Boyd has simplified the anatomy of the subphrenic and subhepatic spaces.[1] He clearly demonstrated that the suspensory ligament of the liver attaches to the posterior abdominal wall and not to the diaphragm. Thus, there is a space beneath the right lobe of the liver, which was formerly labeled the "right posterior subphrenic space." There is one space above the liver on the right and one on the left. Pus beneath the liver, rather than beneath the diaphragm, may not elevate the diaphragm or result in a pleural effusion—two signs considered very important in the diagnosis.

When there is persistent fever, ileus, malaise, and vague upper abdominal pain following an appendectomy for appendicitis, one should suspect a subphrenic abscess. The problem is much more difficult when the child's original appendicitis was overlooked and he or she was treated with antibiotics (Fig. 105–1). In this situation, the abscess may smolder for several weeks while the child is studied for "fever of undetermined origin" and again treated with various antibiotics. An intermittent high fever is the single most important sign of a subhepatic or subphrenic abscess. This may be the only sign when the pus is beneath the liver. A careful physical examination may reveal upper abdominal or posterior tenderness with depressed breath sounds and dullness on the affected side. Either ultrasound or computed tomography (CT) examination will reliably diagnose and localize abnormal collections of fluid or pus in the upper abdomen. A high index of suspicion, combined with frequent physical examination and repeated imaging studies, should lead to the correct diagnosis. It is often necessary to stop administration of all antibiot-

ics to allow the abscess to declare itself. It is as important to know the location of the abscess as it is to know of its existence.

TREATMENT

A subphrenic cellulitis may very well respond to intensive antibiotic therapy. A formed collection of pus requires surgical drainage. One should choose the shortest route to the pus that will allow dependent drainage and that will not transgress the pleural or peritoneal cavity. The right and left subhepatic spaces are easily drained through an oblique incision extending from the tip of the 11th rib medially for several inches.[2] The preperitoneal space is entered after separation of the oblique and transverse muscles. Blunt finger dissection is continued upward until one encounters edema and induration. Needle aspiration is helpful in locating the abscess after the incision has been made. Once the cavity has been entered, all loculations are broken down, and it is irrigated with saline. Large Penrose drains stuffed with gauze are then brought out of the wound.

The suprahepatic or true subphrenic space is most easily found through an incision that traverses the thoracic cavity and diaphragm. The pleura is almost always adherent to the diaphragm, so there is little risk of contamination of the free pleural cavity. If there is a free space, the pleura is sutured to the diaphragm. The pus is located with needle aspiration through the diaphragm, which is then opened directly over the abscess and drained as before. Many intraabdominal fluid collections and abscesses can be managed with percutaneous aspiration and catheter drainage after accurate localization with CT or ultrasonography. This technique is particularly applicable in children who are severely ill after organ transplantation and in those who are immunosuppressed

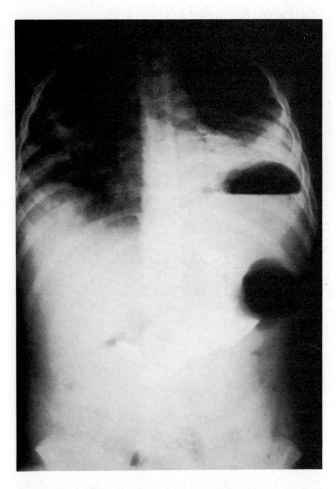

Figure 105–1. This patient's neglected appendicitis was treated with antibiotics, which led to subphrenic abscesses. There is a huge, obvious air–fluid level beneath the left diaphragm that displaces the stomach.

or agranulocytic. Aspiration allows rapid differentiation between sterile fluid collections and pus as well as identification of bacteria.

Imaging studies must identify a route to the abscess that does not traverse loops of bowel or a sterile cavity. The procedure is performed under local anesthesia with the child well sedated. First a 20-gauge needle is advanced into the cavity and fluid is aspirated. Next a guidewire is passed through the needle, and over the guidewire a size 8 French nephrostomy or a 12 French sump catheter is placed. All possible fluid is removed with suction; then the catheter is taped to the skin and left in place until there is no longer drainage and imaging studies demonstrate resolution of the process. Diament et al. successfully treated 16 of 21 patients with this technique.[3] Surgical drainage is necessary for patients who have loculated fluid as demonstrated by CT or ultrasonography. All patients were given specific broad-spectrum antibiotics, based on culture and sensitivity, until the cavity was obliterated and the fever and leukocytocis resolved.

REFERENCE

1. Boyd D: The subphrenic spaces and the emperor's new robes. N Engl J Med 275:911, 1966
2. DeCosse J, Poulin T, Fox P, Condon R: Subphrenic abscess. Surg Gynecol Obstet 138:841, 1974
3. Diament M, Stanley P, Kangarloo H, Donaldson J: Percutaneous aspiration and catheter drainage of abscesses. J Pediatr 108:204, 1986

106
Liver Abscess

In the preantibiotic era of surgical practice, a liver abscess was most often secondary to a perforated appendix. Currently, a pyogenic liver abscess in the neonatal period may be secondary to umbilical vein catheterization.[1-3] Other predisposing factors include chronic granulomatous disease, sickle cell anemia, and intestinal parasites.[4-7] We have also seen liver abscess develop secondary to otitis media, furunculosis, biliary tract surgery, and mycotic emboli from an infected coarctation of the aorta.

PATHOLOGY

The most common organism found in liver abscesses have been *Staphylococcus aureus*, *Streptococcus pyogenes*, and *Escherichia coli*.[8] Other unusual organisms have included *Klebsiella pneumoniae* and *Corynebacterium acnes*.[9,10] Most often, there is a solitary cavity filled with purulent material in the right lobe of the liver. However, 2 of our 6 patients had multiple abscesses throughout both lobes.

DIAGNOSIS

Classically, a liver abscess is heralded by fever, hepatomegaly, and right upper quadrant pain or tenderness. However, these symptoms may not be obvious in a young infant, especially a neonate. There may be only a nonspecific fever, anorexia, and abdominal distention. Jaundice was present in only 3 of our 6 patients. A persistent fever with any suggestion of upper abdominal tenderness or an enlarged liver should lead to a computed tomography (CT) scan or ultrasound examination.[11,12] The diagnosis really rests on the history of a predisposing illness, fever, and upper abdominal tenderness. Imaging studies, particularly CT, will reveal abscess cavities as small as 1 cm.

TREATMENT

A single abscess may be drained with percutaneous aspiration end catheter placement with ultrasound guidance. A transverse upper abdominal incision is made over the suspected abscess. Any suspicious soft areas of the liver are aspirated with a syringe and a needle. If pus is found, the area is walled off with moist pads, and the abscess is unroofed by dividing the overlying liver tissue with the electrocautery. Necrotic tissue within the cavity is debrided, and the area is drained. When there are multiple abscesses, as in chronic granulomatous disease, as many abscesses as possible are unroofed and drained, but the primary treament consists of long-term specific antibiotic treatment after culture of the purulent material.

RESULTS

One of our patients developed hematobilia after drainage of multiple abscesses. This complication required ligation of a branch of the right hepatic artery, but the child survived. One patient, a newborn, died and the abscess was discovered at autopsy. Another child who had a biliary atresia survived drainage of her abscess but died 3 years later of her primary disease. The other three children recovered following drainage of their abscesses and have had no further difficulty.

Chusid has reviewed 5 cases from the Milwaukee Children's Hospital and 61 from the literature.[13] There was a 27 percent mortality in children with chronic granulomatous disease and a 42 percent mortality in those without. The high mortality rate of hepatic abscess makes this an important surgical problem in childhood, particularly when more infants are being treated with umbilical vein catheters and more children are surviving with immunodeficiency diseases.

REFERENCES

1. Tariq A, Rudolph N, Levin E: Solitary hepatic abscess in a newborn infant: A sequel of umbilical vein catheterization and infusion of hypertonic glucose solution. Clin Pediatr 16:577, 1977
2. Kandall S, Johnson A, Gortner L: Solitary neonatal hepatic abscess. J Pediatr 83:567, 1973
3. Williams J, Rittenberry A, Dillard R, Allen R: Liver abscess in newborns: Complications of umbilical vein catheterization. Am J Dis Child 125:111, 1973
4. Quie P, Kaplin E, Page A, et al: Defective polymorphonuclear leukocyte function and chronic granulomatous disease in two female children. N Engl J Med 278:976, 1968
5. Azimis P, Bodenbender J, Hintz R, Kontras S: Chronic granulomatous disease in three female siblings. JAMA 206:2865, 1968
6. Roback S, Weintraub W, Good R, et al: Chronic granulomatous disease of childhood: surgical consideration. J Pediatr Surg 6:601, 1971
7. Shulman ST, Beem M: An unique presentation of sickle cell disease: Pyogenic hepatic abscess. Pediatrics 47:1019, 1971
8. Lazarchick J, deSouza N, Nichols D, Washington J: Pyogenic liver abscess. Mayo Clin Proc 48:349, 1973
9. Fraga J, Javate B, Venkatessan S: Liver abscess and sepsis due to *Klebsiella pneumoniae* in a newborn. Clin Pediatr 13:1081, 1974
10. Balfour H Jr, Minken S: Liver abscess due to *Corynebacterium acnes:* Diphtheroid as pathogen. Clin Pediatr 10:55, 1971
11. Gwinn J, Lee R: Radiological case of the month. Am J Dis Child 123:50, 1972
12. Vicary R, Cusick G, Shirley I, Blackwell R: Ultrasound and amoebic liver abscess. Br J Surg 64:113, 1977
13. Chusid M: Pyogenic hepatic abscess in infancy and childhood. Pediatrics 62:554, 1978

107
Iliac Fossa Abscess

It is difficult to determine if an abscess in the retorperitoneal space arises within the iliac muscle or in the lymph nodes along the iliac vessels. Since there is rarely a history of an infection or trauma in the leg, it is more likely that these abscesses arise in the muscle or nodes secondary to the hematogenous spread of staphylococci.

Once this lesion has been observed, the confusing history and physical findings become obvious.[1] The presenting complaint is an unexplained limp with a fever. The child prefers to lie in bed with the leg and thigh flexed. The child will walk only with reluctance. There may have been an antecedent sore throat or other mild illness. Appendicitis often is initially suspected because when the child walks, he or she is stooped over and has tenderness in a lower quadrant of the abdomen. However, there are no gastrointestinal symptoms other than the mild anorexia associated with fever. The patient will continue to take some food without vomiting, and there is no abdominal distention.

A septic arthritis or synovitis of the hip is next suspected because the child refuses to extend the hip, and passive motion is vigorously resisted. There is no tenderness or direct palpation over the joint and no swelling or edema over the buttock or inguinal region. Roentgenograms of the hip fail to demonstrate a capsular distention or lateral displacement of the proximal femur. When the diagnosis is delayed, the child continues to have intermittent fever and refuses to extend the hip.

An ultrasound examination is an excellent way to image the hip joint, lower abdomen, and iliac fossa, but a computed tomography (CT) examination provides more exact localization of the abscess.[2]

TREATMENT

When the child relaxes under anesthesia, it is possible to palpate a mass. The incision is made either over or lateral to the mass. Most often, a muscle-splitting incision just medial to the anterior superior spine of the ileum can be carried down to the retroperitoneal space by reflecting the peritoneum medially. When pus is encountered, the loculations are broken down and several soft drains are placed in the space.

REFERENCES

1. Maull K, Sachatello C: Retroperitoneal iliac fossa abscess. Am J Surg 127:270, 1974
2. Schwaitzberg S, Pokorney W, Thurston R, et al: Psoas abscess in children. J Pediatr Surg 20:339, 1985

108
Infections in Immunodeficient Children

There are increasing numbers of hospitalized children with impaired immunity who require surgical consultation for infectious complications. Children with malignancy, especially acute lymphocytic leukemia, require multiple bone marrow-suppressing drugs. Some, in fact, have total marrow ablation and transplantation. Biopsy or drainage of possible infectious lesions is frequently indicated in children with congenital immunodeficiency. Leonard et al. have written an excellent review of these diseases, correlating them with the underlying immune mechanisms.[1] Immune suppression also is necessary in children who require solid organ transplantation. Finally, the epidemic of acquired immunodeficiency disease (AIDS) has spread to the pediatric population through the maternal use of intravenous drugs and contaminated blood transfusions.[2]

The usual signs and symptoms of inflammation often are suppressed by steroid therapy and by the absence of neutrophils. Fever may be the only sign of a life-threatening infection and is an indication to search for the site and the offending organism. The physical examination should concentrate on the ears, nose, throat, lungs, perirectal area, and intravenous sites. When an infection is suspected, treatment with multiple broad-spectrum antibiotics is commenced without delay. If nothing is obvious, chest roentgenograms, computed tomography (CT) scans, and nuclear studies are performed on an emergency basis. Cultures are obtained from the nose, throat, and obvious skin lesions. Unusual, resistant organisms, including fungi and normal saprophytes, frequently cause invasive infections in these patients.

SKIN AND SOFT TISSUES

A true subcutaneous abscess develops rarely in neutropenic patients. Pain, redness, and induration are the only signs of infection. Occasionally, it is possible to aspirate a few drops of purulent material or serum for culture, but incision and drainage rarely are indicated. Rapidly advancing necrotizing infections caused by anaerobic organisms require debridement of necrotic tissue together with massive antibiotic therapy for cure. Invasive necrotic infections with *Aspergillus* have been reported.[3] The skin lesion with this organism begins as a black punctate hole with a halo of intense erythema surrounded by a zone of blanching. Aspergillosis requires extensive debridement for cure.

CENTRAL VENOUS LINE INFECTIONS

Central venous access is necessary in these very ill patients, but they are often a nidus for infections. Redness and induration at the skin exit site can be treated with topical and systemic antibiotics. Removal of the catheter is indicated if there is redness and fluctuance along the subcutaneous tunnel or evidence of thrombophlebitis that does not respond promptly. Septicemia alone is not an indication for catheter removal. Colonization of the catheter is diagnosed when there are persistently positive blood cultures obtained through the catheter while peripheral cultures are negative.[4] If catheter sepsis does not respond to antibiotic therapy after 48 hours, it is prudent to remove the catheter. An ultrasound study of the right atrium is indicated to find an infected clot, which may be lysed with enzyme therapy.

LUNG

Acute viral, bacterial, or fungal pulmonary infections may be rapidly progressive and fatal. The initial symptoms are a dry cough and fever. Chest x-rays usually demonstrate a nonspecific interstitial infiltrate. Within a short time, there is progression to tachypnea, dyspnea, and respiratory insufficiency. It is rare that one can find the infecting organism by blood or sputum cultures. Consequently, these children are given broad-spectrum antibiotics and sufficient oxygen to relieve their symptoms. Endotracheal intubation and ventilator support frequently are necessary. Many authors have recommened an open lung biopsy as a diagnostic tool.[5,6] This procedure has been particularly useful in the diagnosis of *Pneumocystis carinii* infections. This organism, a ubiquitous protozoon, is an opportunistic pathogen in debilitated or immunocompromised patients. Fortunately, infections with this organism can be prevented by the prophylactic use of trimethoprim-sulfamethoxazole (TMP-SMZ) in children at risk.[7] Since the introduction of TMP-SMZ at our hospital, the number of children found to have a specific organism has decreased to the point where lung biopsy is of little benefit.[8] Other authors also have found that survival rates have not depended on finding a specific infection by lung biopsy.[9] It is very important to weigh the risk of a biopsy against the need for long-term postoperative ventilator support and possible death. The early enthusiasm for open lung biopsy reflected the urgency in making the diagnosis of *P. carinii* infection. This infection can be prevented or adequately treated with TMP-SMZ, so there is less urgency to perform a biopsy. In children with AIDS, the differential diagnosis of pulmonary disease is often between that caused by *P. carinii* and pulmonary lymphoid hyperplasia. These diseases may be differentiated on the basis of clinical and roentgenographic findings. Infections with *P. carinii* are associated with more tachypnea, wheezing, and rhonchi, whereas lymphoid hyperplasia causes digital clubbing, salivary and lymph node hypertrophy, and a nodular roentgenographic pattern.[10]

It is difficult to state definite indications for open lung biopsy. Every effort should be made to establish a specific diagnosis by sputum culture or bronchial lavage. However, if these procedures are unrewarding or if the child is rapidly progressing into respiratory failure, a lung biopsy is indicated. The risks must be carefully weighed against any potential benefit, and the operation must be discussed clearly with the child's family.

Technique of Open Lung Biopsy

An open lung biopsy requires a general anesthetic and endotracheal intubation. A small anterolateral intercostal incision is made on the side with the most involvement. The biopsy is taken from grossly involved lung by placing a clamp across the anterior edge of a lobe. A 2 × 2 cm segment of lung is then excised. A continuous suture is run beneath the clamp, and after its removal, the suture is run back in an over-and-over fashion. Staples are not reliable in preventing postoperative air leaks from the biopsy site. A small chest tube is inserted,

and while the incision is being closed, the specimen is cut into four or five pieces for cultures and immediate frozen section examination.

The lung may be the primary site of a mycotic infection, especially in children with acute leukemia. Radiographically, these fungal infections are more likely to occur as an isolated or lobar lesion. CT examination may demonstrate a cavity. In the immunodepressed child, treatment with amphotericin B fails to resolve the infection, and surgical resection is necessary to prevent dissemination of the fungus.[11]

GASTROINTESTINAL TRACT

Acute perianal infections commence with a tender, swollen, indurated area that may progress to necrosis and ulceration. These patients are extremely ill with sepsis caused by multiple enteric organisms. Intravenous antibiotic therapy must include clindamycin or metronidazole for anaerobic bacteria. Incision and drainage are of no benefit in neutropenic patients because there is no pus. When there is breakdown of the skin and necrosis, debridement of nonviable tissue together with a completely diverting colostomy is necessary[12] (Fig. 108–1).

Abdominal pain and fever may be secondary to intestinal perforation or pancreatitis as well as any of the usual problems affecting normal children. Plain upright radiographs will demonstrate free air in the peritoneal cavity if there is perforation. An elevation of the serum

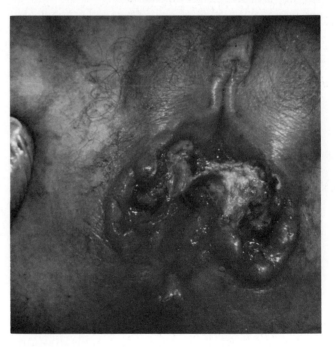

Figure 108–1. Necrotic perineal ulcer in a child with aplastic anemia, which required debridement and a colostomy.

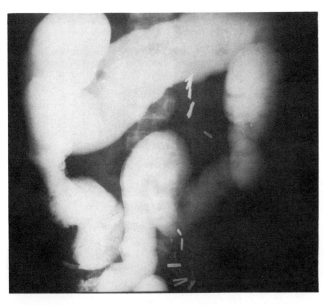

Figure 108–2. Typhlitis in a 13-year-old boy who developed abdominal pain and fever after a renal transplant. There is edema and irregularity of the cecal and ascending colon mucosa.

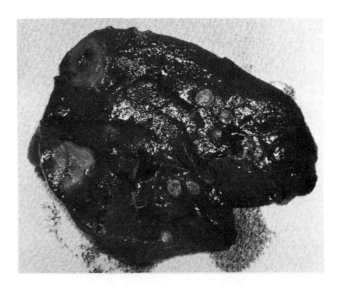

Figure 108–3. Multiple splenic abscess in a child with acute lymphocytic leukemia.

amylase and either CT or ultrasound examination will demonstrate pancreatitis, a pseudocyst, or abscess formation. It is safest to exteriorize intestinal perforations in these children and to carry out the simplest of external drainage procedures for pancreatic cysts or abscesses. Children with renal transplantation, in particular, are susceptible to a phlegmonous inflammation of the cecum. These children have abdominal pain, fever, and tenderness. Their clinical picture resembles acute appendicitis, but there are no definite signs of peritonitis. The history usually extends over several days, and there may be diarrhea. These children should have a barium enema. If there is edema of the cecum and ascending colon, the diagnosis is likely to be typhlitis, and an operation is not indicated (Fig. 108–2). The child should be treated with broad-spectrum antibiotics and bowel rest.

LIVER AND SPLEEN

Chronic granulomatous disease of childhood is a sex-linked recessive defect in neutrophilic functin. During their first 2 years of life, these children have skin and chronic pulmonary infections. Skin biopsies demonstrate a chronic granulomatous reaction in the dermis. As these children grow older, they develop granulomas in the liver, which on either nuclear liver scans or CT scans of the abdomen appear to be abscesses. These do not contain pus that can be incised and drained but rather a grumous, necrotic material. Surgical drainage has little to offer these patients unless there is a single large lesion.

The usual organism is a staphylococcus. If a specific bacterium cannot be obtained by blood culture, aspiration of a lesion under CT guidance may be helpful. Long-term, specific antibiotic therapy is the treatment of choice.

We have now treated five children with acute lymphocytic leukemia who had continuous fever after treatment for septicemia. CT scans of the abdomen demonstrated multiple small splenic abscesses in each. Other than mild shoulder pain in two patients, there were no signs or symptoms pointing to the spleen. All recovered after splenectomy. The cut surface of the spleen demonstrated small, multiple abscesses containing gross pus. There was a variety of organisms, including staphylococci, *Candida,* and *Aspergillus* (Fig. 108–3).

The ultimate recovery of the immunodepressed child with an infectious complication depends not only on our ability to eradicate the infection but also on recovery from the underlying disease. If possible, chemotherapy must be discontinued to allow recovery of the bone marrow. Unfortunately, children who have congenital problems and those who have had organ transplants may never be able to mount an immune defense.

REFERENCES

1. Leonard A, Mulholland M, Filipovich A: Surgery of the immunodeficient child. Surg Clin North Am 65:1505, 1985
2. Rodgers M, Thomas P, Starcher E, et al: Acquired immunodeficiency syndrome in children: Report of the Centers for Disease Control National Surveillance, 1982 to 1985. Pediatrics 79:1008, 1987

3. Golladoy E, Baker S: Invasive Aspergillosis in children. J Pediatr Surg 22:504, 1987

4. Press O, Ramsey P, Larson E, et al: Hickman catheter infections in patients with malignancies. Medicine 63:189, 1984

5. Ballantyne T, Grosfeld J, Knopek R, et al: Interstitial pneumonitis in the immunologically suppressed child: An urgent surgical condition. J Pediatr Surg 12:501, 1977

6. Adeyemi S, Ein S, Simpson J, Turner P: The value of emergency open lung biopsy in infants and children. J Pediatr Surg 14:426, 1979

7. Morgan E: Decreased incidence of nonspecific interstitial pneumonitis in children with acute lymphocytic leukemia treated prophylactically with trimethoprim-sulfamethoxazole. J Pediatr 90:801, 1981

8. Doolin E, Luck S, Sherman J: Emergency lung biopsy: Friend or foe of the immunodeficient child? J Pediatr Surg 21:485, 1986

9. Warner D, Warner M, Divertie M: Open lung biopsy in patients with diffuse pulmonary infiltrates and acute respiratory failure. Am Rev Respir Dis 137:90, 1988

10. Rubinstein A, Moreki R, Silverman B, et al: Pulmonary disease in children with acquired immune deficiency syndrome and AIDS-related complex. J Pediatr 108:498, 1986

11. Shamberger R, Weinstein H, Grier H, Levey R: The surgical management of fungal pulmonary infections in children with acute myelogenous leukemia. J Pediatr Surg 20:840, 1985

12. Hiatt J, Kuchanbecker S, Winston D: Perianal gangrene in the patient with granulocytopenia: the importance of diverting colostomy. Surgery 100:912, 1986

SECTION XV
Endocrine Disorders

The biochemistry of the endocrine secretions and their disorders has become a specialty that is continually changing and advancing. In this section we merely skim the surface of the physiologic mechanisms involved. This is partly because many of the same lesions are encountered more frequently in adults and consequently are known to most surgeons. In children, tumors and other problems of the endocrine glands are so rare that the surgeon is well advised to work closely with a pediatric endocrinologist who is equipped to make a precise biochemical as well as a clinical diagnosis. Further, the endocrinologist will follow the child when surgical ablation requires prolonged substitutional therapy.

The need for cooperation with a well-qualified endocrinologist is nowhere better illustrated than in the care of a baby born with ambiguous genitalia. The decision to rear a child with indeterminate genitalia as a boy or a girl requires rapid, careful clinical evaluation with chromosomal and biochemical analysis and prolonged counseling of the child's family. The endocrinologist is best qualified to assume the major role in this process, whereas the surgeon must be aware of the need for proper timing of surgical therapy. Furthermore, some disorders of sexual development may appear to the surgeon as a simple hernia, and it, therefore, behooves us to be well aware of these problems.

109
Pheochromocytoma

Pheochromocytomas originate from chromaffin cells that are concentrated in the adrenal medulla and the sympathetic paraganglia. Chromaffin cells and, consequently, pheochromocytomas may be found anywhere from the cervical sympathetic chain to the pelvis.[1] These cells produce the vasoactive amines. Epinephrine is produced only in the adrenal medulla and in children in the organ of Zuckerkandl. Norepinephrine originates from the entire sympathetic chain. The biosynthesis of the pressor amines from phenylalanine is as illustrated:

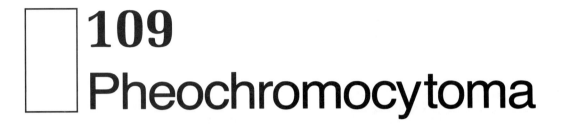

Phenylalanine → tryosine →
dihydroxyphenylalanine (DOPA)
Epinephrine ← norepinephrine ← DOPAmine

The biologic degradation of these compounds is as follows:

Norepinephrine → normetamephrine →
Epinephrine →　　metanephrine ⟶　VMA

PATHOLOGY

Most pheochromocytomas in children measure between 4 and 6 cm by the time they are operated on. On cut section, the lesion is well circumscribed by a rim of normal but compressed adrenal tissue. The lesion is pale tan to yellowish brown in appearance and may have hemorrhagic areas or cystic necrosis. Microscopically, there are islands of plump cells with granular cytoplasm. It is difficult to determine from the microscopic appearance if an individual tumor is malignant, even if one finds nuclear pleomorphism and mitoses. In children, there are fewer malignant tumors but more extraadrenal lesions than in adults.[2] In addition, more cases are familial, and there is a higher association with the multiple endocrine neoplasia (MEN) type II syndrome in children.

The record for multiple tumors appears to be four tumors found in each of two boys in Canada.[3] Bilateral tumors occurred in a startling incidence of 70 percent in 7 children reported by Bloom and Fonkalsrud.[4]

Approximately 30 percent of pheochromocytomas in children are extraadrenal.[5,6] One common extraadrenal site is at the bifurcation of the aorta, the organ of Zuckerkandl.[7] Adrenal and extraadrenal tumors may coexist, and the most important cause for an operative or immediate postoperative death is a second, overlooked tumor.[8–10]

There is a 10 percent incidence of pheochromocytomas or a history of unexplained hypertension in the families of children with this tumor. This appears to be an autosomal dominant characteristic in the involved families. Pheochromocytoma associated with medullary carcinoma of the thyroid is known as Sipple's syndrome. Multiple endocrine adenomatosis, type II (which consists of medullary carcinoma of the thyroid, pheochromocytoma, parathyroid adenomas, and Cushing's disease) appears to be an autosomal dominant trait.[11,12] There is also an increased association of pheochromocytomas with the neuroectodermal dysplasias, von Recklinghausen's disease, tuberous sclerosis, the Sturge-Weber syndrome, and Lindau-von Hippel disease.

DIAGNOSIS

The symptoms of a pheochromocytoma are rather nonspecific and consist of irritability, apprehension, nausea, headaches, and vague chronic pain. It is very easy to pass these symptoms off as being due to "nerves." Later, there are visual disturbances and even convulsions.[13] A detailed family history and the persistence of the symptoms are helpful in at least suggesting an organic rather than a psychosomatic problem. The most important physical finding is a sustained elevation of the blood pressure. Unlike adults whose blood pressure is paroxysmal, a child with a pheochromocytoma will usually have consistent hypertension. Londe reviewed the etiology of secondary hypertension in a series of 563 children.[14] Some 78 percent had a renal abnormality, 12 percent had renal artery stenosis, 2 percent had coarctation of the aorta, and only 0.5 percent had a pheochromocytoma. The initial investigation of a child with sustained hypertension includes a history and physical examination with a urinalysis, urine culture, serum creatinine, BUN, and a rapid sequence intravenous pyelogram. These studies will make the correct diagnosis in almost all children with renal or renal arterial disease. The most commonly measured catecholamine metabolite is vanelmandelic acid, or vanelmandelic acid (VMA), which indicates a tumor originating from the chromaffin cells if the result is abnormal. One or another of the catecholamines or their metabolites (especially metanephrine) will be increased in a patient with a pheochromocytoma.[15] Tests based on these chemicals have superseded the pharmacologic tests, which are potentially dangerous.

In the past, arteriography was used to localize the tumor. This test could precipitate a hypertensive crisis and cardiac arrhythmias. There is no longer any need for arteriography, because the computed tomography (CT) scan will localize both adrenal and extraadrenal tumors with great accuracy. The scan should start below the bifurcation of the aorta and extend up to the apex of the thorax.

PREOPERATIVE PREPARATION

The child's blood pressure should be reduced to normal with alpha-blocking drugs, commencing at least 1 week before the operation. Phenoxybenzamine is the drug of choice. It is started at a dose of 0.2 mg/kg per day and is gradually increased to 1 mg/kg/day or until the blood pressure is reduced to normal.[16] Propranolol may be added to the regimen 3 days before the operation. Since prolonged vasoconstriction may lead to a reduced blood volume, transfusions of plasma or whole blood may be indicated before the operation.

ANESTHETIC MANAGEMENT

Sufficient premedication should be given so the child is brought to the operating room completely relaxed and sedated. Induction is with sodium pentothal and relaxants. The child must be completely monitored, preferably with an intraarterial line to provide sensitive observation and control of the blood pressure. Halothane may cause ventricular arrhythmias and should be avoided. Fortunately, there are many other anesthetics that may be used, including a balanced narcotic muscle-relaxant anesthetic. Innovar and Ethrane are satisfactory.[17,18] Arfonad and nitroprusside are given for intraoperative hypertensive crises, and propranolol or lidocaine may be used for tachycardia or arrhythmias, although, in general, control of the blood pressure will also control arrhythmias. With careful preoperative and intraoperative control there should be no sudden hypotension after removal of the tumor. If this should occur, it should be treated with large volumes of intravenous fluid and a drip of ephedrine or Neo-Synephrine.

SURGERY

Although a thoracoabdominal incision through the base of the eighth rib provides excellent exposure for adrenalectomy, a transverse upper abdominal incision is preferable because each adrenal is thereby easily accessible, and the entire abdomen, including the pelvis, may be explored in the search for a second tumor. The tumor itself is handled as little as possible. On the left side, the spleen, colon, and pancreas are reflected to the right and down to provide complete exposure. Without touching the tumor, the blood supply may be dissected and secured with clips. After ligation and division of the adrenal vein, it is safe to mobilize the mass more extensively. On the right side, the right lobe of the liver and the duodenum are reflected to the left until the inferior vena cava is exposed from the renal veins to the diaphragm. This is effected before the tumor itself is touched. We operated on one boy when he was 9 years old for a large, left-side tumor. There was also a 2 cm tumor in the right gland. A total adrenalectomy was performed on the left, but, in an attempt to preserve adrenal function, only a subtotal resection was performed on the side of the smaller tumor. Five years later, the patient's symptoms recurred, and at a repeat operation the right-side tumor had recurred and extended across the inferior vena cava and the right renal vein. Two of the patients of Bloom and Fonkalsrud also developed recurrences after subtotal resection.[4] From this experience, we prefer to perform a bilateral total adrenalectomy when bilateral tumors are found. Lifelong replacement steroid therapy is then required.

Postoperatively, the blood pressure is continuously monitored until the vital signs are stable. Repeated catecholamine determinations are made during the immediate postoperative period as well as at intervals over several years to detect a second tumor. Long-term follow-up studies indicate that most patients return to a normotensive state.

REFERENCES

1. Crowder RE: The development of the adrenal gland in man with special reference to origin and ultimate location of cell types and evidence in favor of cell migration theory. Carnegie Inst, Contrib Embryol 36:195, 1956
2. Kaufman B, Telander R, Van Heerden J, et al: Pheochromocytoma in the pediatric age group: Current status. J Pediatr Surg 18:879, 1983
3. Marshall D, Ein S: Two boys with four pheochromocytomas each. J Pediatr Surg 21:815, 1986
4. Bloom DA, Fonkalsrud EW: Surgical management of pheochromocytoma. J Pediatr Surg 9:179, 1974
5. Stackpole RH, Melicow MM, Uson AC: Pheochromocytoma in children: Report of cases and review of the first 100 published cases with follow-up studies. J Pediatr 63:315, 1963
6. Fries JG, Chamberlin JA: Extra-adrenal pheochromocytoma: Literature review and report of a cervical pheochromocytoma. Surgery 63:268, 1968
7. Hahn LC, Nadel NS: Angiographic localization of a pheochromocytoma of the organs of Zuckerkandl. J Urol 111:553, 1974
8. Heikkinen ES, Akerblom HK: Diagnostic and operative problems in multiple pheochromocytomas. J Pediatr Surg 12:157, 1977
9. Gibbs MK, Carney JA, Hayles AB, Telander RL: Simultaneous adrenal and cervical pheochromocytomas in childhood. Ann Surg 185:273, 1977
10. Stackpole RH, Melicow MM, Uson AC: Pheochromocytoma in children: Report of 9 cases and review of the first 100 published cases with follow-up studies. J Pediatr Surg 63:315, 1963
11. Funyu T, Shiraiwa Y, Nigawara K, et al: Familial pheochromocytoma: Case report and review of the literature. J Urol 110:151, 1973
12. Steiner AL, Goodman AD, Powers SR: Study of a kindred with pheochromocytoma, medullary thyroid carcinoma, hyperparathyroidism and Cushing's disease: Multiple endocrine neoplasia, type 2. Medicine 47:371, 1968
13. Scwartz DL, Gann DS, Haller JA: Endocrine surgery in children. Surg Clin North Am 54:363, 1974
14. Londe S: Causes of hypertension. Symposium on hypertension in childhood and adolescence. Pediatr Clin North Am 25:56, 1978
15. Gitlow SE, Pertsemlidis D, Bertani LM: Management of patients with pheochromocytoma. Am Heart J 82:557, 1971
16. Perry LB, Gould AB Jr: The anesthetic management of pheochromocytoma: Effect of preoperative adrenergic blocking drugs. Anesth Analg 51:36, 1972
17. Gould AB Jr, Perry LB: The anesthetic management of pheochromocytoma: Cases involving nonexplosive techniques, metastatic tumors, and multiple procedures. Anesth Analg 51:113, 1972
18. Schnelle N, Carney FM, Didier EP, Faulconer A Jr: Anesthesia for surgical treatment of pheochromocytoma. Surg Clin North Am 45:991, 1965

110

Functioning Tumors of the Ovaries and the Adrenals

Hormone-producing tumors create a variety of bizarre syndromes, including sexual abnormalities, Cushing's syndrome, and hypertension. The sexual abnormalities may be classified as isosexual precocity—the early onset of puberty for the sex of the child—or heterosexual precocity, which is virilization in the female or feminization in the male. Sexual maturation and the control of puberty normally commence with the stimulation of the pituitary by the central nervous system and are then controlled by a complex system of feedback mechanisms interrelated among the gonads and the pituitary and adrenal glands.[1]

SEXUAL PRECOCITY IN GIRLS

The onset of puberty is variable in different races and nationalities. The mean age for the appearance of a breast bud was 11.2 years, and menstruation commenced at approximately 13.5 years in a group of British girls. The lowest age for the onset of puberty in this series was 8.4 years.[2] In a similar group of American girls, there was a slightly younger age for the onset of sexual maturity.[3] The appearance of breast enlargement, pubic and axillary hair, growth of the labia minora, or the onset of vaginal bleeding before the age of 8 years must be considered abnormal and is an indication for study of the child. However, the onset of a single abnormality, such as the development of a breast bud, is of less significance than a group of symptoms. Some 15 to 20 percent of girls with sexual precocity show symptoms before they are 2.5 years of age. Vaginal bleeding is the usual first symptom.[4] Reiter and Kulin reviewed several series with a total of 933 girls with precocious puberty.[5] No specific etiology was found in 507, or over half of these children. Some 71 patients had central nervous system disorders that resulted in increased secretion of gonadotropins. A total of 272, or 30 percent, had virilizing adrenal le-

sions, 65 had feminizing ovarian tumors, and only 8 had feminizing adrenal tumors.

DIAGNOSIS

A carefully taken history may offer clues to the correct diagnosis. A specific inquiry must be made about the accidental ingestion of an estrogen-containing medication.[6] Headaches, visual symptoms, or changes in appetite may point to a central nervous system lesion. Lower abdominal pain or swelling is almost diagnostic for an ovarian tumor. The physical examination will confirm hormonal changes. An excess of androgen results in acne, hirsutism, voice changes, increased muscle mass, and clitormegaly. Estrogens cause breast growth, areolar pigmentation, and changes in the vaginal mucosa from a smooth, red surface to a gray-pink, rugated surface with thick secretions. Adrenal tumors are only occasionally palpable, whereas a functioning ovarian cyst or tumor invariably will be palpable on rectal or abdominal examination, provided the child is heavily sedated. Blood pressure elevation is a common finding, especially with virilizing adrenal cortical tumors.

Radiologic studies include a survey of the ossification centers to determine bone age. Both androgens and estrogens hasten osseous maturity. Most children with true sexual precocity will have a significantly advanced bone age.[7] Computed tomography (CT) examination provides the most specific information about the adrenals. Pelvic ultrasound examination has become a routine, valuable procedure for the detection of any ovarian pathology. Skull x-rays and CT are indicated as initial screening tests when there are any associated neurologic signs or symptoms. Endocrine studies may include a cytologic examination of the urinary sediment or a vaginal smear, since estrogen stimulation results in premature cell corni-

TABLE 110–1. DIAGNOSTIC CONSTELLATIONS

History/Physical	Laboratory Results	Most Probable Diagnosis
Isosexual precocity	↑ ↑ Urinary gonadotropins	Chorionic gonadotropin-secreting tumor
Isosexual precocity, hypothyroidism, ± galactorrhea	↓ ↓ T4	Syndrome of sexual precocity and hypothyroidism
Isosexual precocity with irregular vaginal bleeding, pelvic mass	Strong estrogen effect on urocytogram	Ovarian tumor
Isosexual precocity without menses	Elevated urinary pregnanediol, normal urinary gonadotropins	Thecoma
Virilization, no estrogenization	↑ ↑ Pregnanedriol, ↑ ↑ 17 KS, DHA, Dex, suppressible	Congenital adrenal hyperplasia
Virilization, no estrogenization	↑ ↑ 17 KS, ↑ ↑ DHA, not Dex, suppressible	Adrenal tumor

Reiter and Kulin.[5]

fication, and progesterone causes an intermediate cell type.[8,9] Other routine studies include assays for gonadotropins, urinary pregnanediol, 17-ketosteroids, and pregnanetriol.[10] When there is elevation of the 17-ketosteroids, a dexamethasone suppression test is performed. Table 110–1 correlates various clinical syndromes with laboratory findings and the diagnosis.

FUNCTIONING OVARIAN TUMORS

Ovarian tumors that cause isosexual precocity are invariably palpable by rectal and abdominal examination. If there is a question about the pelvic findings, an ultrasound examination will reliably determine ovarian size and consistency.[11] Endocrine studies will demonstrate elevated estrogen levels and cornification of vaginal cells. Granulosa cell tumors are the most common functioning ovarian neoplasms.[12–14] They usually are a mixture of thecal and granulosa cells, with the theca intima cells producing estrogen. Novak et al. found a survival rate of 78 percent over 5 years after resection of granulosa cell tumors.[15] Treatment consists of a total salpingo-oophorectomy with a high ligation of the ovarian vessels. Every effort should be made to resect tumor that extends beyond the ovary. These lesions are radiosensitive. An isolated follicular ovarian cyst may also cause precocious isosexual puberty.[16,17]

Only a few virilizing tumors—arrhenoblastomas or androblastomas—have been reported.[18–20] These are thought to be Seroli-Leydig cell tumors that arise from testislike structures at the hilum of the ovary.[21]

ADRENOCORTICAL TUMORS

In young children, the most important functioning lesions of the adrenal cortex are the adenoma and carcinoma. Cushing's disease and hyperplasia of the adrenals secondary to a pituitary or hypothalamic lesion are unusual, especially in children under 7 years of age.[22] In the review of Hayles et al. of 234 cases, tumors were more frequent in girls (3:1), and two thirds of the tumors produced virilization. The rest of the patients had Cushing's syndrome. Frequently there were signs of both virilization and Cushing's syndrome.[23]

Cushing's Disease

Cushing's sundrome in children consists of the familiar moon face, truncal obesity, acne, hirsutism, and muscle wasting. The affected child will have growth impairment, and arrested growth may be the only sign in mild cases.[24] The physical signs include ecchymoses of the skin (reflecting capillary fragility), hair growth on the temporal areas, back, and arms, striae, and mild hypertension. Although the exact endocrine derangements of Cushing's disease are still not fully understood, there is an overproduction of ACTH, either by a pituitary tumor or because of excessive stimulation of the pituitary by the hypothalamus or higher brain centers.[25] In addition to the clinical findings, the diagnosis of Cushing's disease is made by finding elevation of the 17-hydroxycorticosteroids, elevation of the urinary free cortisol (greater than 85 μg/day), increase of the plasma cortisol, and loss of the normal diurnal variation. These hormones normally are elevated in the afternoon (over morning levels). In addition, there is loss of the normal feedback mechanism between the pituitary and the adrenal because administration of low doses of dexamethasone (1.25 mg/100 pounds per day in four doses over 3 days) fails to suppress the elevated steroids.[26] Higher doses of dexamethasone will suppress steroid production with Cushing's disease, but not if there is an adrenal adenoma or carcinoma.[27] The administration of ACTH will increase steroid levels if there is either Cushing's disease or an adrenal adenome but will have no effect if there is a carcinoma.

Other diagnostic studies include skull CT imaging.[28] The adrenal pathology in Cushing's disease consists of

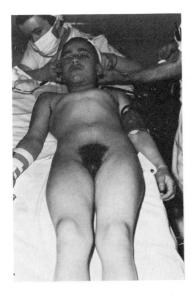

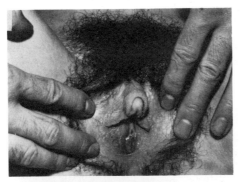

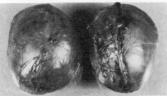

Figure 110–1. Virilization in an 8-year-old girl with a benign adrenal tumor. **Far left.** Muscular development is excellent. **Top Right.** Clitoral hypertrophy with excessive public hair. **Bottom Right.** A well-encapsulated benign adrenal tumor.

bilateral hyperplasia of the adrenal glands, which may contain nodular adenomatosis.[29] There is no completely satisfactory treatment for Cushing's disease in children. A definite pituitary tumor should be removed. However, the radiation therapy used in adults may interfere with secretion of the growth hormone and will prevent normal growth in prepubertal children. Bilateral total adrenalectomy would appear to be the treatment of choice in children. Hardy has demonstrated function in autotransplants of sliced adrenal into muscle after total adrenalectomy.[30] Of a total of 26 patients with autografts in his study, 16 were able to discontinue replacement steroid medication and 3 eventually developed recurrent Cushing's syndrome from the autotransplant.[30] This procedure deserves a trial in children.

Adrenal Adenoma and Carcinoma

Adrenal cortical tumors produce a mixed clinical picture of virilization and Cushing's syndrome, with a predominance of virilization (Figs. 110–1, 110–2, and 110–3). Carcinomas are associated with hemihypertrophy, tumors of the central nervous system, and skin lesions, such as hemangiomas.[31,32] Of Kenny et al.'s 7 patients with virilizing tumors, 4 also had a strong family history of malignant tumors.[33]

Pathology. Adenomas are solitary, well-encapsulated masses that are bright yellow on cut section. Their stroma and vascularity resemble that of the normal adrenal cortex, and the cells are similar to those found in the normal zona glomerulosa. Carcinomas tend to be larger and more readily palpable tumors that infiltrate locally and metastasize to regional lymph nodes, as well as to the lung and liver. Extensive invasion of the inferior vena cava may result in an unresectable tumor.

Diagnosis. Functioning adrenal tumors are more common in females, and although they may occur at any age, they are more common during infancy and have been observed in the neonate.[34] Virilization is most common in both sexes. Girls will have clitoral hypertrophy, whereas in boys the penis and prostate are enlarged. The virilizing influence of androgens counteracts to some extent the protein-wasting effects of cortisol, so growth failure and muscle wasting are not as prominent as in

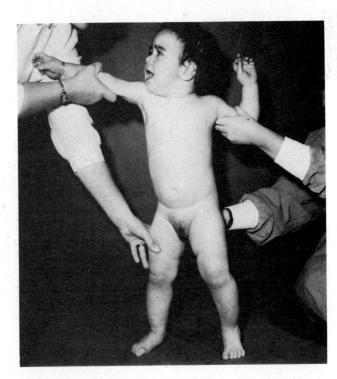

Figure 110–2. Virilization in a 17-month-old child with a benign adrenal tumor. She also had acne.

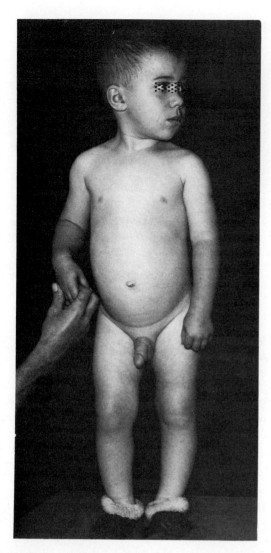

Figure 110–3. Premature virilization in a 2-year-old boy with an adrenal tumor.

tumors are calcified. No single test will differentiate an adenoma from a carcinoma. However, a carcinoma is more likely to secrete a variety of hormones, giving a mixed clinical picture of virilization and Cushing's syndrome, and it tends to be larger than the usual adenoma.

Table 110–2 lists the tests commonly used to distinguish among functional adrenocortical lesions.

Treatment. The functioning adrenal tumors suppress the pituitary. Consequently, the contralateral adrenal is atrophic. The child must be protected against steroid withdrawal after removal of the tumor by providing exogenous hormones before, during, and for several weeks after tumor removal. Cortisone (50 mg/m^2) may be given intramuscularly for 2 days before surgery and on the day of operation. This dose is continued for 2 to 5 days after the operation and is then tapered to a maintenance dose of 25 mg/m^2 by mouth. Cortisone is gradually withdrawn as the contralateral adrenal gland commences to function. Alternatively, intravenous hydrocortisone may be administered during the operation and for several days after. The serum electrolytes must be determined before operation and any deficiencies corrected.

When the tumor can be accurately localized, a posterior-lateral thoracoabdominal incision through the bed of the eighth rib with detachment of the diaphragm peripherally allows excellent exposure. However, each adrenal must be visually and palpably examined, and this may be easier to accomplish through an upper abdominal, transperitoneal incision. On the left side, the spleen and colon are reflected medially with the pancreas to expose the adrenal and kidney. When there is a well-encapsulated tumor, simple removal of the adrenal is all that is required. Otherwise, an extensive retroperitoneal dissection is necessary to remove a carcinoma. On the right side, the liver and duodenum are reflected to expose the superior vena cava and renal vein before dissection of the adrenal.

Recurrent or metastatic carcinoma may respond to radiation or to treatment with adrenolytic drugs, such as ortho-para-DDD. These drugs may reduce the endocrine symptoms, but they are not curative.[40]

Results. Removal of a benign adenoma is curative. The signs of virilization and Cushing's syndrome recede over a period of several months. However, only 3 of 8 patients with virilizing tumors in the series of Burrington and Stephen were alive.[41] Two of these survivors had benign adenomas. The 1 long-term survivor with a carcinoma had 4000 rads administered to the tumor bed following surgical excision. Of the 5 patients operated on by Stewart et al., 4 have survived 1 to 12 years after surgery.[42] Each received 2500 rads to the tumor bed. One of the survivors had an unresectable tumor that disappeared completely after radiotherapy.

a pure case of Cushing's syndrome. Only eight feminizing adrenal tumors have been reported.[35–39] Girls with feminizing tumors have precocious breast enlargement and menstrual bleeding, whereas boys will develop gynecomastia and testicular atrophy. Primary adrenal cortical tumors may arise in the liver or gonad, probably as a result of ectopic adrenal tissue.

Endocrine studies should include serum assays for testosterone and determination of both morning and afternoon levels of cortisol. Determinations are also made of the urinary 17-ketosteroid and 17-hydroxycorticosteroid levels. These levels are all elevated with virilizing tumors. The dexamethasone suppression test will fail to reduce the hormonal secretion, since adrenocortical tumors are not under the influence of ACTH. Intravenous pyelography or CT scan may demonstrate downward displacement of a kidney, and about 20 percent of adrenal

TABLE 110–2. DIAGNOSTIC STUDIES COMMONLY USED IN DISTINGUISHING FUNCTIONING ADRENOCORTICAL LESIONS

	Urinary Steroids	Serum Cortisol	ACTH Level	Decadron Suppression	ACTH Infusion	Comment
Carcinoma	17KS ↑, 17 OHCS ↑	↑ No diurnal variation	Low	No response	No response	Rapid onset of symptoms; usually mixed syndromes
Adenoma	Normal or somewhat elevated	↑ No diurnal variation	Normal or low	Usually minimal response	Marked 17 OHCS ↑	—
Hyperplasia	↑	↑	↑	Reduction in urine output	17 OHCS ↑	Generally pure syndromes

Stewart et al.[42]

Aldosteronomas

Hyperaldosteronism results in muscle weakness, polyuria, and growth failure. The most common signs include arterial hypertension, loss of deep tendon reflexes, and tetany. Many of these symptoms are due to excess loss of potassium in the urine. The hypokalemia may be sufficient to cause depression of the ST segment and inverted T waves on the electrocardiogram. Normally, plasma aldosterone levels are elevated in infancy and decrease to adult levels by 3 to 5 years of age.[43] In childhood, the most common cause for primary aldosteronism is bilateral adrenal hyperplasia. One way to localize a resectable adenoma is by measurement of aldosterone levels from each adrenal vein.[44,45] CT imaging is noninvasive and may provide accurate information. There have been only six cases of aldosteronoma reported in children under 16 years of age. All patients except the most recent, reported by Kafrouni et al., were white and female.[46] The diagnosis was confirmed in this most recent patient by an increased urinary and plasma aldosterone level with a decreased plasma renin. The adenoma was localized by adrenal venography and selective adrenal vein plasma aldosterone levels. There was complete relief of symptoms after removal of the adrenal gland containing the tumor.

REFERENCES

1. Gardner LJ: Endocrine and Genetic Diseases of Childhood and Adolescence, 2nd ed. Philadelphia, Saunders, 1975, p 619
2. Marshall WH, Tanner, JM: Variations in pattern of pubertal changes in girls. Arch Dis Child 44:291, 1969
3. Zacharias L, Wurtman RJ, Schatzoff M: Sexual maturation in contemporary American girls. Am J Obstet Gynecol 108:833, 1970
4. Sigurjonsdottir TJ, Hayles AB: Precocious puberty: A report of 96 cases. Am J Dis Child 115:309, 1968
5. Reiter EO, Kulin HE: Sexual maturation in the female: Normal development and precocious puberty. Pediatr Clin North Am 19:581, 1972
6. Hertz R: Accidental ingestion of estrogens by children. Pediatrics 21:203, 1958
7. Greulich WW, Pyle SL: Radiographic Atlas of Skeletal Development of the Hand and Wrist, 2nd ed. Stanford, CA, Stanford University Press, 1959
8. Preeyasombat C, Kenny FM: Urocytograms in normal children and various abnormal conditions. Pediatrics 38:436, 1966
9. Wied GL, Keebler CM: Vaginal cytology of female children. Ann NY Acad Sci 142:646, 1967
10. Root AW, Moshang T Jr, Bongiovanni AM, Eberlein WR: Concentrations of plasma luteinizing hormone in infants, children and adolescents with normal and abnormal gonadal function. Pediatr Res 4:175, 1970
11. Haller JO, Kassner EG, Staiano BS, Schneider M: Ultrasonic diagnosis of gynecologic disorders in children. Pediatrics 62:339, 1978
12. Busby T, Anderson GW: Feminizing mesenchymomas of the ovary. Am J Obstet Gynecol 68:1391, 1954
13. Zangeneh F, Kelley VC: Granulosa-theca cell tumor of the ovary in children. Am J Dis Child 115:494, 1968
14. Novak ER, Kutchmeshgi J, Mupas RS, Woodrupp JD: Feminizing gonadal stromal tumors. Obstet Gynecol 38:701, 1971
15. Novak ER, Jones GS, Jones HS: Novak's Textbook of Gynecology, 9th ed. Baltimore, Williams & Wilkins, 1975, p 525
16. Steiner MM, Hadawi SA: Sexual precocity, association with follicular cysts of the ovary. Am J Dis Child 108:28, 1964
17. Monteleone JA, Monteleone PL, Danis RK: Pseudoprecocious puberty associated with isolated follicular cysts of the ovary. J Pediatr Surg 8:949, 1973
18. Ammann AJ, Kaufman S, Gilbert A: Virilizing ovarian tumor in a 2½-year-old girl. J Pediatr 70:782, 1967
19. Scully RE: Gonadoblastoma: A gonadal tumor related to the dysgerminoma (seminoma) and capable of sex hormone production. Cancer 6:455, 1953
20. Okun LE: Bilateral arrhenoblastoma of the ovary: Report of a case. Obstet Gynecol 25:448, 1965
21. Teilum G: Arrhenoblastoma-androblastoma: homologous

ovarian and testicular tumors, including so-called "luteo-mas" and "adrenal tumors" of the ovary and interstitial cell tumors of the testis. Acta Pathol Microbiol Scand 23:252, 1946

22. McArthur RG, Cloutier MD, Hayles A, et al: Cushing's disease in children: Findings in 13 cases. Mayo Clin Proc 47:318, 1972

23. Hayles AB, Hahn HB Jr, Sprague RG, et al: Hormone-secreting tumors of the adrenal cortex in children. Pediatrics 37:19, 1966

24. Lee PA, Weldon VV, Migeon CJ: Short stature as the only clinical sign of Cushing's syndrome. J Pediatr 86:89, 1975

25. Feldman JM: Cushing's disease: A hypothalamic flush? N Engl J Med 293:930, 1975

26. Liddle GW: Tests of pituitary-adrenal suppressibility in the diagnosis of Cushing's syndrome. J Clin Endocrinol Metab 20:1539, 1960

27. Eddy RL, Jones AL, Gilliland PF, et al: Cushing's syndrome: A prospective study of six diagnostic methods. Am J Med 55:621, 1973

28. Kandleman M, Grisoli F, Jacquet R: Radio-tomographic study of enclosed pituitary microadenomas. Exerpta Medica 292:218, 1977

29. Neville AM, Symington T: Bilateral adrenocortical hypoplasia in children with Cushing's syndrome. J Pathol 107:95, 1972

30. Hardy J: Surgical management of Cushing's syndrome with emphasis on adrenal autotransplantation. Ann Surg 188:290, 1978

31. Fraumeni JF Jr, Miller RW: Adrenocortical neoplasms with hemihypertrophy, brain tumors and other disorders. J Pediatr 70:129, 1967

32. Haicken BN, Schulman NH, Schneider KM: Adrenocortical carcinoma and congenital hemihypertrophy. J Pediatr 83:284, 1973

33. Kenny FM, Hashida Y, Askari A, et al: Virilizing tumors of the adrenal cortex. Am J Dis Child 115:445, 1968

34. Artigas JL, Niclewicz E, Silva A, et al: Congenital adrenal cortical carcinoma. J Pediatr Surg 11:247, 1976

35. Halmi KA, Lascari AD: Conversion of virilization to feminization in a young girl with adrenal cortical carcinoma. Cancer 27:931, 1971

36. Bacon GE, Lowery GH: Feminizing adrenal tumor in a six-year-old boy. J Clin Endocrinol 25:1403, 1965

37. Gabrilove JL, Nicolis GL, Hausknecht RU, et al: Feminizing adrenocortical carcinoma in a man. Cancer 25:153, 1970

38. Wallach S, Brown H, Englert E, et al: Adrenocortical carcinoma with gynecomastia: A cast report and review of the literature. J Clin Endocrinol 17:945, 1957

39. Howard CP, Takashashi H, Hayles AB: Feminizing adrenal adenoma in a boy: Case report and literature review. Mayo Clin Proc 52:354, 1977

40. Hoffman DL, Mattox VR: Treatment of adrenal cortical carcinoma with O,P'-DDD. Med Clin North Am 56:999, 1972

41. Burrington JD, Stephen CA: Virilizing tumors of the adrenal gland in childhood: Report of eight cases. J Pediatr Surg 4:291, 1969

42. Stewart DR, Jones PH, Jolleys A: Carcinoma of the adrenal gland in children. J Pediatr Surg 9:59, 1974

43. Kowerski AA, Migeon CJ: Aldosterone in childhood. In New MI, Levine L (eds): Juvenile Hypertension. New York, Raven Press, pp 97, 1977

44. Grim CG, McBryde AC, Glenn JF, Gunnells JC Jr: Childhood primary aldosteronism with bilateral adrenocortical hyperplasia: Plasma renin activity as an aid to diagnosis. J Pediatr 71:377, 1967

45. Scoggins BA, Oddie CJ, Hare WSC, Coghlan JP: Preoperative lateralization of aldosterone-producing tumors in primary aldosteronism. Ann Intern Med 76:891, 1972

46. Kafrouni G, Oakes MD, Lurvey AN, DeQuattro V: Aldosteronoma in a child with localization by adrenal vein aldosterone: Collective review of the literature. J Pediatr Surg 10:917, 1975

111
Hyperparathyroidism

_____ *Robert J. Winter*

Hyperparathyroidism in childhood results from adenomatous or hyperplastic changes in the parathyroids or may be secondary to renal disease. The etiology for this aberration is not known, although genetic defects in enzymatic regulation of hormone synthesis, neck irradiation, and coexisting thyroid disease all have been postulated as playing a causative role.[1] The clinical effects of hyperparathyroidism are due to the elevated levels of serum calcium, resulting from elevated levels of parathyroid hormone (the calcium-regulating hormone.) Parathormone acts in several ways to control serum calcium: it increases absorption from the bowel by stimulating the synthesis of the active form of vitamin D (1,25-dihydroxycholecalciferol), it increases reabsorption of calcium by the renal tubules, it acts directly on bone to release calcium into the interstitial fluid, and it reduces renal tubular reabsorption of phosphate.[2]

The calcium ion stabilizes the cell membrane and the inward and outward flux of sodium, therefore regulating action currents and muscular activity. Thus, hypercalcemia is a neuromuscular depressant. The symptoms of hyperparathyroidism in children are more closely related to the effect of calcium on neuromuscular depression and urinary clearance of calcium than to the bone changes and renal calculi that are typically seen in adults. Hypercalcemic infants will demonstrate hypotonia, lethargy, constipation, and retardation of motor development. Unlike other hypotonic infants, those with hypercalcemia may have exaggerated deep tendon reflexes. The depressing effects of calcium also cause bradycardia, with shortening of the Q-T interval on the electrocardiogram. Polyuria and concomitant polydipsia is common, reflecting the osmotic diuresis of excessive calcium. Hypercalcemic infants without access to sufficient fluid will become dehydrated. Chronic hyperparathyroidism, especially that associated with renal disease, is associated with demineralization of bones, increased osteoclastic activity, and eventual formation of bone cysts and pathologic fractures. Metastatic calcification in tissues, especially the formation of renal stones, is another effect of prolonged hypercalcemia.

PARATHYROID ADENOMA IN CHILDREN

Parathyroid adenomas are the most common cause of primary hyperparathyroidism in older children. The reported cases are in children over 8 years of age, and most are in young teenagers.[3-8] Most adenomas are solitary, well-encapsulated, easily recognizable lesions varying from 1 to 1.5 cm in diameter. Different terminology is used to describe the histology, but most adenomas appear to be composed of chief cells. They have been associated with multiple endocrine adenomatosis syndromes type I (pituitary or islet cell tumors, Zollinger-Ellison syndrome, and parathyroid hyperplasia) and type II (medullary thyroid carcinoma, pheochromocytoma, and parathyroid tumor or hyperplasia).[9]

Since the symptoms of hyperparathyroidism in children are nonspecific, the diagnosis will only be suspected when serum calcium and phosphorus levels are determined in children with unexplained abdominal pain, weakness, anorexia, polyuria–polydipsia, weight loss, or constipation. The widespread use of multiphasic screening tests has facilitated the serendipitous diagnosis of

TABLE 111–1. DATA ON PARATHYROID ADENOMAS AT CHILDREN'S MEMORIAL HOSPITAL

Age (years)	Sex	Clinical Data	Laboratory Data	Pathology
8.5	F	Weakness, nervousness, constipation for 6 months with polydipsia, pulse 60, palpable nodule	Serum calcium 13.2 mg/100 ml Phosphate 1.9 mg/100 ml Alkaline phosphatase 27.4 units	Left upper; 1 × 2 cm nodule; small polygonal cells with a rim of normal gland
16.5	F	Muscular pains; swollen, tender ankle joint; polyuria and polydipsia for 5 months	Serum calcium 19.5 mg/100 ml Phosphate 2.9 mg/100 ml Alkaline phosphatase 53.9 units Diffuse subperiosteal bone resorption	Right lower; 2 × 1 cm gland; chief cells with normal thymic tissue
14	M	Recurrent abdominal pain and renal calculi for 1.5 years, palpable nodule	Bilateral renal calculi Serum calcium 15–17 mg/100 ml	Left upper; 1.5 cm in diameter; polygonal cells
9	M	Recurrent abdominal pain, weakness, knee and ankle pain for 6 months, palpable nodule	Serum calcium 15 mg/100 ml Phosphate 3.6 mg/100 ml Alkaline phosphatase 19.3 units	Left upper; 1.5 × 2 cm gland; sheets of polygonal cells

hypercalcemia in centers using such laboratory methods. In the early phases of hyperparathyroidism, serum calcium may be only minimally elevated (11.0 to 12.0 mg/dl). Unlike adults, children have few causes for an elevation of the serum calcium other than hyperparathyroidism. However, malignancy, vitamin D intoxication, Williams' syndrome (in infants), and iatrogenic causes must be considered. Radioimmunoassay of serum parathyroid hormone (PTH) when performed in a reliable laboratory should confirm the diagnosis of hyperparathyroidism. PTH will be grossly elevated in a hyperparathyroid patient, although normally, hypercalcemia should suppress PTH.[10,11]

The clinical and laboratory data of four children operated on for parathyroid adenomas at Children's Memorial Hospital in Chicago are summarized in Table 111–1. The clinical picture in our patients is similar to that reported in the literature. Our patients complained of weakness, anorexia, and recurrent vague abdominal pains, and some had polyuria–polydypsia. Two had joint pains, a symptom found in 17 percent of patients reviewed by Chaves-Carballo and Hayles at the Mayo Clinic.[12] Only one of our patients had kidney stones.

The treatment of a parathyroid adenoma is excision of the tumor with careful identification of the remaining glands to rule out diffuse hyperplasia.

PRIMARY NEONATAL HYPERPARATHYROIDISM

Hyperparathyroidism in infancy is usually due to diffuse hyperplasia of all four glands. This syndrome can be hereditary and has been described in siblings.[13,14] There also may be a family history of hypocalciuric hypercalcemia.[15] The glands in these infants weigh as much as 50 mg, whereas the normal weight is only 4 or 5 mg. Microscopically, there are large, clear cells with small, dark, uniform nuclei.[16]

Symptoms appear soon after birth, but the diagnosis usually is delayed until the infant is several months of age. These babies are seriously ill with hypotonia, poor feeding, constipation, and failure to thrive. Severe dehydration and hypercalcemic crisis occur because the high serum calcium level inhibits the kidney's ability to concentrate urine. Serum calcium levels as high as 27 mg/dl have been recorded. Treatment consists of rehydration (and thereafter a forced diuresis) with normal saline and, if necessary, administration of furosemide, glucocorticoids, and if the hypercalcemia is refractory to that therapy, the use of edetate (EDTA), plicomycin, or calcitonin may be efficacious. An emergency parathyroidectomy may be necessary to control symptoms. Recurrences have occurred after resection of three and a half glands. Therefore, total parathyroidectomy with long-term vitamin D and calcium therapy appears to be the treatment of choice. An alternative would be transplantation of several slices of parathyroid tissue to an accessible muscle, where it could be removed easily if it became hyperplastic.

Idiopathic hypercalcemia of infancy (Williams' syndrome) usually occurs in a less severe fashion. In this syndrome and any other cause of hypercalcemia (at any age), restriction of calcium and vitamin D intake is of paramount importance until the diagnosis is clarified and the hypercalcemia is corrected.[2]

SECONDARY HYPERPARATHYROIDISM

Parathyroid hypersecretion occurs in virtually every patient with chronic renal insufficiency, and hyperplastic glands are found at autopsy. Currently, chronic renal disease is the most common etiology for secondary hyperparathyroidism in children. Declining renal function causes diminished phosphorus excretion, which in turn results in decreased serum ionized calcium. This stimulates secretion of parathormone, which maintains normal calcium levels and increases phosphaturia. With a further decline in renal function, however, maximum phosphaturia is achieved under the influence of high parathormone levels, resulting in further hypocalcemia. If this vicious cycle continues, hyperparathyroid activity results in the full clinical picture of renal osteodystrophy with hypercalciuria.[17] Prevention of renal osteodystrophy consists first of dietary restriction of phosphorus.[2] Since both meat and milk are high in protein and phosphorus, these foods are eliminated from the diet. Oral phosphate binders are useful adjuncts, since they form an insoluble precipitate with phosphate and are eliminated from the gastrointestinal tract. Calcium carbonate is thought to be preferable to aluminum hydroxide for this purpose, since aluminum toxicity is thus avoided. The diet is supplemented with additional calcium and vitamin D in the form of 1,25-dihydroxycholecalciferol (calcitriol) or dihydrotachysterol (Hytakerol). With these measures and a vigorous renal dialysis and transplantation program, parathyroidectomy has rarely been necessary for the control of osteodystrophy at our hospital (R. A. Cohn, personal communication). When these children have progressive bone pain, pathologic fractures, and bone deformity secondary to unremitting renal osteodystrophy, parathyroidectomy will reverse the symptoms and allow bone healing.[18]

PARATHYROIDECTOMY

The superior parathyroids originate from the fourth branchial pouch, and the inferior glands are derived from the third pouch along with the thymus gland.[19] Thus, the glands may be found within the thyroid capsule or almost anywhere in the neck or upper mediastinum. Wang studied the parathyroid glands in 312 patients.[20] Some 77 percent of the superior glands were adjacent to the cricoid cartilage or cricothyroid membrane, 22 percent were behind the upper pole of the thyroid, and 1 percent were retropharyngeal or retroesophageal. Of the lower glands, 57 percent were adjacent to the inferior portion of the thyroid, and 39 percent were in a tongue

of cervical thymus. Two percent were within the mediastinal thymus, and another 2 percent were paratracheal. These variations in the location of the glands have led to techniques for the accurate localization of the enlarged gland or glands. Three adenomas in our series were found on careful physical examination. It would appear that an adenoma is more likely to be palpable in children than in adults. A variety of diagnostic tests are available with which an adenoma may be located. Computed tomography (CT), ultrasonography, and most recently magnetic resonance imaging (MRI) have all been helpful in this regard.[21–23] A thyroid scan may demonstrate an indentation on the thyroid, and an esophagogram may reveal an enlarged adjacent gland. Arteriography and catheterization of the jugular veins to determine parathormone levels from the effluent veins draining each parathyroid also have been recommended to localize adenomas.[24–29] The degree to which these invasive techniques are used depends on one's index of suspicion of hyperparathyroidism and the efficacy of less invasive techniques in localizing an adenoma.

The removal of one or more parathyroid glands is carried out through a conventional collar incision in the lower neck. The platysma is elevated with skin flaps, and the deep cervical fascia is divided in the midline. The strap muscles are transected or, more commonly, retracted. The thyroid gland is then mobilized with the division of the middle thyroid vein and, if necessary, the inferior thyroid artery. The recurrent laryngeal nerve is identified in the lower portion of the neck and traced to the larynx. Adenomas are encapsulated, firm in consistency, and reddish brown in color. When they are in their usual location, they are readily identified. If a bilateral dissection in the region of the thyroid and cricoid fails to demonstrate an adenoma, the superior mediastinum is explored from the cervical incision. A large portion of thymus may be removed through this route. Next, the retroesophageal and retropharyngeal spaces are examined. All suspicious tissue must be submitted for frozen section examination to ensure removal of a parathyroid gland instead of a lymph node. The entire dissection must be performed with great delicacy. Meticulous hemostasis is obtained with the needle-tipped electrocoagulation unit and with fine silk ties. Blood in the field will stain tissues and make identification of the parathyroids much more difficult. After removal of one adenoma, the other glands must be examined to rule out diffuse hyperplasia. Several large series (adults and children) document success with this approach without excessive morbidity. Postoperatively, these patients must be examined at frequent intervals for hypocalcemia. Some will require IV calcium until the remaining parathyroid glands commence to function. Combined therapy with a vitamin D preparation and oral calcium will be necessary if transient hypoparathyroidism is prolonged or in the event that all parathyroid glands are removed.

REFERENCES

1. Aetiology and treatment of hyperparathyroidism (Editorial). Lancet 1:1367, 1983
2. Harrison HE, Harrison HC: Disorders of Calcium and Phosphate Metabolism in Childhood and Adolescence. Philadelphia, Saunders, 1979, pp 15–46, 181–192
3 Bjernulf A, Hall K, Sjogren I, Werner I: Primary hyperparathyroidism in children. Acta Paediatr Scand 59:249, 1970
4. Lund HT: Primary hyperparathyroidism in childhood. Acta Paediatr Scand 62:317, 1973
5. Mannix H Jr: Primary hyperparathyroidism in childhood. Am J Surg 129:528, 1975
6. Verger P, Couraud J, Guillard J, et al: Hyperparathyroidie majeure par adenome parathroidien chez l'enfant. Ann Pediatr 17:17, 1970
7. Rapaport D, Ziv Y, Rubin M, et al: Primary hyperparathyroidism in children. J Pediatr Surg 21:395, 1986
8. Norwood S, Andrassay RJ: Primary hyperparathyroidism in children: a review. Milit Med 148:812, 1983
9. Leshan M: Multiple endocrine neoplasia. In Wilson JD, Foster DW (eds): Williams' Textbook of Endocrinology. Philadelphia, Saunders, 1985, pp 1274–1289
10. Aurbach GD, Marx SJ, Spiegel AM: Parathyroid hormone, calcitonin, and the calciferols. In Wilson JD, Foster DW (eds): Williams' Textbook of Endocrinology. Philadelphia, Saunders, 1985, pp 1175–1179
11. Mallette LE, Bilezlian JP, Heath DA, Aurbach GD: Primary hyperparathyroidism: Clinical and biochemical findings. Medicine 53:127, 1974
12. Chaves-Carballo E, Hayles AB: Parathyroid adenoma in children. Am J Dis Child 112:553, 1966
13. Goldbloom RB, Gillis DA, Prasad M: Hereditary parathyroid hyperplasia: a surgical emergency of early infancy. Pediatrics 49:514, 1972
14. Thompson N, Carpenter I, Kessler D, Nishiyama R: Hereditary neonatal hyperparathyroidism. Arch Surg 113:100, 1978
15. Marx SJ, Attie MF, Spiegel AM, et al: An association between neonatal severe primary hyperparathyroidism and familial hypocalciuric hypercalcemia in three kindreds. N Engl J Med 306:257, 1982
16. Bradford W, Wilson J, Gaede JT: Primary neonatal hyperparathyroidism: An unusual cause for failure to thrive. Am J Clin Pathol 59:267, 1973
17. Bricker NS, Slatopolsky E, Riess E, Avioli L: Calcium phosphorus and bone in renal diseases and transplantation. Arch Intern Med 123:543, 1969
18. Firor H, Moore E, Levitsky L, Galvez M: Parathyroidectomy in children with chronic renal failure. J Pediatr Surg 7:565, 1972
19. Norris EH: Anatomical evidence of prenatal function of the human parathyroid glands. Anat Rec 96:129, 1946
20. Wang CA: The anatomical basis of parathyroid surgery. Ann Surg 183:271, 1976
21. Allen DB, Friedman AL, Hendricks SA: Asymptomatic primary hyperparathyroidism in children. Am J Dis Child 140:819, 1986
22. Sommer B, Welter HF, Spelsberg F, et al: Computed tomography for localizing enlarged parathyroid glands in primary hyperparathyroidism. J Comput Assist Tomogr 6:521, 1982
23. Spritzer CE, Gefter WB, Hamilton R, et al: Abnormal parathyroid glands: High resolution MR imaging. Radiology 162:487, 1987
24. Eisenberg H, Pallotta J, Sherwood L: Selective arteriography, venography and venous hormone: assay in diagnosis and localization of parathyroid lesions. Am J Med 56:810, 1974
25. Gluckman P, Ferguson RS, Osborne D, Evans M: Primary hyperparathyroidism in a child: Use of jugular venous catheterization in diagnosis. Arch Dis Child 52:504, 1977
26. Doppman JL, Marx S, Murray F, et al: The blood supply of mediastinal parathyroid adenomas. Ann Surg 185:488, 1977
27. Salazar J, Dembrow V, Egozi I: A review of 265 cases of parathyroid explorations. Am Surg 52:174, 1986
28. Rudberg C, Akerstrom G, Palmer M, et al: Late results of operation for primary hyperparathyroidism in 441 patients. Surgery 99:643, 1986
29. Paloyan E, Lawrence AM, Oslapas R, et al: Subtotal parathyroidectomy for primary hyperparathyroidism. Arch Surg 118:425, 1983

112
Hypoglycemia

_____ *Robert J. Winter*

Hypoglycemia existing beyond the neonatal period is a rare and serious condition. Prompt diagnosis and therapy are necessary to prevent permanent central nervous system damage. If hypoglycemia persists despite adequate and intense medical management, surgical intervention may be necessary.[1]

The differential diagnosis of hypoglycemia is very much related to the age of the child and the duration over which hypoglycemia occurs. In general, hypoglycemia occurs either because of glucose overuse (e.g., hyperinsulinism) or because of glucose underproduction (e.g., liver disease, resulting in defective glycogenolysis or gluconeogenesis). Normal blood sugar levels vary by age. Premature infants tolerate serum glucose levels of 25 mg/dl or higher,[2] whereas term infants should not fall below 35 mg/dl for the first 24 hours of life or below 45 mg/dl thereafter.[3] It is very important to distinguish between standards for serum and whole blood glucose. The initial standards of Cornblath and Schwartz[2] were reported for whole blood. The standards given here for serum or plasma glucose are 12 to 15 percent higher than levels for whole blood glucose on the same sample when corrections for red cell volumes are made. Although hypoglycemic conditions occur outside the infant age range (e.g., ketotic hypoglycemia), the majority of such cases are well managed medically and do not require surgical intervention. This chapter deals with neonatal and infantile hypoglycemia and the indications for surgical intervention.

Neonatal hypoglycemia usually is transient and responds to intravenous glucose. It commonly occurs in an infant of a diabetic mother (from transient infantile hyperinsulinism stimulated in utero by high maternal glucose) or in the premature or small for gestational age infant (with adequate fuel reserves). When hypoglycemia persists for a week or more, is refractory to constant glucose infusion, or is acquired after discharge from the neonatal nursery, a full endocrine–metabolic investigation is warranted. That investigation is guided by the biphasic differential diagnosis discussed previously. Hormonal abnormalities (insulin excess) cause glucose overuse, and inborn errors of hepatic metabolism, growth hormone, or cortisol deficiency result in glucose underproduction. Hepatomegaly, failure to thrive, and intolerance to certain foods are common in inborn errors of metabolism, whereas hormonal abnormalities often demonstrate no signs or symptoms except hypoglycemia.

The symptoms of neonatal and infantile hypoglycemia are diverse and nonspecific but include apnea, limpness, irritability, seizures, and coma. In older children, hypoglycemia causes nervousness, fatigue, or even seizures. As Whipple and Frantz described in 1935, these symptoms are relieved by eating.[4] A blood sugar measurement should be made during the course of any symptom that is not understood (e.g., seizures, lethargy, irritability). The diagnostic effort for an infant or child with confirmed hypoglycemia must include a simultaneous determination of serum glucose with a radioimmunoassay for serum (or plasma) insulin. Various challenge and tolerance tests may be needed to clarify further the cause of the hypoglycemia. Normal or elevated serum insulin during hypoglycemia is inappropriate and, if confirmed during several studies, is an indication of hyperinsulinism.[2]

TABLE 112–1. USUAL CAUSES OF HYPOGLYCEMIA

Transient (Less than 10–14 Days)		Persistent or Delayed Onset (Intractable)	
Inadequate Glycogen[a] Stores	*Hyperinsulinism[b]*	*Hyperinsulinism[b]*	*Enzyme or Hormone Deficiencies[a]*
Intrauterine growth retardation	Infant of a diabetic mother Erythroblastosis Beckwith syndrome	Insulinoma Islet cell hyperplasia Nesidioblastosis Islet cell secretory	Glycogen storage disease types I, II, VI Fructose 1,6-diphosphatase deficiency Galactosemia Hereditary fructose intolerance Defects in amino acid metabolism: methylmalonic or propionic acidemia, maple syrup urine disease, tyrosinosis Growth hormone or cortisol deficiency

[a] Disorders of glucose underproduction.
[b] Disorders of glucose overuse.

Table 112–1 illustrates the relationship between the child's age and duration of symptoms and the diagnostic approach. Low insulin levels suggest metabolic errors, whereas hyperinsulinemia points to pancreatic lesions. Subtotal pancreatectomy may be required in such hyperinsulinemic conditions if the response to medical management is inadequate.[5] Other causes of hypoglycemia, including growth hormone and cortisone deficiency and hepatic errors of metabolism, are managed with medical therapy alone.

Hypoglycemia of any cause is treated initially by constant infusion of glucose, supplemented when necessary by a bolus of 20 to 25 percent glucose. Because of its extreme hypertonicity, 50 percent glucose has no place in pediatrics. A central venous catheter may be necessary to allow a constant glucose infusion without the danger of hypoglycemia if IV access is a problem. Frequent oral feedings also may be helpful unless the infant is leucine sensitive, in which case, feedings will actually provoke hypoglycemia. The same is true for feedings containing substances an infant is unable to metabolize because of an inborn error, such as fructose or galactose. For hyperinsulinemic conditions, oral administration of diazoxide inhibits insulin secretion. Diazoxide alone or combined with a corticosteroid may help stabilize the serum glucose during prolonged treatment.[2] A long-acting analog of somatostatin has been efficacious in normalizing glucose in neonatal nesidioblastosis.[6] A failure of response to such medical therapy is an absolute indication for surgery in a child with hyperinsulinism.

PATHOLOGY

The islets of Langerhans, arising from the ductal epithelium, contain the beta cells that secrete insulin. Four conditions have been described as the cause of pancreatic

hyperinsulinemic states. These are islet cell hyperplasia, pancreatic adenoma, beta-cell nesidioblastosis, and functional beta-cell secretory defects.[2] In 1971, Yakovac et al. were able to demonstrate, by the use of special staining techniques, a diffuse and random distribution of beta cells throughout the pancreas of an infant with hypoglycemia.[7] The term "beta-cell nesidioblastosis" refers to the condition in which the beta cells, normally found aggregated with the islets of Langerhans, are scattered within the acinar tissue of the pancreas as single cells, clusters of cells, or mini-islets of single cell types. It is thought that these scattered beta cells function autonomously without feedback control from the blood sugar.

Since the initial report from Yakovac et al., the majority of new cases are attributed to nesidioblastosis. Pancreatic adenoma may be aggregates of beta cells. Thus, tiny tumors found in the infant may indeed be nesidioblastomas and not the classic type of tumor found in the adult.[8,9] In the neonate or child under 1 year of age, nesidioblastosis is the most common cause of hyperinsulinism, whereas in the child over 1 year of age, an adenoma is more likely to be found.

After appropriate investigation and treatment, if islet cell pathology is thought to be responsible for the hypoglycemia and medical management has failed, surgical intervention is indicated. Angiographic localization for pancreatic tumors has been used successfully in children.[10–12] However, most hyperinsulinemia in the child under 1 year of age results from diffuse glandular pathology or quite small tumors measuring between 1 and 5 mm. Angiography under these conditions does not seem to have a significant role in diagnosis. The use of computed tomography (CT) also does not seem to be helpful except when a discrete adenoma is present. Indeed, many case reports and collective reviews have emphasized the difficulties in identifying a specific adenoma in the pancreas even at the time of operation.[13–25]

SURGICAL MANAGEMENT

Before operation, the child must be given sufficient intravenous glucose to maintain a euglycemic state. Ongoing glucose monitoring and preparation for treating postoperative hypoglycemia should occur. Celiotomy is performed through an upper abdominal transverse incision with the abdomen hyperextended. The pancreas is exposed by dividing the gastrohepatic omentum and elevating the stomach and is then mobilized by dividing its thin peritoneal attachments to the posterior body wall until the body and tail are completely visualized and can be palpated. Next, the hepatic flexure of the colon and the duodenum are mobilized to the left to expose the head and uncinate process. With this exposure, the entire gland is available for inspection.

Discrete pancreatic adenomas may be no more than a few millimeters in diameter and are pinkish brown in color, with a capillary network. Any suspicious lesion is removed for a frozen section examination. If a discrete tumor is found, it is excised along with a portion of the pancreas so there will be adequate tissue for microscopic study to rule out diffuse disease. If no tumor is present, a 95 percent pancreatectomy is performed, leaving only a portion of the head and the uncinate process intact.

Intraoperative monitoring of the serum glucose does not seem to be a good indicator of the postsurgical success, although such monitoring is important to ensure an intraoperative euglycemic state. Every effort must be made to preserve the spleen.[26]

In the absence of a discrete adenoma, a near-total pancreatectomy for presumed nesidioblastosis should be performed.[21–26] This procedure retains the spleen, duodenum, and bile ducts while promoting better glucose control than can be accomplished with a subtotal pancreatectomy.

With either surgery alone or a combination of medical and surgical treatment, normoglycemia may be achieved. Unfortunately, delay in surgery in instances refractory to medical management frequently leads to permanent brain damage. Therefore, the inability of full medical therapy to achieve euglycemi in 5 to 7 days should lead promptly to surgery. As emphasized by Fonkalsrud et al., the ultimate measure of therapeutic success in this group of infants is the prevention of mental retardation.[27]

Pancreatic exocrine and endocrine function was normal in three patients 9 to 11 years after a 75 percent pancreatectomy, but pancreatic enzyme activity was reduced by half in 7 children 1 to 2 years after a 95 percent resection for nesidioblastosis. Only 1 patient with a 95 percent resection had serious exocrine function failure and growth retardation. Endocrine function was satisfactory in all.[28]

REFERENCES

1. Schwartz R: Hypoglycemia. In Behrman RE, Vaughan VC III (eds): Nelsons' Textbook of Pediatrics 13th ed. Philadelphia, Saunders, 1987, pp 1264–1273
2. Cornblath M, Schwartz JF: Disorders of Carbohydrate Metabolism in Infancy, 2nd ed. Philadelphia, Saunders, 1976
3. Srinivasan G, Pildes RS, Cattamanchi G, et al: Plasma glucose values in normal neonates. A new look. J Pediatr 109:114, 1986
4. Whipple AO, Frantz VK: Adenoma of islet cells with hyperinsulinism: a review. Ann Surg 101:1299, 1935
5. Thomas CG, Underwood LE, Cooney CN, et al: Neonatal and infantile hypoglycemia due to insulin excess. Ann Surg 185:505, 1977
6. Bruining GJ, Bosschaart AN, Aarsen RS, et al: Normalization of glucose homeostasis by a long acting somatostatin analog SMS 201–995 in a newborn with nesidioblastosis. Acta Endocinol (Copenh) [Suppl] 279:334, 1986
7. Yakovac WC, Baker L, Hummerter K: Beta-cell nesidioblastosis in idiopathic hypoglycemia in infancy. J Pediatr 79:226, 1971
8. Carney CN: Congenital insulinoma (nesidioblastoma). Arch Pathol Lab Med 100:352, 1976
9. Dahms B, Lippe B, Dakake C, et al: The occurrence in a neonate of a pancreatic adenoma with nesidioblastosis in the tumor. Am J Clin Pathol 65:462, 1976
10. Case records of the Massachusetts General Hospital. N Engl J Med 299:241, 1978
11. Rickham PP: Islet cell tumors in childhood. J Pediatr Surg 10:83, 1975
12. Cameron GS, Wright H, Tuttle R, et al: Insulinoma diagnosed by insulin immunoassay and angiography. J Pediatr Surg 7:77, 1972
13. Hamilton JP, Baker L, Kaye R, Koop GE: Subtotal pancreatectomy in the management of severe persistent idiopathic hypoglycemia in children. Pediatrics 39:49, 1967
14. Robinson MJ, Clotke AM, Gold H, Connelly JF: Islet cell adenoma in the newborn: Report of two patients. Pediatrics 48:232, 1971
15. Schwartz JF, Zureth GT: Islet cell adenomatosis and adenoma in an infant. J Pediatr 79:232, 1971
16. Woo P, Scopes JW, Polak JM: Idiopathic hypoglycemia in association with morphological evidence of nesidioblastosis of the pancreas. Arch Dis Child 31:528, 1976
17. Boley SJ, Lin J, Schoffmann A: Functioning pancreatic adenomas in infants and children. Surgery 48:592, 1960
18. Liechty RD, Alsever RN, Burrington J: Islet cell hyperinsulinism in adults and children. JAMA 230:1538, 1974
19. Shafney CH, Firage TB: Diagnosis and surgical aspects of insulinoma. Ann J Surg 127:174, 1974
20. Rich RH, Dehner LP, Okmaga K, et al: Surgical management of islet cell adenoma in infancy. Surgery 84:519, 1978
21. Moazam F, Rodgers BM, Talbert JL, Rosenbloom AL: Near-total pancreatectomy in persistent infantile hypoglycemia. Arch Surg 117:1151, 1982
22. Campbell JR, Rivers SP, Harrison MW, Campbell TJ:

Treatment of hypoglycemia in infants and children. Surgical considerations. Am J Surg 146:21, 1983

23. Langer JC, Filler RM, Wesson DE, et al: Surgical management of persistent neonatal hypoglycemia due to islet cell dysplasia. J Pediatr Surg 19:786, 1984
24. Carcassonne M, DeLarue A, LeTourneau JN: Surgical treatment of organic pancreatic hypoglycemia in the pediatric age. J Pediatr Surg 18:75, 1983
25. Simmons PS, Telander RL, Carney JA, et al: Surgical management of hyperinsulinemic hypoglycemia in children. Arch Surg 119:520, 1984

26. Martin LW, Ryckman FC, Sheldon CA: Experience with 95% pancreatectomy and splenic salvage for neonatal nesidioblastosis. Arch Surg 200:355, 1984
27. Fonkalsrud EW, Trout HH III, Lotanchi S: Idiopathic hypoglycemia in infancy. Arch Surg 108:801, 1974
28. Dunger D, Burns C, Ghale G, et al: Pancreatic exocrine and endocrine function after subtotal pancreatectomy for nesidioblastosis. J Pediatr Surg 23:112, 1988

113
Thyrotoxicosis

_____ *Orville C. Green*

Hyperthyroidism is second to diabetes mellitus as the most common disorder encountered in the Endocrine Clinic of the Children's Memorial Hospital. The disorder is now accepted as being of immunologic origin in most cases of diffuse Graves' disease. Genetically susceptible individuals produce thyroid-stimulating immunoglobulins of the IgG class that may separately produce increased hormonal synthesis (TSI) as well as stimulating growth of the gland. These immunoglobulins have been given a variety of names depending on the technique of assay (LATS, TSAL, TSI, TDA, TBII, HTACS). The preferred assay is to determine the ability to increase cyclic AMP (cAMP) activity. Other causes of hyperthyroidism in childhood, such as the hot nodule or toxic adenoma, are almost never encountered. Our only exception to the rule that immunologic disease causes this disorder is one case of hyperthyroidism caused by multiple nodular disease in a patient with Albright's syndrome. Therapeutic efforts used in clinics today do not attack the primary immunologic cause but focus to variable degrees on the thyroid gland itself, the target of these abnormal protein stimulators. Therapy, therefore, is still directed away from etiology, and it is not surprising that several modes of treatment have remained controversial. Three major regimens have been developed: (1) chemical suppression of hormone synthesis with thioamides, (2) thyroidectomy, usually subtotal but sometimes complete, and (3) radiation ablation. Some patients pass through all three therapeutic programs. Our experience indicates that no single method of therapy is wholly effective in achieving the euthyroid state, but we believe that medical therapy provides the best chance for recovery without recourse to lifelong medica-

tions. This chapter presents the results of 15 years' experience.

Seventy-four children have been treated. There were 59 girls and 15 boys, and the age of onset ranged from 10 years to 18 years, with a mean age of onset of 11.2 years. There was a positive family history for thyroid disease for 51 percent of the patients, and 10 percent had one or more affected members in the immediate family. Other diseases were present in 24 of the children. These diseases either were present at the time of diagnosis or developed during the period of treatment. These associations are listed in Table 113–1. Presenting signs and symptoms in this group of patients are in accord with those reported from other clinics and are listed in Figure 113–1. One point of interest is that 7 percent of the children were referred by teachers who insisted that the family see a physician for the child's problems in the school room. The diagnosis can be made on clinical examination in almost all cases. The single laboratory test of circulating thyroxine is all that is necessary for confirmation, but most clinics today perform a battery of assays. We have used radioiodine uptake studies with 4-hour and 24-hour accumulation values, thyroglobulin and thyroid antibody studies, baseline urinary steroid excretion tests, and complete blood counts as initial studies. All of our patients had elevated thyroxine levels, all except three had 4-hour elevations of radioiodine uptake, and 64 percent had elevated antithyroglobulin antibodies. Eight had lymphocytosis greater than 50 percent before therapy, and four had initial white cell counts of less than 4500. Urinary total steroid levels were increased as an index of accelerated metabolism. Hypercalcemia was not found in any patient.

TABLE 113–1. DISEASES ASSOCIATED WITH HYPERTHYROIDISM

Number of Patients	Disease
4	Down's syndrome
3	Diabetes mellitus
3	Vitiligo
2	Enlarged thymus glands
1 for each disease	McCune–Albright syndrome
	Myasthenia gravis
	Familial PAT
	ITP
	Arthritis
	Scoliosis
	Chronic glomerulonephritis
	Spherocytosis
	Chronic urinary tract infections
	Chorioretinitis
	Seizures and microcephaly
	Asthma

In our clinic, all patients are initially administered medical therapy, using either propylthiouracil in a dose of 100 mg three times daily or methimazole in a dose of 10 mg three times daily. When euthyroidism is achieved (usually in 6 to 8 weeks), reevaluation is undertaken, and the option of surgery or prolonged medical therapy is discussed with the family. There is undoubtedly a strong bias among physicians in our clinic toward prolonged medical therapy. Recent data suggest that patients treated with long-term medical therapy will show a 25 percent remission rate every 2 years regardless of the previous number of years of prior therapy.[1]

MEDICAL THERAPY

Medical therapy is advised for a minimum of 2 years unless complete regression in the size of the goiter occurs in less time. After 2 years, withdrawal is undertaken

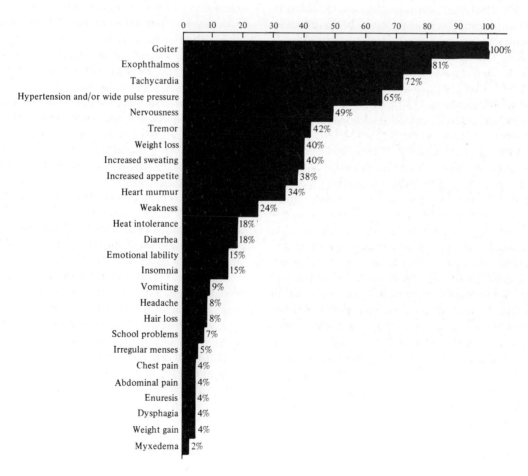

Figure 113–1 Signs and symptoms associated with hyperthyroidism.

TABLE 113–2. COMPLICATIONS OF MEDICAL THERAPY IN PATIENTS WITH HYPERTHYROIDISM

Drug Administered	Reaction	Number of Patients Affected	Length of Therapy for Each Patient
PTU[a]	Nausea	2	0.5 year, 0.5 year
	Rash	3	4 days, 1.16 years, 2.5 years
	Leukopenia < 2000 WBC	2	1.16 years, 4.75 years
	Elevated liver enzymes without jaundice	2	1.6 years, 0.83 year
	Elevated liver enzymes with jaundice	1	0.42 year
	Arthritis	1	2.3 years
Methimazole[b]	Rash	1	2.6 years
	Fever and arthralgia	1	1 month

[a] 68 patients treated—11 had reactions (16 percent).
[b] 17 patients treated—2 had reactions (12 percent).

by tapering the medications over a few months. Of our current patients, 23 (55 percent) are on medical therapy and have been for a mean length of 3.1 years. Three are on a second course, and 1 is on a fourth course of the 2-year program because of recurrence after withdrawal. Nineteen patients (45 percent) are in remission and have been off medications for a mean duration of 4.25 years. Of these 19, 11 have antithyroid antibody titers in excess of 1:32, and 2 have become hypothyroid. Medical therapy was generally well tolerated. Complications are listed in Table 113–2. Of children started on propylthiouracil, 16 percent had reactions, many of which occurred long after therapy had been started. In general, these patients were then switched to methimazole. Two patients (12 percent) developed reactions to methimazole. One of these children had developed serum sickness while receiving propylthiouracil. The other patient developed a rash. All reactions subsided with withdrawal from medication, and the patient with serum sickness was treated by surgery while the other, who had had reactions to both propylthiouracil and methimazole, was treated with radioiodine ablation after she developed concomitant myasthenia gravis. The overall complication rate for our series with medical therapy is 15 percent, and none of the complications were permanent. Table 113–3 summarizes our results with other published series in the literature.[2–6] We have not observed liver disease in the child in our series secondary to propylthiouracil therapy, although 2 patients had elevated transaminase levels.[7]

SURGICAL THERAPY

Poor control secondary to poor compliance was the most common reason for surgery in our series, involving 11 patients. Four additional children were subjected to sur-

gery because of progressive massive thyroid gland enlargement, even though they were on optimal medical therapy. Chronic glomerulonephritis, drug toxicity, and the nodular gland of the child with Albright's syndrome were the indications in the other 4 surgical cases. All of these 19 children had received prior medical treatment for a mean period of 2 years, and Lugol's solution was added to the program for 2 to 3 weeks before surgery. Two patients were treated with propranolol in addition to the other drugs. Mean postoperative follow-up has been 3.4 years. Four patients remain well and euthyroid and require replacement thyroid hormone; 7 (37 percent) have had recurrences of thyrotoxicosis 8 months to 12 years after surgery. The mean time of recurrence was 4.5 years after surgery. At the time of surgery, 3 children showed transient symptomatic hypocalcemia, and 1 additional patient was found to have permanent hypoparathyroidism. One patient developed an abscess, necessitating drainage and resultant revision of the scar tissue. Thus, as a complication of the surgical procedure, 13 of 19 children operated on (68 percent) had some complication of surgery, if one includes hypothyroidism. Pathologic examination of all the glands removed showed diffuse hyperplasia consistent with Graves' disease, except for the gland from the patient with Albright's syndrome, which was interpreted as adenoma. Table 113–4 compares the results of surgery in our 19 patients with other pediatric reports in the literature.[8–12] The incidence of hypothyroidism is related to the aggressiveness of the surgeon in efforts to obtain as much tissue as possible to prevent recurrence. The 7 recurrences in our group were all in patients operated on before 1970, when less radical approaches were taken.

Thyroidectomy

The recurrence rate of thyrotoxicosis is higher in children than in adults. Therefore, a more radical thyroidectomy

TABLE 113-3. RESULTS OF MEDICAL THERAPY IN PATIENTS WITH HYPERTHYROIDISM

Series	Total Number of Patients	Number Receiving Medical Therapy	Patients Gaining Remission			Patients Still on Therapy		No Therapy	Surgery	Radioactive Iodine	Lost to Follow-up	Complications
			Number of Patients[a]	Average Length of Therapy	Average Time of Remission	Number of Patients[a]	Average Length of Therapy					
Hung et al., 1962[2]	34	28	19 (68%)	3.6 years	4 years	9 (32%)	2.3 years		5		1	Perchlorate—2, rash and fever; PTU—3, rash; 2, pharyngitis and granulocytopenia
Root et al., 1963[3]	18	9	7 (78%)	2.8 years	4.7 years	2 (22%)	4 months		8		1	PTU—3, neutropenia, fever, and rash
Hayles 1967[12]	16	9	5 (56%)	2.6 years	3.8 years	4 (44%)	1.8 years		7			PTU—1, rash
Amrhein et al., 1970[4]	38	25	11 (44%)	2.9 years	1.5 years	14 (56%)	1.6 years		8	1	4	PTU—10, leukopenia: 1, SLE; 7, rash; 1, hepatitis; 3, fever and arthralgia; 1, thyroid carcinoma
Vaidya et al., 1974[5]	95	41	23 (56%)	3.2 years	4.2 years	18 (44%)	2 months to 5.75 years	1	32	1	20	PTU—1, rash; 2, neutropenia; 1, fever and purpura
Barnes and Blizzard, 1977[6]	104	67	41 (61%)	12 months	2 years	11	< 12 months		36		16	Perchlorate—2, rash and fever; PTU—1, granulocytopenia, thrombocytopenia, erythema multiforme, drug fever; 2 hepatitis; 8, rash or uricaria
Children's Memorial Hospital	74	42	19 (45%)	4.25 years	4.1 years	23 (55%)	3.1 years	1	19	2	10	PTU—2, nausea; 3, rash; 2, leukopenia; 3, hepatitis; 1, arthritis; Methimazole—1, rash; 1, fever and arthralgia

[a] Numbers in parentheses denote percentage of patients.

TABLE 113–4. RESULTS OF SURGERY IN PATIENTS WITH HYPERTHYROIDISM

Source	Total Patients	Postsurgery Follow-up	Euthyroid	Hypothyroid	Recurrence	Lost To Follow-up	Complications
Arnold et al., 1958[8]	18	5.2 years	9 (50%)	9 (50%)			4, transient hypocalcemia
Hung et al., 1962[2]	5			4 (80%)			1 death
Root et al., 1963[3]	8		3 (38%)	4 (50%)	1 (12%)		1, transient hypocalcemia
Saxena et al., 1964[9]	52	5 years	25 (48%)	18 (35%)	3 (6%)		4, transient hypocalcemia; 5, hypoparathyroidism; 1 death; 2 keloids
Bacon and Lowry 1965[10]	33	2 years	32 (97%)	1 (3%)			1, transient hypocalcemia; 1, hypoparathyroidism; 4, vocal cord paralysis; 2, tracheostomies
Kogut et al., 1965[11]	12		6 (50%)	1 (8%)	2 (17%)	3 (25%)	1, transient hypocalcemia
Hayles et al., 1967[12]	186	10 years	98 (53%)	69 (37%)	19 (10%)		3 deaths; 11, keloids; 4, hypoparathyroidism; 1, vocal cord paralysis
Amrhein et al., 1970[4]	8	2.9 years	6 (75%)	2 (25%)			None
Vaidya et al., 1974[5]	32	3 years	14 (44%)	17 (53%)	1 (3%)		4, transient hypocalcemia; 2, hypoparathyroidism
Barnes and Blizzard, 1977[6]	36	6.2 years	13 (35%)	23 (65%)			6, transient hypocalcemia; 3, vocal cord paralysis; 3, keloids; 1, hypoparathyroidism
Children's Memorial Hospital	19	3.4 years	4 (21%)	8 (42%)	7 (37%)		3, transient hypocalcemia; 1, wound abscess; 1, hypoparathyroidism

is indicated in children. Some surgeons have advocated total thyroidectomy in children to prevent recurrence.[13,14] Weitzman et al. have reported on a series of 66 patients operated on over a period of 14 years. These patients were followed for 2 to 17 years. Eighteen of their patients were euthyroid, 33 were hypothyroid, and hyperthyroidism recurred in only 4 patients. As a result of this extensive experience, the authors observed that relapse of hyperthyroidism was most likely to occur in children who had a significantly enlarged gland at the time of operation. There was no correlation with the size of the remnant left at operation. Furthermore, they did not consider hypothyroidism to be a complication of the operation but rather a desirable objective so that the more serious problem of recurrent hyperthyroidism would be avoided.[15]

We try to leave 1 to 2 g of tissue on one side in the hope of preventing hypothyroidism because one indication for operation is the child's persistent failure to take medication. Obviously, surgically induced hypothyroidism imposes a lifetime of dependence on medication. The technique of subtotal thyroidectomy used in children is identical to that used in adults. However, certain points are worth emphasizing. The incision must be symmetrically curved so that it will disappear into the skin folds of the neck. Meticulous hemostasis with the needle point electrocoagulation unit and 6–0 silk ties is essential. We transect the strap muscles along the incision line without elevating skin flaps. It is necessary to find the correct plane between the sternothyroid muscles and the capsule of the gland. Frequently, fibers of these muscles adhere to the capsule and are torn. This leads to bleeding, which stains tissues and makes identification of the parathyroids and recurrent nerves more difficult. All vessels are triply ligated in continuity with two ligatures left on the vessel side, or else three clamps are applied and the vessels are divided, leaving two proximal clamps. These precautions are essential to preserve a dry field. The recurrent nerves are vulnerable at any point in the dissection but are particularly vulnerable during ligation of the inferior thyroid artery. The nerve must be identified and then traced by opening the jaws of the dissecting scissors parallel with the course of the nerve. If the nerve lies completely behind the artery, the main trunk may be ligated in continuity and divided. On the other hand, in many cases the nerve travels though the vessel's bifurcation. In this situation, it is safer to ligate and divide the branches of the inferior thyroid artery separately, close to the substance of the gland. After division of the inferior vessels and the plexus of veins that drain toward the mediastinum, the inferior poles of the gland may be mobilized from the trachea. The superior thyroid vessels are ligated under direct vision by elevating the strap muscles and by downward traction on the thyroid lobe. It may be necessary to separate the vessels from

the inferior constrictor muscle. When the vessels are clearly in view, the ligature is passed from a medial position to a lateral position, and the vessels are doubly ligated proximally and clamped distally. The lingula and isthmus are removed, but the parathyroids are identified before enucleation of the gland. The superior parathyroids are found at the junction of the upper and middle thirds of the gland, and the inferior glands are closely related to the inferior thyroid arteries. Pretracheal vessels are meticulously suture-ligated with 5–0 silk. The field must be left dry. The wound is closed with interrupted sutures in the platysma, followed by subcuticular polyglyconate and Steristrips. Usually, a small Penrose drain is left for 24 hours.

RADIOACTIVE IODINE ABLATION THERAPY

Hayek et al. and Safa et al. have reported that radioiodine ablation is safe in children, but we have been reluctant to use this mode of therapy.[16,17] We have recommended its use only when both medical and surgical therapy were contraindicated—a rare situation. We used this method only twice: one case where drug therapy resulted in allergic rashes and myasthenia gravis made surgery more risky than use of radioactive iodine and a second case with poor medical compliance and refusal of surgery.

REFERENCES

1. Lippe BM, Landaw EM, Kaplan S: Hyperthyroidism in children treated with long-term medical therapy: Twenty-five percent remission every two years. J Clin Endocrinol Metab 64:1241, 1987
2. Hung W, Wilkins L, Blizzard R: Medical therapy of thyrotoxicosis in children. Pediatrics 30:17, 1962
3. Root A, Bongiovanni A, Harvie F, Eberlein W: Treatment of juvenile thyrotoxicosis. J Pediatr 63:402, 1963
4. Amrhein J, Kenny F, Ross D: Granulocytopenia, lupus-like syndrome and other complications of propylthiouracil therapy. J Pediatr 76:54, 1970
5. Vaidya V, Bongiovanni A, Parks J, et al: Twenty-two years' experience in the medical management of juvenile thyrotoxicosis. Pediatrics 54:565, 1974
6. Barnes H, Blizzard R: Antithyroid drug therapy for toxic diffuse goiter (Graves' disease): Thirty years experience in children and adolescents. J Pediatr 91:313, 1977
7. Fedotin M, Lefer L: Liver disease caused by propylthiouracil. Arch Intern Med 135:319, 1975
8. Arnold M, Talbot N, Cope O: Concerning the choice of therapy for childhood hyperthyroidism. Pediatrics 21:47, 1958
9. Saxena K, Crawford J, Talbot N: Childhood thyrotoxicosis: A long-term perspective. Br Med J 2:1153, 1964

10. Harnburger J: Management of hyperthyroidism in children and adolescents. J Clin Endocrinol Metab 60:1019, 1985

11. Kogut M, Kaplan S, Collipp P, et al: Treatment of hyperthyroidism in children. N Engl J Med 272:217, 1965

12. Hayles C, Chaves-Carballo E, McConaky W: The treatment of hyperthyroidism (Graves' disease) in children. Mayo Clin Proc 42:218, 1967

13. Artman RP: Total thyroidectomy for the treatment of Graves' disease in children. J Pediatr Surg 8:295, 1973

14. Derzik SL: Total thyroidectomy in Graves' disease in children. J Pediatr Surg 2:191, 1976

15. Andrassy RJ, Buckingham BA, Weitzman J: Thyroidectomy for hyperthyroidism in children. Presented at the Section of Surgery, American Academy of Pediatrics, San Francisco, 1979

16. Hayek A, Chapman E, Crawford J: Long-term results of treatment of thyrotoxicosis in children and adolescents with radioactive iodine. N Engl J Med 282:949, 1970

17. Safa A, Schumacher P, Rodriguez-Antrinez A: Long-term follow-up results in children and adolescents treated with radioactive iodine (^{131}I) for hyperthyroidism. N Engl J Med 292:167, 1975

114
Ambiguous Genital Development

Orville C. Green

A neonate with ambiguous genitals requires prompt investigation so that the most suitable sex assignment can be achieved with a minimum of psychologic distress to the parents. If these abnormalities are ignored until later in childhood or adolescence, the entire family may suffer serious difficulties in adjustment if sex reassignment is indicated. This chapter presents a practical clinical approach that has been successful in our hospital in etiologic classification, medical management, and selection of permanent sex assignment.

The family physician or obstetrician delivering the baby is the first to encounter the neonate with ambiguous genitals. His or her comments and explanation of the problem to the parents will determine the degree of anxiety they express when consultation is pursued. We recommend a simple statement that an abnormality of development is present, that tests will be undertaken immediately, and that birth announcements should be delayed until a final decision has been achieved. It is at this point that meticulous laboratory studies are required. Inexperienced laboratories have caused major errors in the decision-making process, with resultant prolonged psychologic problems.

CLINICAL FLOW SHEET FOR DETERMINATION OF ETIOLOGY AND SEX ASSIGNMENT

A simple flow sheet for the progressive investigation of the child born with ambiguous genitals is updated from the flow sheet first described by Green (Fig. 114–1).[1] The process begins with an effort to determine the genetic sex inheritance. The most rapid screening test is

the buccal smear. A chromatin-positive smear indicates the presence of two X sex chromosomes; a chromatin-negative result suggests the absence of the second X sex chromosome normally found in females. False negative buccal smears in neonates are common. The reason for this is obscure, and some centers have stated that neonates do not show Barr bodies (chromatin-positive markers) in the first day of life. Others, including ourselves, have disputed this and attribute variations to methodologic problems. We find that technical problems are the major cause of errors and have established an arbitrary rule that all buccal smears must be performed in two laboratories and that these two must agree before we accept a result. Our endocrinology laboratory uses an aceto-orcein stain, and our pathology laboratory uses the Feulgen technique. Because of this problem, many centers rely only on chromosomal analysis.

CHROMATIN-POSITIVE AMBIGUOUS GENITALS

When the smear is found to be positive for the Barr body or chromosomes are XX female, a presumptive diagnosis of female pseudohermaphroditism may be seriously considered, since true hermaphroditism is so rare. Of our patients with ambiguous genitals, 57 percent have been chromatin-positive. This finding usually allows a gender decision of female, since the majority are genetic females who have suffered virilization due to some source of androgen—either endogenous metabolic defects or steroids transmitted across the placenta from the mother. The rest of these patients will be found to be either entirely normal females with an unexplained genital

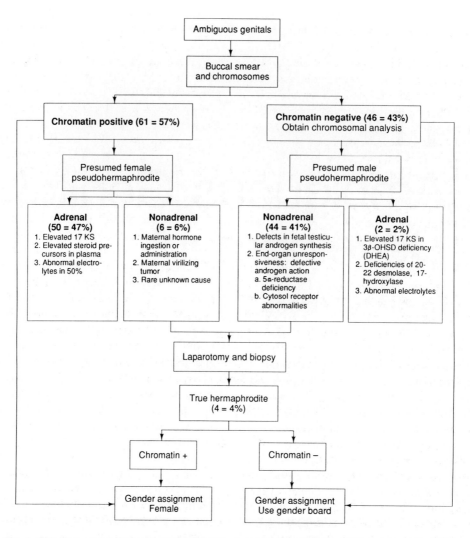

Figure 114–1. This flow sheet diagrams the progressive investigative pathways followed in our institution when confronted with a patient with ambiguous genitals. Numbers in parentheses indicate the number of cases in our files over a 23-year period and the percentages these numbers represent of the entire 107 cases. All 4 cases of true hermaphroditism were chromatin-positive. Of the 44 nonadrenal patients, 22 were raised as females and 22 as males.

anomaly or true hermaphrodites, whose internal structures are usually adequate for assignment of female gender. The exception may (rarely) occur if gonadal structures are palpable in the inguinal or labioscrotal regions. Palpable gonads suggest some form of testicular tissue and are usually found only in male pseudohermaphroditism, but they may also occur in true hermaphroditism. The chromatin-positive Klinefelter's syndrome is almost never associated with ambiguous genitals.

Adrenal Causes for Chromatin-positive Genitals

As seen in Figure 114–1, most infants with chromatin-positive ambiguities have congenital virilizing adrenal hyperplasia (adrenogenital syndrome). The specific enzymatic defect, inherited as an autosomal recessive, can be determined by finding specific steroidal synthetic precursors accumulating in the plasma. A more general diagnosis of adrenal disease can be made by evaluation of total androgen excretion in the urine, the 17-ketosteroid (17-KS) assay. When a diagnosis of adrenal disease is made, medical management of the child requires experienced supervision before surgery. This management is reviewed in detail elsewhere.[2] More than half of these infants will develop serious adrenal insufficiency by the second week of life and should be hospitalized for studies within a few days after birth. Many states are now including a birth screening test for the most common form of this disorder, and, therefore, the disease may be picked up immediately after birth and treatment begun before serious symptoms of adrenal insufficiency develop.

Nonadrenal Causes for Chromatin-positive Ambiguous Genitals

Occasionally, the history will suggest an etiologic cause for the ambiguity. The mother may recall that she inadvertently continued to take oral contraceptive steroids for a few weeks, unaware that a lapse in that program had resulted in pregnancy. Most such oral steroids are commercially synthesized from androgenic precursors and may be readily metabolically reconverted to androgens and thus transmitted to the developing fetus. Very rarely, a mother may have a history of having undergone virilizing changes herself during pregnancy. Some of these mothers have produced virilized female infants. Finally, there have been a few reports of otherwise normal female infants born with ambiguous genitals for which none of the listed virilizing causes have been found. It is at this point on the flow diagram that chromatin-positive babies must undergo laparotomy and gonadal biopsy if no etiologic factors have been found. By following this procedure, we have not yet encountered a case of the rare "unknown cause"—four patients in this series have been demonstrated to be true hermaphrodites with ovotestes at laparotomy.

It is important to recognize that androgenic virilization of a genetic female fetus does not affect development of the internal sexual organs of müllerian derivation (internal portion of the vagina, cervix and corpus of the uterus, and fallopian tubes). When androgenic causes are found (virilizing adrenal hyperplasia, maternal hormone ingestion, or virilization), laparotomy is not necessary. Noninvasive methods of demonstrating internal structures may be as simple as a rectal examination or can involve ultrasonography or other scanning techniques. We caution against vaginograms in the first weeks of life because of the risk of infection and sepsis following the introduction of nonsterile dyes into a vaginal orifice and uterus that may be estrogen-stimulated and highly vascular for a few weeks after birth.

CHROMATIN-NEGATIVE AMBIGUOUS GENITALS

When the buccal smear screening test is negative (absence of Barr bodies), the physician is faced with several difficult decisions about sex assignment. He or she should first be certain that the laboratory is experienced and competent in this technique. A repeat examination, preferably in a second laboratory, is essential. With agreement, it is our recommendation to proceed immediately to chromosomal analysis in the genetics laboratory. In this way, we not only confirm a negative smear but also are able to investigate the possibilities of mosaic genetic conditions, such as XO/XY, XO/XYY, and other combinations that may contribute to genital ambiguity.

Demonstration of the H-Y antigen is a newer method that also will confirm the presence of Y chromosomal material in the patient. The fluorescent technique of demonstrating the Y chromosome on buccal smear has been useful, but this is less reliable methodologically. The finding of chromatin-negative smears, and even of confirmaion of Y chromosomes by the other methods, does not allow the physician to assign a male gender to the baby. Many of these infants will have phallic structures that are so small that there is no reasonable technique to restore a male appearance. Some patients will have severely dysgenetic gonads that can never function, and some will have had severe testicular failure in fetal life and will have intraabdominal müllerian structures. Detailed investigative procedures are indicated before sex assignment can be discussed.

Normal male fetal development depends on fetal testicular production of at least two morphogenetic substances: testosterone and müllerian inhibiting factor (MIF). Fetal testicular testosterone production begins early in the first trimester and is responsible for labioscrotal fusion into a normal scrotum as well as clitoral growth into a normal phallic structure. These external changes from the unaltered female state to a completely structured male state must occur by the fourth month of gestation. Growth in phallic size may continue under adequate testosterone stimulus, but if normal fusion has not occurred before the 16th week, varying degrees of hypospadias will remain. The surgical literature often classifies these defects as hypospadias; the medical literature will classify all cases of third-degree hypospadias (perineal urethral orifice) as male pseudohermaphroditism.

The second responsibility of the fetal testis is to secrete the inhibitor MIF, which acts locally in the region of the developing wolffian and müllerian systems. MIF should inhibit müllerian development. Failure of MIF will result in varying degrees of development of the upper vagina, uterus, and fallopian tubes. It is apparently extremely rare to encounter a human with normal male external genital development but in whom MIF failure has resulted in female internal structures. It is not uncommon, however, to find MIF failure when ambiguous external genitals indicate that fetal testosterone secretion has been inadequate. These combined defects may occur in patients who fall into the category described in Figure 114–1 as nonadrenal. This group should always be subjected to laparotomy and gonadal biopsy.

Male pseudohermaphroditism can, therefore, result from a variety of defects in morphogenesis, occurring at varying times during the first trimester of pregnancy, and will result in a spectrum of external morphologic development failure. The principles of etiologic diagnosis and clinical management as outlined in the flow diagram have been useful. The separation of these patients into adrenal-associated causes and nonadrenal causes will continue to remind the physician that he or she may be dealing with a child who has a life-threatening adrenal disease.

Adrenal Causes for Chromatin-negative Ambiguous Genitals

The steroid hormone-producing cells of the body originate embryologically in a common site and migrate to join other tissues in the formation of the adrenal and gonadal structures, where enzymatic differentiation occurs.[1] It is not unusual, therefore, to find that some enzymes common to both adrenal and gonadal steroid synthesis may be genetically deficient in both organs. Three such enzyme deficiencies have been described, involving 3β-hydroxysteroid dehydrogenase, 20–22 desmolase, and 17-hydroxylase. The first two are essential for synthesis of cortisol and aldosterone as well as testosterone; 17-hydroxylase is essential only for production of cortisol and such androgens as testosterone but is not required for aldosterone synthesis. Variable defects in fuction of these enzymes will produce varying degrees of failure of normal male external development but may also be associated with a life-threatening adrenal insufficiency. The most common is deficiency of 3β-hydroxysteroid dehydrogenase. Some patients with this defect may appear similar to females at birth, whereas others may demonstrate improvement in enzymatic function with age.[3] As with adrenal disease in patients with chromatin-positive pseudohermaphroditism, the physician must be aware that a life-threatening condition may be present that may require medical treatment before the child is 2 weeks of age. Once medical therapy has been stabilized, surgical correction may be enhanced by treatment of the phallic structure with testosterone, since these are responsive tissues.

Nonadrenal Causes for Chromatin-negative Ambiguous Genitals

The majority of babies with chromatin-negative smears will fall into this classification. Two major groups have been defined: (1) those patients whose fetal testes had some defect in synthesis of adequate amounts of testosterone in early fetal life and (2) those infants whose testes secreted adequate testosterone but whose genital tissues failed to respond adequately within the time period allotted for fetal differentiation. With the first group (those with synthetic defects), blood steroid studies at birth may be helpful in clarification. The normal male infant will have adolescent levels of testosterone in his serum at birth, falling to low levels by the fifth day of life but rising again by the tenth day and persisting above 100 ng/ml for at least 2 months. Limited unpublished data from our laboratory suggest that patients with synthetic defects have lower testosterone levels at birth. A variety of enzymatic defects of synthesis have been described in studies involving older patients, and some of the same enzyme deficiencies found in association with adrenal insufficiency may also be found as isolated defects in the testes without necessarily involving adrenal function. These include the 3β-hydroxysteroid dehydrogenase and 17-hydroxylase deficiencies. In addition, specific enzymes involved solely in testosterone synthesis have been described as deficient—17–20 desmolase and 17-ketoreductase. The biochemical studies in such cases have been reviewed by Givens et al.[4] The genital tissues of patients born with defects of testosterone synthesis will respond to testosterone with increase in penile size, thus making surgical reconstruction easier when male gender is selected.

The second group, listed as "androgen insensitive," comprises those patients with defective action of testosterone at the target genital tissues. This group may be subdivided into two categories: (1) those with absence of the specific cytosol and nuclear enzyme 5α-reductase within the target cell, which prevents conversion of testosterone to its active intracellular form, dihydrotestosterone, and (2) those with absence of the specific receptors for testosterone and dihydrotestosterone within the target cells, which prevents initiation of the protein synthesis required for growth and differentiation of the genital tissues (other susceptible body tissues also fail to respond). Separation of patients into these two categories requires sophisticated tissue culture and cell fractionation techniques currently available only in certain research laboratories.[5] The important point in these cases is that testosterone administered in early infancy will not produce further growth of the phallic structure and will not aid in reconstruction toward male appearance. Our experience suggests that half the patients with androgen insensitivity must be raised as females. There is a category of patients with partial deficiency of 5α-reductase who gradually show increasing activity of this intracellular enzyme as they grow, and if the testes are left in place they may virilize at adolescence and show increasing phallic size (the "penis-at-twelve" syndrome).[6] However, since these children have usually been assigned female gender roles in infancy by thir parents, the virilizing changes at adolescence are best avoided by early gonadectomy. Some social groups may accept a role change at adolescence, but experience in the United States suggests such changes may be psychologically disastrous.[7]

TRUE HERMAPHRODITISM

As mentioned earlier, true hermaphroditism is discovered only by gonadal biopsy and proof that ovarian tissue with follicles as well as testicular tissue with tubules is present. These are usually ovotestes, but true lateral

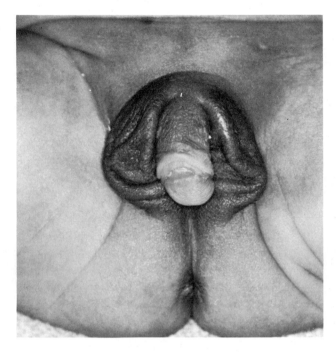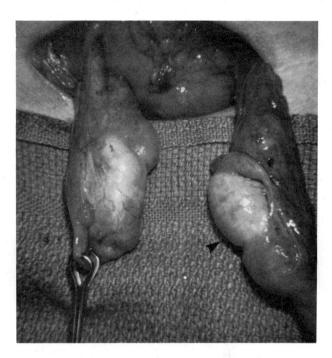

Figure 114–2. Left. True hermaphroditism. There is an enlarged phallus with lax labioscrotal folds and a urogenital sinus at the base of the phallus. This situation is easily misdiagnosed as "hypospadias." **Right.** The gonads were removed at laparotomy at 2 weeks of age. On the right is a testis; the left gonad is an ovotestis (arrow).

hermaphroditism (with an ovary on one side and a testis on the other) has been described (Fig. 114–2). Chromosomal analysis of these gonads has usually shown some mosaic mixtures even if the tissue looks entirely like one or the other type of gonad. Uterine structures are usually present to some degree, and most of these patients are best assigned female gender roles, although this is not an invariable rule. Final judgment regarding sex assignment must depend on local examination (penis size, presence or absence of vagina) and the findings at laparotomy.

OTHER NONENDOCRINE CAUSES

Abnormal differentiation of the entire perineal and genital region may occasionally occur in early fetal life, producing bizarre abnormalities, including true cloacas, complete fusion with abnormal exits for urethral channels and bowels, and imperforate anus. The ambiguous gential findings due to endocrine causes are almost never associated with other anomalies, and when other anomalies of excretory systems are associated, hormonal disorders are not to be expected as etiologic factors. Nevertheless, it is wise to perform a buccal smear and chromosomal analysis in all such infants and to clarify internal structures before sex assignment is irreversible. Normal females have been born with tumors of the clitoris that simulated penile development. Large preputial clitorial folds also

have misled parents in sex assignment, and some children with bladder exstrophy show an ambiguity of genital development that makes chromosomal sex determination imperative. These problems are discussed elsewhere in this text.

SEX ASSIGNMENT

As discussed previously, when a baby with ambiguous genitals is found to be chromatin-positive on buccal smear, a female sex assignment is amost always indicated, with the remote exception of the true hermaphrodite with a well-developed phallus. When the baby is found to be chromatin-negative, major problems must be confronted. In spite of male chromosomes, presence of testes, absence of müllerian structures, and presence of normal amounts of testosterone, it is universally agreed that it is a major error to assign a male gender role if the child has an insignificant penile structure that cannot be reconstructed to a reasonable size. The definitions of "insignificant structure" and "reasonable size" can be the cause of emotional distress in parents and also the child at a later age and may result in litigation. It is for these reasons that we recommend a thorough medical workup with a complete explanation to the parents of all the processes involved in normal genital development. To help them arrive at a joint decision of sex assignment, we involve them in group consultation via a Gender

Board, involving a pediatric surgeon, a urologic surgeon, a psychiatrist, and a pediatric endocrinologist. When possible, the family's physician also is involved. Once a decision is made, it is irrevocable. The major determining factor in agreeing to raise a male pseudohermaphrodite as a boy is a decision as to whether significant penile tissue is present to allow a reasonable reconstruction. Another major consideration is the high risk of malignant degeneration in the testes of such children, and even if the decision has been made to raise the child as a male, castration may become imperative. Most parents will agree with the conclusions of the Gender Board, but we have recently encountered certain ethnic attitudes where babies with insignificant penile development have been raised as males in spite of contrary advice from the Gender Board. Studies of such individuals have indicated that most will suffer extreme emotional disorders thoughout childhood and adult life.[7] In our experience, those children with nonadrenal male pseudohermaphroditism who have been assigned female gender roles have progressed through childhood in a stable emotional environment when parental adjustment has been satisfactory.

SURGICAL MANAGEMENT

The surgical management of the child with ambiguous genitalia includes procedures such as endoscopy and gonadal biopsy, which are helpful in establishing an exact diagnosis. Gonadal biopsy may be performed simultaneously with herniorrhaphy, since the abnormal gonad frequently is found in the inguinal canal. Otherwise, biopsy or gonadal excision is carried out through a small, transverse suprapubic incision. In older children with the testicular feminizing syndrome, we have removed the appendix as well as the gonads, in part so that the child could explain to her friends that she was in the hospital for an "appendectomy." This bit of deception is not necessary when gonadectomy is performed during infancy.

When the female gender has been definitely assigned, surgical therapy is designed to achieve a female appearance and to construct a functioning vagina. In most cases, this consists of a procedure to reduce the size of the phallus and a vaginoplasty.

There is a higher concentration of specialized nerve endings (the genital corpuscles) in the clitoris than elsewhere in the labia or vagina.[8] This anatomic fact confirms the importance of the clitoris in the sexual gratification of normal women as well as those who have undergone one or more operations on their genitalia and require hormonal therapy. Such operations involve complex emotional as well as anatomic problems.[9,10] It is now generally agreed that necessary reduction of the clitoris

by one means or another should be performed during early infancy.[11,12] Total clitoridectomy was the recommended procedure for many years.[13] This procedure produced an excellent cosmetic result. However, in recent years, operations designed to save either the entire clitoris or the glans with its intact nerves and vessels have evolved. The reduction clitoroplasty consists of a dorsal incision between the labial foreskin and the mons veneris. The foreskin is elevated from the shaft of the clitoris distally to within 1 cm of the glans, and then the corpora cavernosa are dissected back beyond the bifurcation well up under the symphysis pubis. Sutures are placed through Buck's fascia just back of the glans and the underside of the pubis. When these are tied down, the clitoris is recessed beneath the pubis.[14,15] It appears to be difficult to obtain a satisfactory cosmetic result with this procedure, and there have been reports of pain and swelling in the retained erectile tissue during sexual stimulation.

Resection of the clitoral shaft with retention of the glans and its blood and nerve supply is a satisfactory alternative to amputation or recession. We prefer this procedure, which has been described by Shaw and by Spence and Allen.[16,17]

Evaluation

The internal anatomy of the vagina is studied by means of injection of the sinus tract and lateral x-rays before the operation. Endoscopy to determine the exact relationship between the urethra and the vagina may be carried out at the same time as the clitoroplasty. If a relatively simple covered vagina exists, it may be opened at the same time. Otherwise it may be wise to delay vaginoplasty. Before surgery, the child's endocrine status will require reevaluation. Children with the adrenogenital syndrome should have their serum electrolyte levels determined and will require increased dosages of steroids before and during surgery.

Technique for Reduction for Clitoroplasty

The child is placed in the lithotomy position. If a perineal vaginoplasty is anticipated, only the perineum need be prepared. If a high vaginal repair is anticipated, the lower abdomen is also draped into the sterile field. The perineum is inspected with a nasal speculum, a Foley catheter is placed in the urethra, and a traction suture is placed through the glans. A dorsal, horseshoe-shaped incision is made in the groove between the clitoris, mons, and upper labia (Fig. 114–3A). This incision must not extend around to the ventral shaft. It is carried down to and through Buck's fascia. The dissection is then carried around the shaft, avoiding the nerves and the deep branch of the pudendal artery to the glans. Once the shaft has been encircled, it is carefully dissected out to

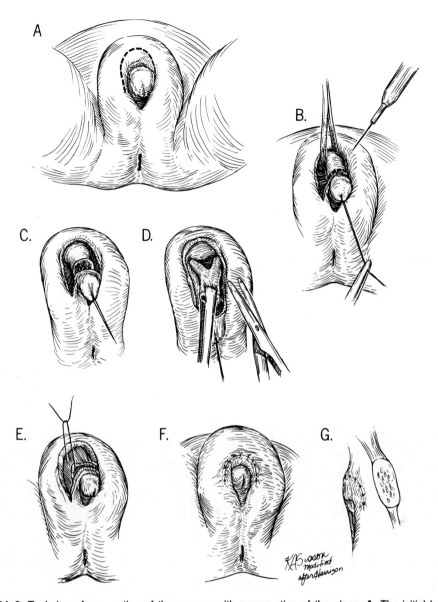

Figure 114–3. Technique for resection of the corpora with preservation of the glans. **A.** The initial horseshoe-shaped incision about the dorsum of the phallus. **B.** Isolation of the fused corpora proximal to the glans. One must be extremely careful to preserve the ventral skin and nerve supply to the glans. **C.** The corpora have been resected. **D.** They are then dissected well back beneath the pubis, where they are again divided and suture-ligated. **E.** The retained glans in then sutured to the undersurface of the pubis. **F, G.** Skin closure with subcuticular 5–0 catgut.

within 1 cm of the glans (Fig. 114–3B). Here it is transected between two clamps, and the distal end is suture-ligated (Fig. 114–3C). The proximal shaft is then dissected proximally (Fig. 114–3D). The suspensory ligament to the pubic symphysis is divided. At this point, it is necessary to ligate the dorsal branch of the internal pudendal artery. Each corpus is dissected out to well under the ischium, where it is amputated and sutured. The remaining stump of the glans is sutured to the periosteum of the inferior edge of the pubis (Fig. 114–3E,F.G). The remainng dorsal redundant skin is then either ex-

cised or saved for construction of labial folds. In most cases, this skin is excised, and a remnant of the foreskin dorsal to the glans is sutured back to the remaining skin over the mons. By leaving a broad base of ventral skin and by keeping the dissection close to the corpora, devascularization of the glans is avoided.

Vaginoplasty

The degree of masculinization of the genitalia is related to the exposure of the fetus to androgen. Most children with female pseudohermaphroditism will have some degree of labia minor fusion. Examination reveals one anterior opening beneath the phallus. Probing of this sinus tract reveals the vagina posteriorly with the urethra in its normal location. With more severe degrees of masculinization, the vagina is at a higher level. Hendren and Crawford described a patient with an entirely male-appearing phallus with a urethra at its tip. The vagina joined the urethra just proximal to the external urethral sphincter.[18] Preoperative roentgenograms of the sinus tract and endoscopy at the time of surgery are indicated to determine if the vaginoplasty should be carried out at the same time as the clitoral recession. The only indication for early repair of the high urogenital sinus type of lesion described by Hendren and Crawford is recurrent urinary tract infection due to urine pooling in the vagina. Early repair may well lead to stenosis and either repeated dilatation or another repair when the child is older.

When there is only a thin membrane between the vagina and the perineum, we prefer to perform the vaginoplasty simultaneously with the clitoral resection. A vertical, longitudinal incision with suture of the vaginal mucosa to the labia is simple, but since the posterior wall of the vagina is somewhat distant from the perineum, there is tension on the suture line that may result in stricture. It is better to bridge the gap between the posterior vaginal wall and the perineum with an inverted U-shaped flap of skin (Fig. 114–4).

Technique. After completion of the clitoral resection, an inverted U-shaped incision is made that is centered at the anterior opening (Fig. 114–5A). This flap of skin is made progressively thicker posteriorly in order to preserve its blood supply. After the flap has been turned back, a curved hemostat is inserted into the vagina. It is essential that a catheter be present in the urethra and the anatomy outlined before the back wall of the vagina is opened! The vagina is then incised down to the junction with the perineal skin slap (Fig. 114–5B,C). It is often necessary to mobilize skin laterally and to dissect back along the vagina for a short distance to bring the skin flaps and vagina together without tension (Fig. 114–5D,E). Absorbable polyglycolic acid sutures are ideal for this repair. At the end of the operation, a wick of petroleum jelly gauze is inserted in the vagina. Postoperatively, the Foley catheter is left in place for 2 or 3 days. The child should be examined under anesthesia 1 month after the operation and again at intervals if there is any tendency for stenosis of the introitus.

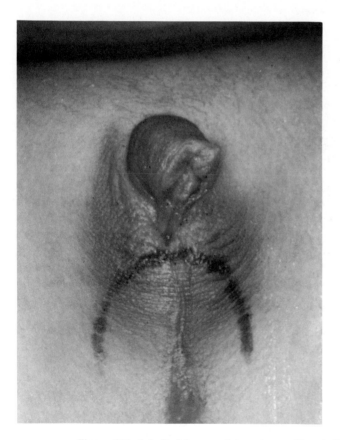
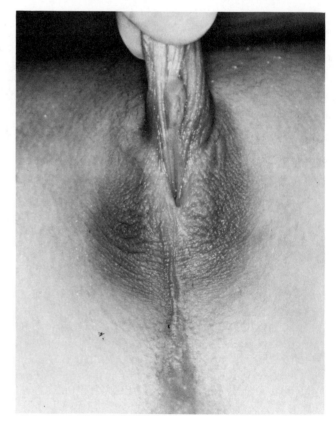

Figure 114–4. Left. Adrenogenital syndrome. The phallus is enlarged, and there is fusion of the skin over the vagina and urethra. This illustrates the inverted U-shaped incision, which creates a flap of skin that is turned up into the posterior wall of the vagina. **Right.** The urogenital sinus beneath the glans.

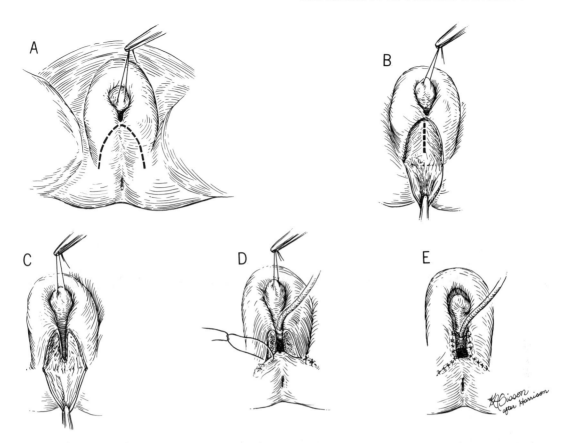

Figure 114–5. Vaginoplasty for adrenogenital syndrome. **A.** The inverted U-shaped incision is made thicker posteriorly in order to preserve the blood supply. **B, C.** The vagina is incised in the midline posteriorly. The urethra must be identified and catheterized. **D, E.** The skin flap is sutured into the vaginal incision, creating a new introitus. This must be examined at intervals under anesthesia for dilatation.

Urogenital Sinus Abnormalities

The high vagina, or urogenital sinus defect, is more often associated with cloacal malformations than with ambiguous genitalia. The technical aspects of separating the urinary tract from the vagina and joining the vagina with the perineum are similar in either case. Before the operation is commenced, the internal anatomy must be completely studied. Often, the urethral orifice can be found and catheterized by examining the urogenital sinus with a long nasal speculum and a fiberoptic headlight. This type of direct examination often provides a better understanding of the lesion than can be obtained with the panendoscope. If the urethral opening is high on the anterior vaginal wall (within 1 or 2 cm of its usual location), a flap vaginoplasty (as was just described) will open the perineum. These children are continent of urine, and once the vagina is opened widely, they no longer have urinary tract infections. Unfortunately, we have not followed any of these children long enough to know if the high urethra will cause problems with intercourse.

Hendren has described repair of the urogenital sinus defect in association with the adrenogenital syndrome through a perineal incision[19] (Fig. 114–6). We have found it difficult and perhaps dangerous to dissect the vagina from the back wall of the urethra and bladder through a deep incision in the perineum. Further, even with long skin flaps, it has been almost impossible to achieve a tension-free anastomosis between the anterior wall of the vagina and the perineum. For this reason, we have used an abdominal approach to separate the vagina from the urethra and bladder. This has allowed much more free mobilization of the vagina and an anastomosis to the perineum with less tension than in other procedures. The perineal dissection is facilitated by placing a metal sound in the urethra for accurate identification and to avoid stricture during the closure of the vaginourethral fistula. The entire urogenital sinus is then left as the urethra and the vagina are brought down to the perineum between the rectum and the urogenital sinus. These are difficult operations that can be performed in young infants, if necessary, although after reviewing our cases, we have decided that, if possible, a major vaginal reconstruction should be left until the child is at least 10 years old. However, clitoridectomy is always performed in infancy.

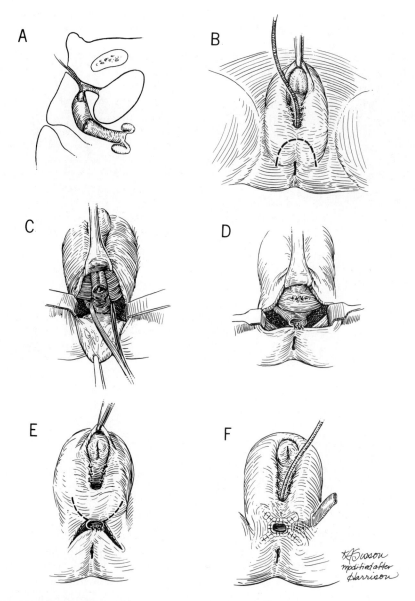

Figure 114–6. Hendren's operation for a severely masculinized child with a high-lying vagina that enters the urethra proximal to the external sphincter. **A.** The internal anatomy. **B.** The same inverted U-incision is made on the perineum. **C.** The perineal incision is deepened until the vagina is exposed and isolated. This facilitated by a metal sound in the urethra or a Foley bag in the vagina. **D.** The vaginal connection with the urethra is divided and sutured. **E, F.** The vagina is then sutured to skin flaps developed on the perineum.

REFERENCES

1. Green OC: Steroid metabolism in the fetus and newborn infant. Pediatr Clin North Am 12:615, 1965
2. White PC, New MI, Dupont BO: Congenital adrenal hyperplasia (2 parts). N Engl J Med 316:1519, 1580, 1987
3. Kenny FM, Reynolds JW, Green OC: Partial 3β-hydroxysteroid dehydrogenase (3β-HSD) deficiency in a family with congenital adrenal hyperplasia: Evidence for increasing 3β-HSD activity with age. Pediatrics 48:756, 1971
4. Givens JR, Wiser WL, Summitt RL, et al: Familial male pseudohermaphroditism without gynecomastia due to defi-
cient testicular 17-ketosteroid reductase activity. N Engl J Med 291, 1974
5. Keenan BS, Kirkland JL, Kirkland RT, Clayton GW: Male pseudohermaphroditism with partial androgen insensitivity. Pediatrics 59:224, 1977
6. Imperato-McGinley J, Guerrero L, Gautier T, Peterson RE: Steroid 5α-reductase deficiency in man: an inherited form of male pseudohermaphroditism. Science 186:1213, 1974
7. Money J, Ehrhardt AA: Man and Woman, Boy and Girl: The Differentiation and Dimorphism of Gender Identity from Conception to Maturity. Baltimore, Johns Hopkins University Press, 1972

8. Erickson KL, Montagna W: New observations on the anatomical features of the female genitalia. J Am Med Wom Assoc 27:573, 1972

9. Sotiropoulos A, Morishima A, Homsy Y, Lattimer JK: Long-term assessment of genital reconstruction in female pseudohermaphrodites. J Urol 115:599, 1976

10. Kumar H, Kiefer JH, Rosenthal IE, Clark SS: Clitoroplasty: Experience during a 19-year period. J Urol 111:81, 1972

11. Canty TG: The child with ambiguous genitalia: A neonatal surgical emergency. Ann Surg 186:272, 1977

12. Platt L, Becker JM: Female adrenogenital syndrome: Early surgical repair. J Pediatr 62:63, 1963

13. Gross RE, Randolph J, Crigler JF Jr: Clitorectomy for sexual abnormalities: Indications and technique. Surgery 59:300, 1966

14. Randolph JG, Hung W: Reduction of clitoroplasty in females with hypertrophied clitoris. J Pediatr Surg 5:224, 1970

15. Fonkalsrud EW, Kaplan S, Lippe B: Experience with reduction clitoroplasty for clitoral hypertrophy. Ann Surg 186:221, 1977

16. Shaw A: Subcutaneous reduction clitoroplasty. J Pediatr Surg 12:331, 1977

17. Spence HM, Allen TD: Genital reconstruction in the female with the adrenogenital syndrome. Br J Urol 45:126, 1973

18. Hendren WH, Crawford JD: Adrenogenital syndrome: the anatomy of the anomaly and its repair. Some new concepts. J Pediatr Surg 4:49, 1969

19. Hendren WH: Surgical management of urogenital sinus abnormalities. J Pediatr Surg 12:339, 1977

Miscellaneous Problems

115
Vaginal Anomalies

LABIAL FUSION

Fusion of the labia minora is commonly observed in 1- to 2-year-old girls. Separation will usually take place if the mother will apply an estrogen cream to the fused skin. If this is unsuccessful, the skin is easily separated under general anesthesia. A petroleum jelly wick is left in place for several days, after which the child is given warm sitz baths. The mother must again separate the skin and apply an estrogen ointment, or the fusion will recur.

VAGINAL OBSTRUCTION

Vaginal obstruction ranges from simple imperforate hymen to agenesis of the vagina and the complex cloacal malformation associated with imperforate anus.

Embryology
The embryology of the female genital tract is difficult to understand, and the various authorities present contradicting theories. The following is derived from Koff's work with the Carnegie collection.[1]

The paired müllerian ducts first appear in a 5-week embryo as a depression in the cranial end of the urogenital ridge. Early in development, they are tubes of epithelial cells that grow caudally beside the wolffian duct. In the pelvis, the müllerian ducts turn in an S-shaped curve, crossing the wolffian duct ventrally until they lie in apposition to and medial to the wolffian duct on the urogenital sinus. Here the ducts fuse to form the uterovaginal canal, or cord, and ultimately the fallopian tubes, uterus, and upper vagina. The junction of the fused müllerian ducts

and the urogenital sinus marks the point at which almost all vaginal obstructions start, regardless of their ultimate levels. The lower vagina and vestibule are derived from the anterior partition of the cloaca, the urogenital sinus. In normal female development, the urogenital sinus undergoes differentiation by combining with the wolffian ducts, producing the ureteric buds and ultimately the ureter and bladder, in addition to the lower vagina.

Vaginal Obstruction in the Neonate
A simple imperforate hymen will result in a hydrocolpos or collection of fluid in the vagina, since the cervix responds to maternal estrogen by secreting a characteristic white mucus. The imperforate hymen is easily recognized on simple examination of the newborn infant. There may be a lower abdominal mass (Fig. 115–1). After the urethra is accurately localized and catheterized, the hymen is incised, and the cut edges are oversewn with 5–0 catgut sutures.

Hydrometrocolpos
Hydrometrocolpos, or fluid in the uterus and vagina, is associated with a persistent urogenital sinus and a high transverse septum (Fig. 115–2). Clinically, these infants at birth have a huge abdominal mass that rises in the midline from the pelvis to reach the costal margin. There may be respiratory distress due to abdominal distention. The mass is palpable anterior to the rectum and is more fixed than an ovarian cyst. The perineum must be examined under a good light while the infant's legs are abducted. The external genitalia appear normal. Specifically, there is no bulge such as the one seen with a simple imperforate hymen. One can easily mistake the urogenital sinus for the vagina; however, there is

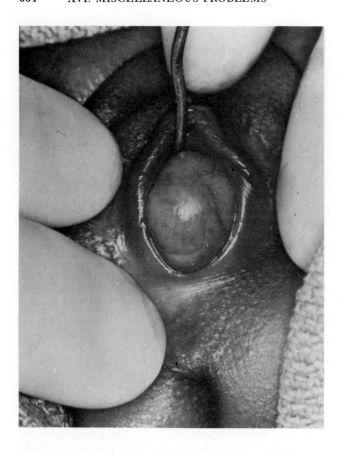

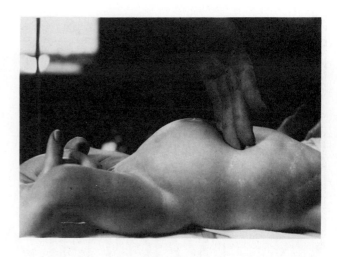

Figure 115–1. Imperforate hymen in a newborn baby. **Left.** The perineum with a bulging membrane. **Above.** The distended vagina extends to above the umbilicus.

no urethra. Catheterization of the perineal opening reveals urine. Roentgenographic studies demonstrate displacement of the bowel by the pelvic mass. Excretory urography reveals wide lateral displacement of the ureters (Fig. 115–3). McKusick et al. have demonstrated that hydrometrocolpos may be a simple, inherited malformation.[2] Kaufman et al. later described a familial syndrome of hydrometrocolpos, polydactyly, and heart disease.[3] The McKusick-Kaufman syndrome has now

been diagnosed by prenatal ultrasonography, and a reveiw of all reported cases suggests that the syndrome may occur in any ethnic group in an autosomal recessive pattern.[4]

Hydrometrocolpos is a surgical emergency because of the severe abdominal distention. In very ill neonates, the vagina may be drained by suturing its anterior wall to the skin. Later, an abdominovaginal pull-through may be carried out. Simple drainage of the vagina through

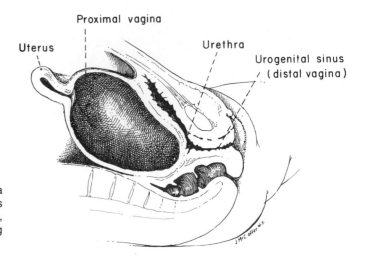

Figure 115–2. Hydrometrocolpos due to a high transverse septum. The urogenital sinus is an extension of the bladder. Consequently, on examination there is only one opening anterior to the anus.

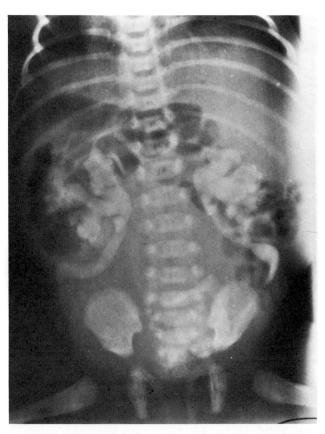

Figure 115–3. An intravenous urogram that shows the intestinal gas displaced upward and the ureters displaced laterally by a mass that rises out of the pelvis.

the urogenital sinus will result in chronic urinary tract infection because of urine reflux into the huge, dilated vagina.[5]

Technique for Abdominovaginal Pull-through

The baby is placed in the lithotomy position, with the abdomen, perineum, and thighs prepared and draped into a single sterile field. A low, transverse abdominal incision exposes the hugely distended vagina with the uterus at its apex. The abdominal cavity is often obliterated with adhesions because of retrograde spillage of secretions from the fallopian tubes. The thick anterior wall of the vagina is opened, and a culture is made of the fluid. Complete exploration of the interior of the vagina is performed to rule out a septate or duplicate vagina. If there are double uteri, one can expect a vaginal septum. This is excised, and the edges are oversewn. An inverted U-shaped flap of skin is then elevated on the perineum just behind the urogenital sinus. This incision is deepened to meet the posterior wall of the vagina. This maneuver is simplified by having an assistant push downward from within the vagina (Fig. 115–4A). When the back wall of the vagina has been well mobilized, it

is opened and sutured to the perineal skin just behind the urogenital sinus (Fig. 115–4B). Cosmetically, it is better to include a bit of the posterior wall of the urogenital sinus so that the relationship of the urethra with the vagina will be more normal. The urogenital sinus is left as the urethra (Fig. 115–4C). An irregular suture line is made that interdigitates flaps of skin with V incisions in the vagina to minimize postoperative stricture.

The child is examined under anesthesia within 1 month of the operation to dilate the skin–vagina anastomosis. She is then followed at intervals for observation of the anastomosis. At or near puberty, a complete gynecologic examination is indicated. Girls with cloacal anomalies have had tuboovarian abscesses, probably as a result of inflammation in and around the fallopian tube.

Vaginal Obstruction in the Older Child

Simple imperforate hymen, transverse vaginal septum, and agenesis of the vagina may not be discovered until the maturing adolescent fails to menstruate. If she has a uterus and a secreting endometrium, there will be recurrent cycles of lower abdominal pain and a lower abdominal mass. If there is a simple imperforate hymen, examination under anesthesia will reveal a bulging membrane. The diagnosis is confirmed by aspirating old blood from the vaginal cavity. A cruciate incision is made through the membrane, extending to the vaginal wall. Care is taken to avoid injury to the urethra. Interrupted catgut sutures join the cut edges of the hymen with the vaginal mucosa. The patient is examined at least once under anesthesia at a later date to make sure there is no stricture.

A high obstructing membrane may bulge with old blood and is visualized with a speculum while the child is under anesthesia. Incision of this membrane is not so simple. Careful aspiration of the bulging membrane is performed while the surgeon has a finger in the rectum to guard against bowel injury and to obtain an idea of its thickness. If there is a gap between the lower and upper vagina, it is well to proceed with a laparotomy and examination of the internal genitalia. The vagina is opened above the obstruction. By approaching the obstruction from above and below, the distended proximal vagina is mobilized until it can be easily sutured to the mucosa of the lower vagina.

Agenesis of the Vagina

Total absence of the vagina results from failure of the distal ends of the müllerian ducts to fuse. Absence of the vagina, with or without the uterus, has been termed the Rokitansky-Kuster-Hauser syndrome.[6] It is associated with a range of müllerian duct anomalies and renal agenesis.[7] The familial incidence indicates a single gene disorder that is not limited to females in the family. Affected males may have renal agenesis with an absence

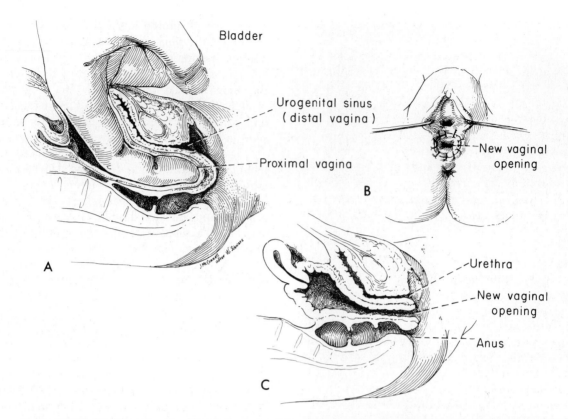

Figure 115–4. Technique for the abdominovaginal pull-through to correct a high hydrometrocolpos. The initial step consists of a low, transverse abdominal incision that exposes the dilated vagina. This is opened, and with downward finger pressure the vagina is found through a second incision in the perineum just posterior to the urogenital sinus. The vagina is sutured to the perineum to create an opening separated from the urogenital sinus, which remains as the urethra.

of the vas deferens or seminal vesicles.[8] The absence of the vagina may be noted at birth, or it may not be noticed until menses are expected. On examination, the perineum between the urethra and the anus is smooth, or there may be a dimple at the usual location of the vagina. A buccal smear should be made to rule out intersex problems.

Ideally, the vaginal agenesis is discovered at birth, the parents are informed of the problem, and a buccal smear, pyelogram, and cystourethrogram are obtained at that time to rule out associated anomalies. Later, laparoscopy or an operation is performed to determine the status of the ovaries, fallopian tubes, and uterus. With vaginal agenesis, the ovaries usually are present but the uterus is absent. The age chosen for vaginal reconstruction is dictated by the presence or absence of the uterus. If there is cyclic pain with a lower abdominal mass, the menstrual secretions from a uterus are dissecting in the alveolar tissue between the bladder and rectum. Construction of an artificial vagina to provide drainage is then indicated. Otherwise, construction of the vagina is delayed until a later age so that regular coitus will provide dilatations.

Many operations have been described for construction of a vagina.[9] Frank, Huffman, and, more recently, Broadbent and Woolf have had the patient apply pressure to the perineal dimple for two 15-minute periods each day.[10–12] Initially, pressure is applied with a Pyrex tube at the perineal dimple. As the skin stretches and a neovagina is created, larger Silastic tubes are used. This simple technique certainly should be attempted because it can be used in conjunction with an inlay split-thickness skin graft and can be commenced during infancy.

The best surgical approach to congenital absence of the vagina is the inlay of split-thickness skin.[13,14] With this technique, a vertical incision is made from 1.5 cm behind the urethra to 2 cm in front of the anus. A cavity is then created by blunt dissection. Absolute hemostasis is necessary. After the cavity is created and obvious bleeders are coagulated, a warm pack is inserted while a skin graft is obtained from the innder side of the thigh. The graft should be 0.015 inches thick and large enough to fit about a mold 10 cm long and 7 cm in circumference. A mold may be formed out of Silastic or material used for dental prosthetic work. The graft is sutured to itself with the raw surface outward. The mold with the graft is then inserted into the cavity, and the perineal skin is sutured to maintain the mold with the graft in place. A small hole is left for drainage. The mold is removed and replaced in 10 days to 2 weeks. Thereafter, the patient must either keep a mold in place or must dilate the neovagina daily.

Alternative techniques include the creation of thin skin flaps from the labia minora or the use of a segment of colon. When there is a uterus and no vagina, it is difficult to connect a split-thickness skin graft to the uterus. In this situation, a combination of a colon segment for the upper vagina, connecting the uterus with a flap from the labia minor, provides the best cosmetic and functional vagina.

Duplication

Failure of fusion of the müllerian ducts may result in a double uterus with a separate vagina. This is asymptomatic because there is an outlet for menstrual secretions. If one side of the vagina is atretic, a hydrocolpos or retention cyst may develop in the neonate. There will be a mass that bulges into the normal vagina. At operation, a clue to the correct diagnosis will be the presence of separate uteri.

This same lesion is more likely to result in a paravaginal mass with the onset of menstruation. The girl will have a normal menstrual flow from the open vagina, but since the separate vagina is obstructed, she will have pain with each period and a mass. A similar problem develops when there is a bicornuate uterus with a rudi-

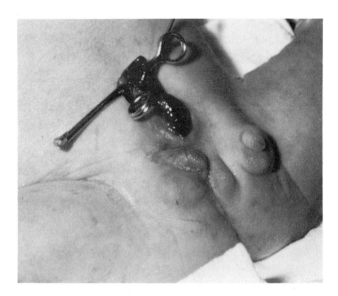

Figure 115–6. This infant had an epispadias (note low-lying umbilicus) and normal-appearing male genitalia lying to the left of her vagina.

mentary horn that does not communicate with the vagina. In this situation, vaginal examination reveals a single vagina with a single cervix, but there is a mass lateral to the uterus. This anomaly is often associated with agenesis of one kidney.[15,16] When the vagina is obstructed, excision of the septum will provide drainage by converting the double vagina into a single chamber with two cervices. Excision is the only possible therapy for a rudimentary obstructed uterine horn.

In our experience, duplication of the external female genitalia has always occurred in association with an ectopic anus, which enters the posterior forchette of the larger vagina. Cystoscopy under anesthesia is indicated to determine the status of the urinary system. The child illustrated in Figure 115–5 had a double bladder and a urethra to each vagina. Figure 115–6 illustrates an infant who had an epispadias with an ectopic anus entering the vagina, which is to the right, whereas on the left there was a phallic structure and scrotum. These were removed, and the imperforate anus was eventually treated with an abdominal-perineal pull-through. Removal of the duplicated external genitalia must be associated with repair or rerouting of the bladder and urethra to the most normal site.

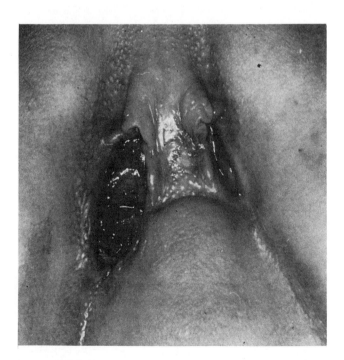

Figure 115–5. Duplication of external genitalia, with two urinary bladders entering into separate urethrae.

REFERENCES

1. Koff AK: Development of the vagina in the human fetus. Carnegie Inst Contrib Embryol 24:59, 1933
2. McKusick VA, Bauer RL, Koop LE, et al: Hydrometrocolpos as a simply inherited malformation. JAMA 189:813, 1964

3. Kaufman R, Hartman F, McAlister W: Family studies in congenital heart disease: II A syndrome of hydrometrocolpos, postaxial polydactyly and congenital heart disease. Birth Defects 8:85, 1972

4. Chitayat D, Hahm S, Marion W, et al: Further delineation of the McKusick-Kaufman hydrometrocolpos-polydactyly syndrome Am J Dis Child 141:1133, 1987

5. Ramenofsky ML, Raffensperger JG: An abdominoperineal-vaginal pull-through for definitive treatment of hydrometrocolpos. J Pediatr Surg 6:381, 1971

6. Griffin J, Edwards C, Madden J, et al: Congenital absence of the vagina: The Mayer-Rokitansky-Kuster-Hauser syndrome. Ann Intern Med 85:224, 1974

7. Leduc B, Van Campenhout J, Simard R: Congenital absence of the vagina: Observations of 25 cases. Am J Obstet Gynecol 100:512, 1968

8. Biedel C, Pagon R, Zapata J: Müllerian anomalies and renal agenesis: Autosomal dominant urogenital dysplasia. J Pediatr 104:861, 1984

9. Goldwyn RM: History of attempts to form a vagina. Plast Reconstr Surg 59:319, 1977

10. Frank RT: The formation of an artificial vagina without operation. Am J Obstet Gynecol 35:1053, 1938

11. Huffman JW: The Gynecology of Childhood and Adolescence. Philadelphia, Saunders, 1968, pp 1053–1055

12. Broadbent TR, Woolf RM: Congenital absence of the vagina: Reconstruction without operation. Br J Plast Surg 30:118, 1977

13. McIndoe A: The treatment of congenital absence and obliterative conditions of the vagina. Br J Plast Surg 2:254, 1949

14. Ortiz-Monasterio F, Serrano A, Barrera G, et al: Congenital absence of the vagina: Long-term follow-up in 21 patients treated with skin grafts. Plast Reconstr Surg 49:165, 1972

15. Yoder IC, Pfister RC: Unilateral hematocolpos and ipsilateral renal agenesis: Report of two cases and review of the literature. Am J Roentgenol Radium Ther Nucl Med 127:303, 1976

16. Stanley-Brown EG, Lavengood RW Jr, Holgersen LO: Hematometria and hematosalpinx in a duplicated uterus with congenital absence of one kidney. J Pediatr Surg 12:745, 1977

116
Conjoined Twins

Louise Schnaufer

We call Monsters, what things soever are brought forth contrary to the common decree and order of Nature. They, for the most part, are very short lived, because they both live and are born, as it were against Nature's consent; to which may be added, they doe not love themselves, by reason they are made a scorne to others, and by that means lead a hated life.[1]

Thus wrote Ambroise Paré, the foremost surgeon of the 16th century, in his book, _Of Monsters and Prodigies_. Teratology, the study of congenital malformations, has always intrigued the mind of man, and the manifestation of doubling of the human form has always been especially fascinating. In his book, Paré lists 11 causes for the birth of monsters, the foremost of which "is the glory of God, that His immense power may be manifested to those which are ignorant of it, by sending of things which happen contrary to nature."[1]

That aspect of teratology that involves duplication or twinning covers a wide range of anomalies. Monozygotic twins, conjoined twins, teratomas, duplications of organs, and even extra digits may be considered types of doubling. Of all of these, the conjoined, or Siamese, twin is perhaps the most challenging to the surgeon, presenting many surgical, medical, and ethical dilemmas in the course of treatment.

HISTORICAL NOTES

In the past, several sets of conjoined twins have survived into adulthood and have led unfortunate lives, often of great notoriety. One of the earliest recorded cases is that of the Biddenden maids, Mary and Eliza Chalkhurst, said to have been born in Biddenden, Kent, in 1100.

They were joined at the hips and lived to the age of 34, at which age one died and was followed 6 hours later by her sister, who refused separation.[2]

Textbooks on monsters and obstetrics and many woodcuts in the 16th and 17th centuries portrayed the various types of conjoining, and many such twins are depicted as adults.

The most famous and well-known twins are Eng and Chang Bunker, born in Siam in 1811. Their father was Chinese, and their mother was half Siamese and half Chinese. The twins were joined by a band of tissue 3.5 inches in width that arose from the lower chest and included their single umbilicus. At the age of 18, they arrived in the United States and were discovered by P. T. Barnum. Soon the whole world knew about Barnum's "Siamese twins," and this term has since persisted as a designation of any type of conjoined twinning.

The band of tissue connecting these two men contained a very thin bridge of liver tissue that was enclosed by a peritoneum-lined canal. Division of this band of tissue would have been a very simple procedure, but surgeons of that day believed that although it was feasible, it would be a very perilous operation, and they did not believe that the twins should submit to it.[3] It is believed that the twins themselves were quite content to remain together. Both twins married, and Eng's wife bore 12 children and Chang's wife 10. In 1874, when they were 63 years old, Chang died of pneumonia. Within 2 hours his brother, who had not been ill, also died of what was described by many as fright, but the description of his death suggests that it was more likely hypovolemic shock. Autopsy of the twins showed that, as stated before, the band of tissue connecting them contained a thin bridge of liver, and it is quite possible that the surviving twin simply bled into his dead brother.[4]

Another set of well-known twins were Rosalie and Josepha Blazek, born in Bohemia in 1878. They were pygopagus, sharing a single broad sacrum and being joined in the lower lumbar region. There was one rectum and one urethra, but each twin had a cervix and uterus. They are distinctive in that in 1910 one sister complained of an abdominal swelling. Although both she and her twin denied the possibility of pregnancy, she shortly thereafter delivered a normal son after an easy labor. At the age of 43, both twins died within 12 minutes of each other from an obscure illness associated with fever and jaundice.[5]

Two more pygopagus twins, Judith and Helena, were born in Hungary in 1701 and lived for 23 years. They were exhibited all over Europe. Another set of twins, Millie and Chrissie, were South Carolina mulattoes born in 1851 and were joined at the sacrum. They also traveled extensively and because of their beautiful voices were called "The Two Headed Nightingale." The pygopagus Gibbs twins, Margaret and Mary, died simultaneously of cancer in 1967.[5]

Embryology

Twins are born in the United States in approximately 1 in 90 pregnancies. Multiple pregnancies are of two varieties: the monovular, in which twins result from the division of a single fertilized ovum, and polyovular, in which two or more ova are fertilized. Since monovular twins arise from a single blastocyst, they have the same chromosomal pattern, the same sex, and are identical in every way. The factors that cause monozygotic twinning are unknown, but it is generally believed that these twins should be considered true terata, since they result from abnormal development of a single zygote. Conjoined twins also arise from a single blastocyst but remain joined by some aberration in the duplication process that normally produces two identical twins. Examples of conjoining may range from two perfectly duplicated individuals joined by a common bridge of tissue to those in which only a small portion of the body is duplicated and is attached as a parasite to the autosite. There may be an amorphous mass of tissue, known as a teratoma, located within the body of the individual.

In 1948, Rock and Hertig, after study of various preimplantation and postimplantation stages of fertilized ova, found that by the 6th day after fertilization, the cluster of cells of the human zygote become the blastocyst.[6] Within the blastocyst, some cells aggregate at one pole and are known as the inner cell mass. It is from this cell mass that the embryo, amnion, and yolk sac develop. In the very early stages, for a short period of time, these cells are considered totipotent and may split and form two germinal discs, which will then develop into two monozygotic individuals. Conjoining is believed to occur when there is incomplete fission of

the inner cell mass. Zimmerman believes that this is caused by interference with the inducers or organizers that determine the formation of body regions and organ systems.[7] Suppression of processes forming and shaping an organ, such as the heart, would prevent its complete differentiation. Therefore, a fused organ would result, such as one sees in the thoracopagus twins. Although this theory is still conjectural because of the unavailability of a series of fetal conjoined twins, it is now accepted that myozygotic twins develop from a single blastocyst and that the common chorion is proof of the splitting of the original inner cell mass.

An alternative theory of conjoining is that of fusion of the embryonic axes after the splitting of the inner cell mass. Areas along the embryonic axes that are in conjunction or overlap during development fuse to produce a particular area of conjoining.[8]

CLASSIFICATION

Although there are many classifications of conjoined twins, the classification proposed by Potter and Craig seems to be the most practical.[9] When the joined twins are complete individuals, fusion may be anterior, posterior, cephalic, or caudal. When doubling is less complete and only parts of the body are duplicated, the attachment of that twin is more often lateral.

Classification of Diploterata

I. Joined twins in which components are equal and symmetrical: Diplopagus (*Pagus* is a Greek word meaning "I fasten").
   A. Each component is complete.
      1. *Thoracopagus*—The connection is in or near the sternal region, and the twins are face to face. Part of the thoracic wall is held in common, and there are fused or shared chest and upper abdominal organs. Variations of this type may be omphalopagus, whereby the twins are united from the umbilicus to the xiphoid cartilage, or sternopagus, whereby only the sterum is shared.
      2. *Pygopagus*—The connection is at the sacrum and lower back, and the twins are back to back. The fusion is usually limited to the pelvic region, in which there is a common sacrum and coccyx. There is a single common rectum and anus and often one bladder and urethra.
      3. *Craniopagus*—The union is in the region of the vertex, occiput, or lateral parietal areas of the skull. The twins may face in the same direction or in opposite directions, and the brains are ordinarily separate.

4. *Ischiopagus*—The connection is in the lower pelvic area, with the axes of the bodies extending in a straight line in opposite directions. The fusion begins at the level of a common umbilicus, the pelvis is fused, and there are shared lower gastrointestinal tracts and genitourinary tracts.

B. Each component is less than an entire individual, and the less complete component is fused in a lateral position.

1. Duplication of the cranial end of the body.
   a. Monocephalus diprosopus: There is a single head with duplication of features of the face.
   b. Dicephalus: Two distinct heads are present, usually with separate necks and one body.

2. Duplication in the caudal region.
   a. Dipygus.
      i. Partial duplication of the pelvis with a third leg—monocephalus tripus dibrachius (Fig. 116–1).
      ii. Four legs—monocephalus tetrapus dibrachius.

3. Duplication of both cranial and caudal regions—dicephalus dipygus.
   a. Common trunk, two to three arms, three legs—dicephalus tripus tribrachius.

II. Unequal and symmetrical conjoined twins in which one is smaller and dependent on the other (heteropagus).

A. The parasite is attached to the visible surface of the autosite and is incomplete, having only arms or a head with arms or legs.

B. The parasite is attached to the back or the sacrococcygeal area. Such parasties are amorphous masses of tissues and are known as teratomas.

C. The parasite has developed in the body cavity and is usually classified as a tumor. If it is farily well developed and recognizable, it is sometimes designated as fetus in fetu.

INCIDENCE

The true incidence of conjoined twins is impossible to ascertain, since the majority are either aborted or stillborn. However, reported incidences are in the range of 1 in 50,000 to 60,000 births. Potter and Craig reported 1 set of symmetrically conjoined twins in 60,000 deliveries at the Chicago Lying-In Hospital.[9] Freedman et al. reported 1 case in 80,000 deliveries at Long Island College Hospital in New York.[10]

Robertson reviewed 117 cases of conjoined twins and cited the incidence as thoracopagus 73.4 percent, pygopagus 18.8 percent, ischiopagus 5.9 percent, and craniopagus 1.7 percent.[11]

Female conjoined twins occur two or three times more commonly than male conjoined twins. It is interesting that although monovular male twins are more common than monovular female twins, 70 percent of conjoined twins are female.

Although some authors have noted that there seems to be a greater number of conjoined twins born of African and Asiatic races, the frequency of monozygotic twinning is constant for all races and is independent of heredity, race, maternal age, and parity. The incidence of dizygotic twinning is, in contrast, greatly influenced by these factors.

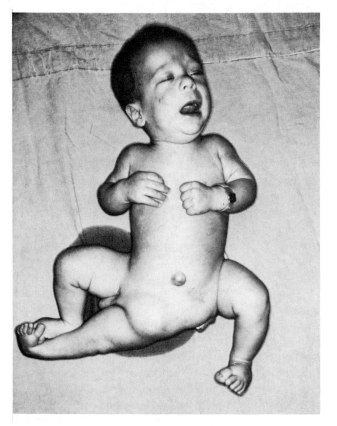

Figure 116–1. Monocephalus tripus dibrachius. Partial duplication of the pelvis, with a third leg.

OBSTETRIC MANAGEMENT

The antepastum diagnosis of cojoined twins is now common because of the routine use of ultrasonography, especially in cases of twinning. Magnetic resonance imaging (MRI) has been used in delineating the cojoining and may become the method of choice in the future.

During delivery of a normal set of monozygotic twins, the first twin is delivered before the amniotic membrane of the second ruptures. In a breech delivery, if three or four legs present, a diagnosis of conjoining can be made. If the diagnosis is suspected, further vaginal examination can be made, and generally the area of fusion can be distinguished by palpation. Spontaneous vaginal delivery occurs in a large number of cases owing to the small size of the twins and premature labor. They rarely weigh more than 500 g. Breech delivery is the most favorable, since the presentation of all four legs permits traction and simultaneous delivery of both trunks if the mother's pelvis is large enough. In vertex presentations, many twins can be delivered in parallel if the head of one is situated under the chin of the other. However, the method of choice is cesarean section if the diagnosis of conjoining has been made.

Dystocia is common, and it is necessary in such a case to proceed to cesarean section or destructive procedures, such as craniotomy or decapitation. Many obstetricians believe that cesarean section should be performed for a set of stillborn twins if they are already partially delivered. In a recent review of 60 sets of conjoined twins, 31 were stillborn and 6 died at delivery.[12]

CLINICAL MANAGEMENT

Surgical separation of a set of conjoined twins is foremost in the minds of everyone caring for these children. The feasibility of separation is another matter, and the location and extent of the conjoining is often the determining factor as to whether both twins can survive as normally functioning individuals. The greater the extent of the conjoining, the greater the possibility of sharing asymmetrical or fused organs.

Both thoracopagus and ischiopagus twins often share portions of the gastrointesinal tract, and the areas of conjunction can be evaluated easily by contrast studies.

Because of the often complex cardiovascular union in thoracopagus twins, evaluation of this system should be done early in the event that emergency separation is made necessary by a deteriorating cardiovascular state. If simultaneously running ECGs show a single heart rate with mirror-image QRS complexes, a conjoined heart is present. Echocardiography will provide important diagnostic information concerning the fused hearts. Selective angiography should be performed in addition to cardiac catheterization to define the extent of liver fusion and the presence or absence of separate extrahepatic biliary systems in thoracopagus twins. It is also helpful in determining the nature of the urinary tract and the blood supply to the bowel. Delayed films following angiography will also produce good nephrograms and visualization of the extrahepatic biliary tree.

Further evaluation of conjoining can be determined by radionuclide scanning. A reliable estimation of the amount of cross-circulation or blood volume exchange between the infants can be made by administering isotope-tagged serum albumin or erythrocytes. The method for calculating the blood volume exchange is described by Spencer et al. in their studies of both the Bayamon and Bay City twins.[13] Organ-specific isotopes may be used to delineate the amount of fusion of the liver if arteriographic studies are not available. Radionuclide scans should be done to rule out the presence of a single biliary excretion system, which is common in thoracopagus twins.

Ischiopagus and pygopagus twins often share a common vagina, bladder, or rectum. Vaginograms and cystograms are very useful in defining anomalies of the urogenital tract and also in determining which twin owns the solitary organ. Computed tomography (CT) scans with three-dimensional reconstruction have proved useful in defining duplicated pelvic organs and bony structures.

In twins with a tetrapus anomaly, the extremity is often shared by both. Although the major blood supply comes from one twin, the vascular contribution to a portion of the skin of the third limb may come from the other child. In order to determine the skin allocation for each child, perfusion fluorometry is a useful technique. Tissue fluorescence can be quantitated by this method and is more sensitive and accurate than the traditional method of fluorescein injection. It is also useful in intraoperative assessment of skin flap viability in reconstructing large defects.[14]

Silastic tissue expanders are useful in the preoperative period to stretch abdominal skin of ischiopagus twins to facilitate skin closure. Multiple injections of saline into the expander to a volume of 1000 ml over a period of 6 to 8 months will often allow sufficient skin coverage so that the use of artificial materials is unnecessary.[15]

There are only two specific indications for separation of conjoined twins in the newborn period. This may be done when (1) one twin is moribund or dead or threatens the life of the other, or (2) there is a condition of one or both that is incompatible with life, such as ruptured omphalocele or an intestinal obstruction.

Gans et al. found only nine sets of twins who were separated in the newborn period reported in the world literature. The majority were separated for the above-mentioned reasons.[16] Other separations were reported for the early neonatal period, by which time the studies had been completed, the children were in good condition, and the surgical team was prepared. In the absence of the absolute indications for separation in the newborn period, there are no definite indications for operating at any particular time. If the babies are to be operated on in an institution that is not equipped to cope with the intricacies of neonatal surgery and postoperative care, the surgery should be postponed until the babies are out of the infancy period. Otherwise, there is no reason to delay elective separation once the studies have been completed and the babies as well as the surgical team are prepared.

The preoperative preparation may be the most significant factor in determining the outcome of the procedure. The surgeon in charge must designate a complete and separate team for each child, with appropriate specialists standing by in case their services are needed. Multiple conferences with the entire team must be held to ensure complete understanding by everyone of the mechanics of the separation procedures. Blackboard sessions and diagramming of the positions and movements of the individuals, a review of the positions of the equipment and tables, and finally a dress rehearsal itself should be carried out. If positioning of the babies is potentially complicated or confusion, they should be brought to the operating room, and a rehearsal with the application of drapes and monitors should be carried out. Finally, tattooing the skin with methylene blue along the proposed line of incision, which can be done the night before surgery, will give much comfort and guidance to the surgeon.

Thorough physiologic monitoring must be carried out during the course of the operative procedure. In addition to ECG and temperature monitoring, multiple routes of vascular access must be provided. These include a central venous and arterial catheter for determination of blood pressure, blood gases, pH, and chemistries. One or more peripheral venous catheters must be available for fluid, albumin, and blood replacement.

Strapping each baby to a wooden frame is helpful in preventing dislodgment of monitors and lines and also in facilitating movement of the babies after separation to another room or operating table. Heat loss must be guarded against, especially during the period of skin preparation, which preparation should be done with warmed solutions. Antibiotic coverage against staphylococcal and gram-negative infections is indicated both preoperatively and intraoperatively, particularly during procedures over 6 hours in duration.

The complexity of the conjoining determines the difficulty of the separation and reconstructive procedures. Thorough knowledge of the configuration and the amount of sharing of viscera in more complicated unions is necessary, and meticulous care must be taken in determining the vascular and nerve supplies of each organ before apportioning it to a twin.

One of the most subtle and mysterious hazards that can develop during a long procedure is the development of hypovolemic shock in one twin, usually the smaller one, either during or at the moment of separation. Even though the blood losses have been carefully monitored during the procedure and replacement has been attended meticulously, one baby may bleed into the other. Large venous channels often exist between shared livers and in the perineum, as described in Koop's pyopagus twins.[17] It seems that the larger twin is capable of capturing the other twin's blood through these channels and thereby producing hypovolemia in the smaller one. If such a vascular communication is known to exist, separation of that conjoined structure should be effected first to prevent vascular shunting while other structures are being divided. Careful monitoring during the procedure may indicate that the smaller infant requires a much greater blood volume replacement than the other twin.

In the postoperative period, hypovolemia may still be a problem and may occur as sudden cardiovascular collapse or anuria. Babies with this problem usually require more fluid and blood replacement than is indicated by the estimated blood loss and their ages and weights. Thoracopagus twins who have had chest reconstructions will quickly exhibit respiratory failure and must be maintained on a ventilator and have their blood gases monitored postoperatively. Sepsis is a hazard if plastic or metal prostheses have been used in reconstruction of the chest or abdominal wall.

ANESTHETIC MANAGEMENT

The administration of anesthesia to a set of conjoined twins presents unique and sometimes difficult problems. The pharmacologic effect of drugs acting in the presence of a crossed circulation depends on the extent of that circulation, the mixing between the twins, and the distribution in the tissues of the agents used. Since the major vascular shunting in most conjoined twins is venous, the administration of an inhalation anesthetic to one twin will have very little effect on the other. The agent would be taken up primarily by the tissues of the one twin, leaving very low venous anesthetic concentrations to affect the other. Intravenous drugs that have a high tissue solubility, such as thiopentol, will also fail to produce a clinical effect in the other twin. Succinylcholine will, however, produce a pharmacologic effect by means of the crossed circulation because it is distributed to both the vascular and the extracellular compartments. It has been noted that the crossover effect of succinylcholine is determined by relation of the dosage to the weight of the twins.[18] However, in cases where there is a conjoined heart or common major arteries, the effect of the drugs should be equal in both infants.

The most difficult mechanical hurdle to overcome is probably that of the intubation of thoracopagus twins. If the conjunction in the thoracic region is quite thick and the infants' heads are close together, there will be an exaggerated cervical lordosis and, in most cases, a receding mandible configuration. This situation requires quick and deft intubation, preferably while the babies are awake. Careful monitoring is necessary during this phase because of the hazard of circulatory collapse while the children are being held in abnormal positions. Hypovolemia can develop if the twins are held in the supine or prone positions because of traction on the great vessels or shunting of blood by gravity from one twin into the other.

SURGICAL SEPARATION

The first successful separation of conjoined twins was effected by Konig in 1689, and the second was performed by Boehm in 1860.[19,20] Both were omphalopagus and were connected only by a narrow skin bridge. The first separation of a more dense and complex union was effected by Biaudet in 1881.[20] A liver bridge was divided, and both twins died. In 1902 a similar set of twins was separated by Chapot-Prevost, with one survivor.[21] The first successful pygopagus separation was performed in 1912 by a naval surgeon in Portsmouth.[21] Before 1950, there were only 10 reported cases of surgical separation of symmetrical conjoined twins.

In 1956, Spencer reported a set of asymmetrical ischiopagus twins, of which one was defective and moribund.[22] An emergency separation was performed successfully, and the other twin survived. In 1957, Koop successfully separated pygopagus twins who had a common anus, uterus, and vagina.[17]

The first successful thoracopagus separation was effected by Peterson and Hill in 1960.[23] In these twins, there was a shared pericardial septum and a broad liver bridge. Separation of thoracopagus twins with a conjoined heart was considered impossible until 1977, when Koop sacrificed the parasitic twin and retained a six-chambered heart in the surviving one (C. E. Koop, personal communication).

THORACOPAGUS TWINS

Thoracopagus twins (those fused in the midportion of the body) represent 75 percent of all symmetrical conjoined twins (Fig. 116–2). Omphalopagus or xiphopagus twins form a subgroup of this classification. The union extends from the umbilicus superiorly to the xiphoid process and may exist as a simple skin bridge or liver bridge or may include fusion of the xiphoid processes. In the true thoracopagus twins, the joining includes the thorax and may extend from the manubrium of the sternum to the umbilicus. An omphalocele may be present also.

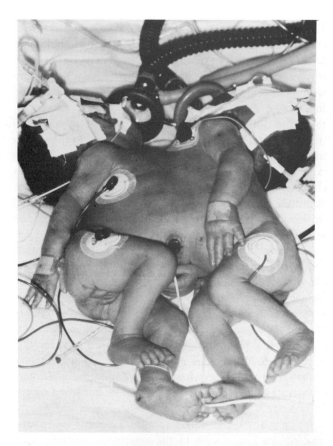

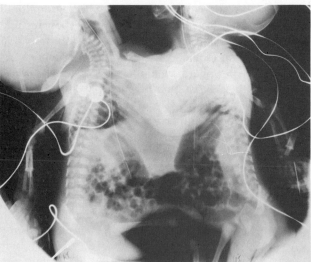

Figure 116–2. Top. Thoracopagus twins sharing a 6-chambered heart and a fused liver. **Bottom.** Lateral film of thoracopagus twins showing communication of peritoneal cavity.

All thoracopagus twins have some abnormality of the heart, and there is a wide range in the complexity of the conjoining of these structures. The simplest type is a shared pericardium that contains two normal hearts.

The most complex cases include bizarre fusions of two or more ventricles and confusing communications of the atria. In a review of 42 cases by Nicholas et al.,[24] the sternum was joined in 100 percent and the pericardium was joined in 90 percent of the twins. Conjoining of the heart to some degree was found in 75 percent of the cases. The presence of separate pulse rates on palpation and the demonstration of individual QRS complexes indicate the presence of two separate hearts. If there is evidence of congenital heart disease or fusion of the chambers, echocardiography, cardiac catheterization, and selective angiography must be performed to delineate the abnormalities and to define the surgical problems involved in separation.

The liver is fused in all thoracopagus twins and the biliary tree is joined in 22 percent.[24] Approximately 50 percent of cases involve conjoining of the gastrointestinal tract, the most common site being the duodenum. If there is a single duodenum, there will be only one common duct draining two gallbladders and two sets of hepatic ducts.

The separation of thoracopagus twins presents several interesting technical problems. Division of the fused liver can be formidable if there is a broad area of union and particularly if there are large vascular channels coursing through the livers. Excessive bleeding during the division can be controlled by placing two Penrose drains around the circumference of the liver to act as a tourniquet and by the use of electrocautery during the division. The use of vascular clips on both the vessels and bile ducts will expedite the procedure. Appropriate resection and anastomosis can be done for a portion of a conjoined gastrointestinal tract, and in the case of a single duodenum and common duct, the duodenum can be given to one twin and a cholecystoenterostomy performed in the other.

In describing the division of the Bay City twins, who had separate hearts enclosed in a single pericardium, Able mentioned cardiac tamponade following closure of the pericardium.[25] This led him to use a siliconized rubber film to fill in the pericardial defect. In addition, he found it necessary to stabilize the thoracic cage with a Kirschner wire because of the formidable chest wall defect that remained. The remaining open sternal and epigastric areas were covered with polypropylene mesh, after which the entire defect was covered with silicone rubber film. Formation of a fibrin layer beneath the plastic permitted the removal of these materials, and the wounds healed quickly by epithelialization over a healthy granulating bed. DeVries closed the large thoracoabdominal defects in the San Francisco twins with a Teflon mesh prosthesis, which was then covered by pedicled skin flaps.[26] Freeze-dried skin homografts were then placed in the lateral skin defects. In Koop's separation

of a set of thoracopagus twins with a conjoined six-chambered heart, a portion of the rib cage of the sacrificed twin was retained, providing adequate space in the remaining twin's chest for the greatly enlarged heart (C. E. Koop, personal communication). Of course, this method can only be used if one twin is to be sacrificed. Otherwise prosthetic materials and metal structs are necessary to stabilize the chest wall and to prevent compression of the heart.

PYGOPAGUS TWINS

Approximately 18 percent of symmetrically conjoined twins are pygopagus. The connection is at the sacrum, and the twins are back to back (Fig. 116–3). The union is usually limited to the pelvic region, and the sacrum and coccyx or portions of them are held in common. There may be a common sacral spinal canal. There are two gastrointestinal tracts terminating in a single rectum. The genitourinary tract may vary, and there may be a shared bladder and urethra or a single vagina and uterus.

In the separation of these twins, the distribution of the solitary organs is determined by their blood and nerve supply. If the vagina is a single structure, it may be divided and half given to each baby. If there is a solitary anus, it is given to the appropriate twin, and a perineal pull-through can be performed on the other twin. This is preferable to a colostomy because the levator sling can be used in the pull-through procedure, as in repairing a high imperforate anus.

ISCHIOPAGUS TWINS

The incidence of ischiopagus twins is approximately 6 percent. The bodies are fused in the region of the pelvis to the level of a common umbilicus (Fig. 116–4). The pelvis of each child is open and fused to the other at the symphysis. Conjoining of the gastrointestinal tract occurs in the terminal ileum and includes a common cecum, colon, rectum, and anus. Two appendices and two sets of taenia are described in the reported cases[22,27] (C.E. Koop, personal communication). There are two vaginas, and the uterus and ovaries are present as mirror images. The urinary tract presents an interesting and consistent configuration because of its mirror image position. There are always two bladders and two urethras, but each bladder receives a ureter from the opposite twin. Therefore, when the pelves are divided, a ureter going to each bladder is also divided. Reconstruction of the urinary tract requires either a ureteroureterostomy or a ureterocystostomy.

The conjoined gastrointestinal tract is apportioned

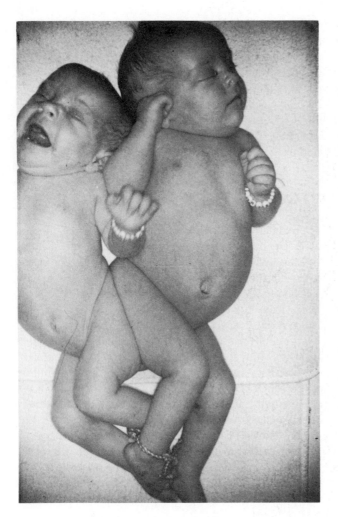 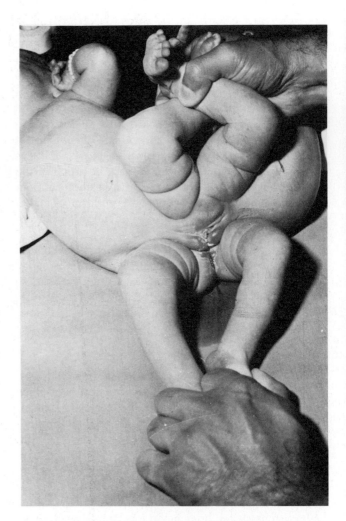

Figure 116–3. Left. Pygopagus twins with fused sacrum and perineum. **Right.** Perineal view showing single anus and vulva.

so that each twin receives half of the colon. After the appropriate resection, one twin will have the normal anus and lower rectum, and the other will have the cecum and upper half of the colon. Here again, a perineal pull-through can be performed with this segment by using the muscles of the levator sling. This technique was used by Koop in the separation of the Rodriguez twins, and the twin who had the pull-through operation had excellent fecal control within 2 years after the separation (C. E. Koop, personal communication). Closure of the abdominal wall defect may be very difficult, and the use of prosthetic materials may be necessary. However, closure can be accomplished by bilateral ileal osteotomies, so that the open ends of the pubic rami may be brought together and sutured in the midline. Often, the skin can be brought together in a fashion similar to closing a large omphalocele, so that a temporary ventral hernia is created. The osteotomies and pelvic reconstruc-

tion can be done as secondary procedures if the abdomen can be closed easily without them.

CRANIOPAGUS TWINS

Craniopagus twins are the rarest of conjoined twins, occurring once in 2,500,000 births. The union is in the region of the vertex, occiput, or lateral parietal areas of the skull, and the babies may face in the same or in opposite directions. The brains are usually separate, and the hazard of separation may lie in the fusion of venous sinuses.

Voris et al. found 40 well-documented cases of craniopagus twins in the literature.[28] Of these, 12 sets of twins have been subjected to surgical separation, with better results and more survivors reported in the recent

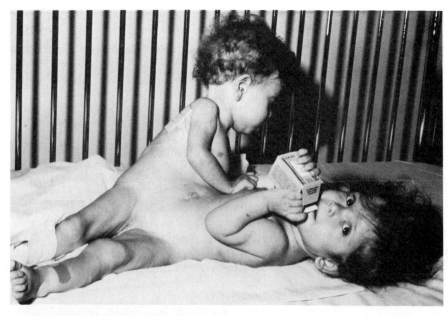

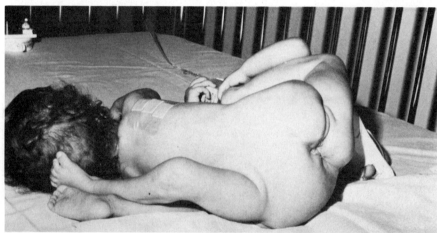

Figure 116–4. Top. Ischiopagus twins fused from umbilicus to perineum. **Bottom.** Perineal view showing single anus.

literature. O'Connell reported that many of the survivors were retarded.[29]

REFERENCES

1. Paré A: Complete Works, Johnson T (trans). 1678
2. Gould GM, Pyle WL: Anomalies and Curiosities of Medicine. Philadelphia, Saunders, 1896, p 175
3. Pancoast WH: Propriety of an operation for separation of Eng and Chang Bunker. Trans Coll Physicians Phil 1:149, 1875
4. Allen H: Report of an autopsy on the bodies of Chang and Eng Bunker. Trans Coll Physicians Phila 1:5, 1875
5. Guttmacher AF: Biographical notes on some famous conjoined twins. Birth Defects 3:10, 1967
6. Rock J, Hertig A: The human conceptus during the first two weeks of gestation. Am J Obstet Gynecol 55:6, 1948
7. Zimmerman AA: Embryologic and anatomic considerations of conjoined twins. Birth Defects 3:18, 1967
8. Stockard CR: Developmental rate and structural expressivity. Am J Anat 28:115, 1921
9. Potter EL, Craig JM: Pathology of the Fetus and the Infant, 3rd ed. Chicago, Year Book, 1975, p 220
10. Freedman HL, Tafeen CH, Harris H: Conjoined thoracopagus twins. Am J Obstet Gynecol 84:1904, 1962
11. Robertson EG: Craniopagus parietalis. Arch Neurol Psychiatr 70:189, 1953
12. Rudolph AJ, Michaels JP, Nicholes BL: Obstetric management of conjoined twins. Birth Defects 3:28, 1967
13. Spencer RP, Rockoff ML, Nichols BL, Johnson PC: Radioisotopic flow studies in conjoined twins. Birth Defects 3:120, 1967
14. Ross AJ, O'Neill JA, Silverman DG, et al: A new technique for evaluating cutaneous vascularity in complicated conjoined twins. J Pediatr Surg 20:743, 1985
15. Zuker RM, Filler RM, Roopnarine L: Intraabdominal tis-

sue expansion: an adjunct in the separation of conjoined twins. J Pediatr Surg 21:1198, 1986

16. Gans SL, Morgenstern L, Gettelman E: Separation of conjoined twins in the newborn period. J Pediatr Surg 3:565, 1968

17. Koop CE: Successful separation of pyopagus twins. Surgery 49:271, 1961

18. Keats AS, Cave PE, Slataper EL, Moore RA: Conjoined twins—a review of anesthetic management for separating operations. Birth Defects 3:80, 1967

19. Scammon RE: The surgical separation of symmetrical double monsters. In Abt IA (ed): Abt's Pediatrics. Philadelphia, Saunders, 1926

20. Kiesewetter WB: Surgery on conjoined (Siamese) twins: case report. Surgery 39:826, 1956

21. Aird I: The conjoined twins of Kano. Br Med J 1:831, 1954

22. Spencer R: Surgical separation of Siamese twins: case report. Surgery 39:826, 1956

23. Peterson D, Hill A: Separation of conjoined thoracopagus twins. Ann Surg 152:717, 1960

24. Nicholas BL, Blattner RJ, Rudolph AJ: General clinical management of thoracopagus twins. Birth Defects 3:38, 1967

25. Able LW: The surgical separation of the Bay City twins. Birth Defects 3:69, 1967

26. deVries PA: Separation of the San Francisco twins. Birth Defects 3:75, 1967

27. Bankole MA, Oduntan SA, Oluwasanmi O, et al: The conjoined twins of Warri, Nigeria. Arch Surg 104:294, 1972

28. Voris HC, Slaughter WB, Christian JR, et al: Successful separation of craniopagus twins. J Neurosurg 14:548, 1957

29. O'Connell JEA: Investigation and treatment of carniopagus twins. Br Med J 1:1333, 1964

☐ INDEX